aspen | LEADING THE SCIENCE AND PRACTICE OF CLINICAL NUTRITION
American Society for Parenteral and Enteral Nutrition

THE A.S.P.E.N. ADULT NUTRITION SUPPORT CORE CURRICULUM
2ND EDITION

EDITOR-IN-CHIEF

Charles Mueller, PhD, RD, CNSD
Clinical and Translational Science Center
Weill Cornell Medical College
New York, NY

SECTION EDITORS

Stephen A. McClave, MD, FASPEN
Division of Gastroenterology/Hepatology
University of Louisville
Louisville, KY

Denise Baird Schwartz, MS, RD, FADA, CNSC
Providence Saint Joseph Medical Center
Burbank, CA

Debra S. Kovacevich, RN, MPH
University of Michigan Home Care Services
Ann Arbor, MI

Sarah J. Miller, RPh, BCNSP
University of Montana School of Pharmacy
Missoula, MT

MANAGING EDITOR

Jennifer M. Kuhn, MPS
Washington, DC

AMERICAN SOCIETY FOR PARENTERAL AND ENTERAL NUTRITION

The American Society for Parenteral and Enteral Nutrition (A.S.P.E.N.) is a scientific society whose members are health care professionals—physicians, dietitians, nurses, pharmacists, other allied health professionals, and researchers—dedicated to ensuring that every patient receives safe, efficacious, and high quality patient care.

A.S.P.E.N.'s mission is to improve patient care by advancing the science and practice of clinical nutrition and metabolism.

NOTE: This publication is designed to provide accurate authoritative information with regard to the subject matter covered. It is sold with the understanding that the publisher is not engaged in rendering medical or other professional advice. Trademarked commercial product names are used only for education purposes and do not constitute endorsement by A.S.P.E.N.

This publication does not constitute medical or professional advice, and should not be taken as such. To the extent the information published herein may be used to assist in the care of patients, this is the result of the sole professional judgment of the attending health professional whose judgment is the primary component of quality medical care. The information presented herein is not a substitute for the exercise of such judgment by the health professional.

ISBN # 978-1-889622-07-1

Printed in the United States

ASPEN — LEADING THE SCIENCE AND PRACTICE OF CLINICAL NUTRITION
American Society for Parenteral and Enteral Nutrition

Contents

Contributors v

Reviewers xi

Foreword xvi

Preface xviii

Acknowledgments xx

PART I Basics of Nutrition and Metabolism

1. **Nutrient Intake, Digestion, Absorption, and Excretion** 3
   Tina Colaizzo-Anas, PhD, RD, CDN

2. **Energy** 22
   Jennifer A. Wooley, MS, RD, CNSC
   David Frankenfield, MS, RD

3. **Carbohydrates** 36
   Pei-Ra Ling, MD
   Karen C. McCowen, MD

4. **Probiotics and Prebiotics** 51
   Gail Cresci, PhD, RD, LD, CNSD

5. **Lipids** 63
   Mary Hise, PhD, RD, CNSD
   John C. Brown, PhD

6. **Protein** 83
   Lorraine S. Young, MS, RD, CNSD, LDN
   Laurel R. Kearns, MS, RD, CNSC, LDN
   Sandra L. Schoepfel, MS, RD, RN, CNSC, LDN
   Nicole Caron Clark, MS, RD, CNSC, LDN

7. **Fluids, Electrolytes, and Acid-Base Disorders** 98
   Ginger Langley, PharmD, BCNSP, BCPS, CPHQ
   Sharla Tajchman, PharmD, BCNSP, BCPS

8. **Vitamins and Trace Elements** 121
   Susan F. Clark, RD, PhD

PART II Clinical Foundations of Nutrition Support

9. **Nutrition Screening and Assessment** 155
   Gordon L. Jensen, MD, PhD
   Pao Ying Hsiao, MS, RD
   Dara Wheeler, RD

10. **Overview of Enteral Nutrition** 170
    Susan L. Brantley, MS, RD, CNSC, LDN
    Mary E. (Beth) Mills, MS, RD, CNSC, LDN

11. **Enteral Formulations** 185
    Gail Cresci, PhD, RD, CNSD, LD
    Jennifer Lefton, MS, RD, CNSD
    Dema Halasa Esper, MS, RD, LD

12. **Enteral Access Devices** 206
    John C. Fang, MD
    Robin Bankhead, CRNP
    Merin Kinikini, RD, RN, FNP

13. **Complications of Enteral Nutrition** 218
    Ainsley M. Malone, MS, RD, LD, CNSC
    David Seres, MD, ScM, PNS
    Linda Lord, NP, MSN, CNSN

14. **Overview of Parenteral Nutrition** 234
    Jay M. Mirtallo, MS, RPh, BCNSP, FASHP
    Meera Patel, PharmD, BCPS

15. **Parenteral Nutrition Formulations** 245
    Jacqueline R. Barber, PharmD, BCNSP, FASHP
    Gordon S. Sacks, PharmD, BCNSP, FCCP

16. **Parenteral Access Devices** 265
    Elizabeth A. Krzywda, APNP, MSN
    Deborah A. Andris, APNP, MSN
    Charles E. Edmiston Jr, PhD

17. **Complications of Parenteral Nutrition** 284
    Vanessa J. Kumpf, PharmD, BCNSP
    Jane Gervasio, PharmD, BCNSP

18. **Drug–Nutrient Interactions** 298
    Carol J. Rollins, MS, RD, CNSD, PharmD, BCNSP

19. **Dietary Supplements** 313
    Joseph I. Boullata, PharmD, RPh, BCNSP
    Michele Nicolo, MS, RD, CDE, CNSD, LDN
    Kathleen W. Stratton, JD, MA, RD, LDN

PART III Nutrition Support of Specific States

20. **Pregnancy and Lactation** 331
Catherine Cimbalik, RN, RD, CNSC
James D. Paauw, MD, PhD

21. **Wound Healing** 348
Joyce K. Stechmiller, PhD, ACNP-BC, FAAN

22. **Nutrition in Neurologic Impairment** 363
Kathryn Ruf, PharmD
Barbara Magnuson, PharmD, BCNSP
Jimmi Hatton, PharmD
Aaron M. Cook, PharmD, BCPS

23. **Critical Care Sepsis** 377
Keith Miller, MD
Laszlo Kiraly, MD
Robert G. Martindale, MD, PhD

24. **Trauma, Surgery, and Burns** 392
Bryan R. Collier, DO, FACS, CNSC
Jill R. Cherry-Bukowiec, MD, MS, FACS
Mary E. (Beth) Mills, MS, RD, CNSC, LDN

25. **Pulmonary Failure** 412
Krista L. Turner, MD, FACS

26. **Gastrointestinal Disease** 426
David Frantz, MD, MS
Craig Munroe, MD
Carol Rees Parrish, MS, RD
Joseph Krenitsky, MS, RD
Kate Willcutts, MS, RD, CNSC
Amy Fortune, RD, PA-C

27. **Liver Disease** 454
Thomas H. Frazier, MD
Benjamin E. Wheeler, MD
Craig J. McClain, MD
Matthew Cave, MD

28. **Pancreatitis** 472
Carol Rees Parrish, MS, RD
Joseph Krenitsky, MS, RD
Stephen A. McClave, MD

29. **Renal Disease** 491
Robert Wolk, PharmD
Charles J. Foulks, MD, FACP, FACN

30. **Short Bowel Syndrome** 511
Sherry Tarleton, RD, CNSC
John K. DiBaise, MD, FACG

31. **Solid Organ Transplantation** 523
Jeanette M. Hasse, PhD, RD, LD, FADA, CNSC
Laura E. Matarese, PhD, RD, LDN, FADA, CNSC

32. **Human Immunodeficiency Virus (HIV) Infection** 536
Peter J. Wasserman, RD, MA
Sorana Segal-Maurer, MD
David S. Rubin, MD

33. **Cancer** 563
Robin B. Mendelsohn, MD
Mark A. Schattner, MD

34. **Nutritional and Medical Management of Diabetes Mellitus in Hospitalized Patients** 580
Laura Newton, MA, RD
W. Timothy Garvey, MD

35. **Obesity** 603
Ryan T. Hurt, MD, PhD
Thomas H. Frazier, MD

36. **Nutrition Support for Older Adults** 620
Charles Mueller, PhD, RD, CNSD
Rena Zelig, MS, RD, CSG

37. **Chylothorax and Chylous Ascites** 630
Thomas H. Frazier, MD
David A. Spain, MD, FACS
Stephen A. McClave, MD

PART IV Management and Professional Issues

38. **Home Nutrition Support** 639
Marion Winkler, PhD, RD, CNSC
Elizabeth Hagan, RN, CNSC, BSN
Jorge E. Albina, MD

39. **Ethics and Law** 656
Cynthia M.A. Geppert, MD, MA, PhD, MPH, FAPM, DAAPM
Albert Barrocas, MD, FACS
Denise Baird Schwartz, MS, RD, FADA, CNSC

40. **Quality Improvement** 677
Naomi E. Cahill, RD, MSc

41. **Application of Research, Derivation of Guidelines, and Evidence-Based Practice** 693
Kelly A. Tappenden, PhD, RD

aspen | LEADING THE SCIENCE AND PRACTICE OF CLINICAL NUTRITION
American Society for Parenteral and Enteral Nutrition

Contributors

Jorge E. Albina, MD
Director, Nutritional Support Service
Rhode Island Hospital
Providence, RI

Deborah A. Andris, APNP, MSN
Adult Nurse Practitioner
Medical College of Wisconsin
Milwaukee, WI

Robin Bankhead, CRNP, MS
Nurse Practitioner
Department of Surgery
Temple University Hospital
Philadelphia, PA

Jacqueline R. Barber, PharmD, BCNSP, FASHP
Pharmacy Clinical Specialist–Nutrition Support
Methodist Hospital–Park Nicollet Health Services
St. Louis Park, MN
Clinical Professor, College of Pharmacy
University of Minnesota, Minneapolis
Minneapolis, MN

Albert Barrocas, MD, FACS
Chief Medical Officer
South Fulton Medical Center
Atlanta, GA

Joseph I. Boullata, PharmD, RPh, BCNSP
Associate Professor
Pharmacology and Therapeutics
Pharmacy Specialist in Nutrition Support
University of Pennsylvania School of Nursing
Hospital of the University of Pennsylvania, Clinical Nutrition Support Services
Philadelphia, PA

Susan L. Brantley, MS, RD, CNSC, LDN
Metabolic Support Nutritionist
University of Tennessee Medical Center–Knoxville
Knoxville, TN

John C. Brown, MS, PhD
Professor Emeritus
Department of Molecular Biosciences
The University of Kansas
Vernon Hills, IL

Naomi E. Cahill, RD, MSc
Project Leader/Doctoral Candidate
Queen's University
Kingston, ON, Canada

Matt Cave, MD
Assistant Professor
Gastroenterology, Hepatology, and Nutrition
University of Louisville
Louisville, KY

Jill R. Cherry-Bukowiec, MD, MS, FACS
Assistant Clinical Professor of Surgery
University of Michigan
Ann Arbor, MI

Catherine Cimbalik, RN, RD, CNSC
Specialty Dietitian Educator
Spectrum Health
Grand Rapids, MI

Nicole Caron Clark, MS, RD, CNSC, LDN
Nutrition Support Dietitian
Boston Medical Center
Boston, MA

Susan F. Clark, RD, PhD
Associate Professor
Virginia Tech
Blacksburg, VA

Tina Colaizzo-Anas, MA, MS, PhD, RD
Assistant Professor
Buffalo State–SUNY
Buffalo, NY

Bryan R. Collier, DO, FACS, CNSC
Section Chief, Trauma
Medical Director, Trauma Center
Director of Surgical Nutrition
Virginia Tech Carilion School of Medicine
Carilion Roanoke Memorial Hospital
Roanoke, VA

Aaron M. Cook, PharmD, BCPS
Clinical Pharmacy Specialist- Neurosurgery/Critical Care
University of Kentucky Chandler Medical Center
Adjunct Assistant Professor
University of Kentucky College of Pharmacy
Lexington, KY

Gail Cresci, PhD, RD, CNSD, LD
Project Research Staff
The Cleveland Clinic
Cleveland, OH

John K. DiBaise, MD, FACG
Professor of Medicine
Mayo Clinic
Scottsdale, AZ

Charles E. Edmiston Jr, PhD
Professor of Surgery
Hospital Epidemiologist
Medical College of Wisconsin
Milwaukee, WI

Dema Halasa Esper, MS, RD, LD
Lecturer
Food and Nutrition Program, Department of Human Ecology
Youngstown State University
Youngstown, OH

John C. Fang, MD
Professor of Medicine
University of Utah
Salt Lake City, UT

Amy Fortune, RD, PA-C

Charles J. Foulks, MD, FACP, FACN
C.S. Lewis, Jr., M.D. Professor of Medicine and Chairman, Department of Medicine
School of Community Medicine
University of Oklahoma College of Medicine
Tulsa, OK

David Frankenfield, MS, RD
Nutrition Support Dietitian/Researcher
Penn State Milton S. Hershey Medical Center
Hershey, PA

David Frantz, MD, MS
Thoracic Surgeon
Lynchburg, VA

Thomas H. Frazier, MD
Assistant Clinical Professor of Medicine
University of Louisville
Three Rivers Medical Center
Louisa, KY

W. Timothy Garvey, MD
Butterworth Professor
Chair, Department of Nutrition Sciences
University of Alabama at Birmingham
Birmingham, AL

Cynthia M. A. Geppert, MD, MA, PhD, MPH, FAPM, DAAPM
Chief, Consultation Psychiatry and Ethics
Ethics, New Mexico Veterans Affairs Health Care System
Associate Professor of Psychiatry
Director of Ethics Education
University of New Mexico School of Medicine
Albuquerque, NM

Jane Gervasio, PharmD, BCNSP
Chair and Associate Professor
Pharmacy Practice
Butler University College of Pharmacy and Health Sciences
Indianapolis, IN

Elizabeth Hagan, RN, BSN, CNSC
Clinical Specialist
Rhode Island Hospital
Providence, RI

Jeanette M. Hasse, PhD, RD, LD, FADA, CNSC
Manager
Transplant Nutrition
Simmons Transplant Institute
Baylor University Medical Center
Dallas, TX

Jimmi Hatton, PharmD
Associate Professor, Pharmacy and Neurosurgery
University of Kentucky College of Pharmacy
Pharmacy Practice and Science
Lexington, KY

Mary Hise, PhD, RD, CNSD
Director, Medical Affairs
Baxter Healthcare Corporation
Deerfield, IL

Pao Ying Hsiao, MS, RD
Doctoral Candidate
Department of Nutritional Sciences
Penn State University
University Park, PA

Ryan T. Hurt, MD, PhD
Assistant Professor of Medicine
Mayo Clinic
Rochester, MN

Gordon L. Jensen, MD, PhD
Professor
Head, Department of Nutritional Sciences
Penn State University
University Park, PA

Laurel R. Kearns, MS, RD, CNSC, LDN
Nutrition Support Dietitian
Boston Medical Center
Boston, MA

Merin Kinikini, RD, RN, FNP
Registered Dietitian and Family Nurse Practitioner
Intermountain Medical Center
Salt Lake City, UT

Laszlo Kiraly, MD
Assistant Professor
Department of Trauma
Oregon Health and Science University
Portland, OR

Debra S. Kovacevich, MPH, RN
Nurse Manager
Home Care Services–HomeMed
University of Michigan Health System
Adjunct Assistant Professor of Pharmacy
University of Michigan College of Pharmacy
Ann Arbor, MI

Joseph Krenitsky, MS, RD
Nutrition Support Specialist
University of Virginia Health System
Charlottesville, VA

Elizabeth A. Krzywda, APNP, MSN
Adult Nurse Practitioner
Medical College of Wisconsin
Milwaukee, WI

Vanessa J. Kumpf, PharmD, BCNSP
Clinical Specialist
Nutrition Support
Vanderbilt University Medical Center
Nashville, TN

Ginger Langley, PharmD, BCNSP, BCPS, CPHQ
Clinical Pharmacy Specialist
University of Texas MD Anderson Cancer Center
Houston, TX

Jennifer Lefton, MS, RD, CNSD
Clinical Nutrition Specialist
Washington Hospital Center
Arlington, VA

Pei-Ra Ling, MD
Assistant Professor of Medicine
Beth Israel Deaconess Medical Center
Harvard Medical School
Boston, MA

Linda Lord, NP, MSN, CNSN
Nutrition Support Nurse Practitioner
University of Rochester Medical Center
Rochester, NY

Barbara Magnuson, PharmD, BCNSP
Nutrition Support Pharmacist
University of Kentucky Healthcare
Lexington, KY

Ainsley Malone, MS, RD, LD, CNSC
Nutrition Support Team
Pharmacy Department
Mt. Carmel West Hospital
Columbus, OH

Robert G. Martindale, MD, PhD
Professor and Chief of Division
Division of General Surgery
Oregon Health and Sciences University
Portland, OR

Laura E. Matarese, PhD, RD, LDN, FADA, CNSC
Associate Professor
Division of Gastroenterology, Hepatology, and Nutrition
Department of Internal Medicine
Brody School of Medicine
Department of Nutrition Science
East Carolina University
Greenville, NC

Craig J. McClain, MD
Professor of Medicine, Pharmacology and Toxicology;
Chief of Research Affairs, Division of Gastroenterology, Hepatology and Nutrition;
Associate Vice President for Translational Research
University of Louisville
Louisville, KY

Stephen A. McClave, MD
Professor of Medicine
Director of Clinical Nutrition
University of Louisville School of Medicine
Louisville, KY

Karen C. McCowen, MD, MRCPI
Physician
Harvard Vanguard Medical Associates
Harvard Medical School
Boston, MA

Robin B. Mendelsohn, MD
Physician
Memorial Sloan-Kettering Cancer Center
New York, NY

Sarah J. Miller, PharmD, BCNSP
Professor, Clinical Pharmacy
Pharmacy Clinical Coordinator
University of Montana Skaggs School of Pharmacy
Saint Patrick Hospital
Missoula, MT

Keith Miller, MD
Surgical Resident
University of Louisville
Louisville, KY

Mary E. (Beth) Mills, MS, RD, CNSC, LDN
Critical Care Dietitian
Vanderbilt University Medical Center
Nashville, TN

Jay M. Mirtallo, MS, RPh, BCNSP, FASHP
Director
MS in Health System Pharmacy
Ohio State University, College of Pharmacy
Columbus, OH

Charles Mueller, PhD, RD, CNSD
Clinical and Translational Science Center
Weill Cornell Medical College
New York, NY

Craig Munroe, MD
General Gastroenterology and Therapeutic Endoscopy
Kaiser Permanente
San Francisco, CA

Laura Newton, MA, RD
Assistant Professor
Department of Nutrition Sciences
University of Alabama at Birmingham
Birmingham, AL

Michele Nicolo, MS, RD, CDE, CNSD, LDN
Clinical Dietitian Specialist
Hospital of the University of Pennsylvania, Clinical Nutrition Support Services
Philadelphia, PA

James D. Paauw, MD, PhD
Director
Nutrition Support
Spectrum Health
Associate Professor
Department of Surgery
Michigan State University
Grand Rapids, MI

Carol Rees Parrish, MS, RD
Nutrition Support Specialist
University of Virginia Health System
Charlottesville, VA

Meera Patel, PharmD, BCPS
Clinical Pharmacist
Moses Cone Health System
Greensboro, NC

Carol J. Rollins, MS, RD, CNSD, PharmD, BCNSP
Coordinator, Nutrition Support Team
Clinical Associate Professor
University Medical Center
The University of Arizona College of Pharmacy
Tucson, AZ

David S. Rubin, MD
Medical Director
AIDS Designated Center
Attending Physician
Infectious Disease Division, Department of Medicine
New York Hospital Queens
Flushing, NY
Assistant Professor of Clinical Medicine
Weill Medical College of Cornell University
New York, NY

Kathryn Ruf, PharmD
Clinical Pharmacist Specialist–Critical Care
Jewish Hospital
Louisville, KY

Gordon S. Sacks, PHARMD, BCNSP, FCCP
Professor and Head
Department of Pharmacy Practice
Harrison School of Pharmacy
Auburn University
Auburn, AL

Mark A. Schattner, MD, FACP
Physician
Memorial Sloan-Kettering Cancer Center
New York, NY

Sandra L. Schoepfel, MS, RD, RN, CNSD, LDN
Clinical Nutrition Support Specialist
Home Solutions Infusion Therapy
Canton, MA

Sorana Segal-Maurer, MD
Chief
Infectious Disease Division
Department of Medicine
New York Hospital Queens
Flushing, NY
Associate Professor of Clinical Medicine
Weill Medical College of Cornell University
New York, NY

David S. Seres, MD, ScM, PNS
Director, Medical Nutrition and Nutrition Support Service
Chair, Nutrition Curriculum
Assistant Professor of Clinical Medicine
Institute of Human Nutrition
New York–Presbyterian Hospital, Columbia University Medical Center
New York, NY

David A. Spain, MD, FACS
The Carol and Ned Spieker Professor and Chief of Acute Care Surgery
Surgical Critical Care Fellowship Program Director and Associate Division Chief, General Surgery Department of Surgery
Stanford University
Stanford, CA

Joyce K. Stechmiller, PhD, ACNP-BC, FAAN
Chair and Associate Professor
University of Florida
Gainesville, FL

Denise Baird Schwartz, MS, RD, FADA, CNSC
Nutrition Support Coordinator
Providence Saint Joseph Medical Center
Burbank, CA

Kathleen W. Stratton, JD, MA, RD, LDN
Clinical Dietitian
Hospital of the University of Pennsylvania, Clinical Nutrition Support Services
Philadelphia, PA

Sharla Tajchman, PharmD, BCNSP, BCPS
Critical Care/Nutrition Support Clinical Pharmacy Specialist
University of Texas MD Anderson Cancer Center
Houston, TX

Kelly A. Tappenden, PhD, RD
Professor of Nutrition and Gastrointestinal Physiology
University of Illinois
Champaign, IL

Sherry Tarleton, RD, CNSC
Gastrointestinal Dietitian
Mayo Clinic
Scottsdale, AZ

Krista L. Turner, MD, FACS
Assistant Professor of Surgery
The Methodist Hospital
Houston, TX

Peter J. Wasserman, RD, MA
Metabolic Support Clinician
Research Associate
Infectious Disease Division, Department of Medicine
New York Hospital Queens
Flushing, NY

Benjamin E. Wheeler, MD
Resident
Department of Internal Medicine
University of Louisville
Louisville, KY

Dara Wheeler, RD
Doctoral Candidate
Department of Nutritional Sciences
Penn State University
University Park, PA

Kate Willcuts, MS, RD, CNSC
Surgical Nutrition Support Dietitian/Assistant Professor
University of Virginia Health System
Charlottesville, VA

Marion Winkler, PhD, RD, CNSC
Surgical Nutrition Specialist
Rhode Island Hospital
Providence, RI

Robert Wolk, PharmD
Manager, Clinical and Education
Department of Pharmacy
Tucson Medical Center
Tucson, AZ

Jennifer A. Wooley, MS, RD, CNSC
Clinical Nutrition Manager
University of Michigan Health Systems
Ann Arbor, MI

Lorraine S. Young, RD, MS, CNSD, LDN
Home Nutrition Support Manager
Boston Medical Center
Boston, MA

Rena Zelig, MS, RD, CSG
Pre-Doctoral Fellow, Graduate Program
University of Medicine and Dentistry of New Jersey
Newark, NJ

aspen | LEADING THE SCIENCE AND PRACTICE OF CLINICAL NUTRITION
American Society for Parenteral and Enteral Nutrition

Reviewers

Jorge E. Albina, MD
Professor of Surgery
Alpert Medical School of Brown University
Director of Nutritional Support Services, Director of Surgical Research
Rhode Island Hospital
Providence, RI

Caroline Apovian, MD
Director, Nutrition and Weight Management
Boston Medical Center
Endocrinology
Professor of Medicine and Pediatrics
Boston University School of Medicine
Boston, MA

David A. August, MD
Professor of Surgery
Chief, Division of Surgical Oncology
UMDNJ/Robert Wood Johnson Medical School and The Cancer Institute of New Jersey
New Brunswick, NJ

Albert Barrocas, MD, FACS
Chief Medical Officer
South Fulton Medical Center
Atlanta, GA

Jeff Binkley, PharmD, BCNSP, FASHP
Maury Regional Medical Center
Columbia, TN

Bruce Ryan Bistrian, MD, PhD
Chief, Clinical Nutrition
Beth Israel Deaconess Medical Center
Professor of Medicine
Harvard Medical School
Boston, MA

Alan L. Buchman, MD, MSPH
Professor of Medicine and Surgery
Division of Gastroenterology
Feinberg School of Medicine
Northwestern University
Chicago, IL

Phila Callahan, RN, CNSC
Home Nutrition Support Nurse
Christiana Care
Surgical & Critical Care Associates
Newark, DE

Pamela Charney, PhD, RD
Affiliate Associate Professor
School of Pharmacy
University of Washington
Nutrition Informatics Consultant
Seattle, WA

Ronni Chernoff, PhD, RD
Associate Director, Education/Evaluation
Central Arkansas Veterans Healthcare System
Geriatric Research Education and Clinical Center
Professor, Geriatrics
University of Arkansas for Medical Science
DW Reynolds Department of Geriatrics
Little Rock, AR

Bryan Collier, DO, FACS, CNSC
Section Chief, Trauma
Medical Director, Trauma Center
Director of Surgical Nutrition
Virginia Tech Carilion School of Medicine
Carilion Roanoke Memorial Hospital
Roanoke, VA

Charlene Compher, PhD
Associate Professor of Nutrition Science
University of Pennsylvania School of Nursing
Philadelphia, PA

Karrie Derenski, BCNSP, CNSC
Metabolic Support Coordinator
CoxHealth
Department of Pharmacy
Springfield, MO

Roland N. Dickerson, PharmD, BCNSP
Professor of Clinical Pharmacy
University of Tennessee Health Science Center
Memphis, TN

Becky Dorner, RD, LD
President
Becky Dorner & Associates, Inc.
Akron, OH

John W. Drover, MD, FACS, FRCSC
Associate Professor Chair and Program Medical Director Critical Care Program
Queen's University
Kingston, ON, Canada

Carrie P. Earthman, PhD, RD, LD
Associate Professor, Clinical Nutrition
University of Minnesota
Department of Food Science and Nutrition
Saint Paul, MN

Eric H. Frankel, MSE, PharmD, BCNSP
Metabolic Support Service & Neonatal Clinical Lead Pharmacist
Truman Medical Center
Department of Pharmacy
Kansas City, MO

Lorraine R Franzi, MS/HSM, RD, LD, CNSC
Dietitian, Specialist/Nutrition Support
University of Pittsburgh Medical Center
Food and Nutrition
Pittsburgh, PA

Juan B. Ochoa Gautier, MD, FACS
Professor of Surgery and Critical Care
University of Pittsburgh
Nestlé Health Care Nutrition, Nestlé Health Science
Medical and Scientific Director
Pittsburgh, PA

Jane Gervasio, PharmD, BCNSP
Chair and Associate Professor of Pharmacy Practice
Butler University College of Pharmacy and Health Sciences
Department of Pharmacy Practice
Indianapolis, IN

Marshall J. Glesby, MD, PhD
Associate Professor of Medicine and Public Health
Weill Cornell Medical College
Medicine/Infectious Diseases
New York, NY

Linda D. Griffith, PhD, RD, CNSC
Clinical Assistant Professor
The University of Kansas Medical Center
Department of Dietetics & Nutrition
Kansas City, KS

Peggi Guenter, PhD, RN
Director of Clinical Practice, Advocacy, and Research Affairs
American Society for Parenteral and Enteral Nutrition
Silver Spring, MD

Kathleen M. Gura, PharmD, BCNSP
Clinical Pharmacy Specialist Gastroenterology/ Nutrition
Children's Hospital Boston
Associate Professor Pharmacy Practice
Massachusetts College of Pharmacy and Health Sciences
Boston, MA

Cindy Hamilton, MS, RD, LD, CNSD
Director, Nutrition
Cleveland Clinic
Center for Human Nutrition, Digestive Disease Institute
Cleveland, OH

Leslie A. Hamilton, PharmD, BCPS
Assistant Clinical Professor
Auburn University
Pharmacy Practice
Birmingham, AL

Michelle Harrington, MS, RD, LDN
Manager, Nutritional Affairs
McNeil Nutritionals, LLC
Fort Washington, PA

Mary Harris, MS, PhD, RD, BC-ADM
Professor of Nutrition, Dietetic Program Director
Colorado State University
Food Science and Human Nutrition
Fort Collins, CO

Lillian Harvey-Banchik, MD, FACS, CNSP
Assistant Clinical Professor of Surgery
Hofstra University School of Medicine in Conjunction with the North Shore LIJ Health Care System
North Shore University Hospital
Department of Surgery
Manhasset, NY

Jeanette M. Hasse, PhD, RD, LD, FADA, CNSC
Manager
Transplant Nutrition
Simmons Transplant Institute
Baylor University Medical Center
Dallas, TX

Wendy D. Heck, PharmD
Manager, Clinical Pharmacy Services
The University of Texas MD Anderson Cancer Center
Division of Pharmacy
Houston, TX

Leslie A. Hourigan, RD, MS, CNSC
Clinical Dietitian
San Antonio Military Medical Center
Department of Nutritional Medicine
San Antonio, TX

Carol Ireton-Jones, PhD, RD, LD, CNSC, FACN
Nutrition Therapy Specialist
Dallas, TX

Khursheed N. Jeejeebhoy, MBBS, PhD, FRCP, FRCPC, AGAF
Emeritus Professor of Medicine and Nutrition
University of Toronto
St. Michael's Hospital
Toronto, ON, Canada

Dong Wook Kim, MD
Instructor of Medicine
Boston University School of Medicine
Division of Endocrinology, Diabetes, and Nutrition
Boston Medical Center
Nutrition and Weight Management Center
Boston, MA

Donald F. Kirby, MD FACP, FACN, FACG, AGAF, CNSC, CPNS
Director, Center for Human Nutrition
Cleveland Clinic
Digestive Disease Institute
Cleveland, OH

Mark G. Klang, PhD
Core Head, Research Pharmacy
Sloan-Kettering Institute
New York, NY

Kenneth A. Kudsk, MD, FACS, FCCM
Professor of Surgery
University of Wisconsin–Madison
Surgery
Madison, WI

Ginger Langley, PharmD, BCNSP, BCPS, CPHQ
Manager, Clinical Pharmacy Services
MD Anderson Cancer Center
Houston, TX

Cynthia L. Lieu, PharmD, BCNSP
Associate Professor of Clinical Pharmacy
Family Department of Clinical Pharmacy and Pharmaceutical Economics & Policy
University of Southern California, School of Pharmacy
Los Angeles, CA

Cynthia Lowen, RD, LD, CNSC, CCRP
Medical Affairs Liaison; Clinical Instructor In Medicine (Gastroenterology and Hepatology)
Nestlé HealthCare Nutrition; University of Louisville
Department of Medicine
Louisville, KY

Barbara Magnuson, PharmD
Nutrition Support Pharmacy Specialist
University of Kentucky HealthCare, Pharmacy Services
Adjunct Associate Professor, University of Kentucky College of Pharmacy
Department of Pharmacy Practice and Science
Lexington, KY

Julie O'Sullivan Maillet, PhD, RD, FADA
Interim Dean
University of Medicine and Dentistry of New Jersey
School of Health Related Professions
Newark, NJ

Ainsley Malone, MS, RD, CNSC
Nutrition Support Dietitian
Mt. Carmel West Hospital
Department of Pharmacy
Columbus, OH

Mary Marian, MS, RD, CSO
Clinical Nutritionist, Lecturer and Faculty
University of Arizona, College of Agriculture and Medicine
Nutrition Science Program in Integrative Medicine
Tucson, AZ

Theresa Mayes, RD, CCRC
Clinical Dietitian
Shriners Hospital for Children
Nutrition Services
Cincinnati, OH

Carol McGinnis, MS, RN, CNSN
Clinical Nurse Specialist
Sanford USD Medical Center
Nutrition Support
Sioux Falls, SD

Gayle Minard, MD
Professor of Surgery
The University of Tennessee Health Science Center
Memphis, TN

Barry A. Mizock, MD
Professor of Medicine
University of Illinois at Chicago
Department of Medicine
Chicago, IL

Steven W. Plogsted, PharmD, BCNSP, CNSC
Clinical Pharmacist
Nationwide Children's Hospital
Nutrition Support Service
Columbus, OH

Mary Russell, MS, RD, LDN
Director, Clinical Nutrition
University of Chicago Medical Center
Chicago, IL

Jose M. Saavedra, MD
Associate Professor of Pediatrics
Johns Hopkins University School of Medicine
Gastroenterology and Nutrition
Baltimore, MD

Edward Saltzman, MD
Chief, Division of Clinical Nutrition, Tufts Medical Center
Chair, Department of Nutrition Sciences,
Friedman School of Nutrition Science and Policy
Tufts University
Boston, MA

John K. Siepler, PharmD, BCNSP, FCCP
Research Specialist
Nutrishare, Inc.
Elk Grove, CA

Janet J. Skates, MS, RD, LDN, FADA
Owner and Nutrition Consultant
Nutrition Consulting Services
Kingsport, TN

Rex A. Speerhas, RPh, BCNSP
Nutrition Support Clinical Specialist
Cleveland Clinic
Cleveland, OH

Ezra Steiger, MD, FACS
Professor of Surgery
Consultant in General Surgery and Gastroenterology
Cleveland Clinic
Nutrition Support Team
Digestive Disease Institute
Cleveland, OH

Charles W. Van Way III, MD
Professor of Surgery
Sosland/Missouri Endowed Chair of Trauma Services
University of Missouri, Kansas City, School of Medicine
Kansas City, MO

Rebecca A. Weseman, RD, CNSC, LMNT
University of Nebraska Medical Center
Department of Surgery
Omaha, NE

Susan J. Whiting, PhD
Professor of Nutrition
College of Pharmacy and Nutrition
University of Saskatchewan
Saskatoon, SK, Canada

Kate Willcutts, MS, RD, CNSC
Surgical Nutrition Support Dietitian/
Assistant Professor
University of Virginia Health System
Patient Care Services/School of Nursing
Charlottesville, VA

Jennifer A. Wooley, MS, RD, CNSC
Clinical Nutrition Manager
University of Michigan Health System
Patient Food and Nutrition Services
Ann Arbor, MI

Yong-Ming Yu, MD, PhD
Assistant Professor of Surgery
Massachusetts General Hospital
Burn Unit, Department of Surgery
Shriners Hospital for Children
Boston, MA

aspen | LEADING THE SCIENCE AND PRACTICE OF CLINICAL NUTRITION
American Society for Parenteral and Enteral Nutrition

Foreword

A.S.P.E.N. is an interdisciplinary society dedicated to improving patient care by advancing the science and practice of clinical nutrition. It is a diverse community of dietitians, nurses, pharmacists, physicians, scientists, students, and other health professionals from every facet of nutrition support clinical practice, research, and education. A.S.P.E.N. is the leader in nutrition support therapy. Strategically, A.S.P.E.N. fosters the discovery of new knowledge and its application, education of health practitioners, and integration of nutrition support into the clinical care of all patients.

The A.S.P.E.N. Adult Nutrition Support Core Curriculum, 2nd Edition (Core) provides the fundamental knowledge necessary to provide optimal nutrition support. It is a must have resource for those individuals that have nutrition therapy as a component of their assigned responsibilities. The diverse backgrounds of the editors and authors, including research (scientist), clinical practice, education, and advocacy enhances the *Core's* usefulness in translating the science of nutrition support to its clinical application. It also fulfills a "high-level" need expressed by respondents to the 2011 A.S.P.E.N. membership survey: improving knowledge and skills, specifically as they relate to incorporating evidence into practice and methods to standardize practice. The *Core* is a resource that may be used by the novice to advance their knowledge and elevate their practice as well as by experienced clinicians preparing for certification in nutrition support. Based on the elements essential to nutrition support practice, it combines in one text the information necessary to practice nutrition support therapy. The chapter structure is conducive to the individual advancing through the hierarchy of knowledge attainment from novice to competent or expert practitioner. Each chapter has a "mini" outline followed by learning objectives and a "Test Your Knowledge" section, which includes questions and answers as a pretest to the chapter content. An important change in the 3rd edition is the evolution from Case Presentations to Practice Scenarios—single teaching questions designed to facilitate critical thinking and application of the content to clinical practice.

This edition of the *Core* continues to focus on the adult. The first section provides principles of basic nutrition and nutritional requirements. The second section includes the fundamentals of nutrition support practice including assessment and basics of enteral and parenteral nutrition. The third section applies nutrition support principles to specific disease conditions such as critical care, gastrointestinal disorders, organ dysfunction, and wound healing. Section four includes professional and management issues and highlights the importance of recognizing nutrition support as not only a therapy but also a "system of care" involving assessment, indication, orders, preparation, delivery, and administration. Also of note are the varieties of health care settings (intensive care, hospital, extended care facility, and home) and age (neonates to elderly). Again, the diversity of the authors and editors of the *Core* reflect the multiple disciplines that collaborate to provide nutrition support and participate in the system of care. As such, nutrition care is interdisciplinary care. Interdisciplinary nutrition care is a thread that appears throughout the *Core*. It is a unique feature of the *Core* that separates it from other nutrition texts.

The strength of the *Core* is in the leadership of the Editor-in-Chief, Charles M. Mueller, PhD, RD, CNSD, who brings a wealth of experience and expertise in nutrition support education, research, and clinical practice. Based on sound principles of nutrition support, the third edition of the *Core* is presented in a manner that facilitates clinical application of the principles and provides a foundation of practice for nutrition support therapy and nutrition in specific diseases using a clear, evidence-based approach to the patient that fosters optimal nutrition outcomes. The editor-in-chief, editors, and contributors have been successful in creating a solid foundation in nutrition support therapy that is evidence based, comprehensive, and reflects the interdisciplinary nature of nutrition support.

Jay M. Mirtallo, MS, RPh, BCNSP, FASHP
President, The American Society for Parenteral and Enteral Nutrition

and

Director, MS in Health System Pharmacy
Professor of Clinical Pharmacy
The Ohio State University, College of Pharmacy
Division of Pharmacy Practice and Administration

aspen | LEADING THE SCIENCE AND PRACTICE OF CLINICAL NUTRITION
American Society for Parenteral and Enteral Nutrition

Preface

The A.S.P.E.N. Adult Nutrition Support Core Curriculum, 2nd Edition is the offspring of the two previous editions of the core curriculum, the previous editions of dietetics and nursing core curriculums, and a selection of case-based study guides published by A.S.P.E.N. pharmacists. Over the years, these texts have become both practice references for professionals, texts for students, as well as study guides for certification and board examinations. The original version of the core published in 2001, *The Science and Practice of Nutrition Support, A Case-Based Core Curriculum,* represented A.S.P.E.N.'s commitment to interdisciplinary organizational, educational, and practice models integrated into one text for all nutrition support professionals. The content of this text was gleaned from a systematic analysis of the MD, RD, and RN National Board of Nutrition Support Certification (NBNSC) examination content outlines and the pharmacy certification in nutrition support offered by the Board of Pharmacy Specialists. Since the publication of the 2007 edition of the Core, in 2007, *The A.S.P.E.N. Nutrition Support Core Curriculum, A Case-Based Approach – The Adult Patient,*[1] NBNSC has discontinued individual professional certifications in nutrition support and replaced them with one credential (and one exam) for all professions. Consideration for this direction was based on the A.S.P.E.N. interdisciplinary model and was confirmed as the best approach to nutrition support practice certification by a practice survey of A.S.P.E.N. members.[2] Subsequently, the content of the single exam was confirmed by a second audit of practice.[3]

When the first edition of the Adult core was published, the A.S.P.E.N. Board of Directors proposed that a three-volume set of cores—pediatric, adult, and older adult—be developed. In 2010, *The A.S.P.E.N. Pediatric Nutrition Support Core Curriculum*[4] was published. Because a core for the older adult has not yet been published, the editors of this 2nd edition of the core decided to include a new chapter (Chapter 36) in the adult core, titled Nutrition Support for Older Adults. Additional new chapters include those on prebiotics and probiotics (Chapter 4), and short bowel syndrome (Chapter 30). The 2nd edition chapter on dietary fiber was incorporated into Chapter 3 (Carbohydrates). These chapters and the rest of the core chapters are authored by recognized experts on the contents of each chapter. Many of the remaining chapter authors have also updated their 2nd edition chapters.

The text is organized into four sections. Part I lays the foundation by providing an overview of nutrient intake digestion and absorption, and by also reviewing specific nutritional requirements and dynamics for fluid, energy, protein, carbohydrate, fiber, and fat and micronutrients. Part II is an overview of enteral and parenteral feeding methods and pharmacotherapeutic considerations. Part III logically progresses to nutrition support during specific states and disorders. Finally, Part IV covers specific management and professional issues relevant to best nutrition support practice.

The general content organization of the chapters covering nutrition support of specific states is also consistent with the previous edition. Chapters on nutrition support for specific states begin with evidence-based, didactic background information that describes core science. Relevant nutrition assessment issues are discussed, including the determination of nutrient requirements. The appropriate route of nutrition support, including oral diet considerations, are also discussed. Monitoring and the recognition of treatment complications are identified and, finally, outcomes relevant to the specific state are addressed. Material is supported by practice recommendations where appropriate and these recommendations are consistent with the most recent A.S.P.E.N. Clinical Guidelines.

A new feature of the text is the Practice Scenario. This feature replaces the more complex case presentation and discussion in previous editions. The Practice Scenarios are directed by a clinical question elucidated by a scenario and answered within the feature format with a provided rationale. Each scenario is referred to in its text chapter as a clinical practice (extension) of text content. The editors of the 2nd edition hope that this new format will provide readers with very specific examples of clinical decision making that extends practical understanding of text content. The scenarios are placed proximate to their referrals in the text, as are tables and figures.

The A.S.P.E.N. Adult Nutrition Support Core Curriculum, 2nd Edition, represents the best efforts of expert nutrition support practitioners using their expertise and A.S.P.E.N.'s collective resources to provide a comprehensive text based on scientific evidence. The editors, authors, and A.S.P.E.N. staff who worked to bring you this edition hope that the text will become a centerpiece of your practice and professional growth.

Charles Mueller
Editor-in-Chief

References

1. Gottschlich MM, ed. *The A.S.P.E.N. Nutrition Support Core Curriculum: A Case-Based Approach — The Adult Patient.* Silver Spring, MD: A.S.P.E.N.; 2007.
2. Schwartz DB, Mirtallo JM, Matarese LE. Practice audit of nutrition support certification. *Nutr Clin Pract.* 2008;23(3):329–340.
3. Materese LE, Chinn RN, Hertz NR, et al. Practice analysis of nutrition support professionals: Evidence-based multidisciplinary nutrition support certification examination. *JPEN J Parenter Enteral Nutr.* 2012. Epub ahead of print. PMID 22368095.
4. Corkins MR, ed. *The A.S.P.E.N. Pediatric Nutrition Support Core Curriculum.* Silver Spring, MD: A.S.P.E.N.; 2010.

aspen | LEADING THE SCIENCE AND PRACTICE OF CLINICAL NUTRITION
American Society for Parenteral and Enteral Nutrition

Acknowledgments

This text represents the effort and hard work of many professional volunteers and A.S.P.E.N. staff over a period of almost 2 years from start to finish. The editors, authors, and reviewers are all volunteers. Without these volunteers, there simply would not be text. In some cases, volunteerism has been equivalent to a part-time job (editors) and in other cases, hours of work and endurance of the editorial and production process.

Before I recognize specific contributors to this text, I would like to thank my mentors in editorial work. Michele Gottschlich was editor-in-chief to my associate editor role on the previous edition *(The A.S.P.E.N. Nutrition Support Core Curriculum: A Case-Based Approach – The Adult Patient)* of this text. Essentially I asked myself throughout the creation of the 2nd edition, "What would Michele do?" In addition, Michele's vision remains intact in the 2nd edition as it should because Michele is one of the most accomplished editors I know. Michele has also inspired me over the years as a singularly creative clinical investigator as well as a superb clinician. And she is funny. My other significant mentor is Peggi Guenter. Peggi was the managing editor of the previous edition and I also was an associate editor to her managing editor on two editions of *The A.S.P.E.N. Nutrition Support Practice Manual.* Peggi is the earth mother of nutrition support. Her humility, kindness, wisdom, humor, and vast clinical and publishing expertise are rarely combined in one woman.

I could not have completed my editorial duties without the assistance of our four associate editors. Denise Schwartz worked with authors, A.S.P.E.N. staff, and her fellow editors with astounding efficiency. When the unexpected happened, Denise forged ahead, thinking only of what to do next to complete a task. I have long admired Denise for her professional and personal qualities in her extraordinary career in clinical dietetics in addition to her long history working as a professional volunteer for A.S.P.E.N. and the National Board of Nutrition Support Certification. Denise doubled as an author as well on Chapter 39. Debra Kovacevich provided nursing expertise to the text and impressed me with her endurance through several lengthy production processes required for some chapters. Sarah Miller was our pharmacy editor and was also my editor when I needed a volunteer to review drafts I was responsible for producing. Her editorial eye is as keen as any I know of. Steve McClave brought new physician talent to the 2nd edition, along with clinical knowledge and editorial skills. Steve helped me keep my sense of humor with his very original emails prodding authors to keep deadlines. Steve also served as an author as well as an editor. Each of these associate editors have a history of professional volunteerism to A.S.P.E.N., ranging from their roles for this text to serving on A.S.P.E.N. committees and task forces to president of the organization (Steve McClave). Egos were left at the door and the work at hand was the singular focus. To them I owe my unqualified gratitude and thanks.

Finally, this text is the product of A.S.P.E.N. and in that capacity I have to thank Patrick McGary, chief operating officer, who oversaw the production of the 2nd edition, especially in the final production stages. Jennifer Kuhn was our managing editor. Jennifer's energy, optimism, efficiency, and work ethic kept me on track when the going got tough. Jennifer has a great career in publishing ahead of her if she chooses. Sara Bazian, publications coordinator, probably ended up doing much more work than she expected, but nevertheless did so with efficiency and good cheer. She was a key player in the production phase of the 2nd edition as well. To each of them, I owe my gratitude and thanks as well.

Charles Mueller
Editor-in-Chief

PART I

BASICS OF NUTRITION AND METABOLISM

1 **Nutrient Intake, Digestion, Absorption, and Excretion** 3
Tina Colaizzo-Anas, PhD, RD, CDN

2 **Energy** 22
Jennifer A. Wooley, MS, RD, CNSC
David Frankenfield, MS, RD

3 **Carbohydrates** 36
Pei-Ra Ling, MD
Karen C. McCowen, MD

4 **Probiotics and Prebiotics** 51
Gail Cresci, PhD, RD, LD, CNSD

5 **Lipids** 63
Mary Hise, PhD, RD, CNSD
John C. Brown, PhD

6 **Protein** 83
Lorraine S. Young, MS, RD, CNSD, LDN
Laurel R. Kearns, MS, RD, CNSC, LDN
Sandra L. Schoepfel, MS, RD, RN, CNSC, LDN
Nicole Caron Clark, MS, RD, CNSC, LDN

7 **Fluids, Electrolytes, and Acid-Base Disorders** 98
Ginger Langley, PharmD, BCNSP, BCPS, CPHQ
Sharla Tajchman, PharmD, BCNSP, BCPS

8 **Vitamins and Trace Elements** 121
Susan F. Clark, RD, PhD

1 Nutrient Intake, Digestion, Absorption, and Excretion

Tina Colaizzo-Anas, PhD, RD, CDN

CONTENTS

Background 4
Nutrient Intake and Appetite 4
Gastrointestinal Motility, Secretion, Circulation, Digestion, and Absorption 7
Motility 7
Types of Movements in the Gut 7
Gastric Motility 9
Small Intestine Motility 10
Colorectal Motility 10
Abnormalities of Gastrointestinal Motility 10
Small Bowel Obstruction/Ileus/Pseudo-obstruction 10
Diarrhea 11
Gastroparesis 12
Constipation 13
Dumping Syndrome 13
Gastrointestinal Secretions 13
Gastric Secretions 14
Bile Secretion 14
Pancreatic Secretions 15
Small and Large Bowel Secretions 15
Gastrointestinal (Splanchnic) Blood Circulation 15
Digestion 16
Digestion of Carbohydrate 16
Digestion of Protein 16
Digestion of Fat 16
Digestion of Nucleic Acids 17
Absorption 17
Mechanisms of Absorption 17
Carbohydrate Absorption 17
Protein Absorption 17
Lipid Absorption 17
Vitamin Absorption 18
Water, Mineral, and Electrolyte Absorption 18
Medium-Chain Triglyceride Absorption 18
Short-Chain Fatty Acid Absorption 18
Alterations in Digestion/Absorption: Starvation, Bowel Rest, Mucosal Atrophy, and Low Flow States 18
Immunity and the Gut 19
References 19

Objectives

1. Translate information on the regulation of appetite to managing transitional feeding regimens.
2. Apply knowledge of the physiology of gastrointestinal (GI) motility to planning enteral nutrition regimens for patients with altered GI motility.
3. Distinguish between different mechanisms of digestion and absorption of various nutrients.
4. Associate the functions of each component of the GI system with their effects on nutrient digestion and absorption and implications for nutrition support.

Test Your Knowledge Questions

1. Which of the following practices is most likely to succeed in improving oral nutrient intake in patients with a prolonged history of weight loss due to poor intake, nausea, and depressed appetite?
   A. Provide a high-calorie oral liquid supplement three times daily
   B. Offer six small, low-fat meals daily
   C. Order fiber supplemented snacks three times daily
   D. Plan primarily solid meals; limit fluids
2. Fermentable fiber is a beneficial addition to enteral formulas because:
   A. Colonic bacteria act on the fiber to produce short-chain fatty acids (SCFAs) that provide an energy source to the intestinal mucosa.
   B. Colonic bacteria act on the fiber to produce SCFAs, which, in turn, exert trophic effects on the intestinal mucosa.
   C. Fermentable fiber may help to control diarrhea by slowing gastric emptying.
   D. All of the above.
3. Which of the following nutrients is added to rehydration liquids to promote sodium (Na^+) absorption in patients with diarrhea?
   A. Glucose
   B. Amino acids
   C. Long-chain fatty acids
   D. Alcohol

Test Your Knowledge Answers

1. The correct answer is **B.** Because of a decline in the stomach's adaptive accommodation function, patients with prolonged negative energy balance may not be able to consume their goal nutrient targets in three regular-sized meals due to feeling of fullness.[1] Six small meals may be more realistic. To address nausea, measures should be taken to prevent slowing of gastric emptying, which could potentiate nausea. These measures may include limiting high-fat foods.[2,3] Providing high-calorie or high-fiber supplements initially may not be the best recommendation because, like fat, caloric density and fiber content can slow gastric emptying.[2–4] Answer D is not a good choice because providing fluids, not limiting them, facilitates gastric emptying.[2]
2. The correct answer is **D.** Although more confirming evidence is needed, the addition of fermentable fibers to enteral formulas likely has multiple beneficial effects, both in the healthy gut and in the malfunctioning gut. Fermentable fibers (eg, pectin, gums, fructooligosaccharides) are metabolized by colonic bacteria to produce SCFAs. SCFAs have multiple benefits for the colonic mucosa. These include providing a significant source of energy for and exerting trophic effects on the intestinal lining.[4,5] However, fiber is not recommended for patients with diarrhea due to *Clostridium difficile* pseudomembranous colitis (PMC) or during low flow states.
3. The correct answer is **A.** The nutrient that is added to rehydration liquids to promote Na^+ and water absorption in patients with diarrhea is glucose. The presence of glucose in the lumen of the small intestines facilitates the absorption of Na^+. When more Na^+ is absorbed, more water from the lumen of the intestines is absorbed. For this reason, oral rehydration fluids that are used to treat Na^+ and water losses from diarrhea include sodium chloride (NaCl) and glucose.[6]

Background

Knowledge of the GI system or gut including its anatomy, physiology, and pathology are central to applying methods of nutrition support. The GI tract is the organ system that allows us to regulate appetite; ingest, digest, and absorb nutrients, phytochemicals, and other food components; and excrete indigestible components of the food we consume. It is also the organ system that serves as one of the body's largest defenses against pathogens as well as a vehicle for nutrients and substances that modulate the immune response. The following discussion will address each of these roles.

Nutrient Intake and Appetite

Blundell and Stubbs have proposed that the physiology of appetite is the physiology of feeding behavior.[1] The physiology of feeding behavior integrates both the physiology of the central nervous system and peripheral nervous system with metabolism. The human appetite system is a redundant system, which means that within it are overlapping subsystems, each of which individually may not be necessary for the system to function normally. This allows feeding behavior to vary in terms of meal size, meal frequency, and food composition. The human appetite system can sense changes in its internal (eg, metabolism of pregnancy) and external (eg, ambient temperature) environments and interacts with other biological systems related to motivation and behavior.[1] A physiological tendency toward overconsumption has evolved and is, therefore, primed to respond to energy/nutrient deficits. The human appetite system exists within equilibrium of energy balance in which energy intake normally equals energy expenditure except when body weight increases or decreases to a new equilibrium. Nonetheless, American adults gain an average of 0.2 to 2.0 kg per year.[7]

As previously suggested, normally food intake adjusts to maintain body weight or to undo changes in weight. When individuals lose weight because of illness, weight is often spontaneously regained during recovery. Likewise, when individuals lose weight while on weight reduction diets, many regain the lost weight. This is also true in animals.[8] The triggers that influence food intake include satiety signals and hunger signals. Overconsumption is likely influenced more strongly by hunger signals as compared to satiety signals. The evidence for the influence of hunger signals on food intake relates to data describing the course of prolonged negative energy balance and significant loss of lean body tissue. It is not clear whether the hunger signals present in prolonged negative energy balance are the same signals that control day-to-day feeding behavior. Data is slowly emerging that describe how these signals influence meal size, frequency, and composition.[1]

Neural and hormonal signals that influence food intake are integrated in the brain, primarily in the arcuate nucleus (ARC) of the hypothalamus and the brainstem. In the ARC, orexigenic (appetite-stimulating) cells express the neurotransmitter, neuropeptide Y (NPY), and agouti-related peptide (AgRP), and anorexigenic (appetite-suppressing) cells express pro-opiomelanocortin (POMC) and cocaine- and amphetamine-regulated transcript (CART). POMC is a natural opioid. ARC signals regulate activity in the paraventricular nucleus (PVN) of the hypothalamus (Figure 1-1).[9] NPY messenger ribonucleic acid (RNA) increases in the hypothalamus during feeding and decreases during satiety. The effects of NPY may be redundant as gene knock-out animals exhibit no significant changes in feeding.[8]

Two major inputs influence appetite regulation: short-term signals related to meal ingestion are transmitted by the "gut-brain axis" and signals associated with energy stores are mediated by leptin. A third system influencing appetite regulation is the circadian rhythm, which will not be discussed in this chapter.[9] The gut-brain axis reflects energy balance via a signaling system between the GI tract and the hypothalamus and brainstem. Both neural (vagal) and gut hormones transmit the signals. The major orexigenic gut hormone is ghrelin, and anorexigenic gut hormones include glucagon-like peptide-1 (GLP-1), oxyntomodulin (OXM), peptide tyrosine-tyrosine (PYY), pancreatic polypeptide (PP), and possibly cholecystokinin (CCK).[10,11] POMC and AgRP expression are regulated by insulin and leptin, insulin via a downstream effector, Forkhead box family transcription factor 01.[12] GLP-1, OXM, PYY, and PP increase in response to feeding. GLP-1, OXM, and PYY are secreted by the distal gut. PP is secreted by the PP cells of the islet of Langerhans in the pancreas. GLP-1 binds GLP-1 receptors in the pancreatic islet cell, heart, lungs, ARC, and PVN. OXM acts as an agonist at glucagon receptors. PYY inhibits NPY and activates POMC. Increased PYY levels also are associated with increased activity of the orbitofrontal cortex (OFC). Increased GLP-1, OXM, PYY, and PP all result in decreased food intake. GLP-1 also delays gastric empyting[9] (Table 1-1). Gut- and fat-derived hormones—ghrelin, leptin, insulin, and peptide YY—are involved in feedback regulation of feeding through signals affecting hunger, satiety, and energy needs.[13] Additionally, ghrelin has been shown to increase when stress hormones increase.[14] Insulin, as well as these gut-derived hormones, affects neural signals in the brain related to acute changes in energy levels. Insulin, along with leptin, inhibits the same neural circuits (dopaminergic) that are stimulated by ghrelin.[13]

FIGURE 1-1 Mechanism of Gut Hormone Action

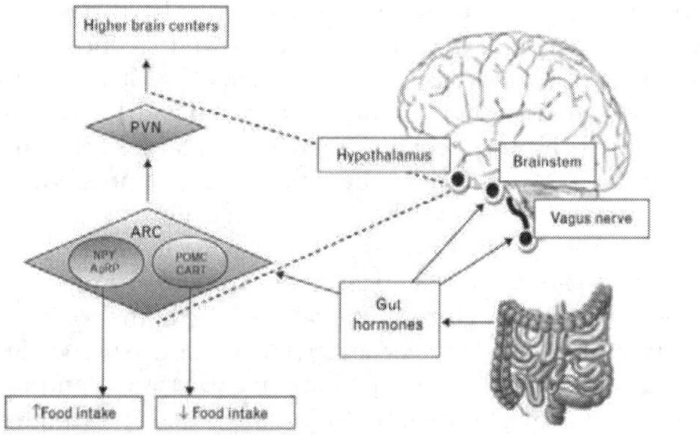

Hormones released from the gut are proposed to act at three sites to influence food intake; the vagus nerve, brainstem, and hypothalamus. PVN, paraventricular nucleus, ARC, arcuate nucleus, NPY, neuropeptide Y, AgRP, agouti-related peptide, POMC, pro-opiomelanocortin, CART, cocaine and amphetamine-regulated transcript. Reprinted with permission from Cegla J, Tan TM, Bloom SR. Gut-brain cross-talk in appetite regulation. *Curr Opin Clin Nutr & Metab Care.* 2010;13(5):588–593.

Gut hormones affect neuronal activity in the central nervous system (CNS) by crossing the blood-brain barrier or by binding to receptors on the afferent vagus, as well as stretch receptors and nutrient chemoreceptors. These signals are channeled through the brainstem and then coordinated with appetite regulation via the ARC (Figure 1-1). End neural signaling in the brain affects "learning about (food) rewards, attending to food rewards, valuation of stimuli in the environment, processing information about energy stores and gastrointestinal contents. Reward pathways motivate food intake and pleasure associated with eating."[13]

Generally speaking, appetite is regulated in two areas of the hypothalamus, a lateral "feeding center" and a medial "satiety center." When the feeding center is stimulated, animals eat. Conversely, when the feeding center is damaged, severe, fatal anorexia can result. When the "satiety center" is stimulated, animals stop eating. Alternatively, when lesions occur in the satiety center, overeating occurs. Some evidence suggests that the satiety center functions by transiently inhibiting the feeding center after food is ingested.[8] When animals gain weight because of lesions in the satiety center, their intake plateaus (after a period of weight gain) and increased weight is thus maintained.

Leptin is a hormone that acts on the hypothalamus to decrease food intake and increase energy expenditure. It provides feedback on the body's fat stores. Serum leptin levels increase in proportion to percentage of body fat. It was originally found in white adipose tissue, but it is also expressed in a variety of other tissues, including the gastric mucosa, which secretes large amounts.[15] Low levels of leptin associated with food deprivation result in increased energy intake and decreased energy expenditure. Additionally, low leptin levels affect not only the ARC, but also centers of the brain that

TABLE 1-1 Gut Hormones and Peptides Influencing Food Intake

Hormone	Site of Secretion	Stimulated by	Mechanism of Action	Effect
GLP-1	Distal gut	Food intake proportional to calorie intake	Binds GLP-1 receptors in pancreatic islet cells, heart, lungs, and brain (ARC and PVC)	- Reduces appetite and calorie intake - Delays gastric emptying - Enhances postprandial insulin release
OXM	L cells of the gut	Food intake	- Agonist at glucagon receptor - Undefined neural effects	- Reduces food intake - Increases energy expenditure
PYY	L cells of the distal gut	Food intake	- Y receptors found throughout the CNS and on vagal afferents - NPY inhibition - POMC activation - Associated with increased activity of OFC	Reduces food intake
Pancreatic polypeptide	Pancreatic polypeptide cells of the islets of Langerhans in the pancreas	- Food intake - Vagal stimulation	- Enters CNS via diffusion in the brainstem and ARC	Reduces food intake
Leptin	- Large amounts from the gastric mucosa -White adipose tissue	Food deprivation is associated with low levels	- Low levels influence ARC - Possibly decreases gene expression of NPY and increases activity of POMC-secreting neurons	Low levels increase energy intake and decrease energy expenditure
Ghrelin	Stomach	- Food intake decreases levels - Fasting increases levels	- Stimulates ARC via receptors - Stimulates GH secretion	Increases food intake

ARC, arcuate nucleus; CNS, central nervous system; GH, growth hormone; GLP-1, glucagon-like peptide-1; NPY, neuropeptide Y; OFC, orbitofrontal cortex; OXM, oxyntomodulin; POMC, pro-opiomelanocortin; PVC, paraventricular nucleus; PYY, peptide-tyrosine-tyrosine.

regulate smelling, tasting, and learning to maximize the rewarding aspects of food.[16] A likely mechanism for the action of leptin is to decrease NPY gene expression in the hypothalamus.[17] It also may increase the activity of POMC-secreting neurons with the effect of decreasing food intake.

Leptin regulates appetite centrally through receptors, which are present in multiple forms. The long form, which is produced by an alternatively spliced leptin receptor gene, is found in the hypothalamus. The short form of the leptin receptor is found in the brain microvessels and may be involved in transporting leptin across the blood-brain barrier. One cause of human obesity may be defects in the leptin receptor gene.[7] Although theoretically it is biologically plausible that the high leptin levels that accompany high-percentage body fat contribute to a negative feedback mechanism resulting in decreased food intake, little evidence exists to document this relationship.

Other factors that may regulate appetite include ghrelin, additional gut peptides, and glucose. Ghrelin is a gastric-synthesized polypeptide that stimulates growth hormone secretion and regulates food intake. Blood levels are decreased when food is eaten and increase during fasting. Ghrelin increases food intake by stimulating the ARC of the hypothalamus. In addition to ghrelin, a number of GI hormones have been implicated in regulating food intake. These include peptide YY (secreted in the small intestine and colon), gastrin-releasing peptide (GRP), glucagon, somatostatin, and CCK, all of which have been proposed to decrease food intake.[8] CCK has been shown to reduce meal size specifically, rather than meal frequency (ie, it seems to be involved in satiation [bringing a meal to an end]).[1]

Glucose is proposed to regulate food intake through its utilization by the neurons in the satiety center. A possible mechanism may be related to low neuronal glucose utilization: when neuronal activity decreases, satiety decreases, and hunger ensues.[8] (Hunger is defined as the "intrinsic desire for food."[18]) Conversely, when glucose utilization is high, the feeding center is inhibited and hunger abates.[8] A decrease in blood glucose is currently considered to be a biomarker for satiety and signals the onset of meal initiation.[19] Appetite can also be influenced by GI distention, which decreases food intake, and contractions of an empty stomach, which increase food intake.

In addition to biological influences on food intake, environmental and cognitive events play major roles. Factors including convenience, price, nutritional beliefs, availability, brand image, and cultural and social influences all serve as determinants of food intake. Palatability, the subjective appreciation of pleasantness, has a positive effect on food intake behavior.

Diet composition plays a role in feeding responses. Some suggest that high-fat diets promote higher energy intake.[20] However, others have demonstrated increased energy intake when the carbohydrate density of the diet was increased.[21] Still others have shown that an isocaloric meal that is higher in fiber and protein than a control meal results in lower calorie intake and decreased hunger scores.[22] Similarly, studies on the effect of sweetness on appetite and the effect of fat on satiety show conflicting results. However, evidence suggests that all three major macronutrients exert effects on satiety to different extents. Protein seems to be more satiating than carbohydrates, which are more satiating than fat. In multiple studies, protein has been shown to significantly increase subjective feelings of satiety[23–25] as well as decrease hunger.[26] Furthermore, certain proteins have been shown to increase satiety more than others. For example, whey protein has been shown to have a significantly stronger influence on satiety compared to casein.[27] Higher protein diets (18% of calories) and associated increased satiety may increase the rate of weight maintenance after weight loss by 50%.[28] Despite the variability in research findings, it seems that dietary fat content is a risk factor for weight gain.[1]

While the influences of macronutrients on appetite control are well-established notions, the role of fiber,[29] especially resistant starch (RS2), is becoming clearer. RS2 is found in native starch granules (B-type X-ray spectrum) in produce such as maize rich in amylase, raw potatoes, and green bananas. Human dietary studies with RS2 have demonstrated increased satiety and associated decreased food intake.[30,31] The effect of fiber on appetite has been demonstrated when enteral formula was used as the sole source of nutrition. Enteral nutrition supplemented with pea-fiber and fructooligosaccharides resulted in increased satiety and feelings of fullness.[32]

In addition to energy value or nutrient content, food weight and volume can be important variables.[1] Weight and volume influence intrameal satiation more than postingestive (between meals) satiety.[33] Viscosity has an inverse effect on hunger.[34]

Stomach size can also influence the amount of food eaten, and its size is related to the amount of food habitually eaten. For this reason, during nutritional rehabilitation of undernourished patients, small frequent meals should be initiated to increase nutrient intake until a time when patients can increase their food intake comfortably at any one sitting.[1] Under normal circumstances, the stomach delivers metered amounts of nutrients to the duodenum often on the basis of number of calories. Subsequently, satiety signals arise from the small intestine as well as the stomach. In fact, it has been documented that the satiating influence of fat is, in part, mediated via signals in the small intestine.[1] Specifically, when infusions of corn oil are infused directly into the jejunum or ileum, bypassing the stomach, gastric emptying is slowed, a feeling of fullness is experienced, and reduced food intake results.[1] These findings regarding macronutrient composition, fiber content, food volume, and viscosity may have implications for the design of transitional feeding regimens.

Clinicians are often faced with having to encourage increased oral food intake in patients who have decreased appetites associated with illness, surgery, or emotional distress. In some instances, pharmacological intervention may serve to stimulate appetite. Megestrol acetate has been studied in neoplastic diseases, human immunodeficiency virus infection, and acquired immunodeficiency syndrome (AIDS).[35] However, additional studies may be needed to prove safety and efficacy. GI side effects occur in 5% of patients with AIDS and 1% to 4% in general.[35] In addition to adverse GI side effects, a variety of reports of adverse side effects have been documented in other major organ systems.[35]

Aging is associated with decreased appetite and food intake. This is likely due to decreased basal hunger rather than increased meal satiety.[36] If the nutrition assessment suggests the need for an enteral supplement, consideration should be given to a liquid, rather than solid, supplement as liquids have been shown to lessen postprandial decline in hunger more than solids with resultant higher calorie intake in a controlled feeding trial.[37]

Gastrointestinal Motility, Secretion, Circulation, Digestion, and Absorption

The assimilation of nutrients occurs as a result of three general and distinct processes. These include (1) the movement of food throughout the GI tract; (2) the digestion of food; and (3) the absorption of nutrients. Each of the structures of the GI tract has specific functions with regard to these three processes. The roles of each of the structures of the GI tract are outlined in the following discussion.

Motility

Normal GI motility is important for optimal digestion and absorption. Each section of the GI tract is structured to handle food of specific physical character and viscosity, and has motor activities that support its specialized function. For example, the esophagus transports small chunks of food, whereas the stomach stores, digests, and grinds solid food into small particles and controls the emptying of food into the small bowel. Sphincters separate sections of the GI tract and act as one-way valves in the forward direction. They both control direction of movement and the amount moved through the GI tract.[38] For example, the lower esophageal sphincter (LES) relaxes in response to swallowing. Between meals, the LES is closed to prevent reflux of gastric contents into the esophagus,[39] which protects the esophageal mucosa from the erosive effects of gastric acid. Chronic acid damage to the esophagus by gastric reflux can result in morphologic changes that, when untreated, can eventually lead to Barrett's esophagus and to an increased risk of esophageal cancer. The closed tone of the LES is under neural control.

Types of Movements in the Gut

The GI tract has two types of movement: propulsive movements and mixing movements. Propulsive movements propel food forward through the GI tract; mixing movements mix food with GI secretions. Peristalsis is the basic propulsive movement.[38,40] Peristalsis occurs in all parts of the GI tract from the esophagus to rectum when the gut wall is stretched by its contents. The stretch stimulus causes a release of serotonin leading to smooth muscle contraction.[39] Other stimuli for peristalsis are chemical or physical irritation of the epithelial lining of the gut. Strong parasympathetic stimulation leads to strong peristalsis.[40] Peristaltic waves in the esophagus and gastric emptying are stimulated by the vagus nerve.[38]

Myogenic, neural, and hormonal factors regulate GI motility. Myogenic control of GI motility is mediated by smooth muscle. Smooth muscle in the GI tract is normally in a polarized state in which the outside of the cell is positively charged relative to the inside of the cell. Contraction of the muscle is associated with depolarization. Conversely, inhibition of contraction is associated with a hyperpolarized state. The depolarized state results from the transfer of positively charged ions (primarily Ca^{2+} with some Na^+ ions) into the cell, the exit of negatively charged (Cl^-) ions out of the cell, and the inhibition of K^+ transfer out of the cell. Hyperpolarization, the state of a muscle cell in which its membrane potential is more negative, is accompanied by an increase of K^+ or decrease of Cl^- transfer out of the cell. The hyperpolarized state inhibits Ca^{2+} channels, preventing Ca^{2+} entry into cells. The hyperpolarized state makes a muscle fiber less excitable. The actions of hormones and neurotransmitters also result in altered intracellular Ca^{2+} concentrations to influence muscle contraction and subsequent GI motility.[38,40]

GI muscle fibers are depolarized in response to (1) stretching the muscle fiber, (2) acetylcholine released by parasympathetic neurons, and (3) gut hormones that will be discussed subsequently. GI muscle fibers are hyperpolarized in response to (1) norepinephrine or epinephrine and (2) sympathetic nerves that secrete norepinephrine.[40]

The neural control of smooth muscle is executed by the enteric nervous system (ENS), which innervates the GI tract from the esophagus to anus. The ENS can function autonomously, but it is connected to the CNS via parasympathetic and sympathetic fibers. Generally, the sympathetic nervous system modulates the activity of the ENS by inhibitory signals. The parasympathetic nervous system stimulates the ENS.[40]

The ENS is organized into two plexuses, the myenteric (Auerbach's) plexus and the submucosal (Meissner's) plexus. GI movement is controlled by the myenteric plexus. The submucosal plexus controls GI secretions and blood flow. The fibers of the parasympathetic neural network that innervate the esophagus, stomach, pancreas, small intestine, and first half of the large intestine are in the vagus nerves. The sympathetic neural fibers arise from the spinal cord and innervate the entire gut. Norepinephrine is the predominant neurotransmitter secreted by the sympathetic nerve endings.[40]

The neurotransmitters of the ENS include acetylcholine, norepinephrine and serotonin, adenosine triphosphate (ATP), dopamine, CCK, substance P, vasoactive intestinal peptide (VIP), somatostatin, leu-enkephalin, met-enkephalin, and bombesin.[40] Acetylcholine is generally excitatory in action (increases muscular activity), whereas norepinephrine exerts inhibitory effects. Epinephrine, which is secreted by the adrenal medullae, is also inhibitory.[40]

Afferent sensory nerve fibers in the ENS are also involved in the neural control of the gut. Sensory stimuli include irritation of the mucosa, excessive distention, or chemical stimuli. Sensory signals are transmitted to the spinal cord, brainstem, or brain medulla, many via afferent fibers of the vagus nerve. These are followed by vagal reflexes to the gut.[40]

While the predominant influence of GI hormones is to regulate GI secretions, GI hormones do influence GI motility. See Table 1-2, which summarizes the actions of intestinal hormones, their stimuli for secretion, and site of secretion. The actions include modulating gastric emptying and the rate of small intestinal transit.[40]

TABLE 1-2 Gastrointestinal Hormone Actions, Stimuli for Secretion, and Site of Secretion

Hormone	Stimuli for Secretion	Site of Secretion	Actions
Gastrin	Protein distention nerve (acid inhibits release)	G cells of the antrum, duodenum, and jejunum	Stimulates gastric acid secretion and mucosal growth
Cholecystokinin	Protein Fat Acid	I cells of the duodenum, jejunum, and ileum	Stimulates pancreatic enzyme secretion, gallbladder contraction, and growth of exocrine pancreas Inhibits gastric emptying
Secretin	Acid Fat	S cells of the duodenum, jejunum, and ileum	Stimulates pepsin, pancreatic and biliary bicarbonate secretion, and growth of exocrine pancreas Inhibits gastric acid secretion
Gastric inhibitory peptide	Protein Fat Carbohydrate	K cells of the duodenum and jejunum	Stimulates insulin release Inhibits gastric acid secretion
Motilin	Fat Acid Nerve	M cells of the duodenum and jejunum	Stimulates gastric motility and intestinal motility

Reprinted with permission from: General principles of gastrointestinal function—motility, nervous control, and blood circulation. In: Hall JE. *Guyton and Hall Textbook of Medical Physiology.* 12th ed. Philadelphia, PA: Elsevier; 2010:753–762.

Gastric Motility

To understand the stomach's role in motility, digestion, and absorption, it is helpful to review relevant aspects of its anatomy and physiology (Figure 1-2). The cardia is the portion of the stomach just distal to the esophagus. Located between the esophagus and the stomach is the LES. At the distal end of the stomach, the pyloric sphincter is positioned between the stomach and the duodenum. The fundus is the uppermost portion of the stomach. Above the fundus is the diaphragm. The body of the stomach begins at horizontal plane of the junction between the stomach and esophagus, the gastroesophageal junction. The antrum, the lower 25% to 30% of the stomach, begins where the lesser curvature of the stomach turns to the right.[2]

The motor functions of the stomach make a significant contribution to digestion of food. These include storage of food, mixing of food with gastric secretions, and emptying of the semifluid mixture (chyme) into the duodenum.[18] Gastric tone is regulated in multiple ways. Intragastric pressure falls in response to the vagal nerve–mediated swallowing reflex and in response to gastric distention by the presence of food. The latter is accomplished by stretch receptors in the gastric wall. Biochemical mediators of proximal gastric relaxation principally include nitric oxide and VIP in addition to dopamine, gastrin, CCK, secretin, GRP, and glucagon. Decreases in gastric tone result from duodenal distention, colonic distention, and ileal perfusion with glucose.[2,38] A relaxed stomach can accommodate 0.8 to 1.5 L. Mixing waves of constriction lead into powerful peristaltic waves that propel the chyme toward the pylorus. Ultimately, this leads to intense peristalsis in the stomach antrum and subsequent gastric emptying.[18]

Gastric emptying is regulated by volume of food, gastrin, enterogastric nervous reflexes from the duodenum, and hormonal feedback from the duodenum. Increased food volume leads to increased gastric distention and release of gastrin. Gastrin has an independent effect on gastric emptying by limiting the activity of the pyloric pump. Three types of inhibitory reflexes arise from the duodenum: (1) from the ENS, (2) from the sympathetic neural fibers, and (3) from the inhibitory fibers of the vagus nerve. These inhibitory reflexes are stimulated by (1) duodenal distention, (2) irritation of the duodenal mucosa, (3) pH less than 3.5 to 4.0, (4) high osmolality, and (5) the presence of breakdown products of protein and fat digestion.[18]

Hormonal feedback from the duodenum has an inhibitory effect on gastric emptying. Dietary fat is the strongest stimulus for hormones of the duodenum and jejunum (eg, CCK). These intestinal hormones act specifically on the pyloric pump and pyloric sphincter. Other probable hormones inhibiting gastric emptying include secretin and gastric inhibitory peptide (GIP).[18]

The tone of proximal stomach influences liquid emptying, whereas the distal stomach is involved in solid emptying. Liquids empty more quickly than solids. The half emptying time of water or isotonic saline is 12 minutes on average. This means that if one drinks 300 mL of water, 150 mL will enter the duodenum in 12 minutes (range 10 to 65 minutes).[41] The emptying time for liquids changes when the composition of the liquid changes. The rate of emptying amounts to about 200 kcal per hour for liquids up to 1 molar concentration. Duodenal osmoreceptors, secretin, and VIP regulate liquid emptying. As mentioned previously, the swallowing reflex influences gastric tone. When the swallowing mechanism is bypassed, as in nasogastric (NG) tube feeding, the rate of gastric emptying is faster. The half emptying time of solids is about 2 hours on average (range 45 to 110 minutes).[41] The rate of solids emptying is influenced significantly by meal particle size, calorie, and fat content.[2f]

Meal composition influences the rate of gastric emptying. Emptying may be slowed by increasing caloric content, fat content, or osmolality of a meal. These effects are mediated by duodenal osmoreceptors, glucoreceptors, and pH receptors via neurohumoral routes.[2,4] Consideration of these factors may be useful in planning medical nutrition therapy for patients who experience nausea. Nausea is defined as an unpleasant sensation felt in the upper abdomen that is associated with the desire to vomit.[42] Limiting high-fat, high-fiber food is recommended to reduce nausea associated with cancer.[3] Carbohydrate-rich foods leave the stomach in a few hours; protein-rich food empties later; fat is the slowest macronutrient to empty.[39] See Practice Scenario 1-1 for a discussion of gastroparesis accompanying type 1 diabetes mellitus.

The primary GI hormone affecting gastric emptying is CCK, which inhibits emptying. This effect of CCK is likely augmented by leptin, which is secreted by cells in the gastric mucosa in addition to fat cells. The volume of gastric contents also influences the rate of gastric emptying. The emptying rate increases as the gastric volume increases.[38]

Gastric motility can influence positioning of nasoduodenal tubes. Often the goal during nasoduodenal intubation for enteral feeding is for peristalsis of the stomach to carry the tube tip through the pylorus. In situations in which the tip fails to pass, prokinetic agents may be used to increase gastric emptying. Because the duodenal mucosa possesses sensory receptors that are associated with neurohumoral reflexes that influence gastric emptying, gastric emptying time after feeding tube placement may decrease significantly if feeding tubes are placed in the jejunum, bypassing the duodenum.[38]

FIGURE 1-2 Anatomic Regions of the Stomach

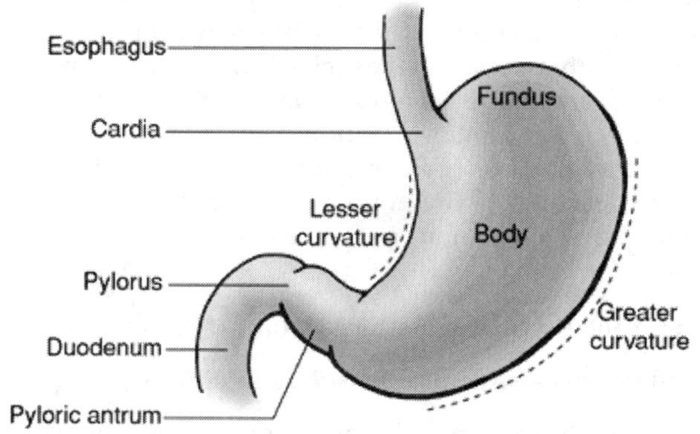

Reproduced with permission from Mercer DW, Liu TH, Castaneda A. Anatomy and physiology of the stomach. In: Zuidema GD, Yeo CJ, eds. *Shackelford's Surgery of the Alimentary Tract.* 5th ed., Vol. II. Philadelphia, PA: Saunders; 2002:3.

Practice Scenario 1-1

Question: What nutrition intervention would you recommend for a patient with gastroparesis who has failed to respond to dietary interventions?

Scenario: A 42-year-old man was admitted with nausea, vomiting, and abdominal pain. He had a 25-year history of type 1 diabetes, diabetic retinopathy, and gastroparesis previously confirmed by a solid phase nuclear medicine gastric emptying scan, and he had been treated with a low-fat diet and promotility agents including metoclopramide. He also had a history of peripheral neuropathy and reflux esophagitis. His diabetes was treated with lispro insulin. Other medications included famotidine 20 mg twice daily. In the previous year, he had five similar admissions. He was made NPO on admission to control vomiting, which was exacerbated by eating. Nutrition assessment data included: weight: 70 kg; BMI: 22; percentage weight loss: 5% in 6 months, electrolytes and hemoglobin were concentrated and suggestive of dehydration. His elevated blood sugar was addressed with sliding scale insulin while NPO. His HgA1c was 7.6%, indicating less than optimal glucose control.

Intervention: He was begun on intravenous feedings and a NG tube was placed to suction. When he demonstrated low NG tube output, a duodenal feeding tube was placed under fluoroscopy. The tip was positioned in the second portion of the duodenum. A 1 kcal/mL enteral standard feeding formula was initiated at 20 mL/hr and advanced every 12 hours by 20 mL/hr increments to a goal of 1.3 × basal energy expenditure (BEE) and 1.2 g/kg protein. He was transitioned to a trial of cycled night-time feedings. The patient demonstrated good tolerance of this regimen with no evidence of abdominal distention, nausea, or vomiting, and acceptable gastric residual volumes and passage of stool.

Answer: The patient was offered the option of a percutaneous endoscopic jejunostomy tube placement for long-term intestinal feedings at night. An oral diet of small amounts of low-fat, low-fiber foods with liquids as tolerated was recommended to address his desire to eat. Given that lispro is a short-acting insulin, a longer-acting insulin was ordered for night-time feedings.

Rationale: The clinical history indicated that this patient was an oral diet failure. His good response to night-time, cycled intestinal feedings suggested that he may be a candidate for a jejunostomy tube for long-term feeding. Jejunal feedings bypass the stomach and obviate the potential of formula intolerance due to delayed gastric emptying. The recommendation of small amounts of low-fat, low-fiber foods taken with fluids may be made to address psychosocial need to eat.

Small Intestine Motility

Movements in the small intestine can be characterized as mixing contractions and propulsive contractions. Mixing contractions are elicited when the small intestine is distended by chyme. The motor functions of the small intestine in the fed state include mixing of food with digestive enzymes secreted from the intestine, pancreas, and biliary system. This mixing aids in digestion as well as absorption.

Typically the rate of mixing contractions is 2 or 3 per minute or maximally 12 per minute. Propulsive movements of the small intestine (peristalsis) move in the direction of the anus at a rate of 0.5 to 2.0 cm per second. Hence, the average time that it takes for chyme to travel from the pylorus to the ileocecal valve is 3 to 5 hours.[18]

Intestinal peristalsis is regulated by neural and hormonal controls. Neural control is partly initiated when chyme stretches the intestinal wall. Additionally, when the stomach is stretched, a gastroenteric reflex initiates intestinal peristalsis.[18]

Hormonal control of intestinal peristalsis includes both inhibitory and stimulatory signals. The stimulatory hormones include gastrin, CCK, insulin, motilin, and serotonin. Inhibitory hormones include secretin and glucagon.[18]

When chyme reaches the end of the terminal ileum, its passage into the cecum is metered by constrictions of the ileocecal sphincter. After a meal, peristalsis increases in the ileum in response to a gastroileal reflex. The volume of chyme that empties into the cecum daily is approximately 1500 to 2000 mL.[18]

Colorectal Motility

The purposes of the motor activities of the colon are to mix, store, concentrate, and eliminate food residues. The ascending colon receives liquid contents through the ileocecal valve. As food residues move through the transverse colon to the descending colon, luminal contents become more solid.[38] As in the stomach and the small intestines, the movements of the colon are mixing and propulsive movements. The mixing movements of the colon result in maximum exposure of feces to the mucosal surface, allowing absorption of fluid and other substances. This concentrating action of the colon results in expulsion of only 80 to 200 mL feces daily. The ileocecal valve prevents backflow of fecal contents into the small intestines. The time that it takes for chyme to move from the ileocecal valve through the colon requires as many as 8 to 15 hours.[18]

Mass movements from the cecum to the sigmoid colon occur one to three times daily, especially during the first hour after eating breakfast. Mass movements occur in response to distention of the stomach and duodenum, which trigger gastrocolic and duodenocolic reflexes. These contractions may occur with or without defecation.[18] Normally, the rectum is empty. Mass movements in the colon propel food residue into the rectum. Distention of the rectum results in the urge to defecate with associated reflex relaxation of the internal and external anal sphincters. Both sphincters contract under voluntary control.[38] In addition, gastric distention by food can stimulate rectal relaxation (gastrocolic reflex) and subsequently, the urge to defecate.[18,38] The normal frequency for bowel movements in developed countries is every 1 to 3 days.[38]

Abnormalities of Gastrointestinal Motility

Small Bowel Obstruction/Ileus/Pseudo-obstruction

Motility of the small bowel is often prohibited by mechanical obstruction or ileus. More than 300,000 hospitalizations per year because of small bowel obstructions (SBOs) are due to adhesions deriving from previous abdominal, including GI and gynecological, surgeries.[43] Intra-abdominal adhesions account for up to 75% of cases of SBO. Management of this condition is discussed in Practice Scenario 1-2. Other etiologies include hernias, Crohn's disease, intestinal malrotation, volvulus, and, uncommonly, tumor.[44] In the colon, obstructions are often caused by tumors.

Ileus, the temporary loss of peristalsis, is another abnormality of GI motility that is the most common cause of delayed discharge after abdominal surgery. Although ileus is commonly associated with abdominal surgery, it can also accompany infection and inflammation, electrolyte imbalances, and the use of certain drugs (especially sedatives, opioid analgesics, α_2-adrenergic receptor agonists, and catecholamine vasopressors). On average, after abdominal surgery, the small intestine regains peristalsis within 24 hours, and motility of the stomach and colon return between 48 hours and 3 to 5 days, respectively.[44] Treatment of ileus includes NG suction, bowel rest, intravenous fluids and electrolytes, and minimal use of sedatives.[45] In some situations, transpyloric feeding may be feasible. PN is warranted if enteral feeding is not possible for 7 days.[46]

Colonic pseudo-obstructions can develop in patients as a complication of narcotic use, bed rest, or disease. Mechanical obstruction is absent in pseudo-obstruction, but the presence of a massively dilated bowel prevents normal bowel function. Treatment includes discontinuation of narcotics, anticholinergics, or other medications that are associated with ileus; strict bowel rest; and intravenous hydration. For prolonged periods of bowel rest, PN may be required. Decompression of the colon is instituted if these measures fail.[47]

Chronic intestinal pseudo-obstruction can be an irreversible disorder of intestinal motility. Treatment often consists of palliation of symptoms including nausea and vomiting, provision of intravenous hydration or PN, and when necessary, withholding oral food. Some patients require a decompressive gastrostomy or small intestinal resections.[44] Small bowel pseudo-obstruction can predispose to bacterial overgrowth with associated diarrhea and steatorrhea. Chronic colonic pseudo-obstruction may lead to significant constipation. Patients may present with abdominal distention and visible bowel loops.[48]

Practice Scenario 1-2

Question: What medical nutrition therapy should be offered to a patient who reobstructs after surgery (lysis of adhesions) for small bowel obstruction?

Scenario: A 59-year-old male was in a normal state of health until he presented acutely with a history of vomiting, abdominal distention, and hyperactive bowel sounds. His height was 170 cm, and his weight was 80 kg. Laboratory findings suggested hypovolemia, hemoconcentration, and electrolyte abnormalities. Past medical history included surgical reduction of an umbilical hernia 5 years prior to admission. Physical examination provided no evidence of hernias in the inguinal or femoral areas, and stools were negative for gross or occult blood. An abdominal series showed dilated small bowel loops greater than 3 cm, air-fluid levels, and limited air in the colon. A computed tomography (CT) scan documented findings of a discrete transition zone with dilation of bowel proximally, decompression of bowel distally, and intraluminal contrast that did not pass beyond the transition zone, and a colon with only a small amount of gas or fluid. A diagnosis of small bowel obstruction was made.

Isotonic intravenous fluids and prophylactic broad-spectrum antibiotics were started. The stomach was decompressed via NG tube. The patient underwent an exploratory laparotomy with lysis of adhesions. Postoperatively, after the initial return of bowel sounds, his NG tube output increased to 1500 mL, and he redeveloped abdominal distention.

Intervention: The patient was placed on bowel rest and parenteral nutrition (PN) was instituted.

Answer: After surgery, it is normal for the stomach and colon to require approximately 48 hours for the return of peristalsis and bowel function. The small bowel takes less time for peristalsis to return (24 hours on average).[44] However, the patient had increasing abdominal distention and increased NG tube output, suggesting reobstruction of the small intestines. Obstruction in the early postoperative period occurs in 0.7% of patients.[44] PN is required because a period of bowel rest of 7 or more days was anticipated.

Diarrhea

Diarrhea refers to an increased frequency and liquidity of stool. The discharge of diarrhea can be characterized many ways: explosive, nocturnal, bacterial, viral, protozoan, osmotic, bloody, chronic, acute, voluminous, fatty, or secretory. Etiologies can range from infection to malabsorption.[49] Watery diarrhea can occur with fecal impaction or obstructing tumor.[50] When transit time is rapid, large amounts of Na^+, potassium, and water pass through the colon. This may lead to severe fluid electrolyte abnormalities, fluid loss, dehydration, hypovolemia, and if untreated, hypovolemic shock and cardiovascular collapse.[39]

When evaluating diarrhea, a left shift with increased white blood cells (WBCs) on a complete blood count may indicate an infectious process. A decreased hemoglobin may indicate anemia from blood loss. Serum sodium and blood urea nitrogen may be increased from dehydration or serum sodium, and potassium may be decreased due to losses. pH may reflect an acidosis related to hyperchloremia or alkalosis related to dehydration. Stool cultures should be ordered to rule out infectious etiologies, and *C. difficile* toxins A and B should be ordered if the patient had been on antibiotics or chemotherapy in recent weeks. Sigmoidoscopy is indicated with bloody diarrhea or when pseudomembraneous colitis (PMC) or ulcerative colitis is suspected. PMC refers to the intestinal inflammation that is accompanied by presence of pseudomembranes on the intestinal mucosa.[51] Most cases of PMC involve the colon (rarely the small intestine) and all are related to *C. difficile* infection. The etiology of up to 20% of cases of antibiotic-induced diarrhea is *C. difficile* infection.[52] See Practice Scenario 1-3 regarding medical nutrition therapy for PMC.

Symptoms of PMC include diarrhea, abdominal pain, fever, elevated WBC, and history of recent use of antibiotics. PMC can lead to life-threatening colitis, which can progress to toxic megacolon and subsequent perforation.[53] When abdominal pain is present or obstruction is suspected, imaging studies may include abdominal radiographs to screen for toxic megacolon and bowel ischemia.

Sigmoidoscopy is indicated with bloody diarrhea or suspected PMC or ulcerative colitis.[46,50] Antiperistaltic agents should be used with caution in patients suspected of having infectious diarrhea or antibiotic-associated colitis.[50] For severe or refractory diarrhea, bowel rest may be recommended. Evidence-based diet recommendations for diarrhea have not been established. However, anecdotal experience suggests early refeeding with initially caffeine-free clear liquids advanced to a low-lactose, low-fat, low-fiber diet. Oral rehydration fluids may be used to restore fluid and electrolyte balance. The World Health Organization has published a standard recipe for an oral rehydration solution: $1/3$ to $2/3$ teaspoon table salt, $3/4$ teaspoon sodium bicarbonate, $1/3$ teaspoon potassium chloride (salt substitute), $1\,1/3$ tablespoon sugar or rice powder, and 1 L bottled or sterile water. Intravenous fluids should be provided if oral intake is less than estimated needs. PN should be reserved for patients who do not tolerate an oral diet or enteral nutrition. Probiotics may be supplemented with lactobacillus or as yogurt with live cultures when diarrhea is related to antibiotic therapy. Some have recommended banana flakes, apple powder, or other pectin sources to thicken the consistency of stools.[54]

In some clinical situations, dietary fiber may be used to control diarrhea. Colonic bacteria ferment fibers (prebiotics: cellulose, pectin, gums, fructooligosaccharides) to form SCFAs. SCFAs, particularly butyrate, are the major energy source for the colonocyte. Fermentable fiber helps to control diarrhea by slowing gastric emptying and by binding bile acids. On the other hand, nonfermentable fibers (lignins) may help to control diarrhea by exerting an osmotic force that absorbs water from the contents of the colon. Soy polysaccharide is a common fermentable fiber in enteral feedings. Fiber supplements have also been used successfully to control diarrhea. One example is psyllium, a nonfermentable fiber. Additional clinical studies are needed to delineate the specific benefits of fiber supplementation in enterally fed patients with diarrhea.[4,55] While acknowledging that large prospective trials are not available, the current A.S.P.E.N. guidelines support the use of soluble fiber–containing or small peptide formulations in the enterally fed patient with diarrhea when the diarrhea is unrelated to hyperosmolar agents or *C. difficile.* Guidelines also state that insoluble fiber should be avoided in critically ill patients. In patients who are at risk for bowel ischemia, both soluble and insoluble fiber should be avoided.[46]

Practice Scenario 1-3

Question: What enteral medical nutrition therapy would you offer to a patient with severe diarrhea related to *C. difficile* PMC?

Scenario: A 56-year-old man was admitted to the hospital for evaluation of crampy abdominal pain and severe diarrhea. The patient had a history of chronic immunosuppression following renal transplantation 3 years prior to admission, gastroesophageal reflux disease, and dyslipidemia. His medications included prednisone, tacrolimus, mycophenolate mofetil, and ranitidine. Four weeks prior to admission, he was diagnosed with sinusitis and treated with a 10-day course of oral trimethoprim-sulfamethoxazole. Several days after completion of his antibiotic, the patient developed crampy abdominal pain and fever. He reported 10 to 12 watery stools per day without blood or mucus. On admission, he had a temperature of 102°F, moderate right-lower quadrant tenderness, and a WBC of 27,000 cells/μL; a stool gram stain showed many leukocytes and fecal flora. A CT scan showed right colon thickening but no abscess. Stool specimens for enteric pathogens and *C. difficile* toxin were obtained, and empiric therapy with 500 mg of metronidazole orally every 6 hours and 250 mg of levofloxacin intravenously every 24 hours was begun. A colonoscopy was performed to evaluate for cytomegalovirus or other opportunistic causes of colitis, and it showed numerous whitish plaques and friable erythematous mucosa consistent with PMC. All subsequent stool cultures for enteric pathogens and viruses were negative. Colon biopsies were negative for viral inclusions. *C. difficile* toxin was found in stool. A diagnosis of *C. difficile* PMC was made, levofloxacin was discontinued, and therapy was switched from oral metronidazole to 125 mg of vancomycin orally every 6 hours. Nutrition assessment data included the following: body mass index (BMI) 28; percentage weight loss after rehydration with intravenous fluids: 3% in one month; percentage of usual body weight: 97%. Electrolytes had normalized by the time the nutrition assessment was completed.

Intervention: The patient was kept on nothing by mouth (NPO) until the diarrhea improved on the vancomycin therapy, about 4 days.

Answer: The patient was started on caffeine-free clear liquids and was advanced to a low-lactose, low-fat, low-fiber diet.

Rationale: While evidence-based diet recommendations for PMC diarrhea have not been established, the goal is to initiate nutrition through the GI tract as early as possible to limit gut mucosa atrophy. Caffeine-free clear liquids are recommended initially to eliminate the stimulatory effects of caffeine on GI motility. A low-lactose, low-fat, low-fiber diet addresses likely transient nutrient intolerances due to suspected loss of brush border enzymes related to diarrhea. American Society for Parenteral and Enteral Nutrition (A.S.P.E.N.) guidelines do not support the use of supplemental fiber in patients with *C. difficile* diarrhea. Intravenous fluids should be provided if oral intake does not keep up with losses. PN would not be offered to this patient as he was not severely malnourished on admission and nutrient intake could be resumed in less than 7 days. Probiotics may be supplemented as lactobacillus or as yogurt with live cultures, but the evidence base for this practice is weak.

Gastroparesis

Gastroparesis refers to a pathological delay in gastric emptying in the absence of obstruction. Its symptoms include fullness after eating and early satiety, and it is often associated with nausea, vomiting, bloating, and abdominal pain. At times, symptoms can result in inadequate nutrient intake. The causes of gastroparesis include diabetes mellitus, complications of surgery, or possible idiopathic reasons. The autonomic neuropathy of prolonged uncontrolled diabetes results in gastroparesis that may affect 50% of diabetic patients, with a smaller percentage of patients reporting symptoms. Diabetic gastroparesis presents difficult challenges in controlling blood glucose with the potential of resultant diabetic ketoacidosis or hypoglycemia. A nuclear medicine gastric emptying study is the diagnostic test of choice for diagnosing gastroparesis as well as for assessing response to treatment. Prokinetic agents such as metoclopramide and domperidone can alleviate gastroparesis as well as symptoms of nausea. Low dose erythromycin can also be used as a promotility agent, although it is not approved by the U.S. Food and Drug Administration.

Postsurgical gastroparesis arises in 2% to 3% of cases after surgeries for gastric outlet obstruction or vagotomy. When medical treatments fail, surgical intervention is offered, with a near-total gastrectomy and Roux-en-Y gastrojejunostomy. Success rates of up to 70% to 80% have been reported.[48]

Dietary treatments for gastroparesis include small, frequent meals, drinking fluids with meals, limiting dietary fat and possibly fiber, maintaining good glucose control, and, when necessary, feeding past the pylorus. See Practice Scenario 1-3 for a discussion of the nutritional management of diabetic gastroparesis.

Constipation

Constipation is a group of syndromes characterized by infrequent and/or difficult bowel movements. Bowel movements are described with a frequency of fewer than three per week, hard stools, excessive straining, prolonged time spent on the toilet, a sense of incomplete evacuation, and abdominal discomfort/bloating. Risk factors include advanced age, low-fiber and low-fluid diet, sedentary lifestyle, and polypharmacy (especially drugs with anticholinergic effects such as antidepressants, narcotics, antipsychotics; calcium and aluminum antacids; and calcium channel blockers). Conditions that are associated with constipation include diabetes mellitus, hypothyroidism, hypercalcemia, dehydration, neurologic disorders, anorectal disease, and collagen vascular/muscular diseases.[56] Treatment includes gradually increasing fiber in the diet to 25 to 30 g individualized to an amount that promotes regularity. Increase fluid to 6 to 8 cups per day.[57,58] When nonpharmacologic approaches fail, first-line medication treatments are the hydrophilic colloids (psyllium, bran methylcellulose, and polycarbophil), stool softeners, and osmotic laxatives (polyethylene glycol, lactulose, sorbitol, and magnesium salts). Second-line medications include stimulants (senna/docusate, bisacodyl/docusate, casanthranol/docusate) and lubricants (mineral oil). Mineral oil has the disadvantages of binding fat soluble vitamins and if aspiration occurs, could produce a lipoid pneumonia.[56] Sometimes when constipation is severe, osmotic laxatives may be combined with suppositories or enemas to loosen stools from a proximal as well as a distal approach.

Dumping Syndrome

Dumping syndrome (DS) is a group of symptoms that develop after gastric surgery that are related to increased gastric emptying following vagotomy and bypass or destruction of the pylorus. DS is accompanied by both GI symptoms and vasomotor symptoms. GI symptoms include a feeling of fullness after eating, crampy abdominal pain, nausea, vomiting, and explosive diarrhea. Vasomotor symptoms include diaphoresis, weakness, dizziness, flushing, and palpitations. Weight loss and food fear may develop. Symptoms can be classified as early or late dumping. Early is defined as within 30 to 60 minutes of eating. Late occurs 2 to 3 hours after eating and usually is limited to vasomotor symptoms. GI symptoms are related to the rapid emptying of hyperosmolar chyme into the small intestine from the stomach, eliciting an osmotic diuresis into the intestinal lumen and subsequent distention. Vasomotor symptoms are related to the rapid delivery of glucose to the upper small intestine, which results in peripheral and splanchnic vasodilation. Rapid delivery of glucose to the small intestines precipitates an increased serum insulin release followed by hypoglycemia and vasomotor symptoms. Dietary modification (see subsequent discussion) controls dumping in most patients. Octreotide, a somatostatin analogue, may be used in patients with severe dumping or in those in whom dietary treatment fails to slow intestinal transit time.[56]

Dietary treatment involves slow introduction of solid food, elimination of simple sugars, frequent small meals, and no liquids with meals. Patients are advised to lie down after eating and to consider adding functional fibers to delay gastric emptying. The initial clear liquid diets should not include simple sugars. Dairy products should be restricted initially due to the frequent occurrence of temporary lactose intolerance. Liquid multivitamins with minerals as well as vitamin B_{12} injections may be warranted in patients who have undergone a gastric resection.[59]

Gastrointestinal Secretions

Before a comprehensive discussion of digestion and absorption can be entertained, a thorough understanding of GI secretions must be established. Secretions in the GI tract serve two primary functions: to supply digestive enzymes and lubricating mucus. Mucus facilitates passage of food through the GI tract and prevents damage to the mucosa. GI secretions are often stimulated by the presence of food, which in turn stimulates the ENS and autonomic nervous system. Likewise, GI hormones contribute to the regulation of volume and type of secretions.[60]

Digestion begins in the mouth. Two major secretions can be found in saliva, mucin for lubrication and ptyalin (α-amylase), an enzyme for starch digestion. Regulation of saliva secretion is primarily under parasympathetic control.[60] Saliva is secreted in response to food in the mouth, stomach, or upper intestine. Conditioned secretion occurs with the sight, smell, and thought of food.

Stretch and chemical receptors mediate the stimulatory influences of saliva in the stomach via parasympathetic neurons that end on parietal cells. Furthermore, peptide products of protein digestion stimulate gastrin production, which augments acid secretion. The presence of carbohydrate, protein, or fat in the duodenum inhibits gastric acid and pepsin secretion and gastric motility. Caffeine and alcohol stimulate acid production.

Gastric Secretions

The gastric glands secrete approximately 2500 mL of gastric secretions, which include hydrochloric acid, each day. Gastric secretions derive from mucus-secreting cells, oxyntic glands (gastric glands), and pyloric glands.[60] Mucus is secreted to protect the gastric lining and duodenum from hydrochloric acid.[2] Oxyntic glands are made up of three kinds of cells including mucus-producing cells, peptic (or chief) cells, which secrete pepsinogen, and parietal cells, which secrete hydrogen chloride (HCl) and intrinsic factor.[60] Parietal cells are located in the body and fundus. The H^+/K^+ ATPases in the membranes of parietal cells pump H^+ against its concentration gradient. When these cells are stimulated, more H^+/K^+ ATPases move to the cell membrane where H^+ is exchanged for K^+. Cl^- moves down its electrochemical gradient. The pH of the gastric acid is approximately 0.8.[60]

Intrinsic factor, required for the absorption of vitamin B_{12}, is secreted by the same cells that also secrete HCl. Therefore, when the parietal cells of the stomach are destroyed (as in chronic gastritis), achlorhydria (the absence of acid) develops in addition to pernicious anemia and vitamin B_{12} deficiency caused by loss of intrinsic factor.[2]

Biochemical stimulants for acid secretion are gastrin, histamine via H_2 receptors, and acetylcholine released by parasympathetic stimulation. Acetylcholine also stimulates pepsinogen and mucus secretion. Pepsinogen is hydrolyzed in the presence of HCl to its active form, pepsin, a protein digestive enzyme.[60] Histamine is secreted in response to gastrin and the ENS by enterochromaffin-like (ECL) cells. Gastrin is secreted in the antrum of the stomach in response to the presence of protein. ECL cells are inhibited by somatostatin. Both histamine-secreting ECL cells and somatostatin-secreting D cells are found in the fundus and the body.

Proton-pump inhibitor drugs exert their effects on acid suppression by interfering with H^+/K^+ ATPase activity. H2-receptor antagonist drugs block histamine stimulation of acid production. H2-blocking drugs can reduce basal acid secretion by 75% to 90%. In the antrum, G cells secret gastrin and D cells secrete somatostatin.[2] Somatostatin inhibits the secretion of pepsinogens.[2]

Acid is secreted in three phases. In the first phase, the cephalic phase, acid is secreted via vagal stimulation in response to the thought, sight, smell, and/or taste of food. The vagus nerve releases acetylcholine, which stimulates the ECL cells and parietal cells. The cephalic phase accounts for 30% of the volume of acid secretion. The gastric phase of secretion begins when food arrives in the stomach. In this phase, amino acids and peptides stimulate the G cells in the antrum to produce gastrin, which enters the general circulation and stimulates parietal cells as an endocrine hormone. Gastric distention also leads to acid secretion via a reflex involving the vagus nerve. Antral distention, in particular, stimulates gastrin secretion, which acts on ECL cells to release histamine. The gastric phase of acid secretion accounts for 60% of the volume of acid secreted.[60]

The final phase of gastric secretion is the intestinal phase. Food in the duodenum continues to stimulate small amounts of gastric secretions, likely related to the small amount of gastrin that is secreted by the duodenal mucosa. The intestinal phase accounts for approximately 10% of gastric acid secretion.[60]

Gastric secretions are inhibited by signals from the intestines in multiple ways. Paradoxically, food in the small intestines not only stimulates gastrin release (which increases secretions), but also initiates a reverse enterogastric reflex that inhibits gastric secretions. Secondly, the presence of acid, fat, products of protein digestion, hyper- or hypotonic fluids, or irritants in the proximal small bowel stimulates the secretion of intestinal hormones. These gastric secretion inhibiting hormones include secretin, GIP, VIP, and somatostatin. During the interdigestive period, gastric secretions can increase in response to emotional stimuli and reach a level high enough to contribute to the development of peptic ulcers.[60]

Bile Secretion

Bile is central to the digestion and absorption of fat because of its role as an emulsifier and its role in aiding absorption of digested fat into the intestinal mucosa. Bile is comprised of water, bile salts, bile pigments, cholesterol, lecithin, fatty acids, and electrolytes. Bile salts are Na^+ and potassium salts of bile acids, which are metabolites of cholesterol. The two principal bile acids are cholic acid and chenodeoxycholic acid. Colonic bacteria convert cholic acid to deoxycholic acid. Chenodeoxycholic acid is converted to lithocholic acid, the secondary bile acids (which are formed after deconjugation and dehydroxylation). Deoxycholate is absorbed. For the most part, lithocholic acid is excreted in the stool.[39]

Bile pigments include bilirubin and biliverdin, which are responsible for the yellow color of bile. Bilirubin is a waste product of the breakdown of hemoglobin. In pathologic conditions when bilirubin accumulates in the blood, skin, sclera, and mucous membranes, it imparts a yellow color and this condition is called jaundice. Jaundice often can be detected when total plasma bilirubin exceeds 2 mg/dL. The brown color of stools derives from pigments formed by colonic bacteria action on bile pigments. Stools become white when bile acids are prevented from entering the colon (eg, biliary obstruction).[39]

Bile production is stimulated by the vagus nerve and by secretin. Bile drains from the liver continually into canaliculi, interlobular septa, and eventually into the right and left hepatic ducts. The right and left hepatic ducts form the common bile duct, which eventually leads to the sphincter of Oddi in the duodenum.[39] Because the sphincter of Oddi remains closed between meals, bile is directed to the gallbladder. The gallbladder contracts after a meal, especially a high-fat meal. The sphincter of Oddi then relaxes (opens), and bile flows into the duodenum.[38] Relaxation of the sphincter of Oddi is mediated by the action of CCK, which also stimulates the gallbladder to contract.[39] CCK secretion is stimulated by the presence of fat in the duodenum.[60]

Bile is concentrated in the gallbladder where water is absorbed. Approximately 500 mL of bile is secreted per day. On the average, 90% to 95% of bile salts are reabsorbed in the terminal ileum. Reabsorbed bile salts and bile pigments are transported to the liver via the portal vein and then are re-excreted in the bile. This process is called enterohepatic circulation. The role of bile salts in the digestion of fat is to act as emulsifiers along with phospholipids and monoglycerides. Without bile, up to 50% of ingested fat can appear in the feces, when, under normal circumstances, nearly 100% of fat is absorbed.[1]

Pancreatic Secretions

The pancreas is an organ that has a variety of functions important to digestion. Pancreatic secretions are produced in response to the presence of chyme in the proximal small bowel. The composition of the pancreatic juice is determined partially by the composition of the chyme. Digestive enzymes are produced in glandular-like cells that secrete the enzymes in zymogen granules via exocytosis into pancreatic ducts. Small pancreatic ducts drain into a large central duct that empties into the common bile duct. About 1500 mL of alkaline, bicarbonate-rich pancreatic juice is secreted daily into the duodenum through the sphincter of Oddi. Pancreatic secretions, along with intestinal secretions and bile, neutralize gastric acid (pH ranges from 1 to 4) to raise the pH of duodenal contents to 6 to 7. Pancreatic juice contains enzymes for digestion of the three major macronutrients: carbohydrate (pancreatic amylase), protein (pancreatic proteases), and fat (pancreatic lipase, cholesterol esterase, and phospholipase). Pancreatic proteases (trypsin, chymotrypsin, and carboxypolypeptidase) are released as inactive proenzymes. The brush border enzyme, enteropeptidase (enterokinase) converts trypsinogen to the active enzyme, trypsin. Trypsin then converts chymotrypsinogen into chymotrypsin and autocatalyzes trypsinogen to produce more trypsin. Under normal circumstances, the pancreas releases small amounts of enzymes into the general blood circulation. However, in acute pancreatitis, serum levels of amylase and lipase rise dramatically and are useful in making a diagnosis.[60]

Secretion of pancreatic juice, particularly high-volume, enzyme-poor, bicarbonate-rich secretions, is stimulated by secretin. CCK promotes the secretion of low-volume, enzyme-rich pancreatic juice from acinar cells. Acinar cells are also stimulated by the vagus nerve and the parasympathetic and enteric nervous systems via acetylcholine.[39,60]

Small and Large Bowel Secretions

Digestion that began in the mouth and stomach is completed in the small intestine, and products of digestion, vitamins, and minerals are absorbed. The small intestine has three regions: the duodenum, the jejunum, and the ileum. The duodenum becomes the jejunum at the ligament of Treitz. The lower 60% of the small bowel that is distal to the ligament of Treitz is designated as the ileum. Between the ileum and the colon is the ileocecal valve. The length of the small bowel can vary from 12 to 20 feet or 350 to 600 cm. When colonic pressure increases, the ileocecal valve shuts. Conversely, when ileal pressure increases or when food exits the stomach (gastroileal reflex), the ileocecal valve opens. When the ileocecal valve is resected, small bowel contents enter the colon quickly and some malabsorption occurs, but the amount may not be significant.[39]

Small bowel secretions begin in the proximal duodenum where Brunner glands secrete mucus, which protects the duodenum from gastric acid. A total of 9 L of fluid enter the small intestine each day, 2 L from dietary sources and 7 L of GI secretions, but only 1 to 2 L normally enter into the colon.[39]

The lining of the small bowel is covered by finger-like projections called villi. Each villus, in turn, is covered by a layer of epithelium and contains capillaries and a lymphatic vessel (lacteal). At the edge of the epithelium of the villi are microvilli that make up the brush border. The so-called brush border enzymes are present on the outer layer of the cell membranes of these mucosal cells, also called enterocytes.[39] An unstirred layer is located between the brush border and mucosal cells, and must be traversed by solutes for them to be absorbed. These substances pass into the enterocytes and then exit into the interstitial fluid.[6]

Lying between the villi are the crypts of Lieberkühn. Lining both the crypts and the villi is an epithelial layer containing goblet cells and enterocytes. The goblet cells secrete mucus throughout the small intestines. Enterocytes secrete large amounts of water (approximately 1800 mL) and electrolytes, and reabsorb water and electrolytes along with products of digestion. Interestingly, the digestive enzymes that are produced by enterocytes are not secreted into the watery secretions. Small bowel enzymes (eg, peptidases, sucrase, maltase, isomaltase, lactase, and intestinal lipase) digest while nutrients are being absorbed through the epithelium.[60]

Undifferentiated cells are formed in the crypts of Lieberkühn. Subsequently, they migrate up the villi, undergo apoptosis (programmed cell death), and are sloughed off into the lumen of the small bowel. The highly proliferative lining of the small bowel turns over every 5 days. The loss of the sloughed cells translates into a loss of protein of about 30 g per day.[39] The small bowel mucosa is particularly susceptible to damage by chemotherapeutic agents that target mitotic cells because it is such a highly proliferating tissue.

The large bowel continues to secrete mucus from crypts of Lieberkühn. Again, the mucus serves to protect the mucosa. However, an additional role of mucus in the colon is to provide an adherent medium for holding feces together. When the large bowel becomes irritated, the mucosa can secrete large volumes of water and electrolytes. This serves to dilute and "wash" the irritant out of the colon.[60]

Gastrointestinal (Splanchnic) Blood Circulation

The network of arteries, veins, and minor blood vessels in the GI tract is referred to as splanchnic circulation. Relatively speaking, the GI tract is a blood-rich area of the body. At rest, 25% of cardiac output is delivered to the splanchnic circulation. This is similar to the amount delivered to the kidneys, but more than is delivered to any other vascular bed, including skeletal muscle. Thirty percent of total body oxygen is consumed by the splanchnic organs at rest, making its oxygen consumption higher than any other area of the body. The demand for oxygen is determined by the large mass of the tissue that is supplied by the splanchnic circulation as well as the high energy demands of absorption, GI secretion, and GI mixing and propulsion. The distribution of the splanchnic blood flow varies disproportionately between organs. Nearly half is supplied to the small intestine.[61]

During feeding, splanchnic blood flow increases 40% to 60%. Oxygen demand in the splanchnic supplied organs increases up to 30%. These facts become important when dealing with states of low pressure, which will be discussed subsequently.

All blood in the GI tract, including the spleen and pancreas, flows to the liver via the portal vein. In the liver, blood encounters reticuloendothelial system (RES) cells in the lining of liver blood vessels (sinusoids). The RES is a system of macrophages that clears the blood of bacteria and other particulate matter to prevent systemic infection when the blood leaves the liver. Blood exits the liver by way of the hepatic vein, which leads to the vena cava.[40]

Blood is delivered to the small intestine by the superior and inferior mesenteric arteries, which branch off the aorta. The celiac artery supplies the stomach. Splanchnic blood vessels branch progressively down to arterioles that supply individual villi lining the intestines. Arterioles empty into venules in each villus with the flow of arterioles opposite in direction to the venules. Normally, 80% of the oxygen in the arterioles may diffuse out into the venules without reaching the tip of the villus. While this shunting of oxygen is not harmful, it can become harmful in low-flow states such as circulatory collapse. In circulatory collapse, the oxygen deprivation in the tips of the villi can result in an ischemic death of the villi, leading to decreased absorptive capacity.[40]

Digestion

Digestion of Carbohydrate

Starches (glucose polymers) and disaccharides must be digested before they are absorbed. The digestion of starch begins in the mouth with the action of salivary α-amylase. When food enters the stomach, the action of salivary α-amylase is gradually inhibited by gastric acid. Starch digestion continues in the more alkaline small intestine where pancreatic α-amylase hydrolyzes 1:4α linkages to form the oligosaccharides: maltose, maltotriose, larger polymers, and α-dextrins, glucose polymers of average chain length of eight glucose molecules. Brush border enzymes are then responsible for further digestion of the oligosaccharides. These include dextrinase (isomaltase), maltase, and sucrase. Sucrase hydrolyzes sucrose into the monosaccharides, glucose and fructose. Another brush border enzyme, lactase, catalyzes the hydrolysis of lactose to the monosaccharides, galactose and glucose. When there is a deficiency of brush border oligosaccharides, diarrhea, bloating, and flatulence may occur. Undigested oligosaccharides are osmotically active and cause a shift of water into the intestinal lumen. The osmotic pressure exerted by luminal contents increases further when colonic bacteria act on remaining oligosaccharides and increase the number of osmotically active particles. Flatulence and bloating are perpetuated because of the formation of CO_2 and H_2 from disaccharides in the small intestine and colon.[6]

Deficiency of the lactase enzyme is common in African Americans, Native Americans, Asians, and individuals of Mediterranean descent; 70% to 100% are deficient and require low-lactose diets, supplemental oral lactase, or lactase-treated food products. Often, yogurt with live bacterial cultures is tolerated because the bacteria produce lactase enzyme.

Digestion of Protein

Protein digestion begins in the stomach with the action of pepsin. In an acid environment, pepsin hydrolyzes the bonds involving aromatic amino acids. This cleavage produces polypeptides of various sizes. When the partially digested chyme enters the alkaline environment of the duodenum, pepsin is inactivated. At this point, trypsin, chymotrypsin, and proelastase—the endopeptidases—hydrolyze internal bonds of the polypeptides. Pancreatic carboxypeptidases—the exopeptidases—hydrolyze the carboxy terminal amino acids of the polypeptides. The majority of protein digestion results from hydrolysis by pancreatic enzymes. Free amino acids and di- and tripeptides are cleaved off by intestinal aminopolypeptidases and dipeptidases in the brush border. These are carried into the interior of the enterocyte where di- and tripeptides are digested to amino acids.[62]

The small intestine digests and absorbs 95% to 98% of the protein in its lumen. Bacteria in the colon digest some of the remaining protein, producing ammonia. Ammonia is absorbed and transported to the liver. The rate of ammonia absorption is dependent on the size of the bacterial population of the colon and the colonic pH. The smaller the number of bacteria (eg, after antibiotic administration) and the lower the pH (eg, after lactulose administration), the lower the amount of ammonia absorbed.[42] Ammonia absorption may be clinically relevant during GI bleeding and in the setting of liver disease, where it may contribute to the development of hepatic encephalopathy. During starvation or during periods of prolonged bowel rest, the peptidase activity of the brush border declines.[6]

Digestion of Fat

Fat digestion begins in the mouth and stomach through the action of lingual lipase and gastric lipase, respectively. The contribution of gastric lipase is small, but lingual lipase hydrolyzes up to 10% of dietary fat. The majority of fat digestion occurs in the duodenum by pancreatic lipase.[62]

The first major step of fat digestion occurs in the duodenum where bile emulsifies fat globules into smaller globules to increase the surface area on which water-soluble lipase enzymes may act. The major sites of action of pancreatic lipase are on the 1- and 3-bonds of triacylglycerols. For this reason, the primary products of digestion by pancreatic lipase are 2-monoglycerides and free fatty acids.[6,62] Hydrolysis by pancreatic lipase is highly reversible; therefore, the next step in fat digestion, the formation of micelles by bile salts, is critical to keep the products of digestion separated. Subsequently, the bile salt micelles transport the monoglycerides and free fatty acids to the brush border where they are absorbed and the micelles are returned to the chyme.[62]

Two other pancreatic enzymes are involved in fat digestion. Cholesterol ester hydrolase hydrolyzes cholesterol esters, and phospholipase A_2 hydrolyzes phospholipids. Again, micelles are required for transport to the brush border.[62] In the setting of pancreatic insufficiency, fat is maldigested and patients have fatty, bulky, clay-colored stools.

Digestion of Nucleic Acids

Ribonuclease/deoxyribonuclease from the pancreas hydrolyze RNA and deoxyribonucleic acid to form mononucleotides. Nucleotides are further cleaved to nucleosides and phosphoric acid by enzymes on the surface of mucosal cells. Finally, nucleosides are cleaved into purines and pyrimidines that are absorbed by active transport.[6]

Absorption

The small intestine is presented daily with approximately 9 L of fluid to absorb, of which 2 L are dietary fluid and 7 L are secretions. All but 1.5 L is absorbed. The rest passes through the ileocecal valve to the colon. Central to the process of absorption is the highly specialized anatomy, histology, and arrangement of the cells and structures of the small intestine. The architecture of the small intestinal mucosa and villi maximizes the potential surface area for absorption. It has been estimated that the absorptive area of the small intestine is approximately the same area as a tennis court. The stomach, on the other hand, does not have the same maximized surface area. Accordingly, the only two substances of note that are absorbed in the stomach in appreciable amounts are alcohol and aspirin.[62]

Mechanisms of Absorption

A variety of mechanisms operate to affect the movement of nutrients from the lumen of the intestine across the mucosal membranes into the cytoplasm. Water is transported by diffusion and obeys the laws of osmosis, which are concentration dependent. Other absorbed substances may move by either passive or active transport. Passive transport is accomplished by diffusion of solutes according to their electrochemical gradients. Transport by passive diffusion may occur across cell membranes or between cells. Negatively charged chloride ions, for example, diffuse along an electrochemical gradient to "follow" positively charged Na^+ ions. Active transport is an energy-requiring mechanism that may be used in the absence of or against an electrochemical gradient.

Active transport is limited to movement across cell membranes. Ions such as Na^+ are actively transported from the chyme through the brush border into the cytoplasm. Na^+ may be co-transported with amino acids or glucose by carrier proteins or may be exchanged with H^+.[62] Endocytosis is a process in which the cell membrane engulfs particles into cells (eg, whole protein allergens). Facilitated diffusion is the movement of nutrients across a semipermeable membrane in conjunction with transport proteins.[44] An example of facilitated diffusion is the transport of Na^+ ions across the basolateral membrane of intestinal epithelial cells into the paracellular space.[62]

Carbohydrate Absorption

Monosaccharides are absorbed rapidly before reaching the terminal ileum. Glucose and Na^+ share common co-transporters. High concentrations of Na^+ in the chyme increase glucose transport. Low concentrations of Na^+ decrease glucose absorption. Na^+ moves into mucosal cells along its concentration gradient and brings glucose along. Glucose is then shuttled into the interstitium by a transporter on into capillaries. The energy for glucose transport is provided for by the active transport of Na^+ out of the cell. The transport of Na^+ out of the cell maintains the concentration gradient needed for Na^+ to shuttle more glucose into the mucosal cells.

Galactose is transported by the same mechanism, whereas the absorption of fructose is independent of Na^+ and glucose. Fructose transport into the mucosal cells is accomplished by facilitated diffusion by GLUT5. GLUT2 mediates facilitated diffusion of fructose out of mucosal cells into the interstitium. Pentoses such as fructose are absorbed by diffusion. From the mucosal cells, these molecules pass into the capillaries, which drain into the portal vein.[6] There are acquired disorders of brush border enzyme deficiency, usually occurring after a bout of gastroenteritis or protracted diarrhea with resultant small bowel villous atrophy. These disorders are usually transient, resolve in a short period of time, and may be addressed temporarily by a low-lactose diet. Additional information regarding carbohydrate absorption may be found in Chapter 3.

Protein Absorption

Amino acid transport can be categorized into processes that require Na^+ and co-transporters and those that are do not require Na^+.[6] Amino acid transport can also be categorized by four different active transport systems. Neutral, basic, and acidic amino acids each have separate transport mechanisms; proline and hydroxyproline share a common transport system. Amino acids are transferred out of mucosal cells by five different transport systems into the portal circulation. Di- and tripeptide absorption into enterocytes requires H^+ instead of Na^+. There is very little absorption of longer-chain peptides.[6] A total of 99% of protein consumed is absorbed by the time it reaches the distal jejunum. Nearly all the protein in stools is from cellular debris or of bacterial origin.[6]

Clinically significant protein deficiencies secondary to enterocyte amino acid transport abnormalities are very unusual. Both inherited and acquired defects exist for protein absorption. An example is Hartnup syndrome. Hartnup syndrome is an autosomal recessive disorder in which neutral amino acids are not absorbed and may present as a pellagra-like syndrome.[63] Additional information regarding amino acid absorption may be found in Chapter 6.

Lipid Absorption

Bile salts form micelles in which their hydrophilic portions face out and their hydrophobic portions face toward the center where lipids collect. Monoglycerides and free fatty acids are transported to the brush border of the intestine, where they diffuse directly into the interior of the epithelial cell.[62] Once inside enterocytes, fatty acids and cholesterol are re-esterified into triglycerides and cholesterol esters. Additional cholesterol and phospholipids, together with protein, envelope these re-esterified products to form chylomicrons. The chylomicrons exit enterocytes and enter the lymphatic circulation. Normally, around 95% to 97% of fat is absorbed on a moderate fat intake.[39,62] Most of the cholesterol that is absorbed is packaged into chylomicrons. Nonabsorbable soy-based sterols reduce cholesterol absorption and are recommended as a serum cholesterol–lowering intervention.[39]

Vitamin Absorption

Generally, vitamins are absorbed from the small intestines via passive diffusion. Fat-soluble vitamin absorption is dependent on normal fat digestion and absorption, because fat-soluble vitamins are carried away from the sites of absorption when fat is malabsorbed. Vitamin E absorption is somewhat obscure. It may share a common mechanism with cholesterol.[64] All water-soluble vitamins except vitamin B_{12} and folic acid require Na^+ co-transporters for absorption.

Vitamin B_{12} requires a unique mechanism for absorption. Intrinsic factor, a glycoprotein that is secreted by the parietal cells of the stomach, binds to cyanocobalamin (vitamin B_{12}) and is taken up by receptors in the distal ileum. Absorption follows by endocytosis. Intracellularly, cyanocobalamin is transferred to transcobalamin II, a transport protein that carries cyanocobalamin to the plasma. Loss of parietal cells for any reason (gastrectomy, pernicious anemia, chronic gastritis) or loss of distal ileum may lead to vitamin B_{12} deficiency and requires monthly supplement injections.[39]

Vitamin K and some B complex vitamins (including folic acid) may be produced by colonic bacteria and are absorbed, sometimes in significant amounts. Additional information regarding vitamin absorption may be found in Chapter 7.

Water, Mineral, and Electrolyte Absorption

Although a small amount of water can be absorbed in the stomach, the small bowel and especially the colon are primarily responsible for water absorption. Water movement is driven to equalize the osmotic pressure between the plasma and intestinal contents. Na^+ moves in and out of the small bowel along its concentration gradient. Na^+ is also actively transported by Na^+/K^+ ATPases along the basolateral membranes of enterocytes. The presence of glucose in the lumen of the small intestines facilitates the absorption of Na^+ just as Na^+ facilitates the absorption of glucose as described previously. For this reason, oral rehydration fluids used to treat Na^+ and water losses from diarrhea include NaCl and glucose.[6]

Water, Na^+, and other minerals are absorbed in the colon. Na^+ is actively transported, and water follows via osmosis. Potassium and bicarbonate are secreted into the colon, potassium along its electrochemical gradient. Enough potassium is secreted into the colon that significant hypokalemia can be associated with ileal or colonic losses due to diarrhea. Potassium is also actively transported from the colon. Thirty percent of the dry weight of fecal matter is made up of bacteria. Feces also contain inorganic material, fiber, and water in addition to bacteria. For this reason, the passage of feces continues during prolonged bowel rest.[6]

Calcium (Ca^{2+}) and iron absorption are dependent on body stores. The amount of Ca^{2+} absorbed is dependent on 1,25-dihydroxycholecalciferol. Ca^{2+} absorption is inhibited by phosphates and oxalates, which form insoluble salts with Ca^{2+}. Protein facilitates both Ca^{2+} and magnesium absorption.

Only 3% to 6% of dietary iron is absorbed under conditions of iron sufficiency. Its absorption is inhibited by phytates in cereal, phosphates, and oxalates. These compounds form insoluble compounds with iron. The ferrous form of iron is the form in which iron must be absorbed. Because most dietary iron is in the ferric form, it must be reduced. This may be accomplished by an iron transporter, Divalent Metal Transporter1 (DMT1), in the brush border. When iron complexes with ascorbic acid, its reduction to the ferrous form is facilitated. Heme iron is absorbed through a different mechanism. Heme complexes with a transport protein in the mucosal cells and is transferred into the cytoplasm. There, HO2, a type of heme oxygenase, dissociates the iron from the heme.[6] Additional information regarding trace element absorption may be found in Chapter 8.

Medium-Chain Triglyceride Absorption

Medium-chain triglycerides (MCTs) (ie, triglycerides with fatty acids with chain lengths of 8 to 12 carbons) do not require the formation of micelles or the action of bile salts because they are water soluble. Medium-chain fatty acids are hydrolyzed and pass through enterocytes directly into the portal circulation. MCTs may be used as a calorie supplement in patients who maldigest or malabsorb fat.

Short-Chain Fatty Acid Absorption

SCFAs, 2- to 5-carbon fatty acids, are produced in the colon by the action of bacteria on dietary fiber. The types of SCFAs formed include acetate, propionate, and butyrate. Once absorbed by the colon mucosal cells, they are metabolized and serve as an energy source for active transport and other cellular processes. Other effects of SCFAs in the colon include their trophic effects on epithelial cells, their anti-inflammatory effects, and their effect on maintaining colonic pH by being absorbed in exchange for H^+.[39]

Alterations in Digestion/Absorption: Starvation, Bowel Rest, Mucosal Atrophy, and Low Flow States

Mucosal atrophy occurs during starvation, stress, PN, and bowel rest.[55] Complete bowel rest results in gut mucosal atrophy that becomes apparent in as little as a few days. PN cannot prevent this change. After 1 week of a protein-deficient diet, the microvilli shorten. This suggests that the bowel mucosa requires luminal nutrients to supply its nutrient needs.[65] Glutamine, in particular, is needed because it is a principal metabolic fuel for intestinal cells,[4] and its absence may directly contribute to mucosal atrophy that accompanies bowel rest. Atrophic changes during bowel rest have been reduced by glutamine-enriched PN.[66] "Trickle" enteral feeding (ie, 10 to 30 mL/h) can prevent mucosal atrophy, but will not achieve desired enteral nutrition clinical outcomes.[46]

Severe metabolic stress that accompanies sepsis or trauma may lead to shock and associated hypoperfusion of the gut splanchnic circulation. In this setting, peristalsis may be decreased or absent, patients may require bowel rest, and consequently, mucosal atrophy may occur. A.S.P.E.N. clinical guidelines advise that enteral nutrition be withheld in patients with hypoperfused gut when patients require a high level of hemodynamic support including high-dose catecholamines (eg, norepinephrine, phenylephrine, epinephrine, dopamine) to maintain cellular perfusion. Enteral nutrition is withheld to avoid ischemic bowel. These patients usually have a mean arterial blood pressure of less than 60 mm Hg. Patients on low doses of pressors may be given enteral nutrition, but they must be monitored closely for signs of intolerance, which could signal development of gut ischemia. Signs of intolerance include abdominal distention, increasing NG tube output or gastric residual volumes, decreased passage of stool, increasing metabolic acidosis, and/or base deficit. [46]

Immunity and the Gut

The GI tract is introduced to many beneficial and pathogenic microorganisms and antigens. A variety of immune defenses operate in the gut. Immune cells including lymphocytes, macrophages, polymorphic granulocytes, and other cells are present throughout the gut. In the small intestines, in addition to immune cells, many proteolytic and lipolytic enzymes secreted by the pancreas degrade pathogens. Mucin, which is produced by the enterocytes, limits the proliferation of bacteria. Additionally, peristalsis acts to propel pathogens out of the gut. Finally, tight junctions between epithelial cells provide a barrier against translocation of pathogens from the lumen to the systemic circulation.[67]

The gut-associated lymphoid tissue (GALT), a term used to refer to the immune system in the small intestines, is one of the largest components of the immune system. Gut epithelial cells and their mucus layer provide defense by trapping pathogens. When the epithelial cells are sloughed off, they are excreted along with the pathogens in the feces. In addition, intraepithelial cytolytic T-lymphocytes are positioned between epithelial cells.

The lamina propria (a layer of connective tissue that together with the epithelium comprises the mucosa) houses many different types of immune cells, including B cells, T-helper cells, mast cells, and eosinophils. The B cells secrete immunoglobulin A (IgA) into the lumen of the gut. Mast cells and eosinophils are involved in allergic and hypersensitivity reactions as well as target parasites. Also present are M cells, which transport antigens to dendritic cells and macrophages and serve as antigen-presenting cells to T-cells in the GALT. This, in turn, results in the production of IgA by plasma cells in the mucosa. Lymphocytes are then activated, enter the lymphatic circulation, and eventually enter into the systemic circulation via the thoracic duct.[67]

The GALT is dependent on luminal nutrition to maintain its integrity. When enteral nutrition is withheld for extended periods, GALT atrophies. Furthermore, in conditions associated with severe metabolic stress, bacteria from the lumen of the gut migrate across the gut barriers and into the mesenteric lymph node and beyond. This bacterial translocation has been implicated as an etiologic factor for septic complications and multiple organ failure.[67] Because enteral nutrition helps to maintain tight junctions between epithelial cells and hence reduces the risk of increased permeability during metabolic stress, A.S.P.E.N. guidelines recommend that enteral nutrition be initiated as early as possible in critically ill patients in whom oral or enteral intake is inadequate.[46]

References

1. Blundell JE, Stubbs J. Diet composition and the control of food intake in humans. In: Bray GA, Bouchard C, eds. *Handbook of Obesity: Etiology and Pathophysiology*. New York, NY: Marcel Dekker; 2004:427–460.
2. Dempsey DT. Stomach. In: Brunicardi FC, ed. *Schwartz's Principles of Surgery*. 8th ed. New York, NY: McGraw-Hill Medical; 2005: 933–996.
3. Dietitians of Canada and American Dietetics Association. Cancer. In: *Manual of Clinical Dietetics*. 6th ed. Chicago, IL: American Dietetics Association and Dietitians of Canada; 2000:236–252.
4. Marino PL. Enteral nutrition. In: Marino PL, ed. *The ICU Book*. 2nd ed. Baltimore, MD: Williams & Wilkins; 1998:737–754.
5. Gottschlich MM. Early and perioperative nutrition support. In: Matarese L, Gottschlich MM, eds. *Contemporary Nutrition Support Practice: A Clinical Guide*. 2nd ed. Philadelphia, PA: Saunders; 2003:276–289.
6. Digestion and absorption. In: Ganong WF. *Review of Medical Physiology*. 22nd ed. New York, NY: McGraw-Hill Lange Medical; 2005:467–478.
7. Kant AK, Graubard BL, Schatzkin A, Ballard-Barbash R. Proportion of energy intake from fat and subsequent weight change in the NHANES epidemiological follow-up study. *Am J Clin Nutr*. 1995;61:11–17.
8. Central regulation of visceral function. In: Ganong WF. *Review of Medical Physiology*. 22nd ed. New York, NY: McGraw-Hill Lange Medical; 2005:232–255.
9. Cegla J, Tan TM, Bloom SR. Gut-brain cross-talk in appetite regulation. *Curr Opin Clin Nutr & Metab Care*. 2010;13(5):588–593.
10. Chaudhri OB, Field BCT, Bloom SR. Gastrointestinal satiety signals. *Int J Obes*. 2008;32(Suppl 7):S28–S31.
11. Zac-Vargheses S, Tan T, Sloom SR. Hormonal interactions between gut and brain. *Discovery Medicine*. 2010;10(55):543–552.
12. Sasaki T, Kitamura T. Roles of FoxO1 and Sirt1 in the central regulation of food intake. *Endocrine Journal*. 2010;57(11):939–946.
13. Blumenthal DM, Gold MS. Neurobiology of food addiction. *Curr Opin Clin Nutr Metab Care*. 2010;13:359–365.
14. Adams CE, Greenway Fl, Brantley PJ. Lifestyle factors and ghrelin: critical review and implications for weight loss maintenance. *Obesity Rev*. 2011;12(5):e211–218.
15. Cammisotto PG, Levy E, Bukowiecki LJ. Bendayan M. Cross-talk between adipose and gastric leptins for the control of food intake and energy metabolism. *Prog Hist & Cytochem*. 2010;45(3): 143–200.

16. Zheng H, Lenard NR, Shi AC, Berhoud HR. Appetite control and energy balance regulation in the modern world; reward-driven brain overrides repletion signals. *Int J Obesity*. 2009;33(Suppl 2):S8–13.
17. Higuchi H, Hasegawa A, Yamaguchi T. Transcriptional regulation of neuropeptide Y gene by leptin and its effect on feeding. *J Pharmacol Sci*. 2005;98:225–231.
18. Propulsion and mixing of food in the alimentary tract. In: Hall JE. *Guyton and Hall Textbook of Medical Physiology*. 12th ed. Philadelphia, PA: Elsevier; 2010:763–772.
19. de Graaf C, Blom WA, Smeets PA, et al. Biomarkers of satiation and satiety. *Am J Clin Nutr*. 2004;79:946–961.
20. Lissner L, Levitsky DA, Strupp BJ, et al. Dietary fat and the regulation of energy intake in human subjects. *Am J Clin Nutr*. 1987;46:886–892.
21. Stubbs RJ, Johnstone AM, Harbron CG, Reid C. Covert manipulation of the energy density of high-carbohydrate diets; effect on ad libitum food intake in "pseudo free-living" humans. *Int J Obes*. 1998;819:11–22.
22. Poortvliet PC, Berube-Parent S, Drapeau V, Lamarche B, Blundell JE, Tremblay A. Effects of a healthy meal course on spontaneous energy intake, satiety and palatability. *Brit J Nutr*. 2007;97(3): 584–590.
23. Halton TL, Hu FB. The effects of high protein diets on thermogenesis, satiety, and weight loss. *J Am Coll Nutr*. 2004; 23(5): 373–385.
24. St-Onge MP, Rubiano F, DeNino WF, et al. Added thermogenic and satiety effects of a mixed nutrient vs a sugar-only beverage. *Int J Obesity Related Metab Dis*. 2004;28(2):248–253.
25. Lejeune MP, Westerterp KR, Adam TC, Luscombe-Marsh ND, Westerterp-Plantenga MS. Ghrelin and glucagon-like peptide 1 concentrations, 24-h satiety, and energy and substrate metabolism during a high-protein diet and measured in a respiration chamber. *Am J Clin Nutr*. 2006;83(1):89–94.
26. Nickols-Richardson SM, Coleman MD, Volpe JJ, Hosig KW. Perceived hunger is lower and weight loss is greater in overweight premenopausal women consuming a low-carbohydrate/high-protein vs high-carbohydrate/low-fat diet. *J Am Diet Assoc*. 2005;105(9): 1433–1437.
27. Hall WL, Millward DJ, Long SJ, Morgan LM. Casein and whey exert different effects on plasma amino acid profiles, gastrointestinal hormone secretion and appetite. *Brit J Nutr*. 2003;89(2): 239–248.
28. Westerterp-Plantenga MS, Lejeune MP, Nijs I, van Ooijen M, Kovacs EM. High protein intake sustains weight maintenance after body weight loss in humans. *Int J Obesity Related Met Dis*. 2004; 28(1):57–64.
29. Lyly M, Liukkonen KH, Salmenkallio-Marttila M, Karhunen L, Poutanen K, Lahteenmaki L. Fibre in beverages can enhance perceived satiety. *Eur J Nutr*. 2009;48(4):251–258.
30. Willis HJ, Eldridge AL, Beiseigel J, Thomas W, Slavin JL. Greater satiety response with resistant starch and corn bran in human subjects. *Nutr Res*. 2009;29(2):100–105.
31. Bodinham CL, Frost GS, Robertson MD. Acute ingestion of resistant starch reduces food intake in healthy adults. *Brit J Nutr*. 2010; 103(6):917–922.
32. Whelan K, Efthymiou L, Judd PA, Preedy VR, Taylor MA. Appetite during consumption of enteral formula as a sole source of nutrition: the effect of supplementing pea-fibre and fructo-oligosaccharides. *Brit J Nutr*. 2006;96(2):350–356.
33. Stubbs J, Ferres S, Horgan G. Energy density foods: effects on energy intake. *Crit Rev Food Sci Nutr*. 2004;40(Supp 6):481–515.
34. Mattes RD, Rothacker D. Beverage viscosity is inversely related to postprandial hunger in humans. *Physiology & Behav*. 2001;74(4–5): 551–557.
35. Megestrol acetate. In: McElvoy GK, ed. *AHFS Drug Information® 2006*. Bethesda, MD: American Society of Health-System Pharmacists; 2006:1129–1131.
36. Sturm K, MacIntosh CG, Parker BA, Wishart J, Horowitz M, Chapman IM. Appetite, food intake, and plasma concentrations of cholecystokinin, ghrelin, and other gastrointestinal hormones in undernourished older women and well-nourished young and older women. *J Clin Endocrin Met*. 2003;88(8);3747–3755.
37. Stull AJ, Apolzan JW, Thalacker-Mercer AE, Iglay HB, Campbell WW. Liquid and solid meal replacement products differentially affect postprandial appetite and food intake in older adults. *J Am Diet Assoc*. 2008;108(7):1226–1230.
38. Goyal RG. Alimentary tract motor function. In: Stein JH. *Internal Medicine*. 5th ed. St. Louis, Mo: Mosby; 1998:1976–1980.
39. Regulation of GI function. In: Ganong WF. *Review of Medical Physiology*. 22nd ed. New York, NY: McGraw-Hill Lange Medical; 2005:479–514.
40. General principles of gastrointestinal function—motility, nervous control, and blood circulation. In: Hall JE. *Guyton and Hall Textbook of Medical Physiology*. 12th ed. Philadelphia, PA: Elsevier; 2010:753–762.
41. Fischbach F. *Manual of Laboratory & Diagnostic Tests*. 7th ed. Philadelphia, PA: Lippincott Williams & Wilkins; 2004: 674.
42. McCallum RW, Soykan I. Nausea, vomiting, and anorexia. In: Stein JH. *Internal Medicine*. 5th ed. St. Louis, MO: Mosby; 1998: 2025–2030.
43. Ray NF, Denton WG, Thamer M, et al. Abdominal adhesiolysis: inpatient care and expenditures in the United States in 1994. *J Am Coll Surg*. 1998;186:1–9.
44. Whang EE, Ashley SW, Zinner MJ. Small intestine. In: Brunicardi FC. *Schwartz's Principles of Surgery*. 8th ed. New York, NY: McGraw-Hill Medical; 2005:1017–1054.
45. Acute abdomen and surgical gastroenterology: abdominal pain. In: Beers MH, Berkow R, eds. *The Merck Manual of Diagnosis and Therapy*. 18th ed. New York, NY: Wiley; 2006:94–108.
46. McClave SA, Martindale RG, Vanek VW, et al., A.S.P.E.N. Board of Directors, American College of Critical Care Medicine, Society of Critical Care Medicine. Guidelines for the provision and assessment of nutrition support therapy in the adult critically ill patient: Society of Critical Care Medicine (SCCM) and American Society for Parenteral and Enteral Nutrition (A.S.P.E.N.). *JPEN*. 2009; 33(3):277–316.
47. Bullard KM, Rothenberger DA. Colon, rectum and anus. In: Brunicardi FC, ed. *Schwartz's Principles of Surgery*. 8th ed. New York, NY: McGraw-Hill Medical; 2005:1055–1118.
48. Tan SA, Sarosi GA. Gastrointestinal motility disorders. In: Mulholland MW, Lillemoe KD, Doherty GM, Maier RV, Simeone DM, Upchurch GR, eds. *Greenfield's Surgery Scientific Principles and Practice*. 5th ed. Philadelphia, PA: Lippincott Williams & Wilkins; 2011:1027–1038.
49. Diarrhea. In: Pugh MB, et. al., ed. *Stedman's Medical Dictionary*. 28th ed. Baltimore, MD: Lippincott Williams & Wilkins; 2006. STAT!Ref Online Electronic Medical Library. http://online.statref.com/document.aspx?fxid=8&docid=11006. Accessed June 7, 2011.

50. Abel C, Grimes JA. Diarrhea. In: Domino FJ, ed. *5-Minute Clinical Consult.* 19th ed. Philadelphia, PA: Lippincott Williams & Wilkins; 2011:394–397.
51. Ros PR, Buetow PC, Pantograg-Brown L, et al. Pseudomembranous colitis. *Radiology.* 1996;198(1):1–9.
52. Kelly CP, Pothoulakis C, LaMont JT. Clostridium difficile colitis. *N Engl J Med.* 1994;330(4):257–262.
53. Kawamoto S, Horton KM, Fishman EK. Pseudomembranous colitis: spectrum of imaging findings with clinical and pathologic correlation. *Radiographics.* 1999;19(4):887–897.
54. The American Dietetics Association. Diarrhea. In: *Nutrition Care Manual.* Chicago, IL: Academy of Nutrition and Dietetics. http://nutritioncaremanual.org/content.cfm?ncm_content_id=88384. Accessed June 20, 2011.
55. Slavin J. Dietary fiber. In: Matarese L, Gottschlich MM, eds. *Contemporary Nutrition Support Practice: A Clinical Guide.* 2nd ed. Philadelphia, PA: Saunders; 2003:173–187.
56. Baldor RA. Constipation. In: Domino FJ, ed. *5-Minute Clinical Consult.* 19th ed. Philadelphia, PA: Lippincott Williams & Wilkins; 2011:306–307.
57. The American Dietetics Association. Constipation recommended foods. In: *Nutrition Care Manual.* Chicago, IL: Academy of Nutrition and Dietetics. http://nutritioncaremanual.org/content.cfm?ncm_content_id=88384. Accessed June 20, 2011.
58. The American Dietetics Association. Constipation. In: *Nutrition Care Manual.* Chicago, IL: Academy of Nutrition and Dietetics. http://nutritioncaremanual.org/content.cfm?ncm_content_id=88384. Accessed June 20, 2011.
59. Academy of Nutrition and Dietetics. Gastric surgery. In: *Nutrition Care Manual.* Chicago, IL: Academy of Nutrition and Dietetics. http://nutritioncaremanual.org/content.cfm?ncm_content_id=88384. Accessed June 20, 2011.
60. Secretory functions of the alimentary tract. In: Hall JE. *Guyton and Hall Textbook of Medical Physiology.* 12th ed. Philadelphia, PA: Elsevier; 2010:773–788.
61. Johnson LR. *Essential Medical Physiology.* 2nd ed. Philadelphia, PA: Lippincott-Raven; 1998.
62. Digestion and absorption in the gastrointestinal tract. In: Hall JE. *Guyton and Hall Textbook of Medical Physiology.* 12th ed. Philadelphia, PA: Elsevier; 2010:788–798.
63. Jepson JB. Hartnup's disease. In: Stanbury JB, Wyngarten JB, Fredrisksno DS, eds. *The Metabolic Basis of Inherited Disease.* 4th ed. New York, NY: McGraw-Hill; 1978:1563–1574.
64. Hacquebard M, Carpentier YA. Vitamin E: absorption, plasma transport and cell uptake. *Curr Opin Clin Nutr Metab Care.* 2005; 8(2):133–138.
65. Bragg LE, Thompson JS, Rikkers LF. Influence of nutrient delivery on gut structure and function. *Nutrition.* 1991;7(4):237–243.
66. Young LS, Stoll S. Proteins and amino acids. In: Matarese LE, Gottschlich MM, eds. *Contemporary Nutrition Support Practice: A Clinical Guide.* 2nd ed. Philadelphia, PA: Saunders; 2003:94–104.
67. Kimchi ET, Gusani NJ, Kaifi JT. Anatomy and physiology of the small intestines. In: Mulholland MW, Lillemoe KD, Doherty GM, Maier RV, Simeone DM, Upchurch GR, eds. *Greenfield's Surgery Scientific Principles and Practice.* 5th ed. Philadelphia, PA: Lippincott Williams & Wilkins; 2011:738–748.

2 Energy

Jennifer A. Wooley, MS, RD, CNSC, and David Frankenfield, MS, RD

CONTENTS

Background 23
Overview of Energy Metabolism 23
Components of Energy Expenditure 23
Basal or Resting Metabolic Rate 23
Thermogenic Effect of Digestion 24
Physical Activity 24
Growth 24
Illness 24
Methods to Determine Energy Expenditure 24
Measurement of Energy Expenditure 24
Direct Calorimetry 24
Indirect Calorimetry 25
Clinical Indications for Indirect Calorimetry 25
Clinical Information from Indirect Calorimetry 25
Technical Aspects of Indirect Calorimetry 25
Interpretation of the Measured Resting Metabolic Rate 25
Interpretation of the Respiratory Quotient 26
Frequency of Conducting Indirect Calorimetry 27
Other Methods of Measuring Energy Expenditure 27
Reverse Fick Equation 27
Doubly Labeled Water 27
Predictive Equations to Determine Energy Expenditure for Healthy Individuals 27
Notes on Validity Testing 27
Harris-Benedict 28
Mifflin-St. Jeor 29
New Equations 29
Predictive Equations for Critically Ill Patients 29
Ireton-Jones 29
Swinamer 30
Penn State 30
Predictive Equations Using kcal/kg 30
Predictive Equations for Acutely Ill (Relatively Stable, Not Critically Ill) Patients 31
Applications to Nutrition Support Therapy 31
Assessing the Metabolic Response 31
Importance of Avoiding Under- and Overfeeding 32
References 32

Objectives

1. Compare energy metabolism during health and illness.
2. Identify evidence-based methods for calculating resting metabolic rate.
3. Review methods for the measurement of energy expenditure.
4. Improve precision in the assessment of the energy expenditure in patients requiring nutrition support therapy.

Test Your Knowledge Questions

1. Which of the following has the greatest influence on total energy expenditure (TEE)?
   A. Resting metabolic rate (RMR)
   B. Thermogenic effect of digestion
   C. Physical activity
   D. Metabolic stress
2. The most commonly used method for assessing energy expenditure is:
   A. Indirect calorimetry
   B. Predictive equations
   C. The Reverse Fick equation
   D. Doubly labeled water
3. Which parameter is measured when using indirect calorimetry?
   A. Heat loss
   B. Catabolic rate
   C. Gas exchange
   D. Free energy balance

Test Your Knowledge Answers

1. The correct answer is **A.** The thermogenic effect of digestion is generally thought to contribute no more than 10% to TEE. Activity contributes 5% to 30% to TEE. With the exceptions of burn (see Chapter 24) and sepsis (see Chapter 23), metabolic stress contributes less than 50% to TEE. However, in almost all situations, RMR constitutes 60% to 75% of TEE.
2. The correct answer is **B.** Most nutrition support feeding regimens are based on predictive equations used to assess energy expenditure. The measurement of energy expenditure via indirect calorimetry is more accurate than predictive equations but is underused because of its expense and the clinical expertise required for use and interpretation of results.
3. The correct answer is **C.** Indirect calorimeters measure respiratory gas exchange. If proper testing conditions are observed, the gas exchange measurement can be converted to resting metabolic rate using the Weir equation.

Background

Acquisition and transformation of energy is one of the most basic characteristics of life.[1] Living things must be capable of consuming chemical energy from the environment, converting it to cellular components and transforming it to a form by which to power work. Energy transformations (metabolism) are necessary for living things to maintain homeostasis and perform the other activities associated with life. In humans, energy metabolism has evolved into a series of interrelated complex biochemical processes by which fuels are consumed from the environment, converted to tissue, oxidized, used to perform work, and ultimately converted to heat, water, and carbon dioxide, which is dissipated back to the environment.

This chapter reviews energy metabolism in healthy subjects as the framework for understanding the alterations in energy metabolism during malnutrition and illness. The energy prescription is a fundamental aspect of the nutrition support regimen. Therefore, emphasis in this chapter is placed on evidence-based methods for determining the energy expenditure of those patients who are unable to meet their needs orally, thus requiring nutrition support therapy.

Overview of Energy Metabolism

The basic fuels of the body are carbohydrate, protein, and fat (ethanol can also be oxidized). Glucose is used preferentially after meals, whereas fat is stored for later oxidation. Protein generally is used for structural and functional rather than oxidative purposes, but during routine protein turnover, some is oxidized (see Chapters 3, 5, and 6). When energy is not available in the form of food, the body cannibalizes its own tissues as an endogenous energy source. This catabolic process is hormonally driven and is reversible by feeding. It is of primary importance to maintain a source of glucose supply while limiting protein loss, and the body has mechanisms to ensure glucose flow if diet sources are unavailable. Glycogen is the immediate store of glucose but is depleted after about 12 hours of fasting. Once glycogen is depleted, protein and glycerol from triglyceride turnover are catabolized to produce new glucose. If starvation continues, other metabolic changes occur that provide alternate fuels that substitute for glucose (ketones from fatty acids) and that recycle glucose rather than oxidizing completely to carbon dioxide. These changes decrease protein catabolism and allow conservation of the body protein mass.[2–4]

Components of Energy Expenditure

TEE can be divided into three major components in healthy, well-nourished adults: basal metabolic rate (BMR) or RMR, energy required for the thermogenic effect of digestion, and energy expenditure associated with physical activity. An underrecognized factor increasing RMR is environmental conditions. At low ambient temperature, body temperature is maintained by insulative and metabolic means. Peripheral vasoconstriction (insulative) limits heat loss, and increased RMR (metabolic) increases heat production (nonshivering thermogenesis). An increase in physical activity (shivering) will also increase the metabolic rate.[5] In some patients, therapeutic hypothermia is induced to limit metabolic rate (eg, in some patients with brain injury), and as long as shivering is prevented with the use of neuromuscular blocking agents, the resting metabolic rate will decrease, along with the body temperature.[6,7] At ambient temperature greater than body temperature, the body will give off heat to the environment to keep itself cool, thus increasing metabolic rate.[8]

Basal or Resting Metabolic Rate

The terms BMR and RMR sometimes cause confusion, partly because they are different but similar terms, and partly because some authors use the terms interchangeably. BMR is metabolic rate measured in a fasting state, immediately upon awakening and before any physical activity is undertaken. RMR also is measured in a fasted state (at least 5 hours)[9] but allows some movement (dressing, walking) before testing. A rest time of 20 minutes is necessary for recovery from this level of activity.[9] Once this rest period is provided, there is only a small difference between RMR and BMR, with RMR usually being slightly higher.[10] Because BMR is a more involved measurement, most studies of human metabolism are made in a resting rather than a basal state. In many nutrition support patients, even the less restrictive RMR standard of measurement is not obtained because so many patients are fed continuously and thus are never in a fasted state. The withholding of feeding in such instances is generally not practiced and instead the resting definition is modified to include the metabolic effect of feeding.

Even in the most physically active people and the most hypermetabolic patients, RMR accounts for the largest portion of TEE (60% to 75%). RMR is determined largely by body size and body composition.[11,12] Gender and age also affect RMR (being lower in females and in the elderly).[12,13] Some of the gender and age effects are indirect, being a result of lower fat-free mass or the amount of high metabolic rate tissue within the fat-free mass rather than gender and age effects per se.[12,13] Composition of the fat-free mass might also explain some racial differences in RMR.[14,15]

Thermogenic Effect of Digestion

The assimilation of macronutrients following the consumption of a meal leads to an increase in metabolism referred to as the thermogenic effect of digestion. This still ill-defined phenomenon was thought originally to be specific to protein (hence, its original name "specific dynamic action").[16] The presence, magnitude, and duration of the thermogenic effect of digestion is believed to be influenced by numerous factors including the size of the meal; ratio of protein, carbohydrate, and fat in the diet; fiber content of the meal; time of day the meal is eaten; degree of psychological stress; age; coffee consumption; smoking; and spiciness of the food eaten.[17] In general, a 5% to 10% increase in TEE is ascribed to the thermogenic effect of digestion.[3,17]

Physical Activity

Physical activity is the most variable and difficult to predict portion of TEE. For critically ill patients, activities of daily living (eg, bathing, turning, wound care, chest physiotherapy) raise metabolic rate, but the cumulative effect of these short-lived activities is usually small, accounting for approximately 5% to 10% of TEE.[18–24] In hospitalized patients who are ambulatory or who display "thrashing" behavior, expenditure of energy caused by activity can be considerably higher.

Growth

In nutrition repletion, pregnancy, and childhood, energy expenditure increases to support tissue growth.[25,26] Tissue growth is a high-energy activity. Not only is the newly synthesized tissue composed of fuel (ie, energy), but the synthesis of the new tissue from individual amino acids, fatty acids, and glucose is an energy-requiring reaction.

Illness

Alterations in energy expenditure occur during illness. While simple starvation is mediated largely by increased counterregulatory hormones and suppression of insulin, stress metabolism is mediated by counterregulatory hormones, prostaglandins, cytokines, and many other factors, leading to increased RMR. A further distinction from starvation is that the metabolic state is not a consequence of feeding status but of disease, so the response is not reversed by feeding but rather by resolution of the illness. Stress metabolism is also marked by gluconeogenesis in the face of insulin resistance, suppression of ketogenesis, increased glutamine synthesis and consumption, and net protein catabolism despite increased protein synthesis in the viscera.

Hypermetabolism is often noted in people with active disease processes.[27,28] Studies of metabolic rate in diseased populations have been carried out since the early part of the 20th century, focusing at first on febrile infectious diseases (eg, malaria, tuberculosis, typhoid) and thyroid conditions, and more recently on a wide range of acute and chronic disease states.[29] Measured rates of metabolism are highly variable among the numerous studies published, for a number of reasons.[18,19,30–35] Some of the variation is related to the disease state being studied, but even among studies of the same disease state there is variation. Another powerful trend is that contemporary studies show a lower metabolic rate than studies performed in the 1960s and 1970s, probably reflecting improvements in patient care. An underappreciated consideration is that the degree of hypermetabolism is not solely determined by the illness but also by the level of inflammation in response to the illness. However, there is probably some interplay between these components.[25,36]

Methods to Determine Energy Expenditure

Measurement of Energy Expenditure

The foundation of nutrition support is to preserve lean body mass and maintain immune function while avoiding complications related to under- or overfeeding. Despite the availability of more than 200 predictive equations to estimate energy expenditure, predicting the needs of an individual critically ill patient remains extremely difficult.[33] Although predictive equations offer various "stress" factors to account for the specific needs of critically ill patients, these factors are often inaccurate and imprecise resulting in either under- or overestimation of energy expenditure.

Direct Calorimetry

Direct calorimetry measures heat released from the subject. Because all energy from macronutrients consumed by a subject is ultimately released as heat, its release is considered a direct measurement of energy expenditure. Direct calorimeters are sophisticated machines that measure changes in temperature of air or water circulating through the insulated walls of an enclosed chamber while the subject resides within. Direct calorimetry is most appropriate in research and academic environments using healthy subjects because this technique is not practical, and the person must remain alone in the chamber without caregivers or life-support equipment during measurements.

Indirect Calorimetry

The inherent limitations of predictive equations have led to the emergence of indirect calorimetry (IC) as the gold standard of nutrition assessment in the intensive care unit (ICU). IC is the most accurate method for determining the energy expenditure of critically ill patients.[34,37–41] Many hospitals have access to metabolic carts to measure RMR. However, this valuable tool remains grossly underutilized because of its expense and the clinical expertise required for use and interpretation of results.

Nutrient requirements vary substantially between patients with altered metabolic states. A major advantage of IC over predictive energy expenditure equations is that it allows the clinician to "match" the nutrition support regimen to the individual patient's needs, at a defined time, based on actual measured energy expenditure.

Clinical Indications for Indirect Calorimetry

Indications for IC can be divided into three general categories. First, Table 2-1 describes several clinical conditions and diagnoses that significantly alter RMR, making predictive equations inaccurate. Second, IC is indicated in patients who fail to respond to nutrition support based on predictive equations during their clinical course. Examples include poor wound healing, failure to wean from mechanical ventilation, and protein malnutrition despite "adequate" support. Third, IC is an effective tool in evaluating whether under- or overfeeding is contributing to metabolic and respiratory derangements in critically ill patients.[34,37–40]

Table 2-1 Factors Affecting Accuracy of Caloric Requirement Estimates[34,41–43]

Acute or chronic respiratory distress syndrome
Large open wounds or burns
Malnutrition with altered body composition:
- Underweight
- Obesity
- Limb amputation
- Peripheral edema
- Ascites

Multiple or neurological trauma
Multisystem organ failure
Postoperative organ transplantation
Sepsis
Systemic inflammatory response syndrome
Use of paralytic or barbiturate agents

Adapted from Wooley JA, Sax HC. Indirect calorimetry: applications to practice. *Nutr. Clin Pract.* 2003;18(5):434–439, with permission from the American Society for Parenteral and Enteral Nutrition.

Clinical Information from Indirect Calorimetry

The basic science and energy dynamics of IC have been extensively studied and reviewed by many authors.[18,34,40,42–45] This chapter focuses on the practical application of the information derived from IC to patient care. IC calculates RMR, and respiratory quotient (RQ) by measuring whole body oxygen consumption (VO_2) and carbon dioxide gas exchange (VCO_2)[34,46] using the abbreviated Weir equation[47] where:

$$(1)\ \text{Energy expenditure} = (3.94 \times VO_2) + (1.11 \times VCO_2)$$

The consumption of oxygen accounts for 80% of RMR despite a relatively small body pool of 1.2 L. Carbon dioxide production accounts for 20% even though the body pool is very large, approximately 16 L.[34,43,45,46] RMR measured by IC is approximately 10% above BMR.[34,47]

IC allows consideration of urinary urea nitrogen (UUN) excretion in an attempt to account for the contribution of protein substrates to energy expenditure. However, measurement of UUN excretion is not essential to ensure accuracy in the determination of RMR.[18,43–47] Even a 100% error in the UUN measurement will only produce an error of approximately 1% to 2% in the true energy expenditure.[43,45] Elimination of cumbersome and often inaccurate 24-hour urine collections will promote both cost and time efficiency in clinical measurement of RMR.

Technical Aspects of Indirect Calorimetry

Accuracy of IC measurements is dependent on patient-, environmental-, and equipment-related factors (Table 2-2). IC can be performed on mechanically ventilated and spontaneously breathing patients. Technical limitations associated with IC are listed in Table 2-3. One key example is the presence of air leaks, which produce a loss of oxygen and carbon dioxide volumes with an associated reduction in the measured RMR.[34,37–40,44,46]

The necessary duration of IC testing is not well defined. Most studies continue until a 5-minute "steady state" period is attained or for a predetermined interval of approximately 30 minutes if it is not.[48–52] Technically, steady state means that the ventilation, acid-base balance, and carbon dioxide production are stable with very little variation. Steady state represents a period of "metabolic equilibrium," where, during a 5-minute interval, VO_2 and VCO_2 change by less than 10%, or the coefficient of variation for these two values is less than 5%.[18,43,44,50,53–55] Achieving steady state may be difficult to attain in the unstable critically ill patient. Increasing the frequency of testing as opposed to extending the duration of an individual study is the most effective way to capture true energy expenditure and minimize error.[53,56]

Interpretation of the Measured Resting Metabolic Rate

The process of interpreting the measured RMR should begin with evaluating the validity of the study by assessing the achievement of steady state, as described previously.[37,41,42] Once the study has been validated, application of the information can begin. If a patient's RMR is measured while fasting, or

Table 2-2 Recommendations for Improving Accuracy of Indirect Calorimetry

- Patients have rested in a supine position (in bed or a recliner) for more than 30 minutes before the study to avoid the effects of voluntary activity on REE.[34,40,46]
- Patients receiving intermittent feedings (ie, bolus enteral feeding, cyclic enteral or parenteral nutrition or meals) are studied approximately 1 hour after the feeding if thermogenesis is to be included in the REE or 4 hours after the feeding if it is not.[34,40]
- The rate and composition of nutrients being infused on a continuous basis are stable for at least 12 hours before and throughout the study.[34,40]
- Measurements are made in a quiet, thermoneutral environment.[34,40,44,46]
- All sources of supplemental oxygen (ie, nasal cannulas, masks, or tracheostomy collars) are turned off during routine room air measurements, if medically feasible.[34,40,46]
- The fraction of inspired oxygen remains constant during the measurement.[34,46]
- The study will be delayed for 90 minutes if changes are required in ventilatory settings.[34,40,44,46]
- The patient has usual patterns of voluntary skeletal muscle activity (movement of the extremities) during the study.[34,40,44,46]
- No leaks are present in the sampling system.[34,40,44,46]
- All data used to derive REE and RQ are taken from a period of equilibrium or steady state that has been identified according to statistically defined guidelines.[34,40,44,46]
- The patient has not received general anesthesia within 6 to 8 hours before the study.[34]
- If the patient is in pain or agitated, analgesics or sedatives will be given at least 30 minutes before the study when clinically possible, and this information will be documented for consideration during the interpretation of the study.[34,40,44]
- The study will be delayed for 3 to 4 hours after hemodialysis.[34,46,103]
- The study will be delayed 1 hour after painful procedures have been performed.[34]
- Routine nursing care or activities involving other health care professionals should be avoided during the study.[34,44]

REE, resting energy expenditure; RQ, respiratory quotient. Adapted from Wooley JA, Sax HC. Indirect calorimetry: applications to practice. *Nutr. Clin Pract.* 2003;18(5):434–439, with permission from the American Society for Parenteral and Enteral Nutrition.

if feedings are intermittent, an additional 5% may be added to account for thermogenesis.[34] However, a thermogenesis factor is usually unnecessary because the majority of patients in the ICU are on continuous feedings. In these instances, the thermogenic effect has been directly measured during IC.

Historically, various multipliers were added to the measured RMR to account for stress or to promote repletion. As mentioned previously, a factor of 5% to 10% was added to the RMR to account for the physical activity of a typical patient in the ICU.[20–24,37,38,40] However, some critically ill patients are unable to use additional substrates designed to offset ICU activities and stress, and promote repletion. In addition, the purpose of measuring RMR is to obviate the use of additional subjective factors. Research has concluded that use of these multipliers should be abandoned.[57] Current recommendations are to feed patients at 100% of the measured RMR without stress or activity factors.[57–59] The measured RMR should be met with total calories as opposed to nonprotein calories with a carbohydrate:lipid:protein ratio of approximately 50%, 20% to 30%, and 15% to 20%, respectively (see Chapters 3, 5, and 6 for further information on carbohydrate, lipid, and protein).

Table 2-3 Technical Factors That Decrease Indirect Calorimetry Accuracy

- Mechanical ventilation with fraction of inspired oxygen ≥ 60
- Mechanical ventilation with positive end expiratory pressure > 12 cm H_2O
- Hyper/hypoventilation (acute changes altering body carbon dioxide stores)
- Leak in the sampling system
- Moisture in the system can affect the oxygen analyzer
- Continuous flow through the system > 0 L/min during exhalation
- Inability to collect all expiratory flow
- Unstable inspiratory fraction of inspired oxygen (> ± 0.01)
- Leaking chest tube (inability to collect all expired gases)
- Bronchopleural fistula (inability to collect all expired gases)
- Supplemental oxygen in spontaneously breathing patients
- Hemodialysis, peritoneal dialysis, or continuous renal replacement therapy in progress
- Errors in calibration of indirect calorimeter

Adapted from Wooley JA, Sax HC. Indirect calorimetry: applications to practice. *Nutr. Clin Pract.* 2003;18(5):434–439, with permission from the American Society for Parenteral and Enteral Nutrition.

Interpretation of the Respiratory Quotient

RQ is defined as the ratio of carbon dioxide production to oxygen consumption. Traditionally, RQ has been used as an indirect measure of substrate utilization (Table 2-4).[34,37,38,40] An RQ < 0.82 suggests underfeeding, or predominant lipid catabolism, indicating the need to increase caloric delivery.[34,37,38,40] An RQ > 1 with excessive carbon dioxide production suggests overfeeding, potential lipogenesis, and increased respiratory demand. The appropriate clinical action would be to decrease total caloric and carbohydrate delivery.[34,37,38,40] An RQ of 0.85 implies mixed substrate utilization—the hallmark of an appropriate nutrition regimen.[34,37,38,40]

Care must be taken when evaluating the RQ in this fashion. Although RQ does correlate to the ratio of percent calories provided/percent calories required, low sensitivity and reduced specificity limit its efficacy as an indicator of under- or overfeeding.[60,61] There are several metabolic causes for an RQ < 0.71, including oxidation of ethanol and ketones, lipolysis, and underfeeding. Diabetes mellitus, ketoacidosis, or

Table 2-4 Traditional Interpretation of Respiratory Quotient

$$RQ = \frac{V_{CO_2}\text{ (carbon dioxide production)}}{V_{O_2}\text{ (oxygen consumption)}}$$

Substrate utilization	*RQ*
Ethanol	0.67
Fat oxidation	0.71
Protein oxidation	0.82
Mixed substrate oxidation	0.85
Carbohydrate oxidation	1
Lipogenesis	1–1.2

RQ, respiratory quotient. Adapted from Wooley JA, Sax HC. Indirect calorimetry: applications to practice. *Nutr Clin Pract.* 2003;18(5):434–439, with permission from the American Society for Parenteral and Enteral Nutrition.

high rates of urinary glucose excretion may also result in low RQ values. An RQ can be falsely measured as < 1 despite overfeeding in the hypermetabolic patient because of substrate shifts caused by inflammatory mediators.[40] Respiratory states such as hypoventilation with high P_{CO_2} levels and technical difficulties may also result in a low RQ but do not reflect substrate utilization.[40]

The clinician needs to bear in mind that gas exchange is a whole body measurement. An RQ of 1 does not necessarily mean that all tissues are burning carbohydrate. It is thought that fat oxidation and lipogenesis can occur simultaneously in two different tissues, resulting in a net RQ of one.[34] Potential metabolic causes for an RQ greater than one include excess carbon dioxide production, the provision of exogenous buffering agents such as sodium bicarbonate, lipogenesis, and overfeeding.

The physiologic range for the RQ in humans is 0.67 to 1.3. A value obtained outside this range should alert the clinician to the possibility of an invalid study.[60,61] The measured RQ should not be used as an indicator of substrate utilization, but rather as a measure of test validity.[43,61]

Frequency of Conducting Indirect Calorimetry

There is no consensus in previous publications on how frequently IC should be done in the critically ill patient. Unfortunately, prospective randomized trials addressing this specific area of IC have been few. Ideally, a baseline study should be followed with measurements at regular intervals to capture changes in energy expenditure during each phase of the metabolic response to stress.[62] When used to guide subsequent modifications in nutrient delivery, IC allows the clinician to respond to changes in a patient's energy expenditure, which can vary ± 15% to 31% on a daily basis.[23,24,43]

Other Methods of Measuring Energy Expenditure

Reverse Fick Equation

Oxygen consumption can be estimated using the Fick principles derived from oxygen content differences in arterial and mixed venous blood multiplied by cardiac output measurements from pulmonary artery catheters.[63] Placement of a pulmonary artery catheter is highly invasive, and the oxygen consumption measurements are poorly correlated with IC oxygen consumption ($R^2 = 0.30$) and biased toward underestimation.[64] Therefore, the Fick equation is not useful for clinical assessment of energy expenditure.

Doubly Labeled Water

The doubly labeled water technique is another option for assessing energy expenditure. This method uses a stable isotope of water (${}^2H_2{}^{18}O$), which is administered to the patient and its disappearance rate is measured over time (days).[65] Disappearance of ${}^2H$ is proportional to water turnover, while the disappearance of ${}^{18}O$ is proportional to water and turnover plus V_{CO_2} production. The difference between the two disappearance rates is the V_{CO_2}. VO_2 is not measured. Instead, V_{O_2} is computed from the "food quotient" (FQ), which is the sum of the carbon dioxide produced from all food eaten divided by the sum of the oxygen consumed during oxidation of all food eaten. From FQ and measured V_{CO_2}, V_{O_2} can be computed ($V_{CO_2}/FQ = V_{O_2}$). Alternately, an RQ can be assumed and V_{O_2} computed as $V_{CO_2}/RQ = V_{O_2}$. The doubly labeled water technique of measuring metabolic rate is useful in field research but is not generally used in clinical care.

Predictive Equations to Determine Energy Expenditure for Healthy Individuals

In most instances when a nutrition support regimen is being formulated, measured RMR is not available and the clinician must rely on an estimate of the energy requirement. Equations for predicting RMR have been in existence since at least 1916.[66] The original purpose of the equations was to develop a standard against which to test whether a measurement of resting metabolic rate fell within the normal range (analogous to determining the laboratory standard for serum sodium concentration in a human being). Over the decades, these standard calculations proliferated and their usage changed to their current purpose of calculating energy prescriptions.

Notes on Validity Testing

Predictive methods should be tested for validity before they are used in practice. Validity is a descriptive term that can be composed of several statistical parameters such as bias, agreement, limit of agreement, and precision. Bias is the tendency for an equation to underestimate or overestimate the true RMR as measured by IC.[67] Agreement is the percentage of estimates that fall within some limit of the true RMR. Typically and historically, this limit is ± 10% of the measured value. Limit of agreement is a term applied by Bland and Altman defined as ± 1.96 standard deviations about the mean difference between two measurements.[68] This statistic is sometimes adopted in the analysis of the difference between a measurement and an estimate of RMR. The limit of agreement should encompass 95% of all the differences measured. Precision is a problematic term that refers to the repeatability of an observation. In its classic connotation, precision of an instrument would be assessed by repeated testing against a reference method under the same conditions, including the same subject. Application of this process to assessment of a metabolic rate equation creates a problem in that the variables used in equations (body weight, body temperature, age, sex, etc.) do not change rapidly enough for repeated measures in rapid succession in the same person to be meaningful. Therefore, the term precision, when used in the testing of a metabolic rate equation, is often defined as the degree to which single estimates in multiple subjects with similar conditions (eg, healthy, critically ill, mechanically ventilated, obese) show the same result.

Note that an estimate can be biased but still have a high agreement and/or a low limit of agreement, and can therefore still be valid. On the other hand, an estimate can be unbiased but the spread of observations can be so wide as to have low agreement and high limit of agreement.

Harris-Benedict

The metabolic rate equations produced by DuBois may be the first standard metabolic equations ever produced.[66] These predate the now more famous Harris-Benedict equations[69] by three years, but have almost been forgotten. The Harris-Benedict equation also is now transitioning from a clinical tool to a historical landmark. This equation is remarkable for three reasons. First, is its longevity, being published in 1919. Second, it represents the first use of regression techniques in physiology.[70] Third, after some initial skepticism, it established linear rather than allometric scaling for calculating resting metabolism, although the argument over which is best continues today.[71] The term allometric describes a change in one biologic parameter that is not linear with another.

Benedict himself recognized that his equations had a tendency to overestimate the true RMR,[72] and this observation has been documented in validation studies since then.[73-77] An evidence review undertaken by the American Dietetic Association (ADA) in 2003 indicated that equations other than the Harris-Benedict were more reliable.[77] Thus, use of the Harris-Benedict equation is waning. One problem with disregarding the equation completely is that most of the descriptive studies of metabolism in illness use the Harris-Benedict equation as the base calculation, so most of the stress factors in use today would need to be recalculated. As Figure 2-1 demonstrates, the differences between Mifflin-St. Jeor and Harris-Benedict are most pronounced at the extremes of RMR range, with Harris-Benedict predicting a higher value in both instances. The low end of the range of metabolic rates tends to be occupied by people with low body mass index, and the high end of the range tends to be occupied by people with high body mass index.

FIGURE 2-1 Difference Between Predicted Resting Metabolic Rate by Mifflin St. Jeor and Harris Benedict Equations

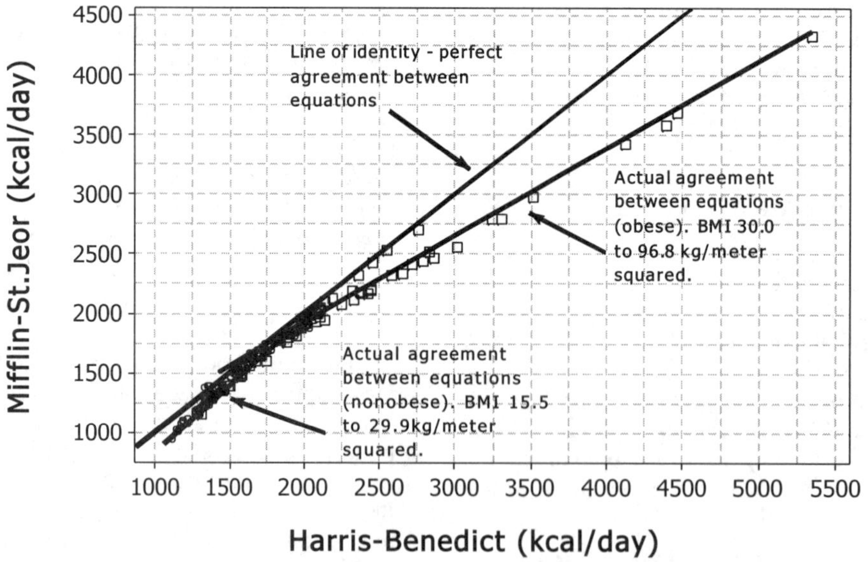

The relationship between the two most common equations for predicting resting metabolic rate in healthy people. Comparison to the line of identity between the methods. The methods tend to disagree at high and low values of metabolic rate. In both high and low values, the Harris-Benedict equation tends to predict a higher metabolic rate than the Mifflin-St. Jeor equation. In the midrange, the two methods agree better. Graph adapted from data in Frankenfield DC, Rowe WA, Smith JS, Cooney RN. Validation of several established equations for resting metabolic rate in obese and nonobese people. *J Am Diet Assoc.* 2003;103:1152–1159.

Mifflin-St. Jeor

In 1990, a study was published in which new predictive equations for RMR were proposed.[76] This study examined 247 women and 251 men, aged 19 to 78 years. Roughly half of the subjects were obese, with a maximum body mass index of 42 kg/m². Fat-free mass was also measured and found to be the strongest single predictor of RMR ($R^2 = 0.64$). However, the combination of body weight, height, age, and gender were found to correlate better than fat-free mass ($R^2 = 0.71$), and being easier quantities to obtain, this combination of factors was chosen to construct the predictive equation. In this way, the Mifflin-St.Jeor equation is in form much like the Harris-Benedict. The highest correlation was obtained when the obese and nonobese subjects were combined into one equation:

(2) Men: Energy expenditure = 5 + 10 (wt in kg) + 6.25 (ht in cm) − 5 (age)

(3) Women: Energy expenditure = −161 + 10 (wt in kg) + 6.25 (ht in cm) − 5 (age)

Whether the combining of obese and nonobese people into one equation is successful because of a statistical artifact (error spread over a wider range of measured values will raise the correlation coefficient) or because it fits physiological reality is debatable, but the Mifflin-St. Jeor equation has been shown to be valid in both populations.[73] The ADA systematic review found more favorable evidence for the Mifflin-St. Jeor equation than for any other,[77] although it is true that accuracy rate falls somewhat when applied to obese people (70% in people with body mass index ≥ 30 kg/m² compared to 82% in people with body mass index < 30 kg/m²) and not every study shows the Mifflin-St. Jeor equation to be the most accurate.[78,79] Because of this evidence analysis, the ADA has recommended the Mifflin-St. Jeor equation in its newest edition of the *Nutrition Care Manual* (online). Research studies since the publication of the systematic review have confirmed that the Mifflin-St. Jeor equation is a reasonable standard for predicting healthy resting metabolic rate in Americans.[80]

New Equations

Livingston[71] resurrected the linear vs. allometric scaling argument with the publication of a new predictive equation in 2005. This equation was calculated from a database composed of the Harris-Benedict data, the Owen data,[72] and from 327 patients measured by the authors (total $n = 670$). The equations are simplified in that they use only weight and age, but computation is made slightly more complex by the presence of a power function:

(4) Men (kcal/d) = 293 × weight$^{0.4330}$ − 5.92 (age)

(5) Women (kcal/d) = 248 × weight$^{0.4356}$ − 5.09 (age)

A validation sample was included in this publication, consisting of 767 individual RMR determinations obtained from the Institute of Medicine. This validation indicated that the Livingston and Mifflin-St. Jeor equations performed about the same in a mixed sample of obese and nonobese individuals. Weijs found the same result, with both Livingston and Mifflin-St. Jeor accurately predicting the resting metabolic rate in 79% of a sample of overweight and obese Americans. (Interestingly, these equations were not as successful at predicting RMR in a sample overweight and obese Dutch.)[80]

Predictive Equations for Critically Ill Patients

Many equations for predicting energy expenditure in hospitalized patients start with one of the calculations discussed previously for healthy individuals (usually Harris-Benedict). A stress factor must then be applied to account for the hypermetabolism of illness. Numerous sets of such factors have been published, and as discussed there is wide variation in the results, even within the same patient types.[35,77]

An alternative to calculations of healthy RMR and multiplication by a stress modifier is to use an equation that includes not only determinants of RMR (body weight, height, age, gender) but modifiers for illness severity, inflammatory state, and respiratory demands.[18,80,81] Because these equations use factors that can change daily (eg, body temperature, minute ventilation), they are more dynamic than typical equations of RMR, which use only static variables such as height, weight, age, gender, and disease type.

Ireton-Jones

The Ireton-Jones equation was one of the first equations that did not approach metabolic rate prediction in the critically ill by adding a stress factor to one of the healthy RMR equations, but neither does it contain physiological variables:

(6) IJEE = 1784–11 (A) + 5 (W) + 244 (S) + 239 (T) + 804 (B)

where IJEE is kcal/day, A is age (years), W is actual body weight (kg), S is sex (male = 1, female = 0), T is diagnosis of trauma (present = 1, absent = 0), and B is diagnosis of burn (present = 1, absent = 0).

Validation studies have shown that this equation has a low accuracy rate in mechanically ventilated critical care patients.[82–87] An update of the ADA Evidence Analysis Library for critical care nutrition does not recommend the use of the Ireton-Jones equation.[88]

There is another Ireton-Jones equation for spontaneously breathing acutely ill patients:

(7) IJEE (s) = 629–11 (years of age) + 25 (kg body wt) − 609 (O)

where O is obesity > 30% above Ideal Body Weight from 1959 Metropolitan Live Insurance Tables or body mass index > 27 (present = 1, absent = 0). This equation could be simplified to:

(8) IJEE (nonobese) = 25 (kg body wt) − 11 (years of age) + 629

(9) IJEE (obese) = 25 (kg body wt) − 11 (years of age) + 20

The Ireton-Jones energy expenditure for spontaneously breathing patients has not been validated, so no recommendation for or against its use can be made.

Swinamer

The Swinamer equation is an early example of an equation that used physiological variables in addition to body size to predict RMR in critically ill patients:

(10) Swinamer[79]: $\text{RMR (kcal/d)} = \text{BSA}\,(941) - \text{age}\,(6.3) + T\,(104) + \text{RR}\,(24) + V_T\,(804) - 4243$

where BSA is body surface area (m^2), T is body temperature (centigrade), RR is respiratory rate (breaths/min), and V_T is tidal volume (L). The Swinamer equation has been found to accurately predict RMR in about 55% of patients and to cause large error (> 15% above measured) 30% of the time.[85]

Penn State

The Penn State equation was first published in 1998. Since then, it has undergone two modifications. The first modification was to substitute the Harris-Benedict equation with the Mifflin-St. Jeor, reflecting contemporary data that validated the Mifflin-St. Jeor equation.[73] The second modification was undertaken when it was found in a validation study that the equation underperforms in older obese patients.[87] In patients who are 60 years or older and who have a body mass index of 30 kg/m^2 or more, the accuracy rate of the Penn State equation was only 53% compared to 72% in other groups, and the rate of large errors was 33% compared to 15% for the other groups. The modification improved the accuracy rate to 74% for these older obese patients and reduced the rate of large errors to 12%.[89]

(11) Penn State[84]: $\text{RMR (kcal/d)} = \text{Mifflin}\,(0.96) + V_E\,(32) + T_m\,(167) - 6212$

(12) Penn State (modified): $\text{RMR (kcal/d)} = \text{Mifflin}\,(0.71) + V_E\,(64) + T_m\,(85) - 3085$

where T_m is maximum body temperature in the previous 24 hours (centigrade), RR is respiratory rate (breaths/min), and V_E is minute ventilation (L/min). The earlier versions of this equation that used Harris-Benedict as the base calculation should not be used and are not shown here in order to foster their disuse.

Predictive Equations Using kcal/kg

The calculation of energy requirements using kcal/kg is often used because of its convenience and wide acceptance by clinicians. American Society for Parenteral and Enteral Nutrition (A.S.P.E.N.) guidelines suggest by consensus a range of 20 to 35 kcal/kg daily for adults.[90] When performing an initial nutrition assessment on a patient, it is generally regarded as adequate to aim for 25 kcal/kg of the appropriate reference weight as long as subsequent adjustments in the caloric goal are made based on the patient's clinical response.[90] The 25 kcal/kg standard has undergone validation study in critically ill mechanically ventilated patients,[87] and it was found to be inaccurate 54% of the time and to produce large errors 43% of the time. This is not a standard upon which to rely for determining energy prescription in critically ill patients.

In summary, methods of predicting energy expenditure can be divided into two categories. The first is aimed at calculating RMR for healthy subjects and modifying for hypermetabolism with a stress factor. The second approach is to calculate RMR from regression equations that incorporate healthy resting metabolism and clinical markers of illness such as body temperature, respiratory rate, or minute ventilation. IC is the most accurate method for determining the energy requirements of the individual patient. However, in the absence of IC, it is incumbent upon the clinician to know the strengths and limitations of each predictive equation and use them judiciously. See Practice Scenario 2-1 for a discussion of energy expenditure prediction in a trauma patient.

Practice Scenario 2-1

Scenario: A 44-year-old woman was flown by helicopter to the emergency department following a high-speed head-on motor vehicle crash. She was a restrained driver, and her injuries included a rapid deceleration closed head injury, subarachnoid hemorrhage, and severe pulmonary contusions with a pneumothorax. The patient was emergently taken to the operating room for a craniotomy and placement of an intracranial pressure monitor. Postoperatively, she remained on a ventilator because of her pulmonary injuries.

The patient's past medical history includes hypertension, Type 2 diabetes mellitus, asthma, hypothyroidism, Class III obesity, and bipolar disorder. Her past surgical history includes an appendectomy, hysterectomy, and oophorectomy. Nutrition parameters are as follows: height, 5 feet 8 inches; actual body weight, 188 kg; body mass index, 62.9 m^2; ideal body weight; 63.6 kg.

Intervention: On hospital day 2, a nasoenteric feeding tube was placed for enteral nutrition. An isotonic, high-nitrogen formula was selected, and feedings were started in a step-wise progression to caloric goal within 72 hours of feeding initiation.

Question 1: If a predictive equation is used to assess energy expenditure, which reference weight should be incorporated into the calculation for obese patients: actual body weight, adjusted body weight [25% rule = (body wt − ideal wt) × 0.25 + (ideal wt)],[101] or adjusted body weight [50% rule = (body wt − ideal wt) × 0.5 + (ideal wt)]?[102]

Answer 1: In this patient's case, use of actual body weight (188 kg) carries a strong predisposition to overestimate her energy expenditure (Table 2-5). Despite the lack of prospective randomized clinical trials demonstrating improvements in accuracy with the use of adjusted body weight with various predictive equations, it is common practice. Significant errors in prediction are possible with all equations regardless of which weight is used. Until more research is available, clinical judgment should be used when choosing the reference weight to be incorporated into calculation methods.

Question 2: Why is this patient a good candidate for IC?

Answer 2: This patient is a perfect candidate for IC for the following reasons: the presence of metabolic stress following traumatic injury, class III obesity, and the use of several medications

Table 2-5 Practice Scenario: Comparison of Measured and Predicted Resting Metabolic Rate

Hospital Day	Measured Metabolic Rate (kcal/d)	Harris-Benedict (RMR × 1.3–1.6)[a] (kcal/d)	Ireton-Jones Equation (kcal/d)	Swinamer Equation (kcal/d)	Mifflin Equation (kcal/d)
5	**2273** (RQ 0.83)[b]	2156–2653	2196	2955	2559
12	**2689** (RQ 0.85)[b]	2156–2653	2196	2955	2559

RMR, resting metabolic rate; RQ, respiratory quotient.
[a]Twenty-five percent rule for adjusted body weight.
[b]Steady state was achieved.

that can alter metabolic rate such as propofol for sedation and cisatracurium as a paralytic to control intracranial pressure, which may have a hypometabolic effect. Every effort should be made to prevent both under- and overfeeding. Indirect calorimetry-based nutrition support has many benefits including promotion of tight glucose control, prevention of infectious complications, and expeditious liberation from mechanical ventilation.

Question 3: What technical factors related to IC should be considered before conducting a measurement?

Answer 3: To achieve accurate results, various technical parameters (Tables 2-2 and 2-3) must be considered before conducting a measurement. Some key factors to consider would be as follows: the ventilator settings should be within acceptable parameters; ventilator settings should not be changed within 90 minutes of the study; the nutrition regimen should be stable for at least 12 hours before the study; painful procedures should be avoided within 60 minutes of the study; the last dose of sedation or analgesia should be noted; and so forth. These factors involve many aspects of the patient's clinical status and daily care, which underscores the value of an interdisciplinary approach to conducting IC.

Question 4: How should the information obtained from IC be used when designing a nutrition regimen?

Answer 4: Upon completion of a valid IC study, the clinician should design a feeding regimen aimed at 100% of the measured REE. Recognizing that the results are a "snapshot" in time, measured REE should be re-evaluated anytime the patient experiences a clinically significant change in her medical status. This approach will capture the natural progression of alterations in metabolism that is unique to each individual patient. Note the upward trend in the patient's measured REE as her clinical course evolved (Table 2-5). This trend is an example of energy expenditure as the patient moved through the stress, catabolic, and anabolic phases of the stress response. Initially, the goal was metabolic support to promote retention of lean body mass and tight glucose control without complications related to overfeeding. As this patient became more stable, the nutrition goals shifted to support repletion and recovery.

Question 5: Based on the data in Table 2-5, what changes should be made to this patient's nutrition regimen over time? If IC weren't available, which predictive equations would have been most appropriate for this patient?

Answer 5: The enteral feeding was adjusted over time to match her measured REE. The patient's ventilatory status improved, and she was weaned from the ventilator. On hospital day 21, the speech pathologist was consulted to evaluate the patient's swallow function. A significant level of dysphagia was present, and the enteral feeding was continued as her primary nutrition mode, but she was allowed sips of fluids for pleasure. A percutaneous endoscopic gastrostomy tube was placed, and the patient's feeding regimen was subsequently transitioned to a bolus regimen to facilitate freedom from the feeding regimen when she transferred to the inpatient rehabilitation center to continue her recovery.

A retrospective analysis of various predictive equations compared to trends in this patient's REE revealed the following conclusions. Initially, the Harris-Benedict equation with adjusted body weight (25% rule) 3 1.3 or the IJEE (v) equation would have been the best match for this patient's actual REE (Table 2-5). As the patient's clinical course evolved and she moved into the anabolic phase of her recovery, the Mifflin-St. Jeor equation or the Harris-Benedict equation with adjusted body weight (25% rule) 3 1.6 would have been the closest approximation to her REE (Table 2-5). Note that the Swinamer equation, which incorporates body surface area into the equation, significantly overestimated the energy expenditure of this patient and should be used cautiously with obese patients.

Predictive Equations for Acutely Ill (Relatively Stable, Not Critically Ill) Patients

The monograph by Taylor is a good single source in which a large portion of the available data in acutely ill patients is reviewed.[35] However, as discussed previously, prediction of RMR in acutely ill, nonventilated patients is hampered by two factors. Most of the available data use the Harris-Benedict equation as the base calculation, and the data are usually divided by disease state, ignoring inflammatory markers such as body temperature, respiratory rate, or heart rate. A third problem occurs in obesity wherein some adjustment to body weight is often substituted into the Harris-Benedict equation. The concept of hypermetabolism being associated with physiology rather than disease description has been demonstrated at least twice in critically ill patients[23,36] and is implied by many of the ICU equations in which disease type is not included as a dependent variable.

Applications to Nutrition Support Therapy

Assessing the Metabolic Response

The metabolic response to critical illness is a highly complex process involving many regulatory systems, which presumably enhances survival.[91] This response has three phases: the stress phase, the catabolic phase, and the anabolic phase. Hemodynamic instability, hypometabolism, surging counterregulatory hormones, and insulin resistance characterize the stress phase (see Chapter 23).[92,93] The stress phase typically lasts 24 hours, but the magnitude and duration of the stress phase is dependent on the severity of the injury or illness. The question of whether to

Table 2-6 Clinical Indications for Consideration of Hypocaloric Feeding[94,95]

Class III obesity (body mass index > 40)
Refeeding syndrome risk
Severe malnutrition
Chronic obstructive pulmonary disease
Acute respiratory distress syndrome
Systemic inflammatory response syndrome
Sepsis with hemodynamic instability
Multiple organ dysfunction syndrome
Persistent elevations in respiratory rate
Hypercapnia
Hyperglycemia
Hypertriglyceridemia

feed at all during this phase arises frequently. Hypocaloric feeding or "permissive underfeeding" where patients are fed below their REE (50% to 75%)[94] has been shown to benefit several populations of critically ill patients (Table 2-6). Overzealous nutrition support may exacerbate hyperglycemia, respiratory failure, and organ dysfunction during the stress phase.[95] Another term for this approach to nutrition is metabolic support.[92,96] The concept of metabolic support represents a distinction from nutrition support that is typically geared toward repletion. The goal of metabolic support is to support cellular metabolic pathways without forcing them in adverse directions secondary to the inability to utilize excess fuel, which can compromise organ structure and function.[92,96]

The catabolic phase occurs after resuscitation and usually lasts for 7 to 10 days.[92,93] It is dominated by fever, hypercatabolism, gluconeogenesis, and increased oxygen demands. Ongoing metabolic support is the focus of nutrition during this phase. High nitrogen feedings (1.5 to 2.0 g protein/kg) with avoidance of overfeeding is desirable.[96] Because the risks of overfeeding are significant, it is prudent to feed patients no more than 100% of the REE during the catabolic phase.[41,53,55]

The anabolic or convalescent phase of the stress response occurs after the acute phase response has resolved and can last for months.[92,93] It is characterized by repletion of lean body mass and adipose tissue. During this phase, the therapeutic goals shift from metabolic support to nutrition support. Caloric delivery during convalescence may be increased to 100% to 130% of the RMR to support tissue repair, repletion, and recovery.[42]

Importance of Avoiding Under- and Overfeeding

The long-term effects of inadequate nutrition in the critically ill are well described (Table 2-7).[62] Underfeeding is common in patients with conditions such as obesity, multiple organ dysfunction syndrome, uncomplicated infection, and hypermetabolism. Underfeeding leads to deterioration of lean body mass, immunosuppression, and poor wound healing, and increases the risk of nosocomial infections.[62] Cumulative deficits in caloric intake have been linked with increased morbidity and mortality.[97–99]

Table 2-7 Consequences of Underfeeding and Overfeeding[43,62,95,97]

Underfeeding:
Decreased respiratory muscle strength
Decreased ventilatory drive
Failure to wean from mechanical ventilation
Impaired organ function
Immunosuppression
Poor wound healing
Increased risk of nosocomial infection
Low transport protein levels in the absence of inflammation or infection
Overfeeding:
Hyperglycemia
Azotemia
Hypertriglyceridemia
Electrolyte imbalances
Immunosuppression
Alterations in hydration status
Hepatic steatosis
Failure to wean from mechanical ventilation

Overfeeding presents a significant threat of negative consequences to patients receiving nutrition support therapy (Table 2-7).[62,100] Nutrition support regimens designed to avoid cumulative caloric deficits can lead to toxic excesses. Patients at particular risk of overfeeding are those with underlying malnutrition, severe traumatic injury, and sepsis. Overfeeding exacerbates respiratory failure by increasing carbon dioxide load, which drives up minute ventilation. Delays in ventilator weaning and long-term ventilator dependence contribute to increased morbidity and mortality risk.[62,95,100]

References

1. Koshland DE. The seven pillars of life. *Science.* 2002;295: 2215–2216.
2. Chandra RK. 1990 McCollum Award Lecture. Nutrition and immunity: lessons from the past and new insights into the future. *Am J Clin Nutr.* 1991;53:1087–1101.
3. Reichard GA, Haff AC, Skutches CL, et al. Plasma acetone metabolism in the fasting human. *J Clin Invest.* 1979;63:619–626.
4. Owen OE, Smalley KJ, D'Alessio DA, et al. Protein, fat, and carbohydrate requirements during starvation: anaplerosis and cataplerosis. *Am J Clin Nutr.* 1998;68:12–34.
5. van Ooijen AMJ, Lichtenbelt VM, van Steenhoven AA, et al. Seasonal changes in metabolic and temperature responses to cold air in humans. *Physiol Behav.* 2004;82:545–553.
6. Bardutzky J, Georgiadins D, Kollmar R, Schwab S. Energy expenditure in ischemic stroke patients treated with moderate hypothermia. *Intens Care Med.* 2004;30:151–154.
7. Badjatia N, Strongilis E, Gordon E, et al. Metabolic impact of shivering during therapeutic temperature modulation. *Stroke.* 2008;39:3242–3247.

8. Charkoudian N. Skin blood flow in adult human thermoregulation. How it works, when it does not, and why. *Mayo Clin Proc.* 2003;78:603–612.
9. Compher CW, Frankenfield DC, Keim N, Roth-Yousey L. Best practice methods to apply to measurement of resting metabolic rate. *J Am Diet Assoc.* 2006;106:881–903.
10. Frankenfield DC, Coleman A. Recovery to resting metabolic state after walking. *J Am Diet Assoc.* 2009;109:1914–1916.
11. Wang Z, Heshka S, Gallagher D, et al. Resting energy expenditure-fat-free mass relationship: new insights provided by body composition modeling. *Am J Physiol Endocrinol Metab.* 2000;279: E539–E545.
12. Muller MJ, Bosy-Westphal A, Kutzner D, Heller M. Metabolically active components of fat-free mass and resting energy expenditure in humans: recent lessons from imaging technologies. *Obes Rev.* 2002;3:113–122.
13. Javed F, He Q, Davidson LE, et al. Brain and high metabolic rate organ mass: contribution to resting energy expenditure beyond fat free mass. *Am J Clin Nutr.* 2010;91:907–912.
14. Gallagher D, Albu J, He Q, et al. Small organs with high metabolic rate explain lower resting energy expenditure in African American than in white adults. *Am J Clin Nutr.* 2006;83:1062–1067.
15. Fukagawa NK, Bandini LG, Young JB. Effect of age on body composition and resting metabolic rate. *Am J Physiol.* 1990;259: E233–E238.
16. Jones A, Shen W, St. Onge MP, et al. Body composition differences between African-American and white women: relation to resting energy requirements. *Am J Clin Nutr.* 2004;79:780–786.
17. Kimm SYS, Glynn NW, Aston CE, et al. Racial differences in the relation between uncoupling protein genes and resting energy expenditure. *Am J Clin Nutr.* 2002;75:714–719.
18. Frankenfield DC. Energy dynamics. In: Matarese LE, Gottschlich MM, eds. *Contemporary Nutrition Support Practice. A Clinical Guide.* Philadelphia, Pa: Saunders; 1998:79–98.
19. James WPT. From SDA to DIT to TEF. In: Kinney JM, Tucker HN, eds. *Energy Metabolism. Tissue Determinants and Cellular Corollaries.* New York, NY: Raven; 1992:163–186.
20. Frankenfield DC, Wiles CE, Bagley S, et al. Relationships between resting and total energy expenditure in injured and septic patients. *Crit Care Med.* 1994;22:1796–1804.
21. Weissman C, Kemper M, Damask MC, et al. Effect of routine intensive care interactions on metabolic rate. *Chest.* 1984;86:815–818.
22. Weissman C, Kemper M, Askanazi J, et al. Day to day variation in the resting metabolic rate of mechanically ventilated critically ill patients. *Crit Care Med.* 1986;14:408.
23. White MS, Shepherd RW, McEniery JA. Energy expenditure measurements in ventilated critically ill children: within- and between-day variability. *J Parenter Enteral Nutr.* 1999;23:300–304.
24. Weissman C, Kemper, M, Elwyn DH, et al. The energy expenditure of the mechanically ventilated critically ill patient: an analysis. *Chest.* 1986;89:254–259.
25. Waterlow JC, Jackson AA. Nutrition and protein turnover in man. *Br Med Bull.* 1981;37:5–10.
26. Hall KD. Predicting metabolic adaptation, body weight change, and energy intake in humans. *Am J Physiol Endocrinol Metab.* 2010;298:E449–466.
27. Fredrix EW, Soeters PB, von Meyenfeldt MF, Saris WH. Resting energy expenditure in cancer patients before and after gastrointestinal surgery. *J Parenter Enteral Nutr.* 1991;15:604–607.
28. Mann S, Westenskow DR, Houtchens BA. Measured and predicted caloric expenditure in the acutely ill. *Crit Care Med.* 1985;13:173–177.
29. Frankenfield DC, On heat, respiration and calorimetry. *Nutrition.* 2010;26:939–950.
30. Hwang TL, Huang SL, Chen MF. The use of indirect calorimetry in critically ill patients—the relationship of measured energy expenditure to Injury Severity Score, Septic Severity Score, and APACHE II Score. *J Trauma.* 1993;34:247–251.
31. Kreymann G, Grosser S, Buggisch P, et al. Oxygen consumption and resting metabolic rate in sepsis, sepsis syndrome, and septic shock. *Crit Care Med.* 1993;21:1012–1019.
32. Roubenoff RA, Borel CO, Hanley DF. Hypermetabolism and hypercatabolism in Guillain-Barré syndrome. *J Parenter Enteral Nutr.* 1992;16:464–472.
33. Foster GD, Knox LS, Dempsey DT, Miller JL. Caloric requirements in total parenteral nutrition. *J Am Coll Nutr.* 1987;6:231–253.
34. McClave S, Snider HL. Use of indirect calorimetry in clinical nutrition. *Nutr Clin Pract.* 1992;7:207–221.
35. Taylor SJ. *Energy and Nitrogen Requirements in Disease States.* London, England: Smith-Gordon Co.; 2007.
36. Raurich JM, Ibanez J, Marse P, Riera M, Homar X. Resting energy expenditure during mechanical ventilation and its relationship with type of lesion. *J Parenter Enteral Nutr.* 2007;31:58–62.
37. Wooley JA, Sax HC. Indirect calorimetry: applications to practice. *Nutr Clin Pract.* 2003;18:434–439.
38. Haugen HA, Chan LN, Li F. Indirect calorimetry: a practical guide for clinicians. *Nutr Clin Pract.* 2007;22:377–388.
39. Moreira da Rocha EE, Alves VGF, da Fonseca RBV. Indirect calorimetry: methodology, instruments and clinical application. *Curr Opin Clin Nutr Metab Care.* 2006;9:247–256.
40. Matarese LE. Indirect calorimetry: technical aspects. *J Am Diet Assoc.* 1997;10(Suppl 2):S154–S160.
41. Porter C, Cohen NH. Indirect calorimetry in critically ill patients: role of the clinical dietitian in interpreting results. *J Am Diet Assoc.* 1996;96:49–54,57.
42. Malone AM. Methods of assessing energy expenditure in the intensive care unit. *Nutr Clin Pract.* 2002;17:21–28.
43. Brandi LS, Bertolini R, Calafa M. Indirect calorimetry in critically ill patients: clinical applications and practical advice. *Nutrition.* 1997;13:349–358.
44. Mullen JL. Indirect calorimetry in critical care. *Proc Nutr Soc.* 1991;50:239–244.
45. Ferrannini E. The theoretical basis of indirect calorimetry. *Metabolism.* 1988;37:287–301.
46. Branson RD. The measurement of energy expenditure: instrumentation, practical considerations and clinical application. *Resp Care.* 1990;35:640–659.
47. Weir JB. New methods for calculating metabolic rate with special reference to protein metabolism. *J Physiol.* 1949;109:1–14.
48. Petros S, Engelmann L. Validity of an abbreviated indirect calorimetry protocol for measurement of resting energy expenditure in mechanically ventilated and spontaneously breathing critically ill patients. *Intensive Care Med.* 2001;27:1164–1168.
49. Frankenfield DC, Sarson GY, Blosser SA, Cooney RN, Smith JS. Validation of a 5-minute steady state indirect calorimetry protocol for resting energy expenditure in critically ill patients. *J Am Coll Nutr.* 1996 Aug;15:397–402.
50. Cunningham KF, Aeberhardt LE, Wiggs BR, Phang PT. Appropriate interpretation of indirect calorimetry for determining energy expenditure in intensive care units. *Am J Surg.* 1994;167:54–57.
51. Smyrnios NA, Curley FJ, Shaker KG. Accuracy of 30-minute indirect calorimetry studies in predicting 24-hour energy expenditure in mechanically ventilated, critically ill patients. *J Parenter Enteral Nutr.* 1997;21:168–174.
52. Behrendt W, Surmann M, Raumanns J, Giani G. How reliable are short-term measurements of oxygen uptake in polytraumatized and long-term ventilated patients? *Infusionstherapie.* 1991;18:20–24.

53. McClave SA, Spain DA, Skolnick JL, et al. Is achievement of steady state required when performing indirect calorimetry? *J Parenter Enteral Nutr*. 1999;23:S8.
54. McEvoy C, Cooke SR, Young IS. A reduced abbreviated indirect calorimetry protocol is clinically acceptable for use in spontaneously breathing patients with traumatic brain injury. *Nutr Clin Pract*. 2009;24:513–519.
55. Barco KT, Smith RA, Peerless JR, et al. Energy expenditure assessment and validation after acute spinal cord injury. *Nutr Clin Pract*. 2002;17:309–313.
56. McClave SA, Snider HL, Green L, et al. Effective utilization of indirect calorimetry during critical care. *Intense Care World*. 1992; 9:194–200.
57. McClave SA, Spain DA, Skolnick JL, et al. Achievement of steady state optimizes results when performing indirect calorimetry. *J Parenter Enteral Nutr*. 2003;27:16–20.
58. Holdy KE. Monitoring energy metabolism with indirect calorimetry: Instruments, interpretation, and clinical application. *Nutr Clin Pract*. 2004;19:447–454.
59. Reeves MM, Capra S. Predicting energy requirements in the clinical setting: are current methods evidence based? *Nutr Rev*. 2003; 61:143–151.
60. McClave SA, Lowen CC, Kleber MJ, et al. Is the respiratory quotient a useful indicator of over or under feeding? *J Parenter Enteral Nutr*. 1997;21:S11.
61. McClave SA, Lowen CC, Kleber MJ, et al. Clinical use of the respiratory quotient obtained from indirect calorimetry. *J Parenter Enteral Nutr*. 2003;27:21–26.
62. McClave SA. The consequences of overfeeding and underfeeding. *J Resp Care Pract*. 1997;10:57–58,60,62–64.
63. Brandi LS, Grana M, Mazzanti T, et al. Energy expenditure and gas exchange measurements in post-operative patients: thermodilution vs. indirect calorimetry. *Crit Care Med*. 1992;20: 1273–1283.
64. Ogawa AM, Shikora SA, Burke LM, et al. The thermodilution technique for measuring resting energy expenditure does not agree with indirect calorimetry for the critically ill patient. *J Parenter Enteral Nutr*.1998;22:347–351.
65. Schoeller DA, VanSanten E. Measurement of energy expenditure in free-living humans by using doubly labeled water. *J Nutr*. 1988;118:1278–1289.
66. Gephart FC, Dubois EF. The basal metabolism of normal adults with special reference to surface area. Clinical Calorimetry Paper XIII. *Arch Intern Med*. 1916;xvii:902–914.
67. Sheiner LB, Beal SL. Some suggestions for measuring predictive performance. *J Pharmacokinetics and Biopharmceuticals*. 1981;9: 503–512.
68. Bland JM, Altman DG. Statistical methods for assessing agreement between two methods of measurement. *Lancet*. 1986;i:307–310.
69. Harris JA, Benedict FG. *A Biometric Study of Basal Metabolism in Man*. Publication No. 279. Washington, DC: Carnegie Institute; 1919.
70. Frankenfield DC, Muth E, Rowe WA. The Harris-Benedict studies of human basal metabolism: history and limitations. *J Am Diet Assoc*. 1998;98:439–445.
71. Livingston EH, Kohlstadt I. Simplified resting metabolic rate – predicting formulas for normal-sized and obese individuals. *Obesity Research*. 2005;13:1255–1262.
72. Benedict FG. Basal metabolism data on normal men and women (series II) with some considerations on the use of prediction standards. *Am J Physiol*. 1928;85:607–620.
73. Frankenfield DC, Rowe WA, Smith JS, Cooney RN. Validation of several established equations for resting metabolic rate in obese and nonobese people. *J Am Diet Assoc*. 2003;103:1152–1159.
74. Owen OE, Kavle E, Owen RS, et al. A reappraisal of caloric requirements in healthy women. *Am J Clin Nutr*. 1986;44:1–19.
75. Owen OE, Holup JL, D'Alessio DA, et al. A reappraisal of the caloric requirements of men. *Am J Clin Nutr*. 1987;46:875–885.
76. Mifflin MD, St. Jeor ST, Hill LA, et al. A new predictive equation for resting energy expenditure in healthy individuals. *Am J Clin Nutr*. 1990;51:241–247.
77. Frankenfield DC, Roth-Yousey L, Compher C. Comparison of predictive equations for resting metabolic rate in healthy nonobese and obese individuals, a systematic review. *J Am Diet Assoc*. 2005; 105:775–789.
78. Melzer K, Laurie K, Genton L, et al. Comparison of equations for estimating resting metabolic rate in healthy subjects over 70 years of age. *Clin Nutr*. 2007;26:498–505.
79. De Oliveira EP, Orsatti FL, Teixeira O, et al. Comparison of predictive equations for resting energy expenditure in overweight and obese adults. *J Obes*. 2011;2011:534714.
80. Weijs PJM. Validity of predictive equations for resting energy expenditure in US and Dutch overweight and obese class I and II adults aged 18-65 y. *Am J Clin Nutr*. 2008;88:959–970.
81. Long CL, Schaffel N, Geiger JW, et al. Metabolic response to injury and illness: Estimation of energy and protein needs from indirect calorimetry and nitrogen balance. *J Parenter Enteral Nutr*. 1979;3: 452–456.
82. Swinamer DL, Grace MG, Hamilton SM, et al. Predictive equation for assessing energy expenditure in mechanically ventilated critically ill patients. *Crit Care Med*. 1990;18:657–661.
83. Frankenfield DC, Omert LA, Badellino MM, et al. Correlation between measured energy expenditure and clinically obtained variables in trauma and septic patients. *J Parenter Enteral Nutr*. 1994;18:398–403.
84. Frankenfield DC, Smith JS, Cooney RN. Validation of two approaches to predicting resting metabolic rate in critically ill patients. *J Parenter Enteral Nutr*. 2004:28:259–264.
85. Flancbaum L, Choban PS, Sambucco S, et al. Comparison of indirect calorimetry, the Fick method, and prediction equations in estimating the energy requirements of critically ill patients. *Am J Clin Nutr*. 1999;69:461–466.
86. MacDonald A, Hildebrandt L. Comparison of formulaic equations to determine energy expenditure in the critically ill patient. *Nutrition*. 2003;19:233–239.
87. Frankenfield DC, Coleman A, Alam S, Cooney RN. Analysis of estimation methods for resting metabolic rate in critically ill adults. *J Parenter Enteral Nutr*. 2009;33:27–36.
88. ADA Evidence Analysis Library. Critical Illness. www.adaevidencelibrary.com/template.cfm?template=guide_summary&key=3200. Accessed May 18, 2012.
89. Frankenfield DC. Validation of an equation for resting metabolic rate in older obese, critically ill patients. *J Parener Enteral Nutr*. 2011;35:264–269.
90. American Society for Parenteral and Enteral Nutrition Board of Directors and the Clinical Guidelines Task Force. Guidelines for the use of parenteral and enteral nutrition in adult and pediatric patients. *J Parenter Enteral Nutr*. 2002;26(Suppl 1):SA22.
91. Wilmore DW. Metabolic response to severe surgical illness: overview. *World J Surg*. 2000;24:705–711.
92. Cerra FB, Hypermetabolism, organ failure, and metabolic support. *Surgery*. 1987;101:1–14.
93. McClave SA, Snider HL. Understanding the metabolic response to critical illness: factors that cause patients to deviate from the expected pattern of hypermetabolism. *New Horiz*. 1994;2:139–146.
94. Dickerson RN, Specialized nutrition support in the hospitalized obese patient. *Nutr Clin Pract*. 2004;19:245–254.

95. Zaloga GD. Permissive underfeeding. *New Horiz.* 1994;2:257–263.
96. Barton R, Cerra FB. The hypermetabolism multiple organ failure syndrome. *Chest.* 1989;96:1153–1160.
97. Bartlett RH, Dechert RE, Mault JR, et al. Measurement of metabolism in multiple organ failure. *Surgery.* 1982;92:771–779.
98. Rubinson L, Diette GB, Song X, et al. Low caloric intake is associated with nosocomial bloodstream infections in patients in the medical intensive care unit. *Crit Care Med.* 2004;32:350–357.
99. Villet S, Chiolero RL, Bollmann MD, et al. Negative impact of hypocaloric feeding and energy balance on clinical outcome in ICU patients. *Clin Nutr.* 2005;24:502–509.
100. Klein CJ, Stanek GS, Wiles CE. Overfeeding macronutrients to critically ill adults: metabolic complications. *J Am Diet Assoc.* 1998;98:795–806.
101. Wilkins K. Adjustment for obesity. *ADA Renal Practice Group Newsletter.* 1984;3:6.
102. Barak N, Wall-Alonso E, Sitrin MD. Evaluation of stress factors and body weight adjustments currently used to estimate energy expenditure in hospitalized patients. *J Parenter Enteral Nutr.* 2002;26:231–238.
103. Blumberg A, Keller G. Oxygen consumption during maintenance hemodialysis. *Nephron.* 1979;23:276–281.

3 Carbohydrates

Pei-Ra Ling, MD, and Karen C. McCowen, MD

CONTENTS

Background 37
Classification of Carbohydrates 37
Digestion and Absorption of Carbohydrates 39
Carbohydrate Metabolism 40
Movement of Glucose into Cells—Glucose Transporters 40
Glycolysis 41
Cell Respiration—Tricarboxylic Acid Cycle 41
Pyruvate-Lactate Pathway 41
Gluconeogenesis 42
Glycogenesis and Glycogenolysis 43
Formation of Precursors for Other Metabolites 45
Plasma Glucose Homeostasis 45
Glucose Regulation During Fasting and Fed States 45
Hormonal Regulation 46
Diabetes Mellitus 47
Stress Hyperglycemia 47
Role of Fiber in Clinical Nutrition 48
Carbohydrate Requirements 48
Healthy Adults 48
Exercise 49
Illness and Injury 49
Summary 49
References 49

Objectives

1. Understand the basic structures of carbohydrates and their digestion and absorption.
2. Describe glucose metabolism inside cells.
3. Analyze the roles of different hormones and organs in the maintenance of normal plasma glucose levels during fasting and fed states.
4. Identify key factors determining carbohydrate requirements.

Test Your Knowledge Questions

1. In the net chemical reaction of glucose catabolism:
   A. Pyruvate is the final product.
   B. Oxygen is required for adenosine triphosphate (ATP) synthesis.
   C. Both water and carbon dioxide (CO_2) are produced.
   D. CO_2 is produced but water is not.
   E. Water is produced but CO_2 is not.

2. Which of the following incorrectly pairs a metabolic process with its site of occurrence?
   A. Glycolysis–cytosol
   B. Tricarboxylic acid (TCA) cycle–mitochondrial membrane
   C. ATP phosphorylation–cytosol and mitochondria
   D. Oxidative decarboxylation of pyruvate–mitochondria
   E. Electron transport chain–mitochondrial membrane
3. Which of the following is least likely to occur during oxygen debt?
   A. Build up of lactic acid
   B. Build up of pyruvate
   C. Decrease in pH
   D. Increased fatigue
   E. Shortage of ATP

Test Your Knowledge Answers

1. The correct answer is **C**. Pyruvate is the final product of glycolysis. It is transported from the cytoplasm into the mitochondrial matrix. Here pyruvate loses CO_2, and the remaining acetyl group is transferred to coenzyme A to form acetyl coenzyme A. Under aerobic conditions (in the presence of oxygen), pyruvate can be further oxidized during cell respiration. Under anaerobic conditions (in the absence of oxygen), pyruvate can be broken down into lactate. Both metabolic pathways can produce ATP. After all of the energy has been released from the glucose moiety, CO_2 and water are the final products.
2. The correct answer is **B**. Glycolysis is a series of reactions that lead to the oxidative breakdown of glucose into pyruvate, the production of ATP, and the reduction of nicotinamide adenine dinucleotide (NAD^+) into reduced form of nicotinamide adenine dinucleotide (NADH). All these reactions occur in the cytoplasm. The TCA cycle is the metabolic reaction of cell respiration, which occurs inside the eukaryotic mitochondrion (not on the mitochondrial membrane). ATP phosphorylation occurs both during glycolysis (in the cytoplasm) and the TCA cycle (in the mitochondrion). The pyruvate formed during glycolysis is transported from the cytoplasm into the mitochondrial matrix where it is decarboxylated. The electron transport chain is a carrier mechanism located on the inside of the inner mitochondrion.
3. The correct answer is **B**. Under anaerobic conditions, pyruvate accepts a hydrogen atom from NADH, forming NAD^+ and lactic acid. At physiological pH, lactic acid is dissociated into lactate and protons. Thus, the local pH decreases. Using this pathway, only two ATPs can be generated. A shortage of ATP is possible, leading to muscle fatigue.

Background

Carbohydrate is a class of organic compounds composed of carbon, hydrogen, and oxygen with the molar ratio of C:H:O as 1:2:1. Carbohydrate is a major energy source in human nutrition, providing approximately 45% to 65% of daily energy. Theoretically, oxidation of 1 g of carbohydrate yields 4 kcal of energy. When hydrated in solution as dextrose, 3.4 kcal of energy results from 1 g. Carbohydrate can be stored as glycogen mainly in liver and muscle for later use. In addition to their role as an energy source, some carbohydrates are sweetening agents such as table sugar, while others are components of dietary fibers such as vegetables. Fiber is a form of carbohydrate that is the remnant of plant cells that resists digestion by intestinal enzymes in humans. Fibers do not provide calories or nutrients by normal digestive processes in the small bowel, but can be fermented by bacteria under anaerobic conditions in the large bowel.

Classification of Carbohydrates

Carbohydrates can be classified as either simple or complex. Simple carbohydrates include monosaccharides (one sugar unit) and disaccharides (two sugar units). A common name of simple carbohydrates is sugar. Most physiological sugars are in the D-isomer form. Glucose, galactose, and fructose are examples of monosaccharides. The monosaccharides are water soluble and have low molecular weight. Glucose and galactose contain a ring with six carbon atoms. Fructose also contains six carbons total, although the ring structure contains five carbons (Figure 3-1). The orientation of the hydroxyl group linked to the first carbon in the ring yields α and β forms. The α form is the hydroxyl group below the hydrogen, whereas the β form has the hydroxyl group above the hydrogen (Figure 3-1). Sucrose (one glucose + one fructose), maltose (two glucose moieties), and lactose (one glucose + one galactose) are three common disaccharides.

Multiple units of glucose monosaccharides and disaccharides can be joined together to form polysaccharides, also called complex carbohydrates. The complex carbohydrates are water insoluble and have high molecular weight. Polysaccharides containing fewer than 10 glucose units are called oligosaccharides. Starch, glycogen, and some fibers (including cellulose) are polysaccharides containing hundreds to many thousands of monosaccharides (usually glucose) connected by straight and/or branched chains. In starch (Figure 3-2), the straight chains are called amylose (about 15% to 20% of the total starch), and branched chains are denoted amylopectin (80% to 85% of the total starch). Amylose is the inner, water-soluble component of starch, whereas amylopectin is a nearly insoluble substance derived from the outer part of starch granules. Plants convert excess glucose into starch for storage, whereas animals store glucose as glycogen. Glycogen has a similar structure to starch, but the branches in glycogen tend to be shorter and more frequent. Cellulose, which is plant fiber, differs from starch and glycogen in that there are no side chains linking glucose units, leading to a long, straight, and rigid molecule.

Food in its natural state contains different types of carbohydrates. About 60% are in the form of starch, 30% in sucrose, and 10% in lactose. The end products of digestion of dietary carbohydrates are the monosaccharides: glucose, fructose, and galactose.

Plant foods contain fibers, mainly as a component of their cell walls. Polysaccharide plant fibers are important in the human diet, in particular cellulose. Other fibers include pectins, lignins, and gums. In general, fiber may be classified as either sol-

FIGURE 3-1 Chemical Structures of Monosaccharide

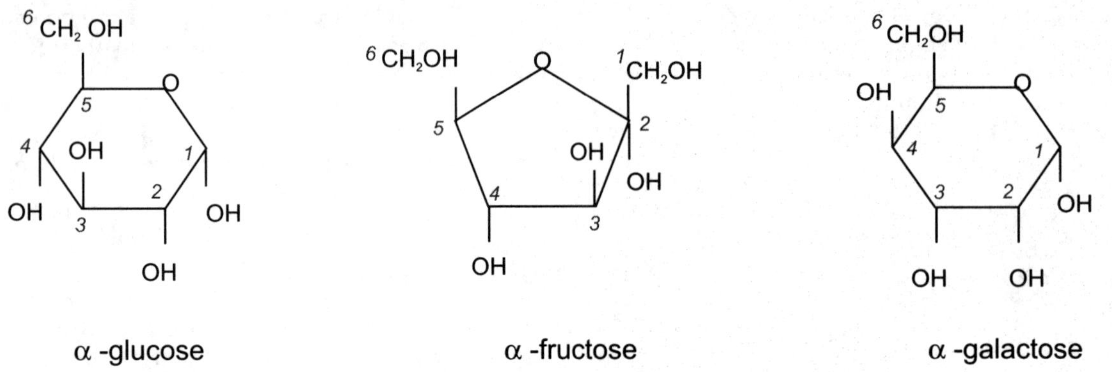

Most physiological monosaccharides are the D-isomer form. Glucose and galactose have a six-membered carbon ring (numbers) and fructose has a five-membered carbon ring (numbers). The ring closure produces α- and β-forms.

FIGURE 3-2 Chemical Structures of Starch

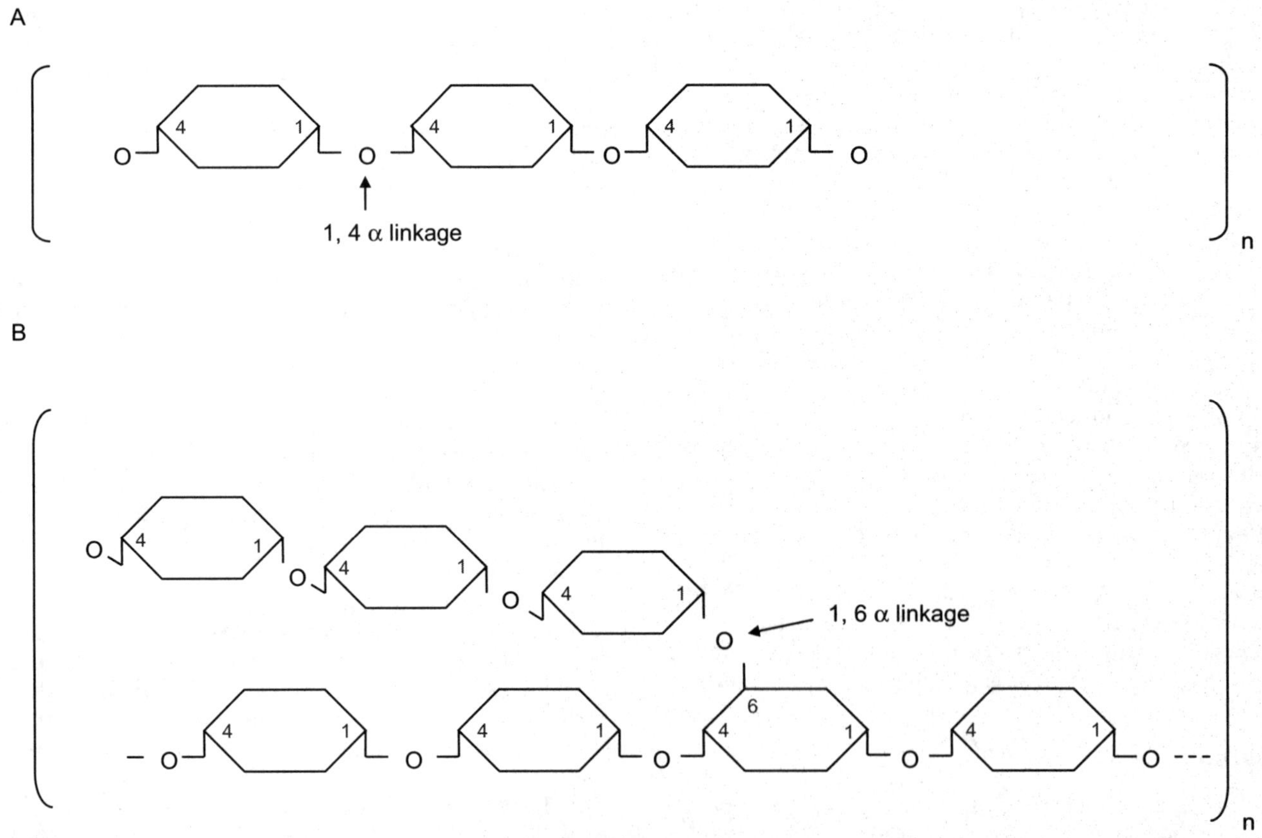

Starch is a mixture of amylose and amylopectin. (A) Amylose has a linear structure of glucose units linked by bonds with α-1, 4 configuration. (B) Amylopectins contain branched structures with α-1, 6 bonds at the branch points.

uble or insoluble based on the degree of dispersion in hot water. Alternatively, fibers can be thought of as either structural or nonstructural in nature. Plant cell walls contain three different types of structural polysaccharide: cellulose, hemicellulose, and pectin. These differ by containing different kinds of simple sugars with different degrees of branching. Soluble fiber includes gums as well as a variety of chemically synthesized compounds. Soluble fibers can be partially digested in the large bowel, whereas insoluble fibers are not.

Digestion and Absorption of Carbohydrates

The process of carbohydrate digestion begins in the mouth where foods are mechanically broken into smaller pieces and mixed with saliva. Salivary amylase acts on the interior α-1,4 linkages of amylose and amylopectin (Figure 3-2) and breaks the polysaccharides into small intermediate forms. In the gut, these molecules are further broken down by pancreatic amylase and by other intestinal enzymes to disaccharides (ie, maltose, sucrose, and lactose). Subsequently, the enzymes maltase, sucrase, and lactase digest these disaccharides into glucose, galactose, and fructose (Figure 3-3). Small amounts of glucose are absorbed directly through the oral mucosa, but most monosaccharides are absorbed in the small intestine.[9]

Glucose and galactose are transported from the intestinal lumen into the enterocyte via the sodium–glucose transporter 1. This protein is present in the apical membrane of the enterocyte. The transport process requires energy provided by hydrolysis of ATP and is, therefore, called an active transport system. Two molecules of sodium are cotransported with one molecule of glucose or galactose. A low intracellular sodium concentration is maintained in the enterocyte by another energy-dependent pump, the ATP-dependent sodium-potassium pump, which is present in the basolateral membrane of the enterocyte. Action of this latter pump maintains an electronegative cell interior, which favors sodium movement across the apical cell membrane from the lumen into the cell (Figure 3-4). Fructose is transported through a special protein called glucose transporter 5, which also is present in the apical membrane.

Glucose, galactose, and fructose are exported into the bloodstream through a different glucose transport protein called glucose transporter (Glut) 2 located in the basolateral membrane of the enterocyte (Figure 3-4). Starch and disaccharides must be digested to monosaccharides for absorption, because transporters cannot carry larger carbohydrate moieties across membranes.

Insoluble fiber, however, is poorly broken down and thus increases the bulk of the stool, rather than contributing to caloric load. Soluble fiber absorbs water to become a gelatinous, viscous substance and is fermented by bacteria in the digestive tract. When soluble fiber is fermented, short-chain fatty acids are produced, which can subsequently be absorbed into the bloodstream. Short-chain fatty acids are involved in numerous physiological processes with potential but currently unproven health benefits.

In the bloodstream, most absorbed compounds pass first through the liver. The liver removes two-thirds of the glucose from the portal vein blood in the fed state. Fructose and galactose are almost totally removed by the liver. The increase in blood sugar that occurs following a meal is one component of the process stimulating release of insulin from the pancreatic islets. However, a complex cascade of neural and gastrointestinal signals that prepares the pancreas for insulin release begins even as anticipation of food intake occurs and is enhanced by every

FIGURE 3-3 Intestinal Digestion of Dietary Carbohydrates

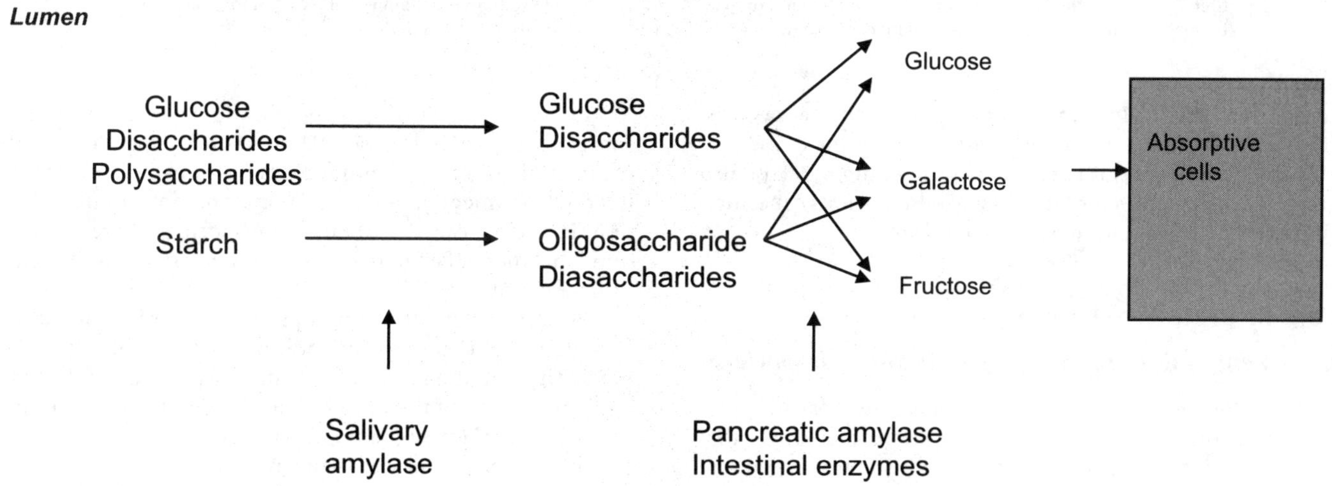

Starch is hydrolyzed by the action of salivary amylase to oligosaccharides, dissacharides, and small amount of monosaccharides, and then to glucose, galactose, and fructose by pancreatic amylase and intestinal enzymes. Monosaccharides are readily absorbed.

FIGURE 3-4 Intestinal Absorption of Dietary Carbohydrates

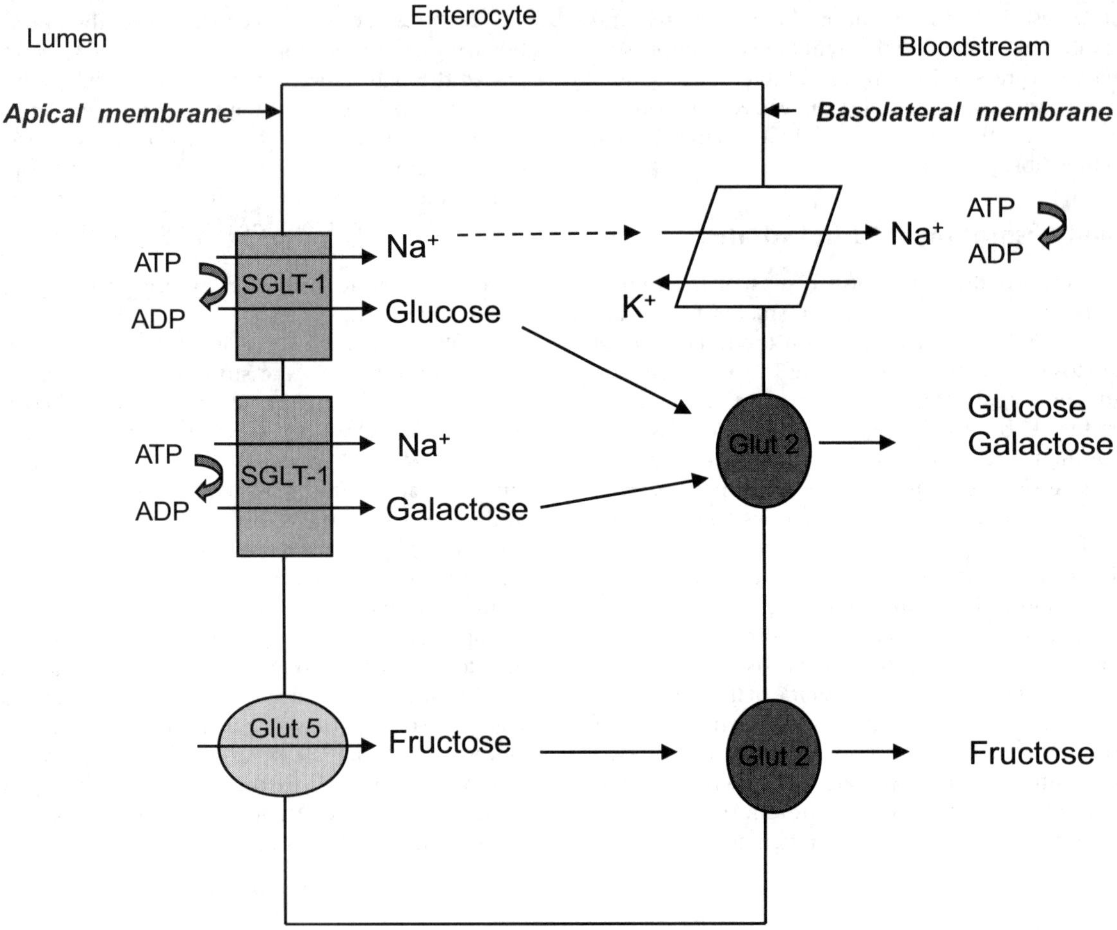

Glucose and galactose enter into enterocytes through sodium glucose transporter 1 (SGLT-1), and adenosine triphosphate (ATP)-dependent active transporter. Fructose is transported by glucose transport 5 (Glut 5), which transports it from the intestinal lumen into enterocytes. Glucose, galactose, and fructose all are exported into the bloodstream through the facilitation of the transporter Glut 2 located in the basolateral membrane of the enterocyte. The ATP-dependent sodium (Na^+)-potassium (K^+) pump located in the basolateral membrane maintains sodium concentration within the cell. ADP, adenosine diphosphate.

step in the process. Insulin promotes glucose uptake by cells, mostly muscle and adipose cells, which reduces the blood glucose concentration toward its basal state. In addition, glucose also can enter other tissues through mass action down its concentration gradient, even in the absence of insulin.

Carbohydrate Metabolism

Movement of Glucose Into Cells—Glucose Transporters[2]

Shifting glucose into cells occurs by means of two classes of glucose transport proteins located in the plasma membrane that serve as channels for glucose. One class, the sodium-dependent glucose transporters, as described previously, is involved in the active, ATP-dependent absorption of glucose from the intestinal lumen into cells. These transport proteins also function in the reabsorption of filtered glucose in the proximal tubule of the kidney.

The second class of cell membrane glucose transporters functions as passive diffusion channels (ie, dependent on the gradient of glucose concentration between extra- and intracellular compartments). These transporters do not require sodium or ATP, and are called facilitative transporters. There are many different types of facilitative glucose transporters distributed in different tissues.

Glut 1 is widely distributed in many tissues, with particularly high concentrations in endothelial and glial cells of the brain. The endothelial cells lining the microvessels of the brain are a major part of the blood–brain barrier. Glut 1 transports glucose and galactose but not fructose.

Glut 2 is mainly located in the liver, small intestine, and kidney. In hepatocytes, Glut 2 has a low affinity but high capacity for glucose, allowing quick equilibration of intra- and extracellular glucose concentrations across the membrane during fasting and fed states. In the small intestine, Glut 2 is important in the transepithelial transport of the absorbed glucose, as described previously. In the kidney, Glut 2 transports the reabsorbed glucose back into the bloodstream from proximal tubular epithelia. In the beta cell of the pancreas, the transport of glucose by Glut 2 serves as part of the glucose-sensing apparatus that controls insulin release.

Glut 3 seems to be present in all tissues, but its highest concentration is seen in the neuronal membranes of the brain. Glut 3 controls the rate of glucose entry into neuronal cells, which is different from the action of Glut 1 in the brain in the transportation of glucose across the blood–brain barrier.

Glut 4 is the major glucose transporter in adipose (brown and white) and in muscle (skeletal and cardiac) tissues. Glut 4 is primarily located in intracellular vesicles of these tissues but can be translocated to the cell surface in response to a rise in plasma insulin concentrations. A rise in circulating insulin results in as much as a 15- to 20-fold increase in Glut 4 on the cell surface of insulin-sensitive cells within minutes, allowing glucose uptake into cells.[3] A dysregulation of Glut 4 translocation in response to insulin is one key defect for the development of type 2 diabetes mellitus.[4] The movement of Glut 4 from vesicles to the cell surface requires ATP. In contrast, action of the other members of this glucose transport family is not sensitive to the prevailing insulin concentrations.

Glut 5 is primarily located in the apical membrane of the jejunum and is the main transporter of fructose from the lumen to the enterocytes. The remaining members of this class of proteins include Glut 6 through Glut 12. The functions of these more newly discovered transporters are less well established.[5]

Once glucose enters cells, the carbon skeleton is broken down through a series of enzymatic reactions, and the energy stored in the carbon–carbon bonds is released. This energy is used for synthesis of other substrates and for a variety of metabolic functions.

The net chemical reaction of glucose catabolism is expressed in the following formula:

$$C_6H_{12}O_2 + 6O_2 \rightarrow 6CO_2 + 6H_2O + \text{Energy}$$

Glycolysis

Glycolysis[6-8] is the process of breakdown of a glucose molecule (6-carbon) into pyruvate molecules (3-carbon) with the release of energy (Figure 3-5). The glycolytic pathway is an anaerobic process occurring in the cytoplasm and is catalyzed by specific enzymes at each step of the reaction.

The net reaction of glycolysis is:

$$1\text{Glucose} + 2\text{adenosine diphosphate} + 2\text{inorganic phosphate} + 2NAD^+ \rightarrow 2\text{pyruvate} + 2ATP + 2NADH + 2H^+ + 2H_2O$$

During the degradation of glucose, adenosine diphosphate and inorganic phosphate combine to form ATP, and the cell uses the coenzyme NAD^+ to shuttle energy between reactions. After a series of reactions, two types of activated energy carrier molecules are produced: ATP and NADH. During glycolysis, the formation of ATP is directly dependent on the dehydration of glucose. This process is called substrate level phosphorylation. During the formation and degradation of ATP, energy is stored in and released from cells. Approximately 7 kcal of energy are released per mole of ATP. In addition, two molecules of NADH are formed from NAD^+ after receiving hydrogen atoms from glucose.

Glycolysis only releases a small fraction of the initial energy stored in the glucose molecule, and the majority of the energy is still present within the chemical bonds of the pyruvate. Pyruvate can be oxidized under aerobic conditions for maximum energy production. During anaerobic glycolysis, pyruvate is reduced to lactate with production of fewer moles of ATP.

In the liver, fructose and galactose also can enter the glycolytic pathway. However, additional enzymes are required to phosphorylate fructose to fructose1,6-phosphate, and convert galactose to glucose1-phosphate before glycolysis.

Cell Respiration—Tricarboxylic Acid Cycle

Under aerobic conditions, pyruvate is transported into the mitochondrial matrix and undergoes a decarboxylation process by which a CO_2 is released and one molecule of ATP is generated. The remaining two carbons (the acetyl group) are then transferred to coenzyme A (CoA) to form acetyl-CoA. The TCA cycle begins with the combination of the two-carbon acetyl group from acetyl-CoA with a four-carbon compound, oxaloacetate, to form citrate. A series of seven complicated reactions follows (Figure 3-6). With the complete oxidation of glucose, two molecules of CO_2 are released and one molecule of oxaloacetate is regenerated to be used in subsequent turns of the TCA cycle. During the TCA cycle, electrons are transferred to NAD^+ and flavin adenine dinucleotide, producing their reduced forms of NADH and reduced flavin adenine dinucleotide, respectively. These coenzymes then transport the electrons to oxygen by a series of carrier molecules located in the inner mitochondrial membrane (called the electron transport chain), leading to the release of free energy for the synthesis of more ATP, a process termed oxidative phosphorylation. A total of 32 molecules of ATP are generated by oxidative phosphorylation, although there is some controversy about the exact number. Thus, the TCA cycle is much more efficient than glycolysis to yield the energy stored in glucose. Mature erythrocytes do not possess mitochondria; therefore, glucose is never oxidized to water and CO_2. Instead, pyruvate is reduced to lactate. The TCA cycle is also known as the Krebs cycle or the citric acid cycle.

To sum up, the oxidation of one glucose molecule produces 4 molecules of ATP via substrate phosphorylation (two from glycolysis and two from pyruvate decarboxylation) plus 32 molecules via oxidative phosphorylation, for a total of 36 molecules of ATP. Approximately 109 moles of ATP are in solution in a typical cell at any instant, and in many cells, all this ATP is turned over (ie, used up and replaced) every 1 to 2 minutes.

Pyruvate–Lactate Pathway

Under anaerobic conditions, pyruvate accepts a hydrogen atom from NADH, forming NAD1 and lactic acid. At physiological pH, lactic acid will be in the form of lactate and protons. Thus, the local hydrogen ion concentration in the muscle increases. Using this pathway, only two ATPs can be generated per molecule of pyruvate.

FIGURE 3-5 Glycolytic Pathway

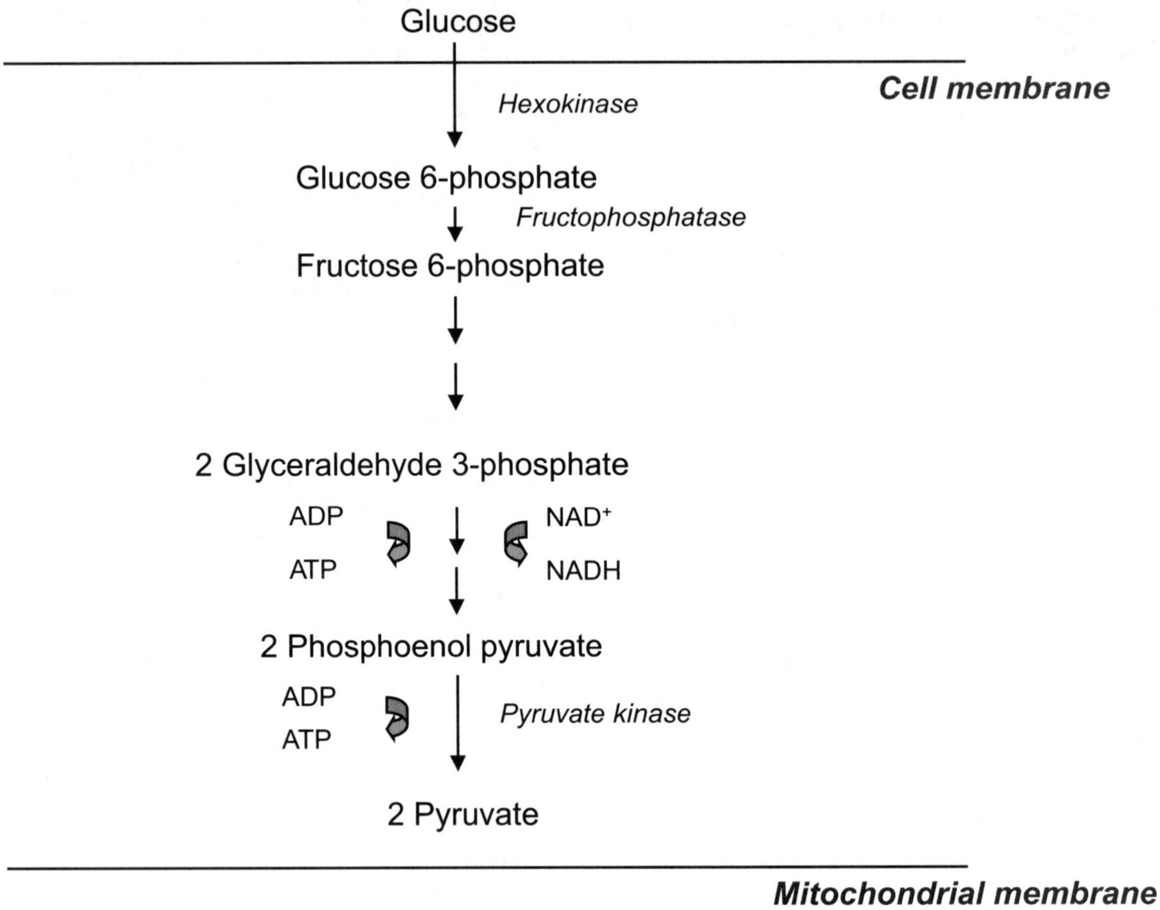

Glycolysis is a key reaction of metabolism. It is an anaerobic process occurring in the cytosol. Glycolysis takes place in almost all liver cells and supplies energy (in the form of two adenosine triphosphate [ATP]/one glucose, substrate phosphorylation); supplies the reduced form of nicotinamide adenine dinucleotide (NADH); and converts carbohydrates into pyruvate. The pathways are shown as they occur in the liver. Each arrow may represent one or more steps in this pathway. There are three major enzymes: glucokinase, phosphofructokinase, and pyruvate kinase. ADP, adenosine diphosphate; NAD^+, nicotinamide adenine dinucleotide.

In most animals and humans, muscle can function for short periods under anaerobic conditions when the energy needs exceed oxygen supply. When lactate accumulates, buffering capacity can be exhausted, and intracellular pH drops in active muscle, which inhibits glycolysis. When the oxygen supply is restored, the lactate can be converted back to pyruvate, and the pH returns toward normal. Oxidative glycolysis predominates again. Although this pathway is an inefficient method of glucose catabolism, it allows some organisms to survive under anaerobic conditions.

Gluconeogenesis

The endogenous formation of glucose is called gluconeogenesis. This step is important to maintain plasma glucose concentration in the normal range during fasting and allows constant provision of energy for metabolic needs.

Gluconeogenesis occurs mainly in the liver and to a more limited extent in the kidney and possibly small intestine under some conditions.[9-10] The pathways of gluconeogenesis are not simply the reverse reactions of glycolysis. There are four new irreversible reactions (Figure 3-7): (1) pyruvate is carboxylated in mitochondria to oxaloacetate; (2) the formed oxaloacetate is phosphorylated in the cytosol to phosphoenolpyruvate; and (3 and 4) special phosphatases hydrolyze fructose 1,6-bisphosphate and glucose 6-phosphate.

During fasting or carbohydrate deprivation, amino acids and fat can provide carbon for gluconeogenesis. All amino acids, except lysine and leucine, are eligible sources because they can be catabolized to pyruvate, oxaloacetate, or precursors of these. Alanine is the most preferred contributor to gluconeogenesis. Glycerol derived from hydrolysis of triacylglycerols in fat cells can also be used for gluconeogenesis because glycerol can be phosphorylated to glycerol 3-phosphate, a glycolytic

FIGURE 3-6 Tricarboxylic Acid Cycle

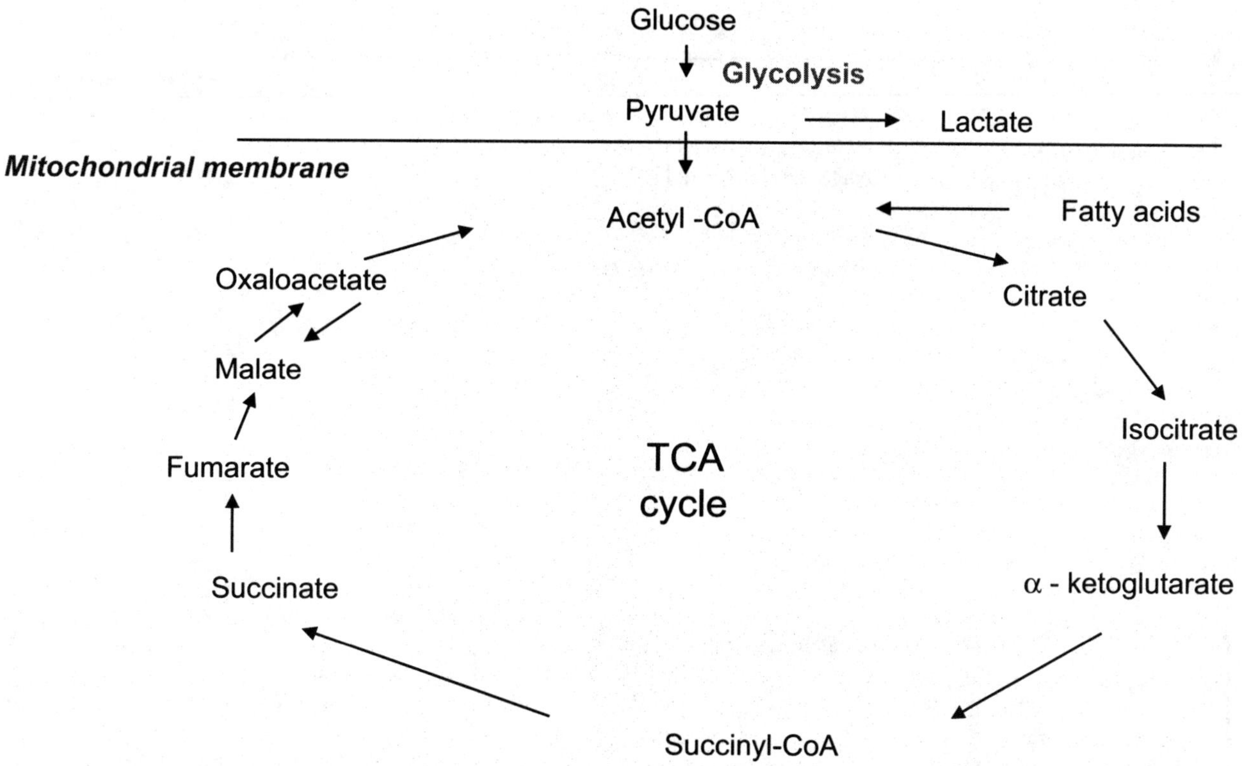

The tricarboxylic acid (TCA) cycle operates only under aerobic conditions and occurs inside of mitochondria. The TCA cycle plays a major role in energy metabolism and also provides intermediates for the synthesis of amino acids and fatty acids. The pathways are shown as they occur in the liver. Each arrow may represent one or more steps in this pathway. A total of 32 adenosine triphosphate is produced through the oxidative phosphorylation in the respiratory chain. CoA, coenzyme A.

intermediate. In addition, fatty acids can be oxidized and transported into the mitochondria and converted to acetyl-CoA. Although oxidation of fatty acids yields enormous amounts of energy on a molar basis, two carbons are lost as CO_2 during the TCA cycle. Thus, fatty acids do not undergo net conversion to carbohydrate via the gluconeogenic pathways.

Gluconeogenesis and glycolysis are strictly controlled by intracellular signals and are constantly coordinated with each other through hormonal regulation. In general, gluconeogenesis and glycolysis do not take place simultaneously in the same cell. Glycolysis occurs under fed conditions, whereas gluconeogenesis occurs under starved conditions.

Three major enzymes, glucokinase, phosphofructokinase, and pyruvate kinase, control the rate of glycolysis and gluconeogenesis. Locally, cells trap glucose by phosphorylation via the enzyme glucokinase, which prevents free glucose diffusing back to the bloodstream. The product of this reaction, glucose 6-phosphate, inhibits glucokinase, which ensures that free glucose does not accumulate within cells. Phosphofructokinase, a rate-limiting enzyme of glycolysis, is inhibited when ATP is plentiful. This step is necessary to prevent further breakdown of glucose and allows the cell to divert glucose to be stored as glycogen for later use. When ATP is limited, phosphofructokinase is activated. Pyruvate kinase, the enzyme that converts phosphoenolpyruvate to pyruvate, also is maximally activated under these conditions, optimizing pyruvate entry to the TCA cycle and allowing maximal ATP production. In addition, a hormone-activated cyclic adenosine monophosphate (cAMP) cascade regulates the activities of these enzymes.

Glycogenesis and Glycogenolysis

Glycogen is the storage form of carbohydrate in the body. In general, only approximately 5% of ingested glucose is polymerized into glycogen, with the majority being oxidized as described previously. Glycogen is present in small amounts in most body tissues but is mainly found in the liver and skeletal muscle. Heart muscle has no glycogen reserves.

In a 70-kg healthy man, the liver contains approximately 100 g of glycogen, which has the potential to provide 390 kcal of energy. Skeletal muscle contains about 300 to 400 g of glycogen, yielding less than 1560 kcal, suggesting that an adult stores only enough glycogen for about a day of normal activities. Because glycogen is stored with water, this is a somewhat bulky depot, and, therefore, an inefficient storage method. Fat is anhydrous and provides a concentrated energy source, so the majority of energy reserves are in adipose tissue.

FIGURE 3-7 Gluconeogenic Pathway

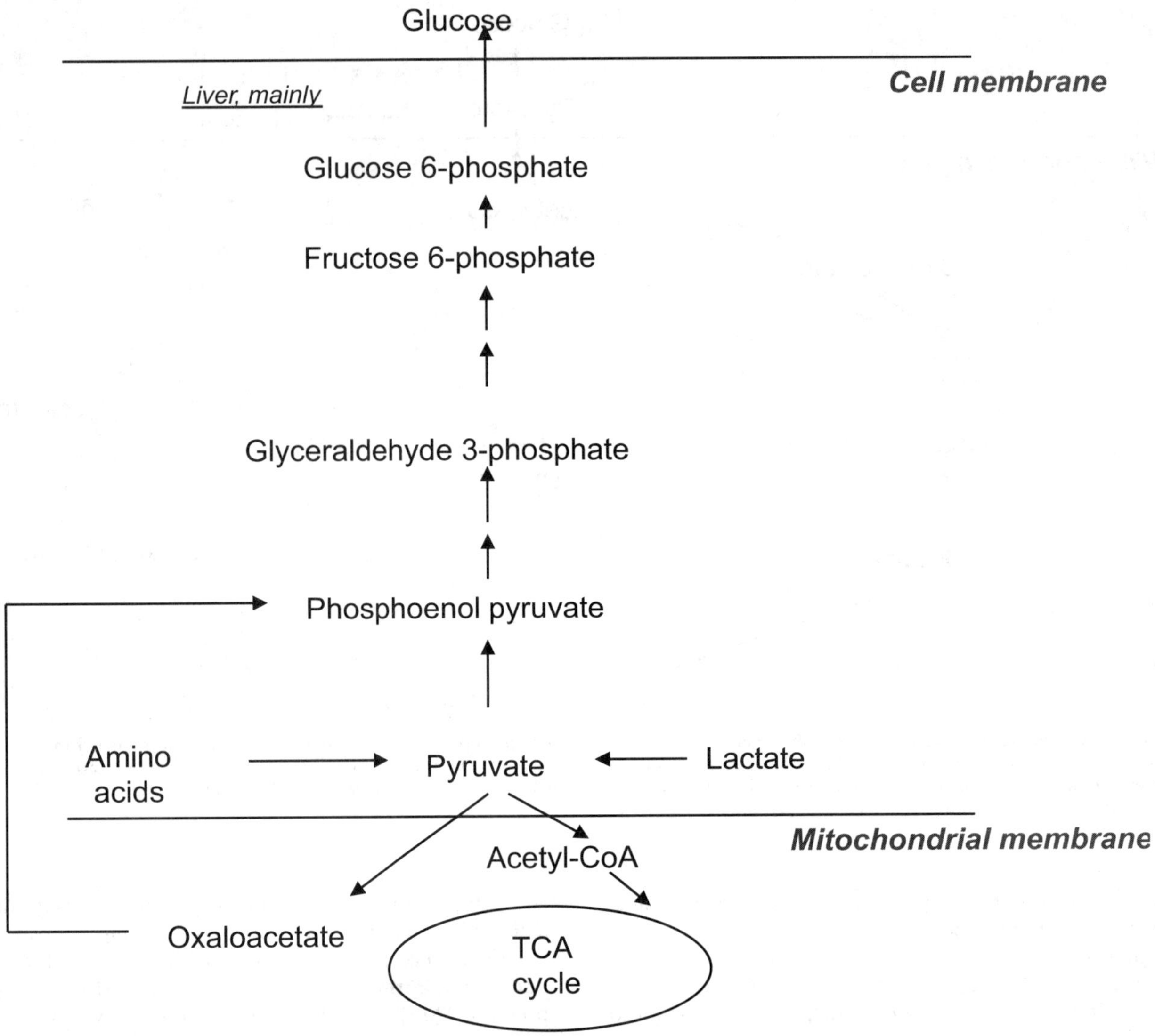

Gluconeogenesis is the formation of glucose. In humans and animals, this takes place in the liver and to a minor extent in the kidney cortex. Most reaction steps are a reversal of the respective glycolysis reaction, with the favored step in the direction of glucose synthesis. The pathways are shown as they occur in the liver. Each arrow may represent one or more steps in this pathway. CoA, coenzyme A; TCA, tricarboxylic acid.

Liver glycogen can be catabolized to provide glucose for use by the whole body. Skeletal muscle glycogen, in contrast, can only be used to provide glucose to the muscle cells themselves. This is because myocytes lack glucose 6-phosphatase and Glut 2 transporters, so that glucose 6-phosphate is the final product and enters glycolysis inside the myocytes. Glucose 6-phosphatase also is present in the kidney and has recently been discovered in the small intestine, so that the kidney and possibly the small intestine may have roles controlling glucose homeostasis. The kidney may contribute up to about 20% of whole body glucose production during fasting.

The formation of glycogen is called glycogenesis, whereas glycogen breakdown is called glycogenolysis. Glycogenesis and glycogenolysis are relatively simple biochemical processes and are regulated according to cellular needs, via the rate-limiting enzymes glycogen synthase and glycogen phosphorylase, respectively. Usually, activation of glycogen synthase occurs only after the inactivation of glycogen phosphorylase in hepatocytes.[11] Three key elements contribute to this glucose-sensing system in the liver. First, glucose 6-phosphatase is not inhibited by its product glucose 6-phosphate, so that glucose 6-phosphate can be converted readily to glycogen if glucose 6-phosphate is in excess inside the cells. Second, there are hormonal influences from insulin, glucagon, and epinephrine. Finally, the concentration of glucose itself can increase and/or inhibit the formation of glycogen by modulating phosphorylation of glycogen synthase and glycogen phosphorylase.

In response to feeding and a rise in plasma glucose concentrations, insulin promotes glycogen synthesis through regulation of the activities of glycogen synthase and glycogen phosphorylase so that glycogenesis is promoted, and glycogenolysis is inhibited. In response to a fall in blood glucose, pancreatic islets release the hormone glucagon, which has many functions opposite to insulin and is usually associated with increased production of glucose. Epinephrine is a hormone released from the adrenal medulla, usually during stress or shock, which also promotes breakdown of glycogen stores to provide energy for the fight-or-flight response. Both glucagon and epinephrine activate a cascade of second messengers through cAMP formation inside cells. The cAMP cascade leads to the phosphorylation and activation of glycogen phosphorylase, even if cellular ATP and glucose 6-phosphate are high. As a result, glucose 1-phosphate in hepatocytes may be converted to glucose 6-phosphate and dephosphorylated, allowing glucose release to the bloodstream in times of need. Insulin antagonizes the glucagon- and/or epinephrine-induced cAMP cascades. With these hormonal interactions, the needs of the organism take precedence over the needs of the cell.

Formation of Precursors for Other Metabolites

Glycolysis and the TCA cycle provide the precursors needed to synthesize many important molecules. Glucose 6-phosphate is required for the synthesis of nucleotides. Pyruvate is a precursor of alanine. Acetyl-CoA can be used for synthesis of triglycerides, and citrate from the TCA cycle is used for the synthesis of cholesterol. Other intermediates from the TCA cycle are the precursors of some amino acids. For example, oxaloacetate and α-ketoglutarate are the precursors of aspartate and glutamate.

Plasma Glucose Homeostasis

Normally, plasma glucose concentrations are maintained in the range of 70 to 120 mg/dL. This level is necessary to provide constant nutrition for the tissues and organs in which metabolic function is regulated primarily by the extracellular glucose concentration.

Glucose Regulation During Fasting and Fed States[6–8]

The liver plays an important role in glucose homeostasis during fasting and fed states. If the blood glucose concentration level is adequate (ie, fed state), the liver metabolizes glucose to fill energy reserves (Figure 3-8). Glucose is metabolized readily to produce ATP, pyruvate, and acetyl-CoA. Acetyl-CoA can be converted to triglycerides and exported in the form of lipoprotein to adipose tissues. Very little glucose is metabolized through the TCA cycle in the liver during the fed state. The primary signal for the metabolic pathways that consume glucose in hepatocytes is the elevated insulin concentration triggered by the rise in blood glucose, in parallel with a very low plasma glucagon concentration.

If blood glucose is lower (ie, fasting state), the first priority of the liver is to generate glucose to maintain blood glucose concentrations (Figure 3-9). Therefore, glucose 6-phosphate is converted to glucose inside hepatocytes and exported to the bloodstream via Glut 2. In the early fasting state, glycogen is an important source of glucose 6-phosphate. Because the hepatic glycogen store is limited, the next source is gluconeogenesis from lactate, amino acids, and glycerol. The primary signal for homeostasis in the fasting state is elevated glucagon concentrations in concert with low plasma insulin.

FIGURE 3-8 Glucose Metabolism in the Fed State

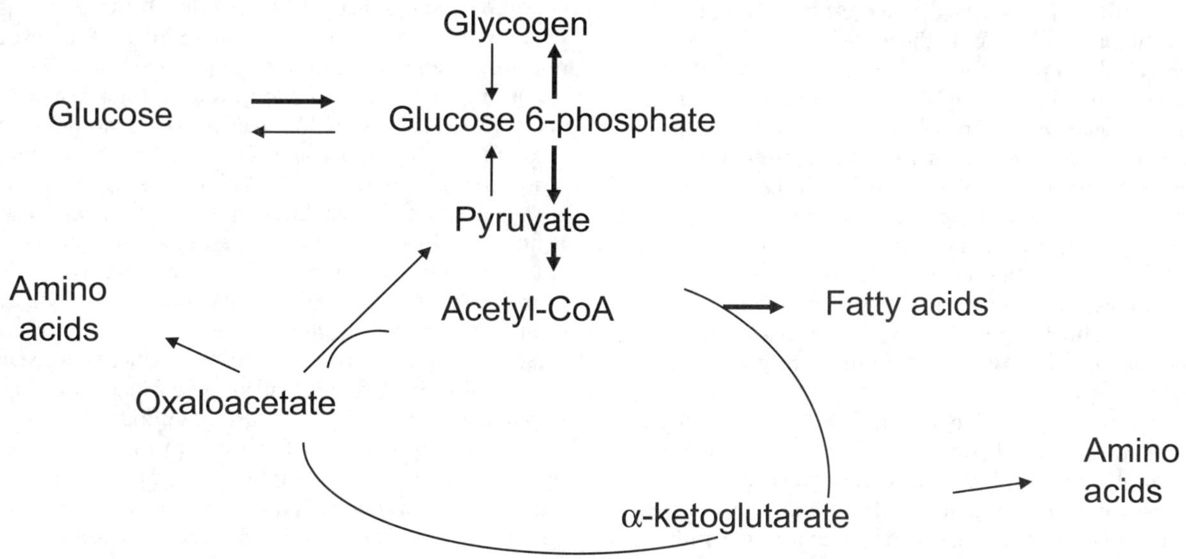

The pathways are shown as they occur in the liver. Each arrow may represent one or more steps in this pathway. The heavy arrow indicates stimulation. The metabolic response to a high glucose level is discussed in the section on the role of the liver during fasting and fed states. CoA, coenzyme A.

FIGURE 3-9 Glucose Metabolism in the Fasting State

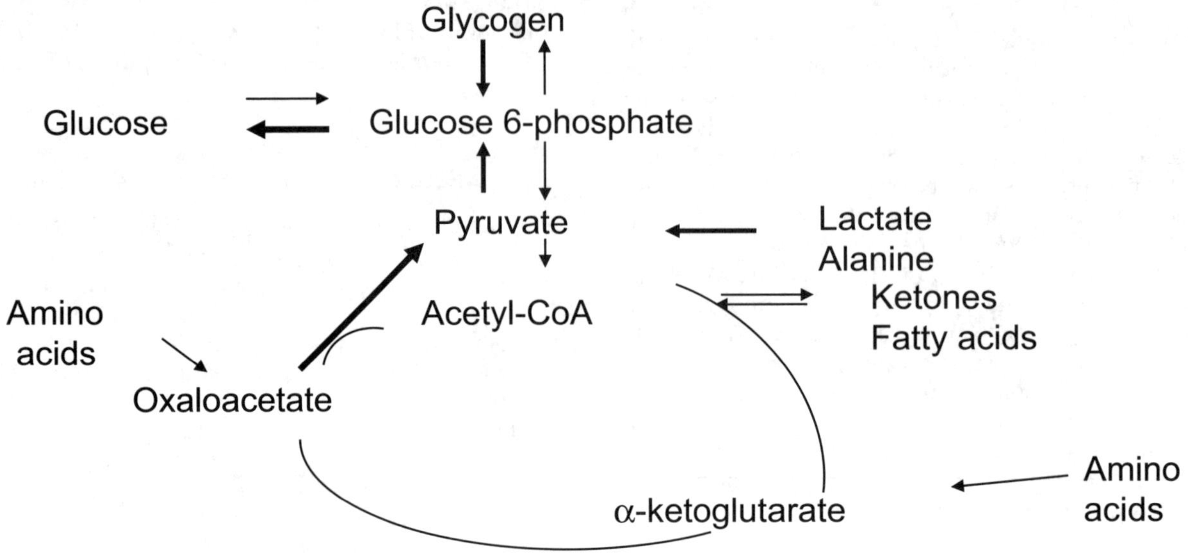

The pathways are shown as they occur in the liver. Each arrow may represent one or more steps in this pathway. The heavy arrow indicates stimulation. The metabolic response to a low glucose level is discussed in the section on the role of the liver during fasting and fed states. CoA, coenzyme A.

Over an extended period of fasting (starvation), glucose utilization is substantially reduced in most tissues and organs because of a reduced supply of glucose and decline in circulating insulin concentration. Higher glucagon concentrations promote fatty acid oxidation. Fat tissue becomes the main energy source for nearly all tissues. After 14 days of fasting, adipose tissue can provide more than 90% of daily energy requirements. Glycerol is transported to hepatocytes and enters the gluconeogenic pathway. When fatty acid oxidation rates are elevated, large amounts of acetyl-CoA are generated, which exceed the capacity of the TCA cycle. Acetyl-CoA is diverted into the ketone synthetic pathway called ketogenesis. Acetoacetate, β-hydroxybutyrate, and acetone (the three ketones formed) are measurable in blood when formed in excess. The rate of ketogenesis is determined by the supply of fatty acids and the regulation of fatty acid oxidation, which is promoted by lower circulating insulin concentrations. In addition, protein catabolism also contributes to gluconeogenesis. In the early phases of fasting, heart and skeletal muscles use ketone bodies as fuel, thereby preserving the limited glucose available for use by the brain. After 1 to 2 weeks of starvation, the brain is able to adapt and use ketones as a source of energy. This metabolic fuel switch is important for preservation of the protein mass in prolonged fasting, as fat stores can be used in preference to protein stores.

Two other conditions, diabetes mellitus (see Chapter 34) and a high-fat, low-carbohydrate diet, often lead to deficient intracellular glucose supplies. In diabetes, glucose entry into insulin-sensitive cells is impaired, related either to deficient insulin concentrations or resistance to insulin action. Similarly, in carbohydrate-restricted diets, the insulin level is relatively low, glucagon level is elevated, fat is plentiful, and ketone production is enhanced.

Hormonal Regulation

Normal blood glucose is regulated by the interplay of multiple hormones. Insulin is of major importance in this homeostasis, but glucagon, glucocorticoids, catecholamines, and growth hormone also have significant effects that are interactive with insulin.

Following a meal, insulin is secreted from pancreatic beta cells in response to increased circulating glucose concentration (> 90 mg/dL). This direct effect of glucose on beta cells is augmented by neural (vagal) and hormonal factors of intestinal origin (eg, glucose-dependent insulinotropic peptide, cholecystokinin, and glucagon-like peptide 1), so that the insulin secretory response to an oral glucose load greatly exceeds the response to an equivalent intravenous glucose infusion.

During fasting, a fall in blood glucose leads to a pronounced decrease in insulin secretion. Under these conditions, the alpha cells of the pancreas become active and deliver glucagon to the bloodstream. Stress, infection, or exercise also can stimulate glucagon secretion. Insulin suppresses glucagon release independent of blood glucose. In response to fasting, increased glucagon stimulates gluconeogenesis and release of the newly formed glucose from the liver to the bloodstream. Muscle proteolysis is stimulated by glucagon, which yields amino acid precursors that can contribute to hepatic gluconeogenesis. Thus, hormonal regulatory mechanisms coordinate glucose metabolism to maintain glucose homeostasis during fasting and feeding.

Comparing metabolic functions of insulin and glucagon, insulin is glycogenic, antigluconeogenic, antilipolytic, and antiketotic in its actions. It favors storage of absorbed nutrients and is, therefore, an anabolic hormone. In contrast, glucagon is glycogenolytic, gluconeogenic, lipolytic, and ketogenic in its actions. Thus, glucagon mobilizes energy storage and is a catabolic hormone.

Diabetes Mellitus

Diabetes mellitus (see Chapter 34) is defined as hyperglycemia (elevated plasma glucose concentrations) caused by deficiency of the action of insulin. Hyperglycemia is the result of the increased production of glucose through gluconeogenesis and glycogen degradation, plus the inhibition of glucose uptake by cells. There are two common types of diabetes: (1) absolute insulin deficiency, called type 1 diabetes, and (2) relative insulin deficiency, called type 2 diabetes.

Compared to type 1 diabetes, patients with type 2 diabetes have milder hyperglycemia and rarely experience ketoacidosis. The majority of people with type 2 diabetes are overweight. Generally, the defect is insensitivity of liver, muscle, and adipose cells to the prevailing insulin concentrations. The symptoms of type 2 diabetes develop gradually and usually are not as noticeable as in type 1 diabetes. Diabetes may also develop during pregnancy (see Chapter 20) because of increased placental hormones, which cause marked insulin resistance, usually in the third trimester. This type of diabetes disappears when the pregnancy is over, but women who have had gestational diabetes have a greater risk of developing type 2 diabetes later. See Practice Scenarios 3-1 and 3-2 for a discussion of gestational diabetes.

Practice Scenario 3-1

Question: How should carbohydrates be prescribed in the management of gestational diabetes?

Scenario: GB is a 28-year-old primigravid Mexican American woman with a prepregancy body mass index of 30. Her mother has history of type 2 diabetes, with onset at age 50. GB has gained 50 pounds when she presents at 28 weeks. Her screening for gestational diabetes is positive. Her obstetrical nurse obtains a history of infrequently consumed very large meals, with little home cooking. The patient explains that she eats at least once daily at a fast food restaurant.

Intervention: The patient is taught to perform fingerstick testing for glucose and instructed to test fasting and 1 to 2 hours after every meal; arrangements are made for diet instruction.

Answer: Although no specific caloric goals are recommended overall, GB is instructed to eat three meals each containing 40 to 60 g carbohydrate along with three to four snacks each containing 15 to 20 g carbohydrate. She is also instructed to increase fiber intake, reduce fat intake, and increase activity by walking as tolerated.

Rationale: The hormonal milieu of pregnancy promotes insulin resistance. Diabetes (usually transient) occurs in up to 10% of pregnant women. Women who have limited ability to secrete insulin in situations of insulin resistance can be diagnosed by screening glucose tolerance tests in the third trimester. Overweight and obese women, particularly ethnic minority women and those with a positive family history of diabetes, are particularly at risk. The cornerstone of therapy is to avoid high glucose (dietary carbohydrate) intake, because the peak postprandial glucose concentrations contribute to fetal overgrowth and other complications. Spreading carbohydrate intake over multiple meals blunts any one peak and allows adequate fetal nutrition without excessive glucose transfer across the placenta.

Practice Scenario 3-2

Question: What should be done if a pregnant patient with gestational diabetes loses weight?

Scenario: LR is a 30-year-old primigravid woman with a prepregnancy body mass index of 30kg/m^2 and a 25-pound weight gain during the first 28 weeks of pregnancy. She was diagnosed with gestational diabetes. She was counseled regarding self-monitoring of blood glucose and her diet. LR reduced her carbohydrate intake to 20 g at lunch and 20 g at dinner. She avoided carbohydrate completely at breakfast because of hyperglycemia particularly at that meal. With this approach, her postprandial glucose values remain in the acceptable range of 130 to 140 mg/dl. However, such marked carbohydrate restriction resulted in a loss of 3 pounds per week over the next 2 weeks.

Intervention: Her obstetrician asks her to test her urine for ketones before each meal and at bedtime for 3 days, and asks her to continue diet counseling where she is counseled to increase her carbohydrate.

Answer: Ketosis and weight loss were caused by carbohydrate avoidance, which is not an uncommon strategy in women given a diagnosis of gestational diabetes. While urine assays for ketones are poor markers of serum ketones, they can serve to reinforce to a patient the importance of balanced carbohydrate nutrition in pregnancy. With liberalized carbohydrate intake, LR may require exogenous insulin and education on the same.

Rationale: Self-starvation during this scenario is due to a misguided effort to avoid hyperglycemia. Adequate carbohydrate intake in this patient may cause hyperglycemia. This, in turn, is appropriately managed with insulin injections before meals and at bedtime. Very low carbohydrate intake leads to reduction in plasma insulin and elevations in circulating glucagon, which permit glycogenolysis, gluconeogenesis, and lipolysis, and increase beta oxidation of fatty acid. This results in ketogenesis. Ketone production during pregnancy leads to ketone transfer across the placenta to the fetus and has been associated with reductions in intelligence quotient in the offspring. Weight loss during pregnancy is controversial, but it is probably acceptable if limited, slow, and not associated with ketone production.

Stress Hyperglycemia

Stress hyperglycemia is a medical term indicating an elevation of the blood glucose in response to the stress of illness. This was previously usually defined as plasma glucose concentration $\geq$ 200 mg/dL.[12,13] Prior to 2001, apathy reigned with regard to control of such hyperglycemia in the hospitalized patient, and even blood sugars > 200 mg/dL were often left untreated. Subsequently, a series of randomized trials addressed the question of whether control of such hyperglycemia into the normal range was beneficial and brought into question what the true definition of stress hyperglycemia should be. The debate has not been fully resolved at this time, although many experts consider blood sugars > 180 mg/dL to be abnormally elevated.[13] This state of hyperglycemia can be aggravated by nutrition support, particularly by the parenteral route. Hyperglycemia varies from mild to severe and disappears when the stress is over.

During periods of illness and trauma, there is increased production of stress hormones such as epinephrine and cortisol, accompanied by an elevation in growth hormone and glucagon. These counterregulatory hormones oppose insulin action, causing increased glucose production by the liver (may exceed 500 g glucose/day) and decreased utilization of glucose in peripheral tissues. This hormonal milieu is also responsible for increased protein breakdown from muscle and enhanced fatty acid oxidation; this is viewed as a metabolic adaptation to provide fuels for heightened demands. Stress also increases production of cytokines such as tumor necrosis factor-α, interleukin-1, and interleukin-6, which further contribute to hyperglycemia through stimulation of counterregulatory hormone release and/or suppression of insulin action (see Chapters 23, 24, and 34 for further discussion of hyperglycemia associated with acute illness and trauma).[14,15]

Role of Fiber in Clinical Nutrition

Most western diets contain inadequate fiber, related largely to the proliferation of fast food intake and insufficient fruit and vegetable intake. However, there is no disease syndrome associated with a fiber-deficient diet. Constipation is the most easily recognized effect of fiber deficiency, although high-fiber diets can produce bloating and excessive gas.

In the upper digestive tract, fibers influence the physical content of the gut and how other foodstuffs are processed and absorbed. Higher fiber in the diet is associated with slowing of gastrointestinal transit.[16] In a patient with diabetes, increased time to empty the stomach may lead to a smaller peak postprandial glucose concentration.[17]

Under anaerobic conditions in the large intestine, dietary fibers are broken to their component sugars and fermentation by bacteria occurs. There is substantial variability in how much resistance to digestion occurs, with soluble fibers undergoing the most complete breakdown. Short-chain fatty acids result from this metabolism. Butyrate, propionate, and acetate (short-chain fatty acids) are absorbed by colonic epithelia, where butyrate may also be metabolized. These short-chain fatty acids then enter the portal vein and are transferred to the liver or eventually to the systemic circulation. The true biological relevance of short-chain fatty acid metabolism, however, remains to be elucidated.

Putative health claims for the benefits of fiber in a variety of primarily bowel disorders remain unproven in large randomized trials.[18] Fibers that resist degradation and fermentation add bulk to the stool, as well as water. Some human trials of addition of fiber to tube feeding in ill patients have shown less diarrhea and more firm stools; however, not all studies have been concordant.[19-21] Use of a high-fiber diet in ambulatory patients to relieve constipation, while theoretically sensible, has not been consistently shown to improve bowel function.[23]

In diabetes, the role of fiber to improve glucose control is better established, although the overall effect is not large and compliance with higher-fiber diets over long periods of time is suboptimal.[24,25] In a randomized cross-over trial of 13 adults with type 2 diabetes, a 50-g fiber diet for 6 weeks was associated with lower 24-hour insulin and glucose concentrations compared with a 24-g fiber diet. Cholesterol, triglycerides, and very-low-density lipoproteins were all reduced in parallel with the high-fiber diet.[26] In the Nurses' Health epidemiological inquiry, more than 7800 women with diabetes were followed over many years.[27] Whole grain and bran intake were associated with lowering of all-cause and cardiovascular mortality. Other large observational studies have largely concurred. In a cohort followed over 7 years, low dietary fiber intake at baseline was associated with a higher risk of developing diabetes.[28] The authors questioned whether the noted inverse association between dietary fiber and inflammatory markers (C-reactive protein and interleukin-6) might have etiologic relevance. Another potential mediator of the fiber effect is magnesium, which may improve insulin sensitivity. In a cohort study of Hawaiian patients without diabetes, the risk of developing diabetes was reduced by 10% in those with the highest intake of either grain fiber or magnesium, and these two intakes were highly correlated.[29] In general, recent reviews concur that dietary fiber supplementation in patients with diabetes is associated with improved glucose metabolism.[24,30]

Dietary fiber has been proposed as a protective factor against colorectal carcinoma as well as adenoma.[31] In some epidemiological studies, fiber consumption is inversely proportional to risk of colonic neoplasia. However, intervention studies do not confirm this.[32] The mechanism whereby fiber lowers cardiovascular disease rates, both in patients with diabetes and those without, is thought to relate to favorable changes in plasma lipid profiles. Meta-analyses have shown that soluble fiber in particular has been associated with improvements in total cholesterol as well as low-density lipoprotein cholesterol.[33,34] High-density lipoprotein cholesterol is usually not influenced by fiber intake. Fiber could reduce lipids by many possible mechanisms, including binding by fibers in the gut to such compounds as sterols that might otherwise be included in cholesterol metabolism, improvements in insulin sensitivity, or impact of hepatic metabolism of short-chain fatty acids on liver production of lipid particles.

Current recommendations from the Institute of Medicine suggest that adults should consume 20 to 35 g of dietary fiber per day, but the average American's daily intake of dietary fiber is only 12 to 18 grams.[35]

Carbohydrate Requirements

Healthy Adults

The amount of dietary carbohydrate that provides optimal health in humans is unknown. The minimal requirement is determined by the brain's need for glucose. A minimum of 50 g of carbohydrates per day is required to avoid ketone production. In a healthy adult, endogenous glucose production, from glycogen or gluconeogenesis, is approximately 2 mg/kg/min following an overnight fast, suggesting that a 70-kg individual has the ability to provide approximately 200 g of glucose per day endogenously.[36] In the nonfed (postabsorptive) state, approximately 50% of glucose production comes from glycogenolysis in the liver and 50% from gluconeogenesis in the liver. Therefore, the required dietary carbohydrate intakes are generally estimated at 200 g/day.[35] Not all carbohydrates lead to the same rise in blood glucose levels following oral ingestion. Glycemic index (Table 3-1) is a system to quantify the glucose response to carbohydrate-containing food. Glycemic index is defined as the area under the curve for the increase in blood glucose during the 2 hours following ingestion of 50 g of food, as compared with ingestion of 50 g of reference food (either white bread or glucose).[37] A food with a low glycemic index will result in a smaller rise in blood glucose than one with a higher glycemic index. Glycemic load quantifies the glucose response to total carbohydrate intake, taking into account both the glycemic index as well as the quantity of carbohydrate ingested. Manipulating carbohydrate intakes according to the values of glycemic index and glycemic load might, in theory, limit postprandial blood glucose concentrations and, hence, insulin excursions. This might be desirable as adjunctive therapy for diabetes, dyslipidemia, and weight control. However, physical forms of a food (such as juice versus whole fruit), methods of cooking (different cooking times), and the presence of other food with a meal influence the glycemic index of a specific food item.[38] In addition, age and gender often cause variations in hormonal release in response to food.[39] The effects of glycemic load from a previous meal also can alter blood glucose response to the current meal.[40] Thus, no standard value of glycemic index is recommended for any medical conditions.

Exercise

The carbohydrate needs of exercise depend on both duration and intensity. A muscle at rest or during low intensity exercise (ie, ≤ 25% maximal oxygen consumption [VO_2 max]) primarily uses fatty acids to spare glucose for the brain. With increasing workloads, glucose becomes more important as fuel. During moderate exercise (ie, ≤ 65% VO_2 max), for example, approximately 60% of the energy is provided by glucose (50% from glycogen, 10% from plasma glucose).[41] Muscle contains limited glycogen, so additional glucose is supplied by liver glycogen breakdown. Extremely hard (ie, ~80% VO_2 max) or prolonged physical work (such as a marathon race) can potentially exhaust glycogen stores.

After exercise, adequate carbohydrate must be eaten to refill glycogen stores in muscle and liver. Studies in athletes have suggested that 50 to 100 g of carbohydrate should be taken immediately after exercise, followed about 2 hours later by a high-carbohydrate meal.[42] When protein is combined with carbohydrate in the immediate postexercise phase, insulin responses are augmented, and glycogen re-storage is enhanced. For those engaged in heavy training, the daily carbohydrate requirement may be as high as 9 to 10 g of carbohydrate per kilogram of body mass to guarantee adequate carbohydrate availability before and during exercise, and to allow full recovery of carbohydrate reserves following exercise. Studies have also shown that consumption of 30 to 60 g of carbohydrate per hour during sustained intensive exercise attenuated the usual increases in exercise-induced stress hormone release and immune depression.[43] Therefore, a low-carbohydrate diet is not advisable for athletes, particularly for those who perform high-intensity anaerobic exercise and resistance training.

TABLE 3-1 Glycemic Index of a Few Common Foods

Food Items	Glycemic Index (white bread = 100)
Rice, white	126
Rice, Uncle Ben's long-grain	72
Corn flakes	119
Cheerios	106
All-Bran cereal	60
Carrots	101
Green peas	68
Kidney beans	42
Cheese pizza	86
Spaghetti (boiled)	83
Banana	76
Orange	62
Apple	52
Orange juice	74
Apple juice	58
Soft drink	97
Skim milk	46

Adapted with permission from Foster-Powell K, Brand Miller J. International tables of glycemic index. *Am J Clin Nutr.* 1995;62:871S–893S.

Illness and Injury

The metabolic response to illness and injury is characterized by hypermetabolism, including negative nitrogen balance, insulin resistance, hyperglycemia, and fatty acid oxidation and mobilization. Provision of energy (carbohydrate or fat) is required to minimize protein degradation and lipolysis in all forms of illness and injury.[44] However, the clearance rate of endogenous and exogenous circulating lipid is decreased during illness, leading to the development of hypertriglyceridemia and hepatic fat accumulation. Thus, carbohydrate should be considered the primary energy source for these patients.[45] However, the capacity for glucose oxidation is also impaired during illness. In burn patients, glucose oxidation rates slow significantly if dextrose is given intravenously at a rate above 5 mg/kg/min.[46] In addition, patients receiving parenteral nutrition who are fed glucose intravenously at rates in excess of 4 mg/kg/min have a substantial incidence of hyperglycemia.[12] Detailed discussion of carbohydrate utilization and requirement in specific disease and trauma conditions is reviewed extensively throughout the text.

Summary

Carbohydrate metabolism is relevant to diverse areas of medical care and research, and is a pivotal part of a prevalent chronic disease, diabetes mellitus. Much has already been well defined; however, as the fields of obesity and exercise science evolve, our knowledge of carbohydrate metabolism will enlarge.

References

1. Gray GM. Carbohydrate digestion and absorption: role of the small intestine. *N Engl J Med.* 1975;292:1225–1230.
2. Pessin JE, Bell SI. Mammalian facilitative glucose transporter family: structure and molecular regulation. *Annu Rev Physiol.* 1992;54: 911–930.

3. Simpson IA, Cushman SW. Hormonal regulation of mammalian glucose transport. *Annu Rev Biochem.* 1986;55:1059–1089.
4. Kotani K, Peroni OD, Minokoshi Y, et al. Glut 4 glucose transporter deficiency increases hepatic lipid production and peripheral lipid utilization. *J Clin Invest.* 2004;114:1666–1675.
5. Joost HG, Thorens B. The extended GLUT-family of sugar/polyol transport facilitators: nomenclature, sequence characteristics, and potential function of its novel members (review). *Mol Membr Biol.* 2001;18(4):247–256.
6. Berg JM, Tymoczko JL, Stryer L, eds. *Biochemistry.* New York, NY: W.H. Freeman; 2002.
7. Nussey SS, Whitehead SA, eds. *Endocrinology: An Integrated Approach.* Oxford, UK: BIOS Scientific Publishers, Ltd; 2001.
8. Cooper GM, Sunderland MA. *The Cell—A Molecular Approach.* 2nd ed. Sunderland, MA: Sinauer Associates; 2000.
9. Battezzati A, Canmo A, Martino F, et al. Nonhepatic glucose production in humans. *Am J Physiol.* 2004;286E:129–135.
10. Ekberg K, Landau BR, Wajngot A, et al. Contributions by kidney and liver to glucose production in the postabsorptive state and after 60 h of fasting. *Diabetes.* 1999;48:292–298.
11. Stalmans W, De Wulf H, Hue L, et al. The sequential inactivation of glycogen phosphorylase and activation of glycogen synthetase in liver after administration of glucose to mice and rats.The mechanism of hepatic threshold to glucose. *Eur J Biochem.* 1974;41: 117–134.
12. McCowen KC, Malhotra A, Bistrian BR. Stress-induced hyperglycemia. *Crit Care Clin.* 2001;17:107–124.
13. Kavanagh BP, McCowen KC. Clinical practice. Glycemic control in the ICU. *N Engl J Med.* 2010;363:2540–2546.
14. Ling PR, Smith RJ, Bistrian BR. Hyperglycemia enhances cytokine production and oxidative responses to a low but not high dose of endotoxin in rats. *Crit Care Med.* 2005;33:1084–1089.
15. McCowen KC, Ling PR, Ciccarone A, et al. Sustained endotoxemia leads to marked down-regulation of early steps in the insulin-signaling cascade. *Crit Care Med.* 2001;29:839–846.
16. Holt S, Heading RC, Carter DC, et al. Effect of gel fibre on gastric emptying and absorption of glucose and paracetamol. *Lancet.* 1979;1(8117):636–639.
17. Jenkins DJ, Jenkins AL. Dietary fiber and the glycemic response. *Proc Soc Exp Biol Med.* 1985;180:422–431.
18. Anderson JW, Baird P, Davis RH Jr, et al. Health benefits of dietary fiber. *Nutr Rev.* 2009;67:188–205.
19. Shimoni Z, Averbuch Y, Shir E, et al. The addition of fiber and the use of continuous infusion decrease the incidence of diarrhea in elderly tube-fed patients in medical wards of a general regional hospital: a controlled clinical trial. *J Clin Gastroenterol.* 2007;41: 901–905.
20. Spapen H, Diltoer M, Van Malderen C, et al. Soluble fiber reduces the incidence of diarrhea in septic patients receiving total enteral nutrition: a prospective, double-blind, randomized, and controlled trial. *Clin Nutr.* 2001;20:301–305.
21. Frankenfield DC, Beyer PL. Dietary fiber and bowel function in tube-fed patients. *J Am Diet Assoc.* 1991;91:590–596, 599.
22. Maffei HV, Vicentini AP. Prospective evaluation of dietary treatment in childhood constipation: high dietary fiber and wheat bran intake are associated with constipation amelioration. *J Pediatr Gastroenterol Nutr.* 2011;52:55–59.
23. Badiali D, Corazziari E, Habib FI, et al. Effect of wheat bran in treatment of chronic nonorganic constipation. A double-blind controlled trial. *Dig Dis Sci.* 1995;40:349–356.
24. Wolfram T, Ismail-Beigi F. Efficacy of high-fiber diets in the management of type 2 diabetes mellitus. *Endocr Pract.* 2011;17: 132–142.
25. Vuksan V, Rogovik AL, Jovanovski E, et al. Fiber facts: benefits and recommendations for individuals with type 2 diabetes. *Curr Diab Rep.* 2009;9:405–411.
26. Chandalia M, Garg A, Lutjohann D, et al. Beneficial effects of high dietary fiber intake in patients with type 2 diabetes mellitus. *N Engl J Med.* 2000;342:1392–1398.
27. He M, van Dam RM, Rimm E, et al. Whole-grain, cereal fiber, bran, and germ intake and the risks of all-cause and cardiovascular disease-specific mortality among women with type 2 diabetes mellitus. *Circulation.* 2010;121:2162–2168.
28. Wannamethee SG, Whincup PH, Thomas MC, et al. Associations between dietary fiber and inflammation, hepatic function, and risk of type 2 diabetes in older men: potential mechanisms for the benefits of fiber on diabetes risk. *Diabetes Care.* 2009;32:1823–1825.
29. Hopping BN, Erber E, Grandinetti A, et al. Dietary fiber, magnesium, and glycemic load alter risk of type 2 diabetes in a multiethnic cohort in Hawaii. *J Nutr.* 2010;140:68–74.
30. Bajorek SA, Morello CM. Effects of dietary fiber and low glycemic index diet on glucose control in subjects with type 2 diabetes mellitus. *Ann Pharmacother.* 2010;44:1786–1792.
31. Sansbury LB, Wanke K, Albert PS, et al. The effect of strict adherence to a high-fiber, high-fruit and -vegetable, and low-fat eating pattern on adenoma recurrence. *Am J Epidemiol.* 2009;170:576–584.
32. Kim Y-I. AGA technical review: impact of dietary fiber on colon cancer occurrence. *Gastroenterology.* 2000;18:1235–1257.
33. Brown L, Rosner B, Willett WW, et al. Cholesterol-lowering effects of dietary fiber: a meta-analysis. *Am J Clin Nutr.* 1999;69:30–42.
34. Talati R, Baker WL, Pabilonia MS, et al. The effects of barley-derived soluble fiber on serum lipids. *Ann Fam Med.* 2009;7:157–163.
35. Institute of Medicine. *Dietary Reference Intakes for Energy, Carbohydrate, Fiber, Fat, Fatty Acids, Cholesterol, Protein, and Amino Acids.* Washington, DC: National Academies Press; 2002. www.iom.edu/Reports/2002/Dietary-Reference-Intakes-for-Energy-Carbohydrate-Fiber-Fat-Fatty-Acids-Cholesterol-Protein-and-Amino-Acids.aspx. Accessed January 13, 2012.
36. Chandramouli V, Ekberg K, Schumann WC, et al. Quantifying gluconeogenesis during fasting. *Am J Physiol.* 1997;273:E1209–1215.
37. Jenkins DJ, Wolever TM, Taylor RH, et al. Glycemic index of foods: a physiological basis for carbohydrate exchange. *Am J Clin Nutr.* 1981;34:362–366.
38. Fernandes G, Velangi A, Wolever TM. Glycemic index of potatoes commonly consumed in North America. *J Am Diet Assoc.* 2005; 105:557–562.
39. Sawaya AL, Fuss PJ, Dallal GE, et al. Meal palatability, substrate oxidation and blood glucose in young and older men. *Physiol Behav.* 2001;72:5–12.
40. Granfeldt Y, Wu X, Bjorck I. Determination of glycemic index, some methodological aspects related to the analysis of carbohydrate load and characteristics of the previous evening meal. *Eur J Clin Nutr.* 2005;60:104–112.
41. Holloszy JO, Kohrt WM. Regulations of carbohydrate and fat metabolism during and after exercise. *Annu Rev Nutr.* 1996;16: 121–138.
42. Hargreaves M. Carbohydrate and exercise. *J Sports Sci.* 1991;9:17–28.
43. Gleeson M, Nieman DC, Pedersen BK. Exercise, nutrition and immune function. *J Sports Sci.* 2004;22:115–125.
44. Blackburn GL, Wollner S, Bistrian BR. Nutrition support in the intensive care unit: an evolving science. *Arch Surg.* 2010;145(6): 533–538.
45. Bistrian BR. Fat versus carbohydrate feeding in the critically ill. *Crit Care Med.* 2001;29(7):1475–1476.
46. Wolfe RR, Allsop JR, Burke JF. Glucose metabolism in man: responses to intravenous glucose. *Metabolism.* 1979;28:210–220.

4 Probiotics and Prebiotics

Gail Cresci, PhD, RD, LD, CNSD

CONTENTS

The Gut Microbiota: An Overview 52
Probiotics 53
Mechanisms of Action 53
Probiotic Sources 54
Prebiotics 54
Synbiotics 56
Prebiotic and Probiotic Applications 56
Potential Candidates for Probiotic Use 56
Type, Timing, and Dosing 56
Safety Issues 56
Contraindications 56
Clinical Evidence with Probiotic Provision 56
Antibiotic-Associated Diarrhea 57
Critical Illness 57
Clinical Evidence with Prebiotic Provision 58
Prebiotic Therapy and Enteral Nutrition 59
Gut Microbiota and Obesity 59
References 60

Objectives

1. Present an overview of the complexity of the human gut microbiota and the factors that influence its development and balance.
2. Provide a working definition for a probiotic and prebiotic.
3. Discuss the proposed mechanisms of action for probiotics and prebiotics including safety considerations.
4. Review available evidence for the application of probiotics and prebiotics in clinical practice relating to common issues surrounding nutrition therapy.

Test Your Knowledge Questions

1. Select the best answer that describes the human gut microbiota.
   A. The human gut microbiota is established by the age of 2 and little influences it.
   B. The human gut microbiota currently is comprised of trillions of bacteria.
   C. The human gut microbiota is highly dependent on the host for survival but provides little to the host.
   D. The human gut microbiota is not influenced by the mode of infant delivery.
2. Select the best answer that describes a probiotic.
   A. A probiotic is a live organism used to make yogurt.
   B. A probiotic is a "live nonpathogenic organism (bacteria or yeast) which when administered in adequate amounts confers a health benefit on the host."
   C. Probiotics are on the generally recognized as safe (GRAS) list and therefore can be safely provided to humans receiving nutrition support therapy.
   D. The mechanisms of probiotics are well known, making probiotic therapy a great addition to nutrition support therapy.

3. Select the best answer that describes a prebiotic.
   A. All fibers are considered prebiotics.
   B. Prebiotics are synthetic compounds.
   C. Prebiotics are dietary polysaccharides that escape digestion by the host enzymes and are fermented by the gut microbiota and influence the gut microbiota pattern in a beneficial manner.
   D. All prebiotics are fermented to yield the same short-chain fatty acids (SCFAs).

Test Your Knowledge Answers

1. The correct answer is **B.** The human gut microbiota is comprised of trillions of bacteria. Humans are sterile in utero and are first sterilized depending on the mode of delivery. The gut microbiota are dependent upon the human diet for survival, primarily undigested polysaccharides that they ferment to produce SCFAs, which serve many biological functions in the host's body. The gut microbiota also has many other positive benefits to the host.
2. The correct answer is **B.** A probiotic is a "live nonpathogenic organism (bacteria or yeast) which when administered in adequate amounts confers a health benefit on the host." While the starter cultures used to make yogurt, *Lactobacillus bulgaricus* and *Streptococcus thermophilus*, are on the GRAS list and therefore considered safe for human consumption, they are not probiotics. There are specific criteria that a bacteria must meet in order to be considered a probiotic. The mechanisms of action of probiotics are still being researched, but what is known is that each strain of bacteria behaves differently, particularly in different environments. Therefore, a general application of probiotic therapy for nutrition support patients is not recommended.
3. The correct answer is **C.** Prebiotics are naturally occurring substances, predominantly dietary polysaccharides, which escape digestion by the host enzymes. They reach the distal intestine where they are fermented by the host gut microbiota to yield SCFAs and beneficially influence the gut microbiota pattern. Commonly thought of as dietary fiber, not all fibers are fermentable, and not all fermentable polysaccharides yield the same molar ratios of SCFAs.

The Gut Microbiota: An Overview

The host's bacterial cells outnumber its eukaryotic cells 10-fold.[1] While mucosal surfaces of humans are colonized with bacteria, the majority of bacteria reside within the gastrointestinal (GI) tract. It has been estimated that there are approximately 800 different bacterial species with over 7000 strains numbering approximately 100 trillion in the human gut; these are predominantly anaerobic bacteria based on the sequencing of the highly conserved 16S region of ribosomal RNA (rRNA).[2] rRNA is the RNA component of the ribosome. rRNA provides a mechanism for decoding messenger RNA into amino acids and interacts with transfer RNAs during translation. Bacterial ribosomes contain about 65% rRNA and 35% protein and consist of two subunits of unequal size, the larger having a sedimentation coefficient of 50S and the small of 30S. The 30S subunit contains one molecule of 16S rRNA and 21 proteins. Multiple sequences of 16S rRNA can exist within a single bacterium.[3] Relatively low densities of bacteria are located in the proximal intestinal tract (stomach, duodenum, and jejunum; 10^2 colony forming units (CFU)/mL of luminal contents) due to an acidic gastric pH, bile, and peristalsis. A marked increase is found in the distal small intestine (10^8/mL) and colon (10^{11} to 10^{12}CFU/mL).[4]

A healthy human fetus develops in a sterile environment. Newborns are first colonized based upon their mode of delivery. The mammalian birth canal is heavily colonized by microbes and thereby provides the initial inoculum for all mammals delivered vaginally. The vaginal ecosystem at the time of delivery is typically comprised of *Lactobacillus*, > 50% of all bacteria present, and *Prevotella* spp.[5] It was recently noted that in nonpregnant, healthy black and Hispanic women, strictly anaerobes rather than lactobacilli dominated vaginal communities.[6] Therefore, these findings indicate that during pregnancy the vaginal community changes to provide newborns with beneficial microbes.[7] A recent community-wide survey using multiplexed 16S rRNA pyrosequencing revealed that vaginally delivered babies acquire, at birth, their own mother's vaginal bacteria.[7] These bacteria can be found on the skin and in the mouth and are already present in the first meconium.[5]

In contrast to vaginal delivery, babies birthed by cesarean section (C-section) harbor bacterial communities that resemble those of the skin, comprising *Staphylococcus*, *Corynebacterium*, and *Propionibacterium* spp.[5,8] Analysis of these communities finds that they are not different from other women's skin, indicating that these most likely are provided by other people with whom the baby is in contact.[7] Because C-section babies do not receive that first vaginal maternal inoculum, it not only affects the development of the GI microbiota,[9,10] but it may also explain the increased vulnerability they have to certain pathogens.[7] Compared to vaginally delivered babies, C-section–delivered babies have a higher incidence of atopic diseases,[11] allergies, and asthma,[12,13] and 64% to 82% of cases of skin infection with methicillin-resistant *Staphylococcus aureus* in newborns occurs in C-section babies.[14] The human host has a mutualistic relationship with its gut microbiota. The gut microbiota plays a role in energy balance,[15–18] metabolism of xenobiotics,[19,20] resistance to pathogen colonization,[21,22] and the maturation of the intestine and immune system.[23,24] A xenobiotic is a chemical that is found in an organism but which is not normally produced or expected to be present in it.

While the newborn's gut microbiota is comprised of relatively few species and lineages, diversity rapidly increases within the first few years of life.[25,26] The exact reason for the increase in diversity is unknown, but is hypothesized to be either from an enlarging intestinal tract that provides a larger habitat for more bacteria, increased exposure to environmental bacteria, and/or dietary changes.[7] Breastfeeding has been shown to enrich vaginally acquired, lactic acid–producing bacteria in the baby's intestine.[27] Breast milk contains bifidobacteria, with *Bifidobacterium longum* the most widely found species followed by *Bifidobacterium animalis*, *Bifidobacterium bifidum*, and *Bifidobacterium catenulatum*; all are *Bifidobacterium* species that may promote healthy microbiota development.[28]

Advancing the diet from simple solid foods (rice cereal) to one including more complex plant polysaccharides (peas) resulted in a change in the relative ratio of bacterial phyla in the GI tract from an unstable community dominated by *Actinobacteria* and *Proteobacteria*, to a stable mixture dominated by *Firmicutes* and *Bacteroidetes*, like that of an adult-like microbiota.[25] Analysis of the gut microbiota from African and Italian children found that African children had an increased abundance and diversity of *Bacteroidetes*.[29] This raises the possibility that the gut microbiota is adapted by local diets, and that the gut microbiota can adapt via genomic changes to changes in the host's diet; this adaption can be achieved by incorporating genes from bacteria in the environment.[30]

The composition of the gut microbiota amongst human family members tends to be similar compared to unrelated individuals,[31] and the same bacterial strains can be shared among family members.[32–34] The gut microbiota pattern varies geographically with the host,[29] as well as with age, noting that elderly gut microbiota varies from younger adults.[35–37] Organisms have defined life spans, playing different roles throughout the life span. Nature has created biologic clocks to monitor the position of an individual in the aging matrix; these clocks are phylogenetically deep and well conserved.[38] One type of clock includes bifunctional genes, which are genes beneficial to young individuals but costly in aging individual.[39] Subsets of endogenous microbiota may have bifunctional genes[7] with evidence for selection of microbes that co-evolve with their host.[40] This could have an impact on drug and nutrient metabolism, making it even more important to perform drug and nutrition trials in age- and location-matched populations to avoid the effects of differences in the metabolic capabilities of the human gut microbiota.[35] This also could influence the outcome after provision of probiotic supplements. Particular species that are beneficial to the young age group (eg, *Lactobacillus* and *Bifidobacterium*) might actually be harmful if provided into the elderly population. These are important topics for study. In addition to diet, age, and geographical residence of the host, the gut microbiota can be altered by other factors such as medications and both physiological and psychological stress.[40]

Probiotics

The literal definition derived from Greek for probiotic is "for life." The Food and Agriculture Organization of the United Nations and the World Health Organization have defined probiotics as "live non-pathogenic organisms (bacteria or yeast) which when administered in adequate amounts confer a health benefit on the host."[41] Currently, the U.S. regulatory framework does not include a definition of probiotics, nor has it established any rules or regulations specific to probiotics. This is concerning because a product can be called a "probiotic" without having substantiated evidence demonstrating that it meets the minimum criteria set forth in guidelines issued by the Food and Agriculture Organization/World Health Organization.[41] Not all bacteria or live cultures found in foods and/or supplements can be characterized as probiotics. In order to be considered a probiotic, the organism must meet very strict criteria (Table 4-1).[41] Ideally, the live, viable organism with strain identification must be able to survive the proximal GI tract environment and reach the distal intestine. Here it must function and/or adhere to the gut epithelial tissue, have a beneficial impact on the gut microbiota pattern, and be scientifically proven to exert a positive health effect. Lastly, it should be safe for human consumption. Even though conventional yogurt is a good food being rich in protein and calcium, the two starter cultures used to produce conventional yogurt, *Streptococcus thermophilus* and *Lactobacillus bulgaricus*, are not probiotics because they do not meet all of these probiotic criteria. Additionally, while it is possible that particular yogurt cultures are probiotic, it is important to have scientific evidence that indicates the yogurt product in question has high amounts of the strains and has demonstrated health benefits. This also should be applied to probiotic supplements.

TABLE 4-1 Probiotic Criteria

- Strain identification
- Human origin
- Live microorganism
- Viable
- Safe for human consumption
- Survive proximal gastrointestinal tract
- Reach distal intestine and colon
- Function/adhere to gut epithelial tissue
- Colonize distal gut impacting microbiome composition
- Scientifically proven health benefits

To appropriately identify a probiotic, one should look at the genus, species, and strain names (eg, *Bifidobacterium* [genus] *lactis* [species] Bb-12 [strain]). Most manufacturers do not include this information in their product labeling such as in yogurts or other fermented milk products. Often, manufacturers have not conducted research on the particular probiotic strain used in their fermented milk product or supplement, and typically generalize health claims from the other research sources for the genus and/or species included in the product. This poses a challenge for the clinician and the consumer regarding whether the product actually confers a health benefit.

Mechanisms of Action

Elie Metchnikoff, a Russian Nobel Prize winner of the 20th century, was the first to propose beneficial effects of probiotics among aging Eastern Europeans. He hypothesized proteolytic microbes in the colon produced toxic substances responsible for the aging process and proposed that consumption of fermented milk would coat the colon with *Lactobacillus*, thus decreasing luminal pH, suppressing proteolytic bacteria, and slowing the aging process.[42] Recent advances in the field are beginning to assist in sorting out the means by which probiotics exert their beneficial effects. Not all probiotic strains exert the same mechanisms of action possessing considerable interstrain diversity. Therefore, properties of one probiotic should not be extrapolated to another. It should not be assumed that probiotic actions in vitro reflect mechanisms of action in vivo. Another issue is whether the same probiotic strain exerts the same mechanism of action in different metabolic environments of the host, such as a patient in the ambulatory care setting versus an intensive care setting.

Probiotic strains may have multiple activities (Table 4-2) and therefore may be influential at various stages.[43] Different probiotics exert their predominant action either in the lumen, at the mucosal surface, by engagement with the mucosal innate immune response, or by action beyond the gut with stimulation of the acquired immune response.[44] An example of a protective luminal action against *Lactobacillus monocytogenes* is via the production of an antimicrobial bacteriocin by the probiotic *Lactobacillus salivarius UCC118*.[45] The same probiotic was effective in protecting against salmonella infection, but by a different mechanism. Another probiotic luminal action is via metabolic alterations of the commensal resident microbiota. Inoculation of germ-free mice with probiotic bacteria resulted in marked changes in gene expression within the resident commensal microbiome.[46]

Probiotics have been shown to have action at the mucosal surface. These effects include induction of mucins (MUC2 and MUC3),[47] with the resultant enhanced mucus layer overlying the gut epithelial lining then serving as an antibacterial shield that prevents the binding of enteric pathogens to mucosal surfaces and increases the clearance of pathogens from the gut.[48] Additionally, mucin-producing cells secrete trefoil factors in response to microbial pathogens, which act together with mucins to prevent their binding to mucosal surfaces.[49] Probiotics also have a direct effect on enhancing gut integrity and its barrier function by preventing changes in tight junction proteins (eg, occludins, claudins) and enhancing the tight junction electrical resistance.[50]

TABLE 4-2 Probiotic Proposed Mechanisms of Action

- Colonization resistance
  - Competitive exclusion
- Intestinal barrier function maintenance
  - Maintain tight junctions
  - Reduce macromolecular permeability and bacterial translocation
- Enhance gut microbiome pattern
  - Enhance ratio of commensal bacteria
- Modulation of inflammatory and immunoregulatory signaling
  - NF-kappa B
  - Interleukin-10
  - Toll-like receptor(s)
- Innate/adaptive immune modulation
  - Increase mucin regulatory genes and mucin production
  - Defensin production
  - Engagement with dendritic cells
  - Immunoglobulin (IgA, IgG, IgM) production
- Metabolic effects
  - Nutrient metabolism
  - Bacteriocins
  - Decrease luminal pH
  - Quorum sensing

NF-kappa B, nuclear factor kappa-light-chain-enhancer of activated B cells.

Probiotics express microorganism-associated molecular patterns capable of engaging with the same pattern recognition receptors as do pathogens, and thus have the means to protect the mucosal surface by competitive exclusion.[50]

The ability to stimulate the innate and acquired immune system via induction of regulatory T-cell function has been exhibited by some probiotics.[51] The secretion of anti-inflammatory (eg, IL-10) and proinflammatory (eg, IL-12) cytokines by immune cells can be affected in a strain-specific manner by some probiotic strains.[43] Some probiotics have also been able to activate specific gut opioid and cannabinoid receptors, thus having the potential to modulate visceral pain.[52]

Probiotic Sources

A challenge to clinicians is finding a commercially available probiotic product that has scientific evidence demonstrating benefit to patients. Many probiotic strains reported in the literature are not commercially available products, limiting the ability to readily translate scientific evidence into clinical practice. Additionally, most manufacturers lack disclosure of strain specificity or quantity of viable organisms (CFU) on products, thus further confusing the clinical application. Table 4-3 lists a select number of commercially available probiotic products.

Prebiotics

The primary food source for commensal microbiota is undigested polysaccharides and sloughed proteins. A prebiotic is defined as "a selectively fermented ingredient that allows specific changes, both in the composition and/or activity in the GI microbiota, that confer benefits upon host well-being and health."[53] Like probiotics, an ingredient must have necessary criteria it must meet to be considered a prebiotic (Table 4-4). In order to selectively stimulate the growth and/or activity of the gut microbiota in a beneficial manner, a prebiotic must be resistant to the host's gastric acidity and digestive enzymes and must be fermented in the distal intestine (ileum and colon) by the commensal anaerobic gut microbiota. Demonstration of prebiotic activity of an ingredient is difficult; therefore it is likely an ingredient may have prebiotic effects, but not yet be called a prebiotic because the necessary criteria have not yet been proven. Prebiotics are simple, naturally occurring or synthetic sugars that vary with their degree of polymerization. A prebiotic is not available to all bacterial species that inhabit GI ecosystems. Currently, *Lactobacillus* and *Bifidobacterium* are considered indicator organisms as currently known prebiotics stimulate the composition and/or activity of these organisms, but not necessarily others in the gut microbiota.

Upon reaching the distal intestine (ileum and colon), prebiotics are fermented by endogenous anaerobic bacteria producing SCFAs, gases (carbon dioxide, hydrogen, and methane) are produced, endogenous bacterial cell mass increases, and endogenous bacterial enzyme activities are altered. This has been shown to cause a drop in intraluminal pH, thus favoring an increase of *Bifidobacteria*, *Lactobacilli*, and nonpathogenic *Escherichia coli* and decreasing *Bacteroidaceae*.[54] As with a high-fiber diet, a prebiotic can produce several unwanted

TABLE 4-3 Some Commercially Available Probiotics

Strain	Initial Product	Supplier	Year Introduced
Lactobacillus casein strain Shirota	Yakult	Yakult	1935
Streptococcus thermophilus	Yogurt	Stoneyfield	1973
Lactobacillus bulgaricus			
Lactobacillus acidophilus			
Bifidus			
Bifidobacterium longum BBS36	Bifidus milk	Moringa Milk Products	1977
Bifidobacterium breve strain Yakult	Mil-Mil (Bifiene)	Yakult	1978
Bifidobacterium lactis BB-12	Yogurt	Chr. Hansen	1988
Lactobacillus rhamnosus GG	Gefilus	Valio	1990
Lactobacillus casei DN-114-001			
(Lactobacillus casei Immunitas)	Actimel (DanActive)	Danone	1994
Lactobacillus johnsonii La-1	LC1	Nestle	1994
Lactobacillus plantarum 299v	ProViva	Probi	1994
Bifidobacterium animalis	BIO (Activia)	Danone	1995
DN-173-010 *(Bifidus regularis)*			
Lactobacillus gasseri LG21	LG21	Meiji Milk Products	2000
Bifidobacterium lactis HN-019	Supplement	Danisco	2001
Lactobacillus casei KW2110	Yogurt	Kirin Holdings	2003
Lactobacillus casei F19	Cultura	Arla Foods	2004

symptoms such as flatulence, bloating, abdominal pain, eructation, and borborygmi,[55] with a wide individual variation found (5 to 20 gm/d). The stoichiometry of fermentation differs for carbohydrates of differing chain lengths and monosaccharide composition, degree of polymerization, and branching, with slower fermentation associated with longer chain length. Prebiotics can also affect bowel habits, resulting in a laxative effect through stimulation of microbial growth and increased bacterial cell mass, leading to stimulation of peristalsis by increased bowel content.[55] However, the effect is small, and there is a need for well-controlled studies to measure an effect. The type of prebiotic influences fecal stool weight with inulin and fructo-oligo-saccharides (FOS) increasing stool weight by 1.3 to 2 g, and wheat bran, fruits, and vegetables increasing stool weight by 5.4 to 4.7 g.[55] Prebiotic inulin-type fructans significantly increase the absorption of both calcium and magnesium in growing animals and in adolescents when added to the diet.[56] In pubertal adolescents, a mixed short and long degree of polymerization inulin-type fructan product (8 g/day) provided daily for 8 weeks significantly increased calcium absorption and enhanced bone mineralization. These effects may be modulated by genetic factors, including specific vitamin D receptor gene polymorphisms.[56]

Prebiotics are fermented by endogenous commensal gut microbiota producing SCFAs, predominantly acetate, propionate, and butyrate.[57] Not all prebiotics yield equal amounts and types of SCFAs.[57] SCFAs are known to serve several biological functions including ion transport (eg, sodium,

TABLE 4-4 Prebiotic Characteristics[104]

Three necessary criteria of ingredients	1. Must be resistant to gastric acidity, to hydrolysis by mammalian enzymes, and to gastrointestinal absorption 2. Must be fermented in the gastrointestinal tract by gut microbiota 3. Must be selective in the stimulation of the gut microbiota growth and/or activity that contribute to health and well-being
Not available to all bacterial species in gut microbiome	*Lactobacilli* and *Bifidobacteria* considered indicator organisms
Simple, naturally occurring or synthetic sugars	– Inulin (chicory, leeks, onion, garlic, artichoke, asparagus: DP 10-60) – Inulin-type fructans (oligofructose or fructo-oligo-saccharide): $DP_{max} < 10$ • Via partial hydrolysis of inulin or synthetically from monomers – Trans-galacto-oligo-saccharides • Enzymatic synthesis based on lactose - Lactulose

DP, degree of polymerization.

bicarbonate), modulation of intracellular pH and cell volume, provision of a metabolic cellular fuel source, and regulation of proliferation, differentiation, and gene expression.[58] Butyrate in particular is known to contribute to differentiation of epithelial cells, enhance water and electrolyte absorption, modulate immune function, exert anti-inflammatory effects, and to posses tumor suppressor effects in the colon through its role as an inhibitor of histone deacetylases and as a ligand for a butyrate transporter and receptor.[59,60]

Synbiotics

A synbiotic is a physical combination of prebiotics and probiotics. Often, candidates for probiotic therapy have inadequate dietary intake of prebiotics and/or their commensal microbiome is altered. Therefore, providing a prebiotic or a probiotic alone may not exhibit a beneficial effect. A synbiotic product may have the advantage of providing substrate (prebiotic) for a potentially beneficial probiotic, which in turn benefits the host (patient).[61] Additionally a synbiotic might maximize the viability and beneficial function of the probiotic before utilization and later as a therapeutic agent in the host GI tract.[62]

Prebiotic and Probiotic Applications

Potential Candidates for Probiotic Use

The gut microbiota is important for intestinal health and is involved with metabolism and immunity. Prebiotic and probiotic therapies may be beneficial for those with poor diets, older age, or stress, or who are taking medications that alter microbiome balance. Potential health benefits from probiotics may vary depending on the type, timing, and dosing of probiotic and/or prebiotic consumed.

Type, Timing, and Dosing

When considering probiotic or prebiotic supplementation, one should first determine the optimal strain for the clinical condition of interest and look for supportive research evidence for justified and cost-effective usage. This can be challenging because the literature contains a variety of probiotic strains and doses that are often not commercially available. Additionally, diverse patient populations, study designs, and small sample sizes have limited the ability to make evidence-based recommendations. Further confusion arises with the lack of knowledge of how probiotic strains behave in various metabolic environments and clinical conditions, the synergy with strain combinations, or when probiotic strains are combined with various prebiotics.[63] However, even though this is frustrating to the clinician, it is imperative to adhere to the concept that a probiotic, identified by strain, should only be provided to a patient with a clinical condition in which the probiotic strain has research evidence to support its use. Probiotics are live viable organisms and may behave differently in various metabolic and environmental milieus. Providing a probiotic strain without these considerations could potentially lead to adverse effects.

The optimal dose for probiotic and prebiotic effect for a specific condition is approximately 10^9 to 10^{12} CFU/d and 5 to 20 g/d for either a probiotic or prebiotic, respectively. Dosing schedules vary from one to two times daily to three to four times per week. Probiotic colonization is transient; therefore, continued dosing may be necessary to maintain a treatment effect for some conditions (eg, *Clostridium difficile* remission).[43]

Safety Issues

Many *Bifidobacteria* (eg, *Bifidobacterium bifidum*, *Bifidobacterium longum*, and *Bifidobacterium infantis*) are common safe species as are many lactic acid bacteria (LAB). Used in foods for many years, LAB are considered harmless, and they fall under the Medical Food and Supplement Act and are afforded GRAS status. LAB that grow as adventitious microflora or which are added to foods as cultures do not pose a health risk to healthy humans. Several strains of LAB species have been isolated from the human GI tract and administered to humans without reported adverse effects. These include *Lactobacillus reuteri*, *Lactobacillus plantarum*, and *Lactobacillus casei* (subspecies *rhamnosus*). However, although probiotics are normal commensals of mammalian microbiota and are generally thought to be without pathologic potential, individual patients may be susceptible to opportunistic infections via normal microbiota. There have been case reports of adverse effects, including sepsis (bacteremia, fungemia), bowel ischemia, and mortality, when probiotics were administered, most of which occurred in patients who had underlying medical conditions.[64–66] Other potential theoretical risks are deleterious metabolic activities related to altered polysaccharide fermentation, lipid metabolism, and glucose homeostasis; immune deviation or excessive immune stimulation; and microbial resistance.[64]

Contraindications

Probiotic use in certain patient populations may not be safe. Studies investigating probiotic benefits typically include strict exclusion criteria that are often not considered by practitioners when using a probiotic in clinical practice. In a review of 92 cases of invasive *Saccharaomyces* infections, treatment with antibiotic therapy and existing intravenous catheters were identified as the most frequent predisposing factors.[66] *Lactobacillus* has been isolated in the blood of patients with short-gut syndrome, leukemia, mitral regurgitation, and cardiac surgery.[64] Risk factors for developing infectious complications associated with the use of probiotics include the presence of a central venous catheter, immunocompromise, administration of the probiotic directly into the small intestine, concomitant administration of broad spectrum antibiotics in which the probiotic is resistant, cardiac valvular disease, and intestinal barrier compromise.[64]

Clinical Evidence with Probiotic Provision

Many clinical conditions can alter the gut microbiota, thus making probiotic therapy attractive, which has led to research trials in a variety of clinical conditions. These include inflammatory bowel diseases, premature infants, diarrhea, critical illness, surgery, and allergy. Two clinical areas most relevant to nutrition support in which probiotic therapy has been investigated are antibiotic associated diarrhea and critical illness.

Antibiotic-Associated Diarrhea

Nearly every hospitalized patient receives one or more doses of antibiotics during their hospital stay.[67] Antibiotic-associated diarrhea (AAD) is a common side effect of antibiotic therapy. The gut microbiota includes both beneficial and pathogenic bacteria, with the pathogenic bacteria outnumbering the beneficial by 10 to 1.[68] Disturbing the normal gut microbiota is believed to predispose the host to pathogenic bacterial colonization.[69] It is estimated that approximately 25% to 30% of cases of AAD in hospitalized patients involve *Clostridium difficile*.[70] *Clostridium difficile* can be debilitating with a high recurrence rate; it can cause pseudomembranous lesions in the colonic mucosa, causing severe inflammation.[68] The most offending antibiotics causing AAD/*Clostridium difficile*–associated disease (CDAD) are the fluoroquinolones. The associated diarrhea typically begins 4 to 9 days following antibiotic cessation, but can occur up to 8 weeks later. Other risk factors include severe illness, advanced age, presence of a nasogastric tube, provision of medications to raise gastric pH, GI surgery or manipulation, immunocompromise, and extended hospital stay.[68] The most effective treatment of AAD/CDAD is to stop the inciting antibiotic. *Clostridium difficile* identified by a positive stool culture is typically treated with metronidazole initially, with correction of fluid and electrolyte imbalance as needed. The treatment is repeated in patients that fail initial treatment; if they relapse again, they are then treated with oral vancomycin. Relapses may occur within 1 to 2 weeks of discontinuing antibiotic treatment. Relapse is believed to be caused by the survival of *Clostridium difficile* spores that later germinate producing vegetative forms and critical illness.[68]

In theory, it makes logical sense to provide probiotics in patients receiving antibiotics to prevent microbiota dysbalance or re-colonize the gut with commensal bacteria. In the past few decades, several strain-specific organisms have been researched in the prevention and treatment of AAD/CDAD. These include *Bifidobacterium*, *Lactobacillus paracasei* subspecies, including *Lactobacillus GG (LGG)*, *Lactobacillus casei*, *Lactobacillus plantarum 299v*, *Enterococcus faecium*, *Saccharomyces boulardii*, *Saccharomyces cerevisiae*, *Bacillus clausii*, *Clostridium butyricum*, and *Lactobacillus acidophilus*.[68] Details on individual studies are presented elsewhere.[68] Heterogeneity in choice of probiotic, lack of criteria for diagnosing CDAD, variation in diarrhea definition, and probiotic dosing, timing, and duration makes it difficult to make a final conclusion for probiotic therapy to prevent and/or treat AAD/CDAD. However, in a meta-analysis of 2810 patients, probiotic provision along with antibiotic therapy showed promise toward alleviating AAD, but not CDAD.[71] *Saccharomyces boulardii*, *LGG*, and probiotic mixtures seemed to exhibit the best protection from AAD. *Saccharomyces boulardii* achieved a significant reduction in *Clostridium difficile* recurrence in patients who were also receiving high-dose oral vancomycin (Practice Scenario 4-1).[71,72]

Practice Scenario 4-1

Question: How do you treat an enterally tube–fed patient with new onset of diarrhea?

Scenario: A 72-year-old woman residing in a long-term care facility for 3 weeks after being discharged from an acute care facility following a stroke is receiving enteral tube feedings via a percutaneous endoscopic gastrostomy and develops diarrhea. Her tube feeding is a fiber-containing standard isotonic formula. She has been receiving her goal volume for 2 weeks with good tolerance until 2 days ago, when she was noted to have excessive, watery, foul-smelling diarrhea. In review of her medical record, she finished a 10-day course of antibiotics 5 days prior to this onset.

Intervention: The dietitian is consulted to change the enteral tube feeding as it is causing this patient to have diarrhea. The dietitian reviews the medical record and notes the previously mentioned information. She rules out osmotic diarrhea from feeds or medications. Noting the onset of diarrhea to be within 7 days of stopping a fluoroquinolone antibiotic, the dietitian is suspicious of AAD/*Clostridium difficile* diarrhea. She recommends that a stool culture be obtained and analyzed for *Clostridium difficile*. It comes back positive for *Clostridium difficile*. Metronidazole is ordered for 10 days at 500 mg three times per day. The dietitian also recommends providing *Saccharomyces boulardii* throughout the course of metronidazole and for 14 days after its cessation.

Answer: Often, the enteral tube feeding is blamed as causing diarrhea in patients. In this case, the patient was receiving an isotonic formula in the stomach and had been tolerating it for several weeks. Medications provided for enteral feeding in stable patients are often liquid but may contain sorbitol or sugar, which can induce an osmotic load in the gut and cause GI intolerance and diarrhea. This patient was not receiving these types of medications. Antibiotics, particularly fluoroquinolones, are the most offending antibiotics that may start the downward spiral of AAD/CDAD.[68] This typically will result 4 to 9 days following the cessation of antibiotics.[68] This patient's course of antibiotics was completed 7 days prior to the onset of diarrhea, so she was highly likely to be experiencing AAD/CDAD. A stool culture was ordered.

Rationale: This patient was positive for *Clostridium difficile* in her stool sample. In addition to treatment with metronidazole, certain probiotics have been shown to be effective in decreasing the duration and symptoms of AAD/CDAD as well as reducing the recurrence of CDAD, with *Saccharomyces boulardii* having the best outcomes against *Clostridium difficile*.[71,72] Providing the probiotic during the course of antibiotics and then for 14 days after is to maintain and reestablish commensal microbiota during this therapy that is known to alter it negatively.

Critical Illness

Critically ill patients are at risk for developing infections and all receive antibiotics. In addition to receiving antibiotics, critically ill patients are recipients of multiple therapies and metabolic conditions that can alter the gut microbiota in a negative manner, thus making probiotic therapy attractive. Probiotic supplementation has been studied in multiple types of critically ill patients. These include those with acute pancreatitis, trauma, major abdominal surgery, liver transplantation, and medical intensive care. Like the studies in AAD, studies in the critically ill vary not only in patient population and underlying disease, but also in probiotic strains and combinations, dosage, duration, delivery method, supplemental feeding, concomitant therapies, and outcome measurements. In a narrative review of 10 randomized controlled trials in which probiotics and/or prebiotics were provided to critically ill patients,[73–83] outcomes included mortality, infections, length of intensive care unit stay, and length of hospital stay. Combining the data from these trials showed no effect of probiotics on mortality. A decreased incidence of infections with probiotic provision was found in nine of the studies; however, methodological bias may have led to this conclusion because when separated by risk of bias scores, effect was diminished. No significant differences were seen in length of stay.

Probiotic provision has been studied in patients with severe acute pancreatitis.[65,84,85] Two of the trials were of high risk for bias and demonstrated a benefit of probiotics in reducing infection.[84,85] However, in a trial with a very low risk of bias, there was an increase in morbidity and mortality associated with the probiotics with nine episodes of intestinal ischemia.[65] This study has led to a major cause for concern regarding provision of probiotics in this patient population.

Barraud et al.[86] performed a double-blind, concealed randomized, placebo-controlled trial in adult patients in the medical intensive care unit (ICU) ventilated for at least 48 hours to evaluate the effects of prophylactic probiotic administration. Patients (n = 167) were provided 2×10^{10} LAB daily, predominantly *Lactobacillus rhamnosus GG*, or a placebo until successful ventilator weaning. Overall, 28-day and 90-day mortality rates were not affected in either group. The incidence of ICU-acquired infections did not differ significantly except for that of catheter-related bloodstream infections, which were lower in the probiotic group. In a prespecified subgroup analysis, 28-day mortality among patients with severe sepsis treated with probiotics was noted with an odds ratio for death at 0.38 (95% confidence interval [CI] 0.16–0.93, $p = 0.035$). However, probiotics were associated with a higher mortality rate in patients with nonsevere sepsis (odds ratio 3.09, 95% CI 0.87–11.01, $p = 0.08$). The authors concluded that despite an acceptable safety profile, daily prophylactic administration of probiotics should not be encouraged in critically ill patients. Seeking to determine if *LGG* would be an effective therapy for diarrhea in enterally fed, critically ill patients (n = 36), Ferrie and Daley[87] conducted a prospective randomized trial in a tertiary referral teaching hospital comparing a placebo (inulin) with 20 billion CFU of *LGG* (an inulin-based probiotic) for 7 days. Overall, there was a trend toward more diarrhea in the probiotic treatment group with a mean of 3.83 days versus 2.56 days ($p = 0.096$). Mean number of loose stools/day did not differ between groups during the 14 days from the first capsule: 1.58/day in the probiotic and 1.1/day in the placebo group. The authors concluded that *LGG* is not effective as a treatment for established diarrhea in critically ill, enterally fed patients.

A meta-analysis of adult patients in the ICU with the use of pre-, pro-, or synbiotics was performed.[88] Randomized controlled trials including eight studies of approximately 1000 total patients were reviewed for evidence that these supplements can reduce rates of nosocomial infection, length of ICU stay, hospital mortality, and incidence of pneumonia. Different supplements were used in the studies including *Lactobacillus plantarum*299v (two patients), synbiotic (six patients), (Synbiotic 2000 [*Lactobacilli, Pediacocci, Leuconostoc* + prebiotics] [two patients], *Lactobacillus plantarum* + fiber [one patient]). Others used different combinations and doses of both. Patient populations included liver transplant (one patient), abdominal surgery (two patients), and general ICU (five patients). Overall, there was no evidence to support use of pre-, pro-, or synbiotics in adult patients in the ICU.

With increased risk of adverse events found in some studies, and limitations and lack of convincing outcomes in available research, the *Guidelines for Nutrition Support in Critically Ill Patients* by the American Society for Parenteral and Enteral Nutrition (A.S.P.E.N.) and the Society of Critical Care Medicine (SCCM) do not provide a recommendation for use of probiotics in the general ICU population or severe acute necrotizing pancreatitis due to the lack of consistent outcome effect.[89] A.S.P.E.N./SCCM Guidelines give a Grade C recommendation for administration of probiotics to improve outcomes (decrease infections) in critically ill patients involving liver transplantation, major abdominal surgery, and severe trauma. Further research on the effects of individual and combined probiotic strains at the molecular and cellular level in a critical care setting would be beneficial and provide insight for future clinical trials and recommendations.

Clinical Evidence with Prebiotic Provision

A number of clinical issues complicate research evidence of beneficial outcomes related to prebiotic use in practice. The gut microbiome is complex, and a number of physiological processes may play a role in treatment effect. These include changes in pH, microbe-microbe interactions, host-microbe interactions, antibiotic activities, and metabolic activities. Knowing the individual's presupplemented microbiota pattern and prebiotic dietary consumption is necessary to be able to detect a change with supplementation; however, this is challenging to accomplish. Studies show that in people that were already consuming fair amounts of prebiotics, little effect was noted with additional supplementation.

Therefore, because of these challenges with the study of prebiotics, the majority of study is in vitro with batch culture studies using fecal slurries incubated with various polysaccharides for certain time periods with an output reading of which bacteria genus is most affected. Other models include continuous culture systems inoculated with fecal slurries to resemble the proximal colon. The best in vivo model is with germ-free rodents inoculated with various prebiotics and/or probiotics for evaluating pattern changes in the gut microbiome. Challenges with human studies include variance in the host's prior diet composition with prebiotics and identifying whether a treatment effect was related to the prebiotic or changes in host-microbe interactions, metabolic milieu, or microbe-microbe interactions.

Prebiotic Therapy and Enteral Nutrition

Diarrhea is a common occurrence among patients being enterally tube fed and can be attributed to many factors including metabolic stress, hyperosmolar formulas or medications, antibiotics, enteropathogenic colonization, and abnormal colonic responses to enteral feeding. Intragastric enteral feeding was found to cause abnormal water secretion into the ascending colon.[90] Infusion of SCFAs into the cecum reverses this abnormal secretion.[91] The exact mechanism is unknown, but it is believed to involve neurohumoral mechanisms initiated in the proximal GI tract. Peptide YY, a polypeptide that promotes colonic water absorption, is not stimulated during intragastric feeding. This causes abnormal colonic water secretion during intragastric feeding, and it may be inhibited by peptide YY. Interestingly, ileal SCFA infusion stimulates peptide YY production.[92]

Enteral feeding is associated with alterations in the gut microbiota. Healthy subjects fed a standard fiber-free enteral formula for 2 weeks were noted to have a decrease in fecal bacteria and SCFA composition, and an increase in fecal pH.[93,94] An evaluation of general hospital patients ($n = 20$) receiving enteral nutrition found those with diarrhea had increased fecal *Clostridia* and decreased fecal *Bifidobacteria*.[93,95] Patients receiving long-term enteral feeding were noted to have an increase in aerobes and decrease in anaerobes but similar SCFA ratios compared to healthy controls.[96] Patients receiving enteral feeding supplemented with $\leq$ 28 g Galactomannan soluble fiber per day had resolution of diarrhea, which was accompanied by decreased fecal aerobes, increased total SCFA ratios, and increased acetate and propionate.

A meta-analysis evaluated the effect of fiber-supplemented enteral feeds on objective and subjective measures of GI function in both healthy volunteers and patients.[97] The analysis included 51 studies, of which 43 were randomized controlled trials. The studies varied in their method of feeding in which subjects were fed orally (13 studies), through a nasogastric feeding tube (18 studies), through a nasojejunal feeding tube (3 studies), or unknown (14 studies). Enteral formulas contained a variety of fiber sources, both insoluble and soluble fibers. The analysis found that in healthy subjects a fiber-feed increased fecal mass and decreased GI transit time compared to a fiber-free feed. In tube-fed patients, a fiber-containing formula decreased the incidence of diarrhea compared to a fiber-free formula.

The effect of prebiotics and enteral feeding affecting the gut microbiota are limited and performed primarily in healthy subjects. One study found that nine subjects fed an enteral formula with FOS (10 g/L) exhibited increased fecal bifidobacteria.[98] A group of 10 healthy subjects fed an enteral formula with short-chain FOS (5.1 g/L) and fiber (8.9 g/L) had increased bifidobacteria, decreased *Clostridia*, but no change in total SCFA ratios.[99] An increase in total SCFA ratio and increased acetate and butyrate ratios was found when healthy subjects received a fiber-FOS enteral feed.[100]

There is limited data on the use of prebiotics to prevent diarrhea during enteral tube feeding. Available studies report fiber-containing formulas with additional but unspecified quantity of FOS, or a compound with uncertain prebiotic characteristics. A prospective randomized trial in elderly patients receiving enteral feeding with fiber (30 g/d) plus an unspecified amount of inulin ($n = 70$) was compared to a group of patients receiving a standard enteral formula ($n = 85$).[101] A decrease in fecal frequency and more formed stools were noted in the fiber-supplemented group (4.1 vs. 6.3 times/wk), but laxative use was also reported. Guar gum[102] or partially-hydrolyzed guar gum[103] have been noted to decrease the incidence of diarrhea in patients receiving enteral feeding. However, these supplements are not typically known as true "prebiotics" because their ability to selectively stimulate the growth of beneficial bacteria in the gut has not yet been demonstrated.

Gut Microbiota and Obesity

The gut microbiota have genetic and metabolic attributes that may play a role in human obesity. Analysis of the bacterial 16S rRNA gene has allowed knowledge regarding variations in the gut microbiota of lean versus obese animals and humans. In a mouse model colonized with the human gut microbiota, the mice became obese when their diet was manipulated from a high carbohydrate diet to a western diet high in fats; this diet also allowed a rapid switch of the microbe community.[91] When this modified gut microbiota was transferred to germ-free mice, known to be lean, they adapted the obese phenotype. A continuation of this line of research to humans analyzing the gut microbiota of lean versus obese adults reveals conflicting results. The first study analyzing stool samples of obese versus matched lean individuals showed a shift in bacterial phyla (lower *Bacteroidetes* and more *Firmicutes*).[90] When weight loss occurred after following a fat-restricted or carbohydrate-restricted low-calorie diet, the ratio of *Bacteroidetes* to *Firmicutes* approached a lean type profile after 52 weeks.[90] However, later work by others shows that either the ratio of *Bacteroidetes* to *Firmicutes* is not altered in obese people,[92] that even more *Bacteroidetes* were detected in obese people compared to normal-weight people,[93] and that surgical manipulation via gastric bypass surgery decreased *Firmicutes*.[93] Discrepancies in results could be related to methodology variations used for bacterial analysis amongst the studies.[96] A large study identifying three robust clusters referred to as "enterotypes" indentified in people from different countries and continents did not reveal any correlation between body mass index and *Firmicutes/Bacteroidetes* ratio.[94] A set of three gene modules have been strongly correlated with the host's body mass index; two are adenosine triphosphatase complexes, which supports a conceptual link between gut microbiota capacity for energy harvest and obesity in a host.[94]

Targeted probiotic therapy with specific strains of *Lactobacillus* has been performed in animals and humans in hopes of decreasing adiposity. Mice fed a high-fat diet supplemented with *Lactobacillus plantarum* or *Lactobacillus paracasein* had reduced adipocyte cell size and body fat.[99,100] When supplemented with *Lactobacillus plantarum*, rats fed a high-energy-dense diet at pregnancy until 6 months of age had lower weight gain and lower retroperitoneal adipose tissue; this was not exhibited in rats fed *Escherichia coli*.[101] Administration of *Lactobacillus gasseri* decreased fat mass (visceral and subcutaneous) and body mass index in obese and patients with type 2 diabetes.[95] Andreasen et al.[97] provided *Lactobacillus acidophilus* NCFM prospectively for 4 weeks to 45 men with type 2 diabetes, impaired glucose tolerance, or normal glucose tolerance and showed preservation of insulin sensitivity as assessed by euglycemic hyperinsulinemic clamp.[97] In young children provided with *Lactobacillus rhamnosus* GG and *Bifidobacterium lactis* Bb12, or a placebo, body mass index was lower in the probiotic treated group during the first years of life (birth to 10 years).[98]

Although limited, there is emerging evidence for the provision of prebiotics in the treatment and/or prevention of obesity. Dietary fructans have been more extensively studied as compared to other compounds with potential prebiotic properties (eg, galacto-oligo-saccharides, xylo-oligo-saccharides, lactulose). Ingestion of inulin-type fructans (8 g/d) for 1 year significantly assisted with body mass index stabilization and fat-mass in nonobese young adolescents.[102] In obese premenopausal women, ingestion of yacon syrup (0.14 g fructans/kg/day for 120 days) increased satiety sensation and decreased body weight, waist circumference, and body mass index.[103] In obese subjects provided with short chain inulin-type fructan supplements for 3 months (21 g/d), food intake, body weight gain, and fat mass development was decreased.[88] These changes were associated with higher postprandial plasma peptide YY levels and decreased ghrelin over a 6-hour meal tolerance test.[88] Modulation of gut peptides by fructan-type prebiotics (16 g/d for 2 weeks) in healthy people increased glucagon-like peptide-1, peptide YY, and gastric inhibitory peptide, and decreased energy consumption.[28]

While these data suggest that an obese phenotype is associated with specific changes in the gut microbiota, there is inconclusive data that targeting one specific bacterial phyla is sufficienrt to improve a complex disease such as obesity. The few interventional studies that have been performed were not aimed to alter a specific "indigenous" bacteria. This is an interesting angle for treatment and/or prevention of obesity and warrants further investigation.

References

1. Hooper L, Midtvedt T, Gordon JI.How host-microbial interactions shape the nutrient environment of the mammalian intestine. *Annu Rev Nutr.* 2002;22:283–307.
2. Ley R, Peterson DA, Gordon JI.Ecological and evolutionary forces shaping microbial diversity in the human intestine. *Cell.* 2006;124:837–848.
3. Lehninger A, Nelson DL, Cox MM, ed. *Principles of Biochemistry.* 2nd ed. New York, NY: Worth Publishers; 1993.
4. Savage D. Microbial ecology of the gastrointestinal tract. *Ann Rev Microbiol.* 1977;31:107–133.
5. Dominguez-Bello M, Costtello, EK, Contreras M, et al. Delivery mode shapes the acquisition and structure of the initial microbiota across multiple body habitats in newborns. *Proc Natl Acad Sci U S A.* 2010;107:11971–119715.
6. Ravel J, Gajer P, Abdo Z, et al. Microbes and health sackler colloquium: vaginal microbiome of reporoductive-age women. *Proc Natl Acad Sci U S A.* 2011;108(Suppl 1):4680–4687.
7. Dominguez-Bello MG, Blaser M, Ley R, Knight R. Development of the human gastrointestinal microbiota and insights from high-throughput sequencing. *Gastroenterology.* 2011;140:1713–1719.
8. Mackie RI, Sighir A, Gaskins HR. Developmental microbial ecology of the neonatal gastrointestinal tract. *Am J Clin Nutr.* 1999;69: S1035–S1045.
9. Biasucci G, Benebati B, Morelli L, et al. Cesarean delivery may affect the early biodiversity of intestinal bacteria. *J Nutr.* 2008;138: S1796–S1800.
10. Biasucci G, Rubini M, Riboni S, et al. Mode of delivery affects the bacterial community of the newborn gut. *Early Human Dev.* 2010;86(Suppl 1):13–15.
11. Penders J, Thijs C, van den Brandt PA, et al. Gut microbiota composition and development of atopic manifestations in infancy: the KOALA Birth Cohort Study. *Gut.* 2007;56:661–667.
12. Bager P, Wohlfhahrt J, Westergaard T. Caesarean delivery and risk of atopy and allergic disease: meta-analyses. *Clin Exp Allergy.* 2008;38:634–642.
13. Negele K, Heinrish J, Borte M, et al. Mode of delivery and development of atopic disease during he first 2 years of life. *Pediatr Allergy Immunol.* 2004;15:48–54.
14. Watson J, Jones R, Cortes C, et al. Community-associated methicillin-resistant Staphylococcus aureus infection among healthy newborns - Chicago and Los Angeles County, 2004. *JAMA.* 2004;296:36–38.
15. Backhed F, Ding H, Wang T, et al. The gut microbiota as an environmental factor that regulates fat storage. *Proc Natl Acad Sci U S A.* 2004;101:1518–1523.
16. Backhed F, Mamchester J, Semenkovich CF, et al. Mechanisms underlying the resistance to diet-induced obesity in germ-free mice. *Proc Natl Acad Sci U S A.* 2007;104:979–984.
17. Samuel BS, Shaito A, Motoike T, et al. Effects of the gut microbiota on host adiposity are modulated by the short-chain fatty acid binding G protein-coupled receptor, Gpr41. *Proc Natl Acad Sci U S A.* 2008;105:16727–16772.
18. Martens EC, Chiang H, Gordon JI. Mucosal glycan foraging enhances fitness and transmission of a saccharolytic human gut bacterial symbiont. *Cell Host Microbe.* 2008;4:447–457.
19. Swann J, Wang Y, Abecia L, et al. Gut microbiome modulates the toxicity of hydrazine: a metabonomic study. *Mol Biosyst.* 2009;5: 351–355.
20. Nicholson JK, Holmes E, Wilson ID. Gut microorganisms, mammalian metabolism and personalized health care. *Nat Rev Microbiol.* 2005;3:431–438.
21. Boullier S, Nougayrède J, Marches O, et al. Genetically engineered enteropathogenic Escherichia coli strain elicits a specific immune response and protects against a virulent challenge. *Microbes Infect.* 2003;5:857–867.
22. Wells C. Relationship between intestinal microecology and the translocation of intestinal bacteria. *Antonie Van Leeuwenhoek.* 1990;58:87–93.
23. Mazmanian S, Liu Ch, Tzianabos AO, et al. An immunomodulatory molecule of symbiotic bacteria directs maturation of the host immune system. *Cell.* 2005;122:107–118.
24. Are A, Aronsson L, Wang S, et al. Enterococcus faecalis from newborn babies regulate endogenous PPAR-gama activity and IL-10 levels in colonic epithelial cells. *Proc Natl Acad Sci U S A.* 2008;105:1943–1948.
25. Koenig J, Spor A, Scalfone N, et al. Microbes and health sackler colloquium: succession of microbial consortia in the developing infant gut microbiome. *Proc Natl Acad Sci U S A.* 2011;108(Suppl 1):4578–4585.
26. Palmer C, Bik EM, DiGiulio DB, et al. Development of the human infant intestinal microbiota. *PLoS Biol.* 2007;5:e177.
27. Zivkovic A, German JB, Lebrilla CB, et al. Microbes and health sackler colloquium: human milk glycobiome and its impact on the infant gastrointestinal microbiota. *Proc Natl Acad Sci U S A.* 2011;108(Suppl 1):4653–4658.
28. Cani P, Lecuort E, Dewulf EM, et al. Gut microbiota fermentaiton of prebiotics increases satietogenic and incretin gut

peptide production with consequences for appetite sensation and glucose response after a meal. *Am J Clin Nutr.* 2009;90: 1236–1243.

29. De Filippo C, Cavalieri D, Di Paola M, et al.Impact of diet in shaping gut microbiota revealed by a comparaitve study in children from Europe and rural Africa. *Proc Natl Acad Sci U S A.* 2010; 107:14691–14696.
30. Hehemann J, Correc G, Barbeyron T, et al. Transfer of carbohydrate-active enzymes from marine bacteria to Japanese gut microbiota. *Nature.* 2010;464:908–912.
31. Turnbaugh P, Hamady M, Yatsunenko T, et al. A core gut microbiome in obese and lean twins. *Nature.* 2009;457:480–484.
32. Vaishampayan P, Kuehl JV, Froula JL, et al. Comparative metagenomics and population dynamics of the gut microbiota in mother and infant. *Genome Biol Evol.* 2010;6:53–66.
33. Falush D, Wirth T, Linz B, et al. Traces of human migrations in Helicobacter pylori populations. *Science.* 2003;299:1582–1585.
34. Moodley Y, Linz B, Yamaoka Y, et al. The peopling of the Pacific from a bacterial perspective. *Science.* 2009;323:527–530.
35. Rajilic-Stojanovic M, Heilig HG, Molenaar D, et al. Development and application of the human intestinal tract chip, a phylogenetic microarray: analysis of universally conserved phylotypes in the abundant microbiota of young and elderly adults. *Environ Microbiol.* 2009;11:1736–1751.
36. Claesson MJ, Cusack S, O'Sullivan O, et al. Composition, variability, and temporal stability of the intestinal microbiota of the elderly. *Proc Natl Acad Sci U S A.* 2011;108(Suppl 1): 4680–4687.
37. Biagi E, Nylund L, Candela M, et al. Through ageing, and beyond: gut microbiota and inflammatory status in seniors and centenarians. *PLoS One.* 2010;5:e10667.
38. Harley C. Telomere loss: mitotic clock or genetic time bomb? *Mutat Res.* 1991;256:271–282.
39. Williams G. Pleiotropy, natural selection and the evolution of senescence. *Evolution.* 1957;11:398–411.
40. Ley R, Lozupone CA, Hamady M, et al. Worlds within worlds: evolution of the vertebrate gut microbiota. *Nat Rev Microbiol.* 2008;6:776–788.
41. Food and Agriculture Organization, World Health Organization. *Guidelines for the Evaluation of Probiotics in Food.* London, Ontario, Canada: Food and Agriculture Organization and World Health Organization.
42. Gordon S. Elie Metchnikoff: father of natural immunity. *Eur J Immunol.* 2008;38:3257–3264.
43. Sherman P, Ossa JC, Johnson-Henry K. Unraveling mechanisms of action of probiotics. *Nutr Clin Pract.* 2009;24:10–14.
44. Shanahan F. Probiotics in perspective. *Gastroenterology.* 2010;139: 1808–1812.
45. Corr S, Li Y, Riedel CU, et al. Bacteriocin production as a mechanism for the antiinfective activity of Lactobacillus salivarius UCC118. *Proc Natl Acad Sci U S A.* 2007;104:7617–7621.
46. Sonnenburg J, Chen CTL, Gordon JI. Genomic and metabolic studies of the impact of probiotics on a model gut symbiont and host. *PLoS Biol.* 2006;4:2213–2226.
47. Mack D, Michail S, Wei S, McDougall L, Hollingsworth MA. Probiotics inhibit enteropathogenic E. coli adherence in vitro by inducing intestinal mucin gene expression. *Am J Physiol.* 1999;276: G941–G950.
48. Linden S, Sutten P, Karlsson NG, et al. Mucins in the mucosal barrier to infection. *Nat Mucosal Immunol.* 2008;1:183–197.
49. Clyne M, Dillon P, Daly S, et al. Helicobacter pylori interacts with the human single-domain trefoil protein TFF1. *Proc Natl Acad Sci U S A.* 2004;101:7409–7414.
50. Lebeer S, Vanderleyden J, De Keersmaecker SCJ. Host interactions of probiotic bacterial surface molecules: comparison with commensals and pathogens. *Nat Rev Microbiol.* 2010;8:171–184.
51. O'Mahony C, Scully P, O'Mahony D, et al. Commensal-induced regulatory T cells mediate protection against pathogen-stimulated NF-kB activation. *PLoS Pathogens.* 2008;4:e1000112.
52. Rousseaux C, Thuru X, Gelot A, et al. Lactobacillus acidophilus modulates intestinal pain and induces opioid and cannabinoid receptors. *Nat Med.* 2007;13:35–37.
53. Gibson GR, Probert HM, Van Loo J, et al. Dietary modulation of the human colonic microbiota: updating the concept of prebiotics. *Nutr Res Rev.* 2004;17:259–275.
54. Damaskos D, Kolios G. Probiotics and prebiotics in inflammatory bowel disease: microflora "on the scope." *British J Clin Pharm.* 2008;65:453–467.
55. Cummings J, Macfarlane GT. Gastrointestinal effects of prebiotics. *Br J Nutr.* 2002;87(Suppl 2):S145–S151.
56. Abrams S, Griffin IJ, Hawthorne KM, et al. A combination of prebiotic short- and long-chain inulin-type fructans enhances calcium absorption and bone mineralization in young adolescents. *Am J Clin Nutr.* 2005;82:471–476.
57. Cummings JH, Macfarlane GT, Englyst HN. Prebiotic digestion and fermentation. *Am J Clin Nutr.* 2001;73:415S–420S.
58. Topping D, Clifton PM. Short-chain fatty acids and human colonic function: roles of resistant starch and nonstarch polysaccharides. *Physiol Rev.* 2001;81:1031–1064.
59. Thangaraju M, Cresci G, Itagaki S, et al. Sodium-coupled transport of the short-chain fatty acid butyrate by SLC5A8 and its relevance to colon cancer. *J Gastrointest Surg.* 2008;12:1773–1782.
60. Thangaraju M, Cresci G, Liu K, et al. GPR109A is a G-protein-coupled receptor for the bacterial fermentation product butyrate and functions as a tumor suppressor in colon. *Cancer Research.* 2009;69:2826–2832.
61. Kolida S, Gibson GR., Synbiotics in health and disease. *Annu Rev Food Sci Technol.* 2011;2:373–393.
62. Bengmark S. Bacteria for optimal health. *Nutrition.* 2000;16: 611–615.
63. Worthington M, Ranz R. Use of probiotics in critically ill patients. *Support Line.* 2009;31(4):8–17.
64. Boyle R, Robins-Browne R, Tang M. Probiotic use in clinical practice: what are the risks? *Am J Clin Nutr.* 2006;83:1256–1264.
65. Besselink M, Van Santvoort HC, Buskens E, et al. Probiotic prophylaxis in predicted severe acute pancreatitis: a randomized double-blind, placebo-controlled trial. *Lancet.* 2008;371:651–659.
66. Enache-Angoulvant A, Hennequin C. Invasive Saccharomyces infection: a comprehensive review. *Clin Infect Dis.* 2005;41:1559–1568.
67. World Health Organization. *Obesity and Overweight.* Fact Sheet Number 311. Geneva, Switzerland: World Health Organization; 2011.
68. Rohde C, Bartolini V, Jones N. The use of probiotics in the prevention and treatment of antibiotic-associated diarrhea with special interest in Clostridium difficile-associated diarrhea. *Nutr Clin Pract.* 2009;24:33–40.
69. Asha N, Tompkins D, Wolcox MH. Comparative analysis of prevalence, risk factors, and molecular epidemiology of antibiotic-associated diarrhea due to Clostridium difficile, Clostridium perfringens, and Staphylococcus aureus. *J Clin Microbiol.* 2006; 44:2785–2791.
70. Mehmet C, Bulent B, Ismail A, et al. Prophylactic Saccharomyces boulardii in the prevention of antibiotic-associated diarrhea: a prospective study. *Med Sci Monit.* 2006;12:119–122.
71. McFarland L. Meta-analysis of probiotics for the prevention of antibiotic associated diarrhea and the treatment of Clostridium difficile disease. *Am J Gastroenterol.* 2006;101:812–822.

72. Surawicz C, McFarland LV, Greenberg RN, et al. The search for a better treatment for recurrent Clostridium difficile disease: use of high-dose vancomycin with Saccharomyces boulardii. *Clin Infect Dis*. 2000;31:1012–1017.
73. Koretz R. Probiotics, critical illness, and methodologic bias. *Nutr Clin Pract*. 2009;24:45–49.
74. Rayes N, Seehofer D, Hansen S, et al. Early enteral supply of lactobacillus and fiber versus selective bowel decontamination: a controlled trial in liver transplant recipients. *Transplantation*. 2002;74:123–128.
75. Jain P, McNaught CE, Anderson ADG, et al. Influence of synbiotic containing Lactobacillus acidophilus La5, Bifidobacterium lactis Bb 12, Streptococcus thermophilis, Lactobacillus bulgaricus and oligofructose on gut barrier function and sepsis in crically ill patients: a randomized controlled trial. *Clin Nutr*. 2004;2:467–475.
76. Alcao de Arruda I, de Aguilar-Nascimento JE. Benefits of early enteral nutrition with glutamine and probiotics in brain injury patients. *Clin Sci*. 2004;106:287–292.
77. McNaught C, Woodcock NP, Anderson ADG, et al. A propsective randomized trial of probiotics in critically ill patients. *Clin Nutr*. 2005;24:211–219.
78. Klarin B, Johansson ML, Molin G, et al. Adhesion of the probiotic bacterium Lactobacillus plantarum 299v onto the gut mucosa in critically ill patients: a randomised open trial. *Crit Care*. 2005;9:R285–R93.
79. Rayes N, Seehofer D, Theruvath T, et al. Supply of pre- and probiotics reduces bacterial infection rates after liver transplantation—a randomized, double-blind trial. *Am J Transplant*. 2005;5:125–130.
80. Kotzampassi K, Giamarellos-Bourboulis EJ, Voudouris A, et al. Benefits of a synbiotic formula (Synbiotic 2000Forte) in critically ill trauma patients: early results of a randomized controlled trial. *W. J. Surg*. 2006;30:1848–1855.
81. Spindler-Vesel A, Bengmark S, Vovk I, et al. Synbiotics, prebiotics, glutamine, or peptide in early enteral nturition: a randomized study in trauma patients. *J Parenter Enteral Nutr*. 2007;31:119–126.
82. Alberda C, Gramlich L, Meddings J, et al. Effect of probiotic therapy in critically ill patients: a randomized, double-blind, placebo-controlled trial. *Am J Clin Nutr*. 2007;85:816–823.
83. Rayes N, Seehofer D, Theruvath T, et al. Effect of enteral nutrition and synbiotics on bacterial infection rates after pylorus-preserving pancreatoduodenectomy. *Ann Surg*. 2007;246:36–41.
84. Olah A, Belagyi T, Poto L, et al. Synbiotic control of inflammation and infection in severe acute pancreatitis: a prospective randomized, double blind study. *Hepatogastroenterology*. 2007;54:590–594.
85. Olah A, Belagyi, T, Issekutz A, Gamal ME, et al. Randomized clinical trial of specific lactobacillus and fibre supplement to early enteral nutrition in patients with acute pancreatitis. *Br J Surg*. 2002;89:1103–1107.
86. Barraud D, Blard C, Hein F, et al. Probiotics in the critically ill patient: a double blind, randomized, placebo-controlled trial. *Intensive Care Med*. 2010;36:1540–1547.
87. Ferrie S, Daley M. Lactobacillus GG as a treatment for diarrhea during enteral feeding in critical illness: randomized controlled trial. *J Parenter Enteral Nutr*. 2011;35:43–49.
88. Parnell JA, Reimer RA. Weight loss during oligofructose supplementation is associated with decreased ghrelin and increased peptide YY in overweight and obese adults. *Am J Clin Nutr*. 2009;89:1751–1759.
89. McClave S, Martindale R, Vanek V, et al. Guidelines for the provision and assessment of nutrition support therapy in the adult critically ill patient. *J Parenter Enteral Nutr*. 2009;33:277–316.
90. Ley R, Turnbaugh PJ, Lkein S, et al. Microbial ecology: human gut microbes associated with obesity. *Nature*. 2006;444:1022–1023.
91. Turnbaugh P, Ridaura VK, Faith JJ, et al. The effect of diet on the human gut microbiome: a megagenomic analysis in humanized gnotobiotic mice. *Sci Transl Med*. 2009;1(6ra):14.
92. Duncan S, Lobley GE, Holtrop G, et al. Human colonic microbiota associated with diet, obesity and weight loss. *Int J Obes (Lond)*. 2008;32:1720–1724.
93. Zhang H, DiBaise JK, Zuccolo A, et al. Human gut microbiota in obesity and after gastric bypass. *Proc Natl Acad Sci U S A*. 2009;106:2365–2370.
94. Arumugam M, Raes J, Pelletier E, et al. Enterotypes of the human gut microbiome. *Nature*. 2011;473:174–180.
95. Kodooka Y, Sato M, Imaizumi K, et al.Regulation of abdominal adiposity by probiotics (Lactobacillus gasseri SBT2055) in adults with obese tendencies in a randomized controlled trial. *Eur J Clin Nutr*. 2010;64:636–643.
96. Hoyles L, McCartney AL. What do we mean when we refer to Bacteroidetes populations in the human gastrointestinal microbiota? *FEMS Microbiol Lett*. 2009;299:175–183.
97. Andreasen A, Larsen N, Pedersen-Skovsgaard T, et al. Effects of Lactobacillus acidophilus NCFM on insulin sensitivity and the systemic inflammatory response in human subjects. *Br J Nutr*. 2010;104:1831–1838.
98. Luoto R, Laitinen K, Nermes M, Isolauri E. Impact of maternal probioitc-supplemented dietary counselling on pregnanacy outcome and prenatal and postnatal growth: a double-blind, placebo-controlled study. *Br J Nutr*. 2010;103:1792–1799.
99. Takemura N, Okubo T, Sonoyama K. Lactobacillus plantarum strain No. 14 reduces adipocyte size in mice fed high-fat diet. *Exp Biol Med (Maywood)*. 2010;235:849–856.
100. Aronsson L, Huang Y, Parini P, et al. Decreased fat storage by Lactobacillus paracasei is associated with increased levels of angiopoietin-like 4 protein (ANGPTL4). *PLoS Biol*. 2010;5: pii–e13087.
101. Karlsson C, Molin G, Fak F, et al. Effects on weight-gain and gut mcirobiota in rats given bacterial supplements and a high-energy-dense diet from fetal life through to 6 months of age. *Br J Nutr*. 2011;6:1–9.
102. Abrams S, Griffin IJ, Hawthorne KM, et al. Effect of prebiotic supplementation and calcium intake on body mass index. *J Pediatr*. 2007;151:293–298.
103. Genta S, Cabrera W, Babib N, et al. Yacon syrup: beneficial effects on obesity and insulin resistance in humans. *Clin Nutr*. 2009;28: 182–187.
104. Roberfroid M. Prebiotics: The concept revisited. *J Nutrition*. 2007; 137:830S–837S.

5 Lipids

Mary Hise, PhD, RD, CNSD, and John C. Brown, PhD

CONTENTS

Background 64
General Lipid Structure 64
Fatty Acid Biochemistry and Nomenclature 65
Enteral Delivery and Metabolism of Dietary Lipids 66
Parenteral Delivery and Metabolism of Intravenous Fat Emulsions 67
Fatty Acid β-Oxidation 68
Lipid and Essential Fatty Acids Recommendations for Healthy Populations 68
Lipid and Essential Fatty Acids Recommendations for Individuals Requiring Specialized Nutrition Support 69
Manifestations of Essential Fatty Acid Deficiency in Patients on Specialized Nutrition Support 72
Eicosanoid Biosynthesis: ω-6 and ω-3 Fatty Acids 73
Clinical Effects of ω-6 Fatty Acids in Parenteral Nutrition 74
Clinical Effects of ω-3 Fatty Acids in Enteral Nutrition 74
Clinical Effects of ω-3 Fatty Acids in Parenteral Nutrition 75
Clinical Effects of ω-9 Fatty Acids in Enteral and Parenteral Nutrition 76
Short-Chain Fatty Acids 76
Medium-Chain Triglycerides 76
Structured Lipids 77
Emerging Data that Concern Intravenous Fat Emulsions and Parenteral Nutrition–Associated Liver Disease 77
References 77

Objectives

1. Describe the nomenclature, route of delivery, and requirements for lipids in the diet of healthy individuals and for those who require specialized nutrition support (SNS).
2. Identify the lipid components in enteral and parenteral formulations.
3. Discuss the clinical effects and biological activity of fatty acids in SNS.

Test Your Knowledge Questions

1. What are the ω-6 and ω-3 fatty acid–derived bioactive mediators that are particularly important to the return to homeostasis during an inflammatory response?
   A. Arachidonic acid (AA) and eicosapentaenoic acid (EPA)
   B. Lipoxins, the E- and D-series resolvins, and protectins
   C. Leukotriene B4 (LTB_4), prostaglandin E2 (PGE_2), leukotriene B5, and prostaglandin E3
   D. Linoleic acid and α-linolenic acid
2. What condition may occur and why, if a parenteral intravenous fat emulsion (IVFE) is provided only as 10% (weight per volume [w/v]) IVFE, such as propofol, or as high amounts of 20% (w/v) IVFE?
   A. Hypercholesterolemia and triglyceridemia may occur due to interference with chylomicron and pseudochylomicron metabolism.
   B. Essential fatty acid deficiency (EFAD) can occur because of the interference with normal lipid uptake.

C. Hyperoxidation of the microvilli of the small intestine may be induced due to the high amount of polyunsaturated fatty acids (PUFAs) in 10% IVFE.
D. Insulin resistance will occur due to the interaction of tocopherol with vitamin A within the emulsions.

3. Which ionized form of a short-chain fatty acid (SCFA; up to six carbons in length) is thought to be the most important to colonic health and why?
   A. Myristate
   B. Caproate
   C. Butyrate
   D. Valerate

Test Your Knowledge Answers

1. The correct answer is **B.** Lipoxins are produced during an inflammatory response by metabolism of AA. Among other properties, lipoxins inhibit chemotaxis of neutrophils and reduce inflammatory activity as a result. The E- and D-series resolvins are generated from EPA and docosahexaenoic acid (DHA), respectively, and serve to slow and eventually resolve inflammation. Protectins are substances derived from DHA that also play an active role in resolution of an inflammatory response. These substances, like lipoxin A_4, inhibit neutrophil migration. Protectins can also reduce the tissue damage due to stroke and help to protect the liver from inflammatory damage.
2. The correct answer is **A.** Hypercholesterolemia and triglyceridemia may occur due to interference with chylomicron and pseudochylomicron metabolism as one result of the presence of liposomes within the IVFE. Liposomes are formed during the emulsification process when parenteral IVFE is produced. These liposomes are usually metabolized similarly to that of pseudochylomicrons, but their presence may lead to the formation of a spherical bilayer of phospholipid and cholesterol known as lipoprotein-X. This lipoprotein inhibits both lipoprotein lipase and hepatic lipase enzymatic activity, and thus can interfere with the proper metabolism of the triglycerides (TGs) that are present as part of the structure of chylomicrons and pseudochylomicrons. This interference and the accumulation of endogenous cholesterol can subsequently lead to an increase in circulating TGs and cholesterol. Because 10% (w/v) IVFE contains a greater number of liposomes relative to 20% (w/v) IVFE as a result of the relative ratio of phospholipid emulsifier to oil, the former formulation places the patient more at risk for triglyceridemia.
3. The correct answer is **C.** SCFAs such as acetate, propionate, and butyrate are primarily produced in the colon by bacteria and can serve as important energy sources for colonic tissue. Butyrate in particular is thought to modify inflammatory activity and to promote colon health. For example, when applied directly to the colon, butyrate can attenuate the inflammatory activity seen in ulcerative colitis. In addition, the fermentation of carbohydrate (fiber) and the production of SCFAs in the colon, especially butyrate production, appear to act as antitumorigenic stimuli. Further, addition of sodium butyrate in vitro to endometrial cancer cell lines activates deoxyribonucleic acid repair systems and suppresses self-renewal of these cells.

Background

Lipids are biological substances that are soluble in organic solvents, such as methanol and chloroform, but insoluble in water. These molecules serve as important dietary sources of energy and in addition provide much of the critical structural and metabolically functional components of all biological membranes. Because of these properties, lipids contribute significantly to a remarkably broad range of cellular functions that are necessary for the maintenance and biological activity of healthy, living cells (Figure 5-1). Indeed, fatty acids such as AA, EPA, and DHA, discussed subsequently, are part of the makeup of membrane lipids. These particular fatty acids are important in development and are sources of critically important metabolic products that include inflammatory mediators (eicosanoids such as prostaglandins, leukotrienes, and thromboxanes), gene regulators, substances that assist in the resolution of an inflammatory response (eicosanoids such as protectins, resolvins, and lipoxins), and substances that regulate overall lipid metabolism.[1-5] In addition to these properties, specific fatty acids are also vitally important to membrane fluidity, membrane and intracellular cell signals, and modulation of apoptotic pathways.[6] This chapter will focus on general lipid structure, fatty acid biochemistry and nomenclature, lipid metabolism, and the clinical aspects of lipid provision in enteral and parenteral nutrition (PN).

General Lipid Structure

The basic TG structure consists of a glycerol backbone and various fatty acids attached in ester linkage at the carbon-1 (*sn*-1), carbon-2 (*sn*-2), and carbon-3 (*sn*-3) positions. TGs are the most abundant lipids in the body, but they do not serve as components of membranes. Instead, these substances serve as an important energy reserve for cells via the enzyme-dependent release, distribution, and oxidation of fatty acids. These energy-dense TGs, when stored as fat in tissues, provide by weight approximately 6-fold the energy available from the same weight of stored carbohydrate such as glycogen. The recoverable energy from a gram of fat versus a gram of carbohydrate stored in tissues is greater because of the lower level of oxidation of TGs relative to carbohydrate and the important fact that the weight contribution of water common to carbohydrates and proteins is missing from lipids. TGs circulate to a limited extent within the bloodstream but are more significantly stored within adipose tissue. The major constituents of the membrane lipid bilayer are phosphoglycerides. Two carbon positions on the glycerol backbone, *sn*-1 and *sn*-2, are esterified by fatty acids with the third available position, *sn*-3, occupied by a phosphate group in phosphoester linkage (1,2-diacylphosphoglycerides). The most abundant phospholipids found within membranes also have a polar group of some kind, such as ethanolamine, serine, or choline, attached to the phosphate moiety. As a consequence, membrane lipids

FIGURE 5-1 The Varied Roles of Fatty Acids in Cell Structure and Function

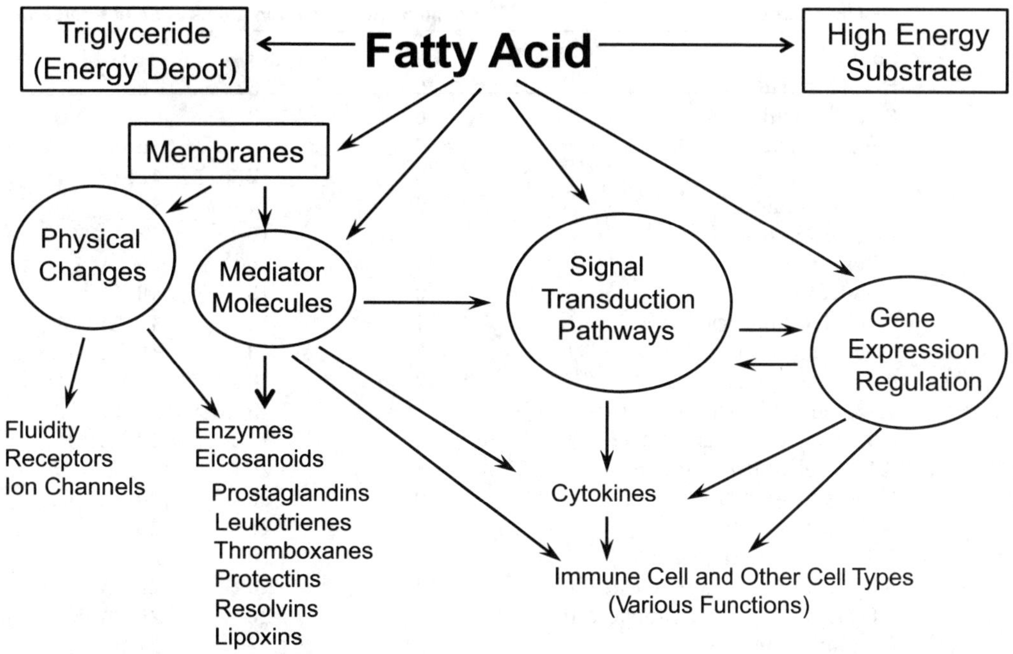

are amphipathic (or amphiphilic, "loving both"), meaning that they simultaneously possess both hydrophobic and hydrophilic characteristics. Thus, lipid bilayer membrane formation is possible when the aqueous environment external to and within cells leads the hydrocarbon portions (tails) of the two fatty acids within the phospholipid to associate in linear rows of phospholipids as opposing leaflets. The linear rows of polar groups face outward (aqueous environment outside the cell) on the external leaflet and inward (aqueous environment inside the cell) on the internal leaflet of the bilayer. Because of their organic solvent solubility, cholesterol and other sterols are classified as lipids. Cholesterol, itself an amphipathic molecule and the precursor of steroid hormones, is an integral constituent of animal cell membranes.

Fatty Acid Biochemistry and Nomenclature

Fatty acids are molecules with an acidic carboxyl group at one end followed by a long chain of hydrogenated hydrophobic carbon atoms (the hydrocarbon chain side group). Each fatty acid is chemically characterized by the number of carbon atoms (chain length) and double bonds (degree of saturation) present. The four general classifications of fatty acids with respect to the number of carbon atoms are short chain (2 to 4 carbons), medium chain (6 to 12 carbons), long chain (14 to 18 carbons), and very long chain (20 or more carbons). Because of the utilization of two carbon units (eg, acetyl-coenzyme A [CoA]) for fatty acid synthesis, almost all fatty acids have an even number of carbon atoms. Double-bond characteristics of fatty acids depend on the level of reduction of the hydrocarbon chain. Saturated fatty acids have all carbon atoms within the hydrocarbon chain completely reduced or "saturated" with hydrogen. In contrast, unsaturated fatty acids contain at least one double bond between two carbon atoms (thus, each carbon atom adjacent to the double bond has lost one hydrogen atom, is less reduced, and therefore less "saturated"). Those fatty acids with two or more double bonds within the hydrocarbon chain are known as PUFAs.

In Table 5-1, the various nomenclatures used to identify some of the more common biological fatty acids are shown. One nomenclature for identification of a particular fatty acid involves a system that reflects a combination of three numerical values, one of which includes the Greek alphabet's uppercase letter Delta (Δ). In this system, the carboxyl group of each fatty acid is considered to occupy the first, or numerical "1" position. For example, the essential, polyunsaturated, 18C-fatty acid, linoleic acid (9,12-octadecadienoic acid) would be designated as $18{:}2\Delta^{9,12}$. An additional system of nomenclature may also be used for PUFAs that in a short-hand fashion helps to identify different fatty acid families based on the last, relative to the carboxyl group, double-bond location. These fatty acid families are known as members of the ω (or *n*) series. In this system, the last double bond that occurs relative to the carboxyl group is designated with the lowercase Greek alphabet's letter omega (ω) (ie, the "last" or "end"). However, in this instance, the numerical position of this double bond is numbered relative to the final methyl group within the molecule. Thus, linoleic acid ($18{:}2\Delta^{9,12}$ in one system) would be denoted as a member of the ω-6 fatty acid family because the last double-bonded carbon atom occurs six carbon atoms from and including the methyl terminus of the hydrocarbon chain. One may also denote such molecules by substitution of

TABLE 5-1 Fatty Acid Nomenclature

Common Name	Chemical Name	Number of Double Bonds	Number of Carbon Atoms	Scientific Δ Double Bond Numbering	*n* and ω Numbering
Butyric acid	Butanoic acid	0	4	4:0	NA
Caproic acid	Hexanoic acid	0	6	6:0	NA
Caprylic acid	Octanoic acid	0	8	8:0	NA
Capric acid	Decanoic acid	0	10	10:0	NA
Lauric acid	Dodecanoic acid	0	12	12:0	NA
Myristic acid	Tetradecanoic acid	0	14	14:0	NA
Palmitic acid	Hexadecanoic acid	0	16	16:0	NA
Palmitoleic acid	9-hexadecenoic acid	1	16	$16{:}1\Delta^{9}$	16:1*n*-7 ω-7
Stearic acid	Octadecanoic acid	0	18	18:0	NA
Oleic acid	9-octadecenoic acid	1	18	$18{:}1\Delta^{9}$	18:1*n*-9 ω-9
Vaccenic acid	11-octadecenoic acid	1	18	$18{:}1\Delta^{11}$	18:1*n*-7 ω-7
Linoleic acid	9,12-octadecadienoic acid	2	18	$18{:}2\Delta^{9,12}$	18:2*n*-6 ω-6
α-Linolenic acid	9,12,15-octadecatrienoic acid	3	18	$18{:}3\Delta^{9,12,15}$	18:3*n*-3 ω-3
γ-Linolenic acid	6,9,12-octadecatrienoic acid	3	18	$18{:}3\Delta^{6,9,12}$	18:3*n*-6 ω-6
Di-homo-γ-linolenic acid	8,11,14-eicosatrienoic acid	3	20	$20{:}3\Delta^{8,11,14}$	20:3*n*-6 ω-6
Arachidic acid	Eicosanoic acid	0	20	20:0	NA
Gadoleic acid	9-eicosenoic acid	1	20	$20{:}1\Delta^{9}$	20:1*n*-9 ω-11
"Mead" acid	5,8,11-eicosatrienoic acid	3	20	$20{:}3\ \Delta^{5,8,11}$	20:3*n*-9 ω-9
Arachidonic acid	5,8,11,14-eicosatetraenoic acid	4	20	$20{:}4\Delta^{5,8,11,14}$	20:4*n*-6 ω-6
Eicosapentaenoic acid	5,8,11,14,17-eicosapentaenoic acid	5	20	$20{:}5\Delta^{5,8,11,14,17}$	20:5*n*-3 ω-3
Behenic acid	Docosanoic acid	0	22	22:0	NA
Erucic acid	13-docosenoic acid	1	22	$22{:}1\Delta^{13}$	22:1*n*-9 ω-9
Docosahexaenoic acid	4,7,10,13,16,19-docosahexaenoic acid	6	22	$22{:}6\Delta^{4,7,10,13,16,19}$	22:6*n*-3 ω-3
Lignoceric acid	Tetracosanoic acid	0	24	24:0	NA

NA, not applicable.

the italicized English alphabet letter *n*, for ω. When the *n* series designation is applied, a combinatorial use of systems is utilized. Thus, linoleic acid would be denoted as 18:2*n*-6 (ω-6 or *n*-6 family member).

Enteral Delivery and Metabolism of Dietary Lipids

Approximately 90% of dietary lipids are ingested in the form of TGs. These hydrophobic substances, because of the secreted presence of bile acids (salts), form micelles in the aqueous environment of the small intestine. Bile acids are amphipathic, detergent-like derivatives of cholesterol produced by the liver that emulsify TGs and esters of long-chain fatty acids (LCFAs). The emulsification process and micelle formation make TGs and fatty acid esters available for hydrolysis by intestinal lipases and esterases. This activity is critical for metabolism of long-chain TGs. Glycerol and fatty acids of up to 10 carbons in length can be absorbed directly via the villi of the intestinal mucosa and can enter the bloodstream through available capillaries. In addition, such fatty acids and glycerol can be directly transported to the liver by lipid carrier proteins. However, long-chain TGs require bile salts for both enzymatic digestion and formation of micelles. Enzymatic activity at the micelle–aqueous interface preferentially releases fatty acids from the *sn*-1 and *sn*-3 positions of the TG to form a mixture of free fatty acids and mono- and diglycerides. Because the presence of bile acids is required for this enzymatic activity to occur, both digestion and absorption of enteral lipids are dependent upon these compounds. Subsequently, the micelles that contain a mixture of free fatty acids and 2-monoacylglycerides are absorbed by the microvilli of the small intestine's epithelial cells. After absorption by the microvilli, the fatty acids within the micelles dissociate, diffuse across the epithelial cell membranes, and enter the cytoplasm. The bile salts are destined to return to the liver via the superior mesenteric and portal veins after reabsorption by the ileum of the small intestine. Inside the cytoplasm, the newly released free fatty acids, monoacylglycerols, and endogenous fatty acids are used for re-esterification into TGs. Circulation of lipids occurs in the form of lipoproteins that include chylomicrons (the largest in size), high-density lipoprotein (HDL), intermediate-density lipoprotein (IDL), low-density lipoprotein (LDL), and very-low-density lipoprotein (VLDL). Intestinal mucosal cells assemble chylomicrons that consist of a combination of dietary TGs, phospholipids, cholesterol, and specialized proteins.

Chylomicrons exit intestinal mucosal cells, enter the tissue lymphatic system, circulate, and eventually enter the bloodstream through the left subclavian vein via the thoracic duct. Acquisition of various apolipoproteins occurs in the blood and allows specific interaction of the chylomicron with various tissues. Lipids are delivered in the form of chylomicrons primarily to the liver and to specialized fat storage cells that comprise adipose tissue and also to the heart, skeletal muscle, and other organs. Lipoprotein lipase within the membranes of the capillary endothelial cells hydrolyzes the TG to free fatty acids and glycerol, which are absorbed by the different tissues. The hydrolysis of the chylomicron TG core over time results in a smaller and smaller circulating chylomicron enriched in cholesterol and proteins. This form of the chylomicron, known as a remnant, is eventually degraded by the liver via specific liver tissue receptors and is thus removed from the circulation. Endogenously (liver) synthesized cholesterol and TGs are converted within the liver to IDLs, LDLs, and VLDLs, enter the bloodstream, and are delivered to tissues. The gradual enzymatic degradation of VLDLs, first to IDLs and then finally to LDLs, occurs. TGs released by this process enter the tissues, and the LDL particles subsequently bind to specific membrane receptors and deliver cholesterol to the tissues. The return of cholesterol and various lipids from tissues to the liver is accomplished via HDLs. Thus, while LDLs deliver cholesterol to the tissues, HDLs scavenge this substance from the tissues and return the material to the liver where conversion of cholesterol to bile acids takes place. Loss of bile acids through intestinal transport effectively removes cholesterol from the tissues. It is for these reasons that LDLs are euphemistically known as "bad" cholesterol and HDLs as "good" cholesterol.

Parenteral Delivery and Metabolism of Intravenous Fat Emulsions

IVFEs are oil and water emulsions consisting of one or more TG-containing oils, glycerin, and a phospholipid emulsifier. Commercial parenteral IVFEs are provided in TG concentrations of 10%, 20%, and 30% (w/v). These emulsions may also contain other lipid-soluble substances such as vitamin E, vitamin K, phytosterols, and cholesterol. A selected list of the oils present in commercially available parenteral emulsions is shown in Table 5-2. These parenteral IVFEs are structurally designed to be similar to natural chylomicrons with respect to size, core TGs, and a monolayer of phospholipid. Similar to natural chylomicrons, these spherical pseudochylomicrons are 200 to 500 nm on average in diameter, and they have a central TGs core surrounded by a phospholipid (emulsifier) envelope.[7] In natural chylomicrons, the core TGs reflect dietary intake, while pseudochylomicrons contain a TGs core that consists of specific commercial oils. In addition to this difference, whereas natural chylomicrons enter the circulation bearing apolipoproteins and further acquire additional apolipoproteins from HDLs, pseudochylomicrons enter the circulation with no apolipoproteins but rapidly acquire them from HDLs.[8] Emulsifying agents, such as egg phosphatide, are used as a barrier to prevent coalescence of oil droplets of the emulsion. Liposomes, a spherical byproduct of the emulsifier used in the emulsification process, are less than 70 nm in diameter and consist primarily of a phospholipid bilayer that surrounds a trapped aqueous phase. Metabolism of each of these entities requires several stages, and the process begins immediately upon entrance into the bloodstream.

Pseudochylomicrons behave similarly to natural chylomicrons with respect to their metabolism. Once in the circulation, pseudochylomicrons acquire apolipoproteins and endogenous cholesterol, and through cell membrane and other lipoprotein interactions, exchange phospholipids. These dynamically changing pseudochylomicrons are efficiently transported in the circulation and engage tissue cell membranes. Cellular interaction (smooth and cardiac muscle and adipose tissue) exposes the pseudochylomicron to lipoprotein lipase activity, the result of which is the release of fatty acids from the TGs core and movement of free fatty acids into the cell. The degradation of the pseudochylomicrons in this manner ultimately results in the appearance of small, TG-poor pseudochylomicrons that are also known as remnants. Similar to natural chylomicron remnants, pseudochylomicron remnants are removed by the liver. Similarly, liposomes acquire apolipoproteins and undergo, in general, metabolic consequences similar to those

TABLE 5-2 Fat Composition of Selected Lipid Emulsions

			Excipients		Oil Content (gm/L)			
Emulsion Product	Lipid (%)	Caloric Content (kcal/L)	Glycerol (gm/L)	Egg Phosphatide (gm/L)	Soybean Oil	Olive Oil	MCT Oil	Fish Oil
ClinOleic®	20	2000	22.5	12	40	160	—	—
Intralipid®	20	2000	22.5	12	200	—	—	—
Ivelip®	20	2000	25	12	200	—	—	—
Lipofundin® MCT	20	1908	25	12	100	—	100	—
Lipofundin® N	20	2008	25	12	200	—	—	—
Lipoplus®	20	1910	25	12	80	—	100	20
Liposyn® III	20	2000	25	12	200	—	—	—
Lipovenoes®	20	2000	25	12	200	—	—	—
Omegaven®	10	1120	25	12	—	—	—	100
SMOFlipid®	20	2000	25	12	60	50	60	30
Structolipid®	20	1960	22	12	64% (w/w) LCT	—	36% (w/w) MCT	—

MCT, medium chain triglycerides; w/w, weight per weight.

of pseudochylomicrons. However, the formation of an abnormal lipoprotein, known as lipoprotein-X, can occur due to the presence of liposomes in the circulation. Lipoprotein-X is essentially a spherical bilayer of phospholipid and cholesterol. This abnormal protein, identified in obstructive jaundice and in congenital lecithin-cholesterol acyltransferase deficiency,[9,10] inhibits lipase activity (both lipoprotein lipase and hepatic lipase) toward natural and pseudochylomicrons. Consequently, a high concentration of lipoprotein-X in the circulation can inhibit lipid metabolism and lead to hypercholesterolemia and triglyceridemia.[6,7] The relative number of liposomes within an IVFE is dependent upon the oil content. Thus, a 10% (w/v) emulsion will contain a larger number of liposomes relative to a 20% (w/v) emulsion, because of the relative ratio of phospholipid emulsifier to oil. And, while most commercial IVFEs are available as 20% (w/v) formulations, other IVFEs used as vehicles for intravenous drug delivery (eg, propofol) are usually 10% (w/v) IVFE. Consequently, lipoprotein-X formation may still occur under certain circumstances and should be considered over the long-term or when high amounts of such lipid emulsions have been provided.

Fatty Acid β-Oxidation

The degradation (ie, catabolism) of fatty acids, whether saturated or unsaturated, even-chain or odd-chain, proceeds by oxidative pathways. As previously addressed, the oxidation of fatty acids (and/or lipid) releases substantially more energy than does oxidation of carbohydrate. This available energy can be used by cells to help meet the enormous energy demands required for various metabolic processes. The oxidation of fatty acids is, therefore, critically important to meeting nutritional energy demands. The most common pathway of oxidative degradation of fatty acids is known as β-oxidation and leads to degradation of fatty acids. The β-oxidation of even-chain fatty acids yields several molecules (equal to one-half the total number of carbons) of the two-carbon compound, acetyl-CoA. For example, complete β-oxidation of the 16-carbon, saturated fatty acid, palmitic acid would yield 8 moles of acetyl-CoA per mole of palmitic acid. Similar oxidation of odd-chain fatty acids also yields several molecules of acetyl-CoA and one molecule of propionyl-CoA (last oxidation step). Acetyl-CoA can directly enter the citric acid (Krebs) cycle, while propionyl-CoA is first converted to succinyl-CoA, which also can directly enter the citric acid cycle. An example of the substantial energy yield afforded by this oxidative process is the net synthesis of 129 moles of adenosine-5′-triphosphate per mole of palmitic acid (aerobic respiration coupled to oxidative phosphorylation) upon the complete β-oxidation of this fatty acid.

For β-oxidation to proceed, free fatty acids in the cytoplasm must first be transported into the mitochondrial matrix. Generally, fatty acids of up to 10 carbons in length may simply cross the mitochondrial membranes and reach the mitochondrial matrix without the requirement for special transport mechanisms. The first step in the β-oxidation of these molecules is the thioester linkage of CoA to the fatty acid by an acyl-CoA synthetase. Acyl-CoA synthetase enzymes are classified by their chain-length specificity. In contrast to the unrestricted movement of SCFAs into the mitochondrial matrix, LCFAs must be shuttled across the membranes by specific carrier and translocase mechanisms that require L-carnitine. The first step in this translocation process is the covalent connection of the fatty acids to CoA by acyl-CoA synthetases. These enzymes are located within the outer membranes of mitochondria. Once the fatty acid is activated in the mitochondrial outer membrane by addition of CoA, the acyl-CoA products enter the intermembrane space and are transported to the mitochondrial matrix by a specific L-carnitine shuttle system. Once the fatty acid-CoA derivative reaches the inner membrane surface, the fatty acid is transferred from CoA in ester linkage to the hydroxyl group of carnitine and subsequently translocated across the inner membrane to the matrix region. Before release from the inner membrane, the fatty acid–carnitine derivative associates with an enzyme that transfers the fatty acid from carnitine to CoA and the fatty acid–CoA derivative is released to the matrix. Carnitine is subsequently transported back across the inner membrane to the intermembrane space, and there can again participate in subsequent shuttles of CoA-activated fatty acids to the mitochondrial matrix. Once in the matrix, the fatty acid–CoA derivative is acted upon by several enzymes that progress down the length of the fatty acid from the carboxyl group to the last methyl group, to oxidize the fatty acid by two carbon lengths at a time (acetyl-CoA is produced). Each round of oxidation yields a remaining fatty acid that is two carbons shorter than the previous molecule. This activity repeats, round after round, until the entire fatty acid has been oxidatively degraded to several molecules of acetyl-CoA (or in the case of odd-numbered fatty acids, several molecules of acetyl-CoA and one molecule of propionyl-CoA). Unsaturated fatty acids undergo identical enzymatic conversion with the only exception being that of additional enzymatic steps to cope with a double bond. The double bond is essentially shifted in position, which allows a two-carbon segment to be oxidized and released as acetyl-CoA.

Lipid and Essential Fatty Acids Recommendations for Healthy Populations

The Dietary Reference Intakes (DRIs) are a comprehensive set of nutrient reference values for healthy populations that can be used for assessing and planning diets. Generally, the DRIs are based on research data from epidemiological, animal, and human studies. The Food and Nutrition Board of the Institute of Medicine determines the DRIs for macronutrients.[11] Specifically, this report provides guidelines that partitions energy sources in the form of an acceptable macronutrient distribution range (AMDR). The AMDR is defined as a range of intake for a particular energy source that is associated with a reduced risk of chronic disease while providing adequate intakes (AIs) of essential nutrients. An AMDR has been set for total fat, ω-6, and ω-3 PUFAs. This evidence-based range was established to ensure sufficient intake of essential lipids and to provide a dietary guide to aid in prevention of chronic diseases that may be associated with diets higher in fat. A tolerable upper intake

TABLE 5-3 Criteria and Dietary Reference Intake Values for n-6 (Linoleic Acid) and n-3 (α-Linolenic Acid)

		Adequate Intake (g/day)[a]	
Age Range	Criterion	Male	Female
19–30 years	Median Intake of linoleic acid from CFSII	17	12
31–50 years	Median Intake of linoleic acid from CFSII	17	12
51–70 years	Median Intake of linoleic acid from CFSII	14	11
19–30 years	Median Intake of α-linolenic acid from CFSII	1.6	1.1
31–50 years	Median Intake of α-linolenic acid from CFSII	1.6	1.1
51–70 years	Median Intake of α-linolenic acid from CFSII	1.6	1.1

CSF II, Continuing Survey of Food Intake by Individuals.
[a]The observed average or experimentally determined intake by a defined population or subgroup that appears to sustain a defined nutrition status, such as growth rate, normal circulating nutrient values, or other functional indicators of health. The adequate intake is used if sufficient evidence is not available to drive an estimated average requirement.

level has not been set for total fat or ω-6 or ω-3 fatty acids because of the lack of a specific intake level that may result in an adverse effect (ie, obesity, immune dysfunction). The AMDR for fat is a dietary intake that meets 20% to 35% of the total energy requirements for adults. In addition to an AMDR, ω-6 and ω-3 fatty acids have an AI level (Table 5-3) based on median intakes of linoleic acid and α-linolenic acid obtained from the Continuing Survey of Food Intakes by Individuals. Adequate intake is defined as "the observed average or experimentally determined intake by a defined population or subgroup that seems to sustain a defined nutrition status, such as growth rate, normal circulating nutrient values, or other functional indicators of health." The AI is used if sufficient evidence is not available to drive an estimated average requirement. The estimated average requirement is defined as "the average daily nutrient intake level estimated to meet the requirement of half the healthy individuals in a particular life stage and gender group."[11]

The presence of either ω-6 or ω-3 fatty acid deficiency is almost nonexistent in a free-living population. For ω-6 fatty acids, a rarity of deficiency may be due to the fact that linoleic acid accounts for 85% to 90% of the ω-6 fatty acids in the western diet.[12] Usual food intakes that meet or exceed the AI for linoleic acid and α-linolenic acid are assumed to be adequate. The lower AMDR boundary level of 5% of total energy will meet the AI for linoleic acid, while the upper boundary level is set at 10% of total energy intake. The percentage value used for the upper boundary limit for linoleic acid intake was determined based on the following information: (1) the usual intake of linoleic acid rarely exceeds 10% of total calories, (2) epidemiological safety data on levels that exceed this range are lacking, and (3) elevated levels of linoleic acid in the diet may create pro-oxidant states that could influence disease development. The average U.S. intake of linoleic acid, according to National Health and Nutrition Examination Survey 2001–2002 data for adults, is 14.8 g/day.[13] If this value is considered with a 2000 kcal/day diet, linoleic acid results in approximately 6.7% of energy intake. Because of the wide variability of linoleic acid content among enteral formulas, however (Table 5-4), dietary intake of linoleic acid among exclusively tube-fed patients may differ significantly from average U.S. intakes. The American Heart Association supports an ω-6 fatty acid intake of 5% to 10% of energy. An AMDR for α-linolenic acid is estimated to be 0.6% (lower limit) to 1.2% (upper limit) of energy requirements. The lower limit of the α-linolenic acid AMDR was based on the lowest level of intake (0.6%) that met the AI level. The upper boundary limit of the AMDR (1.2%) corresponds to the highest α-linolenic acid intake from foods consumed by individuals in the United States and Canada. No DRIs have been established for EPA or DHA at this time.

Lipid and Essential Fatty Acids Recommendations for Individuals Requiring Specialized Nutrition Support

Because the AMDR is designed to be met from a usual diet for healthy individuals, it is not designed to provide lipid and specific fatty acid recommendations for individuals with acute and chronic diseases. Recommendations of percentage and type of lipid provided to persons requiring SNS may differ depending on injury or disease manifestations. Similar to AMDR recommendations to provide adequate intakes of essential fatty acids (EFAs), recommendations to prevent EFAD in persons requiring SNS remain relatively similar (ie, 2% to 4% of total calories in the form of linoleic and 0.25% to 0.5% of total calories in the form of α-linolenic acid). A variety of plant oils have been used as the lipid source to provide essential fatty acids for patients requiring SNS. As shown in Table 5-5, soybean and corn oil are rich sources of linoleic acid that contain, respectively, 54% and 61% of this fatty acid. Soybean and canola oils are each good sources of α-linolenic acid that provide 7% and 10%, respectively, of this EFA. To meet EFAD requirements, commercial enteral formulas employ a variety of these oils in their formula composition, including corn, soybean, safflower, and canola oils (Table 5-4). There is no absolute recommendation for a given enteral formula's lipid content; consequently, as demonstrated by Table 5-4, the lipid content of common enteral formulas varies widely. Generally, elemental products provide the least amount of fat in commercial enteral formulas. In contrast, polymeric enteral products often provide $>$ 25% of calories in the form of fat, and this percentage rises as formulas are concentrated into more calorie-dense solutions. For the provision of PN in the United States, commercially available IVFEs are composed of soybean oil. Soybean oil–based emulsions contain approximately 55% to 60% of total calories as linoleic acid and 3% to 4% of total calories as α-linolenic acid. In other regions of the world, commercial IVFEs are also designed to meet EFA requirements and are composed of soybean oil but may also contain olive, fish, or medium-chain TG oils in varying ratios. By supplying part of the lipid component as soybean oil,

TABLE 5-4 Fat Composition of Selected Enteral Formulas

Formula	Fat (% kcal)	Fat (Source)	Fat (g/L)	Linoleic (g/L)	MCTs (g/L)	n-3 Fatty Acids (g/L)
Compleat	34.0	Canola, residual chicken, soy lecithin	40	8	0	3.1
Diabetisource AC	44.0	Canola, refined menhaden	60	10	0	5.2
Fibersource HN	29.0	Canola, MCTs	39	5.7	7.8	2.1
Glucerna 1.0 Cal	49.0	High-oleic safflower, canola oils	54.4	7.7	0.1	0.7
Impact	25.0	Palm kernel, refined menhaden, safflower, soy lecithin, high oleic sunflower	28.0	2.4	7.6	1.7
Impact with Fiber	25.0	Palm kernel, refined menhaden, safflower, soy lecithin, high oleic sunflower	28.0	2.4	0.0	1.7
Impact with Glutamine	30.0	Palm kernel, refined menhaden, safflower, high oleic sunflower	43.0	3.9	0.0	2.7
Impact Peptide 1.5	38.0	MCTs, fish (anchovy, sardine), canola, soybean, soy lecithin	63.6	8.3	31.8	6.1
Isosource 1.5 Cal	38.0	Canola, MCTs, soybean	65.0	14.0	19.5	3.4
Isosource HN	29.0	Canola, MCTs	39.0	6.3	7.8	2.3
Jevity 1 Cal	29.0	Canola oil, corn oil, medium chain triglycerides, soy lecithin	34.7	10.0	6.6	1.5
Nepro with Carb Steady	48.0	High oleic safflower, canola oils	96.0	14.3	0.0	2.9
Novasource Renal	45.0	Canola, soy lecithin	100.0	18.4	0.0	9.9
Nutren 1.0	33.0	Canola, MCTs, corn, soy lecithin	38.0	7.9	9.5	1.9
Nutren 1.0 Fiber	33.0	Canola, MCTs, corn, soy lecithin	38.0	7.9	9.5	1.9
Nutren 1.5	39.0	MCTs, canola, corn oil, soy lecithin	67.6	10.4	33.8	2.4
Nutren 2.0	45.0	MCTs, canola, soy lecithin, corn	104.0	7.8	7.8	1.7
Nutren Glytrol	42.0	Canola, high oleic safflower, MCTs	47.6	6.7	9.5	1.9
Nutren Pulmonary	55.0	MCTs, canola, corn, soy lecithin	94.8	15.9	37.9	3.9
Nutren Replete	30.0	Canola, MCTs, soy lecithin	34.0	4.9	8.5	2.1
Nutren Replete Fiber	30.0	Canola, MCTS, soy lecithin	34.0	4.9	8.5	2.1
NutriHep	12.0	MCTs, canola, corn, soy lecithin	21.2	2.0	14.0	0.5
Optimental	25.0	Marine oil/MCT structured lipid, canola oil,soybean oil	28.4	4.2	8.0	4.8
Osmolite 1 Cal	29.0	Canola, corn oils, MCTs, soy lecithin	34.7	9.5	6.9	1.8
Oxepa	55.2	Canola, MCTs, marine, borage oils, soy lecithin	93.8	15.0	23.5	11.7
Peptamen	33.0	MCTs, soybean, soy lecithin	39.0	5.1	27.3	0.7
Peptamen 1.5	33.0	MCTs, soybean, soy lecithin	56.0	5.9	39.2	0.8
Peptamen AF	39.0	MCTs, soybean, fish, soy lecithin	54.8	6.5	27.4	3.6
Peptamen Bariatric	33.0	MCTs, fish (anchovy, sardine), high linoleic safflower, soy lecithin, soybean, sunflower	38.0	4.3	18.4	2.4
Peptamen Prebio	33.0	MCTs, soybean, soy lecithin	39.2	5.1	27.4	0.7
Perative	25.0	Canola, MCTs, corn oil, soy lecithin	37.3	6.8	14.9	1.2
Pivot	30.0	Marine oil/MCT structured lipid, soy oil, canola oil, soy lecithin	50.8	10.6	9.5	7.0
Promote	23.0	Soy oil, MCTs, safflower oil, soy lecithin	26.0	10.9	4.9	1.1
Pulmocare	55.1	Canola, MCTs, corn, high-oleic safflower oils, soy lecithin	93.3	18.4	18.7	4.8
RenalCal	35.0	MCTs, canola oils, soy lecithin	82.4	6.2	57.7	1.8
Resource 2.0	40.0	Canola, soy lecithin	88.0	16.0	0.0	8.6
Suplena with Carb Steady	48.0	High-oleic safflower, canola oils	96.0	14.3	0.0	2.9
Tolerex[a]	2.0	Safflower	1.8	1.2	0.0	0.0
Vivonex Plus[a]	6.0	Soybean	6.6	3.4	0.0	0.5
Vivonex T.E.N.[a]	3.0	Safflower	2.6	2.2	0.0	0.0
Vivonex RTF	10.0	Soybean, MCTs	12	3.3	4.8	0.5
Vital 1.0 Cal	33	Canola oil/MCT structured lipid, canola oil, MCT, DATEM	38.1	3.5	18	1.6
Vital 1.5 Cal	33	Canola oil/MCT structured lipid, canola oil, MCT, DATEM	57.1	5.5	27	2.5
Vital AF 1.2 Cal	39	Marine oil/MCT structured lipid, MCT, canola,oil soy oil, DATEM	53.9	6.3	24	7.3
Vital HN[a]	9.5	Safflower oil, MCT, monoglycerides, soy lecithin	10.8	3.6	4.7	0.02
TwoCal HN	40.1	High oleic safflower oil, MCT, canola oil, soy lecithin	90.5	10.8	17.4	1.6

DATEM, diacetyl tartaric acid esters of mono-diglycerides; MCT, medium chain triglycerides.
[a]One-liter reconstituted product.

TABLE 5-5 Comparison of Dietary Fatty Acids in Common Oils

	Breakdown of Fatty Acid Content (Normalized to 100%)			
Dietary Fat	Saturated Fatty Acids	Linoleic Acid	Alpha-Linolenic Acid	Monounsaturated Fatty Acid
Canola oil	6	22	10	62
Safflower oil	10	77	trace	13
Sunflower oil	11	69	0	20
Corn oil	13	61	0	25
Olive oil	14	8	1	77
Soybean oil	15	54	7	24
Peanut oil	18	33	0	49
Palm oil	45	12	1	37
Palm kernel oil	52	10	1	11
Coconut oil	92	2	0	6
Cod liver oil*	23	1	1	47

*Cod liver oil averages approximately 27% eicosapentaenoic acid and docosahexaenoic acid. Wardlaw GM. *Perspectives in Nutrition.* 4th ed. New York: McGraw-Hill; 1999. Adapted with permission from The McGraw-Hill Companies.

requirements of both α-linolenic and linoleic acids may be met concomitantly for individuals requiring SNS.

To meet EFA requirements in PN patients with 100% soybean oil–based IVFEs, a variety of lipid regimens may be prescribed. Often, 500 mL of 20% IVFE may be given weekly or 500 mL of 10% IVFE may be given three times per week to prevent an EFAD.[14] The amount of lipid that should be provided to patients requiring SNS remains controversial. It is recognized that SNS patients require a mixed substrate of carbohydrate and lipids to meet metabolic and energy needs. The ideal amount of lipids to administer to SNS patients remains unknown; however, lipid recommendations usually exceed quantities necessary to prevent EFAD. Reasons for inclusion of higher levels of lipid in the diet have been based on the knowledge that (1) lipids provide the highest energy yield of fuel substrates, (2) oxidative metabolism of lipid produces less carbon dioxide when compared to similar glucose loads, (3) specific fatty acids may potentially modify immune and inflammatory responses, and (4) a "mixed fuel" system may reduce adverse metabolic conditions seen when fat-free PN is administered. In PN, the "mixed fuel" concept decreases risk of exceeding glucose infusion recommendations and improves metabolic tolerance. Fat-free PN products have been associated with larger glucose loads, hyperglycemia, limited glucose oxidation, and hepatic dysfunction.[15] In the literature for SNS, enteral fat recommendations range from 15% to 50% of total calories, depending on disease states.[16] In metabolically stressed patients, an enteral fat range of 25% to 30% of total kilocalories has been proposed.[16]

Animal and human studies in burns have clearly demonstrated that a higher-carbohydrate, lower-fat diet (3% to 15% of total calories) may be associated with decreased protein losses and improved outcomes.[17-20] Additionally, the Society of Critical Care Medicine and American Society for Parenteral and Enteral Nutrition (A.S.P.E.N.) guidelines for critically ill patients recommend not administering soybean-based IVFEs during the first week of hospitalization. The recommendation is based upon limited randomized control trial evidence that suggests soybean-based IVFEs induce immunosuppression and increase morbidity.[21] On the other hand, in enteral studies of patients in the intensive care unit with acute respiratory distress syndrome, clinical benefits were shown with a higher enteral lipid dose when the fat source was significantly shifted toward an ω-3 fatty acid profile.[22-24] Recommendations from A.S.P.E.N. clinical guidelines support the use of a modified enteral formula characterized by an anti-inflammatory lipid profile (containing ω-3 fatty acids, borage oil, and antioxidants) in patients with acute respiratory distress syndrome and patients with severe acute lung injury (Grade A evidence).[21] Historically, higher enteral fat formulas have garnered some interest in pulmonary disease because of theoretical advantages demonstrated with lower carbon dioxide production; however, routine use of higher-fat, lower-carbohydrate enteral formulas in pulmonary disease is not supported at this time.[21] Current enteral fat recommendations are driven primarily by disease state and must be considered in context with the quantity and kind(s) of lipid provided (see disease-specific chapters for further discussion regarding lipid recommendations). In adult patients requiring PN, IVFEs should not exceed 2.5 g lipid/kg/day.[25] In critically ill patients requiring PN, the recommendations are more consistently conservative with some data supporting ≤ 1.0 g lipid/kg per day.[25-27] These recommendations for lipid provision are based on evidence that the potential for metabolic adverse reactions associated with rapid infusion and excessive amounts of parenteral lipids may be reduced while simultaneously improving capacity for lipid clearance. Lipid infused at the maximum recommended rate for the critically ill of 1.0 g/kg/day corresponds to approximately 30% of total calories (Practice Scenario 5-1). Additional recommendations for IVFEs also include an infusion rate not to exceed 0.11 g/kg/h in order to prevent potential adverse reactions or toxicities associated with rapid infusion.[28]

Practice Scenario 5-1

Question: What strategies can prevent adverse metabolic outcomes when propofol is used concomitantly with nutrition support?

Scenario: A 65-year-old female with a past medical history of renal insufficiency and type 2 diabetes mellitus was involved in a motor vehicle accident in which she sustained multiple abdominal injuries including laceration of her spleen and a jejunal tear. On postoperative day 4, her clinical condition declined. The patient required vasopressor administration and was in respiratory failure. Upon examination, her abdomen was firm and distended. A kidney, ureter, and bladder x-ray was consistent with postoperative ileus. Since admission, the patient received a continuous infusion of propofol (Diprivan 1%, Astra Zeneca Pharmaceuticals, Wilmington, DE) for sedation. Average propofol administration was relatively constant at 25 mL/h (3.57 mg/kg/h), providing approximately 60 g of fat, or 660 cal/24 h.

Anthropometrics: height: 165 cm; weight: 70 kg
Metabolic cart: resting energy expenditure: 2100; respiratory quotient: 0.78
Diet order: Trophic enteral feeding
Serum electrolytes: Within normal limits
Serum TGs: Day 4: 300 mg/dl; Day 6: 550 mg/dl

Intervention: On day 5 of admission, the patient has failed trophic enteral feedings and her diet order was changed to a 3-in-1 PN prescription containing 40 g of a 20% IVFE.

Answer: Metabolic cart measurements indicate that propofol alone is currently providing 31.4% of the patient's energy requirements, or 0.86 g lipid/kg of body weight. With the addition of 40 grams of a 20% IVFE as part of the PN prescription, this patient will receive 1.4 g fat/kg/day. Current propofol administration alone provides an acceptable level of lipid dose for this patient (< 1.0 g fat/kg/day). Because of the elevated serum TG level and potential variation in propofol administration, serum TG concentration should be monitored frequently (ie, twice per week). To lower total fat dose and to possibly improve TG clearance, lipids should be removed from the PN solution. Recommendations for acceptable serum TG levels are < 250 mg/dL 4 hours after IVFE infusion for "piggy-backed" lipids and < 400 mg/dL for continuous IVFE infusion.[29]

Rationale: The patient was at significant risk for hypertriglyceridemia by virtue of her history of diabetes, renal insufficiency, critical illness, and propofol infusion. The presence of the higher concentration of phospholipids in 10% IVFE (used as the drug vehicle for propofol) may result in an increase in lipoprotein X particles that compete with TG-rich particles for lipoprotein lipase. This competition for lipase activity may lead to less TG hydrolysis, with the concomitant result of an increase in circulating TGs.

Manifestations of Essential Fatty Acid Deficiency in Patients on Specialized Nutrition Support

EFAD was documented in animals by Burr and Burr in 1929.[30] It was not until the development of PN four decades later that EFAD was demonstrated in humans. During this time period in the early 1970s and 1980s, biochemical and clinical manifestations of EFAD (both linoleic and α-linolenic fatty acids) began to occur in patients requiring PN for extended periods of time (2 to 4 weeks).[31–34] The predominant clinical changes associated with linoleic acid deficiency are characterized by a dry, scaly skin rash. However, other clinical symptoms have been noted including increased susceptibility to infection, impaired wound healing, and immune dysfunction.[35–37] Biochemical changes that occur in response to linoleic acid deficiency are manifested by a fall in both linoleic acid and AA (tetraenoic acid) and a rise in Mead acid (triene acid, 20:3*n*-9; Table 5-1). Mead acid is primarily produced in humans in the absence of EFAs. A triene:tetraene ratio of > 0.2 (Holman Index) has been used to identify the presence of EFAD.[38] The time required to exhibit an EFAD in adults is variable, based upon underlying disease and nutritional status. EFAD may occur rapidly in continuous fat-free PN administration because of elevated insulin levels that prevent adipose tissue lipolysis. Usually, EFAD may be seen in patients after 4 weeks of fat-free PN, although clinical signs may be detected earlier (ie, between 10 and 20 days).[32,39,40] Hypocaloric fat-free PN or a cyclic feeding schedule of fat-free PN may extend the period of time before EFAD is exhibited (Practice Scenario 5-2). When PN is cycled or hypocaloric PN is provided, it is thought that EFAs are mobilized and enter the circulation as a result of increased lipolysis of endogenous fat stores in response to a reduction in serum insulin concentration. In addition, hypocaloric feeding prevents the risk of hepatic dysfunction that may occur if the caloric deficit (caused by the removal of lipids) is corrected by increasing the dextrose or protein calories to maintain energy requirements. When IVFEs are contraindicated, short-term, hypocaloric, fat-free PN has been shown to be safe and appropriate for the critically ill patient.[41] In contrast to linoleic acid, α-linolenic acid deficiency has been less well recognized with clear evidence of deficiency not reported until 1982 in a case study by Holman and colleagues.[31] Unlike the manifestations seen in linoleic acid deficiency, eicosatrienoic acid remains within normal range, and no skin rash is detectable when the diet is deficient of only α-linolenic acid. Deficiency of this nutrient was documented in a 6-year-old female who had been maintained on PN solution lacking α-linolenic acid. The observed symptoms of deficiency were primarily neurological abnormalities that included numbness, paresthesia, blurred vision, and difficulties in walking.

An additional report of α-linolenic acid deficiency appeared several years later that involved elderly nursing home residents who were receiving intragastric feeding of an elemental formula that did not contain α-linolenic acid.[42] With the addition of α-linolenic acid to these elderly patients' diet, clinical symptoms disappeared. Interestingly, Heird and Lapillonne[43] have reported that the metabolites of either linoleic acid metabolism (ie, γ-linolenic acid [GLA], dihomo-γ-linolenic acid [DGLA], and AA) or α-linolenic acid metabolism (ie, EPA and DHA) may correct the clinical symptoms of EFAD. Additionally, recent data suggest that AA, EPA, and DHA alone may satisfy the EFA requirements for humans. In studies of children who received fish oil monotherapy, none of the patients expressed biochemical parameters or other indications of EFAD after a minimum of 30 days of treatment.[44] A review of these and other data is presented by Le et al.[2] However, the issue remains undetermined whether linoleic acid and/or α-linolenic acid per se have specific functional properties that cannot be met by provision of their fatty acid metabolites. Evidence has suggested that the risk of EFAD is increased in some patients who require home PN solutions.[45–47] Evaluation of the EFA status of home PN patients has revealed alterations in fatty acid profiles (decrease of linoleic acid plasma levels, increases in AA plasma levels, and an increase in AA/linoleic acid ratio) and biochemical signs associated with EFAD.[46–49] Intravenous fat emulsions may not be required or provided for all patients receiving home PN, and data are lacking that indicate the optimal amount of EFAs required for these patients. Home PN patients may be at risk for adverse events because of the amount of dietary fat consumed, the degree of intestinal inefficiency, the frequency of IVFE provided in the PN solution, and the availability of endogenous lipid stores. Ling et al[48] have demonstrated that linoleic acid provided at 3.2% of total calories with an average of 0.24 ± 0.13 g fat/kg/day is sufficient to prevent the development of EFAD in home PN patients. Additional data have been reported demonstrating a minimum of 1.0 g fat/kg/body weight weekly or 500 mL of 20% IVFE weekly may be necessary to correct or avoid biochemical alterations associated with EFAD.[46,50]

Practice Scenario 5-2

Question: How can essential fatty acid deficiency be prevented when a lipid-free PN regimen is initiated in the intensive care unit?

Scenario: A 37-year-old male was admitted to a regional hospital due to pneumonia. He has a history of drug abuse and is a heavy smoker (20 to 30 cigarettes/day) and reports very poor food intake for the last month. Family members report that he has lost a significant amount of weight, but the family could not quantify the amount of loss (no scales at home). The patient experienced respiratory failure on hospital day 3 and was transferred to the intensive care unit. On hospital day 4, the patient exhibited clinical signs of an ileus, which was confirmed by x-ray. On hospital day 6, the patient's condition worsened, and a diagnosis of sepsis with acute respiratory distress syndrome was made. Patient failed enteral advancement on hospital day 4, and the tube feeding was discontinued.

Anthropometrics: height: 172 cm; weight: 102 kg; body mass index: 34.5
Serum TG values: Day 3: 598 mg/dl; Day 4: 467 mg/dl; Day 6: 486 mg/dl
Serum glucose: 167 to 232 mg/dl (range during hospitalization)
Metabolic cart Day 6: measured energy expenditure: 2346 kcal; respiratory quotient: 0.80
Protein requirements: 2 g/kg ideal body weight

Intervention: On hospital day 7 of admission, fat-free PN prescription was ordered that met 100% of energy and protein requirements.

Answer: Do not prescribe aggressive caloric regimens in critically ill patients at risk for re-feeding and cardiovascular complications. In this case, to prevent excessive glucose administration and to improve the possibility of mobilizing EFAs from endogenous lipid stores, a fat-free hypocaloric feeding regimen should be initiated slowly (50% of goal calories) with a goal to achieve 80% of estimated energy requirements.[21] After approximately 14 days of a fat-free PN regimen, or when clinical signs and symptoms indicate, plasma fatty acid profiles should be obtained to assess the patient for risk of EFAD. Evidence of EFAD may be detected biochemically in the plasma by an increase in oleic and palmitoleic acids and a decrease in linoleic and arachidonic acids. In EFAD, 5,8,11-eicosatrienoic acid is also present. Excessive percentages of palmitoleic and oleic acids in a fatty acid profile may be indicative of EFAD.

Rationale: Patients should be monitored for EFAD if all sources of lipids are removed from the diet for more than 2 to 4 weeks. Providing 2% to 5% of the caloric requirement as linoleic acid (as little as 8 g/day) may correct EFA insufficiency. In clinical terms, 4% to 10% of total calories from soybean emulsions will provide sufficient EFAs. Initiation of low-dose or trophic enteral feeding may also be used to offset risk of EFAD. A polymeric enteral formula (1.0 kcal/mL, 30% fat) composed of both soybean and a mixture of other high linoleic oils may be used. Providing 10% of total calorie requirements by the enteral formula will supply adequate essential fatty acids.

Eicosanoid Biosynthesis: ω-6 and ω-3 Fatty Acids

Fatty acids are not only necessary for proper membrane and other functions, they are also indirectly involved as metabolic precursors for lipid substances known as eicosanoids that can profoundly affect platelet aggregation, neurotransmitter release, vascular function, infection responses, inflammatory activity, and immune system activity.[16,51,52] Eicosanoids are substances that contain 20 carbons and include prostaglandins, leukotrienes, thromboxanes, prostacyclins, lipoxins, resolvins, and, protectins (neuroprotectins). Consequently, under certain conditions these byproducts of fatty acid metabolism can have far-ranging and potentially detrimental effects. Members of the ω-6 and ω-3 series of fatty acids (AA and EPA, respectively) are the precursors for the intracellular synthesis of inflammatory eicosanoids. The most common dietary sources of ω-6 fatty acids are plants such as soybean, safflower, and corn. Plant dietary sources of ω-3 fatty acids are found in canola oil, flax seed, and leafy vegetables. Other sources are derived from fish and may include tuna, sardines, and salmon. AA may be ingested in the diet via intake of meat and/or organ tissue. However, this lipid is also synthesized when dietary linoleic acid is desaturated by the enzyme Δ6-desaturase to form GLA (18:3*n*-6), which in turn is converted by elongation enzyme 2-carbon addition to form DGLA (20:3*n*-6). This compound is desaturated by Δ5-desaturase to form, in the final reaction of this pathway, AA. The ω-3 fatty acid, α-linolenic acid (18:3*n*-3), is the essential fatty acid that is the precursor of EPA and DHA, although the enzymatic conversion of α-linolenic acid to EPA and DHA is inefficient. Although EPA and DHA may be somewhat enzymatically interconvertible (alternate pathways may exist), the most efficient source of EPA and DHA is via the diet. Both EPA and DHA are critical to development of proper eyesight and brain function, and EPA is the precursor of the less biologically active inflammatory mediators of the 3-series prostaglandins and 5-series leukotrienes eicosanoid series. Other anti-inflammatory prostaglandins and clot-inhibiting thromboxanes of the 1-series, however, may be synthesized from DGLA (ω-6), one of the intermediates in the AA synthesis pathway.

AA, common to membrane phospholipids, usually occupies the *sn*-2 position and is almost always found at this position within the important membrane phospholipid, phosphatidylinositol. During membrane cell signaling events, one possible outcome is the activation of phospholipase A_2, the enzyme that acts upon membrane phospholipids to release fatty acids from the *sn*-2 position.[53] Release of AA sets in motion subsequent intracellular metabolic activity via the cyclooxygenase pathway that leads to the synthesis of the 2-series of prostaglandins, including PGE_2, and thromboxanes, including thromboxane A_2. AA is initially converted to prostaglandin H_2 by the cyclooxygenase enzymes COX-1 and COX-2. Subsequently, prostaglandin H_2, as substrate for prostaglandin synthesis, is converted to the various prostaglandins that include PGD_2, PGE_2, $PGF_{2\alpha}$, PGI_2, and 15-d-PGJ_2. The enzyme COX-1 is generally thought to be constitutively expressed in almost all bodily tissues and is involved in many bodily "housekeeping" activities. The enzyme COX-2, on the other hand, is an inducible enzyme that is directly involved in inflammation.[54,55] Entrance of AA into the lipoxygenase pathway leads to the synthesis of the 4-series leukotrienes that include LTB_4. The 2-series of prostaglandins and thromboxanes are powerful inflammatory mediators that can induce significantly detrimental inflammatory effects. For example, PGE_2 has been extensively studied and is a known immunosuppressant.[56–58] In contrast, ω-3 fatty acid–derived 1- and 3-series prostaglandins and thromboxanes and 5-series leukotrienes (via COX-1 and -2 and lipoxygenases) are less immunosuppressive and less inflammatory. For example, thromboxane A_2 strongly stimulates platelet aggregation and vasoconstriction. In contrast, platelets fail to aggregate and vasoconstriction is mild at best in the presence of thromboxane A_3.[59,60]

Additionally, ω-3 fatty acids are competitive inhibitors of 2- and 4-series eicosanoid formation from AA and thus their physiological availability directly influences synthesis of these substances.[61] Because of these desirable consequences, provision of ω-6 fatty acids such as GLA and/or DGLA in addition to the ω-3 fatty acid EPA in the diet may serve to attenuate inflammatory events.[62] AA, EPA, and DHA are also the precursors of novel anti-inflammatory eicosanoids (ie, lipoxins, resolvins, and protectins) that have critical roles in the active resolution of an inflammatory response. Lipoxins are metabolic derivatives of AA that are generated during an inflammatory response but serve as powerful anti-inflammatory mediators. Through specific receptor signaling, lipoxin A_4, for example, inhibits LTB_4-stimulated neutrophil chemotaxis while at the same time this substance attracts monocytes to apoptotic cells generated as one result of inflammation.[63–65] Resolvins of the E-series, generated from EPA, modify inflammation by, for example, inhibition of polymorphonuclear leukocyte transmigration and protection of the large bowel in colitis. Among other activities, resolvins of the D-series, generated from DHA, protect kidney tissue from ischemic injury. Protectins such as PD1 are substances derived from DHA that also play an active role in resolution of an inflammatory response. When these same substances are produced in neural tissue, they are known as neuroprotectins (ie, NPD1) to denote the tissue of origin. These substances, like lipoxin A_4, inhibit neutrophil migration. In addition, however, protectins reduce the tissue damage due to stroke, and among several other inflammation-resolution activities, help to protect the liver from inflammatory damage.[66] While these substances are clearly critical to physiological processes, their specific role(s) in the clinical aspects of enteral nutrition and PN remain to be determined.

Clinical Effects of ω-6 Fatty Acids in Parenteral Nutrition

Soybean oil IVFEs contain large quantities of linoleic acid. Exclusive provision of soybean oil–based emulsions may therefore greatly exceed the dietary recommendations for ω-6 fatty acids. Fatty acids of the ω-6 family influence the immune system by alteration of membrane structure and function, by modulation of immune function through AA metabolites, and by stimulation of inflammatory cytokines. Intravenous soybean oil emulsions have been shown to depress immune function in both in vitro and ex vivo studies. These types of emulsions have been shown to decrease the cellular immune response in several in vitro studies at varying lipid concentrations. Depression of immunoglobulin M and immunoglobulin A levels, decreases in lymphocyte proliferation, depression of natural killer cell activity, and depression of neutrophil chemotactic motility have been reported with use of soybean oil–based emulsions.[67–71] However, the most significant factor of these in vitro studies seems to be a dose-related response associated with increased immunosuppression in response to increased lipid concentrations. Despite the adverse effects from soybean IVFEs demonstrated in numerous in vitro and ex vivo studies, there is a lack of well-designed prospective randomized clinical trials evaluating the effects of soybean IVFEs upon infections and other clinical outcomes.

In a small prospective randomized study ($n = 57$), trauma patients receiving PN with soybean IVFE had more infections, longer ventilation time, and a longer hospital stay compared to patients receiving lipid-free PN.[72] Unfortunately, this study did not administer equivalent calories to the patients. McCowen et al.[73] performed a randomized study of PN with and without soybean IVFE in 40 critically ill patients and found that infections were more common in the group receiving soybean IVFE (53% vs, 29%; $p = 0.2$). However, the nutritional regimens used in this study were not isocaloric. In a randomized study, Muller et al.[74] administered PN to patients for 10 days prior to surgery for gastrointestinal cancer. A total of 46 patients received soybean IVFE plus glucose and 66 patients received glucose only; all patients received similar amounts of amino acids.[74] Mortality and major complications affecting the site of operation were significantly ($p < 0.05$) higher in the IVFE-containing compared to the lipid-free PN group. The study is confounded by the high energy intake and large amount of lipid (50% of calories) administered to the patients. The quantity of energy and amount of lipid within the IVFE used in the study exceed current A.S.P.E.N. guideline recommendations. The largest trial to evaluate soybean IVFE and infection was performed in bone marrow transplant patients.[75] Patients were randomized to low dose (6% to 8% of energy; $n = 259$) or standard dose (25% to 30% of energy; $n = 253$) IVFE-based PN. There was no association between lipid dose within the IVFE and first infection. Similar numbers of patients in each group developed bacterial and fungal infections. There was no difference between groups for engraftment or graft-versus-host disease, relapse, or survival. In one additional very small study, 15 malnourished patients with advanced gastric or esophageal cancer received 2 weeks of preoperative and 1 week of postoperative isocaloric and isonitrogenous PN with and without soybean-based IVFE.[76] Postoperative infections (13 vs. 15; 87.5% vs. 85.7%) and hospital length of stay (21 vs. 23.7 days) were similar between groups. Overall, the clinical data regarding soybean IVFE and infections are contradictory and there is no clear relationship between the use of soybean IVFE and infections.

Clinical Effects of ω-3 Fatty Acids in Enteral Nutrition

Dietary supplementation with ω-3 fatty acids has recently engendered significant interest with respect to the effect ω-3 supplementation may have on cardiovascular disease (CVD).

Although somewhat conflicting, epidemiological and clinical trial data in general suggest that ω-3 fatty acids reduce the incidence of CVD and benefit individuals at risk for coronary heart disease. Furthermore, reduction in cardiac-associated mortality may occur upon dietary supplementation with both EPA and DHA.[77,78] In addition, there is evidence that the levels of all-cause mortality, stroke, and CVD among individuals examined throughout the world are inversely related to the level of long-chain ω-3 fatty acid dietary intake.[79] The precise mechanisms associated with the effect of ω-3 fatty acid supplementation upon cardiac and other health, however, remain elusive. A systematic review performed by Balk et al.[80] led to the conclusion that, "Overall, little or no effect of fish oil was found for a variety of markers of cardiovascular disease risk." Thus, while there is an indication of cardiac benefit, how this benefit is manifested remains to be determined. The U.S. Food and Drug Administration has ruled that intakes up to 3.0 g/day of EPA and DHA are generally recognized as safe; however, an additional cautionary note based upon ex vivo data comes from the Institute of Medicine that EPA and DHA could particularly affect immunocompromised individuals.[11,80] In contrast to this observation, while in vitro human cell and animal studies have demonstrated suppression of immune-cell activity,[81–84] examination of summary ex vivo data by Fritsche[85] revealed that diets enriched in ω-3 PUFAs showed no effect on ex vivo immune cell activity.

The potential benefit and/or risk of ω-3 fatty acid dietary augmentation has been, and continues to be, of interest. Indeed, experimental animal studies of sepsis showed that mortality declined significantly when a dietary regimen rich in ω-3 fatty acids was followed.[86–88] However, similar to the conflicting clinical data relative to a clearly beneficial effect of ω-3 fatty acids on cardiovascular health, several clinical studies have also led to somewhat conflicting results as to the efficacy of ω-3 dietary supplementation in burn patients. Studies from Gottschlich et al.[18] and Alexander and Gottschlich[89] showed that utilization of an immune-enhancing diet (high-protein, linoleic acid–restricted, ω-3 fatty acid–enriched, low-fat) produced clinical benefit in burn patients. Conclusions in a review by Gerster[90] supported inclusion of ω-3 fatty acids in enteral formula.

In contrast to these studies, no improved clinical benefit of this type of nutrition enriched with ω-3 fatty acids and other components was observed relative to a standard high-protein enteral diet was reported in a randomized trial of 50 burn patients.[91] A separate study by Garrel et al.[17] showed that provision of fish oil in a low-fat (15% of total energy) diet to burn patients did not alter time-to-healing per percent burn or the incidence of pneumonia relative to the group on a similar diet without fish oil. Many of these and other studies and their implications in treatment of burns have been examined in a review by De-Souza and Greene.[92] Beneficial effects of ω-3 fatty acid enteral supplementation have been observed in treatment for acute respiratory distress syndrome.[22] In this study, both EPA and GLA separately and in combination reduced inflammation, improved oxygenation, and improved outcomes in these patients. Enteral diets containing ω-3 fatty acids have also been shown to provide clinical benefit in attenuation of cyclosporine-induced hypertension,[93] in improvement of kidney transplant renal function,[94] in cellular immunity following experimental hemorrhagic shock,[95] and in clinical outcomes associated with the postsurgical and critically ill patient.[96] In addition, a diet enriched in EPA and GLA improved clinical outcomes of ventilated patients with severe sepsis.[97] In contrast to these results, a recent randomized controlled trial that examined the effect of the use of enteral fish oil alone on clinical outcomes in acute lung injury patients showed no reduction of pulmonary or systemic inflammatory biomarkers.[98] Thus, in general, there is some support for the use of enteral or parenteral regimens that are enriched in ω-3 fatty acids, particularly with respect to the potential attenuation effect of such supplementation upon the synthesis of the highly inflammatory eicosanoids along with the increased synthesis of the significantly less inflammatory eicosanoids of the cyclooxygenase and lipoxygenase pathways. However, while this view is supported by promising experimental animal studies, human clinical data are, as yet, much less definitive.[85]

Clinical Effects of ω-3 Fatty Acids in Parenteral Nutrition

With respect to PN, a number of clinical trials and studies have investigated the impact of IVFEs that contain fish oil upon clinical outcomes among adult patients.[99–118] While the data within some of the articles are intriguing, a careful review of this literature reveals that the results remain controversial; there are, to date, only a very limited number of examples of PN studies among the nonchronic disease-associated patients of statistically sound data that support improvement of clinical outcomes by use of ω-3 fatty acids in the form of fish oil (eg, Grimm et al.,[101] Heller et al.,[104] Tsekos et al.,[115] Weiss et al.,[117] and Wichmann et al.[118]). Unfortunately, the study of Heller et al.[104] failed to include a control population, and none of the subjects were randomized. Therefore, in the absence of both randomization and a control group, interpretation of the data in regard to this trial can lead to only general supposition that ω-3 fatty acids had a positive effect. The study by Grimm et al.[101] that examined the effect of ω-3 fatty acids in PN IVFEs upon length of hospital stay reported a significantly shorter length of hospital stay for the ω-3 group relative to the control group. However, the data in this study were apparently generated from a small subgroup of patients (from two participating centers) who were specifically selected from among a much larger patient population involved in the 18-center clinical trial. In contrast to this small subgroup, the results of the entire 18-center trial population failed to show a significant difference in length of hospital stay.[112]

A recent meta-analysis and a systematic review of these and similar literature suggest that ω-3 fatty acids in the form of fish oil within PN improve clinical outcomes.[119,120] In this regard, the studies by Tsekos et al.[115] and Wichmann et al.[118] offer positive results. Although the Tsekos et al.[115] study was entirely a retrospective analysis, and thus suffers somewhat from study design, together with the Wichmann et al.[118] investigation, the data suggest that tandem preoperative and postoperative ω-3 PN provision may impact clinical outcomes. These results also support the positive effect on clinical outcomes provided by preoperative enteral provision of immune-enhancing diets that contain ω-3 fatty acids in fish oil.[21] Therefore, irrespective of inconsistent positive data in this area, there appear to be sufficient suggestive data that beg for more and better-designed clinical trials to determine the efficacy of ω-3 fatty acids use in adult PN.

Clinical Effects of ω-9 Fatty Acids in Enteral and Parenteral Nutrition

Diets containing oils high in ω-9 fatty acids (primary oleic acid within olive oil) have been reported to be beneficial for health due to their lowering effects on cholesterol and TG levels without the negative effects of lipid peroxidation.[121] In an examination of over 7000 individuals, the results of a recent study show that the risk of stroke may be significantly reduced if a diet high in olive oil is used intensively.[122] The high stability of these oils combined with a favorable fatty acid profile has resulted in common use in enteral formulas (Table 5-4). Enteral formulas using engineered sunflower and safflower oils may have an oleic acid content that averages above 70%, a content that is comparable to the oleic acid content in olive oil.[123] Additionally, commercial IVFEs with high olive oil content have been developed to reduce ω-6 content and thus the risk associated with in vivo oxidative stress and the potential for a proinflammatory environment. When compared to soybean oil–based IVFEs, olive oil–based IVFEs have been shown to be less inhibitory of various neutrophil responses including human neutrophil viability,[124] phagocytic activity,[125,126] inflammatory cytokine production,[125,127] and oxidative burst induction.[125,128] These studies generally demonstrate a greater immune-neutral effect of olive oil–based emulsions when compared with soybean IVFEs. However, there is a lack of well designed randomized controlled trials that examine the effect on clinical outcomes of olive oil–based IVFEs.

Short-Chain Fatty Acids

SCFAs play an integral role in colonic health. These fatty acids occur naturally in foods (butter, milk) but only in modest concentrations. The primary source of SCFAs is the large intestine via bacterial anaerobic fermentation of nondigestible dietary carbohydrates and fiber polysaccharides. Fermentation of these carbohydrate compounds produces the following SCFAs: acetate (2C), propionate (3C), and butyrate (4C). SCFAs are absorbed and metabolized primarily by the colon and to a lesser degree by liver, muscle, and brain tissue. The functions of SCFAs are diverse and include (1) a primary energy source for colonocytes, (2) stimulation of water and sodium absorption in the colon, and (3) trophic effects to the intestinal mucosa.[129,130] Butyrate has been shown to be the most important SCFA in regulation and maintenance of colonic tissue. An important role of butyrate may be to modify inflammatory activity by inhibiting the release of the transcription factor, nuclear factor kappa-light-chain-enhancer of activated B cells.[131] In addition, butyrate has been shown to exhibit antitumorigenic effects on cancer cell lines and has been identified with gene regulation involving processes of cellular apoptosis, proliferation, and differentiation.[132,133] Daly and colleagues[133] demonstrated that many of the butyrate-responsive genes are deregulated in colon carcinoma tissue as an apparent result of down-regulation of cellular expression of the butyrate transporter. The data suggest that a reduction in transport of butyrate into the luminal membrane may contribute to sequential genetic alterations that lead to initiation of colorectal cancer.

Additional research has demonstrated reduced levels of butyrate in both patients with inflammatory bowel disease and in patients with ileal reservoirs experiencing pouchitis. The use of butyrate enemas has been shown to decrease symptoms of colitis in small clinical studies.[134–136] Much of the recent nutrition support research has focused on the role of butyrate to alter the gut lumen environment and influence intestinal adaptation in short bowel syndrome. In investigational animal models of PN, the addition of butyrate has been shown to prevent PN-associated mucosal atrophy and improve epithelial surface proliferation.[137] Tappenden and colleagues[138,139] have shown that incorporation of SCFA in PN solutions may modulate the transport capacity of glucose and other nutrients and may further improve intestinal adaptation by the up-regulation of glucagon-like peptide-2. In the future, butyrate-enhanced PN products may offer a mechanism to reduce the length of time that patients require PN by improving intestinal absorption and adaptation, thus reducing the risk of adverse metabolic sequelae associated with PN.

Medium-Chain Triglycerides

Medium-chain TGs (MCTs) are saturated and are 6 to 12 carbons in length. These fatty acids were developed commercially in the 1950s and are one of the first medical foods derived as an alternative to plant oils and other conventional fats. This lipid product is isolated primarily from plants high in MCTs, such as palm kernel and coconut oils. The MCT product does not provide EFAs and has a caloric density of 8.3 kcal/g. When compared to long-chain TGs (LCTs), MCTs are significantly different with respect to absorption, metabolism, and physiological functions. While the saturated LCTs from these sources clearly contribute to coronary heart disease via an increase in LDL cholesterol,[140,141] the effect on LDL cholesterol levels by saturated MCTs from the same sources is not clear, with in some instances an increase,[142] and in other instances, a decrease[143] having been reported. In many of these studies, the contribution and/or specific effect of MCTs alone is difficult to separate from other confounders.[144–146]

MCTs are smaller and more water soluble than LCTs. Liberation of fatty acids through hydrolysis of MCTs in the intestinal lumen is significantly faster relative to LCTs and absorption of medium-chain fatty acids (MCFAs) is more rapid when compared to LCFAs. This rapid absorptive rate may be attributable in part to the fact that MCTs do not require the presence of bile or pancreatic lipases for absorption and are transported directly to the liver via the portal vein (bypassing the traditional LCT pathway). Once in the liver, MCTs are used primarily as an energy source. In comparison to LCTs, MCTs are not stored to any significant degree in adipose tissue, nor do they impact the reticuloendothelial system. Because MCTs are ketogenic, these TGs may provide a useful energy source for enterocytes, lymphocytes, and cells of other tissues that may be increasingly utilized in hypermetabolically stressed patients. Oxidation of MCTs is less affected by glucose and insulin than LCTs.[147] In addition, oxidation of LCTs can be impaired by slow elimination rates from the plasma or by the requirement of carnitine for intracellular transport. In contrast, the metabolism of MCTs is a carnitine independent system for transport into the mitochondria.[148] Because of these metabolic differences, MCTs may be beneficial in attenuating inflammatory stress conditions. The metabolic characteristics of MCTs increase their role as an important lipid source for individuals with impaired and dysfunctional gastrointestinal tracts. For example, individuals who suffer from defects of fat digestion and absorption (ie, patients with pancreatitis) may benefit from MCTs, as well as those individuals with malabsorption secondary to intestinal resections, inflammatory bowel disease, or autoimmune enteropathies.

Many enteral products have been designed with MCTs as a significant lipid component to maximize the absorption, metabolism, and tolerance of these products for use in various disease and metabolic conditions (Table 5-4). MCTs have also been used in PN solutions. LCTs and MCTs may be physically mixed to generate an emulsion that simultaneously provides both LCTs and MCTs in varying ratios and percentages. Physical mixtures of LCTs and MCTs (50:50 weight/weight mixture) have been used in PN solutions for a number of years in Europe and other countries. Research has suggested that these IVFEs may provide benefit by (1) providing a better oxidized energy source, (2) improving nitrogen balance (attenuating protein catabolism in stress), and (3) providing rapid clearance of lipid from the blood. In addition, MCT/LCT emulsions have been shown to produce a fatty acid profile (extracted from cellular phospholipids) that is closer to normal when compared to individuals who receive soybean oil–based IVFEs.[149] However, the use of MCTs in PN may increase the risk of metabolic acidosis and also may lead to a lower level of glucose oxidation relative to LCTs alone,[6] possibilities that are particularly important to the critically ill. Nonetheless, the use of MCTs in nutrition appears to remain a viable alternative for some patients.

Structured Lipids

First developed in the mid-1980s,[150–153] structured lipids (SLs) are "designer" TG molecules that are specifically synthesized in the laboratory via chemical and/or enzymatic methodology, and more recently via genetic engineering.[154] The resulting TG mixture contains a randomly esterified pattern of MCTs and LCTs that can contain within the same TG molecule both MCFAs and LCFAs. In SLs, the MCFAs are predominantly 8 or 10 carbons in length and usually are esterified at the *sn*-1 and *sn*-3 positions, and the LCFA usually is esterified at the *sn*-2 position on the SLs' glycerol backbone. Usually, the LCFAs are predominantly represented as members of the ω-3 family such as GLA, EPA, or DHA. As previously stated, the enzymatic activities of gastric and pancreatic lipases predominantly catalyze the release of fatty acids at the *sn*-1 and *sn*-3 positions from the SLs' glycerol backbone. This catalysis results in formation of 2-LCFA-monoacylglycerols and for *sn*-2 MCFA-structured lipids, free MCFAs. In physical mixtures of LCTs and MCTs, this activity results in 2-monoacylglycerols and a mixture of MCFAs and LCFAs.

Unlike pancreatic lipase, gastric lipase does not require bile salts for enzymatic activity and is more efficiently catalytic against the acyl-MCFA in MCFA-esterified TGs.[155] As previously discussed, these more rapidly liberated MCFAs do not require bile salts for absorption, readily enter the portal system for transport, and enter mitochondria independently of the carnitine membrane transport pathway. Consequently, SLs provide a defined mechanism to rapidly deliver MCFAs and to provide a more rapid availability of EPA and DHA with, as one result, the entire attendant array of nutritionally positive aspects of these substances. It has been demonstrated that fatty acids located at the *sn*-2 position on the glycerol backbone are preferentially absorbed[156,157]; in SLs, both EPA and DHA if esterified at the *sn*-2 position are, indeed, more readily absorbed.[158] Furthermore, in experimental animal studies of intestinally injured rats, SLs prepared with MCTs and fish oils (containing a range of LCFAs from 18:3*n*-3 to 22:*n*-6) infused gastrically were absorbed more quickly in comparison to the physical mixture of the fish oil and MCTs emulsion.[159] Selected human[160,161] and experimental animal enteral nutrition studies[162–164] have investigated SLs and demonstrated the improved physiological effects that result from the use of SLs, including FA absorption and infection rates, as well as hepatic, renal, and immune function. These SLs are approved for inclusion in certain enteral nutrition formulas and find use in many different countries including the United States. In addition, PN formulae that contain SLs are approved for use in Europe.

Emerging Data that Concern Intravenous Fat Emulsions and Parenteral Nutrition–Associated Liver Disease

One of the more difficult nutrition decisions that must be faced by clinicians in treatment of the pediatric population with IVFEs is the occurrence of parenteral nutrition–associated liver disease (PNALD). Since the availability of purified fish oil, studies have shown that use of fish oil as an IVFE monotherapy at 1g/kg/day not only prevents PNALD, but can reverse the condition in the pediatric population.[165–173] However, it remains to be seen whether a similar reduction in the amount of soybean oil–based IVFE would lead to the same effect. Current investigations are underway to examine this issue. Although there are reports, as exampled by a recent individual case study, that the use of fish oil may help to prevent PNALD in the adult patient,[174] an additional investigation concludes there is little effect on hepatobiliary parameters.[175] This area begs for additional well-designed and appropriately powered investigations as randomized controlled trials to determine whether or not fish oil monotherapy, supplemental therapy, or reduced soybean oil–based IVFE can reduce hepatobiliary complications associated with IVFEs in the adult and pediatric populations.

References

1. Serhan CN. Resolvins and protectins: novel lipid mediators in anti-inflammation and resolution. *Scand J Food and Nutr.* 2006; 50(suppl 2):68–78.
2. Le H, Meisel JA, de Meijer VE, et al. The essentiality of arachidonic acid and docosahexaenoic acid. *Prostaglandins Leukot Essentl Fatty Acids.* 2009;81:165–170.
3. Deckelbaum RJ, Worgall TS, Seo T. Fatty acids and gene expresion. *Am J Clin Nutr.* 2006;83(suppl):1520S–1525S.

4. Kopecky J, Rossmeisl M, Flachs P, et al. Symposium on "Frontiers in adipose tissue biology" n-3 PUFA: bioavailability and modulation of adipose tissue function. *Proc Nutr Soc.* 2009;68:361–369.
5. Minihane AM. Nutrient gene interactions in lipid metabolism. *Curr Opinion Clin Nutr Metab Care.* 2009;12:357–363.
6. Wanten GJA, Calder PC. Immune modulation by parenteral lipid emulsions. *Am J Clin Nutr.* 2007;85:1171–1184.
7. Ferezou J, Bach AC. Structure and metabolic fate of triacylglycerol- and phospholipid-rich particles of commercial parenteral fat emulsions. *Nutrition.* 1999;15:44–50.
8. Whittaker JS, Allard JP, Freeman HJ. Nutrition in gastrointestinal disease. In: Thomson ABR, Shaffer EA, eds. *First Principles of Gastroenterology: The Basis of Disease and an Approach to Management.* 5th ed. Toronto, Canada: Janssen-Ortho; 2009:49–78.
9. Seidel D, Alaupovic P, Furman RH, McConathy WJ. A lipoprotein characterizing obstructive jaundice 1. Method for quantitative separation and identification of lipoproteins in jaundiced subjects. *J Clin Invest.* 1969;48:1211–1223.
10. Torsvik H, Berg K, Magnani HN, et al. Identification of the abnormal cholestatic lipoprotein (LP-X) in familial lecithin: cholesterol acyltransferase deficiency. *FEBS Lett.* 1972;24:165–168.
11. Institute of Medicine, Panel on Macronutrients, Panel on the Definition of Dietary Fiber, Subcommittee on Upper Reference Levels of Nutrients, Subcommittee on Interpretation and Uses of Dietary Reference Intakes, Standing Committee on the Scientific Evaluation of Dietary Reference Intakes. *Dietary Reference Intakes for Energy, Carbohydrate, Fiber, Fatty Acids, Cholesterol, Protein and Amino Acids.* Washington, DC: The National Academy Press; 2005.
12. Harris WS, Mozaffarian D, Rimm E, et al. Omega-6 fatty acids and risk for cardiovascular disease: a science advisory from the American Heart Association Nutrition Subcommittee of the Council on Nutrition, Physical Activity, and Metabolism; Council on Cardiovascular Nursing; and Council on Epidemiology and Prevention. *Circulation.* 2009;119:902–907.
13. Moshfegh A, Goldman J, Cleveland L. What we eat in America: NHANES 2001-2002: usual nutrient intakes from food compared to dietary reference intakes. Beltsville, MD: U.S. Department of Agriculture, Agricultural Research Service; 2005.
14. Seidner DL, Mascioli EA, Istfan NW, et al. Effects of long-chain triglyceride emulsions on reticuloendothelial system function in humans. *J Parenter Enteral Nutr.* 1989;13:614–619.
15. Kim H, Son E, Kim J, et al. Association of hyperglycemia and markers of hepatic dysfunction with dextrose infusion rates in Korean patients receiving total parenteral nutrition. *Am J Health Syst Pharm.* 2003;60:1760–1766.
16. Gottschlich MM. Selection of optimal lipid sources in enteral and parenteral nutrition. *Nutr Clin Pract.* 1992;7:152–165.
17. Garrel DR, Razi M, Lariviere F, et al. Improved clinical status and length of care with low-fat nutrition support in burn patients. *J Parenter Enteral Nutr.* 1995;19:482–491.
18. Gottschlich MM, Jenkins M, Warden GD, et al. Differential effects of three enteral dietary regimens on selected outcome variables in burn patients. *J Parenter Enteral Nutr.* 1990;14:225–236.
19. Selleck KJ, Wan JM, Gollaher CJ, et al. Effect of low and high amounts of a structured lipid containing fish oil on protein metabolism in enterally fed burned rats. *Am J Clin Nutr.* 1994;60:216–222.
20. Hart DW, Wolf SE, Zhang XJ, et al. Efficacy of a high carbohydrate diet in catabolic illness. *Crit Care Med.* 2001;29:1318–1324.
21. McClave SA, Martindale RG, Vanek VW, et al. A.S.P.E.N. Board of Directors; American College of Critical Care Medicine; Society of Critical Care Medicine. Guidelines for the provision and assessment of nutrition support therapy in the adult critically ill patient: Society of Critical Care Medicine (SCCM) and American Society for Parenteral and Enteral Nutrition (A.S.P.E.N.). *J Parenter Enteral Nutr.* 2009;33:277–316.
22. Gadek JE, DeMichele SJ, Karlstad MD, et al. Enteral Nutrition in ARDS Study Group. Effect of enteral feeding with eicosapentaenoic acid, gamma-linolenic acid, and antioxidants in patients with acute respiratory distress syndrome. *Crit Care Med.* 1999;27: 1409–1420.
23. Singer P, Theilla M, Fisher H, et al. Benefit of an enteral diet enriched with eicosapentaenoic acid and gamma-linolenic acid in ventilated patients with acute lung injury. *Crit Care Med.* 2006;34: 1033–1038.
24. Pontes-Arruda A, Aragao AM, Albuquerque JD. Effects of enteral feeding with eicosapentaenoic acid, gamma-linolenic acid and antioxidants in mechanically ventilated patients with severe sepsis and septic shock. *Crit Care Med.* 2006;34:2325–2333.
25. A.S.P.E.N. Board of Directors and the Clinical Guideline Task Force. Guidelines for the use of parenteral and enteral nutrition in adult and pediatric patients. *J Parenter Enteral Nutr.* 2002;26: 1SA–138SA.
26. Delafosse B, Viale JP, Tissot S, et al. Effects of glucose-to-lipid ratio and type of lipid on substrate oxidation rate in patients. *Am J Physiol.* 1994;267:E775–E780.
27. Battistella FD, Widergren JT, Anderson JT, et al. A prospective, randomized trial of intravenous fat emulsion administration in trauma victims requiring total parenteral nutrition. *J Trauma.* 1997;43:52–60.
28. Klein S, Miles JM. Metabolic effects of long-chain and medium-chain triglyceride emulsions in humans. *J Parenter Enteral Nutr.* 1994;18:396–397.
29. Guidelines for the use of parenteral and enteral nutrition in adult and pediatric patients. *J Parenter Enteral Nutr.* 1993;17: 1SA–52SA.
30. Burr GO, Burr MD. A new deficiency disease produced by the rigid exclusion of fat from the diet. *J Biol Chem.* 1929;82:345–367.
31. Holman RT, Johnson SB, Hatch TF. A case of human linolenic acid deficiency involving neurological abnormalities. *Am J Clin Nutr.* 1982;35: 617–623.
32. Wene JD, Connor WE, DenBesten L. The development of essential fatty acid deficiency in healthy men fed fat-free diets intravenously and orally. *J Clin Invest.* 1975;56:127–134.
33. Richardson TJ, Sgoutas D. Essential fatty acid deficiency in four adult patients during total parenteral nutrition. *Am J Clin Nutr.* 1975;28:258–263.
34. Fleming CR, Smith LM, Hodges RE. Essential fatty acid deficiency in adults receiving total parenteral nutrition. *Am J Clin Nutr.* 1976;29:976–983.
35. Cederholm TE, Berg AB, Johansson EK, et al. Low levels of essential fatty acids are related to impaired delayed skin hypersensitivity in malnourished chronically ill elderly people. *Eur J Clin Invest.* 1994;24:615–620.
36. Hulsey TK, O'Neill JA, Neblett WR, et al. Experimental wound healing in essential fatty acid deficiency. *J Pediatr Surg.* 1980;15: 505–508.
37. Dupont J, Dowd MK. Eiconsanoid synthesis as a functional measurement of essential fatty acid requirement. *J Am Coll Nutr.* 1990; 9:272–276.
38. Holman RT, Smythe L, Johnson S. Effect of sex and age on fatty acid composition of human serum lipids. *Amer J Clin Nutr.* 1979; 32:2390–2399.
39. Mirtallo J, Canada T, Johnson D, et al. Safe practices for parenteral nutrition. *J Parenter Enteral Nutr.* 2004;28:S39–S70.
40. Dickerson RN, Rosato EF, Mullen JL. Net protein anabolism with hypocaloric parenteral nutrition in obese stressed patients. *Am J Clin Nutr.* 1986;44:747–755.

41. Leung N, O'Brien T, McMahom MM. Parenteral feeding in a patient with hypertriglyceridemia and increased liver enzyme levels. *Endocr Pract.* 1999;5:194–197.
42. Bjerve KS, Mostad I, Thoresen L. Alpha-linolenic acid deficiency in patients on long-term gastric tube feeding: estimation of linolenic acid and long-chain unsaturated n-3 fatty acid requirement in man. *Am J Clin Nutr.* 1987;15:897–904.
43. Heird WC, Lapillonne A. The role of essential fatty acids in development. *Annu Rev Nutr.* 2005;25:549–571.
44. de Meijer VE, Gura KM, Meisel JA, et al. Parenteral fish oil monotherapy in the management of patients with parenteral nutrition-associated liver disease. *Arch Surg.* 2010;145:547–551.
45. Jeppesen PB, Hoy CE, Mortensen PB. Differences in essential fatty acid requirements by enteral and parenteral routes of administration in patients with fat malabsorption. *Am J Clin Nutr.* 1999; 70:78–84.
46. Abushufa R, Reed P, Weinkove C, et al. Essential fatty acid status in patients on long-term home parenteral nutrition. *J Parenter Enteral Nutr.* 1995;19:286–290.
47. Jeppesen PB, Hoy CE, Mortensen PB. Essential fatty acid deficiency in patients receiving home parenteral nutrition. *Am J Clin Nutr.* 1998;68:126–133.
48. Ling PR, Ollero M, Khaodhiar L, et al. Disturbances in essential fatty acid metabolism in patients receiving long-term home parenteral nutrition. *Dig Dis Sci.* 2002;47:1679–1685.
49. Pironi L, Belluzzi A, Miglioli M. Low levels of essential fatty acids in the red blood cell membrane phospholipid fraction of long-term home parenteral nutrition patients. *J Parenter Enteral Nutr.* 1996;20:377–378.
50. Mascioli EA, Lopes SM, Champagne C, et al. Essential fatty acid deficiency and home total parenteral nutrition patients. *Nutrition.* 1996;12:245–249.
51. Goetzl EJ, An S, Smith WL. Specificity of expression and effects of eicosanoid mediators in normal physiology and human diseases. *FASEB J.* 1995;9:1051–1058.
52. Phipps RP, Stein SH, Roper RL. A new view of prostaglandin-E regulation of the immune response. *Immunol Today.* 1991;12:349–352.
53. Janniger CK, Racis SP. The arachidonic acid cascade: an immunologically based review. *J Med.* 1987;18:69–80.
54. Smith WL, Meade EA, DeWitt DL. Pharmacology of prostaglandin endoperoxide synthase isozymes-1 and -2. *Ann NY Acad Sci.* 1994; 714:136–142.
55. O'Banion MK. Cyclooxygenase-2: molecular biology, pharmacology and neurobiology. *Crit Rev Neurobiol.* 1999;13:45–82.
56. Choudhry MA, Ahmed Z, Sayeed MM. PGE(2)- mediated inhibition of T-cell p59 (fyn) is independent of cAMP. *Am J Physiol.* 1999;277:C302–C309.
57. Choudhry MA, Hockberger PE, Sayeed MM. PGE2 suppresses mitogen-induced Ca^{2+} mobilization in T cells. *Am J Physiol.* 1999; 277:R1741–R1748.
58. Cosme R, Lublin D, Takafuji V, et al. Prostanoids in human colonic mucosa: effects of inflammation on PGE(2) receptor expression. *Hum Immunol.* 2000;61:684–696.
59. Herold PM, Kinsella JE. Fish oil consumption and decreased risk of cardiovascular disease: a comparison of findings from animal and human feeding trials. *Am J Clin Nutr.* 1986;43:566–598.
60. Dyerberg J, Bang HO, Stoffersen E, et al. Eicosapentaenoic acid and prevention of thrombosis and atherosclerosis? *Lancet.* 1978; 2:117–119.
61. Palombo JD, DeMichele SJ, Boyce PJ, et al. Metabolism of dietary alpha-linolenic acid vs. eicosapentaenoic acid in rat immune cell phospholipids during endotoxemia. *Lipids.* 1998;33:1099–1105.
62. Fan Y-Y, Chapkin RS. Importance of dietary γ-linolenic acid in human health and nutrition. *J Nutrition.* 1998;128:1411–1414.
63. Maddox JF, Serhan, CN. Lipoxin A4 and B4 are potent stimuli for human monocyte migration and adhesion: selective inactivation by dehydrogenation and reduction. *J Exp Med.* 1996;183: 137–146.
64. Serhan CN, Fiore S, Brezinski DA, Lynch S. Lipoxin A4 metabolism by differentiated HL-60 cells and human monocytes: conversion to novel 15-oxo and dihydro products. *Biochemistry.* 1993;32: 6313–6319.
65. Serhan CN. Lipoxins and aspirin-triggered 15-epi-lipoxin biosynthesis: an update and role in anti-inflammation and proresolution. *Prostaglandins Other Lipid Mediat.* 2002;68-69:433–455.
66. Amiram A, Serhan CN. Resolvins and protectins in the termination program of acute inflammation. *Trends in Immunology.* 2007; 28:176–183.
67. Salo M. Inhibition of immunoglobulin synthesis in vitro by intravenous lipid emulsion (Intralipid). *J Parenter Enteral Nutr.* 1990; 14:459–462.
68. Ladisch S, Poplack DG, Blaese RM. Inhibition of human lymphoproliferation by intravenous lipid emulsion. *Clin Immunol Immunopathol.* 1982;25:196–202.
69. Granato D, Blum S, Rossle C, et al. Effects of parenteral lipid emulsions with different fatty acid composition on immune cell functions in vitro. *J Parenter Enteral Nutr.* 2000;24:113–118.
70. Loo LS, Tang JP, Kohl S. Inhibition of cellular cytotoxicity of leukocytes for herpes simplex virus-infected cells in vitro and in vivo by intralipid. *J Infect Dis.* 1982;146:64–70.
71. Kohelet D, Peller S, Arbel E, Goldberg M. Preincubation with intravenous lipid emulsion reduces chemotactic motility of neutrophils in cord blood. *J Parenter Enteral Nutr.* 1990;14:472–473.
72. Battistella FD, Widergren JT, Anderson JT, et al. A prospective randomized trial of intravenous fat emulsion administration in trauma victims requiring total parenteral nutrition. *J Trauma.* 1997; 43:52–58.
73. McCowen KC, Friel C, Sternberg J, et al. Hypocaloric total parenteral nutrition: effectiveness in prevention of hyperglycemia and infectious complications: a randomized clinical trial. *Crit Care Med.* 2000;28:3606–3611.
74. Muller JM, Keller HW, Brenner U, et al. Indications and effects of preoperative parenteral nutrition. *World J Surg.* 1986;10:53–63.
75. Lenssen P, Bruemmer BA, Bowden RA, et al. Intravenous lipid dose and incidence of bacteremia and fungemia in patients undergoing bone marrow transplantation. *Am J Clin Nutr.* 1998;67:927–933.
76. Dionigi P, Dionigi R, Prati U, et al. Effect of Intralipid on some immunological parameters and leukocyte functions in patients with esophageal and gastric cancer. *Clin Nutr.* 1985;4:229–234.
77. Schmidt EB, Arnesen H, Christensen JH, et al. Marine n-3 polyunsaturated fatty acids and coronary heart disease. Part II. *Thromb Res.* 2005;115:257–262.
78. Kris-Etherton PM, Harris WS, Appel LJ, et al. Fish consumption, fish oil, omega-3 fatty acids, and cardiovascular disease. *Circulation.* 2002;106:2747–2757.
79. Hibbeln JR, Nieminen LR, Blasbalg TL, et al. Healthy intakes of n-3 and n-6 fatty acids: estimations considering worldwide diversity. *Am J Clin Nutr.* 2006;83(suppl):1483S–1493S.
80. Balk EM, Lichtenstein AH, Chung M, et al. Effects of omega-3 fatty acids on coronary restenosis, intima-media thickness, and exercise tolerance: a systematic review. *Atherosclerosis.* 2006;184:237–246.
81. Denys A, Hichami A, Khan NA. Eicosapentaenoic acid and docosahexaenoic acid modulate MAP kinase (ERK1/ERK2) signaling in human T cells. *J Lipid Res.* 2001;42:2015–2020.
82. Versleijen MW, Roelofs HM, te Morsche RH, et al. Parenteral lipids impair pneumococcal elimination by human neutrophils. *Eur J Clin Invest.* 2010;40:729–734.

83. Puertollano MA, Puertollano E, Alvarez De Cienfuegos G, et al. Dietary lipids, modulation of immune functions, and susceptibility to infection. *Nutr Ther & Metab.* 2008;26:97–108.
84. Sadeghi S, Wallace FA, Calder PC. Dietary lipids modify the cytokine response to bacterial lipopolysaccharide in mice. *Immunology.* 1999;96:404–410.
85. Fritsche K. Fatty acids as modulators of the immune response. *Annu Rev Nutr.* 2006;26:45–73.
86. Barton RG, Wells CL, Carlson A, et al. Dietary omega-3 fatty acids decrease mortality and Kupffer cell prostaglandin E2 production in a rat model of chronic sepsis. *J Trauma.* 1991;31:768–774.
87. Peck MD, Ogle CK, Alexander JW. Composition of fat in enteral diets can influence outcome in experimental peritonitis. *Ann Surg.* 1991;214:74–82.
88. Johnson JA III, Griswold JA, Muakkassa FF. Essential fatty acids influence survival in sepsis. *J Trauma.* 1993;35:128–131.
89. Alexander JW, Gottschlich MM. Nutritional immunomodulation in burn patients. *Crit Care Med.* 1990;18:S149–S153.
90. Gerster H. The use of n-3 PUFAs (fish oil) in enteral nutrition. *Int J Vitam Nutr Res.* 1995;65:3–20.
91. Saffle JR, Wiebke G, Jennings K, et al. Randomized trial of immune-enhancing enteral nutrition in burn patients. *J Trauma.* 1997;42:793–800.
92. De-Souza DA, Greene LJ. Pharmacological nutrition after burn injury. *J Nutr.* 998;128:797–803.
93. Ventura HO, Milani RV, Lavie CJ, et al. Cyclosporine-induced hypertension: efficacy of ω-3 fatty acids in patients after cardiac transplantation. *Circulation.* 1993;88:II281–II285.
94. Van der Heide JJH, Bilo HJG, Tegzess AM, et al. The effects of dietary supplementation with fish oil on renal function in cyclosporine-treated renal transplant recipients. *Transplantation.* 1990;49:523–527.
95. Ertel W, Morrison MH, Ayala A, et al. Modulation of macrophage membrane phospholipids by n-3 polyunsaturated fatty acids increases interleukin I release and prevents suppression of cellular immunity following hemorrhagic shock. *Arch Surg.* 1993; 128:15–21.
96. Calder PC. n-3 fatty acids, inflammation, and immunity—relevance to postsurgical and critically ill patients. *Lipids.* 2004; 39:1147–1161.
97. Pontes-Arruda A, Aragão A, Albuquerque J. Effects of enteral feeding with eicosapentaenoic acid, γ-linolenic acid, and antioxidants in mechanically ventilated patients with severe sepsis and septic shock. *Crit Care Med.* 2006;34:2325–2333.
98. Stapleton RD, Martin TR, Weiss NS, et al. A phase II randomized placebo-controlled trial of omega-3 fatty acids for the treatment of acute lung injury. *Crit Care Med.* 2011;39:1655–1662.
99. Berger MM, Tappy L, Revelly JP, et al. Fish oil after abdominal aorta aneurysm surgery. *Eur J Clin Nutr.* 2008;62:1116–1122.
100. Friesecke S, Lotze C, Köhler J, et al. Fish oil supplementation in the parenteral nutrition of critically ill medical patients: a randomised controlled trial. *Intensive Care Med.* 2008;34:1411–1420.
101. Grimm H, Mertes N, Goeters C, et al. Improved fatty acid and leukotriene pattern with a novel lipid emulsion in surgical patients. *Eur J Nutr.* 2006;45:55–60.
102. Grimminger F, Mayser P, Papavassilis C, et al. A double-blind, randomized, placebo-controlled trial of n-3 fatty acid based lipid infusion in acute, extended guttate psoriasis. Rapid improvement of clinical manifestations and changes in neutrophil leukotrienes profile. *Clin Invest.* 1993;71:634–643.
103. Heller AR, Rössel T, Gottschlich B, et al. Omega-3 fatty acids improve liver and pancreas function in postoperative cancer patients. *Int J Cancer.* 2004;111:611–616.
104. Heller AR, Rössler S, Litz RJ, et al. Omega-3 fatty acids improve the diagnosis-related clinical outcome. *Crit Care Med.* 2006;34: 972–979.
105. Katz DP, Manner T, Furst P, et al. The use of an intravenous fish oil emulsion enriched with omega-3 fatty acids in patients with cystic fibrosis. *Nutrition.* 1996;12:334–339.
106. Klek S, Kulig J, Szczepanik AM, et al. The clinical value of parenteral immunonutrition in surgical patients. *Acta Chir Belg.* 2005;105:175–179.
107. Leeb BF, Sautner J, Andel I, et al. Intravenous application of omega-3 fatty acids in patients with active rheumatoid arthritis. The ORA-1 trial. An open pilot study. *Lipids.* 2006;41:29–34.
108. Liang B, Wang S, Ye YJ, et al. Impact of postoperative omega-3 fatty acid-supplemented parenteral nutrition on clinical outcomes and immunomodulations in colorectal cancer patients. *World J Gastroenterol.* 2008;14:2434–2439.
109. Mayer K, Fegbeutel C, Hattar K, et al. Omega-3 vs. omega-6 lipid emulsions exert differential influence on neutrophils in septic shock patients: impact on plasma fatty acids and lipid mediator generation. *Intensive Care Med.* 2003;29:1472–1481.
110. Mayser P, Mayer K, Mahloudjian M, et al. A double-blind, randomized, placebo-controlled trial of n-3 versus n-6 fatty acid-based lipid infusion in atopic dermatitis. *J Parenter Enteral Nutr.* 2002;26:151–158.
111. Mayser P, Mrowietz U, Arenberger P, et al. Omega 3 fatty acid-based lipid infusion in patients with chronic plaque psoriasis: results of a double-blind, randomized, placebo-controlled, multicenter trial. *J Am Acad Dermatol.* 1998;38:539–547. Erratum in: *J Am Acad Dermatol.* 1998;39:421.
112. Mertes N, Grimm H, Fürst P, et al. Safety and efficacy of a new parenteral lipid emulsion (SMOFlipid) in surgical patients: a randomized, double-blind, multicenter study. *Ann Nutr Metab.* 2006;50:253–259.
113. Sabater J, Masclans JR, Sacanell J, et al. Effects on hemodynamics and gas exchange of omega-3 fatty acid-enriched lipid emulsion in acute respiratory distress syndrome (ARDS): a prospective, randomized, double-blind, parallel group study. *Lipids Health Dis.* 2008;7:39.
114. Senkal M, Geier B, Hannemann M, et al. Supplementation of omega-3 fatty acids in parenteral nutrition beneficially alters phospholipid fatty acid pattern. *J Parenert Enteral Nutr.* 2007;31:12–17.
115. Tsekos E, Reuter C, Stehle P, et al. Perioperative administration of parenteral fish oil supplements in a routine clinical setting improves patient outcome after major abdominal surgery. *Clin Nutr.* 2004;23:325–330.
116. Wang X, Li W, Li N, et al. Omega-3 fatty acids-supplemented parenteral nutrition decreases hyperinflammatory response and attenuates systemic disease sequelae in severe acute pancreatitis: a randomized and controlled study. *J Parenter Enteral Nutr.* 2008;32:236–241.
117. Weiss G, Meyer F, Matthies B, et al. Immunomodulation by perioperative administration of n-3 fatty acids. *Brit J Nutr.* 2002;87 (Suppl 1):S89–S94.
118. Wichmann MW, Thul P, Czarnetzki HD, et al. Evaluation of clinical safety and beneficial effects of a fish oil containing lipid emulsion (Lipoplus, MLF541): data from a prospective, randomized, multicenter trial. *Crit Care Med.* 2007;35:700–706.
119. Chen B, Zhou Y, Yang P, et al. Safety and efficacy of fish oil–enriched parenteral nutrition regimen on postoperative patients undergoing major abdominal surgery: a meta-analysis of randomized controlled trials. *J Parenter Enteral Nutr.* 2010;34:387–394.
120. Wei C, Hua J, Bin C, et al. Impact of lipid emulsion containing fish oil on outcomes of surgical patients: Systematic review of

randomized controlled trials from Europe and Asia. *Nutrition.* 2010;26:474–481.
121. Miller M, Stone NJ, Ballantyne C, et al. on behalf of the American Heart Association Clinical Lipidology, Thrombosis, and Prevention Committee of the Council on Nutrition, Physical Activity, and Metabolism, Council on Arteriosclerosis, Thrombosis and Vascular Biology, Council on Cardiovascular Nursing, Council on the Kidney in Cardiovascular Disease. Triglycerides and cardiovascular disease: a scientific statement from the American Heart Association. *Circulation.* 2011;123:2292–2333.
122. Samieri C, Féart C, Proust-Lima C, et al. Olive oil consumption, plasma oleic acid, and stroke incidence: The Three-City Study. *Neurology.* 2011;77(5):418–425.
123. Corbett P. Research in the area of high oleic oils. *Plant Biotechnology Institute Bulletin.* 2002;1:3.
124. Cury-Boaventura MF, Gorjão R, de Lima TM, et al. Effect of olive oil-based emulsion on human lymphocyte and neutrophil death. *J Parenter Enteral Nutr.* 2008;32:81–87.
125. Buenestado A, Cortijo J, Sanz MJ, et al. Olive oil-based lipid emulsion's neutral effects on neutrophil functions and leukocyte-endothelial cell interactions. *J Parenter Enteral Nutr.* 2006;30: 286–296.
126. Versleijen MW, Roelofs HM, te Morsche RH, et al. Parenteral lipids impair pneumococcal elimination by human neutrophils. *Eur J Clin Invest.* 2010;40:729–734.
127. Haase B, Faust K, Heidemann M, et al. The modulatory effect of lipids and glucose on the neonatal immune response induced by *Staphylococcus epidermidis*. *Inflamm Res.* 2011;60:227–232.
128. Jüttner B, Kröplin J, Coldewey SM, et al. Unsaturated long-chain fatty acids induce the respiratory burst of human neutrophils and monocytes in whole blood. *Nutr Metab.* 2008;5:19.
129. Rombeau JL, Kripke SA. Metabolic and intestinal effects of short chain fatty acids. *J Parenter Enteral Nutr.* 1990;14:181S–185S.
130. Cook SI, Sellin JH. Review article: short chain fatty acids in health and disease. *Aliment Pharmacol Ther.* 1998;12:499–507.
131. Segain JP, Raingeard de la Bletiere D, Bourreille A, et al. Butyrate inhibits inflammatory responses through NFkappaB inhibition: implications for Crohn's disease. *Gut.* 2000;47:397–403.
132. Miller SJ. Cellular and physiologicial effects of short-chain fatty acids. *Mini Rev Med Chem.* 2004;4:839–845.
133. Daly K, Cuff MA, Fung F, et al. The importance of colonic butyrate transport to the regulation of genes associated with colonic tissue homeostasis. *Biochem Soc Trans.* 2005;33:733–735.
134. Breuer RI, Buto Sk, Christ ML, et al. Rectal irrigation with short-chain fatty acids for distal ulcerative colitis preliminary report. *Dig Dis Sci.* 1991;36:185–187.
135. Scheppach W, Sommer H, Kirchner T, et al. Effects of butyrate enemas on the colonic mucosa in distal ulcerative colitis. *Gastroenterology.* 1995;103:51–56.
136. Vernia P, Cittadini M, Caprilli R, et al. Topical treatment of refractory distal ulcerative colitis with 5-ASA and sodium butyrate. *Dig Dis Sci.* 1995;40:305–307.
137. Bartholome AL, Albin DM, Baker DH, et al. Supplementation of total parenteral nutrition with butyrate acutely increases structural aspects of intestinal adaptation after an 80% jejunoileal resection in neonatal piglets. *J Parenter Enteral Nutr.* 2004;28:210–223.
138. Tappenden KA, Albin DM, Bartholome AL, et al. Glucagon-like peptide-2 and short-chain fatty acids: a new twist to an old story. *J Nutr.* 2003;133:3717–3720.
139. Tappenden KA. Emerging therapies for intestinal failure. *Arch Surg.* 2010;145:528–532.
140. Subcommittees on Upper Reference Levels, Institute of Medicine of the National Academies. *Dietary Reference Intakes: Energy, Carbohydrate, Fiber, Fat, Fatty Acids, Cholesterol, Protein, and Amino Acids.* Washington, DC: National Academies Press; 2005.
141. Ascherio A, Katan MB, Zock PL, et al. Trans fatty acids and coronary heart disease. *N Engl J Med.* 1999;340:1994–1998.
142. Tholstrup T, Ehnholm C, Jauhiainen M, et al. Effects of medium-chain fatty acids and oleic acid on blood lipids, lipoproteins, glucose, insulin, and lipid transfer protein activities. *Am J Clin Nutr.* 2004;79:564–569.
143. St-Onge MP, Lamarche B, Mauger JF, Jones PJ. Consumption of a functional oil rich in phytosterols and medium-chain triglyceride oil improves plasma lipid profiles in men. *J Nutr.* 2003;133: 1815–1820.
144. Hayes KC. Medium-chain triacylglycerols may not raise cholesterol. *Am J Clin Nutr.* 2000;72:1583.
145. Tsai YH, Park S, Kovacic J, et al. Mechanisms mediating lipoprotein responses to diets with medium-chain triglyceride and lauric acid. *Lipids.* 1999;34:895–905.
146. Hayes KC, Lindsey S, Pronczuk A, et al. Fatty acid modulation of lipoprotein metabolism by natural triglycerides in hamsters: lipoprotein turnover and hepatic mRNA abundance. In: Christophe A, ed. *Structurally Modified Food Fats: Synthesis, Biochemistry, and Use.* Champaign, IL: AOCS Press; 1998:170–181.
147. McGarry JD, Foster DW. The regulation of ketogenesis from octanoic acids. The role of the tricarboxylic acid cycle and fatty acid synthesis. *J Biol Chem.* 1971;246:1149–1159.
148. Bohles H, Akcetin Z, Lehnert W. The influence of intravenous medium- and long-chain triglycerides and carnitine on the excretion of dicarboxylic acids. *J Parenter Enteral Nutr.* 1987;11:46–48.
149. Martin-Pena G, Culebras JM, De P, et al. Effects of 2 lipid emulsions (LCT versus MCT/LCT) on the fatty acid composition of plasma phospholipid: a double-blind randomized trial. *J Parenter Enteral Nutr.* 2002;26:30–41.
150. Bach AC, Babayan VK. Medium-chain triglycerides: an update. *Am J Clin Nutr.* 1982;36:950–962.
151. Mok KT, Maiz A, Yamazaki K, et al. Structured medium-chain and long-chain triglyceride emulsions are superior to physical mixtures in sparing body protein in the burned rat. *Metabolism.* 1984;33:910–915.
152. Babayan VK. Medium chain triglycerides and structured lipids. *Lipids.* 1987;22:417–420.
153. Lee KT, Akoh CC. Structured lipids: synthesis and applications. *Food Rev Int.* 1998;14:17–34.
154. Osborn HT, Akoh CC. Structured lipids - novel fats with medical, nutraceutical and food applications. *Compr Rev Food Sci Food Safety.* 2002;1:93–103.
155. Phan CT, Tso P. Intestinal lipid absorption and transport. *Front Biosci.* 2001;6:299–319.
156. Jensen MM, Christensen MS, Hoy CE. Intestinal absorption of octanoic, decanoic, and linoleic acids: effect of triglyceride structure. *Ann Nutr Metab.* 1994;38:104–116.
157. Stein J. Chemically defined structured lipids: current status and future directions in gastrointestinal diseases. *Int J Colorectal Dis.* 1999;14:79–85.
158. Christensen MS, Hoy CE, Becker CC, Regrave TG. Intestinal absorption and lymphatic transport of eicosapentaenoic (EPA), docosahexaenoic (DHA), and decanoic acids: dependence on intramolecular triacylglycerol structure. *Am J Clin Nutr.* 1995;61: 56–61.
159. Tso P, Lee T, Demichele SJ. Lymphatic absorption of structured triglycerides vs. physical mix in a rat model of fat malabsorption. *Am J Physiol.* 1999;277:G333–340.
160. Swails WS, Kenler AS, Driscoll DF, et al. Effect of fish oil structured lipid-based diet on prostaglandin release from mononuclear cells

in cancer patients after surgery. *J Parenter Enteral Nutr.* 1997;21: 266–274.

161. Kenler AS, Swails WS, Driscoll DF, et al. Early enteral feeding in postsurgical cancer patients. Fish oil structured lipid-based polymeric formula versus a standard polymeric formula. *Ann Surg.* 1996;223:316–333.
162. Lee KT, Akoh CC, Flatt WP, et al. Nutritional effects of enzymatically modified soybean oil with caprylic acid versus physical mixture analogue in obese Zucker rats. *J Agric Food Chem.* 2000; 48:5696–5701.
163. Mu H, Hoy CE. Effects of different medium-chain fatty acids on intestinal absorption of structured triacylglycerols. *Lipids.* 2000; 35:83–89.
164. Straarup EM, Hoy CE. Structured lipids improve fat absorption in normal and malabsorbing rats. *J Nutr.* 2000;130:2802–2808.
165. Gura KM, Duggan CP, Collier SB, et al. Reversal of parenteral nutrition-associated liver disease in two infants with short bowel syndrome using parenteral fish oil: implications for future management. *Pediatrics.* 2006;118:e197–e201.
166. Gura KM, Lee S, Valim C, et al. Safety and efficacy of a fish-oil-based fat emulsion in the treatment of parenteral nutrition-associated liver disease. *Pediatrics.* 2008;121:e678–e686.
167. Ekema G, Falchetti D, Boroni G, et al. Reversal of severe parenteral nutrition associated liver disease in an infant with short bowel syndrome using parenteral fish oil (omega-3 fatty acids). *J Pediatr Surg.* 2008;43:1191–1195.
168. Diamond IR, Sterescu A, Pencharz PB, et al. Changing the paradigm: Omegaven for the treatment of liver failure in pediatric short bowel syndrome. *J Pediatr Gastroenterol Nutr.* 2009;48: 209–215.
169. Calhoun AW, Sullivan JE. Omegaven for the treatment of parenteral nutrition associated liver disease: a case study. *J Ky Med Assoc.* 2009;107:55–57.
170. Cheung HM, Lam HS, Tam YH, et al. Rescue treatment of infants with intestinal failure and parenteral nutrition-associated cholestasis (PNAC) using a parenteral fish-oil-based lipid. *Clin Nutr.* 2009;28:209–212.
171. de Meijer VE, Gura KM, Meisel JA, et al. Parenteral fish oil monotherapy in the management of patients with parenteral nutrition–associated liver disease. *Arch Surg.* 2010;145:547–551.
172. Gura KM, Parsons SK, Bechard LJ, et al. Use of a fish oil-based lipid emulsion to treat essential fatty acid deficiency in a soy allergic patient receiving parenteral nutrition. *Clin Nutr.* 2005;24: 839–847.
173. Gura K, Strijbosch R, Arnold S, et al. The role of an intravenous fat emulsion composed of fish oil in a parenteral nutrition-dependent patient with hypertriglyceridemia. *Nutr Clin Pract.* 2007;22:664–672.
174. Jurewitsch B, Gardiner G, Naccarato M, et al. Omega-3-enriched lipid emulsion for liver salvage in parenteral nutrition-induced cholestasis in the adult patient. *J Parenter Enteral Nutr.* 2011;35: 386–390.
175. Hallay J, Olah AV, Fulesdi B, et al. Hepatobiliary response in postoperative lipid therapy in gastrointestinal surgery. *Hepato-gastroenterology.* 2010;57:1069–1073.

6 Protein

Lorraine S. Young, MS, RD, CNSD, LDN, Laurel R. Kearns, MS, RD, CNSC, LDN, Sandra L. Schoepfel, MS, RD, RN, CNSC, LDN, and Nicole Caron Clark, MS, RD, CNSC, LDN

CONTENTS

Introduction 84
Amino Acids 84
Peptides 86
Functions of Proteins 86
Structure of Proteins 86
Transport Proteins 87
Protein Signaling 87
Digestion and Absorption 87
Protein Synthesis 89
Measurement of Protein Turnover and Breakdown 90
Nitrogen Balance 90
Arteriovenous Amino Acid Differences across Organs 91
Tracer Methodology to Measure Protein Turnover 91
Other Measures of Protein Breakdown 91
Role of the Gastrointestinal Tract 92
Role of the Liver 92
Role of the Skeletal Muscle 92
Role of the Kidney 92
Role of the Brain and Central Nervous System 93
Adaptation to Fasting and Starvation 93
Determining Protein Quality 93
Determining Protein Content in Foods 94
Optimizing Nitrogen-Energy Relationships 94
Protein Requirements in Critical Illness 94
Conditionally Essential Amino Acids 95
References 95

Objectives

1. Compare and contrast the available methods to determine protein and amino acid utilization.
2. Contrast normal, starvation, and injury protein metabolism.
3. Identify the "conditionally essential" amino acids and in what conditions they become essential.
4. Identify the most clinically useful method for assessing protein status.

Test Your Knowledge Questions

1. Which of the following statements is true relating to hydrochloric acid (HCl) and protein digestion?
   A. HCl aids in the conversion of pepsin to pepsinogen.
   B. HCl denatures protein structures to make them more susceptible to enzymatic action.
   C. HCl is secreted by the parietal cells within the duodenum in response to dietary proteins.
   D. HCl's release is stimulated by the hormone insulin.
2. During protein metabolism, branched-chain amino acids (BCAAs):
   A. Are extracted primarily by the liver after a protein-containing meal.
   B. Are released by the skeletal muscle at a higher rate than other amino acids.
   C. Serve as the primary fuel sources for the enterocytes.
   D. Produce oxidative wastes during metabolism within the skeletal muscle which are removed by alanine and glutamine.
3. Proteins perform all of the following physiological functions except:
   A. Provide a major source of calories.
   B. Maintain acid-base balance.
   C. Contribute to immune defense.
   D. Serve as a mode of transport for substances.
4. The rate of protein turnover in catabolic, critically ill patients:
   A. Does not change.
   B. Decreases.
   C. Increases.
   D. Is not affected by nutrition support.

Test Your Knowledge Answers

1. The correct answer is **B**. Denaturing protein structures, making them more susceptible to enzymatic action, is a primary role of HCl. HCl plays several roles in protein digestion, including conversion of the proenzyme pepsinogen to its active form pepsin. HCl is secreted by the parietal cells within the stomach, not the duodenum. HCl secretion is stimulated by gastrin, not insulin.
2. The correct answer is **D**. Nitrogen end products produced during BCAA oxidation within the skeletal muscle are removed by the nitrogen carriers alanine and glutamine. BCAAs are extracted primarily by the skeletal muscle, with minimal extraction by the liver. BCAAs are primarily oxidized in the skeletal muscle (not the enterocytes) and are released from the muscle at a lower rate than other amino acids.
3. The correct answer is **A**. Carbohydrates and fats are the major caloric source in the human diet. Protein is not preferentially used as a source of energy in health. Protein is used as the body's primary buffer to maintain acid-base balance. All cells of the immune system (ie, white blood cells, macrophages, etc.) are made up of proteins. Proteins are the primary carriers for substances such as minerals, vitamins, and hormones.
4. The correct answer is **C**. Protein turnover rates increase dramatically in critical illness. Nutrition support will improve protein synthesis somewhat but has little effect on protein degradation.

Introduction

Proteins are an essential component of all living organisms and are important components of body mass and structure. The word protein is derived from the Greek *protos* meaning "first"; protein is clearly thought of as the most important macronutrient in the body. A thorough knowledge of how proteins are utilized by the healthy body and the changes in protein metabolism that occur with injury and disease is essential in nutrition support practice.

Amino Acids

Amino acids play central roles both as building blocks of proteins and as intermediates in metabolism. The 20 amino acids that are found within proteins convey a vast array of chemical versatility. The content and sequence of the amino acids of a specific protein are determined by the sequence of the bases in the gene that encodes that protein through complex transcription, translation, and posttranslational modifications. The chemical properties of a protein's amino acids and their spatial configurations in a protein determine their biological activity. Proteins not only catalyze most of the reactions in living cells, they control virtually all cellular process.[1] Understanding amino acid structure and properties is key to understanding protein structure and properties.

Dietary proteins are important sources of amino acids. From a nutritional point of view, some are considered essential (indispensable) because they cannot be physiologically synthesized in the human body. Our bodies cannot manufacture them, so they must be obtained exogenously. There are also nonessential (dispensable) amino acids, which are synthesized from available carbon and nitrogen precursors. In addition, there are a few amino acids that can be manufactured by the body under normal circumstances but become "conditionally essential" under certain clinical conditions, meaning the demand exceeds what can be produced. For example, tyrosine is a nonessential amino acid that is normally synthesized from the essential amino acid phenylalanine. But if inadequate phenylalanine is provided, or under certain clinical conditions the tyrosine converted from phenylalanine cannot meet its nutritional requirement, then tyrosine becomes conditionally essential. Other examples of conditionally essential amino acids include cysteine, glutamine, histidine, and taurine.

The classification of an amino acid as essential or nonessential is based on whether this amino acid can be synthesized in the body under physiological conditions. Humans can produce 9 of the 20 amino acids. The others must be supplied exogenously. Failure to obtain enough of even one of the nine essential amino acids results in degradation of the body's proteins, such as muscle, to obtain the one amino acid that is needed. Unlike fat and starch, excessive amino acids are not stored for later use, so amino acids must be consumed from exogenous sources, or the body has to accelerate the breakdown of its own proteins.

The nutritionally essential amino acids are phenylalanine, isoleucine, leucine, lysine, methionine, threonine, tryptophan, valine, and histidine, the latter essential primarily in pediatrics. Foods of animal origin, such as meat, poultry, fish, eggs, and dairy products, are the richest sources of the essential amino acids. Plant sources of protein are often deficient in one or more of the amino acids. It was previously believed that in order for vegetarians to obtain adequate amounts of protein, all of the essential amino acids had to be "balanced" at each meal. For example, a grain and a bean had to be consumed at the same meal. However, more recent research has indicated that while consuming a proper mixture of amino acids is important, it is not necessary to consume them all at the same meal.[2] The structure and classification of the nutritionally important amino acids are listed in Figure 6-1.

The distinctions between essential and nonessential amino acids are not always clearly delineated in all physiological and pathophysiological conditions. The labels "indispensable" and "dispensable" were originally defined not only in dietary terms, but also in relation to the role of amino acids in supporting protein deposition and growth. Reeds examined these labels as they applied to amino acids from three different perspectives. The first perspective comes from a traditional nutritional view that some amino acids are absolute dietary necessities if normal growth is to be maintained. The second perspective comes from a metabolic view that there may be significant limitations on the synthesis of some amino acids, thereby rendering them potential limitations to growth. In addition, a consideration of in vivo amino acid metabolism leads to the definition of a third class of amino acids, termed "conditionally essential," whose synthesis can be carried out by mammals, but is limited by a variety of factors. These factors include the dietary supply of the appropriate precursors, maturity, and the health of the individual. Finally, from a functional perspective, all amino acids are essential, including nonessential and "conditionally essential" amino acids to optimize physiological function.[3]

FIGURE 6-1 Structures of Some of the Nutritionally Important Amino Acids

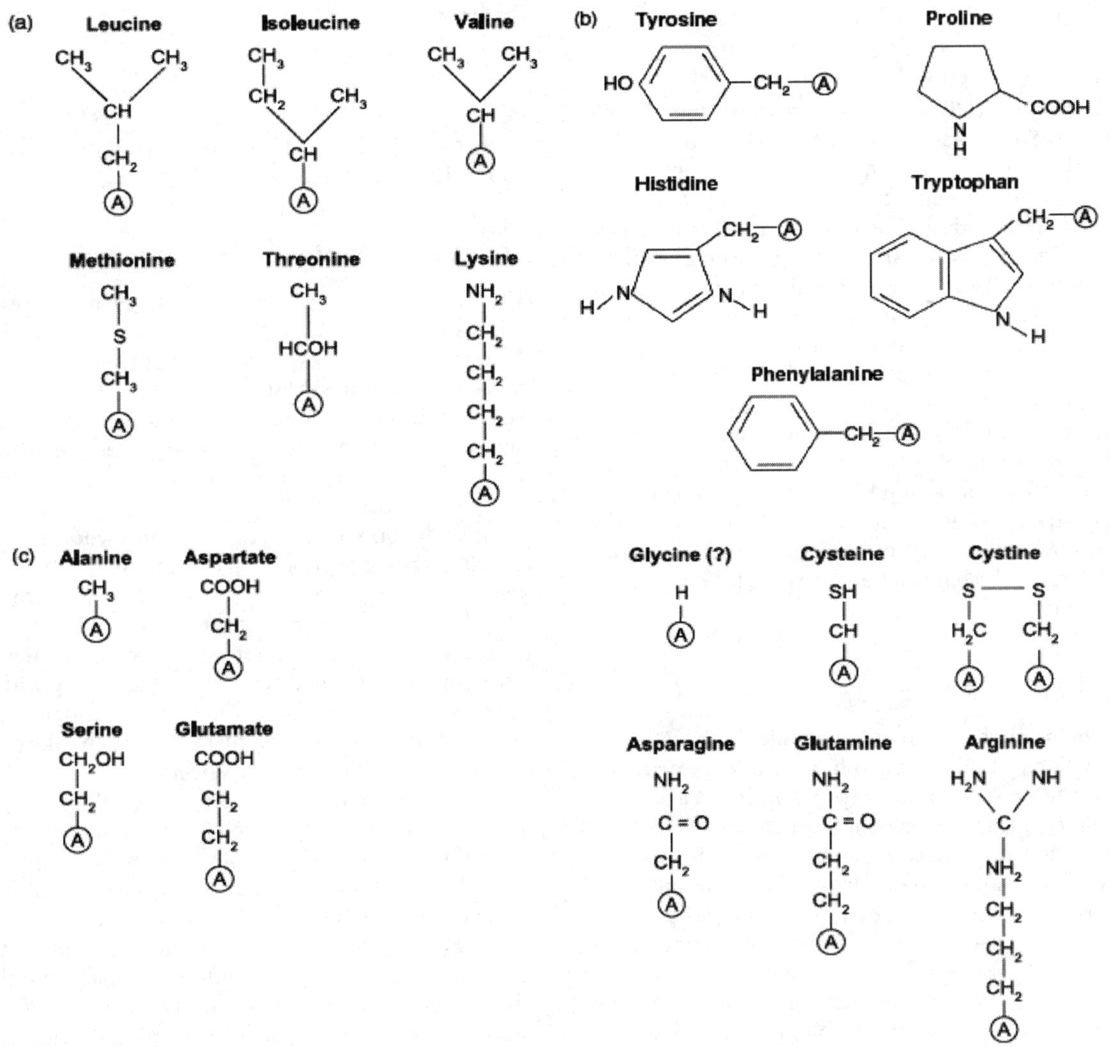

(a) Nutritionally indispensable; (b) nutritionally conditionally indispensable; (c) nutritionally dispensable. (Adapted from Fukagawa and Yu[37]).

Peptides

Peptides are composed of amino acids linked together chemically by peptide bonds. The link between one amino acid residue and the next is an amide bond and is sometimes referred to a peptide bond. The peptide bond always involves a single covalent link between the α-carboxy (oxygen-bearing carbon) of one amino acid and the amino nitrogen of a second amino acid. In the formation of a peptide bond from two amino acids, a molecule of water is eliminated. An amide bond is somewhat shorter than a typical carbon-nitrogen single bond and has a partial double-bond character because the participating carbon atom is double-bonded to an oxygen atom and the nitrogen has a lone pair of electrons available for bonding. Dipeptides are two amino acids bonded together, whereas three amino acids bonded together by peptide bonds are called tripeptides. Polypeptides consist of 10 or more amino acids bonded together by peptide bonds and an intermediate string between 4 and 10 amino acids is an oligopeptide.

Peptides differ from proteins, which are also long chains of amino acids, by virtue of their size. Traditionally, peptide chains that are short enough to be made synthetically from the constituent amino acids are called peptides, rather than proteins. So, in essence, a peptide is a small protein.[4]

The gastrointestinal (GI) tract produces a variety of chemical transmitters (gastrointestinal peptides) that are involved in gastrointestinal motility, secretion, absorption, growth, and development.[5] Dietary protein, for example, is digested in the GI tract to free amino acids and peptides by the action of gastric acid and enzymatic hydrolysis. Multiple amino acid transport systems exist for absorption of the amino acids.[6] While the cells that produce GI peptides are dispersed throughout the GI tract, regulatory peptides are found in the esophagus, stomach, small and large bowel, and the pancreas. Although GI peptides are typically thought of as hormones, not all peptides act via the traditional endocrine pathway by which they are secreted into the bloodstream and act at a distant site. Many of the peptides in the GI tract are also found in the enteric nervous system and the central nervous system. GI peptides can act on the same cells from which they are released, on neighboring cells, via classic endocrine mechanisms, and on cells following their release from nerves.[7]

Functions of Proteins

Proteins are the most abundant organic molecule in cells and are fundamental to cell structure and function. All proteins are constructed from the same basic set of 20 amino acids, covalently linked in characteristic sequences. Because each of these amino acids has a distinctive side chain that lends it chemical individuality, this group of 20 building block molecules may be regarded as the alphabet of protein structure. All proteins contain carbon, hydrogen, oxygen, and nitrogen. Some contain sulfur and others phosphorus, iron, zinc, and copper.

The roles of protein are versatile (Table 6-1). Although these functions are only a few of the many roles proteins play, they convey some sense of the immense variety of proteins and their importance in the body.[8] Newer research reveals increasingly complex roles for protein and amino acids in regulation of body composition and bone health, GI function and bacterial flora, glucose homeostasis, cell signaling, and satiety.[9]

TABLE 6-1 Functions of Proteins and Amino Acids

Growth, maintenance, and movement: Proteins form integral parts of most body structures such as skin, tendons, membranes, muscles, organs, and bones. As such, they support the growth and repair of body tissues.
Enzymes: Proteins facilitate chemical reactions.
Hormones: Functions as messengers and signals. Proteins regulate body processes. Some, but not all, hormones are made of protein.
Immunity: Antibodies, cytokines, chemokines
Regulators of gene transcription and translation through mTOR signaling pathway
Fluid and electrolyte balance: Proteins help to maintain the fluid volume and the composition of body fluids.
Acid-base balance: Proteins help maintain the acid-base balance of body fluids by acting as buffers.
Transportation and storage: Proteins transport substances, such as lipids, vitamins, minerals, and oxygen, throughout the body and storage of micronutrients (ie, ferritin).

mTor, mammalian target of rapamycin.

Structure of Proteins

Understanding protein structure is necessary to understand protein function. Two classes of strong bonds (peptide and disulfide) and three classes of weak bonds (hydrogen, hydrophobic, and electrostatic or salt) stabilize most protein structures. Protein structure is broken down into four levels that include primary, secondary, tertiary, and quaternary structure. These structure levels are explained in the following.

Primary structure refers to the "linear" sequence of amino acids in the polypeptide chain(s) and the location of disulfide bonds, if these are present. In contrast, the higher orders of protein structure (secondary, tertiary, and quaternary) involve mainly noncovalent interactions.

Secondary structure refers to "local" ordered structure brought about via hydrogen bonding mainly within the peptide backbone. The most common secondary structure elements in proteins are the alpha (α) helix and the beta (β) sheet (sometimes called β-pleated sheet).

Tertiary structure refers to the "global" folding of a single polypeptide chain. Hydrogen bonding involving groups from both the peptide backbone and the side chains are important in stabilizing tertiary structure. Disulfide bonds between cysteine residues stabilize the tertiary structure of some proteins.

Quaternary structure refers to the stable association of multiple polypeptide chains resulting in an active unit united by forces other than covalent bonds (not peptide or disulfide bonds). The forces that stabilize these aggregates are hydrogen bonds and electrostatic (or salt) bonds formed between residues on the surfaces of the polypeptide chains.

The protein structure is formed through the processes of translation and posttranslational modification. The configuration of a protein determines the physical property and the function of the protein. Taking enzyme protein as an example, the configuration of an enzyme protein determines the catalytic ability of the individual enzyme.

Transport Proteins

Transport proteins in plasma bind and carry specific molecules or ions from one organ to another. Some transport proteins are not attached to membranes, but move about in the body fluids, carrying nutrients and other molecules. Some examples of proteins acting as transport proteins include hemoglobin carrying oxygen from the lungs to the cells, lipoproteins transporting lipids around the body, and special proteins that carry vitamins (eg, retinol binding protein), minerals (eg, albumin), or hormones (eg, prealbumin). Other kinds of transport proteins are present in cell membranes and are adapted to bind and transport glucose, amino acids, and other nutrients across the membrane into cells. Iron transport provides a good illustration of these proteins' specificity and precision. Dietary iron is mainly absorbed in the duodenum and proximal jejunum where it may be stored bound to ferritin or transported into circulation. As iron is transported from the cell by an export protein into circulation, it is attached to the carrier protein transferrin, which is necessary for transport to other tissues such as bone marrow or other storage sites where it is stored as ferritin or hemosiderin. During periods of physiological need, iron is incorporated into proteins such as those in the red blood cells and muscles that assist in oxygen transport and use.

Protein Signaling

Amino acids and proteins also have important functions as signaling molecules modulating the process of protein synthesis. The "target of rapamycin" is a protein kinase initially discovered in yeast, which is the major signaling pathway regulating messenger ribonucleic acid (mRNA) translation. It is involved in the control of cell growth and proliferation, and is activated by hormones and growth factors as well as amino acids, specifically leucine, and cellular energy status. Research on the mammalian target of rapamycin signaling pathway may help identify the mechanisms involved in the longevity associated with caloric restriction observed in certain species, regulation of cancer cell growth, as well as the role of muscle protein turnover in critical illness.

Digestion and Absorption

Protein and its amino acid components enter the GI tract via both endogenous and exogenous routes. Endogenous sources include desquamated mucosal cells, digestive enzymes, and other glycoproteins such as mucus. Exogenous or dietary protein

FIGURE 6-2 Digestion and Absorption of Dietary Protein in the Intestine

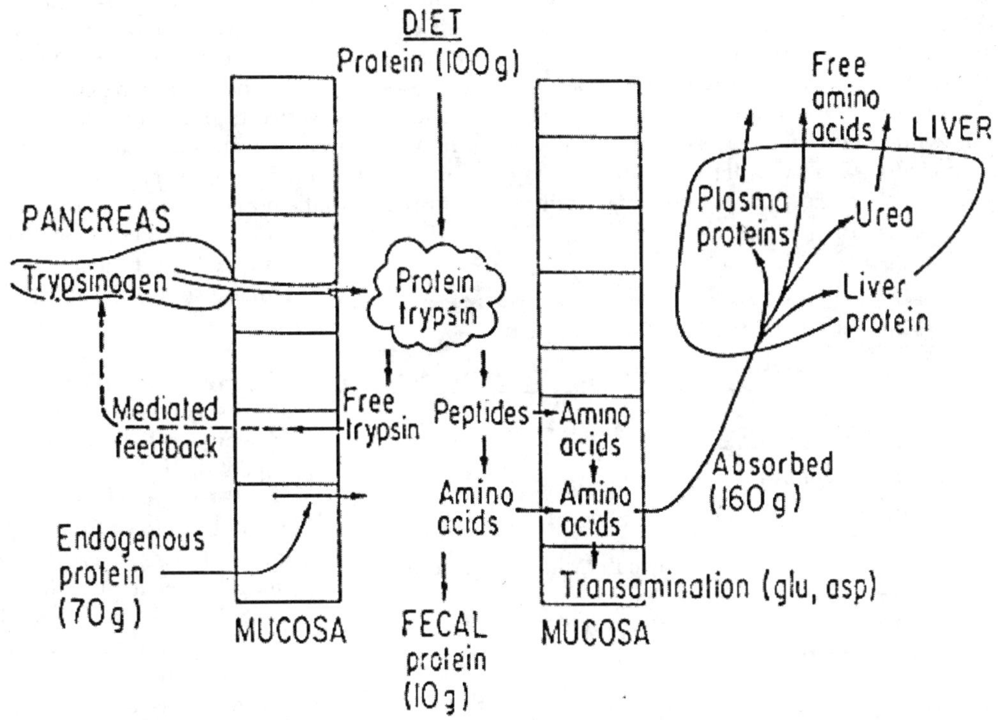

Matthews DE. Proteins and amino acids. *In:* Shils ME, Olson JA, Rose AC, eds. *Modern Nutrition in Health and Disease.* 10th ed. Baltimore, MD: Williams & Wilkins; 2006:23–61, with permission from Wolters Kluwer Health.

sources in the form of meat, poultry, fish, milk products, grains, legumes, and vegetables provide both energy and amino acids essential to the body in roles, as previously described.[9]

As exogenous proteins travel through the GI tract, they are digested into peptides and free amino acids through a series of hydrolytic reactions and feedback mechanisms (Figure 6-2). Minimal protein digestion occurs within the mouth or esophagus. Once proteins reach the stomach, however, HCl is released by the parietal cells of the stomach. HCl release may be stimulated by the hormone *gastrin*, the neurotransmitter *acetylcholine* from vagal nerve stimulation, the neuropeptide *gastrin-releasing peptide*, or the amine *histamine*.[9] HCl denatures protein structures to make them more susceptible to enzymatic action,[10] and converts *pepsinogen*, an inactive *proenzyme* or *zymogen* released by the stomach's chief cells, to its active form, *pepsin*. Pepsin in turn may activate other pepsinogen molecules or hydrolyze specific peptide bonds into the end products of large polypeptides, oligopeptides, and free amino acids.[11]

This mixture, known as acid chyme, next passes into the duodenum and small intestine where the majority of protein digestion takes place. The end products within the acid chyme stimulate the secretion of the hormones, *secretin* and *cholecystokinin* (CCK), which in turn travel through the bloodstream to the acinar cells of the pancreas to stimulate the release of alkaline pancreatic juices. Secretin and CCK also stimulate the release of digestive proenzymes *trypsinogen*, *procarboxypeptidases*, *chymotrypsinogen*, and *proelastase*[11] (Table 6-2). While deactivating pepsin, the higher pH of the duodenum is now optimal for the activity of the pancreatic enzymes.[10,11] By releasing proteolytic enzymes initially in their inactive form, the enzyme-forming cells are protected from self-digestion.[11]

Enterokinase (also known as *enteropeptidase*) is an enzyme secreted from the brush border of the small intestine, also in response to secretin and CCK. Enterokinase serves to activate trypsinogen into *trypsin*, which in turn converts many of the other proenzymes into their respective enzymatic forms for ongoing protein hydrolysis.[11] At this point, endogenous protein sources from sloughing mucosal cells or other secretory proteins are also recycled through the digestive process to form the general pool of amino acids. The presence of protein within the gut signals further enzyme secretions. When the majority of the protein has been digested, the presence of unbound trypsin acts as a feedback mechanism to turn off further secretion of trypsinogen by the pancreas.[12] At this point, the byproducts of pancreatic protease digestion, free amino acids and peptides of two to six amino acid components,[13] now enter the final phases of digestion. The brush border of the small intestine produces a variety of *peptidases*, which allow peptide digestion to continue through the distal small intestine and ileum.[9,14]

The final end products of protein digestion (eg, free amino acids, di- and tripepides) are now ready for absorption within the small intestine. The absorption of intact proteins may occur through leaks in cell junctions to a lesser extent, which accounts for the immune response associated with food allergies.[12,15] However, the majority of amino acids are absorbed in the proximal small intestine, leaving less than 1% of dietary protein to be excreted in the feces.[9,12] Through both sodium-dependent and sodium-independent active transport systems, amino acids pass from the lumen of the small intestine into the enterocyte. The various amino acid carrier systems have an affinity for specific amino acids.[16] The rate of amino acid absorption may vary depending upon the chemical properties of the amino acid. Essential (indispensable) amino acids are absorbed faster than nonessential (dispensable) amino acids. Methionine and the BCAAs leucine, isoleucine, and valine are the most rapidly absorbed.[17] Competition can occur between amino acids for transport by a carrier system.

The active transport of di- and tripeptides across the brush border membrane of the enterocyte also involves a competition for transporters but utilizes different carrier systems than those of the free amino acids. In fact, peptide absorption occurs more rapidly than an equivalent mixture of free amino acid.[18,19] It is estimated that 67% of dietary protein is absorbed as di- and tripeptides with the remaining 33% absorbed as free amino acids.[12,20,21] Once inside the enterocyte, these peptides are finally converted to free amino acids by *peptide hydrolases*. The final phase of amino acid absorption occurs across the basolateral membrane of the enterocyte by diffusion or active transport into the portal circulation (Figure 6-3).[11]

The use of peptide-based enteral formulas for patients with impaired GI function and malabsorption remains controversial. The GI tract has a large reserve capacity for digestive and absorptive processes with a multitude of intestinal folds, villi, and microvilli increasing its surface area. Malabsorption of some nutrients may not be present until 90% of organ function is impaired, such as exocrine pancreatic disease.[22,23] Peptide length may also play a role in effectiveness of GI absorption with di- and tripeptides most readily absorbed. A meta-analysis of elemental (free amino acids) versus polymeric (intact protein) formulas did not show an advantage with the former for patients with Crohn's disease.[24,25] Free amino acid formulas also have a higher osmolality, are less palatable, and cost more, further limiting their application in the clinical setting.[9]

TABLE 6-2 Some Enzymes Responsible for the Digestion of Protein

Zymogen	Enzyme or Activator	Enzyme	Site of Activity
Pepsinogen	HCL or pepsin →	Pepsin	Stomach
Trypsinogen	Enteropeptidase or trypsin →	Trypsin	Intestine
Chymotrypsinogen	Trysin →	Chymotrypsin	Intestine
Procarboxy-peptidases	Trypsin →	Carboxypeptidase A B Aminopeptidases	Intestine

HCL, hydrochloric acid.

FIGURE 6-3 Peptide and Amino Acid Absorption in the Small Intestine

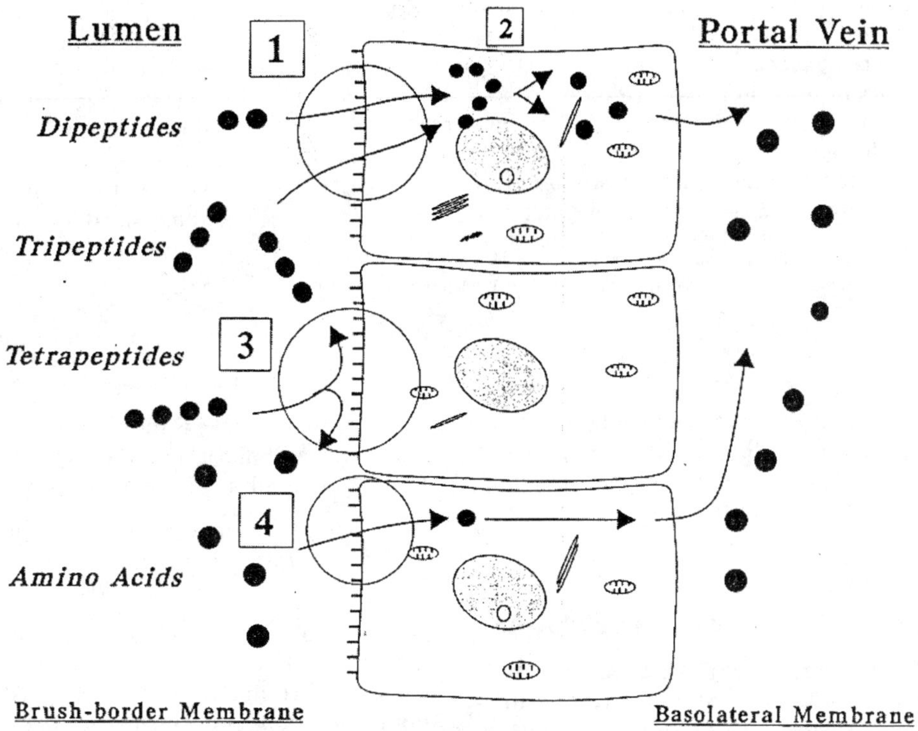

Luminal di- and tripeptides are absorbed by a specific transporter (step 1) and hydrolyzed by intracellular peptidases (step 2). Tetra- and higher peptides are hydrolyzed by brush-border peptidases (step 3). Free amino acids are absorbed by one of the active L-amino acid transporters (step 4). Adapted with permission from Grimble GK. The significance of peptides in clinical nutrition. *Ann Rev Nutr.* 1994;14:419–447.

Protein Synthesis

The human body contains an estimated 10,000 to 50,000 different kinds of proteins. Each protein has a specific function, and that function is determined during protein synthesis. Protein synthesis is a fundamental process for all living organisms. The liver is the major site of amino acid metabolism. The sequence of amino acids in each protein determines its configuration, which supports a specific function. If a genetic error alters the amino acid sequence of a protein, or if a mistake is made in copying the sequence, an altered protein will result, sometimes with dramatic consequences. Because proteins are composed of amino acids, the information necessary for their production resides in the cellular nucleus as deoxyribonucleic acid (DNA). The instructions for protein synthesis are transmitted by genetic information received at conception. There are five major stages in protein synthesis, each requiring a number of components. A brief outline of the different stages follows.[26]

Stage 1: Activation of Amino Acids: To inform a cell of the sequence of amino acids for a needed protein, a stretch of DNA serves as a template for making a strand of RNA that carries a code, listing in order the amino acids that will be needed to make a given protein. Each messenger RNA strand copies exactly the instructions for making some protein that the cell needs.

Stage 2: Initiation of the Polypeptide Chain: The messenger RNA leaves the nucleus through the nuclear membrane. DNA remains inside the nucleus. The messenger RNA, bearing the code for the polypeptide to be made, attaches itself to the protein-making machinery of the cell, the ribosomes.

Stage 3: Elongation: Another form of RNA, transfer RNA, collects amino acids from the cell fluid. Each transfer RNA carries its amino acids to the messenger RNA, which dictates the sequence in which the amino acids will be attached to form the protein strands. Thus the messenger RNA ensures the amino acids are lined up in the correct sequence.

Stage 4: Termination and Release: As the amino acids are lined up in the right sequence and the ribosome moves along the messenger, an enzyme bonds one amino acid after another to the growing protein strand. The transfer RNA is freed to return for more amino acids. When all the amino acids have been attached, the completed protein is released.

Stage 5: Folding and Processing: Finally, the messenger RNA is degraded. To achieve its native biologically active form, the polypeptide must undergo folding into its proper three-dimensional conformation. Before or after folding, the new polypeptide may undergo processing by enzymatic action to remove initiating amino acids; to introduce phosphate, methyl, carboxyl, or other groups into certain amino acid residues; or to attach oligosaccharides or prosthetic groups.

TABLE 6-3 Methods of Measuring Protein Metabolism/Status in Humans
- Nitrogen balance
- Arteriovenous measurement of amino acids and/or tracer across a tissue bed
- End-product method
- Turnover of individual components:
  - Essential amino acids (index of protein breakdown)
  - Nonessential amino acids (de novo synthesis and gluconeogenesis)
  - Urea (amino acid oxidation)
- Tracer *into* a specific protein to measure protein synthesis
- Tracer *from* a specific protein to measure protein degradation

Matthews DE. Proteins and amino acids. *In:* Shils ME, Olson JA, Rose AC, eds. *Modern Nutrition in Health and Disease.* 10th ed. Baltimore, MD: Williams & Wilkins; 2006:23–61, with permission from Wolters Kluwer Health.

Forty to one hundred amino acids can be rapidly added to a growing protein strand in a cell. The completed protein strand is released (Stage 4), the messenger is degraded, and the transfer RNA is freed to return for another load of amino acids.

Measurement of Protein Turnover and Breakdown

Protein turnover is the measurement of protein synthesis and breakdown rates. Protein turnover constantly occurs in the body with all proteins participating at varying rates. The amino acids liberated during protein turnover contribute to the free amino acid pool. There is constant flux of amino acids between muscle and organs, and the turnover rate of individual proteins varies depending on the function of the protein. For example, peptides and hormones have relatively high rates of synthesis and degradation in contrast to structural or plasma proteins. In a normal 24-hour period, dietary intake matches nitrogen output; thus protein breakdown matches synthesis. This process is altered by disease and certain physiological states as well as changes in nutrient intake.[27] Typically, daily protein intake provides only approximately 25% of total nitrogen turnover in the body with other sources coming from muscle, the viscera, and plasma proteins.

Body protein turnover in both healthy individuals and critically ill patients may be determined by several different methods. All of them have some limitations. The methods developed to quantify aspects of protein metabolism are listed in Table 6-3. These range from simple noninvasive measurements that can easily be performed in a clinical setting, such as nitrogen balance (NB), to expensive and more complicated tests such as tracer methodology, arteriovenous differences across tissue beds, and the use of molecular biology techniques.[12]

Nitrogen Balance

NB is calculated in clinical settings to help assess protein requirement and adequacy. This technique is used to determine minimum levels of human protein and amino acid requirements. Determining NB using urinary urea is an approximation based on certain assumptions such as urea accounting for about 80% of the total urinary nitrogen losses. The urinary urea nitrogen concentration is affected by stress and increased urinary excretion of non–urea nitrogen. Nitrogen balance determined with total urinary nitrogen is consistently more reliable. Stool and skin losses are usually estimated to be about 2 g nitrogen/day, unless there is excessive diarrhea or ostomy/fistula losses. In this case, the effluent should also be collected and measured for total nitrogen if possible. There are also negligible losses that are not accounted for clinically, such as menstrual losses and nasal secretion. The nitrogen balance equation used clinically is as follows:

Nitrogen balance = Nitrogen intake − nitrogen output

where nitrogen intake is the total nitrogen intake, enteral and parenteral, and nitrogen output is the sum of nitrogen losses from urine, stool, skin, and body fluids.

Nitrogen output (g/day) = Urinary urea nitrogen (mg/100 mL) × urinary volume (L/day)/100 + 20% of urinary urea losses + 2 g.[28]

In clinical settings, a 24-hour urine collection is required for urea nitrogen measurements. However, others have used shorter collection times and extrapolated those results to a 24-hour collection. Adjustments need to be made in certain patients. Many other factors affect the accuracy of nitrogen balance measurement. In addition to renal dysfunction, errors in estimating intake, or incomplete collections of urine, stool, fistula, or ostomy losses may affect balance results. NB, which may also be affected by changes in the muscle glutamine pool, has been reported to be significantly decreased in critical illness.[29] NB is a poor indicator for characterizing interorgan amino acid flux and changes in protein turnover. More sensitive tools exist for determining substrate balance across an organ and amino acid circulation such as isotopically labeled tracers. Practice Scenario 6-1 discusses the use of NB in a critical care setting.

Practice Scenario 6-1

Question: What are the best ways to evaluate protein adequacy after traumatic injury?

Scenario: A 36-year-old male was admitted to the trauma center after a collision with a tree while riding a motorcycle. He sustained major abdominal injuries including ruptured spleen, severe liver contusions, and small bowel lacerations as well as three fractured ribs, a fractured pelvis, and right femur fracture. He required multiple blood transfusions (10 units) during the first 24 hours in the hospital. After resuscitation and stabilization, he was taken to the operating room for intra-abdominal exploration, splenectomy, and repair of small bowel lacerations, which required two small bowel resections. Also noted was a large right retroperitoneal hematoma, which appeared stable. He also underwent an open reduction internal fixation of his femur fracture and stabilization of his pelvic fracture. His previous medical history is notable for alcohol abuse.

His pertinent objective data include:
Height: 73″
Weight: 95 kg
Ideal body weight: 84 kg
Estimated energy needs (25 to 30 kcal/kg): 2375 to 2850
Estimated protein needs (1.5 g/kg): 142 g

He was initially started on nasogastric feedings on postoperative day 3 with a standard high-calorie, high-protein tube feeding, which was discontinued after 24 hours because of very high gastric residuals (> 250 mL). Parenteral nutrition (PN) was started as a total nutrient admixture to meet the patient's needs until a nasojejunal tube was placed.

Intervention: On day 3 of PN, the nutrition support team was consulted due to worsening azotemia, with his blood urea nitrogen (BUN) rising to 63 mg/dL, creatinine 1.9 mg/dL. His urine output and creatinine clearance were within normal limits. His liver function tests were also elevated, with the transaminases five times normal, total bilirubin 2.9 mg/dL, and direct bilirubin 1.8 mg/dL.

The primary team requested an evaluation of the protein dose provided by the feeding regimen for potential overfeeding.

Answer: A clinically useful and practical tool for assessing protein requirements in hospitalized patients is NB. When PN or tube feeding is the sole source of nutrition intake, accurate determination of nitrogen intake is easier. Collection of output is usually where errors in NB occur. GI losses need to be accounted for but are often difficult to collect and analyze in a clinical setting. If there is significant fluctuation in daily plasma BUN levels (> 10 mg/dL), the change in plasma urea nitrogen generation over the 24-hour collection period should also be included in the output calculations.

Rationale: Although clinical guidelines exist to help define protein requirements in critical illness, it is often necessary to adjust protein intakes depending on the clinical condition of the patient (ie, worsening renal function, where protein may need to be decreased) or results of NB data used in clinical monitoring.[28]

The NB equation was determined as follows:

A 24-hour urine collection was started on day 4 of PN. The patient's BUN was stable, and there were no additional excess GI losses via drains, tubes, etc. The PN solution provided 2450 kcal and 130 g protein over the same 24-hour period as the urine collection. The patient was on nothing by mouth status.

The PN provided 20.8 g nitrogen, urine output was 2870 mL, and urine urea nitrogen was 16 g. Therefore:

$$20.8 - 16 + (20\% \text{ for other urine nitrogen})\ 3.2 + (\text{estimated other nitrogen from skin, GI losses})\ 2 = -0.4 \text{ grams or nitrogen equilibrium.}$$

This NB equation suggests that our feeding regimen is adequate.

Arteriovenous Amino Acid Differences across Organs

A more invasive tool for measuring amino acid flux across tissues and organs is arteriovenous differences. Measurements are made from the amino acids in blood delivered to the tissue and those from the blood leaving the tissue via catheters placed in an artery and vein. Most commonly, these measurements are made across muscle beds, such as the leg or arm, and this method can measure both synthesis and degradation of a protein. A tracer amino acid is given by primed continuous infusion, and replicate samples of blood are obtained from both the arterial and venous catheters once steady-state conditions are met. The net balance of the amino acid is then calculated to determine protein synthesis and protein breakdown of those amino acids not transaminated or metabolized in the muscle.[30] Typically net fluxes of ^{13}C-, ^{15}N-, and ^{2}H-labeled amino acids across tissues are used to investigate changes in protein turnover. Muscle biopsies have also been utilized along with arteriovenous difference measurements to obtain information on the intramuscular pool of amino acids. This allows assessment of intracellular amino acid recycling and transmembrane transport.[30]

Tracer Methodology to Measure Protein Turnover

The first nonradioactive stable isotope tracer amino acids to measure whole body protein turnover were used in the 1950s, but they were fraught with methodological difficulties. It was not until 1969 that a simpler tracer method was developed by Picou and Taylor-Roberts using ^{15}N-glycine. The tracer incorporation methods are based on the rate of incorporation of amino acid tracer into target tissue protein. The tracer was originally administered orally with the metabolite being measured in the urine. However, tracers used currently may be administered orally or intravenously, the latter being preferred to ensure delivery of the tracer throughout the whole body. Labeled tracers are identical to the endogenous metabolites in the body except for the substituted atom that is labeled, which allows detection for measurement.

The constant infusion method is commonly used in human studies utilizing a priming dose of amino acid to achieve plateau labeling rapidly. Major improvements in mass spectrometry have enabled the enrichment of free and protein-bound amino acids to be measured in very small samples of plasma or tissue.[31] To reach plateau labeling, the subject needs to be in a steady state, which can be difficult to achieve in hospitalized patients. A flooding-dose technique is also used to measure protein synthesis rates in isolated tissues and cell cultures; this technique minimizes the intra- and extracellular amino acid enrichment differences. There is no requirement for a steady state, and the measurement period is fairly short. This technique is ideal for measuring acute changes in patients.[31] More recent methodology is being developed using pulse tracer injections, coupled with muscle biopsies, to measure fractional protein breakdown as well as synthetic rates. Tracer methodology is an important research tool for gaining further insight into protein and amino acid flux in health and disease.

Other Measures of Protein Breakdown

Other methods have been used to specifically evaluate muscle protein breakdown such as 3-methyl histidine excretion and creatinine excretion to measure creatinine height index. The amount of urinary creatinine excreted over 24 hours is an indirect measure of muscle mass; however, significant day-to-day variation in creatinine excretion occurs during health and in hospitalized patients with acute illness and renal dysfunction.[27] 3-methyl hisitdine is an amino acid residue formed only by myofibrillar proteins actin and myosin; it is not reutilized for protein synthesis, so its excretion rate from the urine can be used as a measure of protein degradation. However, its accuracy is compromised in hospitalized patients with organ dysfunction, especially those with renal failure. In addition, there are no available objective standards for comparison.[27]

Role of the Gastrointestinal Tract

Because the GI tract is a metabolically active organ, it plays an important role in amino acid homeostasis. The GI tract actively regulates amino acid flow from the diet extracting those amino acids it needs for maintenance and function. Reed and Burrin[32] estimate that a minimum of 25% of protein intake is used within the splanchnic bed, largely by the GI tract. In the presence of a low-protein diet, GI tract growth is preserved over that of other peripheral tissues or muscle.[32,33] A large proportion of the amino acids utilized by the GI tract, especially the small intestine, are used for the synthesis of secretory protein synthesis. Within the intestinal cell, amino acids may also be used for synthesis of nucleic acids, the antioxidant glutathione, apoproteins as components of lipoproteins, or other nitrogen-containing compounds.[32] In addition, amino acids provide an important energy source to the GI tract. Dietary glutamate and aspartate account for a significant proportion of the energy source for the small intestine.[32] Glutamine released by the lung and skeletal muscle is used as a primary source of energy for the enterocyte, and may have trophic effects on the mucosal cells of the GI tract.[34] Glutamine is also used by the immune system, which is abundant within the GI tract as gut-associated lymphoid tissue as a precursor to nucleotide synthesis.[34]

Role of the Liver

The liver is a key organ for protein metabolism due to its high capacity for uptake and metabolism of amino acids. Because of its anatomical relation to the GI tract, the liver plays an essential role in regulating the flow of dietary amino acids and other nitrogenous compounds derived from tissue degradation into the systemic circulation.[35] Approximately 57% of the amino acids extracted by the liver are either oxidized or used to synthesize plasma proteins.[36] Some of these essential plasma proteins made by the liver provided important roles such as maintenance of oncotic pressure in the blood (albumin), transport functions (albumin, prealbumin, transferrin, lipoproteins, some globulins), clotting functions (fibrinogen, prothrombin), and enzymatic reactions (alanine aminotransferase, aspartate aminotransferase). Amino acids are transported across the basolateral membrane of the enterocyte to the portal vein circulation (Figure 6-3). Carrier systems also exist for amino acid transport into the hepatocyte as the only site for oxidation of the essential (indispensable) amino acids, excluding the BCAAs.[9,12]

Another important function of the liver is the metabolism of toxic nitrogenous wastes that have accumulated from exogenous protein intake or from protein breakdown during catabolic states such as trauma or sepsis.[37] The accumulation and elimination of nitrogenous wastes such as ammonia from protein degradation is accomplished by the hepatic ureagenesis. Urea is subsequently excreted in the urine by the kidneys. Carbon skeletons from the degradation of some of the amino acids known as the glucogenic amino acids (alanine, glycine, cysteine, serine, threonine, asparagine, arginine, aspartic acid, histidine, glutamic acid, glutamine, isoleucine, methionine, proline, valine, and phenylalanine) can be metabolized by the liver to glucose. This process of gluconeogenesis provides glucose when supplies are limited in the fasting state, another major homeostatic role of the liver. Also, in critically ill patients, hepatic glucose production is increased, which also contributes to hyperglycemia in these patients.

Role of the Skeletal Muscle

BCAAs are minimally extracted by the liver but instead enter the systemic circulation for metabolism largely by the muscle.[6] Skeletal muscle uptake of amino acids following a protein-containing meal leads to a net protein synthesis within the muscle.[9] The fed state supplies amino acids from dietary protein as a source of energy and helps replenish the amino acid stores. Muscle mass is maintained in a relative steady state with a fraction of the muscle broken down and resynthesized daily (protein turnover).[36] Most amino acids are released from the muscle in proportion to their concentrations within the muscle.[6,38] The release of BCAA is more conservative than that of other amino acids. However, alanine and glutamine release from muscle is higher than their concentrations within the muscle. Alanine and glutamine have a key role in muscle BCAA metabolism by participating in the process to remove the nitrogen wastes that are produced during BCAA oxidation.[6,12,38]

The glucose-alanine cycle is another means for skeletal muscle to eliminate nitrogen waste while replenishing its energy supply. Glycolysis is the process of glucose oxidation within the muscle which produces alanine via the action of alanine transaminase or alanine aminotransferase. Alanine is then transported through the bloodstream to the liver where its carbon atoms are used in gluconeogenesis to produce glucose which is delivered back to the muscle. The amino group from alanine degradation within the liver is converted to urea and eventually excreted by the kidneys.[39]

Within the muscle, leucine is the only amino acid completely oxidized for energy. During a fast, leucine levels rise both in the bloodstream and within the muscle. Leucine oxidation by the skeletal muscle in turn increases, producing acetyl coenzyme A as an energy source for the muscle while simultaneously sparing pyruvate oxidation in the tricarboxylic acid cycle. Pyruvate is then reduced to lactate in the absence of oxygen (anaerobic respiration) by the action of lactate dehydrogenase and released by the muscle. The carbon skeleton of pyruvate is also transferred to liver in the form of lactate as the precursor for gluconeogenesis. Leucine oxidation by the skeletal muscle may have some effect sparing these essential gluconeogenic precursors.[9]

Role of the Kidney

The kidney plays an important role in the interorgan exchange and synthesis of a variety of amino acids.[40] The kidney, preferentially, extracts specific amino acids, such as glycine, alanine, glutamine, glutamate, phenylalanine, and aspartate. The kidney is also a major site for arginine, histidine, and serine production.[9] Additionally, the kidney plays an important role in the conversions of phenylalanine to tyrosine, and glycine to serine.[40] Aside from the liver, the kidney is the only organ with the necessary enzymes for conversion of the gluconeogenic amino acids (see "Role of the Liver") to glucose during the process of gluconeogenesis.

Another major role of the kidney is the removal of nitrogenous waste. Enzymes within the kidney act as catalysts in the removal of ammonia from glutamate and glutamine, promoting the excretion of nitrogenous wastes in the urine. Urea, the hepatic metabolite of ammonia, is excreted by the kidneys, and under normal circumstances, 80% of the body's nitrogenous wastes are excreted as urinary urea nitrogen.[9]

Specialized parenteral glutamine-dipeptides are also thought to require the kidney as a metabolic mediator. The kidney uses some of the glutamine, whereas the remainder is released into the bloodstream.[40] The kidney is also the site of conversion of enterally supplemented glutamine into arginine. Glutamine is first metabolized by the gut to the nonproteinogenic amino acid, citrulline, which in turn is converted by the kidneys to arginine[37,40] (see "Conditionally Essential Amino Acids").

Role of the Brain and Central Nervous System

Essential amino acids are actively transported into the neurons and are present in higher concentrations than within the plasma. These amino acids perform a variety of important functions as neurotransmitters, evoking signals between neurons and other cells. Tryptophan acts as a precursor to the sleep-regulating hormone, melatonin, and the excitatory neurotransmitter, serotonin.[9]

Many nonessential amino acids are required for neurotransmitter synthesis and themselves act as neurotransmitters. Tyrosine is used to synthesize the catecholamines (dopamine, norepinephrine, and epinephrine). Catecholamine levels rise within the blood during stress, causing an increase in heart rate, blood pressure, and blood glucose. Both glycine and taurine act as inhibitory neurotransmitters. In a vitamin B_6–dependent reaction, glutamate is converted to gamma-aminobutyric acid, which acts as an inhibitory neurotransmitter within the central nervous system. Glutamate may also act as an excitatory neurotransmitter or combine with ammonia through the action of glutamine synthetase to form glutamine. Glutamine then diffuses freely into the blood or cerebrospinal fluid, helping to rid the brain of ammonia.[9]

Neuropeptides also act as potent neurotransmitters, primarily in the hypothalamus, and consist of over 100 different peptides. These complex molecules are more potent than other neurotransmitters, thus requiring only small amounts to produce profound effects on hormone release, endocrine function, or modulation of mood and behavior. Neuropeptides are responsible for mediating sensory and emotional responses including hunger, thirst, sex drive, pleasure, and pain. The enkephalins and endorphins are similar to opiates, affecting pain sensation, body temperature, and blood pressure regulation. CCK (see Chapter 1) is one of the most abundant neuropeptides in the central nervous system. Although the function of CCK within the brain is not fully understood, it may play a role in the control of food intake or in the pathogenesis of certain types of anxiety and or schizophrenia. Vasopressin also performs a variety of functions within the body including specific hormonal actions in the brain with respect to memory formation, blood pressure and temperature regulation, and pair bonding.[9,41]

Adaptation to Fasting and Starvation

Protein is the primary substrate for gluconeogenesis during starvation metabolism. The fasting state occurs as blood glucose levels return to a baseline level before the start of the next meal with a decrease in insulin levels and rise in glucagon levels.[42] Tissues such as the brain and red blood cells require a constant supply of glucose whether provided exogenously or not (as during fasting). The breakdown of hepatic glycogen stores (glycogenolysis) for glucose production begins within 2 to 3 hours of fasting but stores are soon depleted in approximately 24 hours.[12] Gluconeogenesis from amino acid substrate occurs in both the liver and the kidney, and begins within 4 to 6 hours of the last meal.[43] After approximately 2 days of starvation, the brain switches its fuel source from glucose to ketone bodies; however, blood cells and the adrenal medulla continue to rely on glucose as the primary source of energy substrate. This adaptation to starvation involves the conversion in the liver of free fatty acids to ketone bodies. As the metabolically active lean mass is diminished with starvation, metabolic processes occurring within these tissues are also reduced, accounting for a reduction in resting energy expenditure. Within approximately 1 week, adaptation to starvation with a ketone-based fuel system minimizes gluconeogenesis and further protein breakdown.[44,45]

Determining Protein Quality

Protein quality is evaluated by calculating the protein digestibility corrected amino acid score (PDCAAS). It was proposed in 1991 by the Food and Agriculture Organization/World Health Organization and has been adopted by the Food and Nutrition Board of the Institute of Medicine.[46] The PDCAAS indicates the overall quality of a protein because it represents the relative adequacy of its most limiting amino acid. The PDCAAS is estimated as follows:

Concentration of the most limiting, digestibility-corrected amino acid in a test protein: PDCAAS = Concentration of that amino acid in the 1991 Food and Agriculture Organization/World Health Organization amino acid scoring reference pattern

For example, if a protein has a PDCAAS of 40 and the lowest amino acid content is for lysine, only 40% of that protein can be utilized for protein synthesis. The highest PDCAAS score any protein can achieve is 100. This would mean that 100% of that protein can be used for protein synthesis or that it contains all essential amino acids. Given that typical diets contain many sources of dietary protein, foods could function as "complementary proteins" if they are higher in the amino acid that is limiting in other protein.[47]

An important benefit to using the PDCAAS score is that this approach uses human amino acid requirements whereas animal bioassays were used in the past.[37] An additional step is added to this method: the lowest amino acid ratio is then multiplied by its true protein digestibility. This ensures that the appropriate levels of essential amino acids are provided in the diet.

Determining Protein Content in Food

Historically, the protein content of foods was determined on the basis of total nitrogen as measured by the Kjeldahl method. Nitrogen content is then multiplied by a factor to arrive at the protein content. This approach is based on two assumptions: that carbohydrates and fats do not contain nitrogen, and that almost all nitrogen in the diet is present as amino acids in proteins. Based on early estimates, an average nitrogen content of proteins was determined to be approximately 16%, which led to the use of the following calculation to convert nitrogen to protein: nitrogen $\times$ 6.25 ($1/0.16 = 6.5$).[48]

Estimating nitrogen content of dietary protein with the use of a single factor may not be an accurate reflection of the true nitrogen content. All nitrogen in foods is not protein-based. For example, nitrogen may be part of amino acids, nucleotides, creatine, and choline, where it is referred to as nonprotein nitrogen. Only a small percentage of nonprotein nitrogen is available to synthesize nonessential amino acids. Moreover, the nitrogen content of specific amino acids varies according to the molecular weight of the amino acid and the number of nitrogen atoms it contains (one to four, depending on the amino acid in question). Based on this information, the nitrogen content of proteins actually varies from 13% to 19%, and nitrogen conversion factors range from 5.26 to 7.69.

Other factors that have been used to determine dietary nitrogen content include "Jones" factors, which are nitrogen conversion factors for specific foods.[49] For example, Jones factors for animal protein such as meat, milk, and eggs are between 6.25 and 6.38, whereas those for vegetable proteins are in the range of 5.7 to 6.25. The difference between the 6.25 factor and the Jones factor is only about 1% for mixed diets. The nitrogen content for enteral and parenteral formulations is also determined by amino acid analysis. The nitrogen content of the enteral and parenteral formula can be calculated according to its amino acid concentrations.

The nitrogen content = the sum of (each amino acid concentration in plasma $\times$ % nitrogen of individual amino acids)

Optimizing Nitrogen-Energy Relationships

Loss of body protein is associated with disability and death when nutrient intake is not sufficient to meet its consumption in starvation and critical illness. However, providing nonprotein calories in amounts to meet energy demands has important effects on nitrogen balance. Calloway and Spector reported nitrogen sparing in early experiments with healthy active men when calories were supplied without protein.[50] Maximum protein sparing occurs at approximately 700 nonprotein calories. Additional increases in calories did not improve NB. However, addition of protein in dietary intake will further improve nitrogen sparing. They concluded that with fixed but adequate protein intake, the energy level is the determinant factor in nitrogen equilibrium, and with fixed and adequate calorie intake, protein intake determines nitrogen equilibrium. The recommended requirement for healthy adults is set at 0.8 g/kg/day based on nitrogen and energy balance studies performed in adult men and women, and adding 25% or two standard deviations to the balance data to meet the needs of 97.5% of a normally distributed population.[46]

Critical illness is associated with increased protein turnover, protein catabolism, and negative NB. The increased metabolic rate and accelerated net protein loss demands a greater energy and protein intake. In fact, protein requirements double in critical illness to approximately 15% to 20% of total calories. For example, the estimated protein requirement for a patient with multiple trauma requiring 2600 calories for maintenance would be at least 98 to 120 g of protein per day. Current practice dictates that energy requirements should be provided to meet energy demands as determined by energy equations or indirect calorimetry and protein intakes of 1.5 g protein/kg/day. There is evidence that protein intakes beyond this level afford no greater advantage in improving nitrogen equilibrium or loss of body protein in sepsis.[51] However, recommendations in trauma and burns suggest an increase in protein requirements up to 2 g/kg/d.[52] NB is difficult to attain in critically ill patients and may not be a realistic goal. Exogenous protein will improve nitrogen retention by increasing synthesis but has little effect on protein catabolic rates.

Protein Requirements in Critical Illness

Nutrient requirements of critically ill patients are remarkably different than in normal individuals because of profound alterations in carbohydrate, lipid, and protein metabolism. Research has focused on providing specific novel nutrients that have the ability to alter the normal response to illness or become "conditionally" essential in certain situations, such as renal or liver dysfunction.

The primary goal of nutritional therapy in critical illness is to preserve lean body mass and support metabolic functions. Lean tissue loss inevitably occurs due to the rapid rates of protein breakdown, mobilization of amino acid from the periphery to the liver for gluconeogenesis, and production of acute phase proteins, to support the immune system in host defense, to the wound to promote healing, and the kidney for acid-base balance. Immobilization after critical illness and in some cases starvation and prolonged bed rest will also contribute to lean tissue wasting. Meeting energy and protein requirements can minimize the loss of lean tissue.

After injury, sepsis, or critical illness, protein turnover rates, synthesis, breakdown, and oxidation of protein is increased. The degree of increase is determined by the severity of the illness and metabolic response.[51] The negative NB seen after minor elective surgery is due primarily to a decrease in protein synthesis. However, with severe sepsis and injury, both synthesis and catabolism are elevated and feeding further increases turnover.[51] Shaw et al.[51] showed that feeding protein in septic patients at 1.1 g/kg/day will decrease net protein loss catabolism; by increasing protein intake further to 1.6 g/kg/day, catabolism was decreased further, but above that intake catabolism increased again. Protein sparing does not typically improve with intakes above 1.5 g/kg/day in critical illness, but the most severe burn patients may require up to 2 g/kg/d.[52] The risks of feeding too much protein can result in prerenal azotemia with the excess protein increasing the burden to the kidneys to work to excrete excess urea nitrogen. Excess protein feeding over the long term can result in kidney stones and increased risk for osteoporosis. Nevertheless, adequately fed, underweight patients may require protein up to 25% more than their normal weight counterparts or 1.9 g/kg/day.[53,54] Clinical studies of underweight critically ill patients have not been performed; however as weight decreases, the more rapidly turning over or metabolically active central protein compartments assume a greater proportion of the lean tissue mass (liver, heart, lungs).[55–58]

Conditionally Essential Amino Acids

Some amino acids may exert pharmacologic action during critical illness when administered at higher doses than normally consumed in food or standard nutrition support. Additionally, requirements for conditionally essential amino acids may change during critical illness due to the altered metabolic demand. For example, glutamine metabolism during critical illness has been extensively investigated over the past 20 years. Glutamine is the most abundant amino acid in the body, accounting for more than 50% of the intracellular free amino acid pool in muscle. It is the vital fuel for rapidly dividing cells such as fibroblasts, reticuloendothelial cells, malignant cells, and gut epithelial cells. Glutamine carries two nitrogen moieties per molecule and along with alanine serves as the body's primary nitrogen shuttle between muscle and visceral organs. In some clinical conditions, such as exercise, trauma, and sepsis, the body's glutamine requirement exceeds the mammalian's ability to synthesize glutamine; this leads to a fall in plasma and intracellular glutamine. This fall in glutamine concentration is associated with atrophy of intestinal mucosa, impairment of immune function, and decreased protein synthesis. Low plasma and muscle concentrations of glutamine in critical illness are correlated with increased mortality, leading to the hypothesis that replenishment of glutamine levels has a therapeutic value in certain clinical conditions.[59,60]

Arginine and cysteine, the former having an important role in immunomodulation, may also have pharmacological properties. Arginine is a semiessential amino acid that has demonstrated importance in immune function and wound healing. It is required exogenously by young mammals but adults can synthesize it de novo. Plasma arginine levels are usually dependent on dietary intake because the rate of endogenous synthesis cannot increase in response to an inadequate supply. Arginine is a urea cycle intermediate. It is deaminated to citrulline. It is also used to synthesize polyamines and, most importantly, nitric oxide, which affects respiratory, cardiovascular, renal, and immunological function. Arginine and cysteine also enhance lymphocyte function and may prove useful in treating inflammatory diseases and acquired immunodeficiency syndrome.[53] Arginine is a key component of some immune-enhancing formulas.[61]

Additional proteins with pharmacological potential include carnitine and choline. Carnitine is a trimethylated amino acid similar in structure to choline, which is required as a cofactor for transformation of free long-chain fatty acids into acylcarnitines and transport into the mitochondria. Although a primary deficiency in carnitine is rare, it has been documented in preterm infants and in chronic renal failure. Carnitine nutrition is discussed in greater detail in Chapter 5.

Choline is also an essential nutrient necessary for proper membrane structure, which is not part of PN formulations. It can be manufactured in the liver from methionine, but synthesis may be impaired in patients on long-term PN or in premature infants. Intravenous methionine is metabolized differently than orally or enterally consumed methionine, which may be partially responsible for the choline deficiency that develops with PN.[62] Small amounts of choline are available in the form of lecithin present in fat emulsions, but despite this, low choline levels have been documented in patients receiving PN.[63] There is some evidence that choline deficiency is partially responsible for the hepatic abnormalities prevalent in patients on long-term PN, specifically hepatic steatosis. There are no available intravenous forms of choline. Repletion, if necessary, needs to be via the oral or enteral route. Finally, creatine and hydroxymethyl butyrate (HMB) have been marketed as ergogenic aids in the sports medicine literature. They have both been extensively studied and have consistently been shown to increase lean body mass and improve strength when combined with resistance training. Creatine has also been studied in diseases associated with muscle wasting (amyotrophic lateral sclerosis, muscular dystrophy). HMB is a metabolite of leucine, but its mechanism of action remains elusive. It has been used as a supplement with glutamine in wasting associated with acquired immunodeficiency syndrome.[64] The ingestion of 3 g/day of HMB in the elderly promotes an increase in strength and lean body mass when combined with resistance exercise.[65,66] Its role in the treatment of the sarcopenia of aging is under current investigation.[67]

References

1. Murray RK, Granner DK, Mayes PA, et al. *Harpers Illustrated Biochemistry*. 26th ed. New York, NY: McGraw-Hill; 2003:14–20.
2. Young VR, Pellett PL. Plant proteins in relation to human protein and amino acid nutrition. *Am J Clin Nutr*. 1994:59(5 suppl): 1203s–1212s.
3. Reeds PJ. Dispensable and indispensable amino acids for humans. *J Nut*. 2000;30:S1835–S1840.
4. Nelson DL, Cox MM. *Lehninger Principles of Biochemistry*. 4th ed. New York, NY: W.H. Freeman; 2005:85–89.
5. Walsh JH, Dochray GJ. *Gut Peptides*. New York, NY: Raven Press; 1994:305–340.
6. Frankenfield D. Energy and macrosubstrate requirements. In: Gottschish MM, ed. *The Science and Practice of Nutrition Support – A Case-Based Core Curriculum*. Dubuque, IA: Kendall/Hunt Publishing Co; 2001:31–52.
7. Solcia E, Fiocca R, Rindi G, et al. The pathology of the gastrointestinal endocrine system. *Endocrinol Metab Clin North Am*. 1993;22: 795–821.
8. Whitney EN, Cataldo CB, Rolfes SR. *Understanding Normal and Clinical Nutrition*. 7th ed. Pacific Grove, CA: Brooks/Cole; 2005: Chapter 6, 180–211.
9. Gropper SS, Smith JL, Groff JL. Protein. In: Gropper SS, Smith JL, eds. *Advanced Nutrition and Human Metabolism*. 5th ed. Belmont, CA: Wadsworth Learning; 2009:179–249.

10. DeLegge MH, Ridley C. Nutrient digestion, absorption, and excretion. In: Gottschlich MM, eds. *The Science and Practice of Nutrition Support: A Case-Based Core Curriculum*. Dubuque, IA: Kendall Hunt; 2001:1–16.
11. Anderson CE. Energy and metabolism. In: Schneider HA, Anderson CE, Coursin DB. eds. *Nutrition Support of Medical Practice*. 2nd ed. Philadelphia, PA; Harper & Row; 1983:10–22.
12. Matthews DE. Proteins and amino acids. In: Shils ME, Olson JA, Rose AC, eds. *Modern Nutrition in Health and Disease*. 10th ed. Baltimore, MD: Williams & Wilkins; 2006:23–61.
13. Trier JS. Intestinal absorption: alimentary tract, liver, biliary tree and pancreas. In: Stein JH, ed. *Internal Medicine*. Vol I. Boston, MA: Little, Brown & Co; 1983:11–16.
14. Beyer PL. Digestion, absorption, transport, and excretion of nutrients. In: Mahan LK, Escott-Stumps S, eds. *Krause's Food, Nutrition, and Diet Therapy*. 10th ed. Philadelphia, PA: WB Saunders; 2000:3–18.
15. Gardner ML. Absorption of intact proteins and peptides. In: Johnson LR, Alpers DH, Christensen J, et al., eds. *Physiology of the Gastrointestinal Tract*. 3rd ed. New York, NY: Raven Press; 1994:1795–1820.
16. Ganapathy V, Brandsch M, Leibach FH. Intestinal transport of amino acids and peptides. In: Johnson LR, Alpers DH, Christensen J, et al., eds. *Physiology of the Gastrointestinal Tract*. 3rd ed. New York, NY: Raven Press; 1994:1773–1794.
17. Adibi SA, Gray S, Menden E. The kinetics of amino acid absorption and alteration of plasma composition of free amino acids after intestinal perfusion of amino acid mixtures. *Am J Clin Nutr*. 1967;20:24–33.
18. Fairclough PD, Hegarty JE, Silk DBA, Clark ML. A comparison of the absorption of two protein hydrolysates and their effects on water and electrolyte movements in the human jejunum. *Gut*. 1980;21:829–834.
19. Silk DBA, Fairclough PD, Clark ML, et al. Use of peptide rather than a free amino acid nitrogen source in chemically defined elemental diets. *J Parenter Enteral Nutr*. 1980;4:548–553.
20. Zaloga GP. Physiological effects of peptide-based enteral formulas. *Nutr Clin Pract*. 1990;5:231–237.
21. Alpers DH. Uptake and fate of absorbed amino acids and peptides in the mammalian intestine. *Fed Proc*. 1986;45:2261–2267.
22. Grimble GK. Thd significance of peptides in clinical nutrition. *Ann Rev Nutr*. 1994;14:419–447.
23. DiMagno EP, Go VLW, Summerskill WHJ. Relations between pancreatic enzyme outputs and malabsorption in severe pancreatic insufficiency. *New Engl J Med*. 1973;288:813–815.
24. Zachos M, Tandeur M, Griffiths AM. A meta-analysis of enteral nutrition as primary therapy of active Crohn's disease: does formula composition influence efficacy? *Cochrane Database Syst Rev*. 2001;3:1–24.
25. Griffiths AM. Enteral nutrition in management of Crohn's disease. *J Parent Enter Nutr*. 2005;29(suppl):S108–S117.
26. Nelson DL, Cox MM. *Lehninger Principles of Biochemistry*. 4th ed. New York, NY: Freeman; 2004:1044–1045.
27. Young LS, Stoll S. Protein in nutrition support. In Matarese LE, Gottschlich MM, eds. *Contemporary Nutrition Support Practice: A Clinical Guide*. 2nd ed. Philadelphia, PA: Saunders; 1998:97–109.
28. Wilmore DW. *Metabolic Management of the Critically Ill*. New York, NY: Plenum Publishing; 1977:193.
29. Walser M. Misinterpretation of nitrogen balances when glutamine stores fall or are replenished. *Am J Clin Nutr*. 1993;5:414–416.
30. Wagenmakers AJM. Tracers to investigate protein and amino acid metabolism in human subjects. *Proc Nutr Soc*. 1999;58:987–1000.
31. Garlick PJ, Wernerman J, McNurlan MA, Heys SD. Organ-specific measurements of protein turnover in man. *Proc Nutr Soc*. 1991;50: 217–225.
32. Reeds PJ, Burrin DG. The gut and amino acid homeostasis. *Nutrition*. 2000;16:666–668.
33. Ebner S, Schoknecht P, Reeds PJ, Burrin DG. Growth and metabolism of gastrointestinal and skeletal muscle tissues in protein-malnourished neonatal pigs. *Am J Physiol*. 1994;266:R1736–R1741.
34. Scheppach W, Loges C, Bartram P, et al. Effects of free glutamine and alanyl-glutamine dipeptide on mucosal proliferation of the human ileum and colon. *Gastroenterology*. 1994;107:429–434.
35. Van de Poll MCG, Siroen MPC, Van Leeuwen PAM, et al. Interorgan amino acid exchange in humans: consequences for arginine and citrulline metabolism. *Am J Clin Nutr*. 2007;85(1):167–172.
36. Ettinger S. Macronutrients: carbohydrates, proteins, and lipids. In: Mahan LK, Escott-Stumps S, eds. *Krause's Food, Nutrition, and Diet Therapy*. 10th ed. Philadelphia, PA: WB Saunders; 2000:31–66.
37. Fukagawa NK, Yu Y-M. Nutrition and metabolism of proteins and amino acids. In: Gibney MJ, Lanham-New SA, Cassidy A, Vorster HH, eds. *Introduction to Human Nutrition*. 2nd ed. Oxford, UK: The Nutrition Society Textbook Series, Wiley-Blackwell; 2009:49–73.
38. Young VR, Meredith C, Hoerr R, et al. Amino acid kinetics in relation to protein and amino acid requirements: the primary importance of amino acid oxidation. In: Garrow JS, Halliday D, eds. *Substrate and Energy Metabolism in Man*. London: John Libbey; 1985:119–134.
39. King MW. Medical biochemistry: glucose-alanine cycle 1996. www.dentistry.leeds.ac.uk/biochem/theme/glucose-alaninecy-cle.html. Accesed April 22, 2006.
40. Van de Poll MCG, Soeters PB, Deutz NE, et al. Renal metabolism of amino acids: its role in interorgan amino acid exchange. *Am J Clin Nutr*. 2004;79:185–197.
41. Cooper PE, Neuroendocrinology. In: Bradley WG, Daroff RB, Fenichel GM, Jankovic J, eds. *Neurology in Clinical Practice. Vol 1: Principles of Diagnosis and Management*. 4th ed. Philadelphia, PA: Elsevier; 2004:849–868.
42. Champe PC, Harvey RA. Metabolism in starvation, diabetes mellitus, and injury. In: Champe PC, Harvey RA, eds. *Lippincott's Illustrated Reviews: Biochemistry*. 2nd ed. Philadelphia, PA: JB Lippincott Co.;1994:291–302.
43. Marks DB, Marks AD, Smith CM. Fasting. In: Smith C, Marks A, Lieberman M, eds. *Basic Medical Biochemistry—A Clinical Approach*. Baltimore, MD: Williams & Wilkins; 1996:27–34.
44. Cahill GF Jr, Aoki TT. Partial and total starvation. In: Kinney JM, ed. *Assessment of Energy Metabolism in Health and Disease: Report of the First Ross Conference on Medical Research*. Columbus, OH: Ross Labs; 1980:129–134.
45. Borum PR. Nutrient metabolism. In: Gottschlich MM, ed. *The Science and Practice of Nutrition Support: A Case-Based Core Curriculum*. Dubuque, IA: Kendall Hunt; 2001:17–29.
46. World Health Organization. *Energy and Protein Requirements. Report of a Joint FAO/WHO/UNO Expert Consultation*. Tech Rep Series 724. Geneva, Switzerland: World Health Organization; 1985:206.
47. Castellanos VH, Litchford MD, Campbell WW. Modular protein supplements and their applications to long-term care. *Nutr Clin Prac*. 2006;21:485–504.
48. Food and Agriculture Organization of the United States: Rome. *Special Report of a Technical Workshop Rome, 3-6, December 2002. Food Energy-Methods of Analysis and Conversion Factors*. 2003. www.fao.org. Accessed September 20. 2005.
49. Jones DB. *Factors for Converting Percentages of Nitrogen in Foods and Feeds into Percentages of Proteins*. Circular No. 183. Washington, DC: United States Department of Agriculture; 1942.
50. Calloway DH, Spector H. Nitrogen balance as related to calorie and protein intake in active young men. *Am J Clin Nutr*. 1954;2: 405–412.

51. Shaw JH, Wildbore M, Wolf RR. Whole body protein kinetics in severely septic patients: the response to glucose infusion and total parenteral nutrition. *Ann Surg*. 1987;205:288–294.
52. Jacobs DG, Jacobs DO, Kudsk KA, et al. Practice management guidelines for nutrition support of the trauma patient. *J Trauma*. 2004;57:660–679.
53. Stehle P. Nutrition support in critical illness: amino acids. In: Cynober L, Moore FA, eds. *Nutrition in Critical Care*. Nestle Nutrition Workshop Series Clinical and Performance Program. Basel, Switzerland: Nestec Ltd.; Vevey/S. Karger AG; 2003: 57–73.
54. Campbell IT. Limitations of nutrient intake. The effect of stressors: trauma, sepsis and multiple organ failure. *Eur J Clin Nutr*. 1999;53 (suppl 1):s143–s147.
55. Hoffer LJ. Protein and energy provision in critical illness. *Am J Clin Nutr*. 2003;78:906–911.
56. Ahmad A, Duerksen DR, Munroe S, Bistrian BR. An evaluation of resting energy expenditure in hospitalized, severely underweight patients. *Nutrition*. 1999;15:384–388.
57. Kurpad AV, Regan MM, Raj T, et al. Lysine requirements of chronically undernourished adult Indian men, measured by a 24-h indicator amino acid oxidation and balance technique. *Am J Clin Nutr*. 2003;77:101–108.
58. Winter TA, O'Keefe SJ, Callahan M, Dip, N, Marks T. The effect of severe undernutrition and subsequent refeeding on whole-body metabolism and protein synthesis in human subjects. *J Parenter Enteral Nutr*. 2005;29:221–228.
59. Griffiths RD, Allen KD, Andrews FJ, Jones C. Infection, multiple organ failure, and survival in the intensive care unit: influence of glutamine-supplemented parenteral nutrition on acquired infections. *Nutrition*. 2002;18:546–552.
60. Alpers DH. Glutamine: do the data support the cause for glutamine supplementation in humans? *Gastroenterology*. 2006;130:S106–S116.
61. McGowen KC, Bistrian BR. Immunonutrition: problematic or problem solving? *Am J Clin Nutr*. 2003;77:764–770.
62. Buchman AL. Choline deficiency during parenteral nutrition in humans. *NCP*. 2003;18:353–358.
63. Chawla RK, Berry CJ, Kutner MH, et al. Plasma concentrations of transulfuration pathway products during nasoenteral and intravenous hyperalimentation of malnourished patients. *Am J Clin Nutr*. 1985;42:577–584.
64. Clark RH, Feleke G, Din M, et al. Nutritional treatment for acquired immunodeficiency virus-associated wasting using beta-hydroxy beta methyl butyrate, glutamine, and arginine: a randomized, double-blind, placebo-controlled study. *J Parenter Enter Nutr*. 2000;24(3):133–139.
65. Flakoll P, Sharp R, Baier S, et al. Effect of beta-hydroxy-beta-methylbutyrate, arginine, and lysine supplementation on strength, functionality, body composition, and protein metabolism in elderly women. *Nutrition*. 2004;20:445–451.
66. Vukovich MD, Stubbs NB, Bohlken RM, et al. Body composition in 70-year old adults responds to dietary beta-hydroxy-beta-methylbutyrate (HMB) similarly to that of young adults. *J Nutr*. 2001;131:2049–2052.
67. Baier S, Johannsen D, Abumrad N, et al. Year-long changes in protein metabolism in elderly men and women supplemented with a nutrition cocktail of beta-hydroxy-beta-methylbutyrate (HMB), L-arginine, and L-lysine. *J Parenter Enter Nutr*. 2009;33:71–82.

7 Fluids, Electrolytes, and Acid–Base Disorders

Ginger Langley, PharmD, BCNSP, BCPS, CPHQ, and Sharla Tajchman, PharmD, BCNSP, BCPS

CONTENTS

Background 99
Fluid Compartments 99
Fluid Balance 100
Fluid and Electrolyte Disorders 101
General Principles for the Management of Electrolyte Disorders 102
Sodium 102
  Hyponatremia 102
  Hypernatremia 104
Potassium 104
  Hypokalemia 106
  Hyperkalemia 107
Magnesium 109
  Hypomagnesemia 109
  Hypermagnesemia 110
Calcium 111
  Hypocalcemia 111
  Hypercalcemia 112
Phosphorus 112
  Hypophosphatemia 112
  Hyperphosphatemia 114
Acid–Base Balance 114
  Acid–Base Physiology 114
    Definitions 114
    Regulation of Hydrogen Ion Concentration 114
    Chemical Buffers 114
    Lungs 115
    Kidneys 115
    Normal Blood Gas Values 115
Analysis of Acid–Base Disorders 115
  Acid–Base Disorders 115
    Respiratory Acidosis 115
    Respiratory Alkalosis 116
    Metabolic Acidosis 116
    Normal Anion-Gap Acidosis (Hyperchloremic Acidosis) 117
    High Anion-Gap Acidosis 118
    Metabolic Alkalosis 118
    Saline-Responsive Metabolic Alkalosis (Urine Chloride $<$10 mEq per Liter) 118
    Saline-Unresponsive Metabolic Alkalosis (Urine Chloride $>$10 mEq per Liter) 118
    Mixed Acid-Base Disorders 118
References 118

Objectives

1. Describe factors that influence fluid movement between the intracellular and extracellular fluid compartments.
2. Calculate replacement and maintenance fluid requirements for various patient populations.
3. Recommend appropriate treatment for common electrolyte abnormalities.
4. Evaluate and treat acid–base disorders based on the clinical presentation and accompanying laboratory data.

Testing Your Knowledge Questions

1. The administration of 1 L of 0.9% sodium chloride to a normonatremic patient will increase the intravascular and interstitial fluid compartments by:
   A. 1000 mL and 0 mL, respectively
   B. 0 mL and 1000 mL, respectively
   C. 750 mL and 250 mL, respectively
   D. 250 mL and 750 mL, respectively
2. Assuming the same weight and serum sodium concentration, which of the following patients has the greatest free water deficit?
   A. A 35-year-old male
   B. A 75-year-old male
   C. A 35-year-old female
   D. A 75-year-old female
3. Which of the following electrolyte derangements is commonly seen in a patient with a high output nasogastric tube?
   A. Hyperchloremia and hyperkalemia
   B. Hyperchloremia and hypokalemia
   C. Hypochloremia and hyperkalemia
   D. Hypochloremia and hypokalemia
4. A patient with severe intractable nausea and vomiting is at risk for which of the following acid–base disorders?
   A. Hyperchloremic metabolic alkalosis
   B. Hyperchloremic metabolic acidosis
   C. Hypochloremic metabolic alkalosis
   D. Hypochloremic metabolic acidosis

Testing Your Knowledge Answers

1. The correct answer is **D**. 0.9% sodium chloride (154 mEq per liter) is isotonic and, therefore, does not contribute to an osmotic gradient. Isotonic saline enters and remains in the extracellular fluid (ECF). Thus, administering 1 L of 0.9% sodium chloride expands the ECF by 1 L. The intravascular volume accounts for 25% of the ECF and will be expanded by 250 mL. The remaining 750 mL will be distributed to the interstitial fluid compartment.
2. The correct answer is **A**. Free water deficit is calculated as follows:

$$\text{Water deficit (L)} = 0.5 \times \text{body weight (kg)} \times \left(\frac{\text{Plasma sodium (mEq/L)}}{140 \text{ mEq/L}} - 1\right)$$

   Given the same body weight and serum sodium concentration, the only variable is the percent of total body water (TBW). The percent of TBW increases as the proportion of lean body mass to adipose tissue increases. In general, the percent of TBW decreases with age and with female gender due to an increase in the proportion of body fat compared to lean body mass. Younger males would be expected to have the highest proportion of lean body mass, the highest percentage of TBW, and therefore the largest free water deficit.
3. The correct answer is **D**. Gastric fluids are composed of hydrochloric acid, sodium chloride, and potassium chloride. Patients who require continuous or intermittent nasogastric suction may lose large amounts of gastric fluids and the electrolytes contained within these fluids. As a result, patients may develop electrolyte derangements such as hypochloremia and hypokalemia.
4. The correct answer is **C**. Gastric fluids contain approximately 130 mEq per liter of chloride and are very acidic with a pH of 1 to 2. Loss of large amounts of gastric fluids via vomiting, especially for a prolonged period of time, can result in a hypochloremic metabolic alkalosis.

Background

Body fluids differ with regard to their distribution and the substances dissolved within them. These substances include electrolytes and nonelectrolytes, such as glucose and proteins. Despite variations in daily intake, fluid and electrolyte balance is maintained through a complex system of regulatory mechanisms to maintain an environment conducive to normal cell function. Cell function is also highly dependent on acid–base homeostasis because nearly all biochemical reactions are influenced by hydrogen ion concentration. In practice, disruption of fluid, electrolyte, and acid–base homeostasis is common, the results of which can have a profound physiological impact on many organ systems. This chapter discusses normal body requirements, the distribution and homeostasis of water and electrolytes, as well as the evaluation and treatment of common fluid, electrolyte, and acid–base disorders.

Fluid Compartments

Water, the most abundant substance in the body, constitutes approximately 50% to 60% of body weight. Total body water (TBW) is a function not only of weight, age, and sex, but also of the relative amount of body fat. Of all body tissues, adipose tissue is least hydrated. Thus, individuals with more body fat have proportionally less TBW content.[1]

Total body water is distributed among three main compartments: the intracellular, the extracellular, and the transcellular fluid compartments. Approximately two thirds of TBW is contained in the intracellular fluid (ICF) and the remaining one third is in the extracellular fluid (ECF). The transcellular fluid compartment accounts for only about 3% of TBW and includes specialized fluids such as cerebrospinal fluid, the aqueous humor of the eye, and secretions of the gastrointestinal tract. Of all fluid compartments, the ECF is the most clinically important, because it contains the intravascular and interstitial spaces.[2]

Osmotic pressure, defined as the pressure required to maintain equilibrium with no net movement of solvent, is of prime importance in determining the distribution of water between the extracellular and intracellular spaces. Each compartment contains one major osmotically active solute that ultimately determines its osmotic pressure. Sodium is the dominant extracellular osmole, which acts to hold water in the extracellular space, whereas potassium is the primary intracellular osmole and acts to hold water within the cells. Activity of cellular sodium-potassium-adenosine triphosphatase (Na^+-K^+-ATPase) pumps allows for the maintenance of these unique solute compositions of the ECF and ICF and plays a key role in the regulation of cell volume.[1]

To better illustrate the dynamics of water distribution between the ICF and ECF, consider the exogenous administration of intravenous fluids. If 1 L of 5% dextrose in water (solute-free water) is infused, the dextrose is metabolized, and the water distributes proportionately to all fluid compartments. That is, two thirds (667 mL) of it will distribute into the ICF and one third (333 mL) will distribute into the ECF. Of the one third distributed into the ECF, 25% (85 mL) will remain in the intravascular space. This is in contrast to the administration of 1 L of 0.9% sodium chloride (isotonic saline), which is distributed completely to the ECF where one quarter (250 mL) will remain in the intravascular space. Alternatively, the addition of hypertonic fluid (eg, 3% NaCl) to the ECF increases its tonicity, establishing an osmotic gradient that results in the movement of water out of cells and into the ECF until osmotic equilibrium is attained. The osmolalities of both compartments will be increased—that of the ECF due to the addition of NaCl and that of the ICF due to water loss. The volume change will be proportional to the degree of increase in ECF osmolality (Figure 7-1).[3]

Although osmotic forces determine the distribution of water between the intracellular and extracellular fluid space, the plasma oncotic and hydrostatic pressure govern the movement of fluid between the plasma and interstitial fluid. These forces are generally balanced such that despite large fluid exchanges between compartments, compartment sizes are maintained in a steady state. Disruption in oncotic and/or hydrostatic pressure results in a net flow of fluid from one compartment to another. When these disruptions favor a plasma-to-interstitial fluid shift, third spacing occurs. Third spacing is the accumulation of excess fluid in the interstices (edema) or in the potential fluid spaces (effusion).[4] Although the fluid will be absorbed back into the extracellular compartment over a period of days to weeks, the acute reduction in blood volume, if not replaced, can lead to severe volume depletion.

This phenomenon is common during critical illness when capillary permeability increases, resulting in the leakage of albumin from the intravascular to the interstitial space. This reduces the plasma oncotic pressure and, thus, favors the movement of fluid from the intravascular to the interstitial space. Specific examples of this phenomenon include intestinal obstruction, severe pancreatitis, crush injuries, bleeding, peritonitis, and obstruction of a major venous system.

Fluid Balance

Fluid gains (input) should be in balance with fluid losses (output) over a period of several days. On average, a healthy adult

FIGURE 7-1 Water Distribution to the Extracellular Fluid and Intracellular Fluid and Composition of Commonly Used Intravenous Fluids

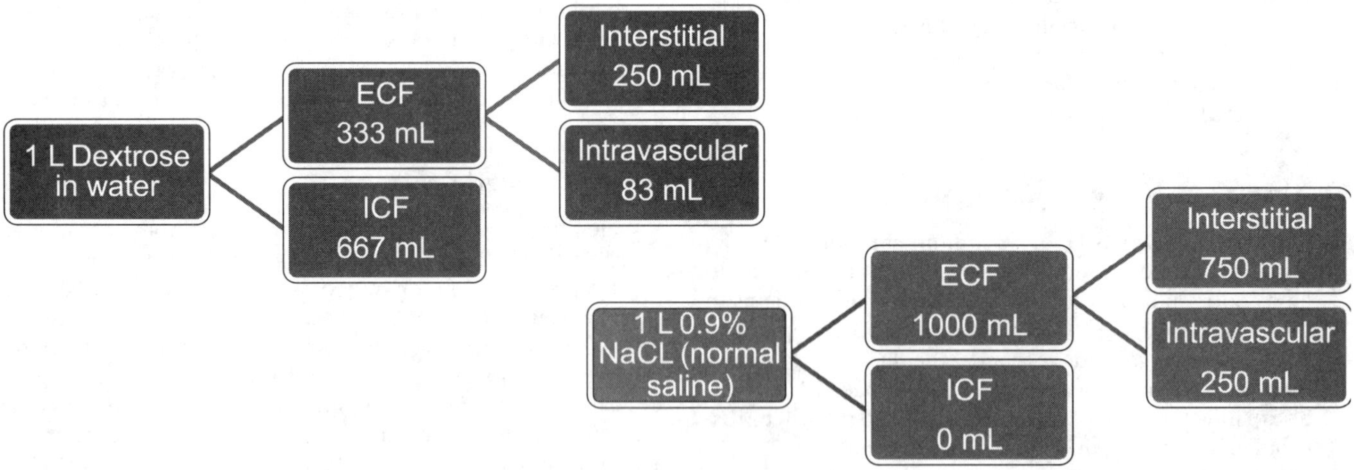

Solution	Dextrose (g/L)	[Na+] (mEq/L)	[Cl−] (mEq/L)	Tonicity	Free Water/L
D5W (5% dextrose)	50	0	0	Hypotonic	1000 mL
0.45% NaCl (½ normal saline)	0	77	77	Hypotonic	500 mL
0.9% NaCl (normal saline)	0	154	154	Isotonic	0 mL
3% NaCl (hypertonic saline)	0	513	513	Hypertonic	−2331 mL
Lactated Ringer's	0	130	109	Isotonic	0 mL

	Weight (kg)	Na+ (mEq/L)	K+ (mEq/L)	Cl− (mEq/L)	HCO_3^- (mEq/L)	BUN (mg/dL)	Creatinine (mg/dL)	Glucose (mg/dL)	Daily Fluid Balance (L)
Day 1	66	134	4	101	26	11	1.1	148	+2.5
Day 3	69	128	3.8	109	32	8	0.9	124	+4
Day 5	62	138	3.5	99	27	15	1.2	137	−6

will require 30 to 40 mL per kilogram per day of fluid to maintain this balance.[5,6] Water intake is derived primarily from the diet (including that generated from the oxidation of carbohydrates, proteins, and fats), whereas various sources of water loss contribute to total fluid output. In most cases, sensible losses from the gastrointestinal tract and kidneys account for the majority of fluid loss, although insensible losses from the lungs and skin can contribute up to 1 L per day.[1] See Practice Scenario 7-1 for a discussion of maintenance fluids in a common clinical condition.

Practice Scenario 7-1

Question: How would you manage maintenance fluids for a patient with heart failure?

Scenario: RA is a 65-year-old male (75 kg; IBW 66 kg) with a past medical history significant for heart failure (HF) and diabetes admitted to your hospital for HF exacerbation. A physical exam reveals jugular venous distention, rales, and 3+ pitting edema in bilateral lower extremities. RA is currently receiving oxygen therapy at 8 L per minute via a nasal cannula and is unable to tolerate an oral diet. 0.9% sodium chloride was initiated at 125 mL per hour. On hospital day 3, RA's oxygen requirements increased necessitating noninvasive positive pressure ventilation and transfer to the intensive care unit (ICU).

Intervention: Upon transfer to the ICU, the intensivist started a furosemide continuous infusion and changed IV fluids to 0.45% sodium chloride at 10 mL per hour to maintain IV access.

Answer: Patients who present with fluid overload secondary to HF exacerbations cannot tolerate normal maintenance fluid requirements. For patients with HF, fluid intake should be between 1.4 and 1.9 L per 24 hours, depending on clinical symptoms (ie, edema, fatigue, shortness of breath). Additionally, sodium should be restricted to less than 2000 mg per day.[7,8] Maintenance fluid requirements for a healthy 75 kg male would be 30–40 mL/kg/day (2250 to 3000 mL per day). Because RA has a history of HF and was admitted with fluid overload and shortness of breath, 3 L per day of maintenance IV fluids contributed to further respiratory decompensation, requiring aggressive diuresis and ICU transfer. The restriction of IV fluids and sodium along with diuresis resulted in decreased oxygen requirements and improvement in other clinical symptoms associated with fluid overload.

Rationale: HF patients with evidence of significant fluid overload should initially be treated with loop diuretics and sodium and fluid restriction. Therapy for hospitalized patients with decompensated HF should begin as soon as possible because early interventions have been associated with better outcomes.[9,10] After admission to the hospital, patients should be carefully monitored in accordance with the severity of their symptoms and the results of initial findings on the physical examination and laboratory assessment.

Plasma osmolality (water balance) is maintained within the normal range of 275 to 290 mOsm per kilogram. This is essential because variations of only 1% to 2% initiate mechanisms to return the plasma osmolality to normal.[1] Two mechanisms regulate water balance: (1) the thirst sensation, and (2) control of renal water excretion by antidiuretic hormone (ADH). The body responds to a water load by suppressing ADH secretion, resulting in decreased collecting tubule water reabsorption and excretion of excess water. The correction of a water deficit requires the intake and retention of exogenous water achieved by increases in thirst and ADH release. Efficiency of this regulatory system is incomplete if any renal impairment or abnormality in the thirst mechanism exists.

Fluid And Electrolyte Disorders

Disorders of fluid balance can be classified as disturbances of volume, concentration, or composition. These disturbances often occur simultaneously in clinical practice. A gain or loss of fluid (ie, water and solute) will alter extracellular fluid volume as determined by physical findings. Such a disturbance is referred to as volume overload or hypervolemia (gain) or conversely as volume depletion or hypovolemia (loss). The gain or loss of water alone is referred to as overhydration or dehydration, respectively, and is recognized by a change in serum sodium concentration and plasma osmolality.[2] Volume depletion describes the loss of sodium and water from the extracellular space (intravascular and interstitial fluid) that occurs after gastrointestinal hemorrhage, vomiting, diarrhea, and diuresis.[11] A disturbance of composition refers to a gain or loss of potassium, magnesium, calcium, phosphate, chloride, bicarbonate, or hydrogen ions.

Knowledge of the composition of specific body fluids is useful in the management of fluid and electrolyte disorders because many causes of water loss also result in significant losses of electrolytes. Table 7-1 shows the volume of fluid secreted and its electrolyte content throughout the gastrointestinal (GI) tract.[12] Abnormalities in renal excretion and excessive losses from the GI tract (ie, vomiting, nasogastric suctioning, diarrhea) are often cited as primary contributors to electrolyte imbalances. Identifying the etiology of the electrolyte imbalance is essential to providing safe and effective treatment.

The therapeutic approach to fluid and electrolyte disorders also requires clinicians to determine the time frame in which the abnormality occurred. Generally, the development of an acute abnormality (<48 hours) is associated with symptoms

TABLE 7-1 Volume and Average Electrolyte Content of Gastrointestinal Secretions

Source/Type of Secretion	Volume (mL/d)	Electrolyte Concentration (mEq/L) Na^+	K^+	Cl^-	HCO_3^-
Saliva	1500	10	26	10	30
Stomach	1500	60	10	130	0
Duodenum	Variable	140	5	80	0
Ileum	3000	140	5	104	30
Colon	Variable	60	30	40	0
Pancreas	Variable	140	5	75	115
Bile	Variable	145	5	100	35

Cl^-, chlorine; HCO_3^-, bicarbonate; K^+, potassium; Na^+, sodium
Adapted with permission from Whitmire SJ. Fluids and electrolytes. In: Matarese LE, Gottschlich MM, eds. *Contemporary Nutrition Support Practice: A Clinical Guide.* 1st ed. Saunders: 1998:130.

that require immediate treatment (ie, altered mental status with a low serum sodium level). The development of a chronic electrolyte disorder is often asymptomatic and harm can occur if corrected too rapidly. In the absence of symptoms, the chronologic trends in electrolyte values are generally more important than the absolute value on any given day.[2] All electrolyte values should be reviewed when available because patients often have more than one electrolyte abnormality present.

General Principles for the Management of Electrolyte Disorders

Several key principles warrant consideration when evaluating and treating electrolyte disorders in clinical practice (Figure 7-2). Upon initial review of laboratory data, clinicians should first determine if the reported electrolyte levels are consistent with the patient's clinical condition. If laboratory results are inconsistent, no further treatment should be considered before validating the accuracy of the specimen collection. This step is crucial to prevent inappropriately treating electrolyte values that may be due to errors in sample collection or handling. If a collection error or specimen mishandling is confirmed, a new specimen should be collected and further analyzed. If the laboratory result is valid, clinicians should then develop a treatment regimen based on the aberrant electrolyte level.

If the electrolyte level is above the normal range, therapy should be directed toward the removal of exogenous sources or facilitating the elimination of the electrolyte. Determining the most appropriate treatment regimen often depends on the severity of the electrolyte disorder and the presence or absence of symptoms. Potential treatments to consider include removing electrolyte supplementation from IV fluids or parenteral/enteral nutrition, discontinuing medications that could be contributing to the electrolyte disorder, and/or inducing renal or GI elimination of the electrolyte.

Electrolyte replacement is the treatment for electrolyte levels below the normal range. To determine if oral or IV electrolyte replacement is appropriate, patient-specific factors should be considered. Intravenous electrolyte replacement is preferred for patients with impaired GI tract function (ie, diarrhea, malabsorption), difficulty swallowing, who are NPO (nothing by mouth), and who have critically low electrolyte levels. Conservative electrolyte replacement is often indicated for patients with impaired renal function unless actively receiving renal replacement therapy. Patients with volume overload should receive volume-restricted electrolyte replacement or oral therapy whenever possible. Peripheral or central IV access should be identified for IV replacement because peripheral administration has limits for volume and the rate of administration. Exceeding these limits can result in tissue damage and potential patient harm. The presence of concurrent electrolyte abnormalities should also be considered to optimize and minimize replacement. For example, to optimize replacement in a patient with hypomagnesemia and hypokalemia, repletion of magnesium should occur prior to potassium because potassium correction rarely occurs if the magnesium deficit is not corrected first. Minimizing electrolyte replacement is best demonstrated with the use of potassium phosphate to correct concurrent hypokalemia and hypophosphatemia. Additionally, clinicians should remain aware of product shortages and availability because dose conservation or alternate therapy may be required.

Sodium

At its normal serum concentration of 135 to 145 mEq per liter, sodium (Na^+) is the principal cation in the ECF. Sodium functions as the major osmotic determinant in regulating ECF volume and water distribution in the body. Other functions include determining the membrane potential of cells and the active transport of molecules across cell membranes.

Hyponatremia

Hyponatremia, defined as a serum sodium concentration less than 135 mEq per liter, occurs in 25% of hospitalized patients.[13] Headache, nausea, vomiting, muscle cramps, lethargy, restlessness, disorientation, and depressed reflexes, as well as severe symptoms including seizures and coma, can all be observed. Clinical manifestations related to central nervous system dysfunction are more likely when the serum sodium concentration drops rapidly and when it falls below 125 mEq per liter.[2] Mortality rates are increased significantly when serum sodium drops below 120 mEq per liter.[14]

FIGURE 7-2 Algorithm for the Management of Electrolyte Disorders

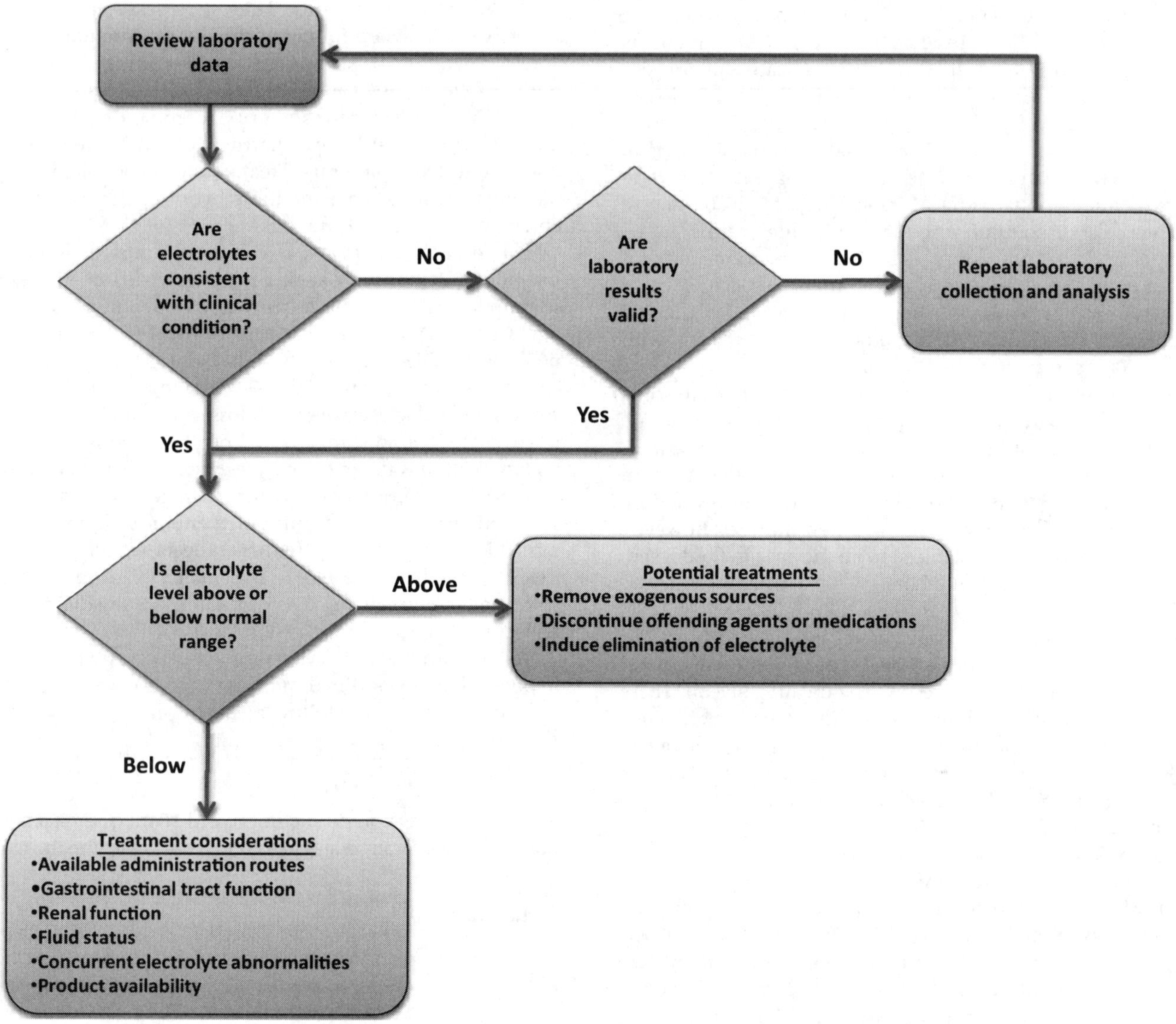

An assessment of the hyponatremic patient is best done with a systematic approach. Upon recognition of clinically relevant hyponatremia (serum sodium $\leq$130 mEq per liter), clinicians should determine (1) serum osmolality and (2) volume status to identify the etiology and appropriate treatment options for patients.

Serum osmolality can be directly measured or calculated with the following equation:

$$\text{Serum osmolality} = 2 \times [\text{Serum Sodium (mEq/L)}] + [\text{Serum Glucose (mg/dL)}] / 18 + [\text{Blood Urea Nitrogen (mg/dL)}] / 2.8$$

Serum and calculated osmolality should be relatively close in value. If there is a difference between the two values, the patient should be assessed for possible ingestion of toxic substances (ethylene glycol, propylene glycol), which can cause a gap in serum versus measured osmolality (referred to as an osmolar gap).

Hypertonic hyponatremia (serum osmolality >290 mOsm per liter) is caused by the presence of osmotically active substances other than sodium in the ECF. Common causes include hyperglycemia and mannitol administration. The correction of serum sodium due to hyperglycemia can be estimated with the following equation:

$$\text{Corrected Sodium} = \text{Serum Sodium (mEq/L)} + 0.016 \text{ Serum Glucose (mg/dL)} - 100$$

Isotonic hyponatremia (serum osmolality within the normal range) occurs when there is a reduction in the fraction of serum that is composed of water (excess of plasma proteins or lipids). With recent advances in laboratory analysis, this is rarely observed. *Hypotonic hyponatremia* (serum osmolality

<275 mOsm per liter) warrants a more detailed assessment of volume status and urine sodium and osmolality.

In *hypovolemic hypotonic hyponatremia*, patients lose more sodium in relation to water. Therefore, it is critical to determine the source of fluid loss. Urine osmolality in these patients is usually >450 mOsm per liter, which is indicative of concentrated urine and the body's attempt to retain fluid. Renal losses are usually caused by diuretic use and identified by a urine sodium <20 mEq per liter. Cerebral salt wasting observed in patients with subarachnoid hemorrhage may also result in hypovolemic hyponatremia. Extrarenal losses can be due to diarrhea, fistula output, excessive sweating, burns, open wounds, and fluid drains (eg, peritoneal, thoracic, pleural, biliary, or pancreatic drains) and are commonly associated with a urine sodium >20 mEq per liter. Both renal and extrarenal fluid losses associated with hyponatremia are treated with isotonic fluids to expand the ECF volume.

In patients with *hypervolemic hypotonic hyponatremia*, some element of end-organ damage (renal failure, hepatic failure with ascites, heart failure) is present resulting in fluid retention or third spacing. These patients retain more water than sodium and treatment consists of both fluid and sodium restriction. Sodium restriction may seem counterintuitive; however, increased sodium intake will lead to an increase in fluid retention, thus worsening hyponatremia.

Euvolemic hypotonic hyponatremia is commonly associated with the syndrome of inappropriate antidiuretic hormone (SIADH). ADH is primarily released from the pituitary gland although a small amount is secreted by the lung alveoli. These patients have stable sodium intake/output but retain large amounts of water due to the excess ADH. Common causes of SIADH include brain or CNS malignancies, head trauma, lung malignancies, and pneumonia. Urine osmolality is >100 mOsm per liter and urine sodium is >20 mEq per liter, indicating the kidneys are appropriately concentrating urine. The mainstay of treatment for SIADH is fluid restriction of 500 to 1000 mL per day and the administration of exogenous salt. Other causes of euvolemic hypotonic hyponatremia are psychogenic polydipsia (the ingestion of large amounts of free water), hypothyroidism, and reset osmostat. Treatment revolves around correcting the underlying disorder and fluid restriction. SIADH refractory to conventional treatment may require pharmacologic therapy with vasopressin-2 receptor antagonists, including conivaptan or tolvaptan.

An algorithm for the evaluation, etiology, and treatment of hyponatremia is outlined in Figure 7-3. Regardless of the severity of symptoms associated with hyponatremia, the targeted rate of sodium correction should not exceed 5 to 10 mEq per liter per day to prevent osmotic demyelination.

Hypernatremia

Hypernatremia (serum sodium >145 mEq per liter) occurs in approximately 2% of hospitalized patients and levels >160 mEq per liter are associated with a significant increase in mortality.[15,16] Similar to hyponatremia, clinical manifestations of hypernatremia are associated with neurologic sequelae that range from mild (headache, dizziness, confusion) to severe (seizures, coma, and death). To determine the etiology of hypernatremia, a similar approach to that of hyponatremia can be used.

In *hypovolemic hypernatremia*, all patients will have an increased serum osmolality. Thus, an assessment of volume status is the first step in diagnosing hypernatremia. In hypovolemic patients, it is important to determine the source of fluid loss. Renal losses are commonly due to diuretic use, solute diuresis due to hyperglycemia or azotemia, or acute tubular necrosis. Extrarenal losses (diarrhea, excessive sweating) can also lead to hypernatremia. Treatment of hypovolemic hypernatremia involves replacing these hypotonic fluids either via enteral or parenteral routes.

Euvolemic hypernatremia is commonly caused by diabetes insipidus (DI). These patients have water losses that exceed sodium losses. DI can be either central or nephrogenic in etiology. Central DI is an impairment of ADH secretion, whereas nephrogenic DI is the inability of the kidneys to respond to ADH circulating in the serum. Table 7-2 lists the causes of DI. Both conditions lead to excessive water losses via urine. Treatment differs for the two disorders but both conditions require the replacement of water either via the enteral or parenteral routes.

Hypervolemic hypernatremia can be iatrogenic in nature (excessive administration of isotonic or hypertonic sodium) or due to mineralocorticoid excess (either exogenous administration, Cushing's syndrome, or adrenal malignancy). Treatment involves correcting the underlying disorder, administering diuretics, and replacing the water.

An algorithm for the evaluation, etiology, and treatment of hypernatremia is outlined in Figure 7-4. Free water deficit can be calculated using the following equation:

$$\text{Free Water Deficit} = \text{Total Body Water} \times 1 - (140 \,/\, \text{Serum Sodium [mEq/L]})$$

Sodium correction should not exceed 10 mEq per liter per day due to the risk of cerebral edema and neurologic impairment.

Potassium

At its normal serum concentration of 3.5 to 5 mEq per liter, potassium (K^+) is the major intracellular cation. In contrast to Na^+, which is restricted primarily to the ECF, 98% of total body K^+ is located within the cells. Potassium plays a critical role in cell metabolism including protein and glycogen synthesis. Additionally, the ratio of potassium concentrations in the cell and the ECF is vital to maintaining resting membrane potential and therefore crucial for normal neural and muscular function. Normal daily potassium requirements range from 0.5 to 1.5 mEq per kilogram per day.

Regulation of the internal distribution of potassium must be extremely efficient, because the movement of only 1.5% to 2% of cellular potassium to the ECF can result in a potentially fatal increase in the plasma potassium concentration to as high as 8 mEq per liter or more.[1] Of all the factors that influence this distribution, the Na^+-K^+-ATPase pump and the plasma potassium concentration are the most important in the daily regulation of potassium balance.[17] Other factors affecting potassium distribution include those regulating the activity of the Na^+-K^+-ATPase pump—specifically insulin and catecholamines—as well as exercise, extracellular pH, and cellular breakdown.

FIGURE 7-3 The evaluation of hyponatremia. ECF, extracellular fluid; BP, blood pressure; SIADH, syndrome of inappropriate antidiuretic hormone secretion; CHF, congestive heart failure

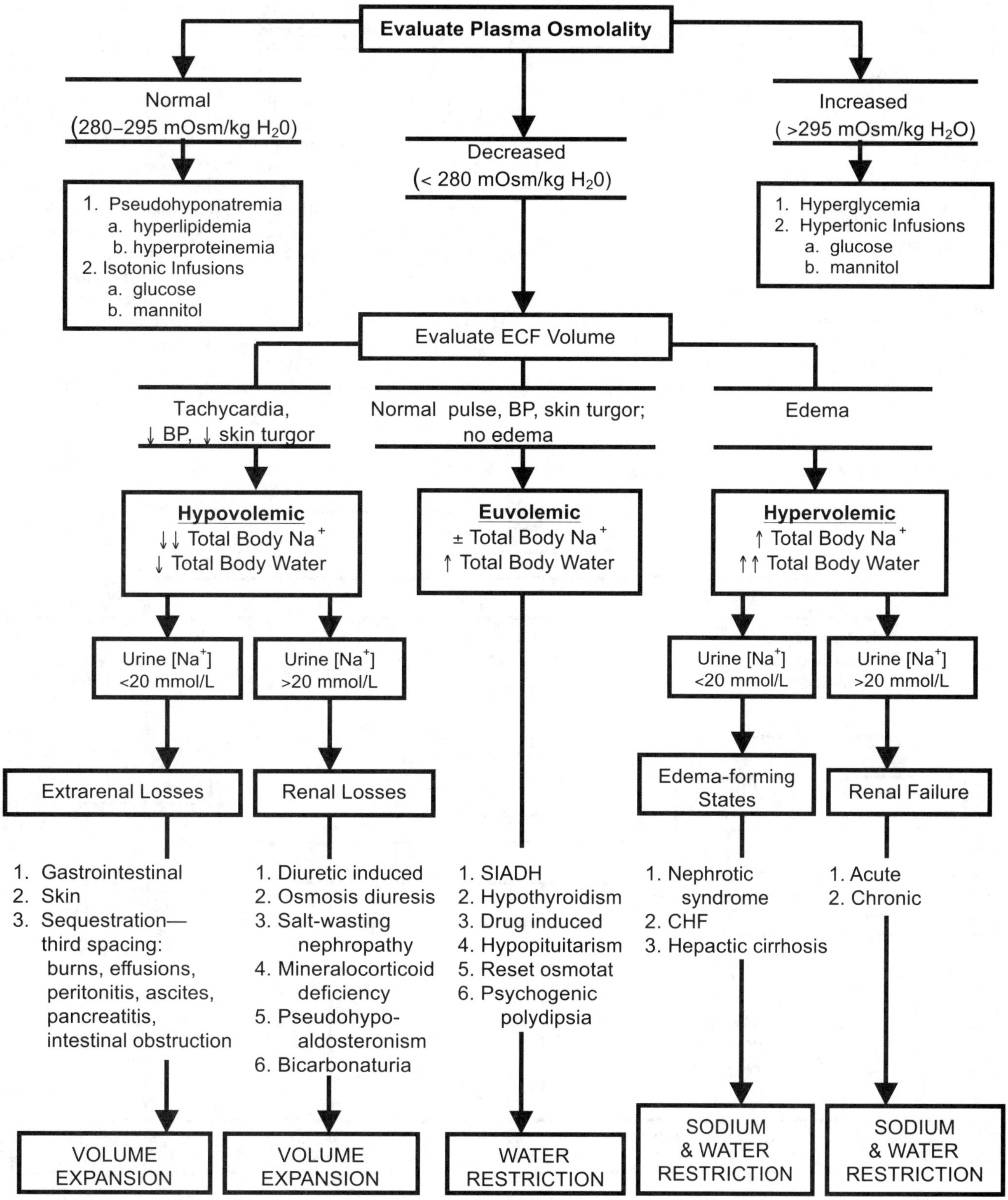

Adapted with permission from Whitmire SJ. Fluids and electrolytes. In: Matarese LE, Gottschlich MM, eds. *Contemporary Nutrition Support Practice: A Clinical Guide*, 1st ed. Saunders: 1998:129.

TABLE 7-2 Causes of Diabetes Insipidus

Nephrogenic	Central
Lithium toxicity	Cerebral hemorrhage
Hypercalcemia	Head trauma
Hypokalemia	Neurosurgery (pituitary)
Polycystic kidney disease	CNS malignancy
Advanced renal disease	Hepatic encephalopathy
Drugs	CNS infection
Cidofovir	
Foscarnet	
Osmotic diuretics	
Demeclocycline	

CNS, central nervous system.

Hypokalemia

Hypokalemia is a common electrolyte abnormality in clinical practice. When defined as a serum potassium concentration less than 3.6 mEq per liter, hypokalemia is found in over 20% of hospitalized patients.[18] Clinical manifestations vary among individuals and are influenced by the rapidity of onset and the degree of hypokalemia. Patients are typically asymptomatic when the disorder is mild (serum potassium 3.0 to 3.5 mEq per liter) but tend to present with nonspecific symptoms such as generalized weakness, lethargy, and constipation with lower serum potassium concentrations. More severe consequences of hypokalemia include muscle necrosis, ascending paralysis, arrhythmias, and possibly, death.[19]

Hypokalemia is almost always the result of abnormal potassium losses via the urine or stool. It can also develop from a transcellular shift of potassium from the ECF into cells or inadequate dietary intake. Metabolic alkalosis and increases in insulin and catecholamines (epinephrine) are potential causes of transcellular shifts of potassium into the cells. Medications are also frequently cited as causes of hypokalemia (Table 7-3).

Goals of therapy for hypokalemia include avoidance or resolution of symptoms, restoring the serum potassium concentration to normal, and preventing hyperkalemia. The administration of oral or IV potassium supplements is the treatment for hypokalemia. Commonly used oral and enteral potassium supplements are listed in Table 7-4. IV potassium supplements are available as chloride, acetate, and phosphate salts. Potassium

FIGURE 7-4 Evaluation of hypernatremia. ECF, extracellular fluid

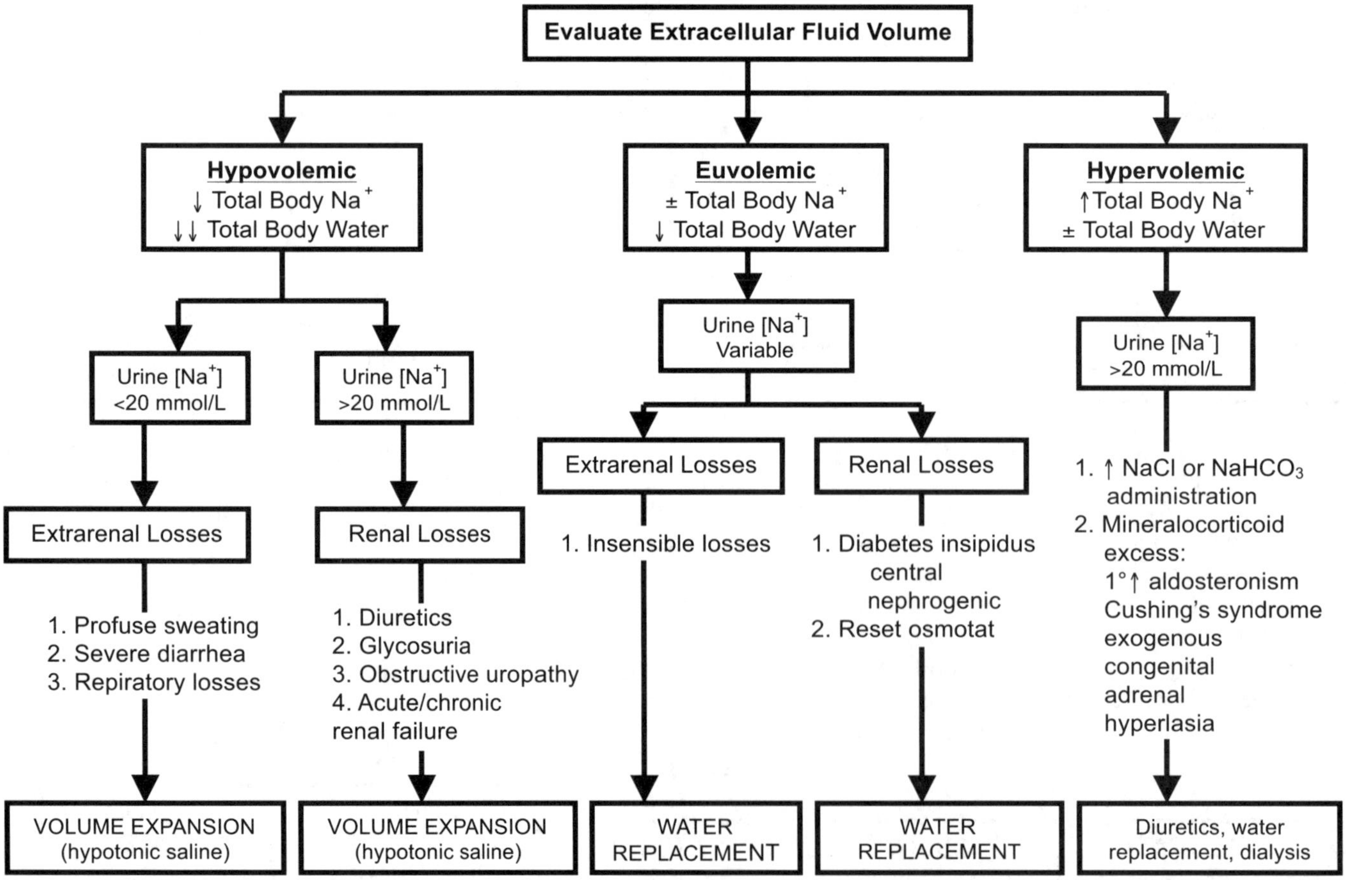

Adapted with permission from Whitmire SJ. Fluids and electrolytes. In: Matarese LE, Gottschlich MM, eds. *Contemporary Nutrition Support Practice: A Clinical Guide*, 1st ed. Saunders: 1998:130.

TABLE 7-3 Drug-Induced Hypokalemia

Increased Renal Potassium Loss	Excess Potassium Loss in Stool	Potassium Shift from ECF to ICF
Diuretics	**Phenolphthalein**	**B_2-Adrenergic agonists**
Acetazolamide	**Sodium polystyrene sulfonate**	Epinephrine
Thiazides		Albuterol
Indapamide	**Sorbitol**	Terbutaline
Metolazone		Pirbuterol
Bumetanide		Salmeterol
Furosemide		Isoproterenol
Torsemide		Ephedrine
Fludrocortisone		Pseudoephedrine
High-dose glucocorticoids		
Drugs associated with magnesium depletion		
Aminoglycosides		**Theophylline**
Cisplatin		**Caffeine**
Foscarnet		**Verapamil intoxication**
Amphotericin B		**Insulin overdose**

ECF, extracellular fluid; ICF, intracellular fluid.

acetate is used as an alternative to potassium chloride in the presence of a metabolic acidosis. Potassium phosphate is used to correct coexisting hypokalemia and hypophosphatemia.

Oral correction of hypokalemia is generally safer and reduces the risk of overcorrection and rebound hyperkalemia. Potassium chloride can be given in a capsule, tablet, or liquid formulation. Although several liquid preparations are available and less expensive, they often have an unpleasant taste and are poorly tolerated. The slow-release tablets are well tolerated but have been associated with ulceration and bleeding of the GI tract.[20] Oral potassium dosages of 40 to 100 mEq daily divided into two to four doses are usually sufficient to correct hypokalemia.[21,22]

IV potassium supplementation is reserved for the treatment of severe hypokalemia or when the GI tract precludes the use of oral agents. Recommendations for IV potassium replacement doses vary according to severity and the presence of renal insufficiency (Table 7-5).[21–25] In general, every 10 mEq of IV potassium administered should increase serum potassium by 0.1 mEq per liter in patients with normal renal function. Infusion rates should generally not exceed 10 to 20 mEq per hour; however, infusion rates as high as 40 mEq per hour have been used for emergent cases or severely symptomatic patients. If an infusion rate exceeding 10 mEq per hour is required, continuous cardiac monitoring is recommended to detect any signs of hyperkalemia. Administration via a central venous catheter is also recommended to minimize phlebitis and burning. Total daily potassium supplementation, in most cases, should not exceed 40 to 100 mEq per day. However, some patients with severe potassium wasting may require doses of 200 mEq per day or higher with additional cardiac monitoring.

Additional caveats to consider when replacing a potassium deficit include the diluent (dextrose versus saline) and the presence of hypomagnesemia. When possible, dextrose solutions should be avoided because they may worsen the hypokalemia by stimulating insulin release that promotes an intracellular shift of potassium.[26] A magnesium deficit should be corrected because hypomagnesemia may result in refractory hypokalemia due to accelerated renal potassium loss or the impairment of Na^+-K^+-ATPase pump activity.[27]

Hyperkalemia

Due to the body's effective regulatory mechanisms, hyperkalemia, defined as a serum potassium greater than 5.0 mEq per liter, rarely occurs in healthy individuals. In contrast to the relatively large decrease in total body potassium needed to effect a slight decrease in serum K^+, even a small excess of total body potassium will elicit a sharp increase in serum potassium.[28] Clinical manifestations of hyperkalemia are related to changes in neuromuscular and cardiac function. Patients are often asymptomatic until the serum potassium concentration exceeds 5.5 mEq per liter.[21] Signs and symptoms of hyperkalemia include muscle twitching, cramping, weakness, ascending paralysis, electrocardiogram (ECG) changes (eg, tall peaked T-waves, prolonged PR-interval, widened QRS complex, shortened QT-interval), and arrhythmias (eg, bradyarrhythmias, ventricular fibrillation, asystole).

Although hyperkalemia can be caused by extracellular shifts of potassium and increased potassium ingestion, it most often occurs in the setting of renal insufficiency. Increased potassium intake alone rarely causes hyperkalemia. Extracellular shifts of potassium are relatively common and are often a result of metabolic acidosis, tissue catabolism, and pseudohyperkalemia. Metabolic acidosis results in an extracellular potassium shift to maintain electroneutrality because some of the excess hydrogen ions are buffered intracellularly.[29] In general, for every 0.1 change in pH, potassium will increase by 0.6 mEq per liter. Tissue destruction or breakdown causes the release of intracellular potassium into the ECF. Pseudohyperkalemia signifies an artifactual increase in serum potassium due to the release of intracellular potassium during or after blood sampling. This is most commonly associated with trauma during venipuncture, but can also occur with the measurement of serum potassium in patients with marked leukocytosis (100,000/mm^3) or thrombocytosis (400,000/mm^3) or when the blood sample is contaminated with infused potassium or hydrolyzed. As such, if a serum potassium level is inappropriately elevated for the clinical situation, a repeat potassium level should be obtained to confirm the diagnosis to avoid unwarranted treatment. Drug-induced causes of hyperkalemia are listed in Table 7-6.[30]

Treatment depends upon the degree of hyperkalemia and the severity of symptoms. Goals of therapy include antagonizing the cardiac effects of potassium, reversing symptoms (if present), and returning the serum K^+ to normal. All sources

TABLE 7-4 Commonly Used Oral Potassium Replacement Products

Dosage Form	Brand Name	Strength	Clinical Considerations
		Enteral/Oral Administration	
Potassium bicarbonate			
Effervescent tablet for solution	Klor-Con/EF, K-Lyte K-Lyte DS	25 mEq 50 mEq 25 mEq	Dissolve tablets in 90 mL water; orange flavor
Potassium chloride			
Effervescent tablet for solution	K-Lor, Klor-Con	20 mEq/packet	Dissolve in 120 mL of water; fruit flavor
Powder for solution	Klor-Con/25	25 mEq/packet	Dilute in 120 mL of cold water or juice for administration; contains sorbitol, which may cause diarrhea
Solution		20 mEq/15 mL 40 mEq/15 mL	
Potassium phosphate			
Tablet for solution	K-Phos	500 mg (3.7 mEq potassium and 3.7 mmol phosphorus per tablet)	Dissolve tablets in 90 mL water
Powder for solution	Phos-NaK	250 mg/packet (7.1 mEq potassium and 8 mmol phosphorus per packet)	Dilute in 75 mL of water; fruit flavor
Tablet	K-Phos No. 2	2.3 mEq potassium and 8 mmol phosphorus per tablet	
		Oral Administration Only	
Potassium chloride			
Capsule, extended release, micro-encapsulated	Micro-K	8 mEq/600 mg 10 mEq/750 mg	Swallow whole; capsules may be opened and contents sprinkled on applesauce and swallowed immediately without chewing
Tablet, extended release		8 mEq/600 mg 10 mEq/750 mg 20 mEq/1500 mg	Swallow whole; do not crush or chew; larger tablet size with higher doses; difficult to swallow; potential noncompliance issues
Tablet, extended release, microencapsulated	Klor-Con M10 Klor-Con M15 Klor-Con M20	10 mEq/750 mg 15 mEq/1125 mg 20 mEq/1500 mg	Tablet may be broken in half; whole tablet may be dissolved in 120 mL of water
Tablet, extended release, wax matrix	Klor-Con	8 mEq/600 mg 10 mEq/750 mg	Do not crush or chew; swallow whole

TABLE 7-5 Empirical Treatment of Hypokalemia

Serum Potassium Concentration (mEq/L)	IV Potassium Dose (mEq)[a]
3–3.4	20–40
2.5–2.9	40–80
< 2.5	80–120

IV, intravenous.

[a]These dosing guidelines are recommended for patients with normal renal function. Patients with renal impairment should receive 50% of the initial empirical dose.

Potassium supplements are best administered orally in a moderate dosage over a period of days to weeks to achieve full potassium repletion. An oral potassium dosage of 20 mEq/day is generally sufficient to prevent hypokalemia, and 40 to 100 mEq/day is sufficient for treatment.

Rate of IV infusion: 10 to 20 mEq potassium per hour; maximum infusion rate: 40 mEq per hour. Continuous cardiac monitoring and infusion via a central venous catheter are recommended for infusion rates > 10 mEq potassium per hour.

of exogenous potassium and other medications that can cause hyperkalemia should be discontinued or dosages should be decreased if feasible. IV calcium gluconate should be given to symptomatic patients or those with ECG changes to restore membrane excitability to normal. Insulin and dextrose, sodium bicarbonate, and alpha$_2$-adrenergic agonists cause potassium to move intracellularly. Loop and thiazide diuretics, cation-exchange resins (ie, sodium polystyrene sulfonate), and dialysis facilitate potassium removal. Serum potassium should be monitored frequently during the treatment of symptomatic patients because many of the therapies employed for acute hyperkalemia redistribute potassium and do not remove it from the body. Upon symptom resolution, continued potassium monitoring is recommended every 4 to 12 hours after therapeutic interventions until potassium levels return to normal. Table 7-7 lists therapies for the treatment of hyperkalemia.[31–33]

TABLE 7-6 Drug-Induced Hyperkalemia

Impaired Renal Potassium Excretion	Increased Potassium Input	Potassium Shift from ICF to ECF
Potassium-sparing diuretics	**Potassium supplements**	**B-blockers**
Spironolactone	**Salt substitutes**	**Succinylcholine**
Triamterene	**Stored packed red blood cells**	**Digoxin intoxication**
Amiloride	**Penicillin G potassium**	**IV amino acids**
Nonsteroidal anti-inflammatory agents		Lysine
ACE-inhibitors		Arginine
Angiotensin-II receptor blockers		
Trimethoprim		
Pentamidine		
Cyclosporine		
Tacrolimus		
Heparin		

ACE, angiotensin-converting-enzyme; ECF, extracellular fluid; ICF, intracellular fluid; IV, intravenous.

Magnesium

At its normal serum concentration of 1.8 to 2.8 mg per deciliter, magnesium (Mg^{2+}) is found predominantly in the ICF.[34] Total body magnesium content is approximately 25 g (2000 mEq), of which 50% to 60% resides in bone.[35] The remainder is located in cardiac muscle, skeletal muscle, and the liver, with only about 2% in the ECF. Magnesium is essential in the activation of over 300 enzymatic reactions including those involved in glucose metabolism, fatty acid synthesis and breakdown, and DNA and protein metabolism.[36] Magnesium is also required for the maintenance of the Na^+-K^+-ATPase pump, and hence, cell membrane action potential. It is a structural component of bone and a factor in parathyroid hormone (PTH) secretion, neuromuscular transmission, cardiovascular excitability, vasomotor tone, and muscle contraction.

Cellular and extracellular magnesium concentrations are carefully regulated by the GI tract, kidney, and bone. Healthy persons absorb approximately 30% to 40% of ingested magnesium. Magnesium absorption occurs primarily in the distal jejunum and ileum and varies inversely with intake. Renal elimination normally accounts for approximately one third of absorbed magnesium. However, with increased magnesium intake, renal magnesium excretion increases to maintain normal serum concentrations.[37]

Hypomagnesemia

Hypomagnesemia, defined as a serum magnesium level of 1.8 mg per deciliter, has been reported in 6.9% to 47% of hospitalized patients,[38–41] and in as many as 65% of patients in ICUs.[42] Neuromuscular hyperexcitability is the primary symptom with magnesium deficiency.[43] Latent tetany, as elicited by a positive Chvostek and Trousseau sign, may be present. Frank, generalized seizures may also occur. Concomitant electrolyte abnormalities in the setting of magnesium deficiency include hypokalemia and hypocalcemia. Both are refractory to treatment until the magnesium deficit is corrected. Hypomagnesemia is present in approximately 38% to 61% of patients with hypokalemia and 22% to 28% of patients with hypocalcemia, respectively.[41,44,45] Magnesium depletion is also associated with cardiac complications, including ECG changes, arrhythmias, and increased sensitivity to cardiac glycosides (digoxin).[46]

TABLE 7-7 Treatment of Hyperkalemia

Treatment	Dose	Onset	Duration	Action
Calcium gluconate[a,b]	1–2 g (4.65–9.3 mEq) IV over 10 min	1–2 min	10–30 min	Antagonizes cardiac conduction abnormalities
Sodium bicarbonate[a]	50–100 mEq IV over 2–5 min	30 min	2–6 h	Shifts potassium intracellularly
Regular insulin with dextrose	5–10 units IV with 50 mL of 50% dextrose injection	15–45 min	2–6 h	Shifts potassium intracellularly
Albuterol	10–20 mg nebulized over 10 min	30 min	1–2 h	Shifts potassium intracellularly
Furosemide	20–80 mg IV push	5–15 min	4–6 h	Promotes renal potassium loss
Sodium polystyrene sulfonate	15–60 g orally or rectally	1 h	4–6 h	Increases fecal potassium elimination
Hemodialysis	Variable	Immediate	Variable	Removes potassium from plasma

[a]First-line therapies in hyperkalemic emergencies.
[b]Repeat dose in 5 minutes if abnormal electrocardiogram persists. Calcium chloride may be used, but calcium gluconate is preferred for peripheral administration (less venous irritation). Calcium chloride (1 g = 13.6 mEq) provides three times more calcium than calcium gluconate (1 g = 4.65 mEq).

TABLE 7-8 Commonly Used Oral Magnesium Replacement Products

Dosage Form	Brand Name	Strength	Clinical Considerations
		Enteral/Oral Administration	
Magnesium gluconate			
Solution	Magonate	4.8 mEq/5 mL (1000 mg/5 mL)	
Magnesium sulfate			
Solution		4 mEq/mL (500 mg/mL)	
		Oral Administration Only	
Magnesium chloride			
Tablet, enteric coated	Slow-Mag	5 mEq	Do not crush or chew; swallow whole; contains 106 mg elemental calcium
Tablet, delayed release	Mag 64	5 mEq	Do not crush or chew; swallow whole; contains 110 mg elemental calcium
Magnesium gluconate			
Tablet	Mag G	2.4 mEq/500 mg	
	Magtrate	2.4 mEq/500 mg	
Magnesium lactate			
Caplet, sustained release	Mag-Tab SR	7 mEq	Do not crush or chew; swallow whole
Magnesium oxide			
Capsule	Mag-Caps	7 mEq	
	Uro-Mag	7 mEq/140 mg	
Capsule, soft gel	MagGel	28.6 mEq/600 mg	
Tablet	Mag-Ox 400	20 mEq/500 mg	Large tablet size; potential noncompliance issues
	MG Plus Protein	11 mEq	Chelated to soy protein; reduced GI side effects

GI, gastrointestinal.

Hypomagnesemia can occur with decreased intake or absorption, excessive losses, or redistribution into the ICF. Protein-calorie malnutrition, prolonged administration of magnesium-free IV fluids or parenteral nutrition, alcoholism, malabsorption syndromes, short bowel syndrome, and intestinal bypass operations are common causes of reduced magnesium intake or absorption. Magnesium losses can occur via the GI tract or the kidneys. Renal losses may be caused by acute tubular necrosis, renal tubular acidosis, Bartter syndrome, hyperaldosteronism, or may be drug-induced (ie, thiazide and loop diuretics, cisplatin, cyclosporine, amphotericin B, aminoglycosides, and foscarnet).[47] Intracellular shifts of magnesium may be seen during refeeding, diabetic ketoacidosis, hyperthyroidism, and myocardial infarction.

Because only about 1% to 2% of total body magnesium is located in the ECF, serum levels may not correlate with intracellular concentrations or total body magnesium levels. As such, treatment of hypomagnesemia is largely empirical. Both oral and IV formulations of magnesium are available to replace estimated deficits. Table 7-8 lists commonly used oral and enteral magnesium supplements. The IV route of administration is often preferred because issues with administration, slow onset of action, and GI intolerance limit the use of oral supplements. Table 7-9 provides recommended dosing regimens for the treatment of hypomagnesemia according to severity.[48–51] Maximal magnesium infusion rates should not exceed 1 g per hour (8 mEq per hour) in asymptomatic patients.[49,51] Similarly, approximately 50% or less of recommended empirical doses should be administered to patients with renal impairment to reduce the risk of hypermagnesemia.

Hypermagnesemia

Hypermagnesemia, defined as serum magnesium levels of 2.8 mg per deciliter, occurs primarily in the setting of renal

TABLE 7-9 Empirical Treatment of Hypomagnesemia

Severity	Serum Magnesium Concentration (mg/dL)	IV Magnesium Dose[a]
Mild to moderate	1.0–1.5	8–32 mEq (1–4 g) magnesium sulfate, up to 1.0 mEq/kg
Severe	< 1.0	32–64 mEq (4–8 g) magnesium sulfate, up to 1.5 mEq/kg

IV, intravenous.
[a]These dosing guidelines are recommended for patients with normal renal function. Patients with renal impairment should receive: 50% of the initial empirical dose. Maximum rate of infusion: 8 mEq (1 g) magnesium sulfate per hour, up to 100 mEq (12 g) magnesium sulfate over 12 hours if asymptomatic; up to 32 mEq (4 g) magnesium sulfate over 4 to 5 minutes in severe symptomatic hypomagnesemia.

insufficiency in combination with increased magnesium intake, often in the form of magnesium-containing antacids. Hypermagnesemia is generally well-tolerated but can affect neurologic, neuromuscular, and cardiac function when magnesium levels exceed 4.8 mg per deciliter.[39] Physical findings include nausea, vomiting, diaphoresis, flushing, sensation of heat, depressed mental functioning, drowsiness, muscular weakness, hypotension, and bradycardia.

IV calcium (chloride or gluconate) should be administered to patients with symptomatic severe hypermagnesemia to reverse the cardiac and neuromuscular effects.[35,52] Therapy for patients with asymptomatic hypermagnesemia includes the removal of exogenous sources of magnesium (eg, parenteral nutrition, IV fluids), magnesium restriction, and loop diuretics.

Calcium

Normal total serum calcium concentrations range from 8.6 to 10.2 mg per deciliter. Calcium is one of the most abundant ions in the body and accounts for 1% to 2% of adult human body weight.[37] It is essential to many physiologic functions, including the preservation of integrity of cell membranes, neuromuscular activity, regulation of endocrine secretory activities, blood coagulation, activation of the complement system, and bone metabolism.[53] Serum calcium concentrations are under hormonal control primarily mediated by PTH, vitamin D, and calcitonin.[1] Low serum calcium concentrations stimulate the release of PTH, which increases bone resorption, augments renal conservation of calcium, and activates vitamin D, which increases intestinal calcium absorption. Calcitonin is released by the thyroid gland in response to elevated serum calcium concentrations and acts to inhibit bone resorption and increase urinary calcium excretion. In healthy individuals, any excess calcium will be excreted in the urine, whereas any decrease in plasma calcium will be met by an increase in calcium mobilization from bone to restore the serum calcium concentration to normal.

About 99% of total body calcium is found in teeth and bones, with less than 1% in the serum.[54] Serum calcium exists in three forms: complexed, protein bound, and ionized. The ionized fraction of calcium, with a normal range of 1.12 to 1.3 mmol per liter, is the metabolically active form and is of greatest physiologic importance.[53] Serum pH, phosphorus, and albumin levels affect the percentage of ionized calcium. A metabolic alkalosis decreases the percentage of ionized calcium, as does an increase in serum phosphorus. Hypoalbuminemia decreases total serum calcium but does not affect ionized calcium levels. For each 1 g per deciliter decrease in albumin below 4.0 g per deciliter total calcium decreases by approximately 0.8 mg per deciliter.[55] Although total calcium can be adjusted for hypoalbuminemia, as noted:

$$\text{Corrected Total Calcium (mg/dL)} = \text{Measured Total Calcium (mg/dL)} + 0.8 \times [4 - \text{Albumin (g/dL)}]$$

the most accurate method for assessing calcium abnormalities is to measure ionized calcium directly. This is especially important in critically ill patients given that this equation often overestimates the corrected calcium concentration.[56]

Hypocalcemia

Hypocalcemia, defined as a total serum calcium concentration of <8.6 mg per deciliter or an ionized calcium concentration <1.12 mmol per liter, frequently occurs secondary to hypoalbuminemia; however, this is usually not significant as long as the ionized calcium concentration remains normal.[16] Causes of hypocalcemia include decreased vitamin D activity (vitamin D deficiency, hyperphosphatemia, pseudohypoparathyroidism), decreased PTH activity (acute pancreatitis, hypomagnesemia, hypoparathyroidism), and hungry bone syndrome (can occur after parathyroidectomy or thyroidectomy). Hypocalcemia is common in critically ill patients and is also associated with sepsis, rhabdomyolysis, and massive blood transfusions (secondary to citrate preservative in the blood bank binding with serum calcium).[57] Drugs implicated in the etiology of hypocalcemia include bisphosphonates, calcitonin, furosemide, foscarnet, and long-term therapy with phenobarbital and phenytoin.[58] Clinical manifestations may be cardiovascular (ie, hypotension, decreased myocardial contractility, or prolonged QT interval) or neuromuscular (ie, distal extremity paresthesias, Chvostek sign, Trousseau sign, muscle cramps, tetany, or seizures).

Severe hypocalcemia (total serum calcium concentration <7.5 mg per deciliter or ionized calcium concentration <0.9 mmol per liter) or acute symptomatic hypocalcemia requires prompt correction with IV calcium gluconate or calcium chloride.[59] Although calcium chloride (10 mL of 10% solution = 270 mg elemental calcium = 13.5 mEq calcium) contains three times more elemental calcium than an equivalent amount of calcium gluconate (10 mL of 10% solution = 90 mg elemental calcium = 4.65 mEq calcium), it may cause tissue necrosis if extravasation occurs.[60–61] Initially, 1 g of calcium chloride (13.6 mEq calcium) or 3 g calcium gluconate (14 mEq calcium) may be given over 10 minutes to control symptoms. Continuous infusions of IV calcium may be required for severe acute hypocalcemia refractory to intermittent bolus doses.[59] Infusion rates should not exceed 0.8 to 1.5 mEq per minute because the potential for cardiac arrhythmias increases with more rapid calcium administration. Guidelines for the acute treatment of hypocalcemia are provided in Table 7-10.[62] If concomitant hypomagnesemia is present, magnesium supplements should be provided to facilitate the correction of hypocalcemia.[63–64] In cases of hypocalcemia due to elevated serum phosphorus levels, treatment with phosphate binders may be warranted prior to calcium replacement to reduce the risk of soft tissue calcification. Chronic or

TABLE 7-10 Empirical Treatment of Acute Hypocalcemia

Serum Ionized Calcium Concentration (mmol/L)	IV Calcium Dose
1–1.12	2 g (9.3 mEq) calcium gluconate over 2 hours
< 1	4 g (18.6 mEq) calcium gluconate over 4 hours

IV, intravenous.

asymptomatic hypocalcemia can be treated with oral calcium supplements and vitamin D.[21] Common calcium supplements are listed in Table 7-11.

Hypercalcemia

Hypercalcemia, defined as a total serum calcium concentration greater than 10.2 mg per deciliter or an ionized calcium concentration greater than 1.3 mmol per liter, most often occurs in hyperparathyroidism and cancer with bone metastases (primarily breast cancer, lung cancer, and multiple myeloma). It can also occur with toxic levels of vitamin A or vitamin D, chronic ingestion of milk and/or calcium-carbonate containing antacids in the setting of renal insufficiency (milk-alkali syndrome), adrenal insufficiency, immobilization, tuberculosis, and various medications including thiazide diuretics and lithium.[53] Early clinical manifestations are nonspecific and include fatigue, nausea, vomiting, constipation, anorexia, and confusion. In more severe causes, cardiac arrhythmias (bradycardia) may be present.

Mild hypercalcemia (total serum calcium concentration of 10.3 to 12.9 mg per deciliter or ionized calcium concentration of 1.31 to 1.49 mmol per liter) usually responds well to hydration and ambulation. Severe hypercalcemia (total serum calcium concentration of 13 mg per deciliter or an ionized concentration of 1.5 mmol per liter or higher) requires immediate treatment because it can lead to acute renal failure, obtundation, ventricular arrhythmias, coma, and death.[54,65] Intravenous hydration using 0.9% sodium chloride should be started promptly at 200 to 300 mL per hour to reverse the IV volume depletion caused by hypercalcemia. After adequate hydration is achieved, furosemide 40 to 100 mg IV can be used to enhance renal calcium excretion with vigilant monitoring to avoid further IV volume depletion. Saline hydration and furosemide can reduce serum calcium levels by 2 to 3 mg per deciliter within the first 48 hours of treatment. Calcitonin can also be used to treat acute hypercalcemia but tachyphylaxis often limits its usefulness. Hemodialysis may be necessary in life-threatening hypercalcemia or in patients with renal insufficiency. Although bisphosphonates have a primary role in the treatment of hypercalcemia of malignancy in the outpatient setting, their delayed onset of action renders these agents as ineffective therapy in the acute care setting.

TABLE 7-11 Common Calcium Supplements

Calcium Salt	Available Dosage Forms	Elemental Calcium (%)
Calcium carbonate	Powder for solution Suspension Chewable tablet Soft chew tablet Tablet	40
Calcium citrate	Granules for solution Capsule Tablet	21
Calcium glubionate	Syrup	6.5
Calcium gluconate	Powder for solution Capsule Tablet	9
Calcium lactate	Tablet	13

Phosphorus

The normal serum phosphorus concentration of 2.7 to 4.5 mg per deciliter reflects less than 1% of total body phosphorus, with the majority existing in bones and soft tissues.[53] Phosphorus is the main intracellular anion (which exists primarily as phosphate in the serum) and has many important functions, including bone and cell membrane composition and maintenance of normal pH. It provides energy-rich bonds in the form of adenosine triphosphate (ATP) and is required in all cellular functions that require energy.[66–68] Adequate total body phosphorus is necessary for glucose use, glycolysis, maintenance of normal pH, 2,3-diphosphoglycerate synthesis and function (which is necessary for oxygen release from hemoglobin and, ultimately, tissue oxygenation), neurologic function, and muscular function (especially the myocardium and diaphragm).[66–72]

Serum phosphate concentrations are determined by intake, intestinal absorption, renal excretion, hormonally regulated bone resorption and deposition, and distribution between intracellular and extracellular compartments. Glucose and insulin administration, catecholamines, and alkalosis are causes of intracellular shifts of phosphorus. Alternatively, cellular destruction and acidosis result in the release of phosphorus from the cell to the ECF.[53]

Hypophosphatemia

Hypophosphatemia (serum phosphorus concentration <2.7 mg per deciliter) can cause a variety of adverse effects. Manifestations may be neurologic (ataxia, confusion, or paresthesias), neuromuscular (weakness, myalgia, or rhabdomyolysis), cardiopulmonary (cardiac and ventilatory failure), or hematologic (reduced 2,3-diphosphoglycerate concentration or hemolysis).[2] Hypophosphatemia is common in chronic alcoholism, critical illness, respiratory and metabolic alkalosis, following the treatment of diabetic ketoacidosis, and in patients receiving phosphate-binding medications.[66–68] The administration of carbohydrate loads or parenteral nutrition (PN) is likely to cause hypophosphatemia if an inadequate amount of phosphate is provided, especially in malnourished patients at risk for developing severe hypophosphatemia and refeeding syndrome.[69,70,73] See Practice Scenario 7-2 for a discussion of prevention of refeeding syndrome.

Practice Scenario 7-2

Question: How can complications be prevented when providing nutrition support therapy to a malnourished esophageal cancer patient?

	Na+ (mEq/L)	K+ (mEq/L)	Cl- (mEq/L)	HCO_3^- (mEq/L)	BUN (mg/dL)	Creatinine (mg/dL)	Glucose (mg/dL)	Mg (mg/dL)	Phos (mg/dL)
Day 1	133	3.6	99	27	3	0.3	89	1.8	2.8
Day 2	132	3.6	98	28	4	0.3	97	1.7	2.6
Day 4	138	2.6	102	21	8	0.4	105	1.2	1.4

Scenario: JR is a 37-year-old male (71 kg; IBW 92 kg) with esophageal cancer status post esophagectomy and chemoradiation. He is admitted to the hospital for progressive weight loss (20 pound weight loss in the previous 2 months) and failure to thrive. On hospital day 2, a percutaneous endoscopic jejunostomy tube is placed and a 1.5 kcal/mL high protein enteral formula is started at 70 mL per hour. On hospital day 4, JR falls attempting to get out of bed and attributes this to new onset muscle weakness and pain.

Intervention: Enteral feeds are reduced to 20 mL per hour. IV electrolyte replacement is ordered to correct electrolyte abnormalities, and serum chemistry monitoring is ordered every 12 hours. Thiamine 100 mg per feeding tube daily is initiated.

Answer: Nutrition support therapy should be advanced cautiously for patients at risk for refeeding. In this case, JR received 2520 kcal per day (35 kcal per kilogram per day) with no enteral feeding titration. This aggressive rate and calorie provision resulted in a massive intracellular shift of potassium, magnesium, and phosphate causing symptomatic hypokalemia and hypophosphatemia. Electrolyte abnormalities should be corrected as soon as identified and nutrition support therapy should be decreased to a safe rate. Thiamine supplementation is also indicated to facilitate efficient carbohydrate metabolism, to correct existing thiamine deficiency, and to prevent potential lactic acidosis and Wernicke encephalopathy. Calories should be advanced to meet estimated nutritional needs as permitted by the resolution of symptoms and normalization of serum electrolyte values.

Rationale: JR was at significant risk for refeeding complications secondary to significant weight loss prior to the initiation of enteral feeds and his low body mass index (BMI). Severely malnourished patients such as those undergoing anticancer treatment, especially radiation to the gastrointestinal tract, are at an increased risk for electrolyte abnormalities and fluid shifts upon the initiation of nutrition support. Electrolyte abnormalities should be corrected prior to nutrition support therapy and should be closely monitored as calories are carefully increased to meet estimated needs.

Treatment of hypophosphatemia varies according to the degree of severity and the presence of symptoms. Asymptomatic mild hypophosphatemia may be treated with oral phosphate supplements if the GI tract is functional. Table 7-12 lists the most commonly used oral and enteral phosphate supplements.[74] Limitations of oral phosphate supplementation include diarrhea and unreliable absorption. Patients with symptomatic, moderate, or severe hypophosphatemia as well as patients unable to tolerate oral phosphorus formulations should receive IV potassium or sodium phosphate to

TABLE 7-12 Common Oral Phosphate Replacement Products

Dosage Form	Brand Name	Clinical Strength	Considerations
Enteral/Oral Administration			
Potassium phosphate			
Tablet for solution	K-Phos	500 mg (3.7 mEq potassium and 3.7 mmol phosphorus per tablet)	Dissolve tablets in 90 mL water
Powder for solution	Phos-NaK	250 mg/packet (7.1 mEq potassium and 8 mmol phosphorus per packet)	Dilute in 75 mL of water; fruit flavor
Sodium phosphate	Fleets Phospho-soda	4.2 mmol phosphate and 4.8 mEq sodium/mL	Saline laxative; available over the counter; concern for renal failure when used for bowel cleansing in high-risk patients (age > 55, dehydration, baseline kidney disease, bowel obstruction, active colitis, medications that affect renal perfusion)

correct serum phosphorus levels.[21] Phosphate boluses should always be ordered as millimoles of phosphate rather than in terms of sodium or potassium content. IV potassium phosphate is preferred unless the potassium concentration is greater than 4 mEq per liter (3 mmol of potassium phosphate = 4.4 mEq of potassium) or renal insufficiency exists. Dosing recommendations (Table 7-13) are largely empirical because serum phosphorus concentrations may not accurately reflect total body stores.[75-77] Reduced phosphorus dosages (approximately 50%) are recommended for patients with renal impairment to prevent the development of hyperphosphatemia. Infusion rates should not exceed 7 mmol per hour because faster infusion rates can often cause thrombophlebitis (ie, potassium phosphate) and soft tissue calcium-phosphate deposition.[78,79]

TABLE 7-13 Empirical Treatment of Hypophosphatemia

Severity	Serum Phosphorus Concentration (mg/dL)	IV Phosphorus Dose (mmol/kg)[a,b]
Mild	2.3–2.7	0.08–0.16
Moderate	1.5–2.2	0.16–0.32
Severe	< 1.5	0.32–0.64

IV, intravenous.
[a]These guidelines are recommended for patients with normal renal function. Patients with renal impairment should receive: 50% of the initial empirical dose. Maximum infusion rate: 7 mmol phosphorus per hour.
[b]Potassium phosphate is preferred over sodium phosphate when the serum potassium concentration is < 4.0 mEq/L.

Hyperphosphatemia

Hyperphosphatemia, defined as serum phosphorus concentrations >4.7 mg per deciliter, most often occurs in the setting of renal insufficiency. Hyperphosphatemia can also be caused by the endogenous release of phosphorus into the ECF from cellular destruction, such as with massive trauma, cytotoxic agents (especially with treatment of lymphomas and leukemias that have large tumor burdens), hypercatabolism, hemolysis, rhabdomyolysis, and malignant hyperthermia. Transcellular shifts of phosphorus from the ICF to the ECF caused by a respiratory or metabolic acidosis may also result in hyperphosphatemia. The administration of large quantities of phosphate-containing laxatives or enemas, especially in the elderly, has been reported to contribute to severe hyperphosphatemia and end-organ damage (renal failure).[80]

The most serious complication of hyperphosphatemia is soft tissue and vascular calcification.[37] Calcification occurs when the calcium-phosphorus product exceeds 55 mg^2 per deciliter.[2,81,82] Additional consequences of hyperphosphatemia include secondary hyperparathyroidism and renal osteodystrophy. Other signs and symptoms are secondary to the development of hypocalcemia and manifest as anorexia, nausea, vomiting, dehydration, and neuromuscular irritability.

Exogenous sources of phosphorus including dietary sources, PN, and phosphate-containing enemas or laxatives should be decreased or eliminated in the setting of hyperphosphatemia. Conventional aluminum- and calcium-based phosphate binders can be used to reduce intestinal absorption of phosphorus. However, recently developed aluminum- and calcium-free binders are at least as effective and without the untoward risks of anemia and osteomalacia seen with use of aluminum-based agents.[83] Dialysis may be required to treat severe hyperphosphatemia associated with renal insufficiency. In patients with normal renal function, volume repletion in conjunction with diuretics is usually sufficient.

Acid–Base Balance

Acid–Base Physiology

Definitions

Nearly all biochemical reactions are influenced by the pH of their fluid environment. Accordingly, the acid–base balance of body fluids is critical and tightly regulated. Alterations in acid–base balance can have adverse consequences and, when severe, can be life-threatening. An understanding of acid–base terminology is critical to accurately diagnose and manage acid–base disorders.

An acid is a substance that can donate hydrogen ions (H^+). A base is a substance that can accept or combine with H^+.[1] The free H^+ concentration determines the acidity of body fluids and is represented by the pH. Because the pH varies inversely with the H^+ concentration, an increase in the H^+ concentration reduces the pH, and a decrease in the H^+ concentration elevates the pH. The pH of arterial blood is normally maintained within the narrow range of 7.35 to 7.45. A pH below 7.35 is called acidemia; a pH greater than 7.45 is called alkalemia.[1] Processes that tend to raise or lower the H^+ concentration are called acidosis and alkalosis, respectively. Recognizing the distinction between these terms is necessary to evaluate acid–base disorders in patients in whom both acidotic and alkalotic processes may coexist (mixed acid–base disorders).

Regulation of Hydrogen Ion Concentration

Although small amounts of acidic substances enter the body via ingested foods, most H^+ originate as by-products or end products of cellular metabolism. Metabolism of carbohydrates and fats alone results in the daily production of approximately 15,000 mmol of carbon dioxide (CO_2), which combines with water to form carbonic acid. Protein metabolism accounts for another 50 to 100 mEq of daily acid (noncarbonic acid) production.[84] A progressive accumulation of acid would occur if these substances were not excreted from the body.

The concentration of H^+ in body fluids must be tightly regulated to maintain a pH compatible with life (6.80 to 7.80).[1] The process of H^+ regulation involves three sequential steps: (1) chemical buffering by extracellular and intracellular mechanisms, (2) control of the partial pressure of carbon dioxide in the blood by alterations in the rate of alveolar ventilation, and (3) control of the plasma bicarbonate concentration by changes in renal H^+ excretion.

Chemical Buffers

Buffering prevents large changes in the H^+ concentration in the body. This process is the body's first line of defense and occurs immediately to resist changes in pH. Buffer systems are primarily weak acids and base pairs able to take up or release H^+ so that changes in the free H^+ concentration are minimized. The principal buffer system is the carbonic acid/bicarbonate (H_2CO_3/HCO_3^-) system. Other buffer systems including proteins, phosphate, and hemoglobin also contribute to the maintenance of normal pH.

Lungs

The principal role of the lungs in maintaining acid–base balance is to regulate the pressure exerted by dissolved CO_2 gas in the blood (PCO_2). Of all the chemicals influencing respiration, CO_2 is the most powerful respiratory stimulant. Both the rate and depth of ventilation can be altered to allow for the excretion of CO_2 generated by diet and cellular metabolism. Adjustments in the rate and depth of ventilation begin to compensate for acid–base disturbances within minutes. Anything that impairs respiratory system functioning has the potential to cause acid–base imbalances.

Kidneys

The final and slowest mechanism by which the body maintains acid–base balance is via alterations in renal H^+ excretion. Two processes achieve this: (1) reabsorption of filtered HCO_3^- and (2) excretion of the H^+ produced daily as a result of protein metabolism. Of all the regulatory mechanisms involved in acid–base homeostasis, only the kidneys have the ability to regulate levels of alkaline substances in the blood and eliminate metabolic acids (organic acids other than carbonic acid) from the body.

Normal Blood Gas Values

Blood gases are used to assess a patient's oxygenation and acid–base status. Arterial blood gases (ABGs) reflect the ability of the lungs to oxygenate blood, whereas venous blood gases (VBGs) reflect tissue oxygenation. Blood gas measurements consist of the pH, PCO_2, PO_2, oxygen saturation (SaO_2), calculated HCO_3^-, and the base excess. Normal values for ABGs and VBGs are given in Table 7-14. ABGs and VBGs have different normal ranges for these measurements and evaluate different aspects of ventilation and perfusion.

As previously described, the pH is a reflection of the degree of blood acidity. The PCO_2 provides information on the lung's ability to excrete CO_2, and changes in PCO_2 are associated with respiratory processes that can lead to acid–base disorders. CO_2 is the acid component of the carbonic acid/bicarbonate buffer system. Increases in PCO_2 represent an acidosis and decreases in PCO_2 represent an alkalosis. The partial pressure of oxygen in the blood (PO_2) reflects the ability of hemoglobin to carry oxygen. The higher the value, the more saturated hemoglobin is with oxygen. This value is related to the SaO_2. When PO_2 is high, the SaO_2 of the blood is high and vice versa. Either the calculated HCO_3^- reported in a blood gas or the serum HCO_3^- can be used to evaluate acid–base status. Changes in HCO_3^- are associated with metabolic processes that can lead to acid–base disorders. HCO_3^- is the base component of the carbonic acid/bicarbonate buffer system. Increases in serum or calculated HCO_3^- represent an alkalosis, and decreases represent an acidosis. Base excess is a calculated value that estimates the metabolic component of an acid–base disorder. An elevated base excess represents a metabolic alkalosis, whereas a base deficit occurs in metabolic acidosis.

TABLE 7-14 Normal Blood Gas Values

	Arterial	Mixed Venous
pH	7.40 (7.35–7.45)	7.36 (7.33–7.43)
PCO_2	35–45 mm Hg	41–51 mm Hg
PO_2	80–100 mm Hg	35–40 mm Hg
O_2 saturation	95%	70%–75%
HCO_3^-	22–26 mEq/L	24–28 mEq/L
Base excess	(−2) – (+2)	(0) – (+4)

HCO_3^-, bicarbonate; O_2, oxygen; PCO_2, pressure of carbon dioxide in the blood; PO_2, partial pressure of oxygen in the blood.

Analysis of Acid–Base Disorders

An analysis of acid–base disorders requires a systematic approach to avoid misdiagnosis and inappropriate treatment. The following stepwise approach is useful in evaluating even the most complex cases:

Step 1: Assess the pH to determine if the patient is acidemic (pH <7.4) or alkalemic (pH >7.4). If the pH is 7.4, the presence of an acid–base disorder cannot be excluded due to the possibility of a mixed acid–base disorder or compensation.

Step 2: Assess the PCO_2 to determine if there is a respiratory process that may contribute to an acid–base disorder. If the PCO_2 is elevated, the patient has respiratory acidosis. If the PCO_2 is low, the patient has respiratory alkalosis (Table 7-15).

Step 3: Assess the HCO_3^- to determine if there is a metabolic process that may contribute to an acid–base disorder. If the HCO_3^- is elevated, the patient has metabolic alkalosis (Table 7-16). If the HCO_3^- is low, the patient has metabolic acidosis (Table 7-17).

Step 4: Calculate the anion gap (refer to section "Metabolic Acidosis" for the equation) to determine if metabolic acidosis is present. This is critical to determine the etiology of the acid–base disorder and to select the appropriate treatment.

Step 5: Determine if the acid–base disorder is acute or chronic in nature. Use the recommended formulas in Table 7-18 to determine if the acid–base disorders are appropriately compensated. If the formulas do not indicate appropriate compensation, a mixed acid–base disorder exists.

Acid–Base Disorders

Respiratory Acidosis

Respiratory acidosis is a clinical disorder characterized by a reduced pH, an elevation in the PCO_2, and a variable increase in the plasma HCO_3^- concentration (Table 7-19).[1] Respiratory acidosis almost always results from decreased effective alveolar ventilation, not an increase in CO_2 production. Hypoventilation can occur when there is interference with any step in the ventilatory process. Table 7-15 includes common causes of respiratory acidosis.

TABLE 7-15 Causes of Respiratory Acid-Base Disorders

Respiratory Acidosis	Respiratory Alkalosis
Central depression of respiration	Central stimulation of respiration
Drugs (opioids, anesthetics, sedatives)	Anxiety
Stroke	Pain
Head injury	Fever
Sleep apnea	Brain tumors
Perfusion abnormalities	Vascular accidents
Massive pulmonary embolism	Head trauma
Cardiac arrest	Pregnancy
Airway or pulmonary abnormalities	Catecholamines
Hypoxemia or tissue abnormalities	Salicylates
Airway obstruction	Peripheral stimulation of respiration
Aspiration	Pulmonary embolus
Asthma	Asthma hypoxemia
COPD	High altitudes
Severe pulmonary edema	Pneumonia
Severe pneumonia	Pulmonary edema
ARDS	Severe anemia
Smoke inhalation	Mechanical ventilator hyperventilation
Pneumothorax	
Neuromuscular abnormalities	
Brainstem or cervical cord injury	
Guillain-Barré syndrome	
Myasthenia gravis	
Multiple sclerosis	
Obesity-hypoventilation (Pickwickian syndrome)	
Mechanical ventilator hypoventilation	
Parenteral nutrition	

ARDS, acute respiratory distress syndrome; COPD, chronic obstructive pulmonary disorder.

Respiratory Alkalosis

Respiratory alkalosis is a clinical disturbance characterized by an elevated pH, a decrease in the PCO_2, and a variable reduction in the plasma HCO_3^- concentration (Table 7-19).[1] Respiratory alkalosis occurs when effective alveolar ventilation is increased beyond the level necessary to eliminate metabolically produced CO_2. Table 7-15 includes common causes of hyperventilation resulting in respiratory alkalosis.

Metabolic Acidosis

Metabolic acidosis is a clinical disturbance characterized by a low pH, a reduced plasma HCO_3^- concentration, and compensatory hyperventilation resulting in a decrease in the PCO_2 (Table 7-19).[1] Metabolic acidosis can be induced by two fundamental mechanisms: (1) an inability of the kidney to excrete the dietary H^+ load or (2) an increase in the generation of H^+ as a result of either the addition of H^+ or the loss of HCO_3^-.

TABLE 7-16 Causes of Metabolic Alkalosis

Saline-Responsive (Urine Chlorine < 10 mEq/L)	Saline-Resistant (Urine Chlorine > 10 mEq/L)
Gastrointestinal loss	Excess mineralocorticoids
Vomiting	Cushing's syndrome
Nasogastric suction	Hyperaldosteronism
Renal loss	Profound potassium depletion
Diuretic therapy	Excessive licorice ingestion
Excessive bicarbonate administration	
Rapid correction of hypocapnia	

Calculating the anion gap is often useful in the differential diagnosis of metabolic acidosis. The anion gap is equal to the difference between the plasma concentrations of the major cation and the major measured anions. Anion gap is calculated as follows:[1]

$$\text{Anion Gap} = [Na^+] - ([Cl^-] + [HCO_3^-])$$

The anion gap represents unmeasured serum anions (proteins, phosphate, sulfate, and organic ions) and is approximately 9 mEq per liter (range 3 to 11 mEq per liter).[85] Albumin accounts for a significant portion of the unmeasured serum anions. For every 1 g per deciliter decrease in serum albumin, the anion gap increases by 2.5 mEq per liter. The anion gap is used to differentiate between the two main types of metabolic acidosis: (1) normal anion gap acidosis (hyperchloremic acidosis) and (2) elevated anion gap acidosis. Common causes of metabolic acidosis with an increased anion gap or a normal anion gap are listed in Table 7-17. See Practice Scenario 7-3 for further discussion of the management of metabolic acidosis.

TABLE 7-17 Causes of Metabolic Acidosis

Normal Anion Gap	Increased Anion Gap
Gastrointestinal loss of HCO_3^-	Increased production of endogenous acid
Diarrhea, pancreatic fistula, small bowel fistula, obstructed ileal loop conduit, ureterosigmoidostomy, anion-exchange resins, ingestion of calcium or magnesium chloride	Lactic acidosis, ketoacidosis (diabetic, starvation, alcoholic), inborn errors of metabolism
Renal loss of HCO_3^-	Failure to excrete acids
Type 2 renal tubular acidosis, carbonic anhydrase inhibitors, hyperparathyroidism, hypoaldosteronism	Renal failure
Ingestions	Ingestion of exogenous acid
Ammonium chloride, parenteral nutrition (chloride salts), sulfur	Salicylates, methanol, ethanol

HCO_3^-, bicarbonate.

TABLE 7-18 Renal and Respiratory Compensation to Primary Acid-Base Disorders

Disorder	Primary Disturbance	Compensatory Response
Metabolic acidosis	HCO_3^-	1.2 mm Hg decrease in PCO_2 for every 1 mEq/L fall in HCO_3^-
Metabolic alkalosis	HCO_3^-	0.7 mm Hg increase in PCO_2 for every 1 mEq/L rise in HCO_3^-
Respiratory acidosis	PCO_2	
Acute		1 mEq/L increase in HCO_3^- for every 10 mm Hg rise in PCO_2
Chronic		3.5 mEq/L increase in HCO_3^- for every 10 mm Hg rise in PCO_2
Respiratory alkalosis	PCO_2	
Acute		2 mEq/L decrease in HCO_3^- for every 10 mm Hg fall in PCO_2
Chronic		4 mEq/L decrease in HCO_3^- for every 10 mm Hg fall in PCO_2

HCO_3^-, bicarbonate; PCO_2, pressure of carbon dioxide in the blood.

Practice Scenario 7-3

Question: How would you alter the electrolyte composition of a parenteral nutrition formula for a patient with a high output ileostomy?

Scenario: BB is a 54-year-old female with a 30-year history of Crohn's disease. Her disease course has included small bowel strictures resulting in multiple small bowel resections, ultimately requiring the creation of an end ileostomy. She is admitted to the hospital for progressive weight loss and fatigue, high ostomy output (between 3 and 4.5 liters per day), and acute renal failure secondary to dehydration. Albumin and prealbumin on admission are 2.1 g per deciliter and 18.6 mg per deciliter, respectively. Intravenous fluids of 0.9% sodium chloride were started at 125 mL per hour in addition to a regular diet. By day 3, BB developed severe metabolic acidosis and continued to experience high-volume ileostomy output. The dietitian reported BB primarily consumed high fat, fried foods and milkshakes.

Intervention: Parenteral nutrition, formulated to correct the metabolic acidosis, was started on hospital day 3. The patient was counseled to restrict her diet to low fat foods only.

	Na+ (mEq/L)	K+ (mEq/L)	Cl^- (mEq/L)	HCO_3- (mEq/L)	BUN (mg/dL)	Creatinine (mg/dL)
Day 1	131	3.3	97	18	69	1.4
Day 2	137	4.1	112	14	30	1.2
Day 3	137	4.1	114	12	23	1.1

Answer: The PN formula for a high-output ileostomy patient should contain maximum amounts of acetate salts to prevent and/or correct a metabolic acidosis. In this patient, PN was started at 50% of estimated caloric needs to prevent possible refeeding syndrome and acetate salts were maximized. Common acetate additives for PN include sodium acetate and potassium acetate. Based on patient laboratory parameters, the amounts of sodium and potassium acetate should be tailored for individual needs/tolerance. In addition, the sodium concentration in the PN should be equal to that of 0.9% NaCl (normal saline) to approximate the sodium concentration of ileostomy fluid.

Rationale: Patients with ileostomies, specifically high output, are at risk for acid–base disturbances secondary to anatomical changes. The management of high-output ileostomies (greater than 1 L per day) should include fluid replacement that approximates the electrolyte composition of ileal fluid (Table 7-1).

Normal Anion-Gap Acidosis (Hyperchloremic Acidosis)

In the setting of normal anion-gap acidosis, there is a milliequivalent-for-milliequivalent replacement of extracellular HCO_3^- by Cl^-; thus, there is no change in the anion gap because the sum of the major measured anions remains constant. Increased GI or renal bicarbonate loss causes this disorder, also known as hyperchloremic metabolic acidosis. Table 7-17 includes common causes of this disorder.

High Anion-Gap Acidosis

The hallmark of this disorder is a metabolic acidosis associated with an accumulation of unmeasured anions, which leads to an elevation in the anion gap. Metabolic acidosis with an elevated anion gap commonly results from increased endogenous organic acid production. Common causes are presented in Table 7-17.

TABLE 7-19 Characteristics of the Primary Acid-Base Disorders

Disorder	pH	Primary Disturbance	Compensatory Response
Metabolic acidosis	↓	↓HCO_3^-	↓PCO_2
Metabolic alkalosis	↑	↑HCO_3^-	↑PCO_2
Respiratory acidosis	↓	↑PCO_2	↑HCO_3^-
Respiratory alkalosis	↑	↓PCO_2	↓HCO_3^-

HCO_3^-, bicarbonate; PCO_2, pressure of carbon dioxide in the blood.

Metabolic Alkalosis

Metabolic alkalosis is characterized by an elevation in the pH, an increase in the plasma HCO_3^- concentration, and compensatory hypoventilation, resulting in a rise in the PCO_2 (Table 7-19).[1] Loss of gastric acid as a result of vomiting or nasogastric suction and loss of intravascular volume and Cl^- as a result of diuretic use are common causes of metabolic alkalosis. This disorder is observed in approximately 33% to 55% of hospitalized patients with acid–base disturbances.[86] Metabolic alkalosis in this setting is often due to the overzealous treatment of metabolic acidosis with bicarbonate or an excess of acetate in PN solutions, which is metabolized to bicarbonate. In addition, the transcellular shift of H^+ that typically occurs with hypokalemia may contribute to the development of metabolic alkalosis.

Under normal circumstances, the kidneys are able to correct a metabolic alkalosis by excreting the excess HCO_3^- in the urine. Therefore, some degree of impairment in renal HCO_3^- excretion must be present for maintenance of metabolic alkalosis.[1] In general, the mechanisms which sustain metabolic alkalosis can be classified into volume-mediated processes (saline responsive) and volume-independent processes (saline unresponsive). The urine chloride concentration is useful in the differential diagnosis of metabolic alkalosis and predicts those patients likely to respond to volume replacement.

Saline-Responsive Metabolic Alkalosis (Urine Chloride, >10 mEq per Liter)

Saline-responsive metabolic alkalosis is by far the more prevalent disorder. Common causes are listed in Table 7-16. In these disorders, the increase in HCO_3^- reabsorption that maintains the alkalosis can be reversed by the administration of half-isotonic or isotonic saline. Although adequate sodium chloride repletion will usually normalize the plasma HCO_3^- concentration, it will not reverse metabolic alkalosis associated with hypokalemia. Only the administration of potassium chloride will correct this disorder.

Saline-Unresponsive Metabolic Alkalosis (Urine Chloride >10 mEq per Liter)

Saline-resistant disorders are commonly associated with hyperaldosteronism and are characterized by a high urinary chloride concentration. Management of these disorders typically consists of the treatment of the underlying cause of the mineralocorticoid excess. Aggressive potassium repletion should also be employed when hypokalemia is present with metabolic alkalosis in primary hyperaldosteronism.

Mixed Acid–Base Disorders

It is not uncommon for a patient to have more than one acid–base disturbance occurring simultaneously resulting in a mixed acid–base disorder. The diagnosis of a mixed disorder requires an understanding of the extent of the renal and respiratory compensations for each of the simple acid–base disturbances (Table 7-18). If a given set of blood gases does not fall within the range of expected responses for a simple acid–base disturbance, a mixed disorder should be suspected. Common examples include: (1) mixed respiratory acidosis and metabolic acidosis, (2) mixed respiratory alkalosis and metabolic alkalosis, (3) mixed metabolic acidosis and respiratory alkalosis, and (4) mixed metabolic alkalosis and respiratory acidosis.

References

1. Rose BD, Post TW. *Clinical Physiology of Acid-Base and Electrolyte Disorders*, 5th ed. New York, NY: McGraw-Hill; 2001.
2. Canada TW, Boullata JI. Fluid and electrolytes. In: Rolandelli RH, Bankhead R, Boullata JI, Compher CW, eds. *Enteral and Tube Feeding*, 4th ed. Philadelphia, PA: Elsevier Saunders; 2005:95–109.
3. Moukarzel A. Understanding and managing fluid and electrolyte abnormalities. In: *A.S.P.E.N. 22nd Clinical Congress Course Syllabus*. Oralando, FL:1999:247–254.
4. Hansen M. Fluid balance. In: Hansen M, ed. *Pathophysiology: Foundations of Disease and Clinical Intervention*. Philadelphia, PA: Saunders; 1998:160–175.
5. Whitmire SJ. Fluids and electrolytes. In: Matarese LE, Gottschlich MM, eds. *Contemporary Nutrition Support Practice: A Clinical Guide*, 1st ed. Philadelphia, PA: Saunders; 1998:129.
6. Mirtallo J, Canada T, Johnson D, et al. Safe practices for parenteral nutrition. *JPEN. J Parenter Enteral Nutr.* 2004; 28:S39–S70.
7. Alvelos M, Ferreira A, Bettencourt P, et al. The effect of dietary sodium restriction on neurohumoral activity and renal dopaminergic response in patients with heart failure. *Eur J Heart Failure.* 2004;6:593–599.
8. Damgaard M, Norsk P, Gustafsson F, et al. Hemodynamic and neuroendocrine responses to changes in sodium intake in compensated heart failure. *Am J Physiol Regul Integr Comp Physiol.* 2006;290:R1294–R1301.
9. Peacock WF, Fonarow GC, Emerman CL, et al. Impact of early initiation of intravenous therapy for acute decompensated heart failure on outcomes in ADHERE. *Cardiology.* 2007;107:44–51.
10. Maisel AS, Peacock WF, McMullin N, et al. Timing of immunoreactive B-type natriuretic peptide levels and treatment delay in acute decompensated heart failure: an ADHERE (Acute Decompensated Heart Failure National Registry) analysis. *J Am Coll Cardiol.* 2008;52:534–540.
11. Mange K, Matsuura D, Cizman B, et al. Language guiding therapy: the case of dehydration versus volume depletion. *Ann Intern Med.* 1997;127:848–853.
12. Whitmire SJ. Fluids and electrolytes. In: Matarese LE, Gottschlich MM, eds. *Contemporary Nutrition Support Practice: A Clinical Guide*, 1st ed. Philadelphia, PA: Saunders;1998:130.
13. Hawkins RC. Age and gender as risk factors for hyponatremia and hypernatremia. *Clinica Chimica Acta.* 2003;337:169–172.
14. Anderson RJ, Chung, HM, Kluge R, et al. Hyponatremia: a prospective analysis of its epidemiology and the pathogenic role of vasopressin. *Ann Intern Med.* 1985;102:164–168.
15. Kumar S, Berl T. Sodium. *Lancet.* 1998;352:220–228.
16. Snyder NA, Feigal DW, Arieff A. Hypernatremia in elderly patients. A heterogeneous, morbid, and iatrogenic entity. *Ann Intern Med.* 1987;107:309–319.
17. Clausen T, Everts ME. Regulation of the Na,K-pump in skeletal muscle. *Kidney Int.* 1989;35:1–13.
18. Paice BJ, Paterson KR, Onyanga-Omara F, et al. Record linkage study of hypokalaemia in hospitalized patients. *Postgrad Med J.* 1986;62:187–191.

19. Gennari FJ. Hypokalemia. *N Engl J Med.* 1998;339:451–458.
20. Strom BL, Carson JL, Schinnar R, et al. Upper gastrointestinal tract bleeding from oral potassium chloride. Comparative risk from microencapsulated vs. waxmatrix formulations. *Arch Intern Med.* 1987;147:954–957.
21. Kraft MD, Btaiche IF, Sacks GS, Kudsk KA. Treatment of electrolyte disorders in adult patients in the intensive care unit. *Am J Health Syst Pharm.* 2005;62:1663–1682.
22. Cohn JN, Kowey PR, Whelton PK, Prisant LM. New guidelines for potassium replacement in clinical practice: a contemporary review by the National Council on Potassium in Clinical Practice. *Arch Intern Med.* 2000;160:2429–2436.
23. Kruse JA, Carlson RW. Rapid correction of hypokalemia using concentrated intravenous potassium chloride infusions. *Arch Intern Med.* 1990;150:613–617.
24. Kruse JA, Clark VL, Carlson RW, Geheb MA. Concentrated potassium chloride infusions in critically ill patients with hypokalemia. *J Clin Pharmacol.* 1994;34:1077–1082.
25. Hamill RJ, Robinson LM, Wexler HR, Moote C. Efficacy and safety of potassium infusion therapy in hypokalemic critically ill patients. *Crit Care Med.* 1991;19:694–699.
26. Agarwal A, Wingo CS. Treatment of hypokalemia. *N Engl J Med.* 1999;340:154–155.
27. Whang R, Whang DD, Ryan MP. Refractory potassium repletion. A consequence of magnesium deficiency. *Arch Intern Med.* 1992;152:40–45.
28. Lutarewych MA, Batlle DC. Disorders of potassium balance. In: Androgue HJ, ed. *Contemporary Management in Critical Care: Acid-Base and Electrolyte Disorders,* Vol. 1, No. 2. New York, NY: Churchill Livingstone; 1991:193–232.
29. Adrogue HJ, Madias NE. Changes in plasma potassium concentration during acute acid–base disturbances. *Am J Med.* 1981;71: 456–467.
30. Perazella MA. Drug-induced hyperkalemia: old culprits and new offenders. *Am J Med.* 2000;109:307–314.
31. Kunau RT, Stein JH. Disorders of hypo- and hyperkalemia. *Clin Nephrol.* 1977;7:173–190.
32. Mandal AK. Hypokalemia and hyperkalemia. *Med Clin North Am.* 1997;81:611–639.
33. Williams ME. Endocrine crises. Hyperkalemia. *Crit Care Clin.* 1991;7:155–174.
34. Connolly E, Worthley L. Intravenous magnesium. *Crit Care Resusc.* 1999;1:162–172.
35. Reinhart RA. Magnesium metabolism. A review with special reference to the relationship between intracellular content and serum levels. *Arch Intern Med.* 1988; 148:2415–2420.
36. Zaloga GP, Roberts PR. Calcium, phosphorus, and magnesium disorders. In: Ayres SM, Grenvik NA, Holbrook PR, Shoemaker WC, eds. *Textbook of Critical Care,* 4th ed. Philadelphia, PA: Saunders; 2000:905–928.
37. Food and Nutrition Board. Dietary reference intakes for calcium, phosphorus, magnesium, vitamin D, and fluoride. The National Academies Press Web site. http://www.nap.edu/openbook.php?isbn50309063507. Accessed September 24, 2011.
38. Whang R. Magnesium deficiency: pathogenesis, prevalence, and clinical implications. *Am J Med.* 1987;82:24–29.
39. Wong ET, Rude RK, Singer FR, Shaw ST. A high prevalence of hypomagnesemia and hypermagnesemia in hospitalized patients. *Am J Clin Pathol.* 1983;79:348–352.
40. Rubeiz GJ, Thill-Baharozian M, Hardie D, Carlson RW. Association of hypomagnesemia and mortality in acutely ill medical patients. *Crit Care Med.* 1993;21:203–209.
41. Whang R, Oei TO, Aikawa JK, et al. Predictors of clinical hypomagnesemia. Hypokalemia, hypophosphatemia, hyponatremia, and hypocalcemia. *Arch Intern Med.* 1984;144:1794–1796.
42. Ryzen E, Wagers PW, Singer FR, Rude RK. Magnesium deficiency in a medical ICU population. *Crit Care Med.* 1985;13:19–21.
43. Rude RK, Singer FR. Magnesium deficiency and excess. *Annu Rev Med.* 1981;32:245–259.
44. Desai TK, Carlson RW, Geheb MA. Prevalence and clinical implications of hypocalcemia in acutely ill patients in a medical intensive care setting. *Am J Med.* 1988;84:209–214.
45. Boyd JC, Bruns DE, Wills MR. Frequency of hypomagnesemia in hypokalemic states. *Clin Chem.* 1983;2:178–179.
46. Rude RK. Magnesium metabolism and deficiency. *Endocrinol Metab Clin North Am.* 1993;22:377–395.
47. Dacey MJ. Hypomagnesemic disorders. *Crit Care Clin.* 2001;17: 155–173,viii.
48. Dickerson RN, Brown RO. Hypomagnesemia in hospitalized patients receiving nutritional support. *Heart Lung.* 1985;14: 561–569.
49. Oster JR, Epstein M. Management of magnesium depletion. *Am J Nephrol.* 1988;8:349–354.
50. Sacks GS, Brown RO, Dickerson RN, et al. Mononuclear blood cell magnesium content and serum magnesium concentration in critically ill hypomagnesemic patients after replacement therapy. *Nutrition.* 1997;13:303–308.
51. Hebert P, Mehta N, Wang J, et al. Functional magnesium deficiency in critically ill patients identified using a magnesium-loading test. *Crit Care Med.* 1997;25:749–755.
52. Van Hook JW. Endocrine crises. Hypermagnesemia. *Crit Care Clin.* 1991;7:215–223.
53. Popovtzer MM. Disorders of calcium, phosphorus, vitamin D, and parathyroid hormone activity. In: Schrier RW, ed. *Renal and Electrolyte Disorders,* 6th ed. Philadelphia, PA: Lippincott Williams & Wilkins; 2003: 216–277.
54. Bushinsky DA, Monk RD. Electrolyte quintet: calcium. *Lancet.* 1998;352:306–311.
55. Singer FR, Bethune JE, Massry SG. Hypercalcemia and hypocalcemia. *Clin Nephrol.* 1977;7:154–162.
56. Dickerson RN, Alexander KH, Minard G, Croce MA, Brown RO. Accuracy of methods to estimate ionized and "corrected" serum calcium concentrations in critically ill multiple trauma patients receiving specialized nutrition support. *JPEN. J Parenter Enteral Nutr* 2004;28:133–141.
57. Zivin JR, Gooley T, Zager RA, Ryan MJ. Hypocalcemia: a pervasive metabolic abnormality in the critically ill. *Am J Kidney Dis.* 2001; 37:689–698.
58. Guise TA, Mundy GR. Clinical review 69: evaluation of hypocalcemia in children and adults. *J Clin Endocrinol Metab.* 1995;80: 1473–1478.
59. Olinger ML. Disorders of calcium and magnesium metabolism. *Emerg Med Clin North Am.* 1989;7:795–822.
60. Jucgla A, Sais G, Curco N, et al. Calcinosis cutis following liver transplantation: a complication of intravenous calcium administration. *Br J Dermatol.* 1995;132:275–278.
61. Semple P, Booth C. Calcium chloride; a reminder. *Anaesthesia.* 1996;51:93.
62. Dickerson RN, Morgan LM, Croce MA, Minard G, Brown RO. Treatment of moderate to severe acute hypocalcemia in critically ill trauma patients. *JPEN.* 2007:31:228–233.
63. Anast CS, Winnacker JL, Forte LR, Burns TW. Impaired release of parathyroid hormone in magnesium deficiency. *J Clin Endocrinol Metab.* 1976;42:707–717.

64. Fatemi S, Rzyen E, Flores J, et al. Effect of experimental human magnesium depletion on parathyroid hormone secretion and 1,25-dihydroxyvitamin D metabolism. *J Clin Endocrinol Metab.* 1991;73:1067–1072.
65. Davis KD, Attie MF. Management of severe hypercalcemia. *Crit Care Clin.* 1991;7:175–190.
66. Peppers MP, Geheb M, Desai T. Endocrine crises. Hypophosphatemia and hyperphosphatemia. *Crit Care Clin.* 1991;7:201–214.
67. Knochel JP. The pathophysiology and clinical characteristics of severe hypophosphatemia. *Arch Intern Med.* 1977;137:203–220.
68. Stoff JS. Phosphate homeostasis and hypophosphatemia. *Arch Intern Med.* 1982;72:489–495.
69. Sheldon GF, Grzyb S. Phosphate depletion and repletion: relation to parenteral nutrition and oxygen transport. *Ann Surg.* 1975; 182:683–689.
70. Travis SF, Sugerman HJ, Ruberg RL, et al. Alterations of red-cell glycolytic intermediates and oxygen transport as a consequence of hypophosphatemia in patients receiving intravenous hyperalimentation. *N Engl J Med.* 1971;285:763–768.
71. Newman JH, Neff TA, Ziporin P. Acute respiratory failure associated with hypophosphatemia. *N Engl J Med.* 1977;296:1101–1103.
72. Aubier M, Murciano D, Lecocguic Y, et al. Effect of hypophosphatemia on diaphragmatic contractility in patients with acute respiratory failure. *N Engl J Med.* 1985;313:420–424.
73. Brooks MJ, Melnik G. The refeeding syndrome: an approach to understanding its complications and preventing its occurrence. *Pharmacotherapy.* 1995;15:713–726.
74. U.S. Food and Drug Administration. Information for Healthcare Professionals: Oral Sodium Phosphate (OSP) Products for Bowel Cleansing (marketed as Visicol and OsmoPrep, and oral sodium phosphate products available without a prescription). FDA Alert 12/11/2008. http://www.fda.gov/Drugs/DrugSafety/PostmarketDrugSafetyInformationforPatientsandProviders/ucm126084.htm. Accessed September 24, 2011.
75. Lentz RD, Brown DM, Kjellstrand CM. Treatment of severe hypophosphatemia. *Ann Intern Med.* 1978;89:941–944.
76. Vannatta JB, Whang R, Papper S. Efficacy of intravenous phosphorus therapy in the severely hypophosphatemic patient. *Arch Intern Med.* 1981;141:885–887.
77. Andress DL, Vannatta JB, Whang R. Treatment of refractory hypophosphatemia. *South Med J.* 1982;75:766–767.
78. Rosen GH, Boullata JI, O'Rangers EA, et al. Intravenous phosphate repletion regimen for critically ill patients with moderate hypophosphatemia. *Crit Care Med.* 1995;23:1204–1210.
79. Clark CL, Sacks GS, Dickerson RN, et al. Treatment of hypophosphatemia in patients receiving specialized nutrition support using a graduated dosing scheme: results from a prospective clinical trial. *Crit Care Med.* 1995;23:1504–1511.
80. Brunelli SM, Lewis JD, Gupta M, et al. Risk of kidney injury following oral phosphosoda bowel preparations. *J Am Soc Nephrol.* 2007;18:3199–3205.
81. Block GA, Port FK. Re-evaluation of risks associated with hyperphosphatemia and hyperparathyroidism in dialysis patients: recommendations for a change in management. *Am J Kidney Dis.* 2000;35:1226–1237.
82. Goodman WG, Goldin J, Kuizon BD, et al. Coronary artery calcification in young adults with end-stage renal disease who are undergoing dialysis. *N Engl J Med.* 2000;342:1478–1483.
83. Ritz E. The clinical management of hyperphosphatemia. *J Nephrol.* 2005;18:221–228.
84. Kurtz I, Maher T, Hulter HN, et al. Effect of diet on plasma acid-base composition in normal humans. *Kidney Int.* 1983;24: 670–680.
85. Winter SD, Pearson JR, Gabow PA, et al. The fall of the serum anion gap. *Arch Intern Med.* 1990;150:311–313.
86. Hodgkin JE, Soeprono FF, Chan DM. Incidence of metabolic alkalemia in hospitalized patients. *Crit Care Med.* 1980;8: 725–728.

8 Vitamins and Trace Elements

Susan F. Clark, RD, PhD

CONTENTS

Background ... **122**
Vitamins ... **123**
Fat-Soluble Vitamins ... **123**
Vitamin A ... **123**
Vitamin D ... **125**
Vitamin E ... **129**
Vitamin K ... **130**
Water-Soluble Vitamins ... **131**
Ascorbic Acid (Vitamin C) ... **131**
Thiamin ... **131**
Riboflavin ... **132**
Niacin ... **133**
Vitamin B_6 (Pyridoxine) ... **133**
Vitamin B_{12} (Cobalamin) ... **134**
Folic Acid (Folate, Folacin) ... **135**
Biotin ... **136**
Pantothenic Acid ... **136**
Choline ... **136**
Trace Elements ... **137**
Iron (Fe) ... **137**
Zinc (Zn) ... **141**
Copper (Cu) ... **142**
Manganese (Mn) ... **143**
Selenium (Se) ... **144**
Iodine (I) ... **145**
Chromium (Cr) ... **145**
Fluoride (F) ... **146**
Molybdenum (Mo) ... **146**
Ultratrace Elements ... **146**
Parenteral Vitamins ... **147**
Parenteral Trace Elements ... **147**
Enteral Vitamins and Mineral Adequacy ... **147**
Best Practice: Clinician's Role in Micronutrient Management ... **147**
Acknowledgment ... **148**
References ... **148**

Objectives

1. Describe the known metabolism, functions, signs of deficiency and toxicity, requirements, and methods of assessment for the vitamins and minerals in human nutrition.
2. Detect how various disease conditions can influence select micronutrient metabolism.
3. Demonstrate, through the use of practice scenarios, clinical examples of potential vitamin and mineral interactions, deficiencies, and/or toxicities.

Test Your Knowledge Questions

1. Which of the following categories is included in the current Dietary Reference Intakes (DRIs)?
   A. Recommended Daily Allowance
   B. Tolerable Upper Intake Level
   C. Estimated Safe Intake
   D. Estimated Mean Requirement
2. What change in circulating serum zinc levels is observed immediately following the systemic inflammatory response syndrome (SIRS)?
   A. Increase by 50%
   B. Decrease by 50%
   C. No change
   D. Increase by 150%
3. Which of the following nutrients modify the demand for choline?
   A. Cyanocobalamin, folic acid, and methionine
   B. B_6, zinc, and arginine
   C. Thiamin, folic acid, and arginine
   D. Cyanocobalamin, zinc, and methionine
4. For which of the following ultratrace elements is there substantial circumstantial evidence to consider it essential for human health?
   A. Aluminum
   B. Boron
   C. Germanium
   D. Tin

Test Your Knowledge Answers

1. The correct answer is **B**. DRI is a generic term that includes four categories: Estimated Average Requirement, Recommended Dietary Allowance, Adequate Intakes, and Tolerable Upper Intake Level. The category Recommended Daily Allowance is incorrect, because this is used for nutritional labeling that tells what percentage of essential nutrients individuals get per serving. It does not differentiate among people of different ages and gender-specific groups as the DRI category, Recommended Dietary Allowance (RDA), does. Answers C and D are incorrect; these terms, Estimated Safe Intake and Estimated Mean Requirement, are old terminologies.
2. The correct answer is **B**. Immediately following the presence of SIRS, circulating serum zinc levels decline to roughly half of normal levels and remain so until the SIRS begins to resolve (generally 7 to 14 days, depending on the etiology of the SIRS).
3. The correct answer is **A**. Vitamin B_{12}, folic acid, and methionine are nutrients involved in metabolic methyl-exchange reactions, which modify the human need for choline.
4. The correct answer is **B**. There is circumstantial evidence that arsenic, boron, nickel, silicon, and vanadium are essential trace elements. Although aluminum, germanium, and tin are considered ultratrace elements, they may not be essential for health.

Background

Although there is a definite role for macronutrients in human nutrition, the need also exists for micronutrients. These include, but are not limited to, vitamins, trace elements, and ultratrace elements. This chapter examines the metabolism, known biochemical functions, signs of deficiency and toxicity, requirements, and methods of assessment for 14 vitamins and 9 trace elements. The clinical conditions that influence the micronutrient status in addition to ultratrace elements are also discussed.

An evaluation of vitamin and trace element status often uses a variety of biochemical measurements. Deficiencies of vitamins and trace elements generally occur in several phases, with alterations in metabolism occurring at a biochemical, clinical, morphological, and/or functional level. Generally, the biochemical alterations occur before evidence of any other changes. In fact, by the time clinical, morphological, or functional alterations occur, the amount of the nutrient in question and the concentration of that nutrient in biological fluids are reduced. Clearly, an early identification of biochemical changes is essential before the appearance of perceivable clinical, morphological, and/or functional alterations due to the deficiency of a particular nutrient. Several different types of biochemical tests can be performed to determine the status of a particular nutrient. In addition, adjustments in micronutrient supplementation may be appropriate for various clinical conditions or diseases. The clinical significance of increasing or decreasing micronutrient levels in appropriate biological samples, the metabolic and clinical effects of supplementation, and determining the optimal dosage and combination of nutrients required to achieve the desired outcomes need to be evaluated. The intake of adequate nutrients and the proper balance of essential micronutrients are critical for maintaining good health.

Because this chapter concerns the appropriate levels of micronutrients to recommend to patients, it is important to understand what serves as the basis for nutrient recommendations or requirements. The *Recommended Dietary Allowances* (RDAs) were published in 1943 to provide "standards to serve as a goal for good nutrition" and have been periodically revised and updated to reflect the latest in scientific knowledge and interpretation.[1] The RDAs are defined as "the levels of intake of essential nutrients that, on the basis of scientific knowledge, are judged by the Food and Nutrition Board to be adequate to meet the known nutrient needs of practically all healthy persons."[1] The RDA for each particular nutrient is generally calculated as two standard deviations above the average requirement for that nutrient except the RDA for energy, which is set at the estimated average requirement. The RDAs were established for the prevention of nutrient deficiencies in a healthy population and are inappropriate for individuals with special nutrition needs. However, the emphasis on nutrition has broadened to include guidelines for a healthy diet and adequate nutrient intakes to reduce the risk of chronic diseases. A series of *Dietary Reference Intake* (DRI) reports have been published by the Food and Nutrition Board of the Institute of Medicine (IOM) in response to this shift in focus. The DRIs expand and replace the series of RDAs that have been published since the 1940s. The DRIs for micronutrients are composed of four categories of reference intakes. These reference intakes are designed to reflect the latest understanding of nutrient requirements based on optimizing health in individuals and groups. The primary goal of having dietary reference values is not only to prevent nutrient deficiencies, but also to reduce the risk of chronic diseases such as osteoporosis, cancer, and cardiovascular disease. The following are definitions and descriptions of the four DRI categories:

- *Estimated Average Requirement (EAR)*—the intake that meets the estimated nutrient needs of 50% of the individuals in that group. It must be derived from scientific studies and it serves as the basis for developing the RDA. It can also be used for evaluating the adequacy of group intakes and planning recommendations for group intakes.
- *Recommended Dietary Allowance (RDA)*—the intake that meets the nutrient need of almost all (97% to 98%) individuals in that group. Depending on the nutrient, the RDA may be two standard deviations above the EAR if the variation in requirement is well defined. For example, the RDA = EAR + 2 SD of EAR or it may be 1.2 times the EAR if the variation is inconsistent or unavailable (ie, RDA = 1.2 × EAR, which assumes a coefficient of variation of 10%).
- *Adequate Intakes (AI)*—the average observed or experimentally derived intake by a defined population or subgroup that seems to sustain a defined nutritional state, such as normal circulating nutrient values, growth, or other functional indicators of health. If no EAR is able to be determined, no RDA can be set; therefore, the AI will serve as a goal for intake.
- *Tolerable Upper Intake Level (UL)*—the maximum intake by an individual that is unlikely to pose risks of adverse health effects in almost all individuals. It must be emphasized that there is no established benefit of consuming nutrients at levels above the RDA or AI, so this UL figure is not intended to be a recommended level of intake. For most nutrients, this figure refers to total intakes from food, fortified food, and nutrient supplements.

DRI reports exist for the following micronutrient groups: (1) calcium, phosphorus, magnesium, vitamin D, and fluoride; (2) folate, vitamin B_{12}, other B vitamins, and choline; (3) vitamin C, vitamin E, selenium, and carotenoids; (4) vitamin A, vitamin K, and trace elements; (5) energy and macronutrients; and (6) electrolytes and water.[2-6] The IOM has recently revised the DRIs for vitamin D and calcium.[6] Debate continues concerning the DRI for several micronutrients as new bioavailability information is gained, which could alter nutrient requirements.[7]

Vitamins

Vitamins are essential organic substances needed in small amounts in the diet to maintain fundamental functions of the body (eg, growth, metabolism, cellular integrity). Vitamins facilitate energy-yielding chemical reactions rather than contribute energy. Thirteen vitamins plus the dietary component, choline, are considered dietary essentials for humans. These include 8 B vitamins (thiamin, niacin, riboflavin, folate, vitamin B_6, vitamin B_{12}, biotin, and pantothenic acid); vitamin C (ascorbic acid); and the fat-soluble vitamins A, D, E, and K. Vitamins are classified as water-soluble or fat-soluble, according to their physical solubility in solvents. The fat-soluble vitamins (A, D, E, and K) dissolve in organic solvents and are less readily excreted than the B vitamins and ascorbic acid, which are water-soluble. The B complex can be further divided according to general function: energy releasing (niacin, riboflavin, thiamin, biotin, and pantothenic acid) or hematopoietic (B_6, B_{12}, and folate). Most vitamins are not related chemically and thus differ in their biochemical and physiological roles.

Malabsorption, medications, certain disease states, or excesses of dietary substances such as alcohol can influence nutrient intake; the digestion, absorption, and transport of vitamins; and consequently, can alter vitamin requirements and status. Clinicians must use a nutrition-focused physical assessment to identify nutrient deficiencies on a physical exam in tandem with the appropriate biochemical assays to determine the adequacy of one's vitamin status. A consultation with multidisciplinary nutrition support teams also improves the nutritional status of patients and the overall safety and efficacy of care.[8]

Fat-Soluble Vitamins

Vitamin A

Vitamin A represents a subgroup of compounds known as retinoids that have biological activity of retinol. Several plant-derived carotenoids, once metabolized, also possess vitamin A activity, so they are also included in the vitamin A family as well. Vitamin A exists in three forms: retinol, retinaldehyde (retinal), and retinoic acid. Beta-carotene, the primary pro-vitamin A carotenoid, can be split into two molecules of retinal and is a dietary precursor of retinol. Retinol can be oxidized reversibly to retinal or it can be further oxidized to retinoic acid, each having unique biochemical functions. Four major processes are involved in the intracellular metabolism of retinol: it may be esterified and stored, converted to active metabolites such as retinoic acid or retinal, form covalent bonds with cell proteins, and be catabolized to an excretory form.

Generally, dietary vitamin A exists as retinoids in animal tissues and carotenoids in plants; however, there are carotenes in butterfat, and some plant-based foods such as breakfast cereals and margarines may be fortified with retinyl ester, the most stable form of vitamin A. Typically, vitamin A is ingested as retinyl ester and must be freed by acidic digestion, the emulsifying action of bile salts, and the subsequent integration of retinol into micelles. The micelles are transported to the intestinal cell, where the retinol is then re-esterified by intracellular binding proteins and packaged into chylomicrons. The chylomicrons enter the mesenteric lymphatic system and pass into systemic circulation where retinol is removed primarily by the liver.[9] Once in the liver, hydrolysis at the membrane and re-esterification within the cell occurs again, as the vitamin enters the hepatocyte for storage. Although the liver is the primary storage site of vitamin A, extrahepatic organs (eg, adipose, kidney, bone marrow, lung, eye) also contain significant amounts of vitamin A.[9]

Approximately 90% of dietary vitamin A is absorbed. In contrast, dietary carotenoids are absorbed primarily in the upper small intestine at a lower efficiency of approximately 8%.[9] Overall, vitamin A absorption is dependent on the amount of dietary fat and factors or disease states that influence fat absorption. Retinol-binding protein (RBP) is a liver-synthesized protein that is required to transport retinol from the liver to the target tissues. Synthesis of this protein is tightly regulated by the availability of retinol and, therefore, is sensitive to the nutritional status of the individual.[9] In the plasma, RBP is bound to another protein called transthyretin (TTR). The protein complex TTR–RBP is responsible for the plasma transport of retinol. Measurement of these binding proteins is used to assess vitamin A status.

Vitamin A is essential for vision, normal reproduction, bone development, and immune function. The biochemical functions of vitamin A are dependent on the particular form. The retinol form is required for reproduction. Retinaldehyde is required for vision, and retinoic acid is required for the normal structure and function of epithelial cells.[9] This last function explains vitamin A significance with wound healing. During the inflammatory phase via synergistic mechanisms, the vitamin increases the number of macrophages and monocytes in the wound, stimulates epithelialization, and increases collagen deposition by fibroblasts.[10] Vitamin A can also reverse the inhibitory effects of corticosteroids on wound healing. Table 8-1 lists the RDA as retinol activity equivalents (RAEs)

TABLE 8-1 Vitamin Dietary Reference Intakes[2–6] and Select Sources

	14–18 Years Male/Female	19–30 Years Male/Female	31–50 Years Male/Female	51–70 Years Male/Female	>70 Years Male/Female
Vitamins					
A (RDA) mcg RAE/d[a]	900/700	900/700	900/700	900/700	900/700
Sources: Liver, fortified milk, eggs, dark green, and yellow-orange vegetables.					
D (RDA) mcg/d[b]	15/15	15/15	15/15	15/15	20/20
Sources: Fish liver oils, fatty fish, fortified milk and breakfast cereals, sunlight.					
E (RDA) mg/d[c]	15/15	15/15	15/15	15/15	15/15
Sources: Vegetable oils, wheat germ, asparagus, and peanuts.					
K (AI) mcg/d	75/75	120/90	120/90	120/90	120/90
Sources: Liver, green leafy vegetables, broccoli, peas, and green beans.					
Thiamin (RDA) mg/d	1.2/1.0	1.2/1.1	1.2/1.1	1.2/1.1	1.2/1.1
Sources: Enriched, fortified, whole grain products, pork products, sunflower seeds, and wheat germ.					
Riboflavin (RDA) mg/d	1.3/1.0	1.3/1.1	1.3/1.1	1.3/1.1	1.3/1.1
Sources: Organ meats, milk, bread products, and fortified cereals.					
Niacin (RDA) mg/d	16/14	16/14	16/14	16/14	16/14
Sources: Meat, fish, poultry, enriched and fortified breads, and fortified cereals.					
B_6 (RDA) mg/d	1.3/1.2	1.3/1.3	1.3/1.3	1.7/1.5	1.7/1.5
Sources: Fortified cereals, organ meats, and whole grains.					
B_{12} (RDA) mg/d	2.4/2.4	2.4/2.4	2.4/2.4	2.4/2.4	2.4/2.4
Sources: Fortified cereals, meat, fish, poultry, and eggs.					
Folate (RDA) mcg/d[e]	400/400	400/400	400/400	400/400	400/400
Sources: Enriched cereal grains, dark green leafy vegetables, and fortified cereals.					
Biotin (AI) mcg/d	25/25	30/30	30/30	30/30	30/30
Sources: Liver and smaller amounts in fruits and meats.					
Pantothenic acid (AI) mg/d	5/5	5/5	5/5	5/5	5/5
Sources: Sunflower seeds, beef liver, mushrooms, peanuts, eggs, broccoli, and milk.					
Choline (AI) mg/d	550/400	550/425	550/425	550/425	550/425
Sources: Milk, liver, eggs, and peanuts.					
C[d] (RDA) mg/d	75/65	90/75	90/75	90/75	90/75
Sources: Citrus fruits and other fruits and vegetables.					

AI, adequate intakes; RAE, retinol activity equivalent; RDA, recommended dietary allowances.
[a]1 RAE = 1 mg retinol, 12 mg beta-carotene, 24 mg alpha-carotene, or 24 mg beta-cryptoxanthin.
[b]Alpha-tocopherol 1 mg = 40 IU vitamin D; to convert IU to mcg, multiply by 0.025.
[c]To convert mg of alpha-tocopherol to IUs, multiply the number of mg by 1.5.
[d]For smokers, recommended intake is an additional 35 mg/d.
[e]As dietary folate equivalents (DFE). 1 DFE = 1 mcg food folate = 0.6 mcg of folic acid from fortified food or as a supplement consumed with food = 0.5 mcg of a supplement taken on an empty stomach.

where 1 RAE = 1 mg retinol, 12 mg beta-carotene, 24 mg alpha-carotene, or 24 mg beta-cryptoxanthin, and sources for vitamin A.[5]

Because the normal liver reserves of vitamin A are adequate for months, signs and symptoms of deficiency in adults take a long time to develop, particularly in conditions associated with fat malabsorption, such as celiac disease, pancreatitis, cystic fibrosis, sprue, biliary atresia, and cholestatic liver disease.[11] Table 8-2 specifies the common signs of a vitamin A deficiency.[9,11] Low circulating levels of vitamin A in critically ill patients have been attributed to decreased hepatic synthesis and the release of RBP during the inflammatory process. Hence, vitamin A transport is diminished, which increases the risk for developing vitamin A deficiency.[12] RBP synthesis is also diminished in patients with liver disease, which results in impaired vitamin A export from the liver. Elevated plasma retinol, RBP, and TTR can occur in chronic renal disease because the kidneys are the primary route of excretion. Serum concentrations of these markers should be monitored to prevent hypervitaminosis A.

There are more than 50 possible signs of vitamin A toxicity (Table 8-2).[9,11] As little as 1800 mcg per day or 6000 IU per day has been reported to cause problems, and pregnant women should always consume less. Other reports have observed toxicity occurring in adults who consumed well above the UL (10,000 and 50,000 IU per day), but they also had a predisposing medical condition such as liver disease, malnutrition, and/or drug or alcohol use. Toxic amounts of vitamin A are known to have negative skeletal effects. The risk of hip fractures in postmenopausal women was almost doubled among women who consumed 2000 mcg/d or 6600 IU/d of retinol, an amount less than the UL of 3000 mcg/d for vitamin A. Thus, chronic intake of retinol may contribute to the development of osteoporotic hip fractures.[13] Elevated serum levels of vitamin A occur in both chronic and acute renal failure because the binding capacity of RBP is exceeded, which allows more of the vitamin to circulate unbound with the potential to damage cell membranes.[14] It is prudent to supplement vitamin A with caution in renal failure and in accordance with standard practice guidelines.[15]

The serum retinol concentration is a practical biochemical test for assessing vitamin A status. A decreased dietary intake of vitamin A correlates well with serum retinol levels. Serum retinol values greater than 1.05 μmol/L (30 mcg/dL) indicate adequate liver stores of vitamin A; serum retinol levels less than or equal to 0.35 μmol/L (10 mcg/dL) may indicate depleted or near depleted liver stores with clinical signs often present.[11] Serum levels greater than 3.5 μmol/L (100 mcg/dL) are suggestive of toxicity. Because retinol circulates attach to RBP and TTR as a complex, the presence of either protein–calorie malnutrition and/or zinc deficiency may compromise circulating serum vitamin A levels. Decreased circulating serum retinol levels may reflect an impaired RBP synthesis and mobilization secondary to inflammatory processes or disease and do not require correction by vitamin A supplementation.[16] Multiple conditions can lead to excess gastrointestinal (GI) losses or malabsorption syndromes that can contribute to low circulating levels of vitamin A. To counter these GI losses, a water-miscible form of vitamin A is routinely supplemented to meet the DRI.

Vitamin A administration is also common to enhance wound healing in patients with comorbidities (diabetes, tumors, and radiation).[10] A wide dosage range of 10,000 to 50,000 IU/d (3 to 5 mg/d) orally or 10,000 IU intramuscularly for 7 days has been recommended to counteract the inhibitory effects steroids have on collagen synthesis and connective tissue repair, although results have been inconsistent.[17] The application of topical vitamin A can minimize delayed wound healing in patients requiring long-term corticosteroid treatment. An oral administration of 10,000 to 15,000 IU/d is recommended to enhance wound healing with concurrent corticosteroid therapy. A careful interpretation of vitamin A status in these populations remains paramount. Newer methods on the horizon to assess vitamin A status include RBP to TTR ratios and a dried blood spot retinol determination, which may assist in a better assessment.[18]

Vitamin D

Vitamin D refers to both ergocalciferol (vitamin D_2) and cholecalciferol (vitamin D_3), which are either consumed in the diet (D_2) or synthesized in the skin from the compound 7-dehydrocholesterol postexposure to solar or artificial ultraviolet (UVB) light (D_3). Vitamin D must undergo hydroxylation on both carbon 25 (in the endoplasmic reticulum of the liver) and on carbon 1 (in the proximal convoluted tubule of the kidney or other tissues that possess 1-hydroxylase) to become biologically active.[19]

About 80% of dietary vitamin D intake is incorporated into a micelle, primarily in the distal small intestine, with uptake more rapid in the duodenum.[19] Vitamin D absorption occurs in tandem with fat and bile salts via passive diffusion into the intestinal cell where it is packaged as chylomicrons for entrance into the lymphatic system, and then into the blood. About 40% of the cholecalciferol is transported via chylomicrons, although some is transferred from the chylomicron to a vitamin D–binding protein (DBP) for export to extrahepatic tissues. The chylomicron remnant that contains vitamin D delivers it to the liver. Cholecalciferol synthesized from the skin is transported to the liver bound to DBP; however, some is deposited in muscle and adipose before its liver uptake. These different mechanisms for vitamin D transport influence the distribution in the body.

Once vitamin D is transported to the liver, it undergoes the first of two hydroxylation steps at carbon 25 via the enzyme 25-hydroxylase to form 25-hydroxy-D_3, its major circulating form that has limited biological activity.[19] Although this enzyme is not tightly regulated, its efficiency is dependent on vitamin D status. Enzymatic conversion is more efficient during vitamin D deprivation. When 25-hydroxy-D_3 is transported to the kidney, it may undergo a second hydroxylation at carbon 1, catalyzed by the enzyme CYP27B1, formerly called 25-OH-D_3-1 alpha-hydroxylase.[20] The product, 1,25-dihydroxyvitamin D, is the active form of the vitamin. Other tissues are capable of expressing CYP27B1 and thus may make 1,25-dihydroxyvitamin D for their own (ie, autocrine) uses.

TABLE 8-2 Vitamin Status[3,9,11,14,24,25,27–29,32,34,35,38,42,45,51,52,55,60,61,66–68,71,82,84,85]

Vitamin	Assay[a]	Deficiency	Toxicity
Vitamin A	Serum vitamin A Normal: >30 mcg/dl	Impaired wound healing, night blindness, Bitot spot, conjunctival xerosis, xerophthalmia	Alopecia, ataxia, muscle and bone pain, cheilitis, headache, conjunctivitis, skin and vision disorders, hepatotoxicity, pruritus, hyperlipidemia, membrane dryness, hip fractures, renal osteodystrophy
Vitamin D	1,25-Dihydroxyvitamin D Normal: 0.7–3.3 IU/dL[23] **25-Hydroxyvitamin D**[25] Normal: 30–70 ng/mL	Hypocalcalcemia Osteomalacia Osteoporosis	Hypercalcemia (nausea, vomiting, weakness, fatigue, diarrhea, anorexia, headache, confusion, psychosis, tremor); hypercalciuria, soft tissue calcification
Vitamin E	Alpha-tocopherol <18 μmol/g; 41.8 μmol/L Plasma vitamin E 0.5–2.0 mg/dL	Increased platelet aggregation, decreased red blood cell survival and hemolytic anemia, neuronal degeneration, decreased creatinine, creatinuria; ataxia, weakness, vision changes	Impaired neutrophil function, abrogated granulocytopenic response to antigen, impaired coagulation; prolonged depletion; skeletal muscle lesions with ceroid deposits in smooth muscle, inclusion bodies in bone marrow
Vitamin K	International normalized ratio: 0.8–1.2 Prothrombin time: 10–15 sec	Bleeding, mild bruising, hemorrhage; low bone density, increased fractures	Prolonged bleeding
Vitamin C	11 μmol/L; 0.2–2.0 mg/dL	Anorexia, fatigue, muscle pain, increased susceptibility to infection; scurvy: anemia, bleeding gums, petechiae, perifollicular hemorrhage, impaired wound healing, joint effusions, weakening of collagen in bone/teeth, sudden death	Nausea, vomiting
Thiamin	Transketolase activity, erythrocyte 1.20 μg/ml/hr	Dry beriberi: paresthesia, anesthesia, weakness in lower extremities; Wet beriberi: high-output cardiac failure, dyspnea, hepatomegaly, tachycardia, oliguria, sodium and water retention; Wernicke-Korsakoff syndrome, Wernicke encephalopathy: mental status changes, global confusion, nystagmus, polyneuritis, gait ataxia, and stupor	Uncommon
Riboflavin	Glutathione reductase, erythrocyte <1.2 IU/g hemoglobin	Sore throat, hyperemia and edema of pharyngeal and oral mucosa, cheilosis, angular stomatitis, glossitis (magenta tongue), seborrheic dermatitis of the face and scrotum, corneal vascularization, photophobia and visual impairment, normochromic and normocytic anemia	Rare
Niacin	N-methylnicotinamide 5.8 μmol/d	Pellagra: dermatitis, diarrhea, and dementia; symmetrical, pigmented rash (sunburnlike) in areas exposed to sunlight; vomiting, diarrhea, and red tongue; apathy, depression, headache, fatigue, and/or memory loss	Flushing of skin; pharmacological doses (3 g/d): vasodilation, itching, sensation of heat, headaches, gastrointestinal irritation, severe hepatitis, glucose intolerance, hepatotoxicity, myopathy

B_6	Pyridoxal 5′–phosphate, plasma 5 ng/ml; 20 nmol/L	Seborrheic dermatitis, microcytic anemia, epileptiform convulsions, confusion, and/or depression; angular stomatitis, glossitis, or cheilosis	Sensory neuropathy: sensory ataxia, areflexia, and impaired cutaneous and deep sensations; dermatologic lesions
B_{12}	24.4–100 ng/dL serum	Cognitive decline, cardiovascular disease, bone fractures; megaloblastic anemia with macrocytosis, neutrophil nuclei hypersegmentation, bone marrow changes, leukopenia, thrombocytopenia; glossitis, constipation, diarrhea; hand/feet paresthesia, diminution of vibration and/or position sense, unsteadiness, confusion, depression, mental slowness, poor memory; delusions and overt psychosis	No toxicity known
Folic Acid	Serum 0.3 μg/dL; 7 nmol/L	Megaloblastic or macrocytic anemia, early indicator neutrophil hypersegmentation; diarrhea, smooth, sore tongue; weight loss, a depression of cell-mediated immunity, nervous instability, and dementia	
Biotin	Serum 100–400 pmol/L. Urinary excretion >6 mcg/d	Hypotonia, anorexia, pallor, glossitis, nausea, vomiting, depression, lethargy, muscle pain, alopecia, erythematous seborrheic dermatitis, visual problems, ketolactic acidosis, elevated cholesterol	No known toxic effects
Pantothenic Acid	Whole blood >1 μmol/L Urinary excretion > 1 mg/d	Listlessness, fatigue, irritability, restlessness, malaise, sleep disturbances, nausea, abdominal cramps, vomiting, diarrhea; neuromuscular disturbances: numbness, paresthesia, muscle cramps, staggering gait, mental depression; hypoglycemia, increased insulin sensitivity; compromised immune function, poor wound healing, diminished engraftment	Rare; mild gastrointestinal distress
Choline	Plasma choline 10 μmol/L	Impairment of verbal and visual memory; hepatic steatosis	Anorexia, fishy body odor, sweating, salivation, hypotension, reduced growth rate, gastrointestinal effects, hepatotoxicity

[a]Estimated and sample normal values; normal ranges will vary by technique and laboratory methodology.

The 1,25-dihydroxyvitamin D that is made by the kidney is released into the circulation, where it is necessary for bone mineralization and intestinal calcium uptake, among other actions. The activity of the enzyme is highly controlled via the vitamin D receptor, and is affected by several factors that influence calcium homeostasis. Accumulation of serum 1,25-dihydroxyvitamin D causes negative feedback on CYP27B1 activity, whereas a decrease in serum concentration increases the activity of the enzyme. Low plasma calcium and the parathyroid hormone both stimulate CYP27B1, whereas high intakes of dietary phosphorus inhibit enzymatic activity. Another metabolite, 24,25-hydroxy-D_3 is formed when excess 25-hydroxy-D_3 is present in the body. Vitamin D can be stored in adipose tissue for later use or converted to 25-hydroxy-D_3 in the liver. Excretion is primarily via bile with minimal amounts lost via urine. New evidence indicates that almost all tissues in the body express vitamin D.

When describing vitamin D functions, it is important to note that it is 1,25-dihydroxyvitamin D that possesses the activity. The principal function of vitamin D is to maintain serum calcium (Ca) and phosphorus (P) levels to support neuromuscular function, bone calcification, and other cellular processes. In its active form, 1,25-dihydroxyvitamin D functions to maintain circulating serum levels of Ca and P within a normal range. It does this by increasing the intestinal absorption of both Ca and P by stimulating osteoclasts to mature, and by increasing Ca and P resorption from bone.[19] It has recently been shown to be involved in the growth and differentiation of hematopoietic and immune cells via gene expression of the vitamin D receptor.[21]

Vitamin D is also emerging as having pleiotropic effects, thus rendering it important in the management of other medical conditions such as musculoskeletal disorders, falls, immunity, autoimmunity, infections, cancer, diabetes or glucose intolerance, and cardiovascular disease.[21–23] The potential effects on the cardio-metabolic system are thought to be mediated by a variety of mechanisms related to the inflammatory response and have been associated with therapeutic doses greater than the current DRI. Although some vitamin D experts are now recommending up to 800 to 1000 IU per day to prevent deficiency in select populations such as the elderly, the new IOM recommendations based on age in adults are 400 to 800 IU per day.[6,21] Table 8-1 lists the RDA and dietary sources for vitamin D.

Vitamin D deficiency or insufficiency has been documented in a variety of populations who have inadequate sun exposure such as the elderly, nursing home residents, dark-skinned individuals, people who wear clothing/veils with little skin exposure, people who are indoors much of the time or who use sunscreen daily, and exclusively breastfed infants.[21–23] Decreased serum concentrations of vitamin D in long-term, parenterally fed patients are associated with metabolic bone disease, a common complication of long-term parenteral nutrition (PN). A high incidence of low serum vitamin D secondary to impaired epidermal vitamin D synthesis has been documented in postburn patients.[24] Other disease states or conditions associated with hypovitaminosis D include malabsorptive diseases such as celiac disease, Crohn's disease, cholestatic liver disease, extensive bowel resection, and antiepileptic therapy (specifically phenytoin and phenobarbital). Deficiencies have been reported in patients after bariatric surgery and partial gastrectomy.[11] See Table 8-2 for other deficiency signs. There is also a reduction in the synthesis of 25-hydroxyvitamin D, and 1,25–dihydroxyvitamin D in hepatic or renal disease, so deficiency is more likely. Patients with renal disease are typically unable to synthesize the active form of vitamin D and often require supplementation to avoid renal osteodystrophy. Hypovitaminosis D has been associated with a higher prevalence of cardiovascular risk factors and disease, including hypertension.[25] Practice Scenario 8-1 discusses the need for vitamin D.

Signs of vitamin D toxicity are found in Table 8-2.[11,25] If allowed to continue, soft tissue calcification may result, increasing the risk for the development of irreversible renal and cardiovascular damage. See Table 8-3 for the tolerable upper intake level of vitamin D.[6]

The measurement of serum 25-hydroxyvitamin D is a reasonable assay to evaluate vitamin D status.[26] Vitamin D adequacy is more clearly defined using surrogate markers such as the PTH and Ca. Normal circulating 25-hydoxyvitamin D levels vary with the degree of sun exposure and range from 135 to 225 nmol/L. Controversy still surrounds the optimal 25-hydoxyvitamin D plasma concentration; however, there is now agreement that plasma concentrations less than or equal to 50 nmol/L is considered a deficiency, whereas levels less than or equal to 75 nmol/L are considered insufficient.[21–23,25,26] When 25-hydroxyvitamin D values fall, decreases in both serum Ca and P levels are observed, which stimulate PTH secretion to increase renal production of vitamin D's active form, 1,25-dihydroxyvitamin D.[23] Consequently, circulating levels of the

TABLE 8-3 Tolerable Upper Intake Level (UL)[2–6]

	14–18 years	19–70 years	> 70 years
Vitamins			
Vitamin A (mcg/d)[a]	2800	3000	3000
Vitamin C (mg/d)	1800	2000	2000
Vitamin D (mcg/d)[b]	100	100	100
Vitamin E (mg/d)[c]	800	1000	1000
Synthetic niacin (mg/d)[d]	30	35	35
Vitamin B_6 (mg/d)	80	100	100
Folic acid (mcg/d)[d]	800	1000	1000
Choline (g/d)	3.0	3.5	3.5
Minerals			
Copper (mg/d)	8	10	10
Fluoride (mg/d)	10	10	10
Iodine (mcg /d)	900	1100	1100
Iron (mg/d)	45	45	45
Manganese (mg/d)	9	11	11
Molybdenum (mcg /d)	1700	2000	2000
Selenium (mcg/d)	400	400	400
Zinc (mg/d)	34	40	40

[a]To convert mcg/d Retinol Equivalents (RE) to International Units (IUs), multiply the mcg RE by 10 for a food of plant origin and by 5 for food of animal origin; UL for preformed only.
[b]1 mcg = 40 IU vitamin D; to convert IU to mcg, multiply by 0.025.
[c]Only from supplement alpha-tocopherol; to convert mg of alpha-tocopherol to IUs, multiply the number of mg by 1.5.
[d]Forms from supplements, fortified foods, or a combination of the two.

active form are often normal or elevated in vitamin D deficiency, making it a less sensitive indicator of vitamin D status. Maintaining 25-hydroxyvitamin D concentrations between 78 and 100 nmol/L is associated with maximum bone health and the prevention of chronic diseases.[23,25,26] It is paramount that long-term PN patients, prone to hypovitaminosis D, are monitored to ensure optimal levels of 25-hydroxyvitamin D; 1,25-dihydroxyvitamin D; PTH; and calcium.

Practice Scenario 8-1

Question: What is the optimal vitamin D requirement and biomarker for nutritional adequacy?

Scenario: On a routine physical exam, a 49-year-old female from New England presents with a family history of breast cancer and coronary artery disease. Regular mammograms have been normal. The patient has borderline hypertension that is closely monitored by her physician; anthropometric measurement is normal (BMI 23.7). The patient is physically active and spends time gardening but limits her sun exposure due to the risk of skin cancer by applying sunblock if spending more than 15 minutes outside during the late spring, summer, and early fall months.

Intervention: The physician ordered routine labs along with assays to assess vitamin D status. These included a bone-mineral density test, a parathyroid hormone (PTH) level, and 25-hydroxyvitamin D level.

Answer: Because of her perimenopausal age as well as family and personal history, there is concern about the patient's vitamin D status. The goal is to achieve optimal vitamin D levels in an effort to reduce her risk of osteoporosis, cancer, and heart disease. Currently, 25-hydroxyvitamin D is still the best-supported means to assess vitamin D status.

Rationale: The role of vitamin D in bone health has been well documented. However, in recent years, vitamin D has been shown to play critical roles in a number of other chronic diseases. Suboptimal vitamin D status has been implicated in the development of hypertension, cardiovascular disease, diabetes, cancer, pulmonary disease, and depression.[22,25] It stands to reason that adequate vitamin D levels can mitigate such conditions. The patient's family history of cancer, heart disease, and personal history of borderline hypertension warrant the evaluation of vitamin D to reduce patient risks. Further, her perimenopausal age places her at risk for bone mineral density loss. The patient's diligent attention to sun exposure and living in northern latitudes minimize cutaneous vitamin D production, further compromising vitamin D status. The current dietary vitamin D intake recommendation for this age group is 15 mcg/d (600 IU/d). The measurement of 25-hydroxyvitamin D level has been the standard method to evaluate vitamin D status; current evidence suggests that it is still the more accurate assay. If the vitamin D blood level is 30 ng/mL (75 nmol/L) and a 40 ng/mL (100 nmol/L) level is desired, then 1000 IU (25 mcg) of vitamin D per day over several months is recommended to achieve a normal blood level (30.0 to 74 ng/mL). Recent research warrants further review regarding optimal requirements, especially given its new emerging relationship to other chronic diseases. The circulating PTH level holds some promise, yet there are still many uncertainties surrounding its use, including calcium intake's tendency to suppress the PTH response to vitamin D supplementation. Bone mineral density has also been suggested as a method to evaluate vitamin D status. However, its use as a marker of functional outcomes has not been validated to date; studies using calcium-tracer and calcium radioisotope techniques have future promise.[26]

Vitamin E

Eight naturally occurring compounds have been found to have vitamin E activity: four tocopherols (alpha, beta, gamma, and delta) and four tocotrienols (alpha, beta, gamma, and delta), each with varying degrees of biological activity.[27] Evidence supports that these eight forms of vitamin E are functionally unique. The most active and naturally occurring form is the RRR isomer of alpha-tocopherol, which exhibits antioxidant activity and also inhibits cell proliferation, platelet aggregation, and monocyte adhesion.[27] Gamma-tocopherol represents the major form of vitamin E in a typical American diet; its functions include anti-inflammatory, antineoplastic, and natriuretic properties.[27,28] Tocotrienols have potent neuroprotective, antioxidant, anticancer, and cholesterol lowering effects that are different from the properties of tocopherols.[28] Some vitamin E molecules, gamma-tocopherols, delta-tocopherols, and alpha-tocotrienols have emerged with roles in health and disease that are distinct from alpha-tocopherols' function. The potential health benefits of alpha-tocopherol supplementation (500 mg/d) in the prevention of cardiovascular disease and cancer may be offset because it significantly reduces the plasma concentration of gamma- and delta-tocopherol. In contrast, supplementation with mixed tocopherols (500 mg/d) increases both serum and cellular alpha- and gamma-tocopherol.[28] Specific protective properties of delta-tocopherol are still unknown; it may have stronger antiproliferative effects on preneoplastic and neoplastic epithelial cells.[28]

Vitamin E absorption is dependent on dietary fat absorption and occurs primarily in the jejunum via nonsaturable, passive diffusion. Absorption varies from about 20% to 50%; however, absorption decreases as intake increases.[27-29] At pharmacological doses (200 mg), absorption drops to less than 10%.[27] Tocopherols are found free in foods; however, the tocotrienols are esterified and must be hydrolyzed before absorption via pancreatic and duodenal esterases located in the lumen. Vitamin E is incorporated into micelles within the lumen of the small intestine. Once taken up by the enterocytes, vitamin E is transported as part of a lipoprotein complex through the lymph into circulation. Adipose tissue, muscle, and the liver serve as the major storage sites. Excretion occurs primarily via the urine and bile. Significant amounts are found in the feces as well because of the limited vitamin E absorption.

The principal biochemical function of vitamin E is the maintenance of membrane integrity in body cells via its action as an antioxidant. By inhibiting lipid peroxidation, vitamin E protects the integrity of all biological membranes.[27] It also acts as an antioxidant by trapping peroxyl free radicals in cell membranes and, by working along with selenium and ascorbic acid, protects against oxidation. The free radical scavenging process produces oxidized vitamin E, which must be regenerated back to the reduced form. This process requires ascorbic acid, reduced glutathione-selenium, and nicotinamide adenine dinucleotide phosphate (NADPH). Thus, vitamin E is critical in the oxidative stress states (chronic inflammation, sepsis, systemic inflammatory response syndrome [SIRS], and organ failure).[29] Table 8-1 lists the RDA and dietary sources for vitamin E.

Early vitamin E deficiency is typically asymptomatic. Table 8-2 describes the signs and symptoms of vitamin E deficiency.[11,28,29] Patients at risk of vitamin E deficiency include those with prolonged steatorrhea, other malabsorptive conditions including Crohn's disease, cystic fibrosis, compromised biliary function, resection of the ileum or small intestine, or long-term PN without vitamin E supplementation. There is a body of evidence, though inconclusive, that indicates an association between vitamin E deficiency and the risk of certain diseases (cancer, cardiovascular, type II diabetes, and hypertension). Coupled with the fact that about 90% of the U.S. population is not currently meeting the DRI for alpha-tocopherol (active form), clinicians should be cognizant that preexisting inadequate vitamin E intake can exacerbate vitamin E status in patients more prone to vitamin E deficiency.[30,31]

Adverse effects of excessive vitamin E are found in Table 8-2.[27,32] Thrombocytopenia and cerebral hemorrhages resulting in death have been reported at pharmacological doses below the UL (50 mg/d and 1000 mg/d).[32,33] Consistent, excessive amounts of vitamin E are contraindicated when a coagulation defect is present.[28] An intake of greater than 1200 mg/d interferes with vitamin K and may be problematic for patients requiring warfarin therapy. An intake of 800 to 1200 mg/d may decrease platelet adhesion.[27,28] The UL is based on the hemorrhagic effects in adults.

Plasma or serum concentrations of alpha-tocopherol are commonly used to evaluate vitamin E status. Values below 11.6 μmol/L (5 mcg/mL) indicate a deficiency state or poor vitamin E status. In addition, a plasma alpha-tocopherol (μmol/L) ratio to plasma cholesterol (mmol/L) below 2.2 indicates a risk for vitamin E deficiency.[31] Many would argue that vitamin E requirements should be reassessed given the prevalence of insufficient intake plus the evidence that vitamin E may play a role in chronic disease risk reduction.[31]

Vitamin K

Vitamin K is a generic name for a family of compounds that include phylloquinone (K_1), which are found in plants, and the menaquinones (K_2), which are found in fish oils, meats, and synthesized by gut microflora in the distal small intestine and colon. Menadione (K_3) is a common synthetic form that is converted to K_2 by intestinal flora. Some of the menaquinones may be synthesized in vivo from vitamin K_1.

Phylloquinone absorption occurs primarily in the jejunum by a saturable, energy-dependent process. Vitamin K absorption is similar to other fat-soluble nutrients and is dependent on the presence of lipids, which stimulate bile salt and pancreatic enzyme release with subsequent incorporation into chylomicrons for transport. Absorption varies from 40% to 80%. With any impairment in the lipid absorption process, such as in the case of a biliary obstruction or a significant small bowel resection, absorption decreases to 20% to 30%.[34,35] The absorption and use of menaquinone synthesized by bacteria is still unknown. Mineral oil and other nonabsorbable lipids interfere with vitamin K absorption. There is no storage form of vitamin K in the body.[34,35]

Vitamin K is involved in a variety of enzymatic reactions within the body, which impact blood coagulation and bone health. The primary biochemical function of vitamin K is as a cosubstrate in the posttranslational carboxylation of proteins at designated glutamic acid residues. As part of a membrane-bound carboxylase system, vitamin K functions in the posttranslational gamma-carboxylation of clotting factors (II, VII, IX, and X), and normally occurring anticoagulant proteins, C and S.[34] In addition, because of its role in promoting the conversion of protein-bound glutamate to gamma-carboxyglutamate (Gla), vitamin K may play a role in skeletal development, because osteocalcin is a bone Gla-protein that facilitates calcium binding to the hydroxyapatite matrix of bone.[36] In fact, emerging evidence in human intervention studies suggests that vitamin K_1 may also benefit bone health, in particular when coadministered with vitamin D.[35]

Several mechanisms have been proposed to explain vitamin K modulation of bone metabolism.[34] One relates to osteocalcin's Gla content, which accounts for up to 80% of the total Gla content of mature bone. Undercarboxylation of osteocalcin secondary to inadequate vitamin K can impair its ability to bind to the bone mineral matrix and thus regulate bone mineralization. There is also increasing evidence that vitamin K positively affects calcium balance, a key mineral in bone metabolism.[35,36] Some researchers contend that the recommendation for vitamin K should be increased given its role in bone health.[35,36] Table 8-1 lists the AI and dietary sources for this vitamin.[4] Another source of vitamin K is from intravenous fat emulsions (IVFE).[37] The vitamin K amount depends on the composition of the IVFE and the manufacturing process.[37] Other conditions that can affect vitamin K requirements include patients receiving long-term PN without lipid emulsion, patients on antibiotic therapy, patients who are receiving nothing by mouth, or patients with significant malabsorption. All of these examples may require additional vitamin K supplementation.[37,38] In addition, vitamin K in lipid emulsions can partially reverse the effects of warfarin.[37,39]

A frank deficiency of vitamin K due to inadequate intake is rare. A deficiency is typically the result of malnutrition, fat malabsorption, antibiotic therapy, inflammatory bowel disease, the use of oral anticoagulants, and/or the result of infant hemorrhagic disease.[40,41] See Table 8-2 for the most common sign of a vitamin K deficiency.[34,35,42] The evidence continues to support an increased recommendation for vitamin K intake to reduce bone loss and fracture risk, especially among the elderly.[43]

Little is known regarding vitamin K (phylloquinone) toxicity.[38] Some adverse side effects have been reported when large doses of this vitamin were given to individuals who had severely compromised liver function.[38] In addition, menadione, a water-soluble synthetic vitamin K analog, has produced fatal anemia, hyperbilirubinemia, and severe jaundice.[37] The most serious consequence has been an anaphylactoid reaction.

Traditional methods using prothrombin time (PT) or activated partial thromboplastin time (aPTT) lack the sensitivity to detect a subclinical vitamin K deficiency. The International Normalized Ratio (INR) is the most common laboratory procedure used to monitor warfarin therapy and to detect potential bleeding problems. A more sensitive indicator of vitamin K status is the measurement of plasma phylloquinone, the major circulating form. Fasting phylloquinone reference values in healthy adults are 0.15 to 1.0 mcg/L and reflect both dietary depletion and repletion.[44]

Water-Soluble Vitamins

Ascorbic Acid (Vitamin C)

The total amount of naturally occurring and biologically active vitamin C is available as ascorbic acid (reduced form) and dehydroascorbic acid (oxidized form). Vitamin C absorption occurs predominately in the ileum, with some absorption in the jejunum via the sodium, energy-dependent active transport system. The transport systems for vitamin C are both saturable and dose dependent; that is, absorption efficiency decreases as intake increases. At pharmacological doses (12 g/d), absorption falls to about 16%, whereas at low intakes (less than 20 mg/d), absorption can reach 98%. At normal intakes (20 to 120 mg/d), absorption is 80% to 90%.[40] Serum ascorbic acid levels rise with dietary intakes of 70 to 140 mg/d, then saturation is reached (at 80 to 90 μmol/L). Once serum levels reach 80 μmol/L, renal clearance sharply increases.[45] This explains why few toxic effects are reported with high vitamin C intakes.

Ascorbic acid serves as an antioxidant, reacting directly with superoxide, hydroxyl radicals, and singlet oxygen.[46] Vitamin C also provides reducing equivalents for a variety of reactions and acts as a cofactor for reactions that require a reduced metal. As a result, vitamin C has very complex functional roles, such as the synthesis of collagen, carnitine, and neurotransmitters; the enhancement of intestinal absorption of nonheme iron; cholesterol hydroxylation into bile acids; the reduction of toxic transition (variable positive oxidative states) metals; the reductive protection of folic acid and vitamin E; and the immune-mediated and antibacterial functions of white blood cells.[45] Table 8-1 lists the RDA and dietary sources for this vitamin.[4]

A vitamin C intake below 10 mg/d over a prolonged period can result in classic deficiency signs and symptoms (Table 8-2).[45,47] Scurvy is rare today because it is preventable with as little 10 mg/d.[4] Supplementation of vitamin C 100 to 200 mg/d is now common in patients who have wounds, including stage I and II pressure ulcers.[9–12] Surgical and burn patients are frequently reported to have ascorbate deficiency.[10,12] It has also been reported that vitamin C statuses deteriorate during hospitalization and from medical or surgical stress, which can negatively impact wound healing.[16] Hyperglycemia is common in acute stress states and prevents vitamin C transport, which is needed for normal leukocyte function.[16] Supplementation improves leukocyte function, but to what extent it influences immune response is unclear.

Reports of vitamin C toxicity are uncommon. People given 5 to 15 g/d, which is well above the TUL, have reported nausea and vomiting. It remains controversial if rebound scurvy occurs following the cessation of large vitamin C doses. Individuals with renal failure, kidney stones, iron overload disease, and/or individuals receiving heparin or warfarin therapy should avoid large vitamin C doses. The relationship between excess vitamin C and oxalate formation can be detrimental in renal failure. Doses in excess of 100 mg/d to 500 mg/d can precipitate oxalate crystals in soft tissues, increasing the risk of kidney stones and further compromising renal function.[15]

Plasma ascorbic acid analysis is the most feasible procedure for evaluating the status of vitamin C in individuals as well as in population groups. Although the concentration of ascorbic acid in leukocytes reflects body stores, this measurement is technically difficult to perform. Plasma/serum levels less than 11 μmol/L (0.2 mg/dL) indicate a "deficient" status of vitamin C; levels 11 to 23 μmol/L (0.2 to 0.4 mg/dL) indicate a "low" status; and levels greater than 23 μmol/L indicates an "acceptable" status of vitamin C.[45]

Thiamin

Thiamin, also known as vitamin B_1, consists of a central carbon to which a nitrogen-containing ring and a sulfur-containing ring are attached. Thiamin is readily inactivated by prolonged exposure to heat or alkaline solutions. Three forms of thiamin exist: (1) thiamin monophosphate (TMP), (2) thiamin triphosphate (TTP), and (3) thiamin pyrophosphate (TPP). TPP, the biologically active coenzyme, is also known as thiamin diphosphate (TDP).

Before absorption, intestinal phosphatases hydrolyze the phosphates, leaving free thiamin. Absorption of thiamin can occur by either active or via passive diffusion, depending on the concentration of intestinal thiamin.[45] At low physiological concentrations, thiamin is absorbed via a specific energy-dependent, saturable, and active transport mechanism. It is mainly absorbed in the proximal small intestine, especially the jejunum, via a carrier-mediated process. Thiamin absorption is passive during high intake. Approximately 30 mg of thiamin is stored in the body as either TPP or TMP, with most found in the skeletal muscle (50%).[48] Alcohol abuse is the most common cause of impaired thiamin absorption. In the blood, thiamin is bound to albumin, with the majority of thiamin present in the red blood cells existing as TDP. Following absorption, most free thiamin is taken up by the liver and is phosphorylated into its coenzyme form, TDP.

Key biochemical functions that require thiamin involve energy transformation, synthesis of pentoses and NADPH, and membrane and nerve conduction. Thiamin, as TDP, serves as a magnesium-coordinated coenzyme for the oxidative decarboxylation of alpha-ketoacids (pyruvate and alpha ketoglutarate), which are involved in carbohydrate metabolism and for the activity of transketolase in the pentose phosphate pathway. As a structural component of nerve membranes, thiamin (TTP) may also function in nerve conduction.[48] Table 8-1 lists the RDA and sources for thiamin.[3]

A deficiency of thiamin affects the central nervous system. Major causes of a deficiency include patients with recurrent vomiting, gastric surgery, alcoholism, or those with an increased demand with marginal nutritional status.[11] A deficiency can occur within 14 days without inadequate intake or increased demand.[49] Some experts recommend prophylactic thiamin dosing when a deficiency is probable, especially in PN patients with a history of alcohol abuse.[49,50] The standard recommendation is 5 to 20 mg/d parenteral thiamin; however, wider ranges between 50 to 300 mg/d (intravenous, intramuscular, or oral) have been advocated.[11,49,50] The classic thiamin deficiency neurological diseases are beriberi and Wernicke encephalopathy (WE), which can develop into Wernicke-Korsakoff syndrome (WKS). Signs of deficiency are found in Table 8-2.[51,52] The prevalence of thiamin deficiency in hospitalized patients with heart failure has been reported to range from 3% to 96%. Such a wide variation is due to a confluence of reasons, such as different techniques for assessing thiamin status, varying nutritional status, comorbidities, and concurrent diuretic medications. Furosemide therapy has been shown to cause thiamin deficiency secondary to the drug's diuretic effect, which results in increased urinary thiamin excretion.[49]

WE caused by thiamin deficiency is generally precipitated by ethanol abuse. The classic triad of symptoms encompasses ocular abnormalities, gait ataxia, and mental status changes (Table 8-2).[11,48] Approximately 80% of patients with WE will develop WKS, resulting in psychosis and memory disturbances. Thiamin deficiency has been associated with chronic alcoholism, long-term PN, refeeding syndrome, malabsorption, dialysis, hyperemesis gravidarum, protracted vomiting after bariatric surgery, and insufficient thiamin supplementation during shortages of injectable multivitamin solutions.[11,53] Severe lactic acidosis can also be a consequence of thiamin deficiency during PN.[54] The first nutritional deficiency often noted when food intake is limited or when absorption is impaired via alcohol abuse is thiamin deficiency because when thiamin status is compromised, a deficiency develops rapidly. Untreated thiamin deficiency can result in fatal lactic acidosis. Acute postgastric reduction surgery neuropathy, also called bariatric beriberi, has become more prevalent as the numbers of bariatric surgeries increase. Although the neuropathy is multifactorial in origin, thiamin deficiencies along with vitamin B_{12} deficiencies have been implicated in 40% of the cases.[53]

Thiamin is remarkably nontoxic. Toxic effects of thiamin have been reported with an excess of 3 g/d (eg, 50 mg/kg body weight); otherwise, it is generally recognized as safe. Hypersensitivity and anaphylactoid reactions are possible, especially if thiamin is given repeatedly via the parenteral route.[11,55] Whether excess intake is given orally or intravenously, the majority of thiamin not used is rapidly excreted in the urine. Because of a lack of suitable data, a UL cannot be set.[3]

The preferred method for differentiating a normal status from subclinical thiamin deficiency is the measurement of erythrocyte transketolase activity (ETKA), with and without the in vivo addition of TDP.[55] This test provides a sensitive, specific, biochemical functional measurement of thiamin status. A normal value, which indicates an acceptable thiamin status, is 0% to 15% stimulation of activity with the additional coenzyme. A low value (or marginally deficient status) is a stimulation of 16% to 24%, whereas a deficient status (or a high risk of deficiency) is a stimulation greater than 25%. Adequacy of thiamin can also be assessed by the measurement of thiamin in whole blood; values less than 1.7 mcg/dL denote deficiency. Prophylactic thiamin supplementation in those patients at risk of a deficiency is warranted given thiamin's low risk of side effects or toxicity.

Riboflavin

Riboflavin (vitamin B_2) chemically contains three linked six-membered rings, with a sugar alcohol attached to the middle ring. It is a precursor to two major coenzyme derivatives, flavin mononucleotide (FMN) and flavin adenine dinucleotide (FAD), which are involved in a wide variety of enzymes in the intermediary metabolism. Dietary sources of riboflavin are primarily in the coenzyme forms, whereas the free form is found in milk and in enriched grain products. All of these forms can be used to meet the requirement for riboflavin.

Before absorption, riboflavin dissociates from the coenzyme derivatives in the stomach via the action of hydrochloric acid. The extent of absorption is proportionate to the dose and occurs predominately in the proximal portion of the small intestine via a saturable, sodium-dependent carrier mechanism. Riboflavin deficiency results in an increased intestinal uptake, whereas high riboflavin intake results in decreased absorption efficiency. The upper limit of absorption is estimated to be approximately 66.4 μmol (25 mg).[56] Several factors can enhance or impair riboflavin absorption. There is evidence that the presence of food increases riboflavin absorption, most likely by delaying the intestinal transit time.[56] Bile salts also increase the absorption of riboflavin. In contrast, several metals and drugs can impede riboflavin. For example, many of the divalent metals such as copper, zinc, iron, and manganese form chelates with riboflavin, and prevent absorption.[56] The clinical significance of this binding may become relevant when deciding the amount of supplementation of these trace elements. Alcohol ingestion can also impair both the digestion and absorption of riboflavin.

Once absorbed into the mucosal cells, riboflavin then enters the portal circulation destined for the liver, where it undergoes phosphorylation into FMN and its other coenzyme, FAD. The synthesis of these coenzymes is under hormonal control; the adrenocorticotropic hormone, aldosterone, and the thyroid hormones stimulate the synthesis of these coenzymes.[56] Riboflavin undergoes little metabolism before it is excreted in the urine. Intake that exceeds plasma saturation levels is lost via the urine primarily as free riboflavin.

The major biochemical function of riboflavin is to serve as a component of FMN and FAD as an electron transport intermediary for oxidation-reduction reactions. As a component of FMN and FAD, riboflavin participates in pyridine and nonpyridine-dependent dehydrogenases, oxygen and mono-oxygen reductases, disulfide reductases, and one-electron transfers. Although seldom recognized, riboflavin also has antioxidant activity because the coenzyme FAD is required for the enzyme glutathione reductase, a pivotal enzyme protecting against lipid peroxides. Riboflavin deficiency has been associated with increased lipid peroxidation, especially in association with excessive ethanol intake.[56] Other micronutrient pathways that require riboflavin include the conversion of vitamin B_6 to its active form (FMN), the synthesis of the active form of folate, and the catabolism of choline. Table 8-1 lists the RDA and sources for riboflavin.[3]

Riboflavin deficiency rarely occurs alone and most often is accompanied by multiple nutrient abnormalities, such as deficits of the other B-complex vitamins. A diet low in dairy products and animal protein can predispose an individual to riboflavin deficiency. Worldwide, it is a commonly observed deficiency, especially in developing countries. A deficiency rarely exists in the general population within the United States, yet suboptimal riboflavin status can be found in critically ill patients.[57] Although it is not associated with a specific deficiency disease, characteristic overt deficiency symptoms do exist (Table 8-2).[55] Populations at risk of riboflavin deficiency include those with thyroid dysfunction, alcoholism, and chronic malabsorption.

Riboflavin toxicity from food or supplements is rare.[1,3] Because of lack of suitable data, a UL cannot be set.[3] The erythrocyte glutathione reductase activity coefficient (EGR-AC) assay is a sensitive, functional indicator of riboflavin status and the method of choice for its analysis.[58] A value less than 1.20 (eg, less than 20% stimulation of activity upon addition of FAD) indicates an acceptable riboflavin status. A value between 1.2 and 1.4 indicates marginal status, and a value greater than 1.4 indicates a riboflavin deficiency.[56,58] This assay is invalid in individuals with a glucose 6-phosphate dehydrogenase deficiency.[3,56]

Niacin

The term niacin (vitamin B_3) is a generic descriptor for two water-soluble active forms, nicotinic acid and nicotinamide. Nicotinamide serves as a component of two coenzymes, nicotinamide adenosine dinucleotide (NAD) and nicotinamide adenosine dinucleotide phosphate (NADP). Niacin occurs mainly in these two forms in dietary sources of animal origin. Other sources are listed in Table 8-1. In addition to dietary sources, NAD can be synthesized from the essential amino acid tryptophan.

Both nicotinic acid and nicotinamide are absorbed rapidly and efficiently from the stomach and intestine by active transport (at low concentrations) or passive diffusion (at high concentrations).[59] Both NAD and NADP are enzymatically hydrolyzed in the intestinal mucosa to release nicotinamide, the major form in the blood. The amount of niacin excreted in the urine, in part, is related to the form of niacin ingested and niacin status of the individual. There is very little excretion of nicotinamide and nicotinic acid because they both are actively reabsorbed from the glomerular filtrate. Excess niacin is methylated in the liver to form methyl-nicotinamide, one of the primary urinary metabolites.

Similar to riboflavin, the nicotinamide portion of NAD and NADP serves as a hydrogen donor or an electron acceptor for over 200 enzymes involved in intermediary metabolism.[59] In this role, niacin functions in the metabolism of amino acids, fatty acids, and carbohydrates. Following hydrolysis, hepatic NAD releases adenosine diphosphate ribose, which, in turn, may be transferred to acceptor proteins and functions in the repair of DNA, as well as calcium mobilization.[3,59] Niacin, as NADPH, is also involved with reducing the antioxidants dehydroascorbate and glutathione. In addition, NADPH is required for activation of folate. Table 8-1 lists the RDA and sources for niacin.[3]

The classic niacin deficiency disease is pellagra, which is rare in developed countries. It can affect the gastrointestinal tract, the skin, and the nervous system, and presents as three D's: dermatitis, diarrhea, and dementia (Table 8-2). A dietary deficiency of niacin is rare in the United States because of the widespread fortification of certain food products with niacin.[55] In addition, niacin can be synthesized from dietary tryptophan, with 60 mg of tryptophan equal to 1 mg of niacin or 1 mg of niacin equivalent (NE).

Pharmacological doses of nicotinic acid used to treat hyperlipidemia may cause vasodilatation as a result of prostaglandin release. Generally, most individuals taking 3 g/d will experience this phenomenon and other effects (Table 8-2).[3,55,59] Low-dose aspirin therapy taken 30 minutes before nicotinic acid helps mitigate these side effects. Treatment using nicotinamide has little if any antihyperlipidemic effect. Advanced stages of pellagra are treated via intramuscular injections of nicotinamide (50 to 100 mg) three times daily for 3 to 4 days followed by oral therapy.[11] See Table 8-3 for the UL for niacin.[3]

The urinary excretion of two major niacin-methylated metabolites, *N*-methylnicotinamide (NMN) and 2-pyridone, are the most commonly used procedures to determine niacin status. A niacin deficiency is defined as urinary levels of NMN less than 5.8 μmol/d and urinary excretion of 2-pyridone less than 2 mg/g of creatinine.[3,59] The measurement of plasma levels of 2-pyridone and/or *N*-methylnicotinamide may also be used to assess niacin status.[3] A decreased concentration of NAD in red blood cells, coupled with a low plasma tryptophan concentration, may also suggest niacin deficiency.[59]

Vitamin B_6 (Pyridoxine)

There are three forms of vitamin B_6: pyridoxine, pyridoxal (PL), and pyridoxamine (PM). These three forms are metabolically, chemically, and functionally related and can be converted to the active coenzymes pyridoxal phosphate (PLP) and pyridoxamine phosphate (PMP). Plant foods contain the more stable pyridoxine, whereas animal products have more PL and PLP. Ingested phosphorylated forms undergo hydrolysis to remove the phosphate group via intestinal phosphatases prior to absorption.[60] Uptake of pyridoxine, PL, and PM by intestinal epithelial cells occurs via a carrier-mediated, pH-dependent mechanism that is both saturable and nonsaturable; their absorption rates range from 71% to 82%.[11,60] Within the intestinal cell, these vitamin B_6 forms are converted back to the phosphorylated forms. Approximately 60% of the vitamin B_6 in the plasma is present as PLP bound to albumin for transport and hemoglobin in the erythrocyte. After uptake by the liver, the hepatocyte converts the dephosphorylated forms into the metabolically active PLP form. Both PLP and PL are released for transport to the extrahepatic tissues, with muscle containing the majority of PLP (75% to 80%).[60] The major excretory metabolite is urinary 4-pyridoxic acid, the oxidation product of PL.

The coenzyme forms of vitamin B_6 participate in over 100 enzymatic reactions. These reactions include, but are not limited to, protein, amino acid, and lipid metabolism; gluconeogenesis; steroid receptor binding, central nervous system development; neurotransmitter synthesis; heme biosynthesis; and normal immune function.[60] Table 8-1 lists the RDA and sources for pyridoxine.[3,11]

Populations at the greatest risk for deficiency include alcoholics, renal patients maintained on dialysis, the elderly, and people receiving medication therapies that inhibit vitamin activity (ie, isoniazid, penicillamine, corticosteroids, and/or anticonvulsants). Recently, a neuromyopathic disorder associated with progressive muscle weakness and gait disturbances postintestinal transplantation (2 years) revealed a PLP deficiency. An assessment of the PLP status is warranted preoperatively in addition to serial long-term monitoring postoperatively in these PN-dependent patients after intestinal transplantation with preemptive replacement treatment when indicated.[61] The clinical deficiency signs are found in Table 8-2.[3,61]

No adverse effects due to high food intakes of B_6 have been reported.[5] However, large oral supplemental doses (greater than 500 mg/d) have resulted in a variety of side effects (Table 8-2). However, doses as low as 100 mg/d have been associated with the Lhermitte sign, which suggests an effect on the spinal cord.[11,60] Negative effects have been related to prolonged intakes of 300 mg/d as well. See Table 8-3 for the UL for this vitamin. Patients undergoing intestinal transplantation given 50 mg/d more than the UL had an accumulation of PLP within the red cells (30 times the upper limit of normal). Clinicians should adopt a cautious approach to B_6 supplementation in this population.[62]

A combination of three tests is recommended to assess vitamin B_6 status because of limits of each individual test.[60] These three tests are (1) direct plasma PLP levels, which respond to intake and reflect liver stores and plateauing in 6 to 10 days; (2) 24-hour urinary excretion of 4-pyridoxic acid, a hepatic B_6 metabolite (greater than 3 μmol/d suggests adequate status); and (3) the activation of erythrocyte aspartate aminotransferase (EAST) and erythrocyte alanine aminotransferase (EALT) by PLP, which is used to evaluate the long-term B_6 status. An EAST value less than 1.6 and an EALT value less than 1.25 reflect adequate B_6 status.[3,60] In the critically ill intestinal transplant patient, intracellular (red cell) PLP concentrations are a more reliable measure of status than are plasma measurements.[62]

Vitamin B_{12} (Cobalamin)

Vitamin B_{12} is found exclusively in foods of animal origin due to microbial synthesis or prior ingestion of the vitamin. These foods provide vitamin B_{12} in the coenzyme forms, methyl-, hydroxyl-, and deoxyadenosyl-cobalamin. The complex structure contains a corrin ring with cobalt incorporated into the center. The only reliable source of vitamin B_{12} comes from animal products. Cyanocobalamin is the form used in supplements and fortified foods. All forms are readily converted into the two biologically active forms, methyl- and deoxyadenosyl-cobalamin. An excess intake of vitamin C (500 mg) can impair the vitamin B_{12} bioavailability from foods and destroy the vitamin.[63]

The digestion and absorption process for vitamin B_{12} is complex and dependent on normal gastrointestinal function. Vitamin B_{12} is released from proteins ingested via the action of hydrochloric acid (HCl) and pepsin in the gastric secretions. The free B_{12} binds to the glycoprotein, haptocorrin (also called R-protein and transcobalamin I [TC I]), which is secreted by the salivary glands and swallowed with food. This complex travels into the small intestine, where pancreatic proteases hydrolyze haptocorrin or R-protein and free B_{12} is released.[63] Free B_{12} encounters another glycoprotein, intrinsic factor (IF) in the duodenum, which is produced by the gastric parietal cells. The IF-B_{12} complex moves into the ileum where it attaches to a specific IF receptor, cubilin, on the GI epithelial cells.[64] Following intestinal absorption 3 to 4 hours later, the vitamin is transferred to a specific transport protein, TC II. This carrier protein enters the portal circulation and is first taken up by the liver and then by bone marrow and erythrocytes. Unlike other water-soluble vitamins, vitamin B_{12} can be stored in the liver.[63]

Adults with normal gastric function absorb approximately 50% of dietary vitamin B_{12}. Vitamin B_{12} is secreted into the bile so most is reabsorbed via enterohepatic circulation. Failure of any of the processes can decrease the absorption of the vitamin. For example, pancreatic insufficiency could interfere with the release of free B_{12} from IF and reduce the amount absorbed. Individuals with impaired HCl production, such as elderly persons or those taking histamine-2 (H_2) antagonists or proton pump inhibitors (PPI) have reduced absorption.[63,65] Patients who have had the removal of a portion or all of the ileum or stomach and patients with chronic malabsorption syndromes also have reduced absorption.

Vitamin B_{12} must be converted to one of its two coenzyme forms, methylcobalamin or 5′-deoxyadenosylcobalamin, to be metabolically active. Methylcobalamin is a cofactor for methionine synthetase, the enzyme that converts homocysteine to methionine. Simultaneously, this conversion of homocysteine to methionine involves the demethylation of 5-methyl-tetrahydrofolate (5-methyl-THF) into its active form, tetrahydrofolate (THF). When vitamin B_{12} is lacking, folate becomes "trapped" in its methyl, or inactive, form. Vitamin B_{12} deficiency often presents as folate deficiency and is, therefore, commonly misdiagnosed. In the deoxyadenosylcobalamin form, vitamin B_{12} is required for the conversion of methylmalonyl coenzyme A to succinyl coenzyme A and for the degradation of certain amino acids and odd chain fatty acids. Table 8-1 lists the RDA and best sources for this vitamin.[3]

Marginal or inadequate vitamin B_{12} status characteristically presents as hematologic, GI, and neurological manifestations, which often appear first. Other common age-related problems include cognitive decline, cardiovascular disease, and bone fractures.[55,66–68] Refer to Table 8-2 for signs of deficiency. Clinical deficiency has been associated with malabsorption syndromes that may occur in patients after gastrectomy, gastric bypass, ileal resection, or those with Crohn's disease. It has also been reported in vegetarian populations. As mentioned earlier, impaired HCl production can lead to a B_{12} deficiency, as can an overgrowth of *Helicobacter pylori*.

Oral vitamin B_{12} is relatively nontoxic in its naturally occurring forms. A rare allergic reaction to crystalline cyanocobalamin, which is the form used in many oral formulations, has been reported.[63] Due to a lack of suitable data, a UL could not be set.[3]

There are four stages of vitamin B_{12} status: stage I, low serum B_{12}; stage II, low cell stores of B_{12}; stage III, a biochemical deficiency; and stage IV, a clinically apparent deficiency.[67] The earliest indicator of a compromise in vitamin B_{12} status is a low serum level of holotranscobalamin II, the primary delivery protein for vitamin B_{12}. The fall in serum vitamin B_{12} levels occurs later and suggests a decline in cellular stores. In fact, serum vitamin B_{12} levels may even be maintained at the expense of its stores.[3] The serum level of methylmalonic acid (MMA) and homocysteine are elevated in greater than 90% of individuals with a vitamin B_{12} deficiency.[67] Homocysteine serum concentrations may also be elevated in folic acid deficiency and, therefore, are not a specific indicator of B_{12} deficiency. Measuring the serum concentration of vitamin B_{12} is the procedure of choice for determining B_{12} status. According to the World Health Organization, serum values of B_{12} less than 150 pg/mL (110 pmol/L) denote a deficiency for all ages. Others suggest that less than either 300 or 350 pg/mL should be considered B_{12} deficient. The goals of treatment lie in mitigating the signs and symptoms. The common dose for treating B_{12} deficiency is 100- or 1000-mcg IM injections at 1-month intervals until corrected. Injections are often initially given more frequently than monthly in symptomatic B_{12} deficiency. Sublingual, nasal spray, oral, and gel B_{12} preparations are also available. Because of the close interrelationships between vitamin B_{12} and folic acid, especially in the presence of megaloblastic anemia, the status of both vitamins should be determined simultaneously. The absence of megaloblastic anemia should not be taken as lack of B_{12} deficiency because folate can mask B_{12} deficiency. Serum homocysteine and MMA are increased in B_{12} deficiency; measurements of both are useful when diagnosing vitamin B_{12} deficiency.[69,70] Normal serum MMA levels are 0.08 to 0.56 μmol/L. Homocysteine levels between 5 and 15 μmol/L are considered normal. Homocysteine and MMA values greater than normal ranges do support vitamin B_{12} deficiency. A standard multivitamin supplement is safe practice for adult vegans and strict vegetarians with normal vitamin B_{12} absorption to avoid a deficiency.

Folic Acid (Folate, Folacin)

Folic acid is also called pteroylglutamate or pteroylmonoglutamate. The metabolically active forms of folate have reduced (tetrahydro) pteridine rings with up to 11 glutamic acids (polyglutamates) attached. Folate in foods, or pteroylpolyglutamates, often contain up to nine glutamate residues.

Prior to absorption, polyglutamates are converted to the monoglutamate form by hydrolytic zinc-dependent enzymes (conjugases) located in the jejunal brush border.[71] Both zinc deficiency and chronic alcohol consumption can impair the conjugase activity and, thus, the absorption of folate. The monoglutamates produced are actively transported via a pH-dependent carrier-mediated mechanism.[71] Any change in luminal jejunal pH secondary to drug therapy or disease can also limit folate absorption. Within the intestinal cell and before entry into the portal circulation, the monoglutamate form of folate undergoes a reduction to THF, which is then converted to either N^5-methyl-THF or N^{10}-formyl-THF. These two forms are secreted into the bile and recirculate via enterohepatic circulation. They may account for as much as 50% of the folate that reaches the peripheral tissues.[71] The predominant form found in the plasma is N^5-methyl-THF, which is loosely bound to albumin and folate-binding proteins (FBPs). Folate transport across membranes into cells of various tissues occurs via a carrier-mediated process. FBPs, also called folate carriers or folate receptors, are found within the intestinal brush border and facilitate cellular folate uptake. Intracellularly, the N^5-methyl-THF is demethylated via a vitamin B_{12}-dependent enzyme and converted back into a polyglutamate form to become the active coenzyme that is capable of transferring one carbon unit. Excretion of folate metabolites is minimal, whereas most of the absorbed dietary folate is reabsorbed via enterohepatic circulation. Conditions or diseases that impair bile secretion may also limit folate recirculation.

The primary biochemical role of folic acid is as a coenzyme in the transfer of single carbon fragments from one compound to another for amino acid metabolism and nucleic acid synthesis.[3,71] Folate (THF) functions as a coenzyme to accept one-carbon groups generated from amino acid metabolism. These THF derivatives serve as donors of one-carbon units for the synthesis of amino acids, purines, and pyrimidines. Table 8-1 lists the RDA and sources for folic acid.[3] Dietary folate equivalents (DFE) are used to express folate requirements and to reflect differences in absorption of food versus synthetic folate (1 DFE = 1 mcg food folate, 0.6 mcg fortified/supplemental folic taken with food, or 0.5 mcg supplemental folate).

An isolated folate deficiency rarely exists and often coincides with other nutrient deficiencies. The classic feature of a folic acid deficiency is megaloblastic or macrocytic anemia, an early indicator of which is hypersegmentation of neutrophils.[3,55,71] Other deficiency signs are found in Table 8-2.

Select populations, medications, and some chronic conditions associated with an increased need for folate can compromise folate status. Folate deficiency is often seen in chronic alcoholism because of decreased dietary folate, as well as the negative effects of alcohol on folate absorption and hepatobiliary metabolism. Many medications, such as phenytoin, cholestyramine, sulfasalazine, and amphotericin B can affect folate absorption and metabolism.[71] Pregnant women are considered to be at greater risk of developing a folate deficiency secondary to the increased demand for DNA synthesis for embryonic development. Because the U.S. Food and Drug Administration (FDA) mandated folate fortification of cereal and grain products in January 1998, the number of reported cases of neural tube defects (NTDs) has declined.[72,73] Low serum folate levels during pregnancy have also been associated with poor pregnancy outcomes.[74] Periconceptional and prenatal supplementation of 400 mcg/d synthetic folic acid is recommended in addition to consuming folate-fortified foods to prevent NTDs.[74,75] A daily dose of 4 mg is recommended if a woman has previously had a pregnancy with an NTD. There is some evidence to support folate treatment of 10 mg/d to improve not only hyperhomocysteinemia but also endothelial dysfunction via improvements in coagulation and free-radical scavenger activity.[76] As mentioned earlier, the metabolism and functions of folate and vitamin B_{12} are interrelated; consumption of large folate amounts can mask a B_{12} deficiency.

Excessive amounts of folic acid (100 times the RDA) may result in seizures in individuals requiring phenytoin therapy. No signs of toxicity were observed when women were given folate 10 mg daily for 4 months.[55] Allergic reactions to oral and parenteral folic acid have been observed.[3,55] Table 8-3 lists the UL for folic acid.

There are four stages of folate deficiency: stage I is early negative balance with serum folate levels less than 3 ng/mL (6.8 nmol/mL); stage II is tissue depletion when red blood cell folate levels are less than 160 ng/mL (362.67 nmol/mL); stage III is folate deficient erythropoiesis, indicated by neutrophil hypersegmentation and an abnormal deoxyuridine (dU) suppression test (correctable by folates in vitro); and stage IV is a clinical folate deficiency, manifested by megaloblastic or macrocytic anemia.[55,60] The goal is early detection and correction. Again, vitamin B_{12} status and homocysteine concentrations should also be determined in tandem with folate. Elevated homocysteine levels have been associated with a risk for cardiovascular disease, stroke, dementia, Alzheimer disease, and osteoporosis.[77–79] The relationship between homocysteine levels, B vitamins, and the risk of these chronic disease conditions is complex and remains unclear. New methodologies to accurately assess folate status via folate derivatives are under development and hold promise for the future.[80]

Biotin

Biotin is ubiquitous in the diet and exists in the free biotin and the protein-bound coenzyme form, biocytin, which is biotin bound to the amino acid lysine. Free biotin is absorbed via facilitated diffusion. Biocytin requires the enzyme, biotinidase, in the small intestine to cleave the protein portion from biocytin, releasing the free vitamin for jejunal absorption.[81] Evidence suggests that biotinidase may also function as a biotin carrier protein.[82]

Biotin functions as a cofactor for four carboxylase enzymes in mammalian systems, which transport carbon dioxide (carboxyl units) to various substrates. These biotin-dependent carboxylases catalyze vital reactions in important metabolic pathways: acetyl-coenzyme A (CoA) carboxylase for fatty acid synthesis, pyruvate carboxylase for gluconeogenesis, propionyl-CoA carboxylase for propionate metabolism, and 3-methylcrotonyl-CoA carboxylase for branched-chain amino acid catabolism. Table 8-1 lists the AI and sources for biotin.[3,82]

Overall, a biotin deficiency is considered rare. However, biotinidase deficiency, an inherited autosomal recessive trait, exists in about 1 in 60,000.[82] These individuals are given pharmacological doses of biotin (5 to 20 mg/d) and improve clinically. The signs and symptoms of an untreated biotin deficiency are found in Table 8-2. Deficiencies have been reported in association with long-term PN, alcoholism, and in patients with partial gastrectomies.

There are no reports of biotin toxicity, and thus, a UL could not be determined.[3] Even at high intakes of biotin, no evidence of toxicity was observed when patients with biotin-responsive inborn errors of metabolism and/or acquired biotin deficiency were treated with daily doses of either 200 mg of biotin orally or 20 mg intravenously.[3,81]

Commonly used methods for determining biotin status include measurement of the serum biotin concentrations and 24-hour urinary excretion of biotin. The most valid indicators of biotin status are an abnormally decreased urinary excretion of biotin and an abnormally increased urinary excretion of 3-hydroxyisovaleric acid.[83] A urinary concentration of less than 6 mcg/d and whole blood or serum biotin concentrations of less than 200 pg/mL indicate biotin deficiency.[55,81]

Pantothenic Acid

Pantothenic acid is a component of the CoA molecule and the acyl carrier protein (ACP) of fatty acid synthetase complex.[84] Dietary CoA is hydrolyzed to pantothenic acid in the intestinal lumen. Absorption is either by passive diffusion or via a saturable, sodium-dependent active transport. Absorbed pantothenic acid is transported via the erythrocytes throughout the body.[84] Most of the pantothenic acid in the body tissues is in the form of CoA, which is hydrolyzed to pantothenic acid before excretion in the urine.[84]

As a component of CoA, pantothenic acid is involved in energy release from fat, carbohydrate, and ketogenic amino acids. In this form, pantothenic acid is also involved in gluconeogenesis, heme and sterol synthesis, and most acetylation reactions. As a part of ACP, pantothenic acid is required for the synthesis of fat. The AI and sources for pantothenic acid are listed in Table 8.3.[3]

Signs and symptoms of a pantothenic acid deficiency have only been observed after the administration of metabolic antagonists (ie, omega methylpantothenate) or feeding a synthetic diet free of this vitamin (Table 8-2).[3,55,84] Deficiency is often in conjunction with multiple nutrient deficiencies or conditions such as diabetes mellitus, inflammatory bowel disease (IBD), and alcoholism. Absorption of pantothenic acid is likely impaired with both IBD and alcoholism.[84] Heavy ethanol drinkers may have an increased requirement for this vitamin. Toxicity due to pantothenic acid is rare. Data were incomplete to develop a UL for this vitamin.[3]

Pantothenic acid status is reflected by both whole-blood assays and urinary excretion determined by a 24-hour urine collection. A blood value less than 1 μmol/L is considered low.[55,84] Urinary pantothenic acid excretion is a more reliable indicator of status because it is closely related to dietary intake and is likely the easiest to conduct and interpret. A urinary pantothenic acid concentration less than 1 mg/d (in adults) indicates a poor status or nutriture of the vitamin.

Choline

Choline is found in a wide variety of foods. Nearly all dietary choline is in the form of choline phosphatides such as lecithin and sphingomyelin. Betaine, the oxidized form of choline, is also present in the diet but it is not able to be directly converted to choline.[85] Dietary choline is absorbed by the small intestine and uptake occurs via choline transporter proteins, and then it is delivered to the liver via the portal vein. It is primarily converted to the major phospholipid, phosphatidylcholine (lecithin). When choline supply is low, it is recycled in the liver and redistributed from the kidneys, lungs, and the intestine to the liver and brain.[86] Very small amounts are excreted in the urine; excess is converted to betaine, a methyl donor providing methyl groups to compounds such as homocysteine.[85]

Choline is needed for neurotransmitter synthesis (acetylcholine), cell membrane signaling (phospholipids), lipid transport (lipoproteins), and methyl-group metabolism (homocysteine production, the betaine-choline-carnitine [BCC] transporter).[85–87] As such, it is essential for cell membrane integrity, methyl metabolism, cholinergic neurotransmission, transmembrane signaling, and the transport and metabolism of lipid cholesterol.[3,86] Endogenous de novo synthesis of choline occurs via the sequential methylation of phosphatidylethanolamine with *S*-adenosylmethionine as the methyl donor.[85] However, this de novo synthesis of choline alone is insufficient to meet human needs. Thus, the demand for choline is influenced by methionine, folic acid, vitamin B_{12}, and betaine, the oxidized form of choline, all of which are involved in metabolic methyl-exchange reactions.[85] Table 8-1 lists the AI and sources for choline.

Whenever the demand for choline is high (during pregnancy, lactation, hypermetabolic states) and supply is low, choline intake is critical. There is also growing evidence calling into question the essentiality of choline specifically related to men and menopausal women, raising the question whether new recommendations are needed to avoid deficiencies.[88,89]

Choline deficiency has been associated with PN support. Humans fed PN formulations without choline developed fatty livers and liver damage, which were corrected in part by giving choline.[3,90] Reductions in plasma choline concentrations observed in long-term PN also correlate with abnormal hepatic aminotransferase levels.[90] Again, there is evidence that choline deficiency may contribute to PN-induced liver dysfunction, causing hepatic steatosis and eventual hepatic failure. Individuals on PN secondary to short-bowel syndrome who develop a choline deficiency are more susceptible to these hepatic consequences. Impairment of verbal and visual memory in choline-deficient PN patients may be related to acetylcholine, a neurotransmitter. Intravenous choline supplementation is needed for optimal long-term PN support to minimize fatty liver infiltration.[90] The UL of choline (Table 8-3) is set to avoid the adverse effects of excessive intakes (Table 8-2).[3,85]

Plasma choline levels reflect dietary intake, yet they do not decline below 50% of normal levels, even following a short fast.[85] Maintaining a plasma choline concentration of 10 μmol/L is desirable in adults for optimal health throughout life.

Significant evidence now exists showing a relationship between choline deficiency and the development of diseases such as liver disease, atherosclerosis, cancer, and possibly neurological disorders (eg, neural tube defects, Alzheimer dementia, memory).[86] These disease relationships and the fact that average American dietary choline intakes are below the AI recommendation warrant establishing a new choline requirement.

Trace Elements

Minerals are required for virtually all aspects of metabolism. The minerals discussed include iron, zinc, copper, manganese, selenium, iodine, chromium, fluoride, and molybdenum. The minerals' absorption, transport, excretion, function, deficiency and toxicity characteristics, and requirements are reviewed. The alterations in metabolism, transport, and excretion that occur with chronic and acute illnesses are emphasized. Subtle physiological changes sometimes associated with trace element deficiency often make a diagnosis difficult. In addition, trace minerals interact with each other and may influence or interfere with the absorption of select minerals.

Iron (Fe)

Iron is a component of every living cell and has been recognized to be essential for the maintenance of health for many centuries. The amount of iron present in an individual varies based on age, sex, weight, and nutritional status. Total body stores contain about 2 to 4 g, with differences between the sexes. Menstruating women average 40 mg/kg, whereas men average 50 mg/kg of body weight.[91]

Normal iron balance is regulated via alterations in absorption. Iron in food occurs in a heme or nonheme form. Approximately 18.5% of iron in the typical diet is from heme iron derived from hemoglobin and myoglobin molecules found in animal flesh. About 40% of ingested heme iron is absorbed. It is more efficiently absorbed compared to nonheme iron found primarily in plant foods. Nonheme iron absorption varies depending on other dietary constituents and is estimated at 10% to 50%. Factors that enhance nonheme iron absorption include organic compounds that increase acidity such as vitamin C, HCl, lactic acid, and the acidic amino acids aspartic and glutamic acid. These components maintain iron in the ferrous form (Fe^{2+}), which is better absorbed compared to ferric iron (Fe^{3+}). A key regulator of iron homeostasis is the peptide hormone, hepcidin, which is synthesized in the liver. It is a key homeostatic regulator of iron metabolism and is involved in pathological regulation of iron in response to infection, inflammation, hypoxia, and anemia.[92,93] Hepcidin regulates both plasma iron concentrations and tissue distribution via the inhibition of dietary iron absorption, iron recycling by macrophages, and the mobilization of iron from hepatic stores.[93] During iron deficiency states, serum hepcidin concentrations are low, whereas concentrations are elevated in the anemia associated with inflammation of chronic disease.

Absorption mechanisms differ for heme versus nonheme iron. Heme iron is absorbed intact into the enterocyte after the globin fraction is removed and then hydrolyzed to ferrous iron by the intestinal cell. In the stomach, nonheme iron is released from food components, usually in the ferric form, and is then converted to ferrous via the action of gastric acid. This ferrous iron can traverse the intestinal cell's glycocalyx and brush border by binding to receptors. The primary sites of iron absorption are in the duodenum and jejunum.

The concomitant use of medications that reduce stomach acidity such as antacids, H_2 antagonists, or PPIs can impair iron absorption. Ineffective iron absorption occurs in malabsorptive states such as celiac disease, Crohn's disease, or pernicious anemia and during frank achlorhydria. Individuals with decreased gastric acid production due to aging are also in jeopardy of absorbing less iron. Dietary factors that reduce nonheme iron absorption by forming insoluble iron complexes include phytic acid in grain fibers; oxalic acid in spinach, chard, tea, and chocolate; polyphenols in coffee, tea, and cocoa; and other nutrients such as calcium, zinc, and manganese.[91] Nutrient–nutrient interactions such as these have clinical significance, especially because increased doses of zinc and manganese are often standard recommendations in critical illness.[94,95] Iron absorption may be competitively impaired when zinc or manganese supplements are provided via the GI tract; these can contribute to compromised iron status.[94,95] In addition, reduced iron absorption occurs following Roux-en-Y gastric bypass, injury, or during inflammation.[16,94–96]

Following absorption into the enterocyte and depending on the body's requirements, iron is either transported in the bloodstream where it is bound to transferrin or stored in the intestinal cell where it binds to apoferritin to form ferritin. Ferritin is a short-term form of iron storage. The iron incorporated into transferrin binds to transferrin receptors on the cell's surface. The number of transferrin receptors is dependent on the cell's iron requirement. An elevated need for iron increases the number of receptors on the cell's surface. Hence, the extent of iron stores in the body determines how much will be absorbed.[91,94] When iron stores are adequate, all of the iron-binding sites for transferrin are saturated and transport into the blood is inhibited. In contrast, when iron stores are low, transferrin receptors increase to allow for more iron binding, thus shifting iron directly from the intestinal cells into the blood. When the amount of iron in the body exceeds the storage capacity of ferritin, some of the ferritin is degraded to the insoluble iron–protein compound, hemosiderin, which also acts as an iron storage site. These mechanisms allow the body to control iron absorption. In addition, the body limits the amount of iron excreted per day because most is conserved and recycled.

The acute phase response (APR) to injury and infection suppresses iron transport. Clinically, serum iron levels are depressed, while serum ferritin levels are increased.[97] Sequestration of iron into a storage form following injury and infection is thought to be physiologically protective to the host on several fronts. It reduces the availability of iron for iron-dependent microorganism proliferation.[98] Iron also reduces free radical production and oxidative damage to membranes and DNA.[91,93] Iron is an essential component of hemoglobin, which is necessary for oxygen transport, and myoglobin, which is necessary for muscle iron storage. Iron is also an important component of cytochromes, which are necessary for the oxidative production of cellular energy as ATP. Table 8-4 lists the RDA and sources for iron.[5]

Iron deficiency presents as an anemia that is usually microcytic and hypochromic. Physical symptoms are listed in Table 8-5.[94,95] Those at risk for developing iron deficiency include women of childbearing age, those hospitalized with excess blood sampling or blood loss, and individuals with malabsorption states such as celiac disease, Crohn's disease, and gastric or intestinal surgery. To determine whether iron malabsorption is present, serum iron levels should be measured before and 2 to 4 hours after the patient is given 325 mg of oral ferrous sulfate. Failure of the iron level to rise over the pretreatment value indicates poor iron absorption.[55,91]

Iron toxicity or overload results from the short- or long-term exposure to iron that exceeds the body's physiological protection mechanisms (Table 8-5).[91,94,95] A serum ferritin value over 150 ng/mL in females and greater than 200 ng/mL in males suggests iron overload; values above 700 ng/mL are usually associated with symptomatic hemochromatosis.[98] Iron therapy in patients with preexisting hemochromatosis is contraindicated. See Table 8-3 for UL.[5]

The diagnosis of iron deficiency and iron deficiency anemia (IDA) is challenging at best. Iron depletion and the development of iron deficiency occur in stages. An assessment includes several hematological indices: hemoglobin, plasma iron, iron-binding capacity, ferritin, transferrin, erythrocyte protoporphyrin, transferrin receptor, and mean cell volume.[91,94,95] An iron status examines these indices in context with the nutritional and medical history. Before a diagnosis of iron deficiency and, in the absence of an inflammatory

TABLE 8-4 Dietary Reference Intakes for Trace Element Intakes[2,4,5]

	14–18 Years Male/Female	19–30 Years Male/Female	31–50 Years Male/Female	51–70 Years Male/Female	>70 Years Male/Female
Mineral					
Chromium (AI) mcg/d	35/24	35/25	35/25	30/20	30/20
Sources: Whole grain products, egg yolks, beer, processed meats, mushrooms, and legumes.					
Copper (RDA) mcg/d	890/700	900/900	900/900	900/900	900/900
Sources: Liver, cocoa, beans, nuts, whole grains, and dried fruits.					
Fluoride (AI) mg/d	3/3	4/3	4/3	4/3	4/3
Sources: Fluoridated water, toothpaste, dental treatments, tea, and seaweed.					
Iodine (RDA) mcg/d	150/150	150/150	150/150	150/150	150/150
Sources: Saltwater fish, seafood, and iodized salt.					
Iron (RDA) mg/d	11/15	8/18	8/18	8/8	8/8
Sources: Meats, seafood, broccoli, peas, bran, and enriched breads.					
Manganese (AI) mg/d	2.2/1.6	2.3/1.8	2.3/1.8	2.3/1.8	2.3/1.8
Sources: Nuts, oats, and other whole grains.					
Molybdenum (AI) mcg/d	43/43	45/45	45/45	45/45	45/45
Sources: Beans, grains, and nuts.					
Selenium (RDA) mcg/d	55/55	55/55	55/55	55/55	55/55
Sources: Fish, meat (organ), eggs, milk, and shellfish.					
Zinc (RDA) mg/d	11/9	11/8	11/8	11/8	11/8
Sources: Seafood, meats, greens, and whole grains.					

AI, adequate intakes; RDA, recommended dietary allowances.

TABLE 8-5 Trace Element Status[2,11,91,94,95,101,106–108,113,115,116,118,123–126,129]

Mineral	Assay[a]	Deficiency Signs	Toxicity Signs
Iron (Fe)	Males: 24–336 mcg/L Females: 11–307 mcg/L Transferrin: 170–340 mg/dL Iron-binding capacity: 240–450 mg/dL	Microcytic, hypochromic anemia; tachycardia, poor capillary refilling, fatigue, sleepiness, headache, anorexia, nausea, pallor; reduced work performance, impaired behavioral and intellectual performance, impaired ability to maintain body temperature in cold environments, decreased resistance to infections, increased lead absorption, and adverse outcomes during pregnancy; koilonychia, glossitis	Organ damage (ie, liver cirrhosis, heart enlargement, pancreatic damage, and/or skin pigmentation)
Zinc (Zn)	Plasma: 70–120 mcg/dL RBC: 1000–1600 mcg/dL	Inadequate growth, acrodermatitis enteropathica (periorificial, over buttocks and perianal regions), hypogonadism, impaired night vision, anorexia, diarrhea, alterations in taste and smell, alopecia, impaired epithelialization, wound healing, impaired immune function	Gastric distress, nausea, and dizziness; decreased immune function and decreased levels of high-density lipoprotein cholesterol
Copper (Cu)	Serum copper: 0.75–1.45 mcg/mL	Sensory ataxia, lower extremity spasticity, paresthesias in extremities, hypochromic microcytic anemia; leukopenia, neutropenia, hypercholesterolemia, decreased ceruloplasmin and erythrocyte Cu/Zn SOD, increased erythrocyte turnover, abnormal electrocardiographic patterns and myeloneuropathy	Rare; liver damage
Manganese (Mn)	Blood: 4.7–18.3 ng/mL Serum: 0.0–2.0 μg/L	Poor reproductive performance, congenital abnormalities in offspring, abnormal bone/cartilage formation, ataxia, growth retardation, and defects in lipid/carbohydrate metabolism	Central nervous system abnormalities: hyperirritability, violent acts, hallucinations, disturbances of libido, ataxia; Mn deposition in the basal ganglia secondary to perioperative parenteral nutrition (PN) support following gastrointestinal surgery; immune system and reproductive dysfunction, nephritis, pancreatitis, hepatic, testicular damage; Parkinsonlike motor dysfunction (ie, tremors, difficulty walking, facial muscle spasms)
Selenium (Se)	Serum Se: 23–190 μg/L Urine: 10–35 mcg/d Plasma glutathione peroxidase: >10.5 U/mL erythrocytes	Oxidative injury, increased susceptibility to mercury exposure, altered thyroid hormone metabolism, increased plasma glutathione levels, Keshan disease	Selenosis: nausea, vomiting, loss of hair and nails, tooth decay, skin lesions, irritability, fatigue; nervous system manifestations: peripheral neuropathy

(continued)

TABLE 8-5 Trace Element Status[2,11,91,94,95,101,106–108,113,115,116,118,123–126,129] *(continued)*

Mineral	Assay[a]	Deficiency Signs	Toxicity Signs
Iodine (I)	Urine: 100–199 mcg/L Serum: 40–92 ng/mL	Jod-Basedow phenomenon: nodular goiter, weight loss, tachycardia, muscle weakness, skin warmth	Depressed thyroid activity, elevated thyroid-stimulating hormone
Chromium (Cr)	Serum: 0.05–0.5 mcg/L Erythrocyte: <20–36 mcg/L Urine: 0.1–2 mcg/L	Weight loss, hyperglycemia refractory to insulin, glycosuria, elevated plasma free fatty acids, peripheral neuropathy, hyperlipidemia	Cr^{3+}: Muscle rhabdomyolysis (1200 mcg/d), liver dysfunction, renal failure (600–1200 mcg/d)
Fluoride (F)	Plasma: 0.01–0.2 mcg/mL; 0.0–4.0 mcmol/L Urine: 0.2–1.1 mg/mL	Increased risk for developing dental caries	Nausea, vomiting, diarrhea, abdominal pain, excessive salivation, lacrimation, pulmonary disturbances, cardiac insufficiency, weakness, convulsions, sensory disturbances, paralysis, coma; enamel and skeletal fluorosis.
Molybdenum (Mo)	Serum: 0.58–0.8 mcg/L; 0.3–2.0 ng/mL	Tachycardia, tachypnea, visual/mental changes, elevated methionine, headache, lethargy, nausea, vomiting	Rare: Hyperuricemia, goutlike symptoms

PN, parenteral nutrition; SOD, superoxide dismutase.
[a]Estimated and sample normal values; normal ranges will vary by technique and laboratory methodology.

response, early stages of iron depletion occur. These changes result in decreased transferrin saturation and are characterized by reduced plasma iron and elevated plasma transferrin. If depletion continues, serum ferritin, which reflects iron body stores, decreases (women less than 10 ng/mL; men less than 20 ng/mL).

The adjustment of plasma ferritin concentrations to remove the effects of inflammation associated with chronic disease is necessary because ferritin is a positive acute-phase protein. It is recommended that both ferritin and C-reactive protein are measured together to discern a more accurate ferritin concentration.[94,95,97,99] Another sensitive indicator of early iron deficiency is elevated levels of erythrocyte protoporphyrin. This iron measure has limitations because it is altered when hemoglobin synthesis is blunted, during situations of hemodilution, or in the presence of inflammation. Given these hematological changes, iron deficiency anemia is subsequently confirmed by a decreased mean corpuscular volume (MCV) and a decreased hemoglobin concentration.[94,95] The currently used indicators of iron status have limitations, especially related to the inflammation of chronic disease. However, serum hepcidin is evolving as a more useful indicator of deficient iron stores.[100] It could significantly aid in the differential diagnosis of anemia of inflammation and IDA. See Practice Scenario 8-2 for more information on the diagnosis of iron deficiency.

The recommended treatment for the iron deficient constitutes a dosage equivalent of 150 to 200 mg of elemental iron per day. Common oral preparations include ferrous sulfate, gluconate, and fumarate. Although the fumarate form has the highest percentage absorption, the preferred forms remain ferrous sulfate and gluconate. These forms are relatively inexpensive and possess good bioavailability. Because oral iron is better absorbed in an acidic environment, it is recommended that iron supplements be taken with a source of ascorbic acid (eg, orange juice). Foods that reduce iron absorption (tea tannins or phytates) or medications that increase the gastric pH (antacids, PPIs, H_2 blockers) should be avoided. Side effects of oral iron preparations include nausea, epigastric discomfort, and constipation. Enteric-coated, delayed release ferric compounds (eg, ferric bisglycinate) are often better tolerated but may be released in the GI tract distal to the site of optimal absorption.

Standard parenteral trace element products do not include iron, in part to avoid potential contribution to microbial growth and damaging oxidative reactions. Parenteral iron preparations should be considered only when a patient does not respond adequately to oral supplementation.[94,99] Five parenteral iron preparations are available and include low-molecular weight iron dextran, high-molecular weight iron dextran, sodium ferric gluconate, iron sucrose, and ferumoxytol. The latter two have been associated with lower rates of adverse side effects. No test dose is required by the package insert information for iron sucrose (Venofer), ferric gluconate (Ferrlecit), or ferumoxytol (Feraheme). A test dose is required for iron dextran to evaluate tolerance and avoid anaphylactic reactions. The dextran formulation, or bound Fe, is the preferable form to add to PN.[98] Iron dextran may be added to dextrose-amino acid solutions, but should not be added to total nutrient admixtures because it can destabilize these emulsions. It seems to be safe, is devoid of lipid peroxide formation, and is the preferred form of addition rather than using free Fe. A parenteral administration of iron may contribute to oxidative reactions that exacerbate tissue damage. In addition, excessive amounts of circulating iron may also stimulate bacterial proliferation, so it is not recommended during acute illness or sepsis. It can be administered during the recovery phase of stress with or without erythropoietin. Additional enteral iron is also not recommended during the acute phase response to an infection due to the same mechanisms as parenteral iron.[98]

Practice Scenario 8-2

Question: What new biomarkers can clinicians use to maximize treatment of iron deficiency in the clinical setting?

Scenario: A 72-year-old female with a history of chronic obstructive pulmonary disease, rheumatoid arthritis (RA), osteoarthritis, lung cancer 10 years ago, and non-Hodgkin lymphoma × 2 within the last 6 years presents with profound weakness, malaise, pallor, and failure to thrive. Admission hemoglobin (Hgb) is 7 g/dL. A physical assessment revealed normal anthropometric measurements: height 167.6 cm and weight 58.6 kg. The patient lives alone and eats relatively healthy meals.

Intervention: The patient's signs and symptoms suggest an anemic state, so an evaluation of her iron status is warranted as well as a search for the underlying cause to diagnose iron deficiency anemia (IDA) versus anemia of chronic disease (ACD). A blood transfusion was ordered to immediately correct the anemic state.

Answer: To discern whether the patient has IDA, ACD, or both, other laboratory assays are necessary, and include ferritin, 66 ng/mL high (H); total iron binding capacity (TIBC), 398 mcg/dL (H); mean corpuscular volume (MCV), 71 fL low (L); transferrin saturation, 17% (L); soluble transferrin receptor (sTfR), 1.9 mg/dL (H); C-reactive protein (CRP), 2.9 mg/L (H); and hepcidin, 10 ng/mL (L). Lab results indicate that the patient exhibits both ACD and IDA with classic microcytic hypochromic characteristics.

Rationale: The type and root cause of anemia must be determined in order for proper treatment and abatement. Ferritin is the first lab value to check when searching for an etiology.[94,99] Levels less than 45 ng/mL likely indicate IDA, whereas levels over 100 ng/mL indicate adequate Fe status. The ferritin level was borderline, prompting further labs. The increased TIBC and decreased transferrin saturation also suggest Fe deficiency. The patient's history of RA and recurrent cancer implicates ACD. C-reactive protein was high, indicating chronic inflammation, which can cause ferritin to be falsely elevated.[93,95,99] The sTfR level can help distinguish between IDA and ACD; levels are usually elevated in IDA. [95,99] A concurrently elevated CRP often indicates that both causes of anemia are present.[94,99] Recent research has provided insight into a new biomarker for determining Fe status: hepcidin. Hepcidin is a "liver-derived protein," which is a critical regulator of Fe homeostasis.[100] Levels are inversely related to demand; expression increases if Fe stores are adequate and decreases if stores are inadequate. Hepcidin regulates the release of Fe into the blood from epithelial cells. Levels are usually higher in ACD than in IDA. Measuring hepcidin levels could become the most reliable method for assessing Fe status. Currently, such assays are expensive and not widely available.[95,100] The hepcidin level is low, suggesting IDA.

The treatment modalities for managing IDA depend on the underlying cause. Once the cause of IDA is determined, either oral or parenteral iron therapy is prescribed to correct the deficiency. Because it was determined that both ACD and IDA were present, oral Fe-replacement therapy can be initiated to treat the IDA while searching for the underlying cause of blood loss, which is often gastrointestinal. Treating the root causes of chronic inflammation will help to correct the ACD.

Zinc (Zn)

Zinc is involved in numerous aspects of cellular metabolism. It is hydrolyzed from amino acids and nucleic acids via the action of gastric HCl and other enzymes in the small intestine before absorption. A reduced gastric acidity can decrease zinc availability for absorption. Zinc is found bound to cellular proteins in virtually all cells in the body. Greater than 95% of the body's zinc content is intracellular.

Approximately 20% to 40% of ingested zinc is absorbed from the small intestine, primarily in the duodenum and jejunum, and to a lesser extent, in the ileum. Absorption occurs by a carrier-mediated (saturable) process and a nonmediated diffusion process.[101] The transcellular movement of zinc into the mucosal cell is modulated by metallothionein (MT), a protein responsible for the regulation of zinc absorption. If zinc is not transferred to the blood or when zinc intake is high, MT synthesis increases.

After the transfer from the intestine, zinc binds to albumin for transport to the liver. The liver releases zinc into the circulation bound to albumin (70%) or alpha-macroglobulins (20% to 40%).[101] Diseases or physiological conditions characterized by hypoalbuminemia can impair hepatic release of zinc. Plasma zinc levels are also subject to a variety of stimuli including dietary zinc intake, fasting, and acute infections. During fasting, plasma zinc concentrations increase. However, during infections, zinc is redistributed, resulting in hypozincemia. Within hours postinjury, plasma zinc levels decrease by 10% to 69%; the extent and type of injury determine the duration and magnitude of this reduction.[16] The stress of acute infection precipitates the secretion of cytokines such as interleukin (IL)-1 and IL-6, which act to increase the hepatic zinc uptake. These acute phase responses are protective to the host and need to be considered when evaluating zinc status.

Various inhibitors of zinc absorption may deplete the zinc status. These include other minerals, vitamins, proteins, phytic acid, alcohol, physiological factors, and disease processes.[101] For example, MT synthesis is stimulated during inflammatory conditions, which can result in reduced zinc absorption. Phytic acid and calcium supplements decrease zinc absorption by as much as 50%. Certain milk proteins may have a negative impact on absorption as well. In addition, the long-term ingestion of large amounts of zinc can compete with copper and iron for absorption. Key excretion routes include the GI tract, the kidney, and the skin.

The overall biochemical functions of zinc can be categorized as catalytic, structural, and/or regulatory in nature. Zinc is important as a catalyst for enzymes in all six enzyme classes, which include over 200 enzymes.[101] Examples of these enzymes include alkaline phosphatase, carbonic anhydrase, alcohol dehydrogenase, and the RNA polymerases I, II, and III. The structural function of zinc includes its role in metalloenzymes and in the zinc-finger motif in proteins (ie, zinc-finger proteins).[101] Zinc also has a regulatory role in gene expression. Zinc is necessary for other physiological processes, such as lipid peroxidation, apoptosis, neuromodulation, cellular proliferation and differentiation, wound healing, insulin synthesis, and action in the pancreas, and hence, glucose control and immune function.[101,102] Zinc may also have mild antimicrobial and anti-inflammatory properties. The RDA and sources for zinc are listed in Table 8-4.[5]

The diagnosis of zinc deficiency is difficult, in part, because of zinc redistribution during the acute phase response to infection, inadequate biomarkers of zinc status, and the diversity of clinical symptoms (Table 8-5).[55,101] Zinc deficiency affects both the innate and adaptive immune systems and thus impacts the immune response, resulting in lymphopenia, impaired phagocytic function, and natural killer cells coupled with an altered secretion of cytokines.[102] Zinc deficiency can have an impact on vitamin A via two mechanisms: (1) by decreasing retinol mobilization from the liver, and (2) by decreasing zinc dependent enzyme conversion of retinol to retinal that is critical to the vision cycle.[101] A zinc deficiency could potentially precipitate a secondary vitamin A deficiency. Zinc deprivation has been reported in a variety of populations including the elderly, alcoholics, postoperative patients, burn patients, patients with malabsorptive diseases or conditions (eg, intestinal bypass or resection, bariatric procedures), and patients with renal disease. Zinc deficiency has also been known to occur in other disease states or conditions such as sickle cell anemia or malignancy, and may contribute to macular degeneration.[40,101] Wound drainage or any clinical condition causing GI zinc losses can further contribute to a declining zinc status. A deficiency can decrease the work capacity of muscles, which can result in detrimental effects on respiratory muscle function, worsen hepatic dysfunction, and cause glucose intolerance. The underlying mechanisms have not been identified.[102,103]

Acute zinc toxicity has been reported when 150 mg of zinc was administered daily (Table 8-5). Death occurred when large IV doses were given. Other toxicities have been associated with chronic oral intakes of 300 mg/d.[101]

Zinc supplementation, although often indicated, can alter the status of other nutrients.[103] Supplements of 50 mg/d of zinc increased urinary zinc excretion, although parenteral doses of 30 mg/d induced an exaggerated acute phase response.[16] Daily zinc doses of 25 to 150 mg can induce a copper deficiency.[101] Prolonged zinc supplementation with amounts greater than 30 mg/d should only be considered under medical supervision. Additional zinc is also recommended in patients with additional losses from thermal injury, hypermetabolic states such as traumatic brain injury (TBI), and in patients with excessive GI losses such as diarrhea, decubitus ulcers, and high fistula outputs.[16] Doses of 80 mg/d of zinc in combination with other antioxidant nutrients can reduce the development of age-related macular degeneration.[104] The standard treatment for TBI now includes zinc sulfate capsules at 220 mg daily or elemental zinc at 6 to 10 mg in a parenteral solution when serum zinc falls below 60 to 130 mcg/mL.[16] Typical recommendations for wound healing are up to 40 mg (176 mg zinc sulfate) for 10 days. The standard oral adult replacement dose is 220 mg twice daily (50 mg elemental zinc).[12] Table 8-6 provides guidelines for additional parenteral zinc supplementation.

In healthy populations, plasma and urinary zinc were recently confirmed as the most reliable biomarkers to assess zinc status.[105] In a clinical setting, the measurement of serum or plasma zinc concentration presents a conundrum. In particular, during SIRS, serum zinc will fall to about half the normal level and will remain depressed until resolved. This decline is secondary to zinc sequestration, which represents a host mechanism to control leukocyte cytokine production.[16] In situations where SIRS is suspected, evaluating serum CRP, an acute phase protein, may help differentiate between a declining serum/plasma zinc level due to an acute phase reaction (APR) and a declining level associated with increased requirements.[16,104] An elevated CRP level is consistent with the APR. Although an analysis of leukocyte zinc and lymphocyte 5′-nucleotidase activities provides more specific and sensitive indicators of zinc status, the current laboratory procedures are too tedious to perform. Serum or plasma zinc concentrations less than 70 mcg/dL (10.7 μmol/L) are considered low, and plasma zinc levels between 70 and 85 mcg/dL (10.7 to 13 μmol/L) generally indicate a marginal zinc status. Clinical manifestations are noted at serum or plasma levels less than 33 mcg/dL. These values should be interpreted cautiously with hypoalbuminemia because zinc transport is dependent on adequate albumin levels.

TABLE 8-6 Daily Parenteral Trace Element Supplementation for Adults (Dose per Day)[50,111,134]

Trace Element	Previous Recommendations (AMA, 1979)[131]	Current Recommendations (A.S.P.E.N., 2004)[132]	GI Losses
Zinc	2.5–4.0 mg	2.5–5 mg[a]	Add[b]
Copper	0.5–1.5 mg	0.3–0.5 mg	500 mcg/d
Chromium	10–15 mcg	10–15 mcg	20 mcg/d[c]
Iron	Not routinely added		
Manganese	150–800 mcg	60–100 mcg	
Selenium	None	20–60 mcg	

[a]Additional 2 mg/d to hypermetabolic patients for a total of 6–12 mg/d.
[b]Add 12 mg/L of small bowel losses and 17 mcg/kg of stool or ileostomy losses.
[c]Check hemoglobin A1C every 6 months.

Copper (Cu)

Copper homeostasis is maintained primarily by excretion rather than by absorption. Most of the copper in food is in the Cu^{2+} ionic state bound to organic compounds such as amino acids. Hence, digestion is necessary to free the copper before absorption. Gastric secretions, HCl, and pepsin assist in the release of bound copper in the stomach, which also has some degree of copper absorption capacity. Most absorption occurs throughout the small intestine, especially in the duodenum. Two mechanisms involved in copper absorption include a saturable, active transport system and a nonsaturable, passive diffusion.[106] Similar to other transport systems, the active transport system operates during low dietary copper intakes, whereas passive diffusion is activated during high dietary intakes. Typically, the intestinal absorption of copper ranges from about 12% to 75%, with higher intakes associated with low absorptive capacity. The reverse is true at low intakes. Hence, the percent of copper absorbed is dependent on dietary copper availability and the body's current copper status. The efficiency of copper absorption changes in order to regulate copper status, with changes in fecal excretion mediating the process. For example, as copper stores increase, biliary copper excretion increases. Dietary factors that negatively influence copper absorption include phytates, dietary fiber, zinc, iron, large doses of calcium gluconate, molybdenum, and large doses of vitamin C. Protein carriers, albumin, and specific trans-cuprein transporters (CTR1, ATP7A) transport copper from the intestinal cell into the hepatocytes and Kupffer cells within the liver.[106,107] Following hepatic uptake, copper is either incorporated into liver enzymes (cytochrome *c* oxidase, superoxide dismutase) or the acute phase protein, ceruloplasmin, which is then either secreted into the blood for transport to extrahepatic tissues, or excreted in bile.

Aside from transporting copper to cells via the specific ceruloplasmin cell surface receptor, ceruloplasmin acts as a scavenger of reactive oxygen species or free radicals. It also catalyzes the oxidation of ferrous ion. Both serum ceruloplasmin and copper levels increase proportionally to the severity of the APR. Elevated serum ceruloplasmin during an infection may occur to increase copper transport to stimulate cuproenzyme synthesis and/or to inactivate inflammation-induced free radicals. These responses are considered a nonspecific host defense mechanism. Postprandially, 60% to 95% of circulating copper exists as a constituent of ceruloplasmin.[106]

Copper is involved in a myriad of biological processes. It primarily functions in oxidation-reduction and electron transfer reactions involving oxygen (eg, cytochrome *c* oxidase).[106] The three copper enzymes that have a role in antioxidant defense are superoxide dismutases (SOD), ceruloplasmin, and copper thioneins. Ceruloplasmin is also responsible for manganese (Mn^{2+}) oxidation and oxidation of ferrous iron (Fe^{2+}) to ferric (Fe^{3+}) iron. Select copper-dependent enzymes and their roles include lysyl oxidase, which forms cross-linkages found in collagen and elastin; dopamine monooxygenase, necessary for the conversion of dopamine to norepinephrine; peptidylglycine α-amidating monooxygenase, necessary for the activation and deactivation of various peptide hormones; and other copper-containing enzymes, which are used for the formation and maintenance of myelin. In addition, copper is necessary for cholesterol and glucose metabolism, and the formation of melatonin pigment.[106,107] Table 8-4 lists the RDA intake and sources for copper.[5]

Clinically evident copper deficiency is uncommon, but can result from poor copper intake, decreased absorption, or increased losses from the GI tract. The clinical presentation of copper deficiency is found in Table 8-5.[11,106–108] Those at greatest risk for developing copper deficiency include those with malabsorptive disorders like celiac disease, those recovering from undernutrition associated with chronic diarrhea, those consuming a milk-based diet, individuals recovering from intestinal surgery or possibly patients after bariatric surgery, or those receiving hemodialysis where copper losses can be excessive. Copper deficiency can be a complication of celiac disease with hematological alterations and rather debilitating and often irreversible neurologic deficits.[109] Copper supplementation is prophylactically advocated in individuals with celiac disease when anemia or neutropenia is present. As noted earlier, overzealous zinc supplementation can hamper copper absorption, as can H_2 antagonist or PPI medications.

Copper toxicity is uncommon because the body regulates copper storage via biliary excretion. As a result, impaired biliary excretion or cholestasis may cause copper retention in the hepatocyte, leading to oxidative damage.[106] Chronic ingestion of excessive copper amounts can result in liver cirrhosis in those with a genetic predisposition (eg, Wilson disease) with an accumulation of copper in the liver and other organs.[106,108] No clinically significant deleterious effects of copper ingestion have been observed with intakes equal to 0.5 mg of copper per kilogram body weight per day. Intakes between 10 to 15 mg can cause a metallic taste, diarrhea, and vomiting. Copper should not be administered, or should be administered with caution, in patients with hepatic dysfunction because it is excreted via the liver. There is a risk of iatrogenic hepatic copper overload in patients receiving PN, which has the potential to do irreparable harm to the liver.[110] Autopsy reports in long-term PN adult patients have revealed some alarming results about copper accumulation. Major elevations in copper (and manganese) were found, which suggests modification to the current parenteral copper recommendations.[111]

The preferred biomarker to assess copper status is serum copper concentration because it reflects changes in both depleted and repleted patients.[112] Serum ceruloplasmin levels are useful as well but may not reflect hepatic Cu stores.[112] Serum ceruloplasmin levels, and subsequently copper, increase in response to SIRS; therefore, the identification of SIRS by the measurement of serum CRP concentration may assist in the interpretation of Cu laboratory findings.[112]

Manganese (Mn)

Manganese is a ubiquitous mineral found in a wide range of oxidative states, yet in humans it occurs only in the divalent state. Although the specific mechanism for manganese absorption is unclear, it seems similar to that of iron absorption. It is absorbed in the Mn^{2+} state equally well throughout the intestine.[113] Approximately 1% to 5% of dietary Mn is absorbed. The absorption process is quickly saturated, such that absorption decreases at high Mn intakes, thus protecting against toxicity. Absorption of Mn can be influenced by iron because iron competes for common binding sites with manganese.[114]

Manganese enters the liver via the portal circulation. There it is oxidized by ceruloplasmin to Mn^{3+}, possibly complexes with transferrin, and is delivered to extrahepatic tissues.[114] Virtually 100% of manganese is excreted via the hepatobiliary system into the feces. Dietary excess is quickly excreted by the liver into bile to maintain manganese homeostasis and to prevent toxicity.

Manganese functions as a constituent of various metalloenzymes and as an activator of certain enzymes. The Mn-containing metalloenzymes include arginase, which is necessary for urea formation; pyruvate carboxylase, which is necessary for carbohydrate synthesis from pyruvate; and Mn SOD, which has antioxidant properties. Mn also activates numerous enzymes such as glycosyltransferases, phosphoenolpyruvate carboxylase, and glutamine synthetase.[113] Table 8-4 lists AI and sources for this mineral.[5]

Manganese deficiency is rare unless the mineral is totally absent in the diet. Symptoms of a manganese deficiency are described in Table 8-5.[1,113]

Because Mn is almost exclusively eliminated via the hepatobiliary system, any patient with hepatobiliary disease such as cholestatic liver disease may be predisposed to Mn toxicity.[115] Manganese toxicity can result in severe abnormalities of the central nervous system (Table 8-5).[113,116] Populations at risk for developing manganese toxicity include those receiving long-term PN (greater than 30 days), who develop obstruction of the biliary duct and are unable to excrete manganese.[116,117] More than 50% of home PN patients have exhibited hypermagnesemia, coupled with clinically significant cerebral and hepatic complications.[115] As previously mentioned, both Mn and Cu levels were elevated in the autopsies of home PN patients.[111] The scientific data continue to accumulate and suggest a reevaluation for prevention of hypermagnesemia and its deleterious consequences. Reports of manganese brain deposition can occur with IV manganese administration of 1.1 mg/d. An oral manganese intake less than 10 mg/d is considered safe.[5]

Reliable biomarkers for determining manganese status have not been identified. Consistent changes in blood/plasma manganese have not been seen in Mn-depleted and Mn-repleted human subjects.[113] Magnetic resonance imaging (MRI) can detect toxicity; however, the procedure is quite expensive.[113] Monitoring whole blood manganese levels is best to monitor trace element status because levels correlate well with MRI abnormalities.

Selenium (Se)

The nonmetal selenium exists in several ionic states, Se^{2-}, Se^{4+}, and Se^{6+}. Selenium content in food depends on soil concentration, which varies widely throughout the world. Most selenium in foods is complexed with derivatives of the amino acids methionine and cysteine. Selenomethionine, the primary dietary form, is derived from plant sources, and selenocysteine is derived from animal sources of food; both are called selenoproteins. The bioavailability of ingested Se is approximately 50% to 100% but can be influenced by luminal factors.[118]

Both forms of Se are well absorbed. Following absorption, selenium is bound to the major plasma protein, selenoprotein P. The role of selenoprotein P in selenium transport remains unclear. Selenium homeostasis is maintained almost equally through urinary and fecal excretion.

The best understood biochemical function of selenium is as a required cofactor in glutathione, iodine, and thyroid metabolism.[118,119] Some Se-dependent enzymes include glutathione peroxidase, iodothyronine deiodinase, and selenoprotein P. Glutathione peroxidase catalyzes reactions to eliminate hydrogen peroxide; iodothyronine deiodinase catalyzes the deiodination of iodine, triiodothyronine, and reverse triiodothyronine; and selenoprotein P is associated with oxidative defense properties.[118-120] The RDA and sources for Se are listed in Table 8-4.[4] Practice Scenario 8-3 discusses the role of selenium in injured and ill patients.

The metabolic effects of a selenium deficiency are outlined in Table 8-5.[118,119] There are several reports of cardiomyopathy and skeletal muscle weakness in patients who received long-term PN without selenium supplementation and in patients with thermal injury.[104,106,120] The statin class of cholesterol-lowering agents inhibit the enzyme 3-hydroxy-3-methylglutaryl coenzyme A reductase and can induce myopathy by interfering with the synthesis of selenoproteins. Depressed serum Se levels in trauma patients postinjury have resulted in decreased thyroxine deiodination, which might explain the changes observed in thyroid metabolism posttrauma.[121]

Selenium toxicity is also known as selenosis and Table 8-5 lists the signs.[106] Because of the potential for selenosis, the consumption of less than 200 mcg of Se per day or no more than 5 mcg/kg body weight each day has been recommended.[118] See Table 8-4 for UL.[4]

Approximately 50% of plasma Se is found as selenoprotein P and 30% as glutathione peroxidase. The plasma or serum Se concentration can be assessed using a variety of methodologies.[122] The plasma or serum selenium concentration reflects the recent intake of selenium, whereas the erythrocyte concentration indicates long-term selenium status. The measurement of plasma glutathione peroxidase reflects the functional status of selenium; values less than 10.5 U/mL erythrocytes denote deficiency. As a general guideline, plasma or serum concentrations of selenium greater than 100 mcg/L represent adequate selenium status.[4] Relationships continue to emerge linking selenium status with numerous chronic diseases (eg, hypertension, cardiovascular disease, cancer, diabetes mellitus) and may alter what is recommended for Se nutriture to avoid deficiency and toxicity.

Practice Scenario 8-3

Question: Is selenium supplementation necessary when parenteral glutamine is administered to the critically ill patient?

Scenario: A 28-year-old male was admitted to the trauma intensive care unit (ICU) after an all-terrain vehicle accident. Injuries include an open tibia/fibula fracture, multiple rib fractures, pneumothorax, lung contusion, and multiple lacerations and abrasions.

Intervention: On hospital day 2, after fluid resuscitation, a high protein enteral formula was initiated with delivery goal of 28 kcals/kg and 1.7 g pro/kg. A preparation consisting of selenium, vitamin C, and vitamin E was administered concurrently with the enteral nutrition (EN) formula plus a glutamine supplement that provided 0.4 g/kg/day. The patient was ventilator dependent for 7 days and made one trip to the operating room for the repair of the complex fracture.

Answer: Both selenium and glutamine have been shown to individually have positive effects in trauma patients. However, evidence-based research fails to validate that Se supplementation is necessary concurrent therapy with enteral glutamine. It remains prudent to provide an antioxidant preparation consisting of selenium, vitamin C, and vitamin E in tandem with enteral glutamine.

Rationale: For patients with multiple trauma, glutamine becomes a conditionally essential amino acid because endogenous production cannot meet metabolic demands, in part secondary to increased losses.[121] Glutamine supplementation in the trauma population has been shown to improve outcomes in multiple ways, including reduced mortality. Intravenous glutamine also produces beneficial antioxidant effects but is not readily available in the United States due to problems with stability.[16,121] Enteral glutamine has been shown to produce positive outcomes, likely secondary to its beneficial role in maintaining gastrointestinal integrity.[16] Selenium has been shown to be a powerful antioxidant.[120,121] A combination of antioxidant nutrients that includes selenium may improve outcomes in critically ill and trauma patients on mechanical ventilation. Both selenium and glutamine have been shown to individually have positive effects in trauma patients. However, one clinical study failed to show a synergistic effect of administrating selenium and glutamine together in PN toward minimizing the incidence of new infections in critically ill patients with GI failure.[121] The role of both of these nutrients in acute care settings is still evolving and needs further investigation.

Iodine (I)

Iodine refers to the element in any ionic form but generally to I_2, the molecular form. The iodide content in foods varies according to the soil concentration and the amount of fertilizer used in plant cultivation. Although the predominant source of dietary iodide comes from iodized salt, the other dietary sources are either bound to amino acids or are found free as iodate (IO_3^-), which is reduced by glutathione to iodide during digestion. Both are rapidly absorbed in the stomach and the upper small intestine.[123,124] Absorbed iodide appears in the portal blood where most is rapidly taken up by the thyroid (70% to 80%) for the synthesis of thyroid hormones. Lesser amounts are found in the kidney, salivary glands, and other tissues. The kidneys are the principal route of excretion.

Iodine functions as an integral component of the thyroid hormones, thyroxine (T_4) and triiodothyronine (T_3).[123] The metabolically active form of T_3 regulates the rate of cell metabolism, as well as the activity and growth in multiple tissues including fetal, neuronal, and those in the periphery.[123] Table 8-4 lists the RDA and sources for iodine.[5]

In an iodine deficiency, insufficient thyroxine is produced, thereby eliminating its negative feedback on thyroid-stimulating hormone (TSH). This results in a constant release of TSH from the pituitary gland, which results in hyperplasia of the thyroid gland or goiter. See Table 8-5 for signs and symptoms of an iodine deficiency.[124]

Iodine is generally well tolerated when thyroid function is normal. If iodine deficiency is present, and iodine intake is increased too rapidly, then normal control mechanisms are ineffective and thyrotoxicosis can occur. Other clinical signs of the so-called Jod-Basedow phenomenon are found in Table 8-5. This phenomenon is especially problematic for the elderly.[123,124] In adults, intakes between 50 and 1000 mcg/d are generally considered safe.[1] See Table 8-4 for the UL.[5] Iodine requirements in adult patients receiving enteral or PN range between 70 and 150 mcg/d.[124] Current parenteral micronutrient formulations do not contain iodine. Hospitalized patients receive iodine primarily from iodine-containing antiseptic preparations absorbed via the skin.

An assessment of iodine status is focused on both the physical exam and biomarkers. Either repeated 24-hour samples or the concentration of iodine in random samples of urine is a reliable biomarker for iodine status.[124] Urinary iodine is a useful indicator of I status and values correlate well with thyroglobulin concentrations, a new biomarker for thyroid function.[124] Data from field studies note that a mean urinary iodine value less than 5 mcg/L suggests a risk for iodine deficiency, whereas a value less than 2 mcg/L implies that there is a serious risk that infants will be born with cretinism.[123,124] Elevated serum levels of total T_3 can also denote deficiency (20 to 50 years old, greater than 24 ng/dL; 50 to 90 years old, greater than 181 ng/dL).

Chromium (Cr)

Chromium is an essential trace metal required for glucose and lipid metabolism. It is ubiquitous within nature and in the food supply and can exist in several oxidation states from Cr^{2+} to Cr^{6+}. The trivalent form seems to be the biologically relevant form. Most Cr in the food supply is in the trivalent form, which is the most stable. The Cr^{6+} compounds are strong oxidizing agents that are readily reduced to Cr^{3+} in an acidic environment.

Absorption of dietary chromium within the intestine is rapid, yet poor, ranging from 0.4% to 3%, whereas the remainder is excreted in the feces.[125] A dose-dependent relationship exists; as intake increases, absorption efficiency decreases. Absorption averages 2% at intakes of 10 mcg, whereas it decreases to 0.5% at doses of 40 mcg. Cr^{6+} is absorbed more readily than Cr^{3+}.[125,126] Some Cr^{3+} is soluble in the stomach and may form complexes with ligands in the acid environment. The remaining chromium is absorbed via nonmediated passive diffusion throughout the intestine, primarily in the jejunum.

Although little is known about the mechanism for Cr^{3+} absorption, the transport modality in the blood is more clearly understood. Trivalent chromium binds competitively with transferrin and is then transported into the blood along with iron. Consequently, Cr uses the Fe transport system for movement from the blood into cells where a rapid transfer from transferrin to the oligopeptide, chromodulin, occurs.[125,126] Chromodulin, formerly called "glucose tolerance factor," binds four Cr^{3+}. Interestingly, increases in serum glucose are accompanied by increases in chromium excretion. This suggests that chromium stored or maintained in the blood is mobilized in response to increases in insulin concentrations and is ultimately excreted in the urine as chromodulin.

Chromium potentiates the action of insulin; therefore, it has a role in glucose, protein, and lipid metabolism and, as such, is required for growth. The biologically active form of chromium is chromodulin, which serves some role in insulin signaling, amplifying the tyrosine kinase activity of the insulin receptor.[125,126] Conditions that lead to increased urinary excretion of Cr include type II diabetes and pregnancy.[125] Thus, individuals with these conditions may benefit from Cr supplementation. Table 8-4 lists the AI and the sources for chromium.[5]

Evidence for Cr deficiency in humans is sparse. A Cr deficiency can result in impaired glucose and amino acid use, increased plasma low density lipoprotein (LDL)-cholesterol levels, and peripheral neuropathy.[104,125] Deficiency has been reported in adult PN patients with massive bowel surgery.[126] To date, the only cases of Cr deficiency in humans have been in patients receiving PN without an adequate chromium replacement. The deficiency signs are found in Table 8-5.[126]

The use of Cr supplements is probably unnecessary for the general population. However, the use of certain Cr forms, such as Cr^{3+} picolinate ($Cr[pic]_3$), the most common product, is potentially harmful.[125] Cr taken as a supplement can cause adverse antioxidant side effects. Potential adverse side effects of $Cr(pic)_3$ supplementation are found in Table 8-5.[126] Iron status can be compromised with Cr supplementation because Cr and iron compete for binding sites on transferrin. Serum ferritin levels decrease at chromium intakes of 200 mcg/d. Improvement in glucose control in type II diabetics taking 200 mcg/d of $Cr(pic)_3$ is one positive health benefit. Individuals with altered glucose metabolism might benefit from pharmacological doses of Cr; however, safety issues of $Cr(pic)_3$ remain a concern.

The determination of Cr status is difficult to perform because the mineral is present in extremely low concentrations in the blood, which approach detection limits.[126] Normal serum, erythrocyte, and urine chromium values are less than 0.05 to 0.5 mcg/L, less than 20 to 36 mcg/L, and 0.1 to 2 mcg/L, respectively.

Fluoride (F)

Fluoride is almost completely absorbed (75% to 90%) from the GI tract, and a significant portion is absorbed from the stomach.[127] Absorption generally occurs via passive diffusion, and is inversely related to pH. Thus, factors that promote gastric acid secretion increase the absorption rate. In contrast, factors that inhibit gastric acid secretion decrease absorption. Fluoride appears in the plasma promptly after absorption, primarily in the ionic form. Removal of fluoride from the circulation occurs via kidney excretion (50%) or by deposition in the calcified tissue (bone and developing teeth).

Although fluoride has not been proven to be an essential trace element in humans, it does have a role in bone mineralization and the hardening of tooth enamel.[127,128] The major biochemical function of fluoride is to protect calcified tissues against pathological demineralization by forming fluorapatite crystals rather than the usual hydroxyapatite crystals. Fluoride is also considered important for minimizing the risk of developing dental caries. Due to fluoride's role in inhibiting and reversing the initiation and progression of dental caries, it is considered to be a "beneficial element for humans."[127,128] Fluoride also stimulates new bone formation by stimulating osteoblasts, and it may reduce the risk for osteoporosis.[2] There are also studies suggesting that it may inhibit the calcification of aorta and soft tissues.[129] Table 8-4 lists the AI and sources for fluoride.[2]

Unequivocal or specific signs and symptoms of fluoride deficiency in humans are nonexistent. When an individual is deficient in fluoride, he or she has an increased risk for developing dental caries.[2] Normal ranges for ionic fluoride are 0.01 to 0.2 mcg/mL in the plasma and 0.2 to 1.1 mg/mL in the urine.

Acute fluoride toxicity may result in a variety of symptoms (Table 8-5).[129] A chronic excessive fluoride intake may result in enamel and skeletal fluorosis. The long-term ingestion of very large amounts of F (greater than 5 mg/d) can lead to skeletal fluorosis, which has several stages. The first is the preclinical stage, which is characterized by slight increases in bone mass and higher fluoride concentrations in the bone.[128] Signs and symptoms of stage 1 include stiffness, joint pain, and some osteosclerosis of the pelvis and vertebra.[128] Stages 2 and 3 present with the calcification of ligaments, osteosclerosis, exostoses, long bone osteoporosis, muscle wasting, and neurological defects.[128] Table 8-4 lists the UL for fluoride.[2]

Molybdenum (Mo)

Molybdenum exists as the ionic states, Mo^{4+} or Mo^{6+}, and is generally bound to either sulfur or oxygen. Human absorption ranges from 85% to 93%. The absorption rate is highest in the proximal small intestine. The transport of Mo occurs by an active carrier-mediated process when Mo blood concentrations are low and via passive diffusion when blood concentrations are high. Molybdenum is transported as molybdate, which is loosely attached to erythrocytes, and tends to bind albumin and/or α-macroglobulin.[127,130] After absorption, Mo elimination occurs as molybdate via the kidney. High dietary intakes increase excretion. Hence, Mo regulation is controlled through excretion rather than absorption.

Biochemically, Mo functions as a cofactor for the metalloenzymes aldehyde oxidase, xanthine oxidase, and sulfite oxidase, and catalyzes the hydroxylation of various substrates.[81,125,130] Molybdenum may also stabilize the steroid-binding affinity of the glucocorticoid receptor.[127] Table 8-4 lists the AI and sources for this mineral.[5]

A Mo deficiency due to diet alone is rare. However, a patient with short bowel syndrome who received prolonged PN developed a syndrome of hypermethioninemia, hypouricemia, hyperoxypurinemia, hypouricosuria, and low urinary sulfate excretion, along with mental disturbances that progressed to a coma.[55,127] Contributing factors included the loss of Mo-dependent enzyme, sulfite oxidase activity, and inadequate Mo.[50,125]

Excessive dietary intake (10 to 15 mg daily) or an environmental contamination may result in a goutlike syndrome with elevated blood levels of Mo, uric acid, and xanthine oxidase.[55,127] Moderate doses (ie, 0.54 mg daily) are associated with losses of copper in the urine.[55,127]

There is no standardized method for Mo analysis. Blood levels vary widely in the literature with normal Mo serum/plasma levels reported from 0.58 ± 0.21 to 0.8 ± 0.2 mcg/L.[127]

Ultratrace Elements

Ultratrace elements are defined as those elements with estimated dietary requirements that are usually less than 1 mcg/g and often less than 50 ng/g of diet for laboratory animals.[131] The ultratrace elements include aluminum, arsenic, boron, bromine, cadmium, chromium, fluorine, germanium, lead, lithium, molybdenum, nickel, rubidium, selenium, silicon, tin, and vanadium. The essentiality of these elements varies, depending on the quality of the experimental evidence.[127,131] Research on the ultratrace element boron is beginning to suggest a relationship between adequate boron intake and health, perhaps making it a more relevant nutritional concern than previously thought.[132] There is also substantial circumstantial evidence for the essentiality of arsenic, nickel, silicon, and vanadium.[5] With the exception of Mo, the DRI process did not address the ultratrace elements.

Parenteral Vitamins

The FDA issued new parenteral multivitamin drug dosing requirements in 2000, which are found in Table 8-7.[133,134] Dosages for vitamins thiamin, B_6, C, and folic acid increased, and vitamin K was added to the multivitamin formulation. The addition of vitamin K raises some concern in patients who receive long-term parenteral multivitamin products and use oral anticoagulant therapy to maintain patency of their IV access devices. Regular monitoring of the INR is needed, and warfarin doses may need adjustment because of the vitamin K content in the multivitamin product. Two products currently exist for adult patients, one with vitamin K and one without vitamin K, but both meet the FDA mandate. Other sources of IV vitamin K are found in IVFE but the amount varies from 0 to 290 mcg/L.[38] Weekly intravenous supply of 250 to 500 mcg phylloquinone is adequate to preserve coagulation in PN patients.[38] It is advisable that clinicians give careful consideration to the impact of the administration of parenteral vitamins outside of these recommendations as well as what impact additional amounts have on other micronutrients.

The parenteral multivitamin supplementation of other select nutrients, such as vitamin D and A, presents clinical challenges. Vitamin D preparations for PN are challenging because of the lack of high-dose parenteral formulas of vitamin D. Currently, patients receiving PN receive a daily multivitamin infusion (MVI) that contains 200 to 400 IU (5 to 10 mcg) of vitamin D. There is an intramuscular form of high-dose vitamin D available outside the United States. It is not currently recommended in the United States because of solubility and absorption inconsistencies, unpredictable clinical response, and significant pain upon administration. An alternative and effective method to ensure vitamin D status for long-term PN patients is simply sunlight exposure or UVB radiation therapy from tanning beds, although concerns regarding the risk of skin cancer cannot be minimized.[135] Other parenteral vitamins have already been previously discussed respective of the nutrient.

The standard practice to avoid the risk of hypervitaminosis A in chronic renal failure patients receiving PN is simply to avoid vitamin A–containing multivitamins, whereas for end-stage renal failure patients, an oral water-soluble vitamin complex is recommended. The dose of vitamin A in the standard PN MVI for adults is 3300 IU.[15]

TABLE 8-7 Parenteral Multivitamin Products[50,133,134]

Vitamin	Amount
Fat-Soluble Vitamins	
Vitamin A (retinol)	1 mg
Vitamin D (ergocalciferol or cholecalciferol)	5 mcg
Vitamin E (alpha-tocopherol)	10 mg
Vitamin K (phylloquinone)	150 mcg
Water-Soluble Vitamins	
B_1 (Thiamin)	6 mg
B_2 (Riboflavin)	3.6 mg
B_6 (Pyridoxine)	6 mg
B_{12} (Cyanocobalamin)	5 mcg
Niacin	40 mg
Folic acid	600 mcg
Pantothenic acid	15 mg
Biotin	60 mcg
Vitamin C (ascorbic acid)	200 mg

Parenteral Trace Elements

The American Medical Association (AMA) and the American Society for Parenteral and Enteral Nutrition (A.S.P.E.N.) have published recommendations for daily parenteral intake of the trace elements zinc, copper, manganese, and chromium.[50,134] Selenium supplementation of 20 to 60 mcg/d is also now recommended for patients receiving PN therapy.[50] The recommended adult daily intake of IV trace elements is found in Table 8-6. Significant alterations in parenteral dosing have previously been mentioned under the respective trace element.

Enteral Vitamins and Mineral Adequacy

Data on the clinical implications regarding micronutrient stability in enteral formulations are limited. Variability in enteral feeding containers, light exposure, hang time, storage temperatures, and shelf life beyond 1 year can cause a reduction in micronutrient value.[136,137] Specific nutrient losses of thiamin, riboflavin, and vitamins A and E have been reported between 20°C and 30°C compared to room temperature (4°C). Storing enteral nutrition (EN) beyond 9 months results in a loss of these nutrients as well.[138] Enteral products hung longer than 6 hours may influence stability of the light sensitive vitamins, riboflavin and thiamin. Currently, enteral formula manufacturers are not required to label products according to the DRI. It would be helpful to require manufacturers to include stability information on EN formulas. Adherence to the EN practice standards mitigates most of the stability issues.[137]

Best Practice: The Clinician's Role in Micronutrient Management

Since the early years of PN and enteral nutrition, clinicians administered trace elements periodically via parenteral infusions or inadvertently through trace mineral contamination found in amino acid solutions. As scientific data accumulated, clinical practice guidelines (CPG) were systematically developed to aid practitioners and patient decisions about appropriate health care for specific clinical circumstances.[50,136,137] These statements offer clinical advice for the management of patients receiving nutrition support therapy. They are the culmination of extensive literature reviews, consultation, and consensus among experts in nutrition support designed to offer recommendations supported by evidence-based research. Such guidelines include the justification, dosage, and the route of delivery for inclusion of vitamins and trace minerals in patients receiving specialized nutrition therapy. Standards for supplementation as well as reformulations of micronutrient products aid clinicians in treating patients on nutrition support. Guideline adherence ensures optimum nutrition care and improves patient outcomes. The original concept of Nutrition Support Teams (NST) was perhaps a prelude to CPGs.

A professional practice consultation during shortages of parenteral vitamins or trace elements is critical. Clinicians involved in the delivery of specialized nutrition therapy should seek the recommendations on usage from A.S.P.E.N., the American Society of Health-System Pharmacists (ASHP) Drug Shortages Resource Center, or the FDA, Drug Shortage Program, and Current Drug Shortages bulletins. Some strategies recommended include reassessing the indication of micronutrient supplementation, providing oral doses, and prioritizing the most vulnerable populations. To avoid micronutrient deficiencies in patients receiving EN or PN, whatever the reason, clinicians with NST, when available, collectively need to continuously monitor and reassess the need for micronutrient supplementation.[139]

Acknowledgement

I would like to generously thank Brittany Cochran, RD, MS, Clinical Dietitian at Carilion Roanoke Memorial Hospital in Roanoke, VA for her contributions in developing the practice scenarios for this chapter.

References

1. Food and Nutrition Board, National Research Council. *Recommended Dietary Allowances*. 10th ed. Washington, DC: National Academy of Sciences; 1989.
2. Food and Nutrition Board, Institute of Medicine. *Dietary Reference Intakes for Calcium, Phosphorus, Magnesium, Vitamin D, and Fluoride*. Washington, DC: National Academy Press; 1998.
3. Food and Nutrition Board, Institute of Medicine. *Dietary Reference Intakes for Thiamin, Riboflavin, Niacin, Vitamin B_6, Folate, Vitamin B_{12}, Pantothenic Acid, Biotin, and Choline*. Washington, DC: National Academy Press; 1998.
4. Food and Nutrition Board, Institute of Medicine. *Dietary Reference Intakes for Vitamin C, Vitamin E, Selenium, and Carotenoids*. Washington, DC: National Academy Press; 2004.
5. Food and Nutrition Board, Institute of Medicine. *Dietary Reference Intakes for Vitamin D and Calcium*. Washington, DC: National Academy Press; 2011.
6. Food and Nutrition Board, Institute of Medicine. *Dietary Reference Intakes for Vitamin A, Vitamin K, Arsenic, Boron, Chromium, Copper, Iodine, Iron, Manganese, Molybdenum, Nickel, Silicon, Vanadium, and Zinc*. Washington, DC: National Academy Press; 2000.
7. Hambidge KM. Micronutrient bioavailability: Dietary Reference Intakes and a future. *Am J Clin Nutr*. 2010;91(5):1430–1432.
8. Delegge M, Wooley JA, Guenter P, et al. The state of nutrition support teams and update on current models for providing nutrition support therapy to patients. *Nutr Clin Pract*. 2010; 25(1):76–84.
9. Ross AC. Vitamin A and carotenoids. In: Shils ME, Shike M, Ross AC, Caballero B, Cousins RJ, eds. *Modern Nutrition in Health and Disease*. 10th ed. Philadelphia, PA: Lippincott Williams & Wilkins; 2006:351–375.
10. Arnold M, Barbul, A. Nutrition and wound healing. *Plast Reconstr Surg*. 2006;117(7 Suppl):42S–58S.
11. Kumar N. Neurologic presentations of nutritional deficiencies. *Neurol Clin*. 2010;28(1):107–170.
12. Stechmiller JK, Cowan L, Logan KM. Nutrition support for wound healing. *Support Line*. 2009;31:2–7.
13. Genaro Pde S, Martini LA. Vitamin A supplementation and risk of skeletal fracture. *Nutr Rev*. 2004;62(2):65–72.
14. Cabral PC, Diniz Ada S, de Arruda IK. Vitamin A and zinc status in patients on maintenance haemodialysis. *Nephrol*. 2005;10(5): 459–463.
15. Brown RO, Compher C. A.S.P.E.N. clinical guidelines: Nutrition support in adult acute and chronic renal failure. *JPEN J Parenter Enteral Nutr*. 2010;34(4):366–377.
16. McClave SA, Martindale RG, Vanek VW, et al. Guidelines for the provision and assessment of nutrition support therapy in the adult critically ill patient: Society of Critical Care Medicine (SCCM) and American Society for Parenteral and Enteral Nutrition (A.S.P.E.N.). *JPEN J Parenter Enteral Nutr*. 2009;33(3):277–316.
17. Stechmiller JK. Understanding the role of nutrition and wound healing. *Nutr Clin Pract*. 2010;25(1):61–68.
18. Tanumihardjo SA. Assessing vitamin A status: past, present and future. *J Nutr*. 2004;134(1):290S–293S.
19. Holick MF. Vitamin D. In: Shils ME, Shike M, Ross AC, Caballero B, Cousins J, eds. *Modern Nutrition in Health and Disease*. 10th ed. Philadelphia, PA: Lippincott Williams & Wilkins; 2006: 376–395.
20. Seifert M, Tilgen W, Reichrath J. Expression of 25-hydroxyvitamin D 1alpha-hydroxylase (1alphaOHase, CYP27B1) splice variants in HaCaT keratinocytes and other skin cells: modulation by culture conditions and UV-B treatment in vitro. *Anticancer Res*. 2009; 29(9):3659–3667.
21. Norman AW. From vitamin D to hormone D: fundamentals of the vitamin D endocrine system essential for good health. *Am J Clin Nutr*. 2008;88(2):491S–499S.
22. Holick MF. Vitamin D: evolutionary, physiological and health perspectives. *Curr Drug Targets*. 2011;12(1):4–18.
23. Pittas AG, Laskowski U, Kos L, et al. Role of vitamin D in adults requiring nutrition support. *JPEN J Parenter Enteral Nutr*. 2011; 34(1):70–78.
24. Lee JO, Benjamin D, Herndon DN. Nutrition support strategies for severely burned patients. *Nutr Clin Pract*. 2005;20(3):325–330.
25. Heaney RP. Vitamin D in health and disease. *Clin J Am Soc Nephrol*. 2008;3(5):1535–1541.
26. Seamans KM, Cashman KD. Existing and potentially novel functional markers of vitamin D status: a systematic review. *Am J Clin Nutr*. 2009;89(6):1997S–2008S.
27. Traber MG. Vitamin E. In: Shils ME, Shike M, Ross AC, Caballero B, Cousins RJ, eds. *Modern Nutrition in Health and Disease*. 10th ed. Philadelphia, PA: Lippincott Williams & Wilkins; 2006:396–411.
28. Zingg JM. Vitamin E: An overview of major research directions. *Molecular Aspects of Medicine*. 2007;28(5–6):400–422.
29. Biesalski HK. Vitamin E requirements in parenteral nutrition. *Gastroenterology*. 2009;137(5 Suppl):S92–S104.
30. Maras JE, Bermudez OI, Qiao N, et al. Intake of alpha-tocopherol is limited among US adults. *J Am Diet Assoc*. 2004;104(4):567–575.

31. Ahuja JK, Goldman JD, Moshfegh AJ. Current status of vitamin E nutriture. *Ann N Y Acad Sci.* 2004;1031:387–390.
32. Bell SJ, Grochoski GT. How safe is vitamin E supplementation? *Crit Rev Food Sci Nutr.* 2008;48(8):760–774.
33. Steiner M. Vitamin E, a modifier of platelet function: rationale and use in cardiovascular and cerebrovascular disease. *Nutr Rev.* 1999; 57(10):306–309.
34. Suttie JW. Vitamin K1. In: Shils ME, Shike M, Ross AC, Caballero B, Cousins RJ, eds. *Modern Nutrition in Health and Disease.* 10th ed. Philadelphia, PA: Lippincott Williams & Wilkins; 2006: 412–425.
35. Bügel S. Vitamin K and bone health in adult humans. *Vitam Horm.* 2008;78:393–416.
36. Cockayne S, Adamson J, Lanham-New S, et al. Vitamin K and the prevention of fractures: systematic review and meta-analysis of randomized controlled trials. *Arch Intern Med.* 2006;166(12): 1256–1261.
37. Fogle P. Vitamin K and lipid emulsions. *Support Line.* 2001;23:3–8.
38. Shearer MJ. Vitamin K in parenteral nutrition. *Gastroenterology.* 2009;137:S105–S118.
39. Dickerson RN, Garmon WM, Kuhl DA, et al. Vitamin K-independent warfarin resistance after concurrent administration of warfarin and continuous enteral nutrition. *Pharmacotherapy.* 2008;28(3):308–313.
40. Marian M, Sacks G. Micronutrients and older adults. *Nutr Clin Pract.* 2009;24(2):179–195.
41. Kuwabara A, Tanaka K, Tsugawa N, et al. High prevalence of vitamin K and D deficiency and decreased BMD in inflammatory bowel disease. *Osteoporos Int.* 2009;20(6):935–942.
42. Nakano T, Tsugawa N, Kuwabara A, et al. High prevalence of hypovitaminosis D and K in patients with hip fracture. *Asia Pac J Clin Nutr.* 2011;20(1):56–61.
43. Booth SL. Vitamin K status in the elderly. *Curr Opin Clin Nutr Metab Care.* 2007;10(1):20–23.
44. Booth SL, Al Rajabi A. Determinants of vitamin K status in humans. *Vitam Horm.* 2008;78:1–22.
45. Levine M, Katz A, Padayatty SJ. Vitamin C. In: Shils ME, Shike M, Ross AC, Caballero B, Cousins RJ, eds. *Modern Nutrition in Health and Disease.* 10th ed. Philadelphia, PA: Lippincott Williams & Wilkins; 2006:507–524.
46. Mandl J, Szarka A, Bánhegyi G. Vitamin C: update on physiology and pharmacology. *Br J Pharmacol.* 2009;157(7):1097–1110.
47. Schleicher RL, Carroll MD, Ford ES, Lacher DA. Serum vitamin C and the prevalence of vitamin C deficiency in the United States: 2003-2004 National Health and Nutrition Examination Survey (NHANES). *Am J Clin Nutr.* 2009;90(5):1252–1263.
48. Butterworth RF. Thiamin. In: Shils ME, Shike M, Ross AC, Caballero B, Cousins RJ, eds. *Modern Nutrition in Health and Disease.* 10th ed. Philadelphia, PA: Lippincott Williams & Wilkins; 2006:426–433.
49. Sica DA. Loop diuretic therapy, thiamine balance, and heart failure. *Congest Heart Fail.* 2007;13(4):244–247.
50. Task Force for the Revision of Safe Practices for Parenteral Nutrition and the A.S.P.E.N. Board of Directors. Safe practices for parenteral nutrition. *JPEN J Parenter Enteral Nutr.* 2004;28: S39–S70.
51. Keith ME, Walsh NA, Darling PB, et al. B-vitamin deficiency in hospitalized patients with heart failure. *J Am Diet Assoc.* 2009; 109(8):1406–1410.
52. Hanninen SA, Darling PB, Sole MJ, Barr A, Keith ME. The prevalence of thiamin deficiency in hospitalized patients with congestive heart failure. *J Am Coll Cardiol.* 2006;47(2):354–361.
53. Kazemi A, Frazier T, Cave M. Micronutrient-related neurologic complications following bariatric surgery. *Curr Gastroenterol Rep.* 2010;12(4):288–295.
54. Cho YP, Kim K, Han MS, et al. Severe lactic acidosis and thiamine deficiency during total parenteral nutrition—case report. *Hepatogastroenterology.* 2004;51(55):253–255.
55. Heimburger DC, McLaren DS, Shils M. Clinical manifestations of nutrient deficiencies and toxicities: a résumé. In: Shils ME, Shike M, Ross AC, Caballero B, Cousins RJ, eds. *Modern Nutrition in Health and Disease.* 10th ed. Philadelphia, PA: Lippincott Williams & Wilkins; 2006:595–612.
56. McCormick DB. Riboflavin. In: Shils ME, Olson JA, Shike M, eds. *Modern Nutrition in Health and Disease.* 10th ed. Philadelphia, PA: Lippincott Williams & Wilkins; 2006:434–441.
57. Gariballa S, Forster S, Powers H. Riboflavin status in acutely ill patients and response to dietary supplements. *JPEN J Parenter Enteral Nutr.* 2009;33(6):656–661.
58. Hoey L, McNulty H, Strain JJ. Studies of biomarker responses to intervention with riboflavin: a systematic review. *Am J Clin Nutr.* 2009;89(6):1960–1980.
59. Bourgeois C, Cervantes-Laurean D, Moss J. Niacin. In: Shils ME, Shike M, Ross AC, Caballero B, Cousins RJ, eds. *Modern Nutrition in Health and Disease.* 10th ed. Philadelphia, PA: Lippincott Williams & Wilkins; 2006:442–451.
60. Mackey AD, Davis SR, Gregory JF. Vitamin B_6. In: Shils ME, Shike M, Ross AC, Caballero B, Cousins RJ, eds. *Modern Nutrition in Health and Disease.* 10th ed. Philadelphia, PA: Lippincott Williams & Wilkins; 2006:452–461.
61. Matarese LE, Dvorchik I, Costa G, et al. Pyridoxal-5′-phosphate deficiency after intestinal and multivisceral transplantation. *Am J Clin Nutr.* 2009;89(1):204–209.
62. Vasilaki AT, McMillan DC, Kinsella J, et al. Relation between pyridoxal and pyridoxal phosphate concentrations in plasma, red cells, and white cells in patients with critical illness. *Am J Clin Nutr.* 2008;88(1):140-146.
63. Carmel R. Cobalamin (Vitamin B_{12}). In: Shils ME, Olson JA, Shike M, eds. *Modern Nutrition in Health and Disease.* 10th ed. Philadelphia, PA: Lippincott Williams & Wilkins; 2006:482–497.
64. Moestrup SK. New insights into carrier binding and epithelial uptake of the erythropoietic nutrients cobalamin and folate. *Curr Opin Hematol.* 2006;13(3):119–123.
65. Laine L, Ahnen D, McClain C, et al. Review article: potential gastrointestinal effects of long-term acid suppression with proton pump inhibitors. *Aliment Pharmacol Ther.* 2000;14(6): 651–668.
66. McCracken C. Challenges of long-term nutrition intervention studies on cognition: discordance between observational and intervention studies of vitamin B12 and cognition. *Nutr Rev.* 2010;68(Suppl 1):S11–S15.
67. VITATOPS Trial Study Group. B vitamins in patients with recent transient ischaemic attack or stroke in the VITAmins TO Prevent Stroke (VITATOPS) trial: a randomised, double-blind, parallel, placebo-controlled trial. *Lancet Neurol.* 2010;9(9):855–865.
68. McLean RR, Jacques PF, Selhub J, et al. Plasma B vitamins, homocysteine, and their relation with bone loss and hip fracture in elderly men and women. *J Clin Endocrinol Metab.* 2008;93(6): 2206–2222.
69. Herrmann W, Obeid R, Schorr H, Geisel J. The usefulness of holotranscobalamin in predicting vitamin B12 status in different clinical settings. *Curr Drug Metab.* 2005;6(1):47–53.
70. Hoey L, Strain JJ, McNulty H. Studies of biomarker responses to intervention with vitamin B-12: a systematic review of randomized controlled trials. *Am J Clin Nutr.* 2009;89(6):1981S–1996S.
71. Carmel R. Folic acid. In: Shils ME, Shike M, Ross AC, Caballero B, Cousins RJ, eds. *Modern Nutrition in Health and Disease.* 10th ed. Philadelphia, PA: Lippincott Williams & Wilkins; 2006:470–481.

72. Food and Drug Administration. *Food Standards: Amendment of Standards of Identity for Enriched Grain Products to Require Addition of Folic Acid* (final rule). Washington, DC: Author; 1996.
73. Stevenson RE, Allen WP, Pai S, et al. Decline in prevalence of neural tube defects in a high-risk region of the United States. *Pediatrics.* 2000;106(4):677–683.
74. Tamura T, Picciano MF. Folate and human reproduction. *Am J Clin Nutr.* 2006;83(5):993–1016.
75. Eichholzer M, Tonz O, Zimmermann R. Folic acid: a public-health challenge. *Lancet.* 2006;367(9519):1352–1361.
76. Mayer O Jr, Simon J, Rosolova H, et al. The effects of folate supplementation on some coagulation parameters and oxidative status surrogates. *Eur J Clin Pharmacol.* 2002;58(1):1–5.
77. McCracken C, Hudson P, Ellis R, et al. Methylmalonic acid and cognitive function in the Medical Research Council Cognitive Function and Ageing Study. *Am J Clin Nutr.* 2006;84(6): 1406–1411.
78. Herrmann M, Kraenzlin M, Pape G, et al. Relation between homocysteine and biochemical bone turnover markers and bone mineral density in peri- and post-menopausal women. *Clin Chem Lab Med.* 2005;43(10):1118–1123.
79. de Bree A, Verschuren MM, Blom HJ, et al. Coronary heart disease mortality, plasma homocysteine, and B-vitamins: a prospective study. *Atherosclerosis.* 2003;166(2):369–377.
80. Shane B. Folate status assessment history: implications for measurement of biomarkers in NHANES. *Am J Clin Nutr.* 2011;94(1): 337S–342S.
81. Mock DM. Biotin. In: Shils ME, Shike M, Ross AC, Caballero B, Cousins RJ, eds. *Modern Nutrition in Health and Disease.* 10th ed. Philadelphia, PA: Lippincott Williams & Wilkins; 2006:498–506.
82. Wolf B. Clinical issues and frequent questions about biotinidase deficiency. *Mol Genet Metab.* 2010;100(1):6–13.
83. Mock NI, Malik MI, Stumbo PJ, Bishop WP, Mock DM. Increased urinary excretion of 3-hydroxyisovaleric acid and decreased urinary excretion of biotin are sensitive early indicators of decreased status in experimental biotin deficiency. *Am J Clin Nutr.* 1997; 65(4):951–958.
84. Trumbo PR. Pantothenic acid. In: Shils ME, Shike M, Ross AC, Caballero B, Cousins RJ, eds. *Modern Nutrition in Health and Disease.* 10th ed. Philadelphia, PA: Lippincott Williams & Wilkins; 2006:462–469.
85. Zeisel SH, Niculescu MD. Choline and phosphatidylcholine. In: Shils ME, Shike M, Ross AC, Caballero B, Cousins RJ, eds. *Modern Nutrition in Health and Disease.* 10th ed. Philadelphia, PA: Lippincott Williams & Wilkins; 2006:525–536.
86. Zeisel SH, da Costa KA. Choline: an essential nutrient for public health. *Nutr Rev.* 2009;67(11):615–623.
87. Perez C, Koshy C, Ressl S, et al. Substrate specificity and ion coupling in the Na+/betaine symporter BetP. *EMBO J.* 2011;30(7): 1221–1229.
88. Fischer LM, daCosta KA, Kwock L, et al. Sex and menopausal status influence human dietary requirements for the nutrient choline. *Am J Clin Nutr.* 2007;85(5):1275–1285.
89. Caudill MA. Pre- and postnatal health: Evidence of increased choline needs. *J Am Diet Assoc.* 2010;110(8):1198–1206.
90. Buchman AL. Choline deficiency during parenteral nutrition in humans. *Nutr Clin Pract.* 2003;18(5):353–358.
91. Wood RJ, Ronnenberg AG. Iron. In: Shils ME, Shike M, Ross AC, Caballero B, Cousins RJ, eds. *Modern Nutrition in Health and Disease.* 10th ed. Philadelphia, PA: Lippincott Williams & Wilkins; 2006:248–270.
92. Young MF, Glahn RP, Ariza-nieto M, et al. Serum hepcidin is significantly associated with iron absorption from food and supplemental sources in healthy young women. *Am J Clin Nutr.* 2009;89(2):533–538.
93. Muñoz M, García-Erce JA, Remacha AF. Disorders of iron metabolism. Part 1: molecular basis of iron homoeostasis. *J Clin Pathol.* 2011;64(4):281–286.
94. Clark SF. Iron deficiency anemia. *Nutr Clin Pract.* 2011;23(2): 128–141.
95. Muñoz M, García-Erce JA, Remacha ÁF. Disorders of iron metabolism. Part II: iron deficiency and iron overload. *J Clin Pathol.* 2011;64(4):287–296.
96. Ruz M, Carrasco F, Rojas P, et al. Iron absorption and iron status are reduced after Roux-en-Y gastric bypass. *Am J Clin Nutr.* 2009;90(3):527–532.
97. Thurnham DI, Mccabe LD, Haldar S, et al. Adjusting plasma ferritin concentrations to remove the effects of subclinical inflammation in the assessment of iron deficiency. *Am J Clin Nutr.* 2010; 92(3):546–555.
98. Forbes A. Iron and parenteral nutrition. *Gastroenterology.* 2009;137(5 Suppl):S47–54.
99. Clark SF. Iron deficiency anemia: diagnosis and management. *Curr Opin Gastroenterol.* 2009;25(2):122–128.
100. Pasricha SR, McQuilten ZK, Westerman M, et al. Serum hepcidin as a diagnostic test of iron deficiency in premenopausal female blood donors. *Haematologica.* 2011;96(8):1099–1105.
101. King JC, Cousins RJ. Zinc. In: Shils ME, Shike M, Ross AC, Caballero B, Cousins RJ, eds. *Modern Nutrition in Health and Disease.* 10th ed. Philadelphia, PA: Lippincott Williams & Wilkins; 2006:271–285.
102. Heyland DK, Jones N, Cvijanovich NZ, Wong H. Zinc supplementation in critically ill patients: a key pharmaconutrient? *JPEN J Parenter Enteral Nutr.* 2011;32(5):509–519.
103. Wiernsperger N, Rapin J. Trace elements in glucometabolic disorders: an update. *Diabetol Metab Syndr.* 2010;2:70–79.
104. Fuhrman MP. Micronutrient assessment in long-term home parenteral nutrition patients. *Nutr Clin Pract.* 2006;21(6):566–575.
105. Lowe NM, Fekete K, Decsi T. Methods of assessment of zinc status in humans: a systematic review. *Am J Clin Nutr.* 2009;89(6): 2040–2051.
106. Turnlund JR. Copper. In: Shils ME, Shike M, Ross AC, Caballero B, Cousins RJ, eds. *Modern Nutrition in Health and Disease.* 10th ed. Philadelphia, PA: Lippincott Williams & Wilkins; 2006: 286–299.
107. Uauy R, Maass A, Araya M. Estimating risk from copper excess in human populations. *Am J Clin Nutr.* 2008;88(3):867S–871S.
108. Shike M. Copper in parenteral nutrition. *Gastroenterology.* 2009;137(5 Suppl):S13–S17.
109. Halfdanarson TR, Kumar N, Hogan WJ, Murray JA. Copper deficiency in celiac disease. *J Clin Gastroenterol.* 2009;43(2): 162–164.
110. Blaszyk H, Wild PJ, Oliveira A, Kelly DG, Burgart LJ. Hepatic copper in patients receiving long-term total parenteral nutrition. *J Clin Gastroenterol.* 2005;39(4):318–320.
111. Howard L, Ashley C, Lyon D, Shenkin A. Autopsy tissue trace elements in 8 long-term parenteral nutrition patients who received the current U.S. Food and Drug Administration formulation. *JPEN J Parenter Enteral Nutr.* 2007;31(5):388–396.
112. Harvey LJ, Ashton K, Hooper L, Casgrain A, Fairweather-Tait SJ. Methods of assessment of copper status in humans: a systematic review. *Am J Clin Nutr.* 2009;89(6):2009S–2024S.
113. Buchman AL. Manganese. In: Shils ME, Shike M, Ross AC, Caballero B, Cousins RJ, eds. *Modern Nutrition in Health and Disease.* 10th ed. Philadelphia, PA: Lippincott Williams & Wilkins; 2006:326–331.
114. Aschner JL, Aschner M. Nutritional aspects of manganese homeostasis. *Mol Aspects Med.* 2005;26(4–5):353–362.

115. Dickerson RN. Manganese intoxication and parenteral nutrition. *Nutrition.* 2001;17(7–8):689–693.
116. Dobson AW, Erikson KM, Aschner M. Manganese neurotoxicity. *Ann N Y Acad Sci.* 2004;1012:115–128.
117. Hardy G. Manganese in parenteral nutrition: who, when, and why should we supplement? *Gastroenterology.* 2009;137(5 Suppl):S29–S35.
118. Burk RF, Levander OA. Selenium. In: Shils ME, Shike M, Ross AC, Caballero B, Cousins RJ, eds. *Modern Nutrition in Health and Disease.* 10th ed. Philadelphia, PA: Lippincott Williams & Wilkins; 2006:312–325.
119. Boosalis MG. The role of selenium in chronic disease. *Nutr Clin Pract.* 2008;23(2):152–160.
120. Shenkin A. Selenium in intravenous nutrition. *Gastroenterology.* 2009;137(5 Suppl):S61–S69.
121. Andrews PJ. Selenium and glutamine supplements: where are we heading? A critical care perspective. *Curr Opin Clin Nutr Metab Care.* 2010;13(2):192–197.
122. Ashton K, Hooper L, Harvey LJ, et al. Methods of assessment of selenium status in humans: a systematic review. *Am J Clin Nutr.* 2009;89(6):2025S–2039S.
123. Dunn JT. Iodine. In: Shils ME, Shike M, Ross AC, Caballero B, Cousins RJ, eds. *Modern Nutrition in Health and Disease.* 10th ed. Philadelphia, PA: Lippincott Williams & Wilkins; 2006: 300–311.
124. Zimmermann MB, Crill CM. Iodine in enteral and parenteral nutrition. *Best Pract Res Clin Endocrinol Metab.* 2010;24(1): 143–158.
125. Stoecher BJ. Chromium. In: Shils ME, Shike M, Ross AC, Caballero B, Cousins RJ, eds. *Modern Nutrition in Health and Disease.* 10th ed. Philadelphia, PA: Lippincott Williams & Wilkins; 2006: 332–337.
126. Moukarzel A. Chromium in parenteral nutrition: too little or too much? *Gastroenterology.* 2009;137(5 Suppl):S18–S28.
127. Nielsen FH. Boron, manganese, molybdenum, and other trace elements. In: Bowman BA, Russel RM, eds. *Present Knowledge in Nutrition.* 8th ed. Washington, DC: ILSI Press; 2001:384–400.
128. Warren JJ, Levy SM. Current and future role of fluoride in nutrition. *Dent Clin North Am.* 2003;47(2):225–243.
129. Eren E, Ozturk M, Mumcu EF, Canatan D. Fluorosis and its hematological effects. *Toxicol Ind Health.* 2005;21(10):255–258.
130. Schwarz G, Mendel RR. Molybdenum cofactor biosynthesis and molybdenum enzymes. *Ann Rev Plant Biol.* 2006;57:623–647.
131. Eckhert CD. Other trace elements. In: Shils ME, Shike M, Ross AC, Caballero B, Cousins RJ, eds. *Modern Nutrition in Health and Disease.* 10th ed. Philadelphia, PA: Lippincott Williams & Wilkins; 2006:338–350.
132. Nielsen FH. Is boron nutritionally relevant? *Nutr Rev.* 2008; 66(4):183–191.
133. Food and Drug Administration. Parenteral multivitamin products (notices). *Federal Register.* 2000;65(77):21200–21201.
134. American Medical Association Department of Foods and Nutrition. Multivitamin preparation for parenteral use: a statement by the Nutrition Advisory Group. *JPEN J Parenter Enteral Nutr.* 1979;3(4):258–262.
135. Koutkia P, Lu Z, Chen TC, Holick MF. Treatment of vitamin D deficiency due to Crohn's disease with tanning bed ultraviolet B radiation. *Gastroenterology.* 2001;121(6):1485–1488.
136. A.S.P.E.N. Board of Directors. Clinical Guidelines for the use of parenteral and enteral nutrition in adult and pediatric patients. *JPEN J Parenter Enteral Nutr.* 2009;33(3):255–259.
137. A.S.P.E.N. Board of Directors. Enteral nutrition practice recommendations. *JPEN J Parenter Enteral Nutr.* 2009;33:122–167.
138. Frias J, Vidal-Valverde C. Stability of thiamine and vitamins E and A during storage of enteral feeding formula. *J Agric Food Chem.* 2001;49(5):2313–2317.
139. Guenter P. Safe practices for enteral nutrition in critically ill patients. *Crit Care Nurs Clin North Am.* 2010;22(2):197–208.

PART II

CLINICAL FOUNDATIONS OF NUTRITION SUPPORT

9. **Nutrition Screening and Assessment** 155
Gordon L. Jensen, MD, PhD
Pao Ying Hsiao, MS, RD
Dara Wheeler, RD

10. **Overview of Enteral Nutrition** 170
Susan L. Brantley, MS, RD, CNSC, LDN
Mary E. (Beth) Mills, MS, RD, CNSC, LDN

11. **Enteral Formulations** 185
Gail Cresci, PhD, RD, CNSD, LD
Jennifer Lefton, MS, RD, CNSD
Dema Halasa Esper, MS, RD, LD

12. **Enteral Access Devices** 206
John C. Fang, MD
Robin Bankhead, CRNP
Merin Kinikini, RD, RN, FNP

13. **Complications of Enteral Nutrition** 218
Ainsley M. Malone, MS, RD, LD, CNSC
David Seres, MD, ScM, PNS
Linda Lord, NP, MSN, CNSN

14. **Overview of Parenteral Nutrition** 234
Jay M. Mirtallo, M.S., RPh, BCNSP, FASHP
Meera Patel, PharmD, BCPS

15. **Parenteral Nutrition Formulations** 245
Jacqueline R. Barber, PharmD, BCNSP, FASHP
Gordon S. Sacks, PharmD, BCNSP, FCCP

16. **Parenteral Access Devices** 265
Elizabeth A. Krzywda, APNP, MSN
Deborah A. Andris, APNP, MSN
Charles E. Edmiston, Jr., PhD

17. **Complications of Parenteral Nutrition** 284
Vanessa J. Kumpf, PharmD, BCNSP
Jane Gervasio, PharmD, BCNSP

18. **Drug–Nutrient Interactions** 298
Carol J. Rollins, MS, RD, CNSD, PharmD, BCNSP

19. **Dietary Supplements** 313
Joseph I. Boullata, PharmD, RPh, BCNSP
Michele Nicolo, MS, RD, CDE, CNSD, LDN
Kathleen W. Stratton, JD, MA, RD, LDN

9 Nutrition Screening and Assessment

Gordon L. Jensen, MD, PhD, Pao Ying Hsiao, MS, RD, and Dara Wheeler, RD

CONTENTS

Introduction—Concepts of Screening and Assessment 156
Malnutrition Syndromes 156
Nutrition Assessment 161
Historical Data 161
Weight History 161
Medical/Surgical History 161
Medication History 161
Physical Examination 161
Anthropometric Data 162
Height 162
Body Weight 162
Skin Folds and Circumferences 162
Other Body Composition Assessment Tools 162
Laboratory Data 162
Dietary Data 162
Functional Outcomes 165
Multi-Item Nutrition Screening and Assessment Tools 165
Conclusion 167
References 167

Learning Objectives

1. Introduce a new approach to characterizing malnutrition syndromes that incorporates a current understanding of the contributions of inflammatory response.
2. Appreciate that there is no single clinical or laboratory indicator of comprehensive nutritional status.
3. Highlight practical nutrition screening and assessment techniques suitable for routine clinical applications.
4. Promote an approach to assessment of patients that incorporates data from the historical, clinical signs/physical examination, anthropometric, laboratory, dietary, and functional domains.

Test Your Knowledge Questions

1. An example of a patient condition that would be anticipated to manifest severe systemic inflammatory response would be which of the following?
   A. Anorexia nervosa with body mass index (BMI) of 15 kg/m^2
   B. Major depression with compromised dietary intake and 5% loss of body weight
   C. Homebound elder with restricted access to food and 10% loss of body weight
   D. Thermal burn injury of second and third degrees covering 15% body surface area

2. A physician tells you a patient has reduced serum albumin of 2.8 g/dL and prealbumin of 14 mg/dL and asks whether these laboratory findings mean the patient is malnourished. Appropriate response or responses would be?
   A. The patient's protein intake must be inadequate, and the patient should receive prompt nutrition support.
   B. Additional evidence suggesting loss of body cell mass or compromised dietary intake is warranted in order to appropriately diagnose a malnutrition syndrome.
   C. Evaluation of clinical and laboratory signs of inflammatory response would be helpful in interpreting these laboratory findings.
   D. Review of the medical history and clinical diagnosis may help to discern whether inflammatory response and/or malnutrition are likely to be present.
3. One of the best validated screening indicators for malnutrition risk is what?
   A. Patient reports a nonvolitional weight loss of 10% of usual body weight.
   B. Patient reports following a low-carbohydrate weight loss diet.
   C. Patient is 2 days status post laparoscopic cholecystectomy.
   D Patient reports a recent flu-like febrile illness.

Test Your Knowledge Answers

1. The correct answer is **D**. The burn injury is significant and will be associated with severe systemic inflammatory response. The diagnosis, clinical signs/physical examination, and laboratory indicators of such a patient will all support this conclusion. The other patient conditions are all states of starvation that are not likely to be associated with severe systemic inflammatory response.
2. The correct answers are **B**, **C**, and **D**. By themselves, these proteins should be interpreted with caution because they lack specificity and sensitivity as indicators of nutritional status. Both albumin and prealbumin may be reduced by the systemic response to injury, disease, or inflammation. Patients with low albumin or prealbumin may or may not be malnourished. Responses B, C, and D will all help to clarify whether inflammation is present and whether the patient is malnourished.
3. The correct answer **A**. The only well-validated indicator of the options provided to screen for malnutrition risk is a nonvolitional weight loss of 10% of usual body weight. The other options might all be noted in screening and assessment but do not in and of themselves confer validated measures of malnutrition risk.

Introduction—Concepts of Screening and Assessment

Malnutrition among hospitalized patients has been a documented concern for many years.[1,2] Prevalence as high as 30% to 50% has been described depending upon the setting and criteria that are used. Malnutrition has been associated with increased complications that include poor wound healing, compromised immune status, impairment of organ functions, and increased mortality. Of particular concern, malnutrition is also associated with increased health care resource use.

The poor recognition and treatment of malnutrition has been linked to a general lack of practitioner awareness.[3] It is therefore essential that practitioners increase their recognition of malnutrition through the use of appropriate screening and assessment methods. Screening is a process to identify an individual who is malnourished or at risk to become malnourished, whereas assessment is a more comprehensive evaluation to make a diagnosis of a malnutrition syndrome and to guide intervention and expected outcomes.[4] This chapter will introduce a new approach to understanding adult malnutrition syndromes that incorporates a modern understanding of the contributions of inflammatory response. Practical nutrition screening and assessment techniques suitable for routine clinical applications will be highlighted.

Malnutrition Syndromes

Recent evidence suggests that varying degrees of acute or chronic inflammation are key contributing factors in the pathophysiology of malnutrition that is associated with disease or injury.[5] Historic nutritional assessment parameters like albumin and prealbumin have been revealed to be impacted by inflammatory response. The presence of inflammation can also blunt favorable responses to nutrition therapies. An International Guideline Committee has recently proposed the following nomenclature for nutrition diagnosis in adults in the clinical practice setting.[6] "Starvation-associated malnutrition" when there is chronic starvation without inflammation, "chronic disease–associated malnutrition" when inflammation is chronic and of mild to moderate degree, and "acute disease– or injury-associated malnutrition" when inflammation is acute and of severe degree. Selected examples are shown below with additional examples presented in Table 9-1.

- Starvation-associated malnutrition: Anorexia nervosa or compromised intake in the setting of major depression (Practice Scenario 9-1).
- Chronic disease–associated malnutrition: Organ failure, pancreatic cancer, rheumatoid arthritis, or sarcopenic obesity (Practice Scenarios 9-2 and 9-3).
- Acute disease– or injury-associated malnutrition: Major infection, burns, trauma, or closed head injury (Practice Scenario 9-4).

A patient may be appropriately diagnosed with one or more of these syndromes or may change from one to another. It is useful to discern whether inflammation is present and if so, to clarify whether it is mild/moderate or severe in severity, and transient or sustained. Assessment of patients can be facilitated using the indicators of malnutrition and inflammation that follow.

- *History and clinical diagnosis* can be a helpful guide to raise suspicion for presence of inflammation and malnutrition.
- *Clinical signs and physical examination:*
  - Clinical indicators of inflammation may include fever or hypothermia as well as other nonspecific signs of systemic inflammatory response like tachycardia.
  - Physical examination can reveal signs of edema, weight gain/loss and specific nutrient deficiencies.

- *Anthropometric data:*
  - Weight loss and underweight status are well-validated indicators of malnutrition. Height, weight, skin folds, circumferences, and other assessments of body composition are helpful.
- *Laboratory indicators* of inflammatory response and possible protein malnutrition (albumin, prealbumin) should be interpreted with caution. Other useful laboratory indicators of inflammation can include elevated C-reactive protein, white blood cell count, and glucose. Negative nitrogen balance and elevated resting energy expenditure may also be used to support the presence of systemic inflammatory response.
- *Dietary data* may be obtained in practical fashion using a modified diet history and/or 24-hour recall.
- *Functional outcomes* like strength and physical performance may also be tested as additional supportive findings.

TABLE 9-1 History and Physical Examination Elements

Element	Notes
Historical Data	
Body weight	Ask about usual weight, peak weight, and deliberate weight loss. A 10-lb weight loss over 6 months is noteworthy and a weight loss of > 10% of usual body weight is prognostic of clinical outcomes.[27, 28] Use medical records, family, and caregivers as information resources.
Medical and surgical conditions; chronic disease	Look for medical or surgical conditions or chronic disease that can place one at nutritional risk secondary to increased requirements, or compromised intake or assimilation like critical illness, severe burns, major abdominal surgery, multitrauma, closed head injury, previous gastrointestinal surgery, severe gastrointestinal hemorrhage, enterocutaneous fistula, gastrointestinal obstruction, mesenteric ischemia, severe acute pancreatitis, chronic pancreatitis, inflammatory bowel disease, celiac disease, bacterial overgrowth, solid or hematologic malignancy, bone marrow transplant, acquired immune deficiency syndrome, and organ failure/transplant of the kidney, liver, heart, lung, or gut. A number of conditions or diseases are characterized by severe acute inflammatory response including critical illness, major infection/sepsis, adult respiratory distress syndrome, systemic inflammatory response syndrome, severe burns, major abdominal surgery, multitrauma, and closed head injury. Many conditions or diseases are more typically associated with mild to moderate chronic inflammatory response. Examples include cardiovascular disease; congestive heart failure; cystic fibrosis; inflammatory bowel disease; celiac disease; chronic pancreatitis; rheumatoid arthritis; solid tumors; hematologic malignancies; sarcopenic obesity; diabetes mellitus; metabolic syndrome; cerebrovascular accident; neuromuscular disease; dementia; organ failure/transplant of the kidney, liver, heart, lung, or gut; periodontal disease; pressure wounds; and chronic obstructive pulmonary disease. Note that acute exacerbations, infections, or other complications may superimpose acute inflammatory response on such conditions or diseases. Examples of starvation-associated conditions that generally have little or no inflammatory component include anorexia nervosa or compromised intake in the setting of major depression.
Constitutional signs/symptoms	Fever or hypothermia can indicate active inflammatory response. Tachycardia is also common. Anorexia is another manifestation of inflammatory response and is also often a side effect of treatments and medications.
Eating difficulties/ gastrointestinal complaints	Poor dentition or problems swallowing can compromise oral intake. Vomiting, nausea, abdominal pain, abdominal distension, diarrhea, constipation, and gastrointestinal bleeding can be signs of gastrointestinal pathology that may place one at nutritional risk.
Eating disorders	Look for distorted body image, compulsive exercise, amenorrhea, vomiting, tooth loss, dental caries, and use of laxatives, diuretics, or ipecac.
Medication use	Many medications can adversely affect nutrient intake or assimilation. Review potential drug–drug and drug–nutrient interactions. A pharmacist consultant can be helpful.
Dietary practices and supplement use	Look for dietary practices including therapeutic, weight reduction, vegetarian, macrobiotic, and fad diets. Also record use of dietary supplements, including vitamins, minerals, and herbals. Ask about dietary intake. Recall, record, and food frequency tools are available. It is estimated that 50% of adults take dietary supplements.[29]
Influences on nutritional status	Ask about factors such as living environment, functional status (activities of daily living[30] and instrumental activities of daily living[31]), dependency, caregiver status, resources, dentition, alcohol or substance abuse, mental health (depression or dementia), and lifestyle.

(continued)

TABLE 9-1 History and Physical Examination Elements *(continued)*

Element	Notes
Physical Examination Data	
Body mass index	BMI = weight (kg)/(height (m))^2 BMI < 18.5 kg/m^2 proposed screen for malnutrition per National Institutes of Health guidelines.[9] BMI ≤ 15 kg/m^2 or less is associated with mortality. Comparison with ideal body weight for stature can also be determined from reference tables. Note hydration status and edema at the time body weight is determined.
Weight loss	Look for loss of muscle mass and subcutaneous fat. Temporal and neck muscle wasting may be readily observed. Anthropometrics including skin folds and circumferences can be useful but require training to achieve reliability.
Weakness/loss of strength	Decreased hand-grip and leg extensor strength have been related to loss of muscle mass in malnourished states.[32–34] Lower extremity weakness may be observed in thiamin deficiency.
Peripheral edema	Peripheral edema may confound weight measurements and is often observed with reduced visceral proteins as well as inflammatory states. Edema may also be observed with thiamin deficiency.
Hair exam	Hair findings are indicative of certain nutrient deficiencies.[35] Loss: protein, B_{12}, folate Brittle: biotin Color change: zinc Dry: vitamins A and E Easy pluckability: protein, biotin, zinc Coiled, corkscrew: vitamins A and C Alopecia is common in severely malnourished persons. Ask about excessive hair loss on pillow or when combing hair.
Skin exam	Skin findings are indicative of certain nutrient deficiencies.[35,36] Desquamation: riboflavin Petechiae: vitamins A and C Perifollicular hemorrhage: vitamin C Ecchymosis: vitamins C and K Xerosis, bran-like desquamation: essential fatty acid Pigmentation, cracking, crusting: niacin Acneiform lesions, follicular keratosis, xerosis: vitamin A Acro-orificial dermatitis, erythematous, vesiculobullous, and pustular: zinc Characteristic nutritional dermatitis and skin findings may be observed with a number of nutrient deficiencies. Wounds and pressure sores should also be noted as indicators of compromised nutritional status.
Eye exam	Ocular findings are indicative of certain nutrient deficiencies.[35] Bitot spots: vitamin A Xerosis: vitamin A Angular palpebritis: riboflavin Also ask about difficulties with night vision/night blindness; indicates vitamin A deficiency.
Perioral exam	Perioral findings are indicative of certain nutrient deficiencies.[35] Angular stomatitis and cheilosis: B complex, iron, and protein Glossitis: niacin, folate, and vitamin B_{12} Magenta tongue: riboflavin Bleeding gums, gingivitis, tooth loss: vitamin C Angular stomatitis, cheilosis, and glossitis are associated with vitamin and mineral deficiencies. Note poor dentition, caries, and tooth loss.[37] Difficulty swallowing and impairment of gag should also be recognized.
Extremity exam	Extremity findings indicate certain nutrient deficiencies. Arthralgia: vitamin C Calf pain: thiamin Extremities may also exhibit loss of muscle mass and/or peripheral edema. Neurological findings in the extremities may also result from deficiencies described in the following.

(continued)

TABLE 9-1 History and Physical Examination Elements *(continued)*

Element	Notes
Mental status/nervous system exam	Mental and nervous system findings indicate certain nutrient deficiencies. Ophthalmoplegia and foot drop: thiamin Paresthesia: thiamin, vitamin B_{12}, and biotin Depressed vibratory and position senses: vitamin B_{12} Anxiety, depression, and hallucinations: niacin Memory disturbance: vitamin B_{12} Hyporeflexia, loss of lower extremity deep tendon reflexes: thiamin and vitamin B_{12} Conduct formal cognitive[38] and depression[39,40] assessments as appropriate. Dementia and depression are common causes of malnutrition among older persons. Wernicke-Korsakoff syndrome may be observed with severe thiamin deficiency.
Functional assessment	Observe and test physical performance as indicated: gait, chair stands, stair steps, and balance. These provide complex measures of integrated neurological status, coordination, and strength.[41]

BMI, body mas index.
Adapted with permission from Jensen G, *Nutritional Syndromes*. Philadelphia, PA: American College of Physicians, 2011. http://pier.acponline.org/physicians/diseases/d270/d270.html. Accessed June 3, 2011.

Practice Scenario 9-1

Question: What malnutrition syndrome would you anticipate in a patient who presents with anorexia nervosa, and how would you confirm this?

Scenario: A 26-year-old female was admitted to the hospital with a diagnosis of anorexia nervosa and a longstanding history of restrictive eating behavior without purging. She had lost one-third of her body weight over 6 months. Upon admission the patient was 5′6″ (167.6 cm) in height and weighed 82 pounds (37.2 kg), with a BMI of 13.2 kg/m^2. Her resting heart rate was 50 beats per minute. She was afebrile. Laboratory values included C-reactive protein 0.7 mg/dL, white blood cell count 6200/mm^3, albumin 4.0 g/dL, prealbumin 25 mg/dL, and fasting blood glucose 75 mg/dL. She exhibited generalized loss of muscle and subcutaneous fat. Other physical findings included lanugo hairs. Marked underweight status was evident with weight loss of 42 pounds (19.1 kg) over 6 months. Mid-arm muscle circumference measurement was below the fifth percentile.

Intervention: Resuscitate patient cautiously to avoid refeeding syndrome (see Chapter 24).

Answer: Malnutrition syndrome: Starvation-associated malnutrition

1. History and clinical diagnosis: Anorexia nervosa is consistent with starvation without significant inflammatory component.
2. Clinical signs/physical examination: Consistent with severe malnutrition without inflammatory response.
3. Anthropometric data: Weight loss, underweight status, and mid-arm muscle circumference consistent with severe malnutrition.
4. Laboratory indicators: Do not suggest active inflammation.
5. Dietary intake: Severely compromised for months.
6. Functional outcomes: Would be likely to have diminished grip strength and physical performance.

Rationale: Resuscitation should begin with decreased macronutrients to reduce risk of complications. Close monitoring is indicated because refeeding concerns in the resuscitation of the severely malnourished may include fluid retention and falling potassium, phosphate, and magnesium. In the setting of pure starvation, it is feasible to resuscitate individuals from even life-threatening malnutrition with appropriate nutrition intervention. In the absence of inflammation, albumin and prealbumin will often remain normal or near normal unless malnutrition is quite advanced.

Practice Scenario 9-2

Question: What malnutrition syndrome would you anticipate in a patient who presents with cirrhosis with portal hypertension and ascites, and how would you confirm this?

Scenario: A 52-year-old male presented for a follow-up clinic appointment with an established history of cirrhosis and portal hypertension in the setting of long-term ethanol abuse. He had gained 10 pounds (4.5 kg) over the prior 2 weeks and exhibited massive ascites. Additional findings included mild encephalopathy (grade 1) with poor concentration, asterixis, and scleral icterus. A family member reported that his food intake had been severely compromised for weeks. At presentation, the patient was 5′8″ (172.7 cm) in height and weighed 161 pounds (73.0 kg) (usual weight ~150 pounds, 68.0 kg). He was afebrile. Laboratories included total bilirubin 3.8 mg/dL, aspartate aminotransferase 96 IU/L, alanine aminotransferase 111 U/L, alkaline phosphatase 162 IU/L, albumin 1.7g/dL, prothrombin time 18 seconds, white blood cells 3700/mm^3, C-reactive protein 27 mg/L, prealbumin 6.8 mg/dL, hemoglobin 8 g/dL, hematocrit 32%, and fasting glucose 107 mg/dL. Physical findings were notable for ascites and extensive loss of muscle and subcutaneous fat.

Intervention: Promote adequate caloric intake with balanced macronutrients and sodium restricted diet. The patient may benefit from protein-energy supplements.

Answer: Clinical malnutrition syndrome: Chronic disease–associated malnutrition

1. History and clinical diagnosis: Cirrhosis is consistent with malnutrition and chronic inflammation of mild to moderate degree.
2. Clinical signs/physical examination: Consistent with malnutrition in setting of chronic liver disease/cirrhosis.
3. Anthropometric data: Ascites and weight gain mask true underweight status and loss of body cell mass. Other body composition measures may demonstrate loss of muscle.
4. Laboratory indicators: Consistent with cirrhosis and cannot be reliably interpreted to support malnutrition or inflammation.
5. Dietary intake: Severely compromised for weeks.
6. Functional outcomes: Would be likely to have diminished grip strength and physical performance.

Rationale: Albumin and prealbumin levels are decreased by liver failure and so serve as poor indicators of nutritional status in this setting. Elevated C-reactive protein levels have been described in patients with hepatic encephalopathy. It has been suggested that they may represent the inflammatory response to subclinical infection. In this patient, malnutrition is identified on the basis of clinical diagnosis, history of compromised intake, and physical findings. Chronic inflammation is consistent with the clinical diagnosis and may not be revealed by available laboratory indicators. Mild encephalopathy is generally not an indication for severe protein restriction.

Practice Scenario 9-3

Question: What malnutrition syndrome would you anticipate in an older patient who presents to your clinic with obesity and frailty, and how would you confirm this?

Scenario: A 70-year-old female presented for a follow-up clinic appointment with longstanding obesity and metabolic syndrome. She has been receiving medications that include a statin, a diabetes oral agent, and a nonsteroidal anti-inflammatory for her hypercholesterolemia, diabetes mellitus, and painful destructive joint disease of the knees, respectively. Her chief complaint is worsening limitations in function that include compromised mobility. She lives in her own home and is effectively housebound. She reports limited financial resources and difficulty obtaining regular meals. She indicates that she may have lost some 10 to 20 pounds (4.5 to 9.0 kg) over the past 6 months without trying to lose weight. An adult daughter accompanies the patient and reports that she checks on her mother once a week and drops off some meals during those visits. Upon evaluation her height was 5 ft 2 inches (157.5 cm) and weight was 200 lbs (90.7 kg) (BMI 37 kg/m^2). Prior records confirm a 20-pound (9.0 kg) weight loss compared to her last visit a year before. She was afebrile with blood pressure 135/85 and pulse 72. Laboratories included fasting glucose 130 mg/dL, hemoglobin A1c 7.0%, cholesterol 180 mg/dL, high-density lipoprotein cholesterol 45 mg/dL, triglyceride 125 mg/dL, albumin 4.1 g/dL, white blood cells 5100/mm^3, and C-reactive protein 48 mg/L. Physical examination revealed truncal adiposity with waist circumference of 96 cm. She had difficulty arising from a chair and ambulating with evidence of generalized loss of strength and knee discomfort.

Intervention: Encourage diabetic diet regimen with regular high-quality meals and snacks. In view of her malnutrition and lipid profile on statin therapy, there is little indication to be overly restrictive of cholesterol or fat while her malnutrition is addressed. Supplement a daily multivitamin with minerals. Promote strength and flexibility training to improve function and mobility. Consider consultations to social services, dietitian, Agency on Aging, Meals on Wheels, physical therapy, and orthopedic surgery. Encourage family engagement. If available, consider evaluation by comprehensive geriatric assessment and endocrine/diabetes management teams. Knee replacement surgery may be a consideration once malnutrition and other concerns are suitably addressed.

Answer: Clinical malnutrition syndrome: Chronic disease–associated malnutrition

1. History and clinical diagnosis: Longstanding obesity and metabolic syndrome with compromise in dietary intake and weight loss are consistent with malnutrition and chronic inflammation of mild to moderate degree. A clinical diagnosis of sarcopenic obesity is suspected.
2. Clinical signs/physical examination: Consistent with obesity and limitations in mobility associated with painful destructive joint disease of the knees and loss of strength.
3. Anthropometric data: BMI and waist circumference are consistent with obesity. Loss of muscle mass will be difficult to appreciate by simple anthropometric measures in this patient. Other body composition measures like DEXA, CT, and MRI may be used to demonstrate loss of muscle and to confirm the diagnosis of sarcopenic obesity.
4. Laboratory indicators: Fasting glucose and hemoglobin A1c are consistent with diabetes mellitus, lipid profile is consistent with statin-controlled hypercholesterolemia, and the elevated C-reactive protein is typical of the inflammation observed with obesity.
5. Dietary intake: Likely compromised secondary to homebound status and limited resources. It will be appropriate to confirm poor-quality diet with diet recall or history.
6. Functional outcomes: A physical performance test battery will be helpful to confirm the degree of functional impairment. Assessment of strength measures may also be useful.

Rationale: In an older person with obesity and frailty, an emphasis on promoting strength and flexibility rather than weight loss may be most appropriate. Prior to embarking on any weight loss intervention, this patient's malnutrition must be addressed. Weight loss intervention remains controversial in older persons, though improvements in metabolic syndrome parameters, inflammatory status, and function have been described for selected cohorts. In this particular patient, once she has been stabilized, modest weight reduction would offer potential benefits to her obesity-related comorbidities as well as decrease her risks for possible elective knee replacement surgery. Malnutrition is in this case identified on the basis of clinical history of compromised intake and nonvolitional weight loss. Compromised strength and function provide additional supporting data. Chronic inflammation is consistent with the clinical diagnoses and elevated C-reactive protein. Obesity is a major risk factor for destructive joint disease of the knees. Moderate weight loss has been found to reduce disability for obese individuals with knee osteoarthritis. Sarcopenic obesity is characterized by muscle loss in the setting of obesity and is common among obese older persons and those obese persons with significant disease burden or injury. Dropout of α-motor neurons, changes in anabolic hormones, and malnutrition may be contributing factors, but inflammation-promoted erosion of muscle mass as well as the synergy of physical inactivity, increased adiposity, and accumulated disease burden are likely important as well.

Practice Scenario 9-4

Question: What malnutrition syndrome would you anticipate in a multiple trauma victim early in his or her course, and how would you confirm this?

Scenario: A 38-year-old male suffered multitrauma secondary to a motor vehicle accident. His injuries included ruptured spleen, Grade III liver laceration, left femur fracture, and bilateral pulmonary contusions. He is status post damage control celiotomy, splenectomy, and packing of the liver. He was transferred to the trauma intensive care unit on a ventilator where he continued to be resuscitated. Clinical and laboratory criteria for systemic inflammatory response syndrome (SIRS) include temperature > 38°C or < 36°C, heart rate > 90 beats/min, respiratory rate > 20 breaths/min, white blood cell count > 12K/mm^3, and Pco_2 < 32 mm Hg. Post-surgery day 2 of admission this patient had temperature 39°C, heart rate 98 beats per minute, respiratory rate 26 breaths per minute, white blood cell count 25,000/mm^3, and carbon dioxide partial pressure 28 mm Hg. He was markedly edematous with weight gain of 15 pounds (6.8 kg) above his usual body weight. His open abdomen was dressed. Additional laboratories consistent with active inflammation included C-reactive protein 45 mg/dL, albumin 2.6 g/dL, prealbumin 11.0 mg/dL, and glucose 220 mg/dL. He had an increased metabolic rate by indirect calorimetry with a resting energy expenditure of 3000 kcal. Dietary intake was anticipated to be compromised for a week or greater. He was reported to have been well nourished with suitable dietary intake prior to his injury.

Intervention: Enteral feedings were initiated within 24 hours of admission (see Chapters 7, 13, and 17).

Answer: Malnutrition syndrome: Acute disease—or injury-associated malnutrition

1. History and clinical diagnosis: Multiple trauma is consistent with severe acute systemic inflammatory response and high nutritional risk.
2. Clinical signs/physical examination: Consistent with severe acute inflammatory response.
3. Anthropometric data: Body weight gain consistent with appreciable edema.
4. Laboratory indicators: Supportive of presence of severe acute inflammation.
5. Dietary intake: At risk for extended duration of compromise.
6. Functional outcomes: Grip strength and physical performance testing is not feasible in acutely injured and sedated patient.

Rationale: Signs of severe acute systemic inflammatory response are caused by hormonal, metabolic, and immunological mediators that include cytokines. Nutrition intervention is intended to support vital immune system, wound healing, and organ system functions to help the patient through this phase of acute inflammatory response. Trauma victims are often not malnourished at baseline, and they are at risk to become severely malnourished due to acute metabolic dysregulation and associated catabolism. In addition, those with severe injury may be unable to eat for extended periods. Even with aggressive nutrition support, during this acute phase such patients will likely remain in negative nitrogen balance and have low albumin and prealbumin due to the marked proinflammatory state.

Nutrition Assessment

Because there is no single clinical or laboratory indicator of comprehensive nutritional status, an assessment requires collection of information from a variety of sources including the historical, clinical signs/physical examination, and anthropometric, laboratory, dietary, and functional domains.

Historical Data

Weight History

One of the most important historical elements is prior weight loss (including volitional weight reduction). Clinical relevance varies according to the degree and duration of weight loss. Table 9-1 gives more details on weight history.

Medical/Surgical History

Many medical and surgical diagnoses and associated interventions are known to impact inflammatory and nutritional status, and are often associated with characteristic malnutrition syndromes. The inflammatory milieu, especially if severe, may alter nutrient requirements by raising resting energy expenditure and promoting nitrogen excretion. Anorexia often accompanies inflammation, further compromising nutritional status. Some disorders and interventions may precipitate malnutrition because they adversely impact the inability to ingest or absorb nutrients, or they impose dietary restrictions or other limitations. The presence of inflammation may reduce the effectiveness of nutritional interventions, and the associated malnutrition may in turn blunt the effectiveness of medical therapies. Table 9-1 gives examples of some of the most common medical or surgical diagnoses and conditions that are associated with nutritional risk as well as their characteristic inflammatory components.

Medication History

Review of medications is warranted. Practitioners should aim to be familiar with the potential nutrient interactions of drugs that they commonly use to treat their patients. A pharmacy consultant can be helpful. Nutritional status may be adversely impacted by drugs that interfere with food intake or with the absorption, metabolism, and excretion of nutrients. Drug levels may also be altered by foods and nutrients that modify drug absorption, metabolism, and excretion.

Physical Examination

Malnutrition can broadly affect organs and tissues, resulting in physical findings that may be detected by the knowledgeable practitioner. Among the most key of the physical findings are signs of weight loss (loss of body cell mass). Highlighting the importance of the physical examination, edema that might otherwise go undetected may mask weight loss. It is important to note that peripheral edema is often associated with reduced albumin in the setting of inflammatory response and is not necessarily a manifestation of poor protein nutrition. Particular attention should be given to the examination of parts of the body where high cell turnover occurs (eg, hair, skin, mouth, tongue) as they are among the most likely to show signs of malnutrition. Notable physical examination elements for malnutrition appear in Table 9-1.

Anthropometric Data

Anthropometric measures (height, weight, skin folds, and circumferences) are relatively simple physical measurements that provide an indirect assessment of body size and composition. Findings are compared with standards (for the same gender and age) and/or with previous measurements taken on the same individual. Trends can be particularly useful in assessment.

Height

Accurate measurement of height is indicated as a variety of anthropometric measures are standardized for height. For those who are able to stand without assistance, height should be measured in a standing position without shoes using a wall-mounted stadiometer. For adults who are unable to stand, height can be estimated by doubling the arm span measurement (from the patient's sternal notch to the end of the longest finger). Stature in older persons can also be estimated by measuring knee height using a caliper device.[7]

- Men: Stature (cm) = $[2.02 \times \text{knee height (cm)}] - (0.04 \times \text{age}) + 64.19$
- Women: Stature (cm) = $[1.83 \times \text{knee height (cm)}] - (0.24 \times \text{age}) + 84.8$

Body Weight

Actual measured body weight and weight change trends are particularly important components of nutrition assessment. Those who can stand should be weighed in a consistent manner without shoes or overgarments. Chair and bed scales are available for those who cannot stand. Reliance on self-reported weights or weights abstracted from medical records may be unreliable. Reference tables of standards for body weight relative to height such as the Metropolitan Height and Weight Tables[8] are often used, but suffer notable limitations that include subjective interpretation of frame size and inadequate availability of reference data for many population groups.

A practical measure of body size and an indirect measure of body fatness is provided by BMI, defined as weight (kg)/(height (m))^2. The National Institutes of Health guidelines[9] for interpretation of BMI are:

- BMI < 18.5 = underweight, at risk of malnutrition
- BMI 18.5 to 24.9 = desirable
- BMI 25 to 29 = overweight
- BMI ≥ 30 = obese

Skin Folds and Circumferences

Anthropometric measurements such as skin folds and circumferences can be quite helpful, but they have had limited practical application in patient care settings because appropriate training is required to achieve acceptable practitioner reliability. The practitioner who would like to learn these methods can find an educational description of procedures in the NHANES III Anthropometric Procedures video.[10]

Other Body Composition Assessment Tools

Other body composition assessment tools are often used in research but generally have had limited availability or portability for routine clinical applications. They include water displacement, bioelectrical impedance analysis, dual-energy x-ray absorptiometry (DEXA), computed tomography (CT), magnetic resonance imaging (MRI), total body counting of the naturally occurring potassium isotope, and air plethysmography. Table 9-2 describes each of them in more detail.

Laboratory Data

Laboratory studies can be useful in the diagnosis and interpretation of a patient's nutritional status. There is, however, no single laboratory test or panel that allows one to make a diagnosis of malnutrition, so laboratory findings must be used with other assessment data, such as clinical history and physical examination, to make a diagnosis of a malnutrition syndrome.

Serum albumin or prealbumin should be obtained to evaluate any patient with a suspected malnutrition syndrome. However, these proteins should be interpreted with caution because they lack specificity and sensitivity as indicators of nutritional status.[5,11] Both albumin and prealbumin may be reduced by the systemic response to injury, disease, or inflammation. Patients with low albumin or prealbumin may or may not be malnourished. C-reactive protein is a positive acute phase reactant and may be measured to help clarify whether active inflammation is present. If C-reactive protein is elevated and albumin or prealbumin reduced, then an inflammation is likely to be manifest. Leukocytosis and hyperglycemia are additional nonspecific indicators that may suggest inflammatory response. Further findings that may be used to support the presence of inflammatory response include negative nitrogen balance and elevated resting energy expenditure. In order to diagnose a malnutrition syndrome, additional evidence suggesting loss of body cell mass or compromised dietary intake is warranted. Table 9-2 addresses a variety of laboratory and other tests used to evaluate nutritional disorders.

Dietary Data

Dietary assessment can be used to detect inadequate or imbalanced food or nutrient intakes, which can lead to nutrient deficiencies or excesses. There are a number of methods with which to assess dietary intake, and the choice depends on the population of interest, availability of resources, skills of the

TABLE 9-2 Body Composition, Laboratories, and Other Studies

Test	Notes
Body Composition Studies	
Anthropometrics	Skin folds and circumferences require training for reliability.[42,43] Typical coefficient of variation is 10% or greater.
Bioelectrical impedance	Based upon differential resistance of body tissues.[44,45] Equipment easily portable. Good measure of body water. Requires population specific validation of regression equations.[46]
Water displacement	Impractical for most clinical settings. Weighed in water tank. Historic reference measure.[47]
Whole body counting and isotope dilution techniques	Research methodologies. Naturally occurring ^{40}K isotope to measure body cell mass by whole body counting.[48] Total body water measurement by dilution volume of tritium, deuterium, or ^{18}O-labeled water.[49,50]
Air plethysmography	Research methodology.[51] Subject sits inside moderately sized BodPod chamber. (Life Measurement, Inc., Concord, CA) Validated against water displacement and impedance.[52]
Dual energy x-ray absorptiometry	Often used for bone density but can be used for soft tissue measurements with appropriate software.[53,54] Can compare truncal and appendicular components. Modest x-ray exposure.
Imaging with computed tomography or magnetic resonance imaging	State-of-the-art research methods for visualizing body tissue compartments.[55,56] Can quantify visceral fat. Costly and computed tomography entails x-ray exposure.
Laboratories and Other Studies	
Albumin	Lacks sensitivity and specificity for malnutrition.[5,11] Potent risk indicator for morbidity and mortality.[57–59] Proxy measure for underlying injury, disease, or inflammation.[60] Half-life is 14 to 20 days. Useful screening indicator may be < 38 gm/L for older persons.[61] Also consider liver disease, nephrotic syndrome, and protein-wasting enteropathy.
Prealbumin	Sensitive to short-term changes in inflammation and protein nutrition with half-life of 2 to 3 days.[62–65] Otherwise suffers the same limitations of albumin with limited sensitivity and specificity for malnutrition. Levels may be decreased in liver failure and increased in renal failure.[66]
Transferrin	Acute phase reactant also altered by perturbation in iron status.[67–69] Half-life is 8 to 10 days. Lacks sensitivity and specificity for malnutrition.
Retinol-binding protein	Responds to very short-term changes in nutritional status but utility is also limited by response to stress and inflammation.[70–72] Half-life is 12 hours. Also affected by vitamin A deficiency[73] and renal disease.[66]
C-reactive protein	C-reactive protein is a positive acute phase reactant.[74,75] It is generally elevated if an active inflammatory process is manifest.
Cholesterol	Low cholesterol (< 160 mg/dL) is often observed in malnourished persons with serious underlying disease.[76,77] It is unrelated to dietary intake in many clinical settings.[78] Increased complications and mortality are observed. It appears that low cholesterol is again a nonspecific feature of poor health status that reflects cytokine-mediated inflammatory condition.[79] Vegans may also exhibit low cholesterol.
Carotene	Nonspecific indicator of malabsorption and poor nutritional intake.
Cytokines	Research is exploring prognostic use of cytokine measurements as indicators of inflammatory status.
Electrolytes, blood urea nitrogen, creatinine, and glucose	Monitor for abnormalities consistent with under- or overhydration status and purging (contraction alkalosis). Blood urea nitrogen may also be low in the setting of markedly reduced body cell mass. Blood urea nitrogen and creatinine are elevated in renal failure. Hyperglycemia may be nonspecific indicator of inflammatory response.
Complete blood count with differential	Screen for nutritional anemias (iron, B_{12}, and folate), lymphopenia (malnutrition), and thrombocytopenia (vitamin C and folate). Leukocytosis may be observed with inflammatory response.
Total lymphocyte count	Relative lymphopenia (total lymphocyte count $< 1200/mm^3$) is a nonspecific marker for malnutrition.[80–83]
Helper/suppressor T-cell ratio	Ratio may be reduced in severely undernourished patients. Not specific for nutritional status.[84]

(continued)

TABLE 9-2 Body Composition, Laboratories, and Other Studies *(continued)*

Test	Notes
Nitrogen balance	Twenty-four-hour urine can be analyzed for urine urea nitrogen to determine nitrogen balance and give indication of degree of catabolism and adequacy of protein replacement. Requires accurate urine collection and normal renal function. Nitrogen balance = (protein/6.25) − (urine urea nitrogen + 4). Generally negative in the setting of acute severe inflammatory response.
Urine 3-methylhistidine	Indicator of muscle catabolism and protein sufficiency.[85,86] Released upon breakdown of myofibrillar protein and excreted without reutilization. Urine measurement requires a meat-free diet for 3 days prior to collection.
Creatinine height index	Creatinine height index = (24-hour urinary creatinine excretion/ideal urinary creatinine for gender and height) × 100. Indicator of muscle depletion. Requires accurate urine collection and normal renal function.[2,87]
Prothrombin time/international normalized ratio	Nonspecific indicator of vitamin K status. Prolonged in liver failure.
Specific micronutrients	When suspected a variety of specific micronutrient levels may be measured: thiamin; riboflavin; niacin; folate; pryridoxine; vitamins A, C, D, E, and B_{12}; zinc; iron; selenium; carnitine; and homocysteine—indicator of B_{12}, folate, and pyridoxine status.
Skin testing—recall antigens	Delayed hypersensitivity testing.[80,88] While malnourished patients are often anergic, this is not specific for nutritional status.
Electrocardiogram	Severely malnourished patients with reduced body cell mass may exhibit low voltage and prolonged QT interval.[89–91] These findings are not specific for malnutrition.
Video fluoroscopy	Helpful to evaluate suspected swallowing disorders.
Endoscopic and x-ray studies of gastrointestinal tract	Useful to evaluate impaired function, motility, and obstruction.
Fat absorption	Seventy-two-hour fecal fat can be used to quantitate degree of malabsorption.
Schilling test	Identifies the cause for impaired vitamin B_{12} absorption.
Indirect calorimetry	Metabolic cart can be used to determine resting energy expenditure for accurate estimation of energy needs.[92,93] Elevated resting energy expenditure is a sign of systemic inflammatory response.

Adapted with permission from Jensen G, *Nutritional Syndromes.* Philadelphia, PA: American College of Physicians, 2011. http://pier.acponline.org/physicians/diseases/d270/d270.html. Accessed June 3, 2011.

health professional, feasibility, and purpose. Broadly speaking, dietary assessments can be divided into prospective and retrospective methods. Common dietary assessment methods are described in Table 9-3. In contrast to the research setting, the clinician is generally interested in evaluating food intake at the individual (versus population) level. Both the 24-hour recall and a modified version of the diet history are commonly used in clinical settings. Originally developed by Burke and Stuart,[12] the diet history, in the most general sense, refers to obtaining information about an individual's past diet and can include queries of information about both types and frequencies of intake of various foods. While the original Burke diet history method included a detailed interview about usual food intake, a food frequency checklist, and a 3-day diet record, this level of detail is often omitted in the clinical setting and a modified diet history is obtained. It is a priority to query a history of dietary practices when completing any nutritional assessment. Use of dietary supplements should also be specifically questioned. Dietary practice history elements appear in Table 9-1.

Once dietary data has been collected, it can then be entered into a nutrition software program that provides an analysis of the energy and nutrients of the diet. The analysis is typically based on information from a database containing values for food ingredients derived from the U.S. Department of Agriculture National Nutrient Database for Standard Reference. Although a number are available, some of the more widely used programs are Nutritionist Pro (Axxya Systems, Stafford, TX), Nutrition Data System for Research (University of Minnesota, Nutrition Coordinating Center, Minneapolis, MN), and Food Processor (ESHA Research, Salem, OR). Selection of diet analysis software will depend on cost, system requirements, usability, and available features.

Reports of nutrient intake generated by the diet analysis software can then be compared to recommendations. Recently updated, the Dietary Reference Intakes[13] are a set of nutrient recommendations established by the Food and Nutrition Board of the Institute of Medicine. These include adequate intakes (AI), recommended dietary allowances (RDA), upper tolerable intake levels (UL), and estimated average requirements (EAR). Caution

TABLE 9-3 Dietary Assessment Methods

Method	Procedure	Characteristics	Limitations
Diet record/ food diary	Subject is asked to record food and beverage intake usually for a brief period of time (1 to 7 days)	Prospective; food portions may be weighed or estimated using household measurements; can be used to record compliance to a dietary regimen or used to self-monitor food intake; does not rely on subject recall	Captures recent intake which may or may not reflect usual intake; high subject burden; act of recording can influence food intake; analysis can be cumbersome
Twenty-four hour recall	Subject is asked to recall exact food and beverage consumption for previous/past 24 hours	Retrospective; low subject burden; trained interviewer using probes will result in collection of more detailed information; can be administered via telephone or in-person by trained interviewer; can be inexpensive and quick; does not influence food intake	Accuracy dependent upon subject's ability to recall and estimate portion size; multiple recalls may need to be conducted to capture usual food intake
Food frequency questionnaire	Subject asked to report frequency of consumption of a selected list of foods	Retrospective; provides assessment of long-term diet intake patterns; may or may not query portion size; low subject burden; can be easily self-administered; commonly used with large-scale populations	Use with special populations should be validated; intake often misreported
Diet history	Original approach included three elements: detailed interview of food intake, checklist of foods, and a 3-day diet record	Retrospective and prospective; often modified in clinical settings; the three elements can be used to cross-check reported intake	High interviewer burden/time-consuming; relies on subject recall and portion size estimation
Direct observation	Visual examination of meal before and after being served to capture/ estimate food intake	Prospective; most used with hospitalized patients or those in residential facilities and includes a "calorie count" to assess if subject is likely meeting nutrient needs; cost-effective; quick	If meal tray is removed/discarded before clinician can observe, food intake cannot be estimated; relies on clinician ability to estimate portion size

should be used when evaluating nutrient intakes of individuals with diseases as Dietary Reference Intake values were intended to define amounts that support most healthy individuals.

As with any other information, dietary data should not be considered in isolation, but rather should be used in combination with other components of a nutrition assessment to evaluate the patient's nutritional status. Each approach to dietary assessment is subject to both systematic (eg, recall ability of subject, ability to accurately estimate portion size) and random (eg, misreporting of true intake by certain population groups) errors. Measurement of nutrient intake is complex. While potential sources of error cannot be eliminated entirely, it is essential that the practitioner understand the nature of the errors and how they may affect analysis and interpretation of the data.[14] Special consideration should be given to dietary assessment of certain populations, including infants, children and adolescents, the older adult population, and ethnic populations.[15] In some cases, caregivers can often be used as a proxy to report dietary intake. Obtaining dietary information from ethnic populations might require special modifications, such as population-specific food frequency questionnaires or use of translators. It is also important that the food database used contains foods and preparation methods relevant to the target population.

Functional Outcomes

Measurable declines in strength and physical performance will be associated with the loss of muscle mass and function that accompany advanced malnutrition syndromes. Contributing factors to functional decline may include nutrient deficiencies and impairment of organ system functions. The most commonly used measure for routine clinical assessment is handgrip strength. Physical performance batteries that include measures like timed gait, chair stands, and stair steps are sometimes used in the comprehensive assessment of frail older persons. Additional details are found in Table 9-1.

Multi-Item Nutrition Screening and Assessment Tools

Nutrition screening programs are required for most health care facilities (eg, acute care, long-term care) by The Joint Commission for the purpose of systematically identifying individuals at nutritional risk.[16] The screening process typically involves use of an instrument or set of standardized criteria that aids in determining whether or not additional information is required to warrant an intervention. The Joint Commission mandates

TABLE 9-4 Selected Nutrition Screening and Assessment Instruments

Instrument	Anthropometry and/or Diet Related	Severity of Illness	Other Variables
Screening tools			
Birmingham Nutrition Risk Score[94]	Weight loss, BMI, appetite, ability to eat	Stress factor, (severity of diagnosis)	
Malnutrition Screening Tool[18]	Appetite, unintentional weight loss		
Malnutrition Universal Screening Tool[20]	BMI, change in weight	Presence of acute disease	
Maastricht Index[95]	Percentage ideal body weight	Albumin, prealbumin, lymphocyte count	
Nutrition Risk Classification[96]	Weight loss, percentage ideal body weight, dietary intake		Gastrointestinal function
Nutritional Risk Index[97]	Present and usual body weight	Albumin	
Nutritional Risk Screening 2002[21]	Weight loss, BMI, food intake	Diagnosis (severity)	
Prognostic Inflammatory and Nutritional Index[98]		Albumin, prealbumin, C-reactive protein, α1-acid glycoprotein	
Prognostic Nutritional Index[99]	Triceps skin fold	Albumin, transferrin, skin sensitivity	
Simple Screening Tool[100]	BMI, percentage weight loss	Albumin	
Short Nutrition Assessment Questionnaire[19]	Recent weight history, appetite, use of oral supplement or tube feeding		
Nutrition Screening Initiative DETERMINE Checklist[24]	Poor eating pattern, tooth loss/ mouth pain, weight loss/gain	Disease	Economic hardship, reduced social contact, need assistance for self-care, older than 80 years, "polypharmacy"
Mini Nutritional Assessment Short Form[22]	Appetite, weight loss, BMI or calf circumference		Mobility, psychological/neuropsychological status, dementia
Nutrition assessment tools			
Mini Nutritional Assessment[25, 26]	Weight data, height, mid-arm and calf circumferences, diet history, appetite, feeding mode	Albumin, prealbumin, cholesterol, lymphocyte count	Self-perception of nutrition and health status
Subjective Global Assessment[23]	Weight history, diet history	Primary diagnosis, stress level	Physical symptoms (subcutaneous fat, muscle wasting, ankle edema, sacral edema, ascites), functional capacity, gastrointestinal symptoms
Nutrition Screening Initiative Level I Screen[24]	Measures of height and weight as well as additional assessment items regarding weight change and dietary habits		Functional status, living environment
Nutrition Screening Initiative Level II Screen[24]	All items from Level I plus additional laboratory and anthropometric measures	Albumin, cholesterol	Functional status, living environment; provision for more detailed physical examination and evaluation of depression and mental status

BMI, body mass index.
Adapted from Mueller C, Compher C, Druyan ME, ASPEN Board of Directors. A.S.P.E.N. Clinical guidelines: nutrition screening, assessment, and intervention in adults. *J Parenter Enteral Nutr*. 2011;35(1):16–24, with permission from the American Society for Parenteral and Enteral Nutrition.

that each individual be screened for nutritional risk within 24 hours of admission. Each individual is assigned a level of nutritional risk based on a set of standardized guidelines. Risk levels guide how quickly the individual must be rescreened or assessed. According to a recent survey,[17] most facilities use a two-level or three-level risk classification system (eg, risk/no-risk, or low, moderate, or high risk, respectively). Screening is often conducted by nursing staff. For the sake of expediency, many facilities are using instruments and criteria that are not evidence-based and/or lack established validity for the applications for which they are being used. It must also be highlighted that most instruments have not been specifically validated for use with malnourished obese individuals.

Multi-item screening and assessment instruments (Table 9-4) have been developed as indicators of nutritional status because no single measures have validity for this purpose. These instruments range from brief and simple screening tools that use self-reported queries of variables that include weight loss and poor appetite (eg, Malnutrition Screening Tool[18] and Short Nutrition Assessment Questionnaire[19]); to more robust screening tools that require additional time to obtain height and weight, calculate BMI, determine percentage of weight loss, and evaluate severity of disease (eg, Malnutrition Universal Screening Tool,[20] Nutrition Risk Screening 2002,[21] and Mini Nutritional Assessment Short Form[22]); to even more comprehensive and time-consuming assessment tools (eg, the Subjective Global Assessment,[23] the Nutrition Screening Initiative Level I and Level II Screens,[24] and the Mini Nutritional Assessment[25,26]).

Conclusion

This chapter has introduced a new approach to understanding malnutrition syndromes in adults and has highlighted some practical nutrition screening and assessment methods suitable for routine clinical applications. The lack of any single clinical or laboratory measure that provides a comprehensive assessment of nutritional status requires a systematic approach that gathers information from historical, clinical signs/physical examination, and anthropometric, laboratory, dietary, and functional components.

References

1. Bistrian BR, Blackburn GL, Hallowell E, Heddle R. Protein status of general surgical patients. *JAMA*. 1974;230:858–860.
2. Bistrian BR, Blackburn GL, Sherman M, et al. Therapeutic index of nutritional depletion in hospitalized patients. *Surg Gynecol Obstet*. 1975;141:512–516.
3. Roubenoff R, Roubenoff RA, Preto J, et al. Malnutrition among hospitalized patients. A problem of physician awareness. *Arch Intern Med*. 1987;147:1462–1465.
4. Mueller C, Compher C, Druyan ME, American Society for Parenteral and Enteral Nutrition (A.S.P.E.N.) Board of Directors. A.S.P.E.N Clinical Guidelines. Nutrition screening, assessment and intervention in adults. *J Parenter Enteral Nutr*. 2011;35:16–24.
5. Jensen GL. Inflammation as the key interface of the medical and nutrition universes: a provocative examination of the future of clinical nutrition and medicine. *J Parenter Enteral Nutr*. 2006;30: 453–463.
6. Jensen GL, Mirtallo J, Compher C, et al. Adult starvation and disease-related malnutrition: a proposal for etiology-based diagnosis in the clinical practice setting from the International Consensus Guideline Committee. *J Parenter Enteral Nutr*. 2010;34: 156–159.
7. Chumlea WC, Roche AF, Steinbaugh ML. Estimating stature from knee height for persons 60 to 90 years of age. *J Am Geriatr Soc*. 1985;33:116–120.
8. Society of Actuaries and Association of Life Insurance Medical Directors. *1979 Build Study*. Chicago, IL: Metropolitan Life Insurance Company; 1980.
9. National Institutes of Health. *Clinical Guidelines on the Identification, Evaluation, and Treatment of Overweight and Obesity in Adults*. Bethesda, MD: National Institutes of Health; 1998.
10. Centers for Disease Control and Prevention. NHANES III Anthropometric Procedure Videos. www.cdc.gov/nchs/nhanes/nhanes3/anthropometric_videos.htm. Accessed May 29, 2011.
11. Jensen GL, Bistrian B, Roubenoff R, et al. Malnutrition syndromes: a conundrum versus continuum. *J Parenter Enteral Nutr*. 2009;33: 710–716.
12. Burke BS, Stuart HC. A method of diet analysis: application in research and pediatric practice. *J Pediatrics*. 1938;12(4):493–503.
13. Institute of Medicine. *Dietary Reference Intakes Tables and Application*. www.iom.edu/Activities/Nutrition/SummaryDRIs/DRI-Tables.aspx. Accessed May 29, 2011.
14. Smiciklas-Wright H, Mitchell DC, et al. Dietary intake assessment: methods for adults. In: Berdanier CD, Dwyer J, Feldman EB, eds. *Handbook of Nutrition and Food*. 2nd ed. Boca Raton, FL: CRC Press; 2007:497–500.
15. Thompson FE, Subar A. Dietary assessment methodology. In: Coulston AM, Boushey CJ, eds. *Nutrition in the Prevention and Treatment of Disease*. New York: Academic Press; 2008:16–18.
16. The Joint Commission. www.jointcommission.org. Accessed June 13, 2011.
17. Chima CS, Dietz-Seher C, Kushner-Benson S. Nutrition risk screening in acute care: a survey of practice. *Nutr Clinical Prac*. 2008;23(4):417–423.
18. Ferguson M, Capra S, Bauer J, et al. Development of a valid and reliable malnutrition screening tool for adult acute hospital patients. *Nutrition*. 1999;14:458–464.
19. Kruizenga HM, Tulder MW, Seidell JC, et al. Effectiveness and cost effectiveness of early screening and treatment of malnourished patients. *Am J Clin Nutr*. 2005;82:1082–1089.
20. Elia M. *The "MUST" Report, Nutritional Screening of Adults: A Multidisciplinary Responsibility*. Redditch, UK: British Association for Parenteral and Enteral Nutrition; 2003. www.bapen.org.uk/pdfs/must/must_exec_sum.pdf. Accessed May 29, 2011.
21. Kondrup J, Rasmussen HH, Hamberg O, et al, Ad Hoc ESPEN Working Group. Nutritional risk screening (NRS 2002): a new method based on an analysis of controlled clinical trials. *Clin Nutr*. 2003;22:321–336.
22. Kaiser MJ, Bauer JM, Ramsch C, et al. Validation of the Mini Nutritional Assessment short-form (MNA-SF): a practical tool for indentification of nutritional status. *J Nutr Health Aging*. 2009;13: 782–788.
23. Detsky A, McLaughlin, Baker J, et al. What is subjective global assessment of nutritional status? *J Parenter Enteral Nutr*. 1987; 11(1):8–13.
24. Nutrition Screening Initiative. *Nutrition Interventions Manual for Professionals Caring for Older Americans*. Washington, DC; Nutrition Screening Initiative; 1992.
25. Guigoz Y. The Mini Nutritional Assessment review of the literature - what does it tell us? *J Nutr Health Aging*. 2006;10:466–485.

26. Kaiser MJ, Bauer JM, Ramsch C, et al. Frequency of malnutrition in older adults: a multinational perspective using the Mini Nutritional Assessment. *J Am Geriatr Soc.* 2010;58:1734–1738.
27. Stanley KE. Prognostic factors for survival in patients with inoperable lung cancer. *J Natl Cancer Inst.* 1980;65:25–32.
28. Dewys WD, Begg C, Lavin PT, et al. Prognostic effect of weight loss prior to chemotherapy in cancer patients. *Am J Med.* 1980;69: 491–497.
29. Ervin RB, Wright JD, Kennedy-Stephenson J. Use of dietary supplements in the United States, 1988–94. *Vital Health Stat 11.* 1999;i-iii: 1–14.
30. Katz S, Downs TD, Cash HR, et al. Progress in development of the index of ADL. *Gerontologist.* 1970;10:20–30.
31. Lawton MP, Brody EM. Assessment of older people: self-maintaining and instrumental activities of daily living. *Gerontologist.* 1969;9:179–186.
32. Russell DM, Leiter LA, Whitwell J, et al. Skeletal muscle function during hypocaloric diets and fasting: a comparison with standard nutritional assessment parameters. *Am J Clin Nutr.* 1983;37: 133–138.
33. Windsor JA, Hill GL. Weight loss with physiologic impairment. A basic indicator of surgical risk. *Ann Surg.* 1988;207:290–296.
34. Bassey EJ, Fiatarone MA, O'Neill EF, et al. Leg extensor power and functional performance in very old men and women. *Clin Sci.* 1992;82:321–327.
35. McLaren DS. *Color Atlas of Nutritional Disorders.* Chicago, IL: Year Book Medical Publishers; 1981.
36. Miller SJ. Nutritional deficiency and the skin. *J Am Acad Dermatol.* 1989;21:1–30.
37. Sullivan DH, Martin W, Flaxman N, et al. Oral health problems and involuntary weight loss in a population of frail elderly. *J Am Geriatr Soc.* 1993;41:725–731.
38. Folstein MF, Folstein SE, McHugh PR. "Mini-mental state." A practical method for grading the cognitive state of patients for the clinician. *J Psychiatr Res.* 1975;12:189–198.
39. Beck AT, Beck RW. Screening depressed patients in family practice. A rapid technic. *Postgrad Med.* 1972;52:81–85.
40. Yesavage JA, Brink TL, Rose TL, et al. Development and validation of a geriatric depression screening scale: a preliminary report. *J Psychiatr Res.* 1982;17:37–49.
41. Reuben DB, Siu AL. An objective measure of physical function of elderly outpatients. The Physical Performance Test. *J Am Geriatr Soc.* 1990;38:1105–1112.
42. Lean ME, Han TS, Deurenberg P. Predicting body composition by densitometry from simple anthropometric measurements. *Am J Clin Nutr.* 1996;63:4–14.
43. Hall JC, O'Quigley J, Giles GR, et al. Upper limb anthropometry: the value of measurement variance studies. *Am J Clin Nutr.* 1980; 33:1846–1851.
44. Elia M. The bioimpedance "craze." *Eur J Clin Nutr.* 1993;47: 825–827.
45. Jebb SA, Elia M. Techniques for the measurement of body composition: a practical guide. *Int J Obes Relat Metab Disord.* 1993;17: 611–621.
46. Roubenoff R, Baumgartner RN, Harris TB, et al. Application of bioelectrical impedance analysis to elderly populations. *J Gerontol A Biol Sci Med Sci.* 1997;52:M129–M136.
47. Durnin JV, Womersley J. Body fat assessed from total body density and its estimation from skinfold thickness: measurements on 481 men and women aged from 16 to 72 years. *Br J Nutr.* 1974;32: 77–97.
48. Kehayias JJ, Fiatarone MA, Zhuang H, et al. Total body potassium and body fat: relevance to aging. *Am J Clin Nutr.* 1997;66:904–910.
49. Pierson RN Jr, Wang J, Colt EW, et al. Body composition measurements in normal man: the potassium, sodium, sulfate and tritium spaces in 58 adults. *J Chronic Dis.* 1982;35:419–428.
50. Schoeller DA. Changes in total body water with age. *Am J Clin Nutr.* 1989;50(Suppl 5):1176–1181; discussion 1231–1275.
51. Dempster P, Aitkens S. A new air displacement method for the determination of human body composition. *Med Sci Sports Exerc.* 1995;27:1692–1697.
52. Biaggi RR, Vollman MW, Nies MA, et al. Comparison of air-displacement plethysmography with hydrostatic weighing and bioelectrical impedance analysis for the assessment of body composition in healthy adults. *Am J Clin Nutr.* 1999;69: 898–903.
53. Pietrobelli A, Formica C, Wang Z, et al. Dual-energy X-ray absorptiometry body composition model: review of physical concepts. *Am J Physiol.* 1996;271(6 Pt 1):E941–E951.
54. Rubiano F, Nunez C, Heymsfield SB. A comparison of body composition techniques. *Ann NY Acad Sci.* 2000;904:335–338.
55. Sjostrom L. A computer-tomography based multicompartment body composition technique and anthropometric predictions of lean body mass, total and subcutaneous adipose tissue. *Int J Obes.* 1991;15(Suppl 2):19–30.
56. Selberg O, Burchert W, Graubner G, et al. Determination of anatomical skeletal muscle mass by whole body nuclear magnetic resonance. *Basic Life Sci.* 1993;60:95–97.
57. D'Erasmo E, Pisani D, Ragno A, et al. Serum albumin level at admission: mortality and clinical outcome in geriatric patients. *Am J Med Sci.* 1997;314:17–20.
58. Friedmann JM, Jensen GL, Smiciklas-Wright H, et al. Predicting early nonelective hospital readmission in nutritionally compromised older adults. *Am J Clin Nutr.* 1997;65:1714–1720.
59. Corti MC, Guralnik JM, Salive ME, et al. Serum albumin level and physical disability as predictors of mortality in older persons. *JAMA.* 1994;272:1036–1042.
60. Rall C, Roubenoff R, Harris T. Albumin as a marker of nutritional and health status. In: Rosenberg IH, ed. *Nutritional Assessment of Elderly Populations: Measure and Function.* 1st ed. New York, NY: Raven; 1995:1–17.
61. Reuben DB, Moore AA, Damesyn M, et al. Correlates of hypoalbuminemia in community-dwelling older persons. *Am J Clin Nutr.* 1997;66:38–45.
62. Ingenbleek Y, Young V. Transthyretin (prealbumin) in health and disease: nutritional implications. *Annu Rev Nutr.* 1994;14: 495–533.
63. Carpentier YA, Barthel J, Bruyns J. Plasma protein concentration in nutritional assessment. *Proc Nutr Soc.* 1982;41:405–417.
64. Boles JM, Garre MA, Youinou PY, et al. Nutritional status in intensive care patients: evaluation in 84 unselected patients. *Crit Care Med.* 1983;11:87–90.
65. Goldberg DM, Brown D. Advances in the application of biochemical tests to diseases of the liver and biliary tract: their role in diagnosis, prognosis, and the elucidation of pathogenetic mechanisms. *Clin Biochem.* 1987;20:127–148.
66. Smith FR, Goodman DS. The effects of diseases of the liver, thyroid, and kidneys on the transport of vitamin A in human plasma. *J Clin Invest.* 1971;50:2426–2436.
67. Roza AM, Tuitt D, Shizgal HM. Transferrin—a poor measure of nutritional status. *J Parenter Enteral Nutr.* 1984;8:523–528.
68. Fletcher JP, Little JM, Guest PK. A comparison of serum transferrin and serum prealbumin as nutritional parameters. *J Parenter Enteral Nutr.* 1987;11:144–147.
69. Spiekerman AM. Proteins used in nutritional assessment. *Clin Lab Med.* 1993;13:353–369.

70. Carpentier YA, Barthel J, Bruyns J. Plasma protein concentration in nutritional assessment. *Proc Nutr Soc.* 1982;41:405–417.
71. Boles JM, Garre MA, Youinou PY, et al. Nutritional status in intensive care patients: evaluation in 84 unselected patients. *Crit Care Med.* 1983;11:87–90.
72. Winkler MF, Gerrior SA, Pomp A, et al. Use of retinol-binding protein and prealbumin as indicators of the response to nutrition therapy. *J Am Diet Assoc.* 1989;89:684–687.
73. Sachs E, Bernstein LH. Protein markers of nutrition status as related to sex and age. *Clin Chem.* 1986;32:339–341.
74. Pepys MB. C-reactive protein fifty years on. *Lancet.* 1981;1:653–657.
75. Deodhar SD. C-reactive protein: the best laboratory indicator available for monitoring disease activity. *Cleve Clin J Med.* 1989; 56:126–130.
76. Noel MA, Smith TK, Ettinger WH. Characteristics and outcomes of hospitalized older patients who develop hypocholesterolemia. *J Am Geriatr Soc.* 1991;39:455–461.
77. Rudman D, Feller AG. Protein-calorie undernutrition in the nursing home. *J Am Geriatr Soc.* 1989;37:173–183.
78. Goichot B, Schlienger JL, Grunenberger F, et al. Low cholesterol concentrations in free-living elderly subjects: relations with dietary intake and nutritional status. *Am J Clin Nutr.* 1995;62:547–553.
79. Ettinger WH Jr, Harris T, Verdery RB, et al. Evidence for inflammation as a cause of hypocholesterolemia in older people. *J Am Geriatr Soc.* 1995;43:264–266.
80. Bistrian BR, Blackburn GL, Scrimshaw NS, et al. Cellular immunity in semistarved states in hospitalized adults. *Am J Clin Nutr.* 1975;28:1148–1155.
81. Law DK, Dudrick SJ, Abdou NI. Immunocompetence of patients with protein-calorie malnutrition. The effects of nutritional repletion. *Ann Intern Med.* 1973;79:545–550.
82. Seltzer MH, Fletcher HS, Slocum BA, et al. Instant nutritional assessment in the intensive care unit. *J Parenter Enteral Nutr.* 1981;5: 70–72.
83. Mitchell CO, Lipschitz DA. The effect of age and sex on the routinely used measurements to assess the nutritional status of hospitalized patients. *Am J Clin Nutr.* 1982;36:340–349.
84. Kaiser FE, Morley JE. Idiopathic CD4+ T lymphopenia in older persons. *J Am Geriatr Soc.* 1994;42:1291–1294.
85. Ballard FJ, Tomas FM. 3-Methylhistidine as a measure of skeletal muscle protein breakdown in human subjects: the case for its continued use. *Clin Sci.* 1983;65:209–215.
86. Iapichino G, Radrizzani D, Solca M, et al. Influence of total parenteral nutrition on protein metabolism following acute injury: assessment by urinary 3-methylhistidine excretion and nitrogen balance. *J Parenter Entreal Nutr.* 1985;9:42–46.
87. Heymsfield SB, Arteaga C, McManus C, et al. Measurement of muscle mass in humans: validity of the 24-hour urinary creatinine method. *Am J Clin Nutr.* 1983;37:478–494.
88. Christou NV, Meakins JL, MacLean LD. The predictive role of delayed hypersensitivity in preoperative patients. *Surg Gynecol Obstet.* 1981;152:297–301.
89. Simonson E, Henschel A, Keys A. The electrocardiogram of man in semi-starvation and subsequent rehabilitation. *Am Heart J.* 1948;55:584–602.
90. Isner JM, Roberts WC, Heymsfield SB, et al. Anorexia nervosa and sudden death. *Ann Intern Med.* 1985;102:49–52.
91. Heymsfield SB, Bethel RA, Ansley JD, et al. Cardiac abnormalities in cachectic patients before and during nutritional repletion. *Am Heart J.* 1978;95:584–594.
92. Makk LJ, McClave SA, Creech PW, et al. Clinical application of the metabolic cart to the delivery of total parenteral nutrition. *Crit Care Med.* 1990;18:1320–1327.
93. Compher C, Frankenfield D, Keim N, et al, The Evidence Analysis Working Group. Best practice methods to apply to measurement of resting metabolic rate in adults: a systematic review. *J Am Diet Assoc.* 2006;106:881–903.
94. Reilly HM, Martineau JK, Moran A, et al. Nutritional screening - evaluation and implementation of a simple nutrition risk score. *Clin Nutr.* 1995;14:269–273.
95. Kuzu MA, Terzio lu H, Gene V, et al. Preoperative nutritional risk assessment in predicting postoperative outcome in patients undergoing major surgery. *World J Surg.* 2006;30:378–390.
96. Kovacevich DS, Boney AR, Braunschweig CL, et al. Nutrition risk classification: a reproducible and valid tool for nurses. *Nutr Clin Pract.* 1997;12:20–25.
97. The Veterans Affairs Total Parenteral Nutrition Cooperative Study Group. Perioperative total parenteral nutrition in surgical patients. *N Eng J Med.* 1991;325:525–532.
98. Ingenbleek Y, Carpentier YA. A prognostic inflammatory and nutritional index scoring critically ill patients. *Intl J Vitam Nutr Res.* 1985;55:91–101.
99. Buzby GP, Mullen JL, Matthews DC, et al. Prognostic nutritional index in gastrointestinal surgery. *Am J Surg.* 1980;139:160–167.
100. Laporte M, Villalon L, Thibodeau J, et al. Validity and reliability of simple nutrition screening tools adapted to the elderly population in healthcare facilities. *J Nutr Health Aging.* 2001;5: 292–294.

10 Overview of Enteral Nutrition

Susan L. Brantley, MS, RD, CNSC, LDN, and Mary E. (Beth) Mills, MS, RD, CNSC, LDN

CONTENTS

Background 171
Indications for Enteral Nutrition 171
Patient Selection 171
Benefits 171
Contraindications 173
Timing of Enteral Nutrition 173
Dosing of Enteral Nutrition 173
Enteral Nutrition Administration 173
Enteral Access Devices 173
Enteral Order Sets and Protocols 174
Delivery Methods 175
Continuous Infusion 175
Cyclic Feeding 175
Intermittent Feeding 175
Bolus and Gravity Drip Feeding 176
Transitional Feeding 176
Enteral Formulations 176
Monitoring During Enteral Nutrition 176
Confirming and Monitoring Feeding Tube Placement 176
Medication Administration 177
Meeting Nutritional Goals 177
Gastrointestinal Issues 178
Aspiration 179
Metabolic Monitoring 179
Enteral Nutrition Safety 180
Contamination 180
Enteral Misconnections 181
Enteral Nutrition Outcomes 181
Summary 182
References 182

Objectives

1. Identify the indications and contraindications for initiating enteral nutrition (EN) support in certain patient populations.
2. Explain how the timing of enteral nutrition support can affect patient care.
3. Identify and define the safety issues associated with enteral nutrition.

Test Your Knowledge Questions

1. Utilizing the normal route of digestion and absorption of the gastrointestinal (GI) tract supports maintenance of the:
   A. Functional integrity of the gut
   B. Gut barrier functions
   C. Gut-associated and mucosa-associated lymphoid tissues
   D. All the above

2. In critically ill patients, EN should be initiated early within _____ of admission to the intensive care unit (ICU).
   A. 24 to 48 hours
   B. 3 to 5 days
   C. 12 hours
   D. First hour
3. The entire enteral feeding system, from the feeding tubes to the bags and sets, has been reviewed and is being redesigned in an effort to avoid any potentially dangerous complications associated with medical misconnections. Medical misconnections are primarily associated with _________ connectors.
   A. Syringe
   B. Luer
   C. Y-port
   D. Dialysis catheter

Test Your Knowledge Answers

1. The correct answer is **D**. The presence of nutrients in the small intestine maintains normal gallbladder function by stimulating the release of cholecystokinin, reducing the risk of cholecystitis that may occur with parenteral nutrition. Besides the benefit of maintaining normal digestive and absorptive capabilities, luminal nutrients provide structural support and also aid to maintain the gut-associated and mucosa-associated lymphoid tissues vital to gut-associated immune function. Immunoglobulin A (IgA), secreted within the GI tract, can prevent bacterial adherence and translocation. IgA production is reduced when intraluminal nutrients are not present.[1]
2. The correct answer is **A**. For critically ill patients, EN should be initiated early within 24 to 48 hours of admission to the ICU.[2–5] McClave and Heyland propose that there is a "window of opportunity" in which the benefits of early EN (EEN) can be obtained.[6] It has been noted that the early delivery of EN affects the functional and structural integrity of the GI tract. They looked at 14 prospective, randomized controlled clinical trials comparing the provision of early enteral nutrition (initiated 48 hours after admission) to delayed enteral nutrition. There was a reported significant 24% reduction in infectious complications and a 32% reduction in mortality.[4,6]
3. The correct answer is **B**. At the center of the catheter/tubing misconnections in health care are the Luer connector systems. These Luer connectors are called Luer-Lok, Luer-Slip, Luer tip, or small-bore connectors.[7] As a part of the new 2013 enteral standards developed by the International Organization for Standardization, female Luer connectors will no longer be found on feeding tubes. This will force the use of a compatible oral/enteral syringe to give oral medications via a feeding tube.[8]

Background

EN is defined as "nutrition provided through the gastrointestinal tract via a tube, catheter, or stoma that delivers nutrients distal to the oral cavity."[9] EN is the preferred method of feeding patients who are unable to maintain volitional intake.[2,3] The ancient and fascinating history of EN from the first rectal feedings[10]; the early "formula" mixtures of wine, eggs, milk, and other food substances[11]; and the growth and utilization of EN as routine care in modern day critical care units can be found elsewhere.[11,12] Today, enteral formulas are formulated from a variety of sources of macronutrients and contain micronutrients and water in various amounts per specific formula (see Chapter 11). In some clinical situations, adjunctive therapy with additional specific amino acids, probiotics, enhanced amounts of vitamins, and trace minerals along with soluble and insoluble fiber sources may be considered.[2] Currently, proactive utilization of EEN therapy, along with appropriate glycemic control, is seen as a therapeutic strategy to reduce disease severity by attenuating the metabolic response to stress, diminishing complications by preventing oxidative cellular injury, and favorably modulating the immune response thereby showing trends of decreasing ICU length of stay and favorably impacting patient outcomes.[2–5]

Indications for Enteral Nutrition

Patient Selection

Boullata and colleagues[1] indicate individuals with a functional GI tract, along with clinical situations in which oral intake is deemed unsafe, insufficient, or impossible, are candidates for EN support. Prior to initiating EN, clinicians should consider ethical issues of the patient and/or family's wishes, quality of life, and risks and benefits of EN therapy together with the patient's prognosis, diagnosis, and clinical status.[13] Considerations of these issues are necessary to determine if aggressive EEN in the patient in the ICU is warranted and/or if delaying initiation of EN for a few days in the noncritically ill patient is the most appropriate approach to providing care (Figure 10-1).[1,13]

Benefits

If patients are unable to consume nutrients orally, EN offers a wealth of benefits. Utilizing the normal route of digestion and absorption of the GI tract supports maintenance of the functional integrity of the gut (see Chapter 1). EN is the preferred route of feeding[3] due to the benefits of supporting the components of the gut barrier functions.[14] Nutrients provided via the enteral route undergo first-pass metabolism, promoting efficient utilization of the nutrients. The presence of nutrients in the small intestine maintains normal gallbladder function by stimulating the release of cholecystokinin, reducing the risk of cholecystitis that may occur with parenteral nutrition. Besides the benefit of maintaining normal digestive and absorptive capabilities, luminal nutrients provide structural support and also aid to maintain the gut-associated and mucosa-associated lymphoid tissues vital to gut-associated immune function. IgA, secreted within the GI tract, can prevent bacterial adherence and translocation. IgA production is reduced when intraluminal nutrients are not present. Additionally, EN has been shown to reduce infectious complications associated with pneumonia, sepsis, intravenous line sepsis, and intra-abdominal abscess in several prospective randomized clinical trials. Finally, in

FIGURE 10-1 Route of Administration Algorithm

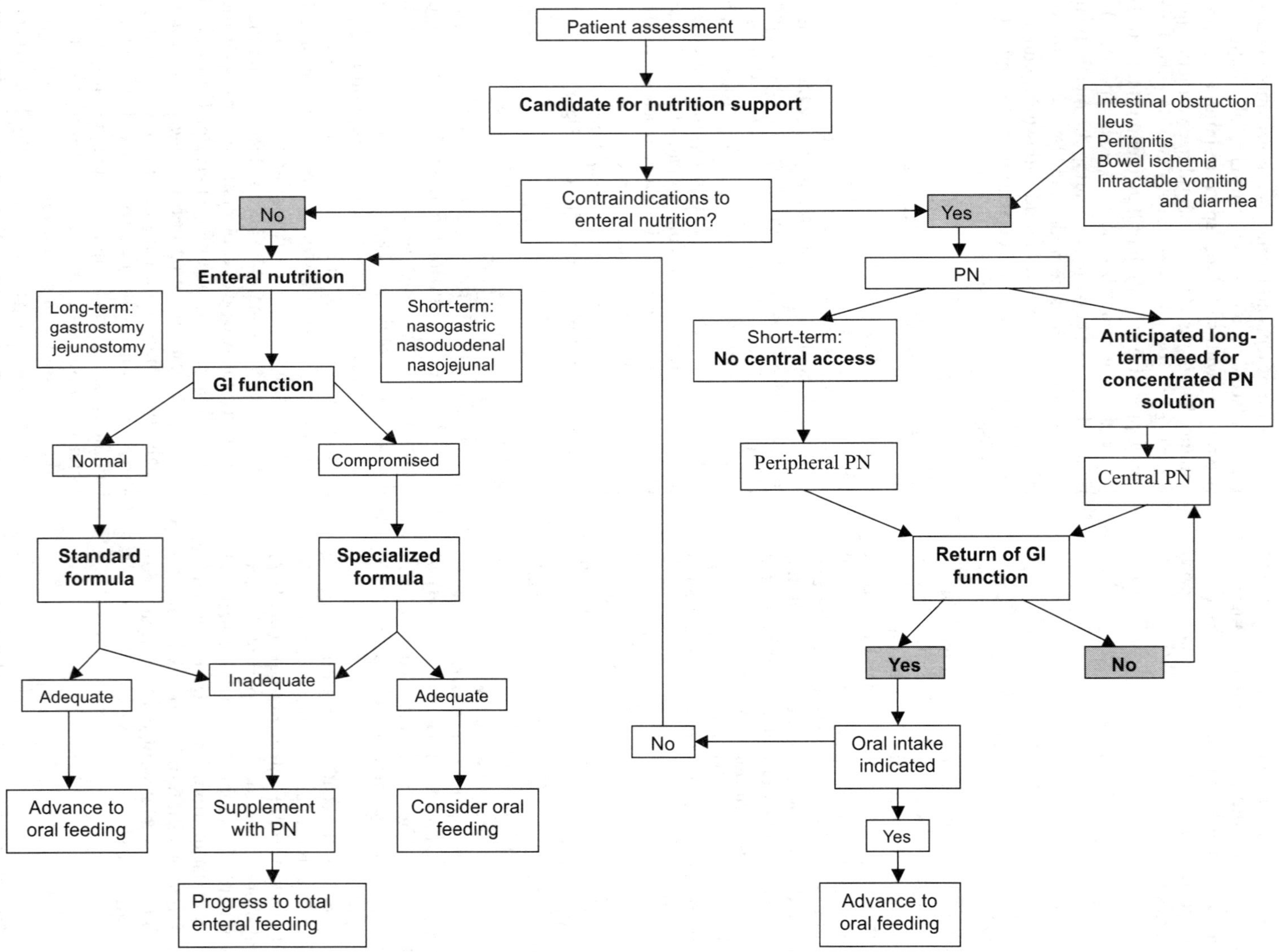

GI, gastrointestinal; PN, parenteral nutrition.
Reprinted from A.S.P.E.N. Board of Directors. *Clinical Pathways and Algorithms for Delivery of Parenteral and Enteral Nutrition Support in Adults*. Silver Spring, MD: American Society for Parenteral and Enteral Nutrition; 1998:4.

© 2012 A.S.P.E.N. www.nutritioncare.org

general from a cost standpoint, the overall provision of EN is less expensive than parenteral nutrition.[1]

Contraindications

Although EN is the preferred route of nutrition support, it may be contraindicated in certain circumstances (Table 10-1).[1]

EN is contraindicated if the expected duration of EN therapy is for less than 5 to 7 days in the malnourished adult patient or less than 7 to 9 days in the adequately nourished adult patient, or if EN support is not desired or warranted.[1] Patients with severe short bowel syndrome (< 100 cm remaining small bowel), severe GI bleed, severe GI malabsorption, distal high-output fistulas, intractable vomiting and/or diarrhea refractory to medical management or paralytic ileus, with nonoperative mechanical obstructions, or in the clinical situation of the inability to gain access to the GI tract may require parenteral nutrition support (see Chapters 21–36).[1]

Timing of Enteral Nutrition

The most recent American Society for Parenteral and Enteral Nutrition (A.S.P.E.N.) guidelines[3] do not specifically address the timing of EN in the noncritically ill patient; however, the 2002 "Guidelines for the Use of Parenteral and Enteral Nutrition in Adult and Pediatric Patients"[15] stated that specialized nutrition support "should be initiated in patients with inadequate oral intake for 7 to 14 days, or in those patients in whom inadequate oral intake is expected over a 7- to 14-day period." Therefore, in the previously well-nourished noncritically ill patient, initiation of EN support may be delayed until the patient demonstrates insufficient oral intake, unless the clinical situation is highly indicative for expected insufficient oral intake and the anticipated need for EN therapy is for > 7 days duration.

For critically ill patients, EN should be initiated early within 24 to 48 hours of admission to the ICU.[2–5] The 2006 European Society of Parenteral and Enteral Nutrition guidelines on EN agree that hemodynamically stable patients with a functional GI tract should be fed early. In the critically ill patient population, the European Society of Parenteral and Enteral Nutrition defines early enteral feeding as within < 24 hours.[16] These recommendations for early enteral feedings are supported by the Canadian Guidelines for Nutrition in the Critically Ill.[4] McClave and Heyland propose that there is a "window of opportunity" in which the benefits of EEN can be obtained.[6] Based on a review of the literature, they further postulate that a "cumulative caloric deficit" is associated with longer lengths of ICU stay, more days on mechanical ventilation, and more complications.[6] The occurrence of adult respiratory distress syndrome, renal failure, need for surgery, development of pressure ulcers, and total complication rate was highly correlated with negative cumulative energy balance.[6] During the first week of the patients' ICU stay a cumulative caloric deficit of >10,000 kcal was found to be associated with worse clinical outcomes.[6] Owens and Fang,[16] after a literature review on the benefits of EEN,[17] stated that "Diet (ie, enteral nutrition support) should be viewed as the next step in the resuscitation of patients after airway, breathing, and circulation needs have been addressed in an 'ABCD' mnemonic approach to critically ill patients."

TABLE 10-1 Contraindications to Enteral Nutrition Support

- Nonoperative mechanical GI obstruction
- Intractable vomiting/diarrhea refractory to medical management
- Severe short-bowel syndrome (< 100 cm small bowel remaining)
- Paralytic ileus
- Distal high-output fistulas (too distal to bypass with feeding tube)
- Severe GI bleed
- Severe GI malabsorption (eg, enteral nutrition failed as evidenced by progressive deterioration in nutritional status)
- Inability to gain access to GI tract
- Need is expected for < 5–7 days for malnourished adult patients or 7–9 days if adequately nourished
- Aggressive intervention not warranted or not desired

GI, gastrointestinal.
Reprinted from Enteral Access Devices: Selection, Insertion, Maintenance, and Complications. In: Boullata J, Nieman Carney L, Guenter P, eds. *The A.S.P.E.N. Enteral Nutrition Handbook*. Silver Spring, MD: A.S.P.E.N.; 2010: 164,165 with permission from the American Society for Parenteral and Enteral Nutrition (A.S.P.E.N.).

Dosing of Enteral Nutrition

The A.S.P.E.N. guidelines[3] recommend that, in order to derive clinical benefit from EEN, achievement of greater than 50% to 65% of goal calories during the first week of hospitalization is desired.

Until a universal definition of effective EN delivery is determined, Parrish[18] has suggested defining effective EN delivery as consistent infusion of > 90% of a calculated caloric goal.

Enteral Nutrition Administration

Enteral Access Devices

When considering the type of enteral access that is most appropriate for the patient, decisions should be based on disease state, GI function, duration of EN support therapy, and the available expertise for placement of the access.[13] Options include short-term placement through the nose or mouth into the stomach, past the pylorus, or distal to the ligament of Trietz. More permanent feeding tube placement options are available. Gastrostomy, jejunostomy, and gastrojejunostomy tubes are used when feeding tubes will be required for nutrition support for a period of more than 4 to 6 weeks.

The type of tube needed as well as the technique utilized to obtain enteral access must be determined by careful evaluation of the patient's needs and the institutional resources available. Surgical methods include open methods such as laparotomy and laparoscopy. The gastroenterological method of percutaneous, endoscopically guided tubes is often used as a minimally invasive method, while radiological methods such as with the use of fluoroscopy, ultrasound, or computed tomography are also possible placement procedures (Figure 10-2; for more information, see Chapter 12).[18,19]

Enteral Order Sets and Protocols

The Society of Critical Care Medicine (SCCM)/A.S.P.E.N. and the Canadian Clinical Practice Guidelines support the use of protocols and enteral order sets to maximize the safe delivery of EN.[4,20] These order sets can be designed to meet the needs of the institution and can be paper- or computer-based protocols. They should include the four elements of (1) patient identifier, (2) formula name, (3) enteral access device and site, and (4) administration method and rate.[21] Protocols and order sets should include strategies to minimize the risk of enteral feeding contamination and the risk of regurgitation and aspiration.[17] To promote optimal EN delivery and maximize tolerance, the protocol should be evidence-based and should clearly outline what the nurse should do in specific clinical situations. For example, initiating EN and advancing to the goal

FIGURE 10-2 Enteral Access Decision Tree

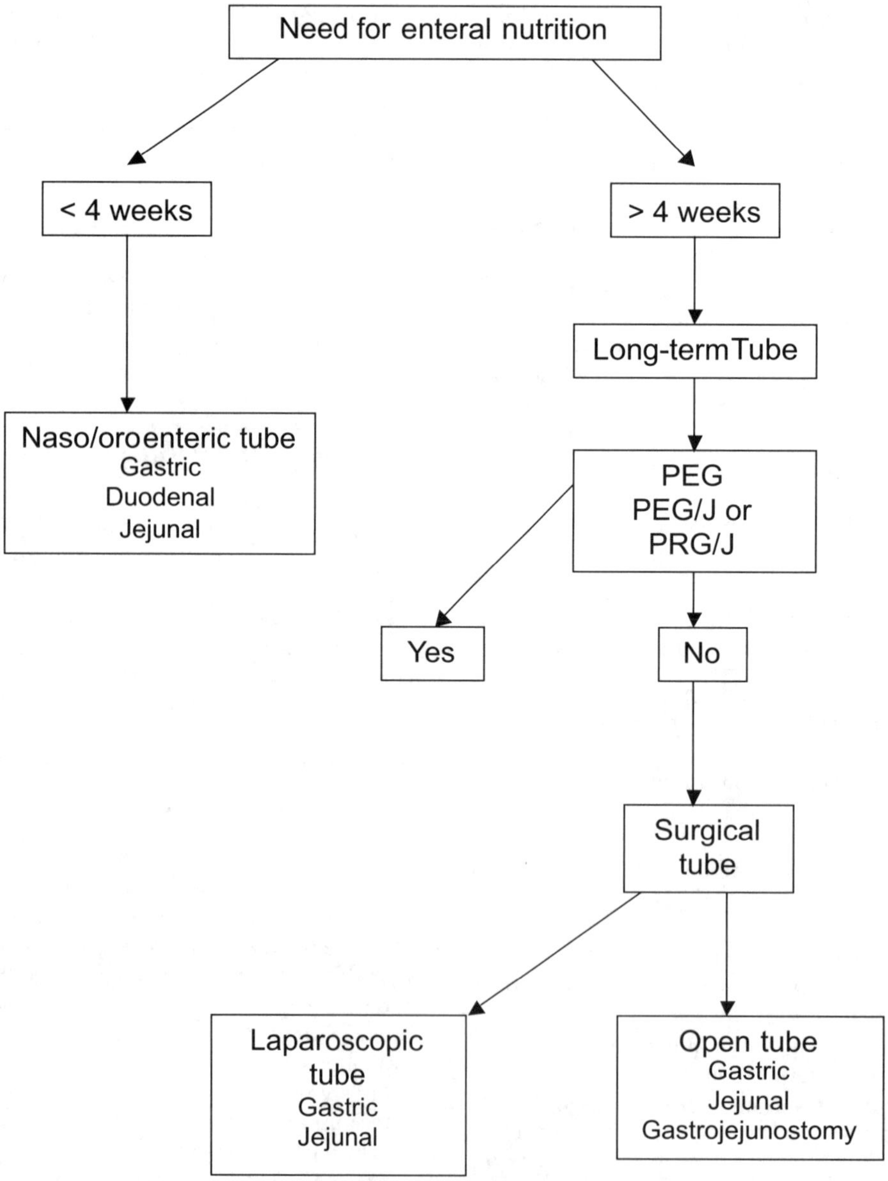

PEG, percutaneous endoscopic gastrostomy; PEG/J, percutaneous endoscopic gastrojejunostomy; PRG/J, percutaneous radiographic gastrostomy with a jejunal extension.

in a timely manner are important elements to include in a nurse-driven protocol. The inclusion of more recent evidence-based recommendations can empower the nurse to make changes to improve the delivery of EN. Order sets can assist in decision making by allowing a more consistent gastric residual volume (GRV)[22] of two consecutive checks of 250 mL or one check of more than 500 mL before EN is discontinued.[2,21] They could incorporate prokinetics if a patient is experiencing persistently elevated GRVs.[4,22] In a recent observational study, sites using an EN protocol achieved better nutrition practice. They had increased use of EN and received it earlier in their hospital stay. These institutions provided a higher percentage of goal calories than sites lacking a protocol.[22]

Delivery Methods

Enteral feeding may be administered using either the continuous, intermittent drip, or the bolus method. Factors such as the patient's preexisting and current medical conditions, location of the feeding tube tip, and the patient's expected tolerance to tube feedings should be considered when selecting the delivery method.[23] The patient's current location of care, whether in the acute care setting with critical illness, a stable ward patient, a patient residing in a long-term care facility, or a patient at home will also impact the choice of feeding method. Patients may be fed with one method or utilize a combination of methods to improve quality of life. Some patients in the acute care setting will transition from one method of feeding administration to another as their clinical status evolves.

Continuous Infusion

Pump-assisted continuous drip infusions are the preferred method of choice for feeding patients that are critically ill, intubated for respiratory failure, at risk for refeeding syndrome, have poor glycemic control, are being fed via jejunostomy tube, or have demonstrated intolerance to intermittent gravity drip feedings.[23] The gravity drip method may be utilized to provide continuous drip feedings to the noncritically ill patient. Dividing the total daily formula volume desired by the number of hours per day of administration will yield the goal feeding rate.[24] Typically, continuous feedings are initiated at 20 to 50 mL/hr and advanced as tolerated by 10 to 25 mL/hr every 4 to 24 hours until the goal rate per hour is achieved.[18] Figure 10-3 shows a sample calculation of a continuous EN prescription.[1] In the continuous feeding method, volume prospective was provided by Parrish,[18] in that 60 mL/hr = one-quarter cup or 4 tablespoons of formula infused over an entire hour, or 1 mL per minute. In some stable patients, enteral feedings may be initiated at the goal rate per hour.[1] There are a variety of enteral feeding pumps available on the market allowing for lightweight portable pumps for home use to more durable pumps for health care facilities (see Chapter 12).

Cyclic Feeding

Cycle feeding is essentially providing feedings by pump in less than a 24-hour time period. Depending on the patient's volume tolerance, infusion times may be decreased from 24 hours per day down to as little as 8 hours.[25] As a patient recovers from illness, this method may be used to transition from the 24-hour continuous feeding method to 12-hour or less nocturnal feedings in an effort to increase the patient's volitional intake during the day and increase mobility providing time free from tubing and pump connections.[25]

FIGURE 10-3 Calculation of Enteral Nutrition Prescription: Adult Patient

Calculations:

Select formula for this patient.
Example: Standard 1.0 kcal/mL formula

Determine required kcal/day.
Example: Patient needs 2000 kcal/day

Divide total number of kcal required by kcal/mL to determine mL per day needed.
Example: 2000 kcal needed ÷ 1.0 kcal/mL = 2000 mL/day

To determine protein dose, multiply daily formula in mL by grams of protein/L
Example: 2000 mL/day × 44 g/L = 88 g/day protein

Assure that this volume of the selected EN formula will provide adequate micronutrient dosing.

Determine required fluid in mL/day. Multiply percent water in formula times daily formula in mL to determine water contribution of EN. Subtract formula water from total fluid requirements to determine water flushes.
Example: Patient needs 2200 mL fluid. 2000mL formula × 84% water − 1680 mL water. 2200 mL − 1680 mL = 520 mL additional water. (Some of which may already be met by IV fluid or medication dilution.)

Determining Administration Rate:

Take total mL per day of formula and divide by 24 hours to determine continuous feeding goal rate.
Example: 2000 ml ÷ 24 hours = 83 mL/hour

EN, enteral nutrition.
Reprinted from How to Write Enteral Nutrition Orders. In: Boullata J, Nieman Carney L, Guenter P, eds. *The A.S.P.E.N. Enteral Nutrition Handbook*. Silver Spring, MD: A.S.P.E.N.; 2010: 230 with permission from the American Society for Parenteral and Enteral Nutrition (A.S.P.E.N.).

Intermittent Feeding

Intermittent feedings can be delivered by infusion pump or by the gravity drip method. This feeding regimen is usually selected for patients with feeding catheters that terminate in the stomach to accommodate the larger volumes administerered per feeding. Volumes can range from 240 to 720 mL (1 to 3 cups), be administered over a time period ranging from 20 to 60 minutes, and be provided anywhere from four to six times per day depending on the volume of formula required to meet the patient's specific needs.[23] It is important to let the home patient know that intermittent feeding can occur entirely during the waking hours and that it is not necessary to administer intermittent feedings during the sleeping hours. Some home patients have tried to mimic what was done at the hospital, setting alarms to awaken and administer feeds every 4 to 6 hours, even during the night. Therefore, as tolerated, some alert and mobile patients may choose to increase the volume and decrease the number of feeding times required per day to improve their quality of life.

Bolus and Gravity Drip Feeding

Bolus or gravity drip feedings are accomplished by providing a set volume of formula at specified time intervals over a very short period of time. A typical feeding regimen might provide 240 mL of formula over a 4- to 10-minute timeframe infused three to six times per day.[25] A too rapid infusion can cause GI intolerance and discomfort.[21,26] The rate of formula infusion using a gravity drip bag is regulated by adjusting a roller clamp. When utilizing a syringe without a plunger as a funnel, the rate of delivery of formula is controlled by raising or lowering a formula-filled syringe or adjusting the rate of pressure applied when using the syringe plunger.[25] Bolus feedings mimic normal feedings, provide freedom of movement, and are usually the least expensive delivery option.[25]

Transitional Feeding

Enteral feedings can be transitioned from continuous feedings to bolus or intermittent feedings. This is usually done through a series of steps to evaluate if the patient can tolerate a larger volume given periodically while still providing adequate nutrition with limited continuous feedings. Enteral feedings are sometimes changed from continuous feedings to cyclic feedings. This may be accomplished by increasing the rate while decreasing the hours of infusion. When transitioning from enteral feeding to an oral diet, it is important to consider the individual formula volume tolerance of each patient to the intermittent or cyclic infusion regimen. After the patient has been clinically cleared to begin an oral diet and the required, safe consistency has been determined, the diet is advanced. The enteral feedings may be held prior to meals to encourage intake, or they may be infused only during the evening hours to further stimulate the appetite. When the patient is meeting two-thirds to three-quarters of their nutrient needs through the oral route, EN may be discontinued. Monitoring oral intake should continue, however, to assure adequacy.[26]

Enteral Formulations

Current enteral formulas are more specialized to specific disease state and conditions than in the early years of feeding by tubes. Formulas have evolved from milk-based concoctions, to blenderized diets, to defined formulas with elemental components. New products are constantly being developed based on recent controlled studies, clinical practice guidelines, and recommendations.[12] Formulas are categorized based on their formulations: standard or polymeric, elemental or defined formula, and specialized. Standardized formulas are used for the majority of patients. They have a caloric density of 1.0 to 2.0 calories/mL. Some formulas contain fiber.[27] Disease-specific formulas are designed for a particular disease state or condition. These include formulas designed for patients with renal disease, hepatic disease, diabetes, pulmonary disease (chronic obstructive pulmonary disease and acute respiratory distress syndrome), and immunocompromised patients. Finally, the elemental or defined formulas were formulated to require minimal digestion. They were designed to benefit those patients with malabsorption and/or pancreatic insufficiency.[28] Although homemade blenderized formulas can be used, they are more susceptible to contamination.[27]

Modular components can be added to the nutritional regimen to increase the caloric content by the addition of hydrolyzed cornstarch and maltodextrin as a carbohydrate component. The fat composition can also be increased through the addition of oils such as fish oils, medium-chain triglycerides, and safflower oils. The protein content can be increased as well through the addition of powdered calcium caseinates and whey protein concentrates. Other amino acids such as glutamine and arginine are available and can be added via the enteral route as well.[29] It is important to never add medications or any other additive directly to an enteral feeding formula. When adding any modular, particularly through a feeding tube, the tube should be flushed adequately both before and after administration to avoid the risk of clogging the tube. Proper techniques to avoid contamination should be adhered to such as the use of gloves and clean technique when handling the enteral sets.[21]

Monitoring During Enteral Nutrition

Confirming and Monitoring Feeding Tube Placement

Before using any feeding tube placed blindly into the GI tract, correct placement should be confirmed radiographically. This practice is used more consistently in adults than children due to the higher radiation risk in this vulnerable pediatric patient population. The ausculatory method to determine correct placement, either gastric or small bowel, is inadequate in adults.[21] Radiography remains the only reliable method to accurately determine placement, even though there are concerns about both financial and time constraints using this method. According to research and expert opinion, secondary confirmation using pH or carbon dioxide testing or by visualization of tube at exit site should be included as a regular reassessment of tube location.[30]

The exit site of a feeding tube, whether it is at the nare or the skin, should be marked at the time of the initial radiograph.[21] This practice can help determine if the tube position should be checked with another radiograph should the patient vomit or gag, or if the tube is pulled as a result of being improperly secured.[30]

One of the most common problems associated with the provision of EN is clogged or obstructed feeding tubes. Feeding tubes clog for a variety of reasons. This can occur with small bore feeding tubes, with crushed or powdered medications, and with acidic or alkaline medications. Without regular flushing, tubes can collect residue on the inner lumen from the formula and from medication administration.[31] Tube occlusions can also occur as a result of GRV checks.[32] Prevention of tube occlusions is best practice. For example, routine water flushes of 20 to 40 mL every 4 hours during a continuous feeding and before and after each bolus feeding can decrease the incidence of clogging.[21,33] Water, and more specifically sterile water, is superior to other liquids for flushing and maintaining patency of feeding tubes.[21,31,34,35] This is especially true for patients who are critically ill and immunosuppressed.[36,37] In addition, finding other routes of medication administration should be investigated if an appropriate enteric form of a medication cannot be obtained. Enteral formulas with intact protein are more susceptible to a change in the consistency of the formula when exposed to a medication or other liquid with a more acidic pH. This can result in thickening of the formula and clogging of the feeding tube. This is the potential reason that flushing a tube with cranberry juice or soda is inferior to using water as a flush medium. Utilizing feeding tubes with a larger inner lumen can also be an effective method of avoiding frequent clogging.[38]

Once the feeding tube is clogged, only two options are available: remove the tube or clear the clog. Warm water is the optimal medium for attempting to clear tube occlusions. In the past, a mixture of pancrelipase and sodium bicarbonate have proven successful in dissolving tube obstructions[35]; however, the short-acting, crushable tablets are not currently available. Enteric-coated tablets formulated for sustained release are not recommended for this use. Recently, an in vitro study indicated that the release of these enteric-coated pancreatic enzymes dissolved with sodium bicarbonate in water will still disrupt smaller clogs.[39] At present, however, no information exists to describe the preferred dose or method of administration of these extended-release products for clearing clogged enteral feeding tubes.[38] In addition, stylets used for feeding tube placement, unclogging kits, endoscopy brushes, and other small tubes have been used to break up clogs.[31]

Different solutions used to unclog tubes can damage the materials of the tube surface. When both silicone and polyurethane tubes were tested, damage to the surface of the feeding tubes were seen with papain syrup, sodium bicarbonate solutions, and digestive enzymes. Orange juice and colas did result in some damage to the polyurethane tubes, while water and pineapple juice did not affect the surfaces of these tubes.[40]

Medication Administration

Often, the feeding tube must be utilized for medication administration. If the patient is unable to swallow safely or when the medication is not available in an intravenous form, the enteral access must be used as a medication administration device. In order to avoid tube obstruction and assure adequate drug delivery, it is important to adhere to specific techniques during administration via the enteral route.[21]

The dosage form of the medication must be considered before administering the drug through a feeding tube. Dosage forms include liquids or solids such as capsules and tablets. Immediate-release tablets are the most common and can be crushed or opened and diluted before administering down the feeding tube. On the other hand, delayed or extended-release tablets or capsules are usually difficult to crush due to the surface coating. They should not be opened or crushed and diluted to be administered, as this will alter the drug efficacy.[21] Liquid dosage forms may not always be the best option for delivery through a feeding tube. It can depend upon the properties of the specific drug such as viscosity and the type, size, and placement of the tube.[41]

The preferred diluent for medication administration is purified water (used for sterile irrigation) or saline.[21] Tap water should not be used to prepare medication for administration through feeding tubes. Tap water may contain heavy metals, medication residues, pesticides, and other contaminants that can react with the crushed medication. These interactions could change the bioavailability and effectiveness of the medication.[21,42]

There is also potential for drug–drug interactions if two or more drugs are crushed and/or diluted together to be given enterally. Drug stability can be affected when the dosage form is altered: "Mixing two or more dosage forms creates a new entity; it's unknown how each drug would be released."[43] This pertains to mixing two or more liquid medications as well: "It's also often unknown how a particular mixture of liquid dosage forms might behave in the body."[43] As a result, when more than one drug is prescribed for administration through a feeding tube, the drugs must be given separately.[7]

The site of the termination of the feeding tube should be determined and the medications evaluated to assure they do not bypass the area of the bowel intended for optimal absorption of the drug. There may be unknown sites of dissolution and absorption for certain drugs. A pharmacist should be consulted to determine if the drug "requires gastric acid, bile, pancreatic secretions, or a combination of these for adequate dissolution, as well as where in the GI tract most of the drug is absorbed."[7]

Drugs should never be added to the EN formula. Mixing the drug and the formula can increase the potential for drug–nutrient interactions. This can occlude the tube, interfere with the drug and nutrient bioavailability, and affect GI function. If the drug is mixed with the enteral formula, it is unknown how much of the drug actually will reach its site of action.[7]

Finally, medications should be delivered through syringes intended for oral or enteral use. These oral syringes can be used to measure and administer a medication safely as the tips are too wide to fit into Luer ports. These syringes should be clean and used only once.[21]

Meeting Nutritional Goals

One of the most important parts of monitoring a patient receiving enteral feeding is to assess achievement of estimated nutritional needs. An astute clinician should evaluate whether or not the patient has attained prescribed enteral feeding goals. If not, one should determine impediments, then troubleshoot and develop new recommendations for attainment of goals. Many methods have been utilized to improve the daily amount of calories and protein provided to patients. Examples include compensatory goal feeding rate increases,[44] avoidance of unnecessary cessation of tube feedings for repositioning patients,[45] reduction in the time patients with protected airways are made nothing by mouth prior to procedures or surgeries,[46] and the bridling of feeding tubes.[47] Utilizing the compensatory feeding rate method, Lichenberg et al. significantly reduced caloric deficits from frequent EN holding, promoting optimal nutrient delivery by calculating and prescribing a higher EN infusion rate assuming duration of 20 hours/day instead of the standard 24-hour infusion duration.[44] Metheny concluded that cessation of enteral feeding when lowering a patient's bed for repositioning is not necessary but in fact is counterproductive.[45] However, it is important to quickly elevate the head of the bed to the desired 30- to 45-degree angle after repositioning the patient.[45] In critically ill, mechanically ventilated trauma patients, Pousman et al. tested and then adopted a reduced fasting protocol as results showed trends toward faster attainment of targeted nutrition goals and greater total EN delivered in the intervention arm of their study.[46] Normally, patients are made nothing by mouth after midnight prior to planned procedures or surgeries. The reduced fasting protocol was utilized in patients receiving enteral feeding with endotracheal tubes (protected airways) in place. In this protocol, infusion of EN in small bowel–fed patients is continued up to the time of the procedure and in gastric-fed patients until 45 minutes prior to the procedure, unless the planned procedure or surgery is intra-abdominal or requires prone positioning. Seder et al. reported that patients in a surgical ICU with bridled nasoenteric feeding tubes received a higher percentage of goal calories by decreasing the occurrences of feeding tube dislodgement.[47] Recently, Heyland et al. have completed a pilot study assessing a new feeding protocol known as "The PEP uP protocol."[48] This protocol, driven by the bedside nurse, utilizes daily volume-based goals, liberalization of the gastric residuals volume threshold, and initiation of protein supplementation and motility agents on day 1 of a patient's ICU stay. The results of this trial showed trends toward enhanced delivery of EN. Instructions were given to nurses on how to set the hourly rate for EN infusion based upon the 24-hour volume prescribed. If EN infusion were disrupted, beside nurses would recalculate the hourly rate based upon the required volume and time remaining to achieve the prescribed 24-hour volume. At the beginning of the next day, the targeted goal rate would be reset to the rate needed to achieve the required volume for infusion duration of 24 hours. In addition, another method to promote adequate enteral provision is early initiation of EN infusions after percutaneous endoscopic gastrostomy tube placement. In adults, current practice recommendations indicate that after a percutaneous endoscopic gastrostomy tube is placed, it may be utilized for feeding within 2 hours instead of the routine 24-hour delay (Practice Scenario 10-1).[21]

Practice Scenario 10-1

Question: What is the best method to achieve a goal feeding rate in a critically ill patient?

Scenario: An intubated 25-year-old man status post a pedestrian versus car accident is admitted to a trauma unit with the following injuries: bilateral pneumothorax, pneumomediastinum, left diaphragm rupture along with sternum, right scapula and left-sided rib fractures, and a T12 burst fracture with retropulsion into the spinal canal with resultant paraplegia. On hospital day 1 due to planned surgical procedures requiring prone positioning, patient remained nothing by mouth. On hospital day 2, patient underwent T10-L4 posterior spinal fusion; EN was initiated postoperatively but was again held at midnight for planned thoracic surgery. On hospital day 3, patient underwent bilateral chest wall reconstruction, sternum repair, and primary repair of lung with bilateral placement of two chest tubes. On hospital day 4, EN was held for planned extubation; patient failed and therefore was reintubated with EN reinitiated. On hospital day 5, EN was briefly held for bronchoscopy. On hospital day 7, EN was briefly held for tracheostomy placement.

Intervention: For a minimum formula volume required per day, a calorically dense, high-protein, immune-enhancing formula was prescribed to meet the patient's estimated caloric and protein need. Despite multiple infusion interruptions from hospital day 2 to 7, EN infusions achieved 58% of caloric and 57% of protein needs as estimated thus meeting A.S.P.E.N.'s recommendation to meet 50% to 65% of energy needs during the first week of hospitalization.[2]

Answer: Goal feeding rate in a enterally fed, critically ill patient is achieved by a standard protocol for the implementation of EN. In an effort to meet the patient's nutritional needs, protocols were put in place that promoted early initiation of EN and accepted GRVs of 500 mL without clinical signs of intolerance prior to holding of EN and reduced times of holding EN prior to procedures.

EN was initiated within 48 hours of injury and quickly advanced to goal rate per hour, anticipating EN infusion interruptions for planned surgical repairs.

Rationale: Traumatic injury patients have been shown to benefit from early enteral feeding,[35] along with other critically ill patients when attainment of > 50% to 65% of goal calories is achieved during the first week of hospitalization.[2] Efforts should be made to ensure EEN occurs and that a patient's dosing requirements are achieved. This can be achieved by following accepted practice guideline recommendations and complying with protocols designed to enhance protein and energy provision via the enteral route.[45]

Gastrointestinal Issues

Upper and lower GI motility disturbances are frequently seen in patients receiving EN support. Because there are limited therapeutic options available to treat motility disorders, monitoring to prevent them is the key to successful delivery of adequate EN.[49]

Enteral feeding fails most often as a result of gastric intolerance. This can be related to esophageal motility disorders, which can occur with diabetes, alcoholism, and other systemic diseases. A decrease in the pressure of the lower gastroesophageal sphincter can result in the regurgitation of gastric contents and potential aspiration.[49] Impaired gastric emptying in the critically ill patient is affected by age, illness severity, and diagnosis. For example, patients with burns, multiple trauma, head injury, and sepsis frequently experience delayed gastric emptying.[50] Historically, GRVs have been used as a marker to determine risk of aspiration due to regurgitation of enteral feedings. There have been no adequately powered studies that demonstrate a direct relationship between aspiration pneumonia and GRVs. Elevated GRVs cannot be correlated with pneumonia after enteral feedings are initiated, ICU, or hospital mortality.[51] Recommended practice is to avoid holding enteral feeding if the GRV is ≤ 500 mL in the absence of other signs or symptoms of intolerance (see Chapter 13 for a detailed discussion of gastric residuals).[20,52]

Lower GI motility disorders can lead to microbial overgrowth and bacterial translocation. These disorders can also contribute to the high incidence of diarrhea in the critically ill patient population.[49] Contrary to past practice, documentation of the presence of bowel sounds in a hemodynamically stable patient is not necessary before initiating enteral feeding. Likewise, the passage of flatus and/or stool is not required to begin EN.[20,21] In addition, patients can be fed through a mild to moderate ileus.[20]

One of the most common GI complications associated with enteral tube feeding is diarrhea. Because of the low osmolarity and the presence of fiber in many formulas, diarrhea is seldom a direct result of the formula itself. It may be associated with drugs such as H_2 blockers, proton pump inhibitors, antibiotics, and liquid medications with fillers such as sorbitol. Because contamination can also be a cause of infectious diarrhea, strict adherence to guidelines when handling the formula and sets can reduce the risk. Fat malabsorption may also result in diarrhea in the tube-fed patient. This may occur in patients with pancreatic deficiency, biliary obstruction, or small bowel resection. Some formulas contain low amounts of fat or may have a larger percentage of the total fat as a medium-chain triglyceride. Medium-chain triglycerides do not require micelle formation and are absorbed directly into the lymphatic system.[53]

Aspiration

Patient position aids in minimizing the risk for aspiration. Keeping the head of the bed elevated to 30 to 45 degrees during the infusion of EN has been shown to reduce aspiration risk and improve tolerance to enteral feeding. If the patient is unable to tolerate the elevation of the backrest of the bed due to diagnosis, prone positioning, or medical procedures, a reverse Trendelenburg position should be considered.[54]

Clinical practice continues to vary regarding the benefits and limitations of the placement of feeding tubes transpylorically or gastrically. Research is inconclusive to support feeding into the small bowel to decrease the risk of aspiration. Part of this controversy exists because it is known that patients can aspirate oropharyngeal secretions as well as gastric contents.[55,56] Attempts to control the aspiration of gastric contents have historically been the focus in tube-fed patients, however. Metheny and colleagues performed a retrospective analysis on tube-fed patients to evaluate aspiration risk as a function of enteral tube site in high-risk, critically ill patients.[57] They found that the percentage of patients with evidence of aspiration decreased as the terminal end of the feeding tube progressed from the stomach to the first, second/third, and fourth portions of the duodenum. This group concluded that "the findings support feeding critically ill patients with numerous risk factors for aspiration in the mid-duodenum and beyond to reduce the risk as aspiration and associated pneumonia."[57]

Metabolic Monitoring

The potential of developing metabolic complications with the initiation and provision of EN is not uncommon, particularly in the critically ill patient population. Electrolyte disturbances, fluid status, and glycemic control should be monitored frequently following initiation of EN support and on a regular basis during the duration of nutritional therapy. Prevention of refeeding syndrome, characterized by significant electrolyte disturbances (decreased phosphorous, magnesium, and potassium), is as important as repletion of those electrolytes when it does occur. Patients who are at high risk of developing refeeding syndrome should be identified and treated before starting nutrition support and monitored carefully as EN is slowly increased to goal.[21,58]

Fluid requirements must be considered when EN is prescribed for any patient. The amount of free water supplied through the provision of the EN formula should be considered when estimating any additional fluid needed to meet needs and losses.[59] Figure 10-4 shows methods of including fluid requirements when calculating an EN prescription.[1]

FIGURE 10-4 Calculation for Fluid-restricted Adult Enteral Nutrition Regimen

Calculations:

Select formula for this patient.
Example: Calorically dense 1.5 kcal/mL formula

Determine required kcal/day.
Example: Patient needs 2000 kcal/day

Divide total number of kcal required by kcal/mL to determine mL per day needed.
Example: 2000 kcal needed ÷ 1.5 kcal/mL = 1333 mL/day

To determine protein dose, multiply daily formula in mL by grams of protein/L
Example: 1333 mL/day × 64 g/L = 85 g/day protein

Determine required fluid in mL/day. Multiply percent water in formula times daily formula in mL to determine water contribution of EN. Subtract formula water from total fluid requirements to determine water flushes.
Example: Patient can only tolerate 1200 mL fluid.
1333 L formula × 76% water = 1013 mL water.
1200 mL − 1013 mL = 187 mL water (would use this small water allowance for medication delivery).

Determining Administration Rate:

Take total mL per day of formula and divide by 24 hours to determine goal rate.
Example: 1333 mL ÷ 24 hours = 56 mL/hour

EN, enteral nutrition.
Reprinted from How to Write Enteral Nutrition Orders. In: Boullata J, Nieman Carney L, Guenter P, eds. *The A.S.P.E.N. Enteral Nutrition Handbook*. Silver Spring, MD: A.S.P.E.N.; 2010: 230 with permission from the American Society for Parenteral and Enteral Nutrition (A.S.P.E.N.).

Finally, glycemic control can become a challenge with the initiation of EN support. Hyperglycemia should be treated before starting the EN infusion and should be treated with an established protocol as nutrition support continues. Episodes of hypoglycemia may occur with feeding when EN is stopped suddenly in a patient who is being treated for hyperglycemia with insulin or with oral hypoglycemic agents.[59] The controversy remains to determine how tightly blood glucose should be controlled in the critically ill patient.[60] For detailed discussion of glycemic control during EN support, refer to Chapter 34.

Enteral Nutrition Safety

Effective EN interventions are facilitated by safe provision of EN in all aspects of care.[21] Contamination of the formulas during the manufacturing processes, during preparation, and during the actual infusion is a concern with all patients, but particularly with those who are immunocompromised. The entire enteral feeding system, from the feeding tubes to the bags and sets, has been reviewed and is being redesigned in an effort to avoid any potentially dangerous complications associated with medical misconnections. The placement of the feeding tubes is another area where it is of utmost importance to adhere to protocols based on best practice. The procedures for the placement of nasogastric or nasoduodenal feeding tubes and reliable methods to assure and maintain proper placement remain controversial. The decision to percutaneously or surgically place gastrostomy tubes and jejunostomy tubes is based on many factors, and the procedures to place them vary as widely as the many types of tubes available. The safety and efficacy of EN support in different patient populations is of concern to practitioners. Vulnerable patient populations include neonates,[61–63] infants,[43,64,65] and children[66]; patients with pancreatitis[67] and pancreatic fistulas[68]; patients with open abdomen[69]; the elderly[70,71]; patients with head and neck cancer requiring gastrostomies[72–74]; mechanically ventilated patients[75,76]; and patients in the shock phase of injury and disease.[77,78]

Contamination

One potential problem that must be considered in the provision of EN is the issue of contamination. Although less likely, contamination of enteral feedings can occur at the manufacturing level. This can include steps during the preparation, decanting, packaging, and storing processes. Sterile, liquid formulas are preferred in the clinical setting as powdered formulas requiring reconstitution are not sterile and can result in increased bacterial growth upon reconstitution.[21] At the clinical level, contamination can be related to the use and maintenance of the equipment needed to deliver the formula, poor maintenance of the feeding tube, additives added to the formula, poor hand hygiene, and improper handling of the feeding during setup and administration of the enteral feeding. In order to minimize these potential issues and avoid symptoms of contamination such as GI-related problems and infection, all components of the enteral system must be evaluated and protocols established to ensure minimal risk.[79]

Equipment used in the provision of EN includes enteral feeding pumps, the administration sets and containers, and the syringes used for flushing and medication administration. Pumps should be centrally stored. They should be cleaned and carefully checked to assure they are safe to use before sending to a patient. Daily cleaning of the pump is important during use.[79] Feeding pumps for adult enteral formula delivery should be accurate within 10% for adults and 5% for neonatal and pediatric patients. Current pumps on the market can be programmed to safely and accurately deliver enteral feeding by continuous drip or by bolus feeds.[21]

The administration set used should be compatible with the design of the enteral feeding system used and the feeding pumps. These should be labeled prior to use with each patient. It is during this process of setting up and manipulating the enteral feeding system that the potential is greatest for contamination. Standardized precautions including handwashing and donning clean gloves should be observed routinely when manipulating enteral feedings and the associated equipment.[21] To minimize contamination and potential bacterial overgrowth, the set should have a recessed spike so no part of the set is touched prior to being connected to the formula container during setup or changing of the formula container.[79] The feeding hub and Y-port of the tubes should be cleaned with alcohol wipes when accessed either to initiate or change enteral feeding.[80] On the other hand, a separate port for medication administration and water flushes may contribute to contamination. Mathus-Vliegen et al. found that handling the Y-ports on feeding tubes improperly can contribute to bacterial proliferation by retrograde growth from the distal end of the feeding tube upward into the delivery set.[81] It has also been suggested that the presence of a drip chamber in the administration set can retard or prevent the retrograde movement of bacteria. At present, it is recommended that administration sets for enteral feedings be changed every 24 hours for open systems.[21]

The type of enteral formula container also can affect bacterial growth. As mentioned previously, a recessed spike set limits the possibility of contamination by touch and is recommended by A.S.P.E.N.'s "Enteral Nutrition Practice Recommendations." They further suggest that formulas decanted with a flip top may be at greater risk of bacterial contamination than those from a screw top container. Closed systems have a longer hang time of 24 hours when compared to open systems, and the risk of touch contamination is less.[21] It should be noted, however, that the safety of the whole system is affected most significantly by the appropriate handling of the delivery set rather than the container.[81]

Reconstituted enteral formulas must be prepared aseptically and by trained personnel. All equipment used in the process of preparation must be sanitized.[13] Aseptic technique should be used when filling open system containers. The top of the can or the bottle lids should be wiped with isopropyl alcohol and allowed to dry before pouring them into the container. Any unused portions should be refrigerated immediately. After the formula container is sealed, it should be labeled with the formula name and the time prepared. Hang time is limited to 4 hours at room temperature for reconstituted powdered formulas and to 8 hours for canned or bottled sterile, liquid formulas. Any formula remaining after the designated time must be discarded.[21]

Oral medications and the water flushes associated with them require the use of syringes. Following the publication of the National Patient Safety Agency alert, oral/enteral syringes, as opposed to Luer syringes, should be used for this purpose.[82] These syringes are sterile and for single use only to decrease contamination risk.[79]

Enteral Misconnections

Enteral misconnections are connections between any part of an enteral feeding system and a nonenteral system such as intravenous lines, dialysis catheters, and other connections involving intravenous connections. Simmons et al. reviewed a total of 116 case studies reported in the literature involving enteral misconnections. At total of 60 cases involved adults, 30 cases involved infants and children, and 26 cases did not report the age of the patients. Patient death was reported in 21 of the cases.[83] In 2007, a National Patient Safety Alert was released calling attention to the design of intravenous syringes and their potential use in the delivery of oral medication through an intravenous route. As a result, health care organizations were advised to "review the design and supply of the oral/enteral syringes and enteral feeding systems being used, as well as the way in which they are used."[82] It was suggested that changes be made to correct this potential fatal mistake through the development of new policies and procedures.[82,84]

At the center of the catheter/tubing misconnections in health care are the Luer connector systems. These Luer connectors are called Luer-Lok, Luer-Slip, Luer tip or small-bore connectors.[83] As stated in a recent Institute for Safe Medication Practices alert, "At the center of one of the most commonly reported problems is the fact that some manufactured enteral catheters still have ports that only accept parenteral administration sets and syringes."[8] The EN system can also lend itself to misconnections between the administration set and a prefilled container, particularly if that system allows intravenous tubing to be used instead of an enteral administration set. To create a safer environment for patients, these connections must be made physically incompatible. Design changes by manufacturers would prevent misconnections forcing the user to reexamine a connection that simply will not fit.[84] As a part of the new 2013 enteral standards developed by the International Organization for Standardization, female Luer connectors will no longer be found on feeding tubes. This will force the use of a compatible oral/enteral syringe to give oral medications via a feeding tube.[8] Change in the device design to force enteral/intravenous connector is the best way to prevent accidental tubing misconnection (Practice Scenario 10-2).[83]

Practice Scenario 10-2

Question: What are the potential consequences of administration of a medication or supplement through the intravenous route rather than through a feeding tube?

Scenario: An 86-year-old female was admitted to the hospital secondary to a cerebral vascular accident. She was a resident of a nursing home due to a past history of dementia. After being in the hospital for several days, she was seen by the speech therapist who documented a new onset of an inability to swallow resulting from the cerebral vascular accident. A percutaneous endoscopic gastrostomy tube was placed for EN support. The enteral feeds were initiated using a standard formula; however, the patient developed diarrhea. Believing the cause to be a lack of fiber in the diet, the physician ordered a product containing pectin as powdered banana flakes to be administered three times daily via the tube. Her nurse was a new graduate and being mentored by another assigned nurse. The patient's nurse asked the new graduate to mix the fiber product in sterile water and give it through the "tube." The new graduate misunderstood the directions and mixed the product in sterile water using a Luer slip tip 60 mL syringe and infused the diluted fiber product through the peripheral intravenous line in the patient's arm. Within the hour, the patient went into respiratory failure. She was not intubated due to a previous Do Not Intubate/Do Not Resuscitate order in the chart.

Intervention: Feeding tubes were obtained that are not compatible with Luer syringes and connectors. Sixty milliliter Luer syringes were replaced with a smaller (30 mL) size strictly for IV administration. All 60 mL syringes have either a catheter or oral tip for feeding tube administration. These are not compatible with intravenous sets.

Answer: This scenario represents an inadvertent misconnection involving a Luer syringe. The product or supplement was designed to be given through an enteral route. In this case, the product was prepared in a syringe that can be used as an intravenous connector as well as an enteral connector. Institutions should obtain enteral syringes or catheter tip syringes to be used for the mixing and administration of oral medications or supplements through a feeding tube.

Rationale: Because Luer syringes are compatible with both enteral systems and nonenteral systems such as an intravascular system or catheter, this is an example of an enteral misconnection that can result in significant harm or death to a patient.

Enteral equipment that can mate with female Luer connectors should not be used in this situation. Oral syringes should be purchased and used instead of Luer syringes to draw up and deliver medications intended to be administered through the GI tract. Any product delivered for administration should be clearly labeled with the correct syringe type, along with dispensing instructions and proper labeling. Large catheter tip syringes can also be used for product delivery through feeding tubes.[21]

Enteral Nutrition Outcomes

A number of systemic reviews and meta-analyses have been published summarizing the outcomes of EN.[85–90] Available literature investigating and advocating EEN indicates trends toward reduced ICU and hospital mortality,[85–89] shorter ICU length of stays,[90] shorter time on the ventilator,[85,86] lower incidents of new pneumonia,[85] reduced wound infection risk,[90] and decreased complication rates.[88] However, in Kortez's controversial critical review of the available trials comparing EN with no nutrition therapy, he concludes that the efficacy of

EN has not been proven.[91] The randomized, controlled trials reviewed showed that "the study designs have failed to use methods to prevent bias from interfering with the observations . . . limiting any positive conclusions."[91] In contrast, Delegge states, "Although we may never have the appropriately powered prospective, randomized trial for all nutrition interventions, best practice can often be created from a review of the combined literature including retrospective, prospective observational and small randomized trials. The lack of a definitive prospective randomized trial does not mean a therapy does not work or should not be attempted. The potential benefit of that therapy must be weighed against the potential risk and cost of that therapy."[92]

Summary

Best practice, based on the current available evidence-based guidelines, indicates that EN can be an effective nutritional intervention. The benefits derived from the use of EN have been demonstrated in many patient populations. EN can maintain the functional integrity of the gut. EN also improves GI and systemic immune function and can attenuate the infectious complications associated with disease and trauma. Both the timing of initiation and the adequacy of dosing are fundamental to effective outcome of EN. In addition, safe EN practices help ensure the highest quality of care by preventing misconnections, bacterial contamination, metabolic abnormalities, mechanical (feeding tube device) complications, and monitoring for aspiration and GI complications.

References

1. Boullata J, Nieman Carney L, Guenter P, Eds. *The A.S.P.E.N. Enteral Nutrition Handbook*. Silver Spring, MD: American Society for Parenteral and Enteral Nutrition; 2010.
2. McClave SA, Martindale RG, Vanek VW, et al. Guidelines for the provision and assessment of nutrition support therapy in the adult critically ill patient: Society of critical care medicine and American Society for Parenteral and Enteral Nutrition: Executive summary. *Crit Care Med*. 2009;5:1757–1761.
3. Martindale RG, McClave SA, Vanek VW, et al. Guidelines for the provision and assessment of nutrition support therapy in the adult critically ill patient: Society of Critical Care Medicine (SCCM) and American Society for Parenteral and Enteral Nutrition (A.S.P.E.N.). *J Parent Enteral Nutr*. 2009;33:277–316.
4. Heyland DK, Dhaliwal R, Drover JW, et al. Canadian clinical practice guidelines for nutrition support in mechanically ventilated, critically ill adult patients. *J Parenter Enteral Nutr*. 2003;27(5): 355–373.
5. Critical Illness Work Group. Critical illness. 2009. http://adaevidencelibraru.com/topic.cfm?cat=3016. Accessed June 2011.
6. McClave SA, Heyland DK. The physiologic response and associated clinical benefits from provision of early enteral nutrition. *Nutr Clin Pract*. 2009;24(3):305–315.
7. Boullata J. Drug administration through an enteral feeding tube. The rationale behind the guidelines. *Am J Nurs*. 2009;109(10): 34–42.
8. Institute of Safe Medication Practices. Preventing catheter/tubing misconnections: Much needed help is on the way. www.ismp.org/newsletters/acutecare/articles/20100715.asp. Accessed July 5, 2011.
9. Teitelbaum D, Guenter P, Howell WH, et al. Definition of terms, style, and conventions used in ASPEN guidelines and standards. *Nutr Clin Pract*. 2005;20:281.
10. McCamish MA, Bounous G, Geraghty ME. History of enteral feedings: past and present perspectives. In: Rombeau JL RR, ed. *Clinical Nutrition Enteral and Tube Feeding*. 3rd ed. Philadelphia, PA: WB Saunders; 1997:1–11.
11. Bartlett RH. Nutrition in critical care. *Surg Clin N Amer*. 2011;91: 595–607.
12. Skipper A. Enteral nutrition. In: Skipper A, ed. *Dietitian's Handbook of Enteral and Parenteral Nutrition*. 3rd ed. Sudbury, MA: Jones & Bartlett Learning; 2012:259–280.
13. Ukleja A, Freeman KL, Gilbert K, et al. Standards for nutrition support: adult hospitalized patients. *Nutr Clin Pract*. 2010;25: 403–414.
14. Magnotti LJ. Mechanism and significance of gut barrier function and failure. In: Rolandelli RH, Bankhead R, Boullata J, et al, ed. *Clinical Nutrition Enteral and Tube Feeding*. 4th ed. Philadelphia, PA: WB Saunders; 2005:23–31.
15. August D, Teitelbaum D, Albina J, et al. Guidelines for the use of parenteral and enteral nutrition in adult and pediatric patients. *J Parent Enteral Nutr*. 2002;26(1):S1–19SA.
16. Kreymann KG, Berger MM, Deutz NEP, et al. ESPEN guidelines on enteral nutrition: intensive care. *Clin Nutr*. 2006;25:210–223.
17. Owens CFJ. Decisions to be made when initiating enteral nutrition. *Gastrointest Endoscopy Clin N Am*. 2007;17:687–702.
18. Parrish CR. Enteral feeding: the art and science. *Nutr Clin Pract*. 2003;18:76–85.
19. Cresci G. Enteral access. In: Charney PMA, ed. *ADA Pocket Guide to Enteral Nutrition*. Chicago, IL: American Dietetic Association; 2006:26–62.
20. McClave SA, Martindale RG, Vanek VW, et al. Guidelines for the provision and assessment of nutrition support therapy in the adult critically ill patient. *J Parenter Enteral Nutr*. 2009;33(3): 277–316.
21. Bankhead R, Boullata J, Brantley S, et al. Enteral nutrition practice recommendations. *J Parenter Enteral Nutr*. 2009;33(2):122–167.
22. Heyland DK, Cahill NE, Dhaliwal R, et al. Impact of enteral feeding protocols on enteral nutrition delivery: results of a multicenter observational study. *J Parenter Enteral Nutr*. 2010;34(6): 675–684.
23. Clohessy SRJ. Administration of enteral nutrition: initiation, progression, and transition. In: Rolandelli RH, Bankhead R, Boullata J, Compher CW, ed. *Clinical Nutrition Enteral and Tube Feeding*. 4th ed. Philadelphia, PA: WS Saunders; 2005:243–247.
24. Bloch AS. Enteral and parenteral nutrition support. In: Mahan LK ES, ed. *Krause's Food, Nutrition and Diet Therapy*. 10th ed. Philadelphia, PA: Saunders; 2000:461–482.
25. Lord LM, Harrington M. Enteral nutrition implementation and management. In: Merritt R, DeLegge MH, Holcombe B, ed. *The ASPEN Nutrition Support Practice Manual*. Silver Spring, MD: ASPEN; 2005:76–89.
26. Thompson C. Initiation, advancement, and transition of enteral feedings. In: Charney P, ed. *ADA Pocket Guide to Enteral Nutrition*. Chicago, IL: American Dietetic Association; 2006:123–154.
27. Malone A. Enteral formula selection. In: Charney P and Malone A, ed. *ADA Pocket Guide to Enteral Nutrition*. Chicago, IL: American Dietetic Association; 2006:63–122.
28. Chen Y, Peterson S. Enteral nutrition formulas: Which formula is right for your adult patient? *Nutr Clin Pract*. 2009;24(3):344–355.
29. Fussell ST. Enteral formulations. In: Matarese LE GM, ed. *Contemporary Nutrition Support Practice: A Clinical Guide*. 2nd ed. Philadelphia, PA: Saunders; 2003:188–214.

30. Bourgault AM, Halm MA. Feeding tube placement in adults: safe verification method for blindly inserted tubes. *Am J Crit Care.* 2009;18(1):73–76.
31. Beyer PL. Complications of enteral nutrition. In: Matarese LE, Gottschlich MM, ed. *Contemporary Nutrition Support Practice: A Clinical Guide.* 2nd ed. St. Louis, MO: Saunders; 2003: 215–226.
32. Powell KS, Marcuard SP, Farrior ED, et al. Aspirating gastric residuals causes occlusion of small-bore feeding tubes. *J Parenter Enteral Nutr.* 1993;17(3):243–246.
33. Bourgult AM, Ipe L, Weaver J, et al. Development of evidence-based guidelines and critical care nurses' knowledge of enteral feeding. *CCN.* 2007;27(4):17–29.
34. Marcuard SP, Perkins AM. Clogging of feeding tubes. *J Parenter Enteral Nutr.* 1988;12(4):403–405.
35. Marcuard SP, Stegall KS. Unclogging feeding tubes with pancreatic enzymes. *J Parenter Enteral Nutr.* 1990;14(2):198.
36. Rogues AM, Boulestreau H, Lasheras A, et al. Contribution of tap water to patient colonisation with pseudomonas aeruginosa in a medical intensive care unit. *J Hosp Infect.* 2007;67:72–78.
37. Anaissie EJ, Penzak SR, Dignani MC. The hospital water supply as a source of nosocomial infections: a plea for action. *Arch Intern Med.* 2002;162:1483–1492.
38. Dandeles LM, Lodolce AE. Efficacy of agents to prevent and treat enteral feeding tube clogs. *Ann Pharmacother.* 2011;45(5): 676–680.
39. Arriola TAD, Hatashima A, Klang MG. Evaluation of extended-release pancreatic enzyme to dissolve a clog. *Nutr Clin Pract.* 2010; 25(5):563–564.
40. Rucart PA, Boyer-Grand A, Sautou-Miranda V, et al. Influence of unclogging agents on the surface state of enteral feeding tubes. *J Parenter Enteral Nutr.* 2011;35(2):255–263.
41. Boullata J. Medication administration through feeding tubes. *Am J Health-Syst Pharm.* 2010;67(1):23.
42. United States Pharmacopoeial Convention. *United States Pharmacopoeia/National Formulary.* Edition 31/26. Rockville, MD: United States Pharmacopoeia; 2008.
43. Jirapaet K, Jirapaet V, Sritipsukho S. Safety of initiating early enteral feeding with slow volume advancement in preterm infants. *J Med Assoc Thai.* 2010;93(10):1177–1187.
44. Lichtenberg K, Guay-Berry P, Piptone A, et al. Compensatory increased enteral feeding goal rates: a way to achieve optimal nutrition. *Nutr Clin Pract.* 2010;25:653–657.
45. Metheny N. Turning tube feeding off while repositioning patients in bed. *Crit Care Nurse.* 2011;31(2):96–97.
46. Pousman RM, Pepper C, Pandharipande P, et. al. Feasibility of implementing a reduced fasting protocol for critically ill patients undergoing operative and non-operative procedures. *J Parent Enteral Nutr.* 2009;33:176–180.
47. Seder CW, Stockdale W, Hale L, et al. Nasal bridling decreases feeding tube dislodgement and may increase caloric intake in the surgical intensive care unit: a randomized, controlled trial. *Crit Care Med.* 2010;38:797–801.
48. Heyland DK, Cahill NE, Dhaliwal R, et al. Enhanced protein-energy provision via the enteral route in critically ill patients: a single center feasibility trial of the PEP uP protocol. *Crit Care.* 2010; 14(2):R78.
49. Fruhwald S, Holzer P, Metzler H. Intestinal motility disturbances in intensive care patients: pathogenesis and clinical impact. *Intensive Care Med.* 2007;33(1):36–44.
50. Chapman MJ, Nguyen NQ, Fraser RJ. Gastrointestinal motility and prokinetics in the critically ill. *Curr Opin Crit Care.* 2007;13(2): 187–194.
51. McClave SA, Lukan JK, Stefater JA, et al. Poor validity of residual volumes as a marker for risk of aspiration in critically ill patients. *Crit Care Med.* 2005;33(2):324–330.
52. Bankhead RR, Fisher CA, Rolandelli RH. Gastrostomy tube placement outcomes: comparison of surgical, endoscopic, and laparoscopic methods. *Nutr Clin Pract.* 2005;20(6):607–612.
53. Stroud M, Duncan H, Nightingale J. Guidelines for enteral feeding in adult hospital patients. *GUT.* 2003;52(Suppl VII):vii1–vii12.
54. Metheny NA, Clouse RE, Chang YH, et al. Tracheobronchial aspiration of gastric contents in critically ill tube-fed patients: frequency, outcomes, and risk factors. *Crit Care Med.* 2006; 34:1–9.
55. Zaloga GP. Aspiration-related illnesses. *J Parent Enteral Nutr.* 2002;26(6 Suppl):S2–S7.
56. Metheny NA. Preventing respiratory complications of tube feedings: evidence-based practice. *Am J Crit Care.* 2006;15:360–369.
57. Metheny NA, Stewart BJ, McClave SA. Relationship between feeding tube site and respiratory outcomes. *J Parent Enteral Nutr.* 2011;35:346–355.
58. Kraft MD, Btaiche IF, Sacks GS. Review of the refeeding syndrome. *Nutr Clin Pract.* 2005;20:625–633.
59. Russell MK. Monitoring complications of enteral feedings. In: Charney P, ed. *ADA Pocket Guide to Enteral Nutrition.* 1st ed. Chicago, IL: American Dietetic Association; 2006:155–192.
60. Elia M, De Silva A. Tight glucose control in intensive care units: an update with an emphasis on nutritional issues. *Curr Opin Clin Nutr Metab Care.* 2008;11:465–470.
61. Corpeleijn WE, Vermeulen MJ, van den Akker CH, et al. Feeding very-low-birth-weight infants: our aspirations versus the reality in practice. *Ann Nutr Metab.* 2011;58(Suppl 1):20–29.
62. Ziegler EE, Carlson SJ. Early nutrition of very low birth weight infants. *J Matern Fetal Neonatal Med.* 2009;22(3):191–197.
63. Willis L, Thureen P, Kaufman J, et al. Enteral feeding in prostaglandin-dependent neonates: Is it a safe practice? *J Pediatr.* 2008;153(6):867–869.
64. Tyson JE, Kennedy KA, Lucke JF, et al. Dilemmas initiating enteral feedings in high risk infants: how can they be resolved? *Semin Perinatol.* 2007;31(2):61–73.
65. Parish A, Bhatia J. Early aggressive nutrition for the premature infant. *Neonatology.* 2008;94(3):211–214.
66. Evans S, MacDonald A, Daly A, et al. Home enteral tube feeding in patients with inherited metabolic disorders: safety issues. *J Hum Nutr Diet.* 2007;20(5):440–445.
67. Al Samaraee A, McCallum IJ, Coyne PE, et al. Nutritional strategies in severe acute pancreatitis: a systematic review of the evidence. *Surgeon.* 2010;8(2):105–110.
68. Klek S, Sierzega M, Turczynowski L, et al. Enteral and parenteral nutrition in the conservative treatment of pancreatic fistula: a randomized clinical trial. *Gastroenterology.* 2011;141(1):157–163.e1.
69. Dissanaike S, Pham T, Shalhub S, et al. Effect of immediate enteral feeding on trauma patients with an open abdomen: protection from nosocomial infections. *J Am Coll Surg.* 2008;207(5): 690–697.
70. Finucane TE, Christmas C, Leff BA. Tube feeding in dementia: how incentives undermine healthcare quality and patient safety. *J Am Med Dir Assoc.* 2007;8(4):205–208.
71. Hitchings H, Best C, Steed I. Home enteral tube feeding in older people: consideration of the issues. *Br J Nurs.* 2010;19(18): 1150–1154.
72. Clavel S, Fortin B, Despres P, et al. Enteral feeding during chemoradiotherapy for advanced head-and-neck cancer: a single-institution experience using a reactive approach. *Int J Radiat Oncol Biol Phys.* 2011;79(3):763–769.

73. Gomes CA Jr, Lustosa SA, Matos D, et al. Percutaneous endoscopic gastrostomy versus nasogastric tube feeding for adults with swallowing disturbances. *Cochrane Database Syst Rev.* 2010;(11): CD008096.
74. Paleri V, Patterson J. Use of gastrostomy in head and neck cancer: a systematic review to identify areas for future research. *Clin Otolaryngol.* 2010;35(3):177–189.
75. Guidroz AD, Chaudhary AJ. Enteral access in mechanically ventilated patients. *Nutr Clin Pract.* 2004;19(6):610–621.
76. Haslam D, Fang J. Enteral access for nutrition in the intensive care unit. *Curr Opin Clin Nutr Metab Care.* 2006;9(2):155–159.
77. Thibault R, Pichard C, Wernerman J, et al. Cardiogenic shock and nutrition: safe? *Intensive Care Med.* 2011;37(1):35–45.
78. Rowan CJ, Gillanders LK, Paice RL, et al. Is early enteral feeding safe in patients who have suffered spinal cord injury? *Injury.* 2004;35(3):238–242.
79. Best C. Enteral tube feeding and infection control: How safe is our practice? *Br J Nurs.* 2008;17(16):1036,1038–1041.
80. Matlow A, Jacobson M, Wray R, et al. Enteral tube hub as a reservoir for transmissible enteric bacteria. *Am J Infect Control.* 2006; 34(3):131–133.
81. Mathus-Vliegen EM, Bredius MW, Binnekade JM. Analysis of sites of bacterial contamination in an enteral feeding system. *J Parenter Enteral Nutr.* 2006;30(6):519–525.
82. National Patient Safety Agency. *Promoting Safer Measurement and Administration of Liquid Medicines via Oral and Other Enteral Routes.* Updated March 28, 2007. www.nrls.npsa.nhs.uk/alerts/. Accessed July 6, 2011.
83. Simmons D, Symes L, Guenter P, et al. Tubing misconnections: normalization of deviance. *Nutr Clin Pract.* 2011;26(3): 286–293.
84. Guenter P, Hicks RW, Simmons D. Enteral feeding misconnections: an update. *Nutr Clin Pract.* 2009;24(3):325–334.
85. Woo SH, Finch CK, Broyles JE, et al. Early vs delayed enteral nutrition in critically ill medical patients. *Nutr Clin Pract.* 2010;25: 205–211.
86. Barr J, Hecht M, Flavin KE, et al. Outcomes in critically ill patients before and after the implementation of an evidence-based nutritional management protocol. *Chest.* 2004;125: 1446–1457.
87. Doig GS, Heighes PT, Simpson F, et. al. Early enteral nutrition reduces mortality in trauma patients requiring intensive care: a meta-analysis of randomized controlled trials. *Injury.* 2011;42: 50–56.
88. Stratton RJ, Elia M. Who benefits from nutritional support: what is the evidence? *Eur J Gastroenteral Hepatol.* 2007;19:353–358.
89. Khalid I, Doshi P, DiGiovine B. Early enteral nutrition and outcomes of critically ill patients treated with vasopressors and mechanical ventilation. *Am J Crit Care.* 2010;19:261–268.
90. Mosier MJ, Pham TN, Klein MB, et al. Early enteral nutrition in burns: Compliance with guidelines and associated outcomes in a multicenter study. *J Burn Care Res.* 2011;32:104–109.
91. Koretz RL. Enteral nutrition: a hard look at some soft evidence. *Nutr Clin Pract.* 2009;24(3):316–324.
92. DeLegge MH. Enteral feeding. *Curr Opin Gastroenterol.* 2008;24: 184–189.

11 Enteral Formulations

Gail Cresci, PhD, RD, CNSD, LD, Jennifer Lefton, MS, RD, CNSD, and Dema Halasa Esper, MS, RD, LD

CONTENTS

Introduction ... 186
Formula Composition ... 186
Carbohydrate ... 186
Fiber ... 187
Fat ... 187
Protein ... 188
Vitamins and Minerals ... 188
Electrolytes ... 188
Water ... 188
Osmolality ... 188
Food Allergies/Intolerances ... 189
Oral Products ... 189
Formulations Marketed for Specific Diseases or Conditions ... 189
Diabetes/Glucose Intolerance ... 189
Gastrointestinal Disorders/Malabsorption ... 192
Hepatic Failure ... 192
Immune Modulating ... 192
Pulmonary Failure/Acute Respiratory Distress Syndrome ... 196
Renal Failure ... 197
Wasting Conditions ... 199
Wound Healing ... 200
Bariatric Formulations ... 200
Modular Products ... 201
Developing an Enteral Product Formulary ... 202
Open versus Closed Systems ... 202
Formula Safety ... 202
References ... 203

Objectives

1. Identify and evaluate enteral formulas for nutrition support of the general patient on tube feeding.
2. Recognize enteral product attributes for the patient with food allergies or intolerances.
3. Analyze and appraise evidence associated with the selection of enteral products marketed for specific diseases or conditions.
4. Design an enteral formulary based upon patient populations.

Test Your Knowledge Questions

1. A 62-year-old patient with chronic kidney disease requires hemodialysis three times weekly. Her most recent laboratory work shows a blood urea nitrogen of 65 mg/dL, creatinine 3.2 mg/dL, potassium 3.9 mEq/L, and phosphorus 4.4mg/dL. Which of the following formulas would best meet her nutrient needs?
   A. A formula restricted in fluid, protein, and electrolytes.
   B. A formula not restricted in protein but restricted in fluid and electrolytes.
   C. A formula restricted in fluid but not restricted in protein or electrolytes.
   D. A formula not restricted in fluid or protein but restricted in electrolytes.

2. A 55-year-old critically ill patient has been tolerating a standard 1 cal/mL feeding formula well over the past week. She begins having frequent bouts of loose stools. What should be the clinician's next suggestion?
   A. Change to a peptide-based formula
   B. Determine the cause of diarrhea
   C. Add pre- and probiotics
   D. Change to a fiber-supplemented formula
3. All of the following are recommended to prevent formula contamination except:
   A. Use aseptic technique when preparing formula
   B. Use formula decanted from a flip top container
   C. Change administration sets every 24 hours
   D. Allow sterile decanted formula to hang for no longer than 8 hours

Test Your Knowledge Answers

1. The correct answer is **C**. Not all renal failure patients require fluid restrictions, but of the answers provided, a formula restricted in fluid but not protein or electrolytes is the best option. There is no need to restrict protein in patients that are dialyzed. Additionally, electrolytes such as potassium and phosphorus need only be restricted when serum levels are chronically high.
2. The correct answer is **B**. Determining the cause of acute diarrhea is the correct answer. The feeding formula that she had been tolerating fine over the past week is the least likely cause of the diarrhea. Assessing for newly ordered medications that can cause diarrhea or ruling out infections such as *Clostridium difficile* may help to determine the cause of diarrhea. If no obvious cause of diarrhea can be found, then a different feeding formula may be trialed.
3. The correct answer is **B**. Using formula decanted from a screw cap container instead of a flip top container has resulted in less contamination. Aseptic technique for formula preparation, changing administration sets daily, and allowing sterile formula to hang for 8 hours or less are all recommended to prevent formula contamination.

Introduction

One of many decisions when initiating enteral nutrition (EN) is identifying an appropriate enteral formulation that will meet the patient's needs. Approximately 200 different commercially prepared enteral formulations are currently available. Limited data is available regarding the efficacy and outcomes associated with the use of many of these enteral formulations. This chapter reviews the composition of current enteral formulations that are available and their indications for use.

Enteral formulations are considered "medical foods" by the U.S. Food and Drug Administration (FDA).[1] The FDA defines medical foods as "a food which is formulated to be consumed or administered enterally under the supervision of a physician and which is intended for the specific dietary management of a disease or condition for which distinctive nutrition requirements, based on recognized scientific principles, are established by medical evaluation."[1] Therefore, their labels can make "structure and function" claims without the approval of the FDA. A structure and function claim is a claim that a specific nutrient is intended to affect the normal structure or function in humans. The mere quantity of formula options and lack of clinical research to support structure and function claims make it challenging for clinicians to select an optimal enteral formula. The American Society for Parenteral and Enteral Nutrition (A.S.P.E.N.) "Enteral Nutrition Practice Recommendations"[1] include the following statements regarding enteral formulation selection:

1. The veracity (accuracy, credibility) of adult enteral formula labeling and product claims is dependent on formula vendors.
2. Nutrition support clinicians and consumers are responsible for determining the veracity of adult enteral formulations.
3. Interpret enteral formulation content/labeling and health claims with caution until such time as more specific regulations are in place.

These practice recommendations were based on expert opinion and editorial consensus.[1]

Formula Composition

Carbohydrate

Carbohydrate (see Chapter 3) is the primary macronutrient and principal energy source in most enteral formulations. Enteral formulations typically offer 40% to 90% of their calories as carbohydrate.[2] Carbohydrates contribute to osmolality, digestibility, and sweetness of enteral formulations.[3]

Most formulations contain oligosaccharides or polysaccharides.[3,4] Polymeric formulas use primarily corn syrup solids as their source of carbohydrate; hydrolyzed formulas use maltodextrin or hydrolyzed cornstarch (Tables 11-1 and 11-2).[4,5] Oral products contain simpler or less complex carbohydrates, such as sucrose, to increase the palatability of the product. Due to the prevalence of lactose intolerance, most formulations do not contain lactose.[2,3]

TABLE 11-1 Classification of Enteral Formulation: Common Terms and Definitions[4–6]

Common Terms	Definitions
Standard, polymeric	Formula containing intact nutrients
Elemental and semielemental	Contains partially or completely hydrolyzed nutrients (protein) and altered fats
Blenderized	Used for patients that cannot tolerate semisynthetic formulas; formulated with a mixture of blenderized food sources
Disease-specific	Targeted for organ dysfunction or specific metabolic conditions
Modular	Used for supplementation to create a formula or enhance nutrient content of a formula or diet

TABLE 11-2 Macronutrient Sources in Enteral Formulations

Enteral Formulation	Carbohydrate	Fat	Protein
Polymeric	Corn syrup solids Hydrolyzed cornstarch Maltodextrin Sucrose Fructose Sugar alcohols	Borage oil Canola oil Corn oil Fish oil High-oleic sunflower oil Medium-chain triglycerides Menhaden oil Mono- and diglycerides Palm kernel oil Safflower oil Soybean oil Soy lecithin	Casein Sodium, calcium, magnesium, and potassium caseinates Soy protein isolate Whey protein concentrate Lactalbumin Milk protein concentrate
Hydrolyzed	Cornstarch Hydrolyzed cornstarch Maltodextrin Fructose	Fatty acid esters Fish oil Medium-chain triglycerides Safflower oil Sardine oil Soybean oil Soy lecithin Structured lipids	Hydrolyzed casein Hydrolyzed whey protein Crystalline L-amino acids Hydrolyzed lactalbumin Soy protein isolate

Adapted from Malone A. Enteral formula section: a review of selected product categories. *Pract Gastro.* 2005;24:44–74.

Fiber

Fiber, both insoluble and soluble forms, is a polysaccharide found in plant foods that is not digested by humans. Soluble-fermentable fiber is fermented by the gut microbiota in the distal intestine to produce short-chain fatty acids (SCFAs). The SCFAs are a source of energy for colonocytes, and they help to increase intestinal mucosal growth and promote water and sodium absorption (see Chapter 4).[6] Insoluble fiber is not effectively fermented by the gut microbiota.

Fiber (see Chapter 3) is added to some enteral formulations. Most enteral formulations contain a combination of both soluble and insoluble fiber. Soluble fiber may help control diarrhea due to its ability to increase sodium and water absorption via its fermentation byproducts, the SCFAs. Insoluble fiber may help to decrease transit time by increasing fecal weight.[6] Some studies of enteral formulations supplemented with soluble fiber have been shown to reduce the incidence of diarrhea.[7,8] Current A.S.P.E.N. and Society of Critical Care Medicine (SCCM) guidelines suggest that formulas with soluble fiber may be beneficial for critically ill patients with diarrhea as long as the patient is fully resuscitated and hemodynamically stable.[9] Because there is little evidence to support this recommendation, the patient's medical condition and the clinician's expertise play a bigger role in deciding whether to use a fiber-supplemented formula. Infections, such as *Clostridium difficile*, and hyperosmolar medications often lead to diarrhea and should be ruled out as the cause before changing the enteral formula to treat diarrhea.[9] Studies of formulations supplemented with insoluble fiber have not shown any benefit.[10]

The use of fiber-supplemented enteral formulations should be monitored closely, particularly in critically ill patients. Cases of bowel obstruction from the use of these formulations have been reported.[11,12] It may be safer to use a fiber-free formulation for critically ill patients that are at risk for gut dysmotility or bowel ischemia.[9,13]

Some enteral formulations contain fructo-oligo-saccharides, a nondigestable oligosaccharide, or prebiotic, that helps promote growth of beneficial bacteria (*Lactobacilli* and *Bifidobacterium*) in the distal bowel and is fermented to produce SCFAs.[14] Although fructo-oligo-saccharides add sweetness to products, it provides fewer direct calories due to lack of absorption and indirectly may increase caloric harvest due to SCFA yield (see Chapter 4 for further information on prebiotics).

Fat

Fat (see Chapter 5) added to enteral formulations serves as a concentrated energy source and provides essential fatty acids (linoleic and linolenic acid). A mixture of long-chain triglycerides (LCTs) and medium-chain triglycerides (MCTs) is often used in enteral formulations. Corn and soybean oil are the most common sources of LCTs used; however, safflower, canola, and fish oils are also used.[2,3,14]

Palm kernel and coconut oil may be added to enteral formulations as a source of MCTs, which offers several advantages. They are absorbed directly into the portal circulation and do not require chylomicron formation for absorption. They also do not require pancreatic enzymes or bile salts for digestion and absorption. MCTs are cleared from the bloodstream rapidly and cross the mitochondrial membrane without the need for carnitine, where they are oxidized to carbon dioxide (CO_2) and water and therefore not stored.[3] However, MCTs do not provide essential fatty acids and therefore most enteral formulations contain a mixture of LCTs and MCTs.

Some enteral formulations contain structured lipids as their fat source. Structured lipids are a chemical re-esterification of LCTs and MCTs on the same glycerol backbone, offering advantages of MCTs while including enough LCTs to meet essential fatty acid needs. Considerable attention has been devoted to omega-3 fatty acids in recent years due to their health benefits. Although both omega-6 and omega-3 fatty acids share the same enzyme systems as they are desaturated and elongated, their end products are different. Omega-3 fatty acids are metabolized to prostaglandins of the 3 series and leukotrienes of the 5 series, which are associated with anti-inflammatory effects, slowing of platelet aggregation, immune enhancement, and antiarrhythmic properties. Omega-6 fatty acids are metabolized to prostaglandins of the 2 series and leukotrienes of the 4 series, which are involved in inflammation, platelet aggregation, and immunosuppression. Some enteral formulations have altered the ratio of omega-6 to omega-3 fatty acids to include more omega-3 fatty acids due to their anti-inflammatory effects. Research done on enteral formulations supplemented with omega-3 fatty acids is discussed in the immune modulating and pulmonary section of this chapter.

Protein

Protein (see Chapter 6) is a source of nitrogen and energy in enteral formulations. Enteral formulations may have intact proteins, hydrolyzed proteins, or free amino acids.[3] Intact protein refers to whole protein or protein isolates. Casein and soy protein isolates are most commonly used. Lactalbumin, whey, and egg albumin are also sources of intact protein.[15] Formulations with intact proteins require normal levels of pancreatic enzymes for digestion and absorption.

Formulations with hydrolyzed protein, small peptides (more than three amino acid residues), di- and tripeptides, and free amino acids are referred to as semielemental or elemental formulations. The intestine expresses both free amino acid and peptide transport systems so it is able to absorb both free amino acids and di- and tripeptides. Any peptide greater than three amino acid residues requires further hydrolyzation prior to absorption.[16] Some research has suggested greater nitrogen absorption with peptide-based formulations rather than those containing only free amino acids.[16,17] Semielemental or elemental formulations are intended for patients with gastrointestinal (GI) dysfunction such as short bowel syndrome, malabsorption, or pancreatic exocrine insufficiency (see GI Disorders/Malabsorption section later in chapter).

Some enteral formulations add specific amino acids at pharmacologic level to function in wound and muscle repair (eg, glutamine and arginine) (see Chapter 6 for detailed information on glutamine and arginine).

Vitamins and Minerals

Most enteral formulations provide adequate amounts of vitamins and minerals to meet the Dietary Reference Intake (DRI) when provided in volumes of 1000 to 1500 mL daily.[15] Supplementation should be provided for patients when the enteral formulation does not meet their vitamin and mineral needs, or the volume provided inadequately meets the minimum intake for the DRI of vitamins and minerals.

Some disease-specific enteral formulations may have low or high amounts of specific vitamins and minerals.[3] Practitioners should pay close attention to the vitamin and mineral content of the enteral formulations used to avoid adverse clinical outcomes associated with inadequate or excessive micronutrient intakes. This may be of particular interest now that higher amounts of antioxidants and trace minerals such as selenium have been recommended for critically ill patients.[9]

Electrolytes

Standard enteral formulations contain modest amounts of electrolytes, typically enough to meet daily needs in most patients when the formula is provided in adequate amounts to meet the DRI. Disease-specific formulations may be altered because of the amounts of electrolytes they contain due to the disease process targeted (eg, renal failure). When recommending an enteral formulation, attention should be made to the disease or medical condition of the patient and the medical therapy provided.

Water

Enteral formulas contain roughly 70% to 85% free water.[3,18] In general, the more calorically dense the formula, the less free water it contains. Enteral formulations are not intended to meet the patient's total fluid needs. The percentage of water from enteral formulations should be included in the patient's total fluid intake. Most patients receiving EN require an additional source of water to meet their fluid needs. Water is often provided through the feeding tube for hydration and also as flushes to maintain feeding tube patency. Intravenous fluids have to be accounted for and adjusted as required when EN is implemented.

Osmolality

Osmolality of enteral formulation is the concentration of free particles, molecules, or ions in a given solution, and it is expressed as milliosmoles per kilogram water (mOsm/kg).[3] The osmolality of enteral formulations ranges from 270 to 700 mOsm/kg. Therefore, the more free particles, ions, or molecules in the product, the higher the osmolality will be. For instance, formulas containing sucrose have a higher osmolality than those with corn starch or maltodextrin; formulas with single amino acids or high amounts of di- and tripeptides have a higher osmolality than those with intact proteins. Hypertonic enteral formulations (osmolality $>$ 320 mOsm/kg) have frequently been blamed for formula intolerance (eg, diarrhea). When hyperosmolar formulas containing sucrose are delivered directly into the small intestine, dumping syndrome can occur, but this is unlikely to occur when peptide or single amino acids are provided in a similar manner. Other than simple sugar–related hyperosmolality, the osmolality of an enteral formulation has little to do with formula tolerance. Formula tolerance or diarrhea is most often related to the severity of illness, comorbid conditions, enteric pathogens, or the concomitant use of medications administered through the enteral access device.[19-21] Additionally, the average gastric tube–fed patient will dilute the enteral formula with 1 to 2 L of saliva and gastric juices. The osmolality of several items on a clear liquid diet and many medications given via the enteral route is much higher than the osmolality of enteral formulations. Further information on enteral feeding complications and tolerance is covered in Chapter 13.

Food Allergies/Intolerances

Fifteen million Americans may have food allergies.[22] It is important that the clinician complete a diet history including any food intolerances or allergies as part of the nutrition assessment. This can be helpful in determining whether a reported allergy is simply intolerance or a true food allergy. For example, some patients report a milk allergy that in fact is really just lactose intolerance.

Enteral formulations may contain milk, soy, corn, or egg products, all of which are common allergens. However, most enteral formulations are lactose free and gluten free. Clinicians must be knowledgeable about the ingredients in enteral formulations that may not be suitable for those with food allergies.

Oral Products

Enteral formulations used as oral supplements are available as either a liquid or a powder that must be reconstituted to form a liquid. These products are used for individuals who are unable to ingest adequate nutrients in the form of a standard oral diet.[23] Additional oral products are also available in the form of juices, nutrient-dense bars, cookies, puddings, and soups. These products provide approximately 40% to 60% of total calories from carbohydrates, 15% to 25% from protein, and 15% to 35% from fat. The recommended daily allowance for vitamins and minerals can be met when ingesting a portion of these oral supplements daily. These products may contain a blend of soluble and insoluble dietary fiber.

The efficacy of oral supplements has been studied mostly in older adults. Nutritional supplements containing protein and energy are often prescribed in this population because they are vulnerable to malnutrition and deterioration of nutrition status due to acute and chronic illnesses. Two reviews assessed the effectiveness of these supplements on anthropometric indexes, muscular skeletal strength, and functional status. They reported that supplementation produces a small but consistent weight gain in older adults and that mortality may be reduced in older adults who are undernourished.[24,25] Reduction of length of hospital stay and improved functional status was not seen in these reviews; further clinical trials are needed to determine additional benefits from oral nutrition supplementation.

A previous review indicated those with chronic obstructive pulmonary disease or a body mass index < 20 kg/m² seemed to show the greatest weight gain with the use of oral supplementation.[26] Patients with muscle wasting diseases (eg, cancer, acquired immunodeficiency syndrome [AIDS], and sarcopenia) may also benefit from oral nutrition supplements containing added amino acids and anti-inflammatory agents to attenuate lean muscle loss and improve immune function.[27] However, it appears early intervention with an oral nutrition supplement is imperative to gain the benefit.

Varieties of supplements are available in different flavors, textures, and consistency, and ultimately should be used on a daily schedule that is suitable for each individual; however, supplementation should not replace the benefits of eating a balanced diet but rather augment calories and nutrients that can be received with whole foods.

Formulations Marketed for Specific Diseases or Conditions

Just like standard EN formulations, there are numerous disease-specific EN formulations on the market. Enteral formulations are classified as medical foods, so unlike medications, these formulations are not regulated by the FDA; therefore, they do not require rigorous research prior to market availability to determine if they are indicated for various clinical conditions. Research that has been conducted with these formulations is typically performed by private investigators, and the funding may or may not be supported by the formula company. This leaves the evaluation for efficacy of the disease-specific formulations up to the clinician. When evaluating the efficacy of a disease-specific enteral formula, several considerations should be made (Table 11-3). It is important to recognize the quality of the research study and the patient populations included in the study to determine the value of the research results and whether the study endpoints are applicable to clinical practice. Many of the disease-specific formulas lack rigorous study and therefore have limitations when recommending their use in all clinical practice areas. For example, a disease-specific formula may have been studied in an ambulatory care setting and shown some benefit but has little to no studies available for the acute care setting; therefore, it should not be recommended for use in that practice area. There are multiple practice guidelines now available to help guide the clinician with use of disease-specific enteral formulas.

Diabetes/Glucose Intolerance

Research supports maintenance of blood glucose levels in a range of 80 to 150 mg/dl to improve patient morbidity and outcomes.[9] Recent guidelines for nutritional management of type II diabetes state there is no dietary intervention other than one that achieves weight loss for those who are overweight or obese.[28] Diets that are low in saturated fat and high in unsaturated fat, have low glycemic index/load and are higher in fiber

TABLE 11-3 Considerations When Evaluating Specialized Enteral Formulas

- In vitro versus in vivo study (animal versus human)
- Quality of study design
  - Prospective randomized controlled trial
  - Retrospective review
  - Case reports
  - Patient population studied (homogeneous, same clinical environment, etc.)
  - Generalized results

and whole grain foods, contain low-fat dairy foods, green leafy vegetables, coffee, and moderate intakes of alcohol are associated with a reduced risk of type II diabetes.[28] For optimal glycemic control, the focus should be made on total energy intake rather than macronutrient source of the energy. But the total amount of carbohydrate for both type I and type II diabetes is a strong predictor of glycemic response, and monitoring its intake remains a key strategy for maintaining glycemic control.[28] Previous practice guidelines stated that the diet should be composed of 45% to 60% of total calories as carbohydrates.[29] However, recent updates in guidelines recommend active carbohydrate management in terms of glycemic control or weight loss rather than prescribing absolute carbohydrate amounts.[28] For the acute care setting, practice guidelines recommend glycemic control protocols in the form of insulin therapy to assist with improving patient outcomes (see Chapter 34 for detailed discussion of diabetes and enteral nutrition).[9]

Enteral formulations designed to optimize glycemic control typically contain less carbohydrate (34% to 40% of total calories), higher amounts of fat (40% to 49% of total calories), and have 10 to 15 g/L of fiber (Table 11-4) compared to standard polymeric formulations. The premise for these formulations relates to the concept that reduced carbohydrates and increased fats and fiber will result in better glycemic control.

There are a limited number of studies evaluating a standard enteral formula with a formula targeted for better glycemic control. Pohl et al. conducted a randomized control trial, which was the second stage of a two-part study evaluating neurological patients with dysphagia ($n = 105$) that had preexisting hyperglycemia and elevated hemoglobin A1c (HbA1c) levels.[30] Patients were randomized to a diabetic formula or a standard enteral formula and provided with 27 kcal/kg/day for up to 84 days. Outcome parameters included total insulin requirements, fasting and afternoon blood glucose levels, and HgbA1c levels, which were assessed on days 1, 28, 56, and 84. Of the 55 patients that completed study through day 84, those that received the diabetic formula had decreased total insulin requirements (eight versus two units/day; $p = 0.001$), decreased fasting glucose (39 versus 12 mg/dl; $p = 0.001$), and decreased hypoglycemic episodes (five versus one). The authors concluded that the diabetic formula resulted in improved glycemic control and reduced insulin requirements compared to the standard formula.

A meta-analysis including 23 studies compared diabetes-specific to standard enteral formulas.[31] Results of this analysis found that people that received the diabetic formula had a decreased postprandial rise in blood glucose levels (1.03 mmol/L [95% confidence interval (CI) 0.58–1.47]), decreased peak in blood glucose concentration (1.59 mmol/l [95% CI 0.86–2.32]), and reduced HgbA1C levels in long-term care patients, but there was a lack of power for statistical significance. Caveats of this analysis are that most of the studies were short-term single meal studies with < 24-hour follow-up, only one short-term study looked at enteral feedings in critically ill patients, and all but two of the long-term studies used formulas as oral supplements. The Academy for Nutrition and Dietetics *Evidence Analysis Library* states "there is insufficient evidence to determine whether the nutrient composition of EN has an impact on mortality in critically ill patients with diabetes."[32] Overall, practice guidelines are to minimize overfeeding, use a standard enteral formula, and to consider a diabetic formula if glucose control becomes problematic despite insulin use.[32] There is a need for further research in the form of well-designed, adequately powered prospective randomized controlled trials that will determine the role of enteral nutritional support and diabetes-specific formulas on the management, clinical outcome, and quality of life of malnourished patients with diabetes or stress-induced hyperglycemia (see Practice Scenario 11-1 for a discussion of the best approach to enteral formula selection and glycemic control in a critical care setting).

Practice Scenario 11-1

Question: How do you enterally feed a patient postoperative with type 2 diabetes? What is the best approach to enteral nutrition management in a postoperative patient with type 2 diabetes?

Scenario: A 56-year-old male (MM) is admitted to the surgical intensive care unit (ICU) following an aortic valve replacement. On postoperative day 1, MM is intubated and chemically sedated. His past medical history is significant for type 2 diabetes, gastroparesis, and hypertension. MM is 5′10″ (178 cm) and weighs 80 kg, which is 10 kg less than what he weighed 3 months prior to admission. The ICU team wants to begin enteral feedings. In review of laboratory values, they are all insignificant except for blood glucose levels, which have been consistently elevated above 170 mg/dl since his admission to the ICU. MM has been receiving regular insulin subcutaneously every 4 hours when his glucose levels have been monitored. MM's medications are also significant for intravenous fluid of 5% dextrose with half-normal saline at 100 mL/hr, propofol at 5 mL/hr, and metoprolol. He has a nasogastric tube to lower intermittent wall suctioning, and it has removed ~750 mL of gastric contents over the past 24 hours. His abdomen is soft and nondistended, and he has no bowels sounds or bowel movements. His estimated energy requirements are ~1800 calories and protein requirements are 120 gm/day (1.5 gm/kg).

Intervention: A small bowel feeding tube is placed to initiate enteral feedings. A soluble fiber–containing, standard enteral formulation is recommended. An intravenous insulin infusion is recommended per an insulin protocol established within the ICU to maintain blood glucose levels within the range of 80 to 150 mg/dl. Recommendations are made to omit the dextrose from the intravenous fluid and to decrease the rate of intravenous fluid as the enteral feeding advances toward goal.

Answer: EN is indicated at this time as MM is critically ill, is at 88% of his usual body weight, is within 24 to 48 hours of ICU admission, and likely will remain on the ventilator for several more days. Because his gastric output is elevated and MM has a history of gastroparesis, he would benefit with a small bowel feeding tube for enteral feedings.

A standard formula is indicated for MM as evidence supporting a diabetic formula in critically ill patients to control blood glucose levels is lacking. His current intravenous fluids provide him ~720 calories (dextrose and propofol), which likely is exacerbating his hyperglycemia. Providing regular insulin on an "as needed" basis is not effective in controlling blood glucose within 80 to 150 mg/dl, which practice guidelines indicate is beneficial to minimize complications and improve patient outcomes.[9]

TABLE 11-4 Select Enteral Formulations Marketed for Use in Patients with Diabetes/Glucose Intolerance

		Protein		Carbohydrate		Fat	
Product (Company)	**kcal/mL**	**g/L (% kcal)**	**Source**	**g/L (% kcal)**	**Source**	**g/L (% kcal)**	**Source**
Diabetisource® AC (Nestle Nutrition)	1.2	60 (20)	Soy protein isolate, L-arginine	100 (36)	Corn syrup, fructose, tapioca dextrin, vegetables, fruits, FOS	60 (44)	Canola and menhaden oils
Glucerna® 1.0 Cal (Abbott Nutrition)	1	41.8 (16.7)	Sodium, calcium caseinates	95.6 (34.3)	Corn maltodextrin, soy fiber, fructose	54.4 (49)	High-oleic safflower and canola oils, soy lecithin
Glucerna® 1.2 Cal (Abbott Nutrition)	1.2	60 (20)	Sodium caseinate, soy protein isolate, milk protein concentrate	114.5 (35)	Maltodextrin, isomaltulose, fructose, sucromalt, FOS, oat and soy fiber	60 (45)	Safflower and canola oils, marine oil
Glucerna® 1.5 Cal (Abbott Nutrition)	1.5	82.5 (22)	Sodium, calcium caseinates, soy protein isolate	133.1 (33)	Corn maltodextrin, isolmaltulose, fructose, sucromalt, FOS, oat and soy fiber	75 (45)	Safflower and canola oil
Nutren® Glytrol® (Nestle Nutrition)	1.0	45.2 (18)	Calcium, potassium caseinate	100 (40)	Maltodextrin, modified cornstarch, pea fiber, gum Arabic, oligofructose, inulin	47.6 (42)	Canola, high-oleic safflower and MCT oils, soy lecithin

Product (Company)	**Osmolality (mOsm/kg)**	**100% RDI (mL)**	**% H_2O**	**Fiber (g/L)**	**Comments**
Diabetisource® AC (Nestle Nutrition)	450	1250	82	15	Arginine 3.2 g/L Vitamin E 96 units/L Vitamin C 240 mg/L Chromium 140 mcg/L
Glucerna® 1.0 Cal (Abbott Nutrition)	355	1422	85.3	14.4	Vitamin A 6300 units/L Vitamin C 215 mg/L Chromium 85 mcg/L
Glucerna® 1.2 Cals (Abbott Nutrition)	720	1250	80.5	16.1	Vitamin A 7730 units/L Vitamin E 39 units/L Vitamin C 260 mg/L Chromium 160 mcg/L
Glucerna® 1.5 Cal (Abbott Nutrition)	875	1000	75.9	16.1	Vitamin A 8660 IU/L Vitamin E 48 IU/L Vitamin C 325 mg/L Chromium 200 mcg/L
Nutren® Glytrol® (Nestle Nutrition)	280	1400	84	15.2	Vitamin A 5080 units/L (55% β-carotene) Vitamin E 30 units/L Vitamin C 140 mg Chromium 124 mcg/L

FOS, fructo-oligo-saccharides; MCT, medium-chain triglyceride; RDI, Reference Daily Intake.

Gastrointestinal Disorders/Malabsorption

GI disorders, particularly those affecting the lower GI tract, can impair nutrient utilization and absorption. Additionally, exocrine pancreatic function may be reduced in various clinical conditions, which can lead to altered digestion and absorption of intact proteins and long-chain lipids. Persistent feeding intolerance or malabsorption can compromise nutrition status warranting specialized nutrition support. Historically, patients were kept on nothing by mouth orders when they experienced malabsorption; however, current research indicates it important to enterally feed patients to maintain gut integrity and immunity.[9,33]

Due to the increasing knowledge of the immunologic and barrier functions of the intestine, enteral formulations specific for GI disorders have emerged (Table 11-5). These products contain hydrolyzed proteins (peptides, amino acids) and MCTs to aid in nutrient digestion and absorption. A few of these available products contain omega-3 fatty acids, which affect inflammatory metabolism (see Chapters 5 and 24). Prebiotics, such as synthetic fructo-oligo-saccharides and inulin, have been added to some of the formulations to support growth of beneficial colonic bacteria (eg, *Lactobacilli* and *Bifidobacteria*) along with increased production of SCFAs,[34] which have been shown to enhance fluid and electrolyte absorption. Further review of prebiotics can be found in Chapter 4.

Peptide-based formulas as a group have not been extensively evaluated, and the results of the available studies have been contradictory.[35–38] A reduced incidence and/or frequency of diarrhea using a peptide-based formula were shown in two studies,[35,36] a higher frequency of diarrhea was shown with a similar formula,[37] and another study found no difference in the incidence of diarrhea with a peptide-based formula.[38] Even though it makes theoretical sense to provide a peptide-based formula routinely in a patient with diarrhea or malabsorption, the lack of clinical evidence for support has led to no recommendation for this use of these formulas at this time as indicated by A.S.P.E.N. and European Society of Parenteral and Enteral Nutrition practice guidelines.[9,39] A thorough evaluation of a patient with diarrhea and/or malabsorption (eg, medications, too rapid rate of formula or fluid infusion into small intestine, small intestinal bacterial overgrowth [eg, *Clostridium difficile* infection]) should be made rather than assuming the enteral formula is the cause.[40] These formulations, however, warrant further and more detailed investigation due to their other newer added components (prebiotics, omega-3 fatty acids).

Hepatic Failure

Patients with liver failure often have other comorbidities including malnutrition, and their energy and protein requirements are elevated (see Chapter 27). To complicate provision of adequate nutrition to liver failure patients, they may be intolerant to protein. Liver failure patients may have impaired hepatic deamination, which lends to an increase in serum aromatic amino acid (AAA), which includes tyrosine, tryptophan, and phenylalanine. Branched-chain amino acids (BCAAs), leucine, valine, and isoleucine are metabolized by skeletal muscle; although depleted in these patients, skeletal muscle is still functioning. Thus, patients with liver failure may exhibit an altered AAA:BCAA ratio. This amino acid imbalance allows for AAA to cross the blood-brain barrier, producing false neurotransmitters with increases in neuropsychiatric symptoms of hepatic encephalopathy (HE).[41,42]

Based on this rationale, liver failure formulations were developed containing a lower total protein content but a higher amount of BCAA and lower amount of AAA to assist in restoring the amino acid balance and potentially improve the neurological symptoms of HE. These formulations are also calorically dense and low in sodium due to ascites caused by advance liver disease. They are also low in fat-soluble vitamins and other minerals due to liver and other organ failure, and the potential for these vitamins to accumulate in the liver and/or exacerbate other organ damage. In critically ill patients with HE, there is no evidence to support use of high BCAA formulations to alter patient outcomes compared to provision of a standard enteral formula.[9] Supplementation with oral BCAA formulations may be useful in slowing the progression of liver disease or failure, thus increasing survival in long-term (12 to 24 months) outpatients.[9] Coma grade may be improved in patients refractory to conventional treatment of HE (neomycin, lactulose) with provision of a high BCAA formula rather than a standard formula.[9,43]

Immune Modulating

Since the 1990s, immune-modulating formulations (IMF) have been investigated and are the most studied category of enteral formulations. Key immune-modulating nutrients in these complete EN formulas include arginine, glutamine, nucleotides, and omega-3 fatty acids either alone or in combination. It is beyond the scope of this chapter to discuss these nutrients in detail. Summarily, they have been included in these formulations due to their effects on the immune system (eg, T-cell, macrophage, neutrophil function), wound healing, inflammation, and energy transfer.[44] While there is biochemical and physiological basis for adding these nutrients, extensive clinical trials evaluating each nutrient individually has not been done. Comparing the IMFs against each other is problematic because they vary in the amounts of these key ingredients and therefore cannot necessarily be considered equivalent (Table 11-6). In addition, comparing the outcomes from research studies of IMFs is problematic because formulations vary from study to study and some formulations used in published studies are not commercially available. Population heterogenicity, study design variability and quality (not all prospective, randomized, blinded), and timing of feeding variation (preoperative, 24 to 96 hours of admission) also contribute to difficulties in applying outcomes to clinical practice. Some studies have included supplemental parenteral nutrition, and data analysis techniques vary amongst the studies.

Nine published meta-analysis or systematic reviews[45–53] have evaluated outcomes of IMFs in predominantly surgical

TABLE 11-5 Gastrointestinal Disorders/Malabsorption

		Protein		Carbohydrate		Fat	
Product (Company)	**kcal/mL**	**g/L (% kcal)**	**Source**	**g/L (% kcal)**	**Source**	**g/L (% kcal)**	**Source**
Optimental® (Abbott)	1.0	51.3 (20.5)	Whey protein hydrolysate, partially hydrolyzed sodium caseinate	139 (54.5)	Maltodextrin, sucrose, FOS	28.4 (25.0)	Structured lipid (MCT/fish oil)
Peptamen® (Nestle)	1.0	40 (16)	Enzymatically hydrolyzed whey protein	127 (51)	Maltodextrin, corn starch	39 (33)	MCT, soybean oil
Peptamen 1.5® (Nestle)	1.5	67.6 (18)	Enzymatically hydrolyzed whey protein	188 (49)	Maltodextrin, corn starch	56 (33)	MCT, soybean oil
Peptamen AF® (Nestle)	1.2	75.6 (25)	Enzymatically hydrolyzed whey protein	107 (36)	Maltodextrin, corn starch, oligofructose (FOS), inulin	54.8 (39)	MCT, fish oil, soybean oil (EPA/DHA 2.4 g/L)
Peptamen with Prebio® (Nestle)	1.0	40 (16)	Enzymatically hydrolyzed whey protein	127 (51)	Maltodextrin, corn starch, oligofructose (FOS), inulin	39.2 (33)	MCT, soybean oil
Peptamen Bariatric	1.0	93.3 (37)	Partially hydrolyzed whey protein concentrate	77.8 (30)	Maltodextrin, corn starch, oligofructose, inulin, guar gum	38 (33)	MCT, fish oil, high linoleic safflower oil
Tolerex® (Nestle)	1.0 (3.3 packets)	20.5 (8.0)	100% free amino acids L-glutamine 3.5g/L, L-arginine 2.4 g/L	224 (90)	Maltodextrin, modified food starch	1.8 (2.0)	Safflower oil
Vital 1.0 Cal® (Abbott)	1.0	40 (16)	Whey protein hydrolysate, partially hydrolyzed sodium caseinate	130 (51)	Maltodextrin, sucrose, short-chain FOS	38.1 (33)	Structured lipid (canola oil/MCT)
Vital 1.5 Cal® (Abbott)	1. 5	67.5 (18)	Whey protein hydrolysate, partially hydrolyzed sodium caseinate	187 (49)	Maltodextrin, sucrose, short-chain FOS	57.1 (33)	Structured lipid (canola oil/MCT)
Vital AF 1.2 Cal® (Abbott)	1.2	75 (25)	Whey protein hydrolysate, hydrolyzed sodium caseinate	110.6 (36)	Corn maltodextrin, short-chain FOS	53.9 (39)	Structured lipid (canola oil/MCT)

(continued)

TABLE 11-5 Gastrointestinal Disorders/Malabsorption *(Continued)*

		Protein		Carbohydrate		Fat	
Product (Company)	**kcal/mL**	**g/L (% kcal)**	**Source**	**g/L (% kcal)**	**Source**	**g/L (% kcal)**	**Source**
Vital HN® (Abbott)	1.0	41.7 (16.7)	Partially hydrolyzed protein blend (soy, collagen), whey protein concentrate, whey protein hydrolysate	185 (73.8)	Corn maltodextrin, sucrose	10.8 (9.5)	Safflower oil, MCT
Vivonex T.E.N.® (Nestle)	1.0 (3.3 packets)	35.7 (15)	100% free amino acids L-glutamine 4.8 g/L L-arginine 3.9 g/L	204 (82)	Maltodextrin, modified food starch	2.6 (3.0)	Safflower oil
Vivonex RTF® (Nestle)	1.0	50 (20)	100% free amino acids L-arginine 5.3 g/L	12 (70)	Maltodextrin, food starch modified	12 (10)	Soybean oil, MCT
Vivonex Plus® (Nestle)	1.0 (3.3 packets)	45 (18)	100% free amino acids L-glutamine 9.5 g/L L-arginine 6.3 g/L	57 (76)	Maltodextrin, modified food starch	6.6 (6)	Soybean oil

Product (Company)	**Osmolality (mOsm/kg)**	**100% RDI (mL)**	**% H_2O**	**Soluble Fiber (g/L)**	**Vitamin A (IU/L)**	**Vitamin C (mg/L)**	**Vitamin E (IU/L)**	**MCT:LCT (ratio)**	**n6:n3**
Optimental (Abbott)	585	1422	83.2	5.0	8290	215	215	28:72	0.81:1
Peptamen (Nestle)	270	1500	85	0	1075	340	30	70:30	7.4:1
Peptamen 1.5 (Nestle)	550	1000	77	0	6460	512	45	70:30	7.4:1
Peptamen AF (Nestle)	300	1000	84.5	5.2	8000	384	120	50:50	1.8:1
Peptamen with Prebio (Nestle)	300	1500	85	4.0	6670	320	100	70:50	7.4:1
Peptamen Bariatric	345	1500	84	4.3	6670	320	100	50:50	1.8:1
Tolerex (Nestle)	550	1800	84	0	2750	33	17	Minimum calories from fat	NA
Vital 1.0 Cal (Abbott)	390	1422	84.2	4.2	4570	350	70	47.5:52.5	2.1:1
Vital AF 1.2 Cal (Abbott)	425	1185	81.1	5.1	5485	422	253	45:55	0.9:1
Vital 1.5 Cal (Abbott)	610	1000	76.4	6.0	6500	500	100	47.5:52.5	2.1:1
Vital HN (Abbott)	500	1500	86.7	0	3332	200	30	45:55	48:1
Vivonex T.E.N. (Nestle)	630	2000	83	9.8	2500	60	15	Minimum calories from fat	NA
Vivonex RTF (Nestle)	630	1500	85	0	3300	67	20	40:60	6.7:1
Vivonex Plus	650	1800	83	0	2750	66	21.5	100% LCT minimal fat	NA

DHA, docosahexaenoic acid; EPA, eicosapentaenoic acid; FOS, fructo-oligo-saccharides; LCT, long-chain triglyceride; MCT, medium-chain triglyceride; RDI, Reference Daily Intake.

TABLE 11-6 Select Enteral Formulations Marketed for Immune Modulating: Products for Feeding Tube Use

		Protein		Carbohydrate		Fat	
Product (Company)	**kcal/mL**	**g/L (% kcal)**	**Source**	**g/L (% kcal)**	**Source**	**g/L (% kcal)**	**Source**
Crucial® (Nestle Nutrition)	1.5	94 (25)	Enzymatically hydrolyzed casein, L-arginine	134 (36)	Maltodextrin, cornstarch	67.6 (39)	MCT, fish oil, soybean oil, soy lecithin
Impact® (Nestle Nutrition)	1	56 (22)	Sodium, calcium caseinates, L-arginine	130 (53)	Maltodextrin, hydrolyzed cornstarch	28 (25)	Palm kernel, safflower, menhaden oils
Impact® with Fiber (Nestle Nutrition)	1	56 (22)	Sodium, calcium caseinates, L-arginine	140 (53)	Maltodextrin, soy fiber, guar gum	28 (25)	Palm kernel, safflower, menhaden oils
Impact® 1.5 (Nestle Nutrition)	1.5	84 (22)	Sodium, calcium caseinates, L-arginine	140 (38)	Maltodextrin, corn syrup solids	69 (40)	MCT, palm kernel, menhaden fish oils, safflower oils
Impact® Glutamine (Nestle Nutrition)	1.3	78 (24)	Wheat protein hydrolysate, sodium caseinate, L-arginine	150 (46)	Maltodextrin, hydrolyzed guar gum, soy fiber	43 (30)	Palm kernel, menhaden, safflower oils
Impact® Peptide 1.5 (Nestle Nutrition)	1.5	94 (25)	Hydrolyzed casein, L-arginine	140 (37)	Maltodextrin, corn starch	63.6 (38)	MCT oil, fish, canola, soybean oil
Optimental® (Abbott Nutrition)	1	51.3 (20.5)	Whey protein hydrolysate, hydrolyzed sodium caseinate, L-arginine	139 (54.5)	Corn maltodextrin, sucrose, FOS	28.4 (25)	Sardine/MCT structured lipid
Perative® (Abbott Nutrition)	1.3	66.7 (20.5)	Partially hydrolyzed sodium caseinate, whey hydrolysate, L-arginine	180.3 (54.5)	Corn maltodextrin, FOS	37.3 (25)	Canola, MCT and corn oils, soy lecithin
Pivot™ 1.5 (Abbott Nutrition)	1.5	93.8 (25)	Partially hydrolyzed sodium caseinate, whey hydrolysate, L-arginine	172.4 (45)	Corn syrup solids, FOS	50.8 (30)	Sardine/MCT structured lipid, soybean, canola oils, soy lecithin

FOS, fructo-oligo-saccharides; MCT, medium-chain triglyceride.

and critical care populations. Patients that received an IMF had decreased risk for infections/infectious complications,[45-51] reduced length of stay,[45-51] and reduced mortality.[50] Nutrition guidelines published recently by the SCCM and A.S.P.E.N. recommend the use of IMFs in surgical ICU patients (Grade A) and medical ICU patients (Grade B).[9] The European Society for Parenteral and Enteral Nutrition guidelines for intensive care suggest, "Immune modulating formulae (formulae enriched with arginine, nucleotides, and omega-3 fatty acids) are superior to standard enteral formula in patients without severe sepsis."[39] However, updated guidelines from May 2009 by the Canadian Practice Group recommends that formulas supplemented with arginine not be used in critically ill patients.[54] Similarly, the Academy of Nutrition and Dietetics *Evidence Analysis Library* also does not recommend routine use of IMFs in critically ill patients.[55]

Continued clinical research is necessary for a better understanding of IMFs, particularly since studies evaluating each immune-modulating nutrient individually as well as in various combinations, at various doses, and in defined patient populations, would lend to better evidence-based practice guidelines. At this time, there is enough evidence to support the use of IMFs in the elective surgical patient populations, but the provision in critically ill septic patients warrants further investigation.

Pulmonary Failure/Acute Respiratory Distress Syndrome

Respiratory failure is associated with decreased compensation to elevated CO_2 levels. When oxidized, macronutrients yield different amounts of CO_2; therefore, the respiratory quotient (RQ), a value that describes CO_2 production in relation to oxygen consumption, varies for carbohydrate (1.0), protein (0.8), and lipid (0.7); RQ for lipogenesis is 8.0.[23] In the 1980s, it was noted that high carbohydrate–containing parenteral nutrition formulations were associated with CO_2 retention, and when the carbohydrate content was decreased, respiration improved.[56-58] This led to the development of pulmonary failure–specific enteral formulas.

Pulmonary failure enteral formulas should have two classifications: those for ambulatory, noncritically ill patients and those for critically ill patients with acute respiratory distress syndrome (ARDS)/acute lung injury (ALI) (Table 11-7). In general, pulmonary failure formulas are calorically dense as these patients typically have a fluid restriction, are low in carbohydrate (27% calories) and high in lipid (55% calories), and contain moderate amounts of protein. The formulas for ambulatory and critically ill patients vary by the type of lipid they contain; the noncritically ill formula contains corn and safflower oils (omega-6 fatty acids) and the ARDS/ALI formulation contains marine oil and borage oil (omega 6:omega 3 fatty acid ratio is 1.8:1) in addition to added antioxidants.

While the theoretical basis may be sound, the reality of manipulating macronutrient composition with omega-6 fatty acids has not shown a consensus benefit. The early parenteral nutrition and EN studies revealed that patients were overfed, and that simply avoiding overfeeding improved oxygenation.[59] Practice guidelines do not recommend use of pulmonary formulas rich in omega-6 fatty acids for critically ill patients and recommend that overfeeding should be avoided.[9] Although studies of ambulatory patients with chronic obstructive pulmonary disease have reported reduced CO_2 production and RQ when patients were given higher fat formulations orally, improved clinical outcomes were not seen.[60-62]

A persistent pulmonary and systemic inflammation occurs in ARDS/ALI. The development of the ARDS/ALI formula was to potentially counteract this inflammatory state by manipulating the lipid profile to yield "less inflammatory" prostaglandins (PGE1 and 3), thromboxane (TXA3), and leukotriene (LTB5). Several high-quality clinical trials have shown benefit when providing this formula versus the noncritically ill pulmonary formula to patients with ARDS/ALI. A recent meta-analysis evaluated three of these trials.[63] The use of an eicosapentaenoic acid (EPA)/γ-linolenic acid (GLA) diet was associated with a 60% reduction in the risk of 28-day in-hospital all-cause mortality (odds ratio [OR] = 0.40, 95% CI = 0.24–0.68; $p = 0.001$) in the evaluable patients ($n = 296$). A 49% reduction in the risk of 28-day in-hospital all-cause mortality was evident (OR = 0.51, 95% CI 0.33–0.79; $p = 0.002$) in the EPA/GLA diet group on the basis of intent-to-treat (ITT) analysis ($n = 411$ patients). Additionally, a significant reduction in the risk of developing new organ failures (OR = 0.17; 95% CI = 0.08–0.34; $p < 0.0001$), time on mechanical ventilation, and ICU stay was seen.

These studies have been criticized for choice of the control diet: a diet rich in omega-6 fatty acids, which are known to exacerbate inflammation. A recent prospective, multicenter, randomized, double-blinded, controlled trial evaluated the ARDS/ALI formula in comparison to a standard, calorically dense, moderate fat-containing formula (29% calories) in patients with early stages of sepsis without any organ dysfunction.[64] Overall, patients receiving the ARDS/ALI formula exhibited less severe sepsis and/or septic shock (26.3% versus 50%, respectively; $p = 0.0259$), developed cardiovascular failure less often (21% versus 36.2%, $p = 0.0381$), and respiratory failure less often (24.6% versus 39.6%, $p = 0.0362$) than the control group.

Patients receiving the ARDS/ALI formula had fewer ICU days (ITT patients: 21.1 ICU-free days versus 14.7 ICU-free days, respectively; $p < 0.0001$; evaluable patients: 20.8 ICU-free days versus 14.3 ICU-free days, respectively; $p < 0.0001$) and fewer hospital days (ITT patients:19.5 hospital-free days versus 10.3 hospital-free days, respectively; $p < 0.0001$; evaluable patients: 19.1 hospital-free days versus 10.2 hospital-free days, respectively; $p < 0.001$) (all numbers expressed as means). There was no significant difference in 28-day all-cause mortality observed (ITT patients: 26.2% ARDS/ALI diet versus 27.6% control diet, respectively; $p = 0.72$; evaluable patients: 26.4 ARDS/ALI diet versus 30.18 control diet, respectively; $p = 0.79$).

Current practice guidelines for the provision of nutrition support in the critically ill recommend that patients with

TABLE 11-7 Select Enteral Formulations Marketed for Use in Patients with Pulmonary Failure: For Feeding Tube or Oral Use

		Protein		Carbohydrate		Fat	
Product (Company)	**kcal/mL**	**g/L (% kcal)**	**Source**	**g/L (% kcal)**	**Source**	**g/L (% kcal)**	**Source**
Nutren® Pulmonary (Nestle Nutrition)	1.5	68 (18)	Calcium, potassium caseinates	100 (27)	Maltodextrin	94.8 (55)	Canola, corn, MCT oil
Pulmocare (Abbott Nutrition)	1.5	62.6 (16.7)	Sodium, calcium caseinates	105.7 (28.2)	Sucrose, maltodextrin	93.3 (55.1)	Canola, corn, safflower, MCT oil

Product (Company)	**Osmolality (mOsm/kg)**	**100% RDI (mL)**	**% H_2O**	**Fiber (g/L)**
Nutren® Pulmonary (Nestle Nutrition)	330 (450 vanilla flavor)	1000	78	0
Pulmocare® (Abbott Nutrition)	475	947	78.5	0

MCT, medium-chain triglyceride; RDI, Reference Daily Intake.

Select Enteral Formulations Marketed for Use in Patients with Acute Respiratory Distress Syndrome/Acute Lung Injury: For Feeding Tube Use

		Protein		Carbohydrate		Fat	
Product (Company)	**kcal/mL**	**g/L (% kcal)**	**Source**	**g/L (% kcal)**	**Source**	**g/L (% kcal)**	**Source**
Oxepa® (Abbott Nutrition)	1.5	62.7 (16.7)	Sodium, calcium caseinates	105.3 (28.1)	Sugar, maltodextrin	93.8 (55.2)	Canola oil, MCT, marine oil, borage oil

Product (Company)	**Osmolality (mOsm/kg)**	**100% RDI (mL)**	**% H_2O**	**Fiber (g/L)**	**Additional**
Oxepa® (Abbott Nutrition)	535	946	78.5	0	Vitamin A 11,910 IU/L Vitamin E 320 IU/L Vitamin C 850 mg/L Selenium 74 mcg/L

MCT, medium-chain triglyceride; RDI, Reference Daily Intake.

ARDS and ALI should be fed with a formula that has an anti-inflammatory lipid profile (omega-3 fatty acids, fish oils, borage oil) and antioxidants.[9] However, these guidelines may be downgraded because a more recent randomized, double-blind, placebo-controlled, multicenter trial showed that twice-daily enteral supplementation of n-3 fatty acids, GLA, and antioxidants compared with an isocaloric control in addition to enteral feeding per protocol provided no benefit to patients with ALI.[65] In fact, the study was stopped early for futility after 143 and 129 patients were enrolled in the n-3 and control groups, respectively. Despite an eightfold increase in plasma EPA levels, patients receiving the omega-3 (n-3) supplement had more days on the ventilator (14.0 versus 17.2; $p = 0.02$) (difference, −3.2 [95% CI, −5.8 to −0.7]) and more days in the ICU (14.0 versus 16.7; $p = 0.04$). Patients in the n-3 group also had more nonpulmonary organ failure days (12.3 versus 15.5; $p = 0.02$). Sixty-day hospital mortality was 26.6% in the n-3 group versus 16.3% in the control group ($p = 0.054$), and adjusted 60-day mortality was 25.1% and 17.6% in the omega-3 and control groups, respectively ($p = 0.11$). Additionally omega-3 supplementation resulted in higher incidence and duration of diarrhea (29% versus 21%; $p = 0.001$).

Renal Failure

Patients with acute renal failure are typically critically ill, hypermetabolic and hypercatabolic, and have other organ dysfunctions; patients with chronic renal failure are often malnourished.[66] Therefore, these two states of renal dysfunction should be approached differently clinically. In addition to evaluating the patient's comorbidities and metabolic state, the clinician should evaluate the nutrition implications of decreased kidney function in relation to the medical therapy the patients are receiving (eg, continuous renal replacement therapy versus hemodialysis). Optimal nutrition management in acute kidney injury includes providing adequate macronutrient support to correct underlying conditions and prevent ongoing loss, supplementing micronutrients and vitamins during renal replacement therapy, and adjusting electrolyte replacement based on the degree and extent of renal dysfunction (see Chapter 29).

Nutrition-related functions of the kidney include filtration and excretion of fluid and nitrogenous waste products, and electrolyte, vitamin, and mineral homeostasis. Therefore, renal enteral formulations are altered in the amounts of free water, protein, electrolytes, vitamins, and minerals they contain (Table 11-8). Table 11-9 contains standard, fluid-restricted enteral formulas that can often be used instead of renal formulas. These formulations are available for use as oral supplements or as tube feeding formulations.

The biggest variation amongst the renal formulations is the protein content, which varies depending on the intended use. Formulas marketed for patients with kidney dysfunction not yet on dialysis are protein restricted, whereas those marketed for patients on dialysis have higher protein content as dialysis is catabolic and protein wasting to the patient, making the protein requirements higher despite organ dysfunction. Patients

TABLE 11-8 Select Enteral Formulations Marketed for Use in Patients with Renal Failure: For Feeding Tube or Oral Use

		Protein		Carbohydrate		Fat	
Product (Company)	**kcal/mL**	**g/L (% kcal)**	**Source**	**g/L (% kcal)**	**Source**	**g/L (% kcal)**	**Source**
Nepro® with Carb Steady® (Abbott Nutrition)	1.8	81 (18)	Sodium, calcium, magnesium caseinates, milk protein isolate	161 (34)	Corn syrup solids, sucrose, corn maltodextrin, FOS	96 (48)	Safflower and canola oil
Novosource® Renal (Nestle Nutrition)	2.0	90.7 (18)	Sodium, calcium caseinates, soy protein	183 (37)	Corn syrup, sugar	100 (45)	Canola oil
RenalCal® (Nestle Nutrition)[a]	2.0	34.4 (7)	Whey protein concentrate, amino acid blend	290.4 (58)	Maltodextrin	82.4 (35)	MCT and canola oil
Suplena® with Carb Steady® (Abbott Nutrition)[b]	1.8	45 (10)	Milk protein isolate, sodium caseinates	196 (42)	Corn maltodextrin, isomaltulose, sucrose, FOS	96 (43)	Safflower and canola oil

Product (Company)	**Osmolality (mOsm/kg)**	**100% RDI (mL)**	**% H_2O**	**Fiber (g/L)**	**Sodium (mg/L)**	**Potassium (mg/L)**	**Magnesium (mg/L)**	**Phosphorus (mg/L)**
Nepro® with Carb Steady® (Abbott Nutrition)	745	944	72.7	12.6	1060	1060	210	720
Novosource® Renal (Nestle Nutrition)	800	1000	72	N/A	945	945	197	819
RenalCal® (Nestle Nutrition)[a]	600	1000	70	N/A	740	1256	200	700
Suplena® with Carb Steady® (Abbott Nutrition)[b]	780	944	73.8	12.7	802	1139	215	717

FOS, fructo-oligo-saccharides; MCT, medium-chain triglyceride; RDI, Reference Daily Intake.

[a]Per manufacturer's product handbook, RenalCal is intended for oral supplementation and short-term tube feeding. It is not intended for use as a sole source of nutrition and use of the product requires careful monitoring due to negligible electrolyte content.

[b]Suplena® is marketed for individuals with renal failure that are not receiving dialysis.

TABLE 11-9 Select Enteral Formulations Marketed for Use in Patients Requiring Fluid Restriction: For Feeding Tube Use

		Protein		Carbohydrate		Fat	
Product (Company)	**kcal/mL**	**g/L (% kcal)**	**Source**	**g/L (% kcal)**	**Source**	**g/L (% kcal)**	**Source**
Nutren® 2.0 (Nestle Nutrition)	2.0	80 (16)	Calcium and potassium caseinates	196 (39)	Corn syrup solids, maltodextrin	104 (45)	MCT, canola, corn oil
TwoCal® HN (Abbott Nutrition)	2.0	83.5 (16.7)	Sodium, calcium, soy protein isolate	218.5 (43.2)	Corn syrup solids, maltodextrin, sucrose, FOS	90.5 (40.1)	Safflower, canola, MCT oil

Product (Company)	Osmolality (mOsm/kg)	100% RDI (mL)	% H_2O	Fiber (g/L)	Sodium (mg/L)	Potassium (mg/L)	Phosphorus (mg/L)	Magnesium (mg/L)
Nutren® 2.0 (Nestle Nutrition)	745	750	70	0	1300	1920	1340	536
TwoCal® HN (Abbott Nutrition)	725	948	70	5	1450	2440	1050	425

FOS, fructo-oligo-saccharides; MCT, medium-chain triglyceride; RDI, Reference Daily Intake.
Adapted from Bankhead R, Boullata J, Brantley S, et al. A.S.P.E.N. Enteral Nutrition Practice Recommendations. *J Parenter Enteral Nutr.* 2009;33(2):122–167 with permission from the American Society for Parenteral and Enteral Nutrition (A.S.P.E.N.).

on renal replacement therapy have higher protein needs due to loss of protein to exchange fluids.

There is a lack of evidence supporting the general use of a renal formula in kidney dysfunction. One group of authors concluded that there is insufficient data available to complete a meta-analysis comparing outcomes in patients receiving renal formulations compared to standard enteral formulations.[67] Current practice guidelines for critically ill patients state that patients with acute renal failure or kidney injury should be placed on standard enteral formulations consistent with recommendations that apply to the critically ill for protein and calorie provision. A renal formulation may be considered if significant electrolyte abnormalities exist or develop.[9]

Wasting Conditions

Wasting disorders, such as cancer and AIDS, contribute to patient morbidity and mortality. Tumor-induced and host-derived products facilitate wasting (eg, proinflammatory cytokines cause metabolic and neuroendocrine disturbances in the host).[68] Proteolysis-inducing factor has been identified to cause protein catabolism, which contributes to the skeletal muscle mass depletion seen in cancer cachexia.[69–71] In addition to the disease process, many factors contribute to loss of lean body mass and malnutrition, and vary depending on the type of cancer, including anorexia, pain, malabsorption, early satiety due to ascites, bowel or gastric outlet obstruction, and GI toxicities related to chemotherapy and medication side effects.[72]

Muscle loss is associated with an imbalance between protein synthesis to protein degradation, with the latter being greater. The conditionally essential amino acids glutamine (Gln) and arginine (Arg) are associated with improving immune function and wound complications when supplemented at pharmacological levels.[49,52] β-hydroxy-β-methylbutyrate (HMB), a metabolite of the BCAA leucine, is a dietary supplement that when provided with or without arginine and glutamine, results in positive patient outcomes. HMB promotes anabolism by increasing protein synthesis and inhibiting the ubiquitin-proteasome pathway controlling protein degradation, thereby conserving and even promoting accretion of lean body mass.[73] Trauma patients receiving only HMB supplementation had improved (less negative) nitrogen balance compared with patients receiving an isonitrogenous placebo and an isonitrogenous combination of HMB, arginine, and glutamine.[74] HMB helps preserve lean body mass in patients with sarcopenia,[75,76] cancer cachexia,[77] and AIDS.[78] Additionally, HMB supplementation is associated with improved immune status with surrogate markers cluster of differentiation 3 and cluster of differentiation 8 levels as well as decreased viral load in patients with AIDS.[78]

Enteral formulations have evolved to include these amino acids and are marketed to enhance muscle mass and improve wound healing (Table 11-10). There is limited supportive data for the routine use and effectiveness of these supplements in patients with wasting syndrome. May et al. evaluated a combined supplement of HMB/Arg/Gln against a control supplement in Stage IV cancer patients ($n = 24$). After 4 weeks of supplementation, the HMB/Arg/Gln group gained 0.95 ± 0.66 kg of body mass (1.12 ± 0.68 kg fat-free mass) and the controls lost 0.26 ± 0.78 kg (1.34 ± 0.78 kg fat-free mass), which was maintained over 24 weeks of evaluation.[77] A more recent phase III trial was unable to adequately test the ability of HMB, Gln, and Arg to reverse or prevent lean body mass wasting among patients with cancer.[79] The

TABLE 11-10 Select Enteral Formulations Marketed for Use in Patients with Wound Healing and Muscle Repair: Products for Oral Use

		Protein		Carbohydrate		Fat	
Product (Company)	**kcal/237 mL**	**g/L (% kcal)**	**Source**	**g/L (% kcal)**	**Source**	**g/L (% kcal)**	**Source**
Ensure® Clinical Strength	350	13 (15)	Sodium, calcium, milk protein concentrate	51 (57)	Corn maltodextrin, sucrose, short-chain FOS	11 (28)	Canola and corn oil
Juven® (Abbott)	80 per serving	14 g/pkt (71/75)	L-arginine, L-glutamine	7.9 g/pkt (25/29)	Sucrose	0	None
Arginaid® (Nestle)	0.11	4.5	L-arginine	4 (47)	Citric and malic acids	0	None
RESOURE Arginaid® EXTRA	250	10.5 (17)	Whey protein isolate, L-arginine	52 (83)	Sucrose, corn syrup solids	0	None

Product (Company)	**Osmolality (mOsm/kg)**	**Water g/mL/cc**	**Fiber (g)**	**Vitamin A IU**	**Vitamin C (mg)**	**Zinc (mg)**	**Comments**
Ensure® Clinical Strength	850	180	3.0	1250	36	3.8	1.5 g of CaHMB per 8 fl oz
Juven® (Abbott)	451	-	0	7 g/pkt	7 g/pkt	0	Mix with 8 fl oz water 1.5 g of CaHMB per packet
Arginaid® (Nestle)	170 (mixed in 237 mL)	-	0	-	156	-	Mix with 237 ml water. 4.5 g L-arginine per packet
RESOURE Arginaid® EXTRA (Nestle)	1340	83	0	1000	250	15	4.5 g L-arginine per 237 mL

CaHMB, Calcium Beta-hydroxy-Beta-methylbutyrate; FOS, fructo-oligo-saccharides.

study results are impacted by the fact that many patients were unable to complete the 8-week trial and therefore were lost to follow-up, as well as that weight loss was associated with lack of appetite rather than cancer cachexia. Further research is needed in this area to determine if the in vitro and animal models of this supplementation translate to humans.

Wound Healing

Patients with malnutrition are likely to have poorer outcomes than nonmalnourished patients, including poor wound healing or accelerated development of wounds (see Chapters 9 and 21). Certain nutrients, beyond calories and protein, have been linked with improving patient outcome including Gln, Arg, omega-3 fatty acids, zinc, selenium, and vitamins A, C, and E (see Chapter 21).[80]

Pharmacologic dosing of various nutrients is linked with improved wound healing.[81] EN formulations and supplements are available and targeted for wound healing (Tables 11-6, 11-10, and 11-11). These formulations may or may not provide complete nutrition in addition to these wound healing nutrients.

As discussed previously, provision of the IMFs, which contain Arg, omega-3 fatty acids, ± Gln, and antioxidants, decreases patient complication incidence including anastomotic wound strength. These effects have been demonstrated in GI surgery and trauma populations.[49,51,52] A systematic review and meta-analysis examined the impact of EN support, enteral tube feeding, or oral nutrition supplements on pressure ulcer incidence and healing.[82] Five randomized controlled trials were reviewed to compare nutrition support to routine care (usual diet and pressure ulcer care). The use of high-protein oral nutrition supplements reduced the risk of developing pressure ulcers by 25% in high-risk patients (eg, elderly, postsurgical, and chronically hospitalized patients). This review and others have suggested a high-protein diet, along with adequate serum levels of vitamin A and zinc, can assist patients at risk for pressure ulcers (nursing home, spinal cord patients, those with wounds) as long as other protective behaviors like weight control, exercise, and healthy lifestyle are involved (see Chapter 21).[81]

Bariatric Formulations

The 2009 Critical Care Practice guidelines state that critically ill obese people should receive patient, permissive hypocaloric feeding.[9] The target for all people with a body mass index > 30 kg/m^2 is to deliberately provide 60%% to 70% of target energy requirements and ≥ 2.0 gm/kg ideal body weight of protein per day for Class I and ≥ 2.5 g/kg ideal body of protein for Class II patients (body mass index 30 to 40). The rationale is that severe obesity increases risks of insulin resistance, sepsis, infections,

TABLE 11-11 Select High Protein Containing Enteral Formulations: Products for Feeding Tube Use

		Protein		Carbohydrate		Fat	
Product (Company)	kcal/mL	g/L (% kcal)	Source	g/L (% kcal)	Source	g/L (% kcal)	Source
Nutren® Replete (Nestle)	1.0	62.4 (25)	Calcium, potassium caseinate, soy lecithin	113 (45)	Maltodextrin	34 (30)	Canola oil, MCT
Nutren® Replete Fiber (Nestle)	1.0	62.5 (25)	Calcium, potassium caseinate	113 (45)	Maltodextrin, corn syrup	35 (30)	MCT
Perative® (Abbott)	1.3	66.7 (21)	Partially hydrolyzed sodium caseinate, whey protein hydrolysate	180 (54.5)	Corn maltodextrin, FOS	37.5 (25)	Canola oil, MCT
Promote® (Abbott)	1.0	62.5 (25)	Sodium, calcium caseinates	130 (52)	Corn maltodextrin	26 (23)	High oleic safflower, canola, and MCT
Promote® with Fiber (Abbott)	1.0	62.5 (25)	Sodium, calcium caseinates, soy protein isolate	138 (50)	Corn maltodextrin, oat fiber	28 (25)	Safflower oil, soy oil, and MCT

Product (Company)	Osmolality (mOsm/kg)	100% RDI (mL)	% H_2O	Fiber (g/L)	Vitamin A IU/L	Vitamin C mg/L	Zinc mg/L
Nutren® Replete (Nestle)	300	1000	85	0	5000	340	24
Nutren® Replete Fiber (Nestle)	310	1000	84	14	5000	340	24
Perative® (Abbott)	460	1155	79	9.8	8675	260	20
Promote® (Abbott)	340	1000	83.9	0	7250	345	24
Promote® with Fiber (Abbott)	375	1500	86.8	14.4	12.5	340	24

FOS, fructo-oligo-saccharides; MCT, medium-chain triglyceride; RDI, Reference Daily Intake.

organ failure, and deep venous thrombosis. These comorbidities, as well as ease of nursing care, may be improved with weight loss. Studies showing provision of > 2.0 gm/kg/day of protein with hypocaloric feeding is adequate to achieve nitrogen balance in the morbidly obese patient.[83]

An EN formulation that targets the critically ill morbidly obese patient is available (Table 11-12). The profile of the formula follows the 2009 A.S.P.E.N. guidelines and is high in protein (37% of calories) and contains omega-3 fatty acids. Providing this combination of nutrients enterally to patients is problematic and requires the use of modular protein supplements (see subsequent discussion), which can clog feeding tubes and/or cause and increase osmotic load into the small intestine resulting in diarrhea. No clinical studies have been published as yet utilizing this formulation, but it certainly is an area that needs further research.

Modular Products

Modular products are typically single nutrient products and are available for use in addition to the selected enteral formulations. Protein powders are the most common modular components. Modular protein products have been evaluated based on their amino acid profile and the protein digestibility corrected amino acid score. The protein digestibility corrected amino acid score assesses the bioavailability of essential amino acids of a protein module.[84] Manufacturers have used these scores to suggest that one modular protein product is superior to another. Modular products are also available for carbohydrate powders, MCT oil, and amino acids (eg, Gln, Arg). Modular products are commonly used to fortify tube feedings and/or food trays. The powders may be mixed into beverages and/or tube feeding oral supplements. Liquid variations of

TABLE 11-12 Formulas Marketed for Obese Patients

		Protein		Carbohydrate		Fat	
Product (Company)	**kcal/mL**	**g/L (% kcal)**	**Source**	**g/L (% kcal)**	**Source**	**g/L (% kcal)**	**Source**
Peptamen Bariatric	1.0	93.3 (37)	Partially hydrolyzed whey protein concentrate	77.8 (30)	Maltodextrin, corn starch, oligosaccharides	38 (33)	MCT, fish oil, high linoleic safflower oil

Product (Company)	Osmolality (mOsm/kg)	100% RDI (mL)	% H_2O	Fiber (g/L)	Vitamin A (IU/L)	Vitamin C (mg/L)	Vitamin E (IU/L)	MCT:LCT (ratio)	n6:n3 Ratio
Peptamen Bariatric	345	1500	84	4.3	6670	320	100	50:50	1.8:1

MCT, medium-chain triglyceride; LCT, long-chain triglycerides; RDI, Reference Daily Intake.

modular products are available but often are hyperosmolar, so caution should be made when administering them into a feeding tube. On occasion, modular products may be combined to prepare a tube feeding formula for special circumstances (eg, no LCT feeding for chylothorax). Caution should be made to assure adequate vitamins, minerals, and electrolytes are also supplemented in these circumstances.

Developing an Enteral Product Formulary

Many health care facilities choose to develop an enteral formulary. The benefits of a formulary are inventory control and cost savings. Additionally, a formulary simplifies product selection competency by professional staff.[1]

To develop a product formulary, one should evaluate the facility's patient population, current utilization, and contractual requirements. Selection of appropriate products for an enteral formulary by clinicians should be based on the best available evidence. Simply matching a medical diagnosis to a formula that is specifically marketed for that diagnosis could lead to inappropriate nutrition support provision as well as significantly increased costs to the facility.[1] The following should be considered when developing an enteral formulary[85,86]:

- Patient acuity
- Digestive and absorptive capacity, organ dysfunction, and metabolic requirements of most patients
- Formulation components that may be contraindicated
- Needs for fluid restriction
- Need for added formulation components

Enteral formulary contracts should include a clause that allows for a noncompeting product if it better meets the nutritional needs of the patients.[1]

Open versus Closed Systems

Enteral formulations are available as liquids ready to feed, liquids ready to hang, or powders that must be reconstituted. Each of these systems has advantages and disadvantages. With ready-to-feed products, enteral formulations must be transferred from a can, bottle, or brick pack to a refillable administration set or bag before delivery. This "open system" method, in theory, increases the risk of formula contamination. In addition, more nursing time is required with an open system.

Ready-to-hang, or closed system, enteral formulations are packaged in sealed bags or rigid containers that hold volumes of 1000, 1500, or 2000 mL. Administration tubing (eg, "spike sets") must be attached to the container before use, but no further manipulation of the formulation should occur, thus potentially reducing opportunities for contamination. Hang times for closed systems for enteral formulations range from 24 to 48 hours. In addition to reducing the potential for contamination, these systems offer greater convenience to both nurses and patients. Less nursing time is required to administer enteral formulations through a closed system. Despite their obvious advantages, closed system containers do have some drawbacks. Increased wastage of formulas may take place in situations where feeding intolerance is common or in unstable patients where changes in the formula occur frequently. A more serious concern with closed systems is the potential for misconnection errors. Container design may allow the insertion of an intravenous spike set and inadvertent intravenous administration of enteral formulation, a life-threatening medical error.[87] A sentinel event alert from The Joint Commission has raised awareness of this potentially deadly error and emphasized the importance of appropriate staff education concerning proper use of these products.[88] Powdered formulas require the addition of water to reconstitute the formula. This must be done in a sanitary environment with accurate measurements of formula and water to ensure proper nutrient concentration and delivery. Powdered formulas are susceptible to contamination because they require more manipulation during preparation.

Formula Safety

Safety concerns focus on enteral formula contamination. *Clostridium difficile* colonization has been reported in tube-fed patients.[89] Approximately 30% to 75% of formulations prepared in the hospital have been found to be contaminated with bacteria and at

TABLE 11-13 American Society for Parenteral and Enteral Nutrition Practice Recommendations for Adult Enteral Formula Safety

1. Each institution should define an ongoing quality control process for EN formula preparation, distribution, storage, handling, and administration. (B)
2. Institutions should maintain written policies and procedures for safe EN formula preparation and handling, as well as maintain an ongoing surveillance program for contamination. These should be based on HACCP and the USP good compounding practices. (B)
3. EN formulas should be prepared to patient use in a clean environment using aseptic technique by specially trained personnel. Strict aseptic technique (done under sterile conditions) should be used in the preparation and administration of enteral formulas. (A)
4. All personnel involved in preparing, storing, and administering EN formulas should be capable and qualified for the tasks, and follow accepted best practices. (C)
5. Sterile, liquid EN formulas should be used in preference to powdered, reconstituted formulas whenever possible. (A)
6. Store unopened commercially available liquid EN formulas under controlled (dark, dry, cool) conditions. (B)
7. Maintain a rapid enteral feeding formula inventory turnover well within the product's expiration date. (C)
8. Formulas reconstituted in advance should be immediately refrigerated, and discarded within 24 hours of preparation if not used; formulas should be exposed to room temperature for no longer than 4 hours, after which they should be discarded. (B)
9. Use a purified water or sterile water for irrigation supply, formula reconstitution, and medication dilution. Consider purified water for enteral access device flushes in at-risk patients. (B)
10. Strict adherence to manufacturer's recommendations for product use results in less contamination of EN. (A)
11. Use of disposable gloves is recommended in the administration of EN. (A)
12. Formula decanted from a screw cap is preferable instead of a flip top because formula poured from a screw cap was associated with less microbial growth. (A)
13. A recessed spike on a closed system container is preferable. (B)
14. A feeding pump with a drip chamber prevents retrograde contamination of the EN formula from the feeding tube. (A)
15. Sterile, decanted formula should have an 8-hour hang time. (B)
16. Administration sets for open system enteral feedings should be changed at least every 24 hours. (B)
17. Powdered, reconstituted formula, and EN formula with additives should have a 4-hour hang time. (C)
18. Closed-system EN formulas can hang for 24 to 48 hours per manufacturer's guidelines. (A)
19. Administration sets for closed-system EN formulas should be changed per manufacturer guidelines. (A)

EN, enteral nutrition; HACCP, hazard analysis and critical control points; USP, U.S. Pharmacopeial Convention.
Adapted from Bankhead R, Boullata J, Brantley S, et al. A.S.P.E.N. Enteral Nutrition Practice Recommendations. *J Parenter Enteral Nutr.*2009;33(2):122–167 with permission from the American Society for Parenteral and Enteral Nutrition (A.S.P.E.N.).

least half of those had bacterial counts in excess of federal limits ($> 10^4$ colony-forming units/mL).[1] Although there is not a strong link between formula contamination and formula tolerance in the literature, employing methods to reduce formula contamination is recommended as a best practice.[1] Storage, preparation, handling, administration, and hang time of the formulations should all be considered when evaluating the potential for contamination. Current practice recommendations to avoid enteral formulation contamination are in Table 11-13.

References

1. Bankhead R, Boullata J, Brantley S, et al. Enteral nutrition practice recommendations. *J Parenter Enteral Nutr.* 2009;33:1–46.
2. Charney P. Enteral nutrition: indications, options, and formulations. In: Gottschlich MM, ed. *The Science and Practice of Nutrition Support: A Case Based Core Curriculum.* Dubuque, IA: Kendall/Hunt Publishing Co.; 2001:141–166.
3. Trujillo E. Enteral nutrition: a comprehensive overview. In: Matarese LE, Gottschlich MM, eds. *Contemporary Nutrition Support Practice: A Clinical Guide.* Philadelphia, PA: W.B. Saunders Company; 1998:192–201.
4. Malone AM. Enteral formulations. In: Cresci GA, ed. *Nutrition Support for the Critically Ill Patient: A Guide to Practice.* Boca Raton, FL: CRC; 2005:253–277.
5. Matarese LE. Enteral nutrition. In: Lysen LK, ed. *Quick Reference to Clinical Dietetics.* Gaithersburg, MA: A.S.P.E.N. Publishers; 1997: 198–225.
6. Malone A. Enteral formula selection: a review of selected product categories. *Pract Gastroenterol* 2005;24:44–74.
7. Spagen H, Diltoer M, Malderen CV, et al. Soluble fiber reduces the incidence of diarrhea in septic patients receiving total enteral nutrition: a prospective, double blind, randomized, and controlled trial. *Clin Nutr.* 2001;20:301–305.
8. Rushdi TA, Pichard C, Khater YH. Control of diarrhea by fiber-enriched diet in ICU patient on enteral nutrition: a prospective randomized controlled trial. *Clin Nutr.* 2004;23:1344–1352.
9. McClave SA, Martindale RG, Vanek VW, et al. Guidelines for the provision and assessment of nutrition support therapy in the adult critically ill patient: Society of Critical Care Medicine and American Society for Parenteral and Enteral Nutrition. *J Parenter Enteral Nutr.* 2009;33:277–316.
10. Frankenfield DC, Beyer PL. Soy-polysaccharide fiber: effect on diarrhea in tube-fed, head injured patients. *Am J Clin Nutr.* 1989; 50:533–538.

11. Scaife CL, Saffle JR, Morris SE. Intestinal obstruction secondary to enteral feedings in burn trauma patients. *J Trauma*. 1999;47:859–863.
12. McIvor AC, Meguid MM, Curtas S, et al. Intestinal obstruction from cecal bezoar: a complication of fiber-containing tube feedings. *Nutrition*. 1990;6:115–117.
13. McClave SA, Chang WK. Feeding the hypotensive patient: does enteral feeding precipitate or protect against ischemic bowel? *Nutr Clin Pract*. 2003;18:279–284.
14. Ettinger S. Macronutrients: carbohydrates, proteins, and lipids. In: Mahan K, Escott-Stump S, eds. *Krause's Food, Nutrition, and Diet Therapy*. 11th ed. Philadelphia, PA: Saunders; 2004:37–74.
15. Charney P, Russell MK. Enteral formulations: standard. In: Rolandelli RH, ed. *Clinical Nutrition: Enteral and Tube Feeding*. 4th ed. Philadelphia, PA: Elsevier Saunders; 2005:216–223.
16. Silk DB, Fairclough PD, Clar ML, et al. Use of peptide rather than free amino acid nitrogen source in chemically defined enteral diet. *J Parenter Enteral Nutr*. 1980;4:548–553.
17. Craft IL, Geddes D, Hyde CW, et al. Absorption and malabsorption of glycine and glycine peptides in man. *Gut*. 1968;9:425–437.
18. Lipp J, Lord LM, Scholer LH. Fluid management in enteral nutrition. *Nutr Clin Pract*. 1999;14:232–237.
19. Edes TE, Walk BE, Austin JL. Diarrhea in tube-fed patients: feeding formula not necessarily the cause. *Am J Med*. 1990;88:91–93.
20. Eisenberg PG. Causes of diarrhea in tube-fed patients: a comprehensive approach to diagnosis and management. *Nutr Clin Prac*. 1993;8:119–123.
21. Fuhrman MP. Diarrhea and tube feeding. *Nutr Clin Prac*. 1999;14:83–84.
22. The Food Allergy and Anaphylaxis Network. www.foodallergy.org. Accessed October 2011.
23. A.S.P.E.N. Board of Directors and the Clinical Guideline Task Force. Guidelines for the use of parenteral and enteral nutrition in adult and pediatric patients. *J Parenter Enteral Nutr*. 2002; 26:1SA–128SA.
24. Milne AC, Potter J, Vivanti, et al. Protein and energy supplementation in elderly people at risk from malnutrition. *Cochrane Database Syst Rev*. 2009;15:CD003288.
25. American Dietetic Association Evidence Analysis Library. Unintentional weight loss in Older Adults. www.adaevidencelibrary.com/conclusion.cfm?conclusion_statement_id=250778&auth=1. Assessed on October 25, 2011.
26. Stratton RJ, Marinos E. Are oral nutrition supplements of benefit to patients in the community? Findings from a systematic review. *Curr Opin Clin Met Care*. 2000; 3:311–315.
27. Lynch GS, Schertzer JD, Ryall JG. Therapeutic approaches for muscle wasting disorders. *Pharamcology & Therapeutics*. 2007;113:461–487.
28. Dyson PA, Kelly T, Deakin T, et al. Diabetes UK position statements and care recommendations. Diabetes UK evidence-based nutrition guidelines for the prevention and management of diabetes. *Diabet Med*. 2011;28:1282–1288.
29. Sheard NF, Clark NG, Brand-Miller JC, et al. Dietary carbohydrate (amount and type) in the prevention and management of diabetes. *Diabetes Care*. 2004;27:2266–2271.
30. Pohl M, Mayr P, Mertl-Roetzer M, et al. Glycemic control in patients with type 2 diabetes mellitus with a disease specific enteral formula: stage II of a randomized, controlled multicenter trial. *J Parent Ent Nutr*. 2009;33:37–49.
31. Elia M, Ceriello A, Laube H, et al. Enteral nutritional support and use of diabetes-specific formulas for patients with diabetes: a systematic review and meta-analysis. *Diabetes Care*. 2005;28(9):2267–2279.
32. ADA Evidence Analysis Library. www.adaevidencelibrary.com/evidence.cfm?format_tables=0&evidence_summary_id=250992. Last accessed February 6, 2012.
33. Santarpia L. Gut flora in the intestinal and extra intestinal diseases: a general overview and the effects of artificial nutrition. *Curr Nutr and Food Science*. 2009:180–192.
34. Guarner F, Malagelada JR. Gut flora in health and disease. *Lancet*. 2003;361:512–519.
35. Mowatt-Larssen CA, Brown RO, Wojtysiak SL, et al. Comparison of tolerance and nutritional outcome between a peptide and a standard enteral formula in critically ill, hypoalbuminemic patients. *J Parenter Enteral Nutr* 1992;16:20–24.
36. Brinson RR, Kolts BE. Diarrhea associated with severe hypoalbuminemia: a comparison of a peptide-based chemically defined diet and standard enteral alimentation. *Crit Care Med*. 1988;16:130–136.
37. Heimburger DC, Geels VJ, Bilbrey J, et al. Effects of small-peptide and whole-protein enteral feedings on serum proteins and diarrhea in critically ill patients: a randomized trial. *J Parenter Enteral Nutr*. 1997; 21:162–167.
38. Meredith JW, Ditesheim JA, Zaloga GP. Visceral protein levels in trauma patients are greater with peptide diet than with intact protein diet. *J Trauma*. 1990;30:825–828.
39. Kreymann KG, Berger MM, Deutz NEP, et al. ESPEN guidelines on enteral nutrition: intensive care. *Clinical Nutrition*. 2005:210–223.
40. Edes TE, Walk BE, Austin JL. Diarrhea in tube-fed patients: feeding formula not necessarily the cause. *Am J Med*. 1990;88:91–93.
41. Ong JP, Mullen KD. Hepatic encephalopathy. *Eur J Gastroenterol Hepatol*. 2001;13:325–334.
42. Fischer JE, Rosen HM, Ebeid AM, et al. The role of normalization of plasma amino acids on hepatic encephalopathy in man. *Surgery*. 1976;80:77–91.
43. Blei AT, Cordoba J, The Practice Parameter Committee of the American College of Gastroenterology. Hepatic encephalopathy. *AJG*. 2001;96:1968–1975.
44. Worthington M, Cresci G. Immune-modulated diets: who wins the meta-analysis race? *Nutr Clin Pract*. 2011;26:650–655.
45. Heys SD, Walker LG, Smith I, et al. Enteral nutritional supplementation with key nutrients in patients with critical illness and cancer: a meta-analysis of randomized controlled clinical trials. *Ann Surg*. 1999; 229:467–477.
46. Beale RJ, Bryg DJ, Bihari DJ. Immunonutrition in the critically ill: a systematic review of clinical outcome. *Crit Care Med*. 1999;27:2799–2805.
47. Heyland DK, Novak F, Drover JW, et al. Should immunonutrition become routine in critically ill patients? A systematic review of the evidence. *JAMA*. 2001;286:944–953.
48. Montejo JC, Zarazaga A, Lopez-Martinez J, et al. Immunonutrition in the intensive care unit: a systemic review and consensus statement. *Clin Nutr*. 2003;22:221–233.
49. Waitzberg DL, Saito H, Plank LD, et al. Postsurgical infectious are reduced with specialized nutrition support. *World J Surg*. 2006;30:1592–1604.
50. Marik PE, Zaloga GP. Immunonutrition in critically ill patients: a systematic review and analysis of the literature. *Intensive Care Med*. 2008;34:1980–1990.
51. Marik PE, Zaloga GP. Immunonutrition in high-risk surgical patients: a systematic review and analysis of the literature. *J Parenter Enteral Nutr*. 2010;34:378–386.
52. Cerantola Y, Hubner M, Grass N, et al. Immunonutrition in gastrointestinal surgery. *Br J Surg*. 2010;98:37–48.

53. Drover JW, Dhaliwal R, Weitzel L, et al. Perioperative use of arginine-supplemented diets: a systematic review of the evidence. *J Am Coll Surg.* 2011; 212:385–399.
54. Canadian Practice Group. *Critical Care Clinical Practice Guidelines.* Kingston, Ontario, Canada: 2009. www.criticalcarenutrition.com/docs/cpg/srrev.pdf. Last accessed February 6, 2012.
55. American Dietetic Association. *Critical Illness Guideline.* www.adaevidencelibrary. Accessed February 4, 2012.
56. Askanazi J, Elwyn DH, Silverberg PA, et al. Respiratory distress secondary to a high carbohydrate load: a case report. *Surgery.* 1980; 87:596–598.
57. Dark DS, Pingleton SK, Kerby GR. Hypercapnia during weaning: a complication of nutritional support. *Chest.* 1985;88:141–143.
58. Covelli HD, Black JW, Olsen MS, et al. Respiratory failure precipitated by high carbohydrate loads. *Ann Intern Med.* 1981;95: 579–581.
59. Talpers SS, Romberger DJ, Bunce SB, et al. Nutritionally associated increased carbon dioxide production: excess total calories vs. high proportion of carbohydrate calories. *Chest.* 1992;102: 551–555.
60. Angelillo VA, Sikhdarshan B, Durfee B, et al. Effects of low and high carbohydrate feedings in ambulatory patients with chronic obstructive pulmonary disease and chronic hypercapnia. *Ann Intern Med.* 1985;103:883–885.
61. Kuo CD, Shiao GM, Lee JD. The effects of high fat and high carbohydrate diet loads on gas exchange and ventilation in COPD patients and normal subjects. *Chest.* 1993;104:189–196.
62. Akrabawi SS, Mobarhan S, Stoltz RR, et al. Gastric emptying, pulmonary function, gas exchange, and respiratory quotient after feeding a moderate versus high fat enteral formula meal in chronic obstructive pulmonary disease patients. *Nutrition.* 1996;12: 260–265.
63. Pontes-Arruda A, DeMichele SJ, Seth A, et al. The use of an inflammation-modulating diet in patients with acute lung injury or acute respiratory distress syndrome: a meta-analysis of outcome data. *J Parenter Enteral Nutr.* 2008;32:596–605.
64. Pontes-Arruda A, Martins LF, Maria de Lima S, et al. Enteral nutrition with eicosapentaenoic acid, g-linolenic acid and antioxidants in the early treatment of sepsis: results from a multicenter, prospective, randomized, double-blinded, controlled study: the INTERSEPT Study. *Crit Care.* 2011;15:R144.
65. Rice TW, Wheeler AP, Thompson BT, et al. Enteral omega-3 fatty acid, gamma-linolenic acid, and antioxidant supplementation in acute lung injury. *JAMA.* 2011:306(14):1574–1581.
66. Gervasio JM, Garmon WP, Holowatyj M. Nutrition support in acute kidney injury. *Nutr Clin Pract.* 2011;26(4):374–381.
67. Stratton RJ, Bircher G, Fongue D, et al. Multinutrient oral supplements and tube feeding in maintenance dialysis: a systematic review and meta-analysis. *Am J Kidney Disease.* 2005;46: 387–405.
68. Tisdale MJ. Inhibition of lipolysis and muscle protein degradation by EPA in cancer cachexia. *Nutrition.* 1996;12:S31–S33.
69. Smith HJ, Lorite MJ, Tisdale MJ. Effect of a cancer cachectic factor on protein synthesis/degradation in murine C2C12 myoblasts: modulation by eicosapentaenoic acid. *Cancer Res.* 1999;59: 5507–5513.
70. Smith KL, Tisdale MJ. Mechanism of muscle protein degradation in cancer cachexia. *Br J Cancer.* 1993;68:314–318.
71. Lorite MJ, Smith HJ, Arnold JA, et al. Activation of ATP-ubiquitin-dependent proteolysis in skeletal muscle in vivo and murine myoblasts in vitro by a proteolysis-inducing factor (PIF). *Br J Cancer.* 2001;85:297–302.
72. Falconer JS, Fearson KC, Plester CE, et al. Cytokines, the acute-phase response, and resting energy expenditure in cachectic patients with pancreatic cancer. *Ann Surg.* 1994;93:380–383.
73. Siddiqui R, Pandya D, Harvey K, et al. Nutrition modulation of cachexia/proteolysis. *Nutr Clin Pract.* 2006;21:155.
74. Kuhls DA, Rathmacher JA, Musngi D, et al. β-hydroxy-β-methylbutyrate supplementation in critically ill trauma patients. *J Trauma.* 2007;62:125–132.
75. Flakoll P, Sharp R, Baier S, et al. Effect of β-hydroxy-β-methylbutyrate, arginine, and lysine supplementation on strength, functionality, body composition, and protein metabolism in elderly women. *Nutrition.* 2004;20:445–451.
76. Baier S, Johannsen D, Abumrad N, et al. Year-long changes in protein metabolism in elderly men and women supplemented with a nutrition cocktail of β-hydroxy-β-methylbutyrate (HMB), L-arginine, and L-lysine. *J Parenter Enteral Nutr.* 2009;33(1): 71–82.
77. May PE, Barber A, D'Olimpio JT, et al. Reversal of cancer-related wasting using oral supplementation with a combination of β-hydroxy-β-methylbutyrate, arginine, and glutamine. *Am J Surg.* 2002;183:471–479.
78. Clark RH, Feleke G, Mehraj D, et al. Nutritional treatment for acquired immunodeficiency virus-associated wasting using β-hydroxy-β-methylbutyrate, glutamine, and arginine: a randomized, double-blind, placebo-controlled study. *JPEN J Parenter Enteral Nutr.* 2000; 24:133–139.
79. Berk L, James J, Schwartz A, et al. A randomized, double-blind, placebo-controlled trial of a beta-hydroxyl beta-methyl butyrate, glutamine, and arginine mixture for the treatment of cancer cachexia (RTOG 0122). *Support Care Cancer.* 2008;16(10):1179–1188.
80. Scholl D, Langkamp-Henken B. Nutrient recommendations for wound healing. *J Intraven Nurs.* 2001;24:124–132.
81. Hayes GL, McKinzie BP, Bullington WM, et al. Nutritional supplements in critical illness. *AACN Advanced Critical Care.* 2011;22: 301–316.
82. Stratton RJ, Ek AC, Engfer M, et al. Enteral nutritional support in prevention and treatment of pressure ulcers: a systematic review and meta-analysis. *Ageing Res Rev.* 2005;4:422–450.
83. Choban PS, Dickerson RN. Morbid obesity and nutrition support: is bigger different? *Nutr Clin Pract.* 2005;20:480–487.
84. Castellanos VH, Litchford MD, Campbell WW. Modular protein supplements and their application to long-term care. *Nutr Clin Pract.* 2006;21:485–504.
85. Gottschlich MM. Adult enteral nutrition: formulary and supplements. In: Buchman A, ed. *Clinical Nutrition: A Guide for Gastroenterologists.* Thorofare, NJ: Slack Incorporated; 2006:505–520.
86. Russell MK. Establishing an enteral formulary for adults. *Future Dimensions in Clinical Nutrition Management.* 2004;23(1):1–8.
87. Neven A, Wilson R, Kochevar M, et al. Compatibility of IV administration sets with closed enteral nutrition containers. *J Parenter Enteral Nutr.* 2000;24:369.
88. Joint Commission on Accreditation of Healthcare Organizations. Tubing misconnections—a persistent and potentially deadly occurrence. www.jointcommission.org/assets/1/18/SEA_36.PDF. Accessed February 6, 2012.
89. Bliss DZ, Johnson S, Savik K, et al. Acquistion of clostridium difficile and clostridium difficile-associated diarrhea in hospitalized patients receiving tube feeding. *Ann Intern Med.* 1998;129: 1012–1019.

12 Enteral Access Devices

John C. Fang, MD, Robin Bankhead, CRNP, and Merin Kinikini RD, RN, FNP

CONTENTS

Introduction **207**
Enteral Device Selection **207**
Tube Selection **208**
Physical Characteristics **208**
Tube Types **208**
Methods of Access **209**
Nasal Tubes **209**
Enterostomy Tubes **211**
Gastrostomy Tubes **211**
Gastrojejunal Tubes **212**
Jejunostomy Tubes **212**
Skin-Level Devices **212**
Postinsertion Catheter Care **212**
Skin Care **212**
Prevention of Clogging **213**
Exchange and Removal of Enterostomy Tubes **213**
Complications of Enteral Access Devices **214**
Nasal Tubes **214**
Enterostomy Tubes **214**
Gastrojejunal and Jejunal Tubes **215**
Conclusion **215**
References **215**

Objectives

1. Define the patient and tube selection criteria for various enteral access devices.
2. Outline the insertion techniques for the different types of enteral access devices.
3. Describe proper maintenance for enteral access devices.
4. List the complications of enteral access devices.

Test Your Knowledge Questions

1. If an enteral access tube cannot be unclogged using warm water flushes, what is the next most reliable method for unclogging the tube before being replaced?
   A. Administer cola through the tube, and let it sit for a few hours.
   B. Administer Clog Zapper (CORPAK MedSystems, Wheeling, IL) and flush within 30 to 60 minutes.
   C. Wait a few hours to see if the clog dissolves spontaneously.
   D. Administer a mixture of pancreatic enzymes and bicarbonate solution, allow it to sit for 1 to 2 hours, and then flush with warm water.

2. You perform a telephone evaluation on a patient who relates increased redness, pain, and swelling around their existing low-profile gastrostomy tube. They have not been seen in the clinic for over 6 months and when asked, state they have been doing quite well on their enteral tube feeds. In fact, the patient states he has gained over 20 pounds. You would proceed as follows:
   A. Congratulate him on gaining the weight and tell him to continue his present tube feeding plan.
   B. If possible, have him come into clinic or call his physician managing the tube for a possible buried bumper syndrome.
   C. Direct him to put some triple antibiotic around the site and call back in a couple of weeks if the discomfort continues.
   D. Tell him to put hot packs on it, take acetaminophen, and rest for a few days.

Test Your Knowledge Answers

1. The correct answer is **D.** The first suggestion is a common misconception: administering an acidic solution can actually make formula and many medication clogs much worse. Clog Zapper is a commercial mixture of papain, alpha amylase, and citric acid solution. It has a lower success rate when compared to pancreatic enzyme solutions. The correct answer is not C, as waiting longer will not help a tube become unclogged. Pancreatic enzyme solutions have been studied and in one report had a 90% success rate when the tube was allowed to sit for 2 hours. The mixture of one tablet of pancrelipase (6000 units, protease 19,000 units, amylase 30,000 units) and sodium bicarbonate 325 mg (half of a 650-mg tablet) is crushed and mixed with 5 mL of warm water and instilled into the feeding tube for 30 minutes to 2 hours. This can be tried an additional time if the shorter waiting period is ineffective.
2. The correct answer is **B.** Whenever a patient with a low-profile feeding tube gains or loses a significant amount of weight, there is a chance his or her tube is no longer sized correctly. This is the most problematic with weight gain, as this can cause abnormal internal pressure from the bolster or balloon, which can erode the gastric mucosa. If this process continues, buried bumper syndrome may develop. It results from growth of the gastric mucosa partially or completely over the internal bumper, usually because of excessive tension between the internal and external bumpers. Poor wound healing and significant weight gain without adjusting the external bumper or changing to a longer low-profile feeding tube can contribute as well. Patients are often unaware of this until the tube site becomes extremely painful. As the skin becomes irritated and swells, it magnifies the problem. This patient needs to be evaluated soon and have the feeding tube exchanged for either a longer low-profile tube or a standard tube. If the process has progressed too far, more intensive treatment with antibiotics and tube removal may be required.

Introduction

Enteral nutrition (EN) is the preferred method of feeding in the presence of a functional gastrointestinal (GI) tract and requires an enteral access device. The type of enteral access device is dependent on many factors. Ethical considerations, risk factors related to tube placement, the patient's disease state, gastric and small bowel function, short- and long-term goals, and length of therapy are all considered in the decision to feed the patient via the enteral route. Selecting the best enteral access device within the limits of your own institution's resources and expertise, placing the device in the optimal location within the GI tract, and communicating with and involving the patient and family in the decision-making process is essential for the successful delivery of enteral feedings in the hospital or at home. Nutrition support providers should also provide the appropriate postplacement care of feeding tubes to prevent complications of enteral access devices.

Enteral Device Selection

There are several factors that assist the clinician in determining the optimal type of enteral access device to place. A clear rationale for enteral feedings, potential length of therapy, and a plan for enteral access placement must be determined. A thorough history including the patient's current and past medical and surgical conditions and a focused physical assessment including the anatomy and function of the upper airway, esophagus, and digestive tract is imperative in the selection of the appropriate enteral access device.

The estimated duration of enteral therapy is the main factor in determining nasal tube placement versus tube enterostomy. Generally, tubes used for short-term therapy (< 4 weeks) are placed nasally (or in some cases orally) at the bedside blindly, endoscopically, or fluoroscopically in interventional radiology.[1] These tubes include nasogastric, nasoduodenal, nasojejunal, and nasogastric-jejunal tubes. For long-term placement, greater than 4 to 6 weeks, percutaneous enterostomy tubes are placed into the stomach and small bowel using endoscopic, fluoroscopic, laparoscopic, and open laparotomy techniques (Practice Scenario 12-1).

When long-term access is needed, the condition of the external abdominal wall, ability to correct coagulopathies, and patient tolerance to anesthesia must be assessed. Long-term access devices can be placed with local anesthesia of the abdominal wall and intravenous conscious sedation, and may be a better option than those placed under general anesthesia, especially in the patient who may not tolerate general anesthesia. Direct jejunal tube placement in some hospitals may be limited to the surgical setting. Assessment of the abdominal wall for open wounds and fistula, the presence of or future requirements for ostomies, percutaneous or intra-abdominal infusion devices, and peritoneal dialysis catheters must be known and become part of the decision-making process.

The decision to place an enteral access device for gastric or small bowel feedings is based on gastric motility, gastric aspiration risk, alterations in GI anatomy (ie, postsurgical), and coexisting medical conditions. Gastric feeding is generally reserved for the patients with normal gastric emptying and a low risk of gastric aspiration. Small bowel feedings are the preferred choice in the presence of conditions such as gastric outlet obstruction, gastroparesis, patients at increased risk of aspiration, and pancreatitis. The use of gastrojejunal tube systems, which allow for simultaneous gastric decompression and small bowel feedings, may be indicated for gastric outlet obstruction, severe gastroesophageal reflux, gastroparesis, and early (postoperative) feeding.[8,9] Use of small bowel feeding to reduce aspiration pneumonia is controversial, though recent data suggests this may be of benefit.[10–12]

Practice Scenario 12-1

Question: Is a patient with head and neck cancer a candidate to receive an enteral feeding device? If so, what type of enteral feeding tube?

Scenario: A 64-year-old male was diagnosed with squamous cell carcinoma of the tongue. He is scheduled to receive a 6-week course of combination of chemotherapy and radiation therapy followed by reassessment of tumor response. Physical exam reveals thin male who weighs 80 kg and has lost approximately 11 kg over the past 3 months, which represents 14% of overall body weight. His electrolytes, complete blood count, liver function tests, and albumin are within normal limits.

Intervention: Patient received a percutaneous gastrostomy tube using the introducer method technique performed by an interventional radiologist.

Answer: This patient could benefit from an enteral feeding tube to address both his existing malnutrition as well as likely further decreases in oral intake due to mucositis, nausea, and vomiting from chemoradiation. As the expected duration of therapy will be > 4 weeks, the preference would be to place a percutaneous gastrostomy over a nasoenteric feeding tube.

Rationale: During radiation and chemotherapy treatment for head and neck cancer, there is near-universal development of dysphagia, odynophagia, and mucositis. In fact, this problem is so prevalent that some advocate placing "prophylactic" gastrostomy tubes prior to starting treatment.[2,3] This type of therapy can help the patient maintain hydration and caloric and protein goals while his or her dysphagia is severe. One study showed that patients who had a prophylactic gastrostomy tube placed before treatment lost 5% less weight than the control group.[3] In addition to the timing of gastrostomy placement, there is also controversy surrounding the type of feeding tube to place in head and neck cancer patients. Some centers feel that keeping a nasogastric tube (vs. percutaneous gastric tube) will preserve the muscles of swallowing and allow the patient to independently feed more quickly after their therapy is completed.[4,5] In this case, a percutaneous feeding tube is chosen because of the preexisting malnutrition, the expected development of further nutritional impairment with chemoradiotherapy, and the estimated length of time a feeding tube will be required.

There has also been concern that by utilizing the pull technique for PEG placement, there will be tumor implantation due to dragging the gastrostomy tube through the cancer field, potentially seeding the gastrostomy tract with tumor cells.[6] In order to avoid this, the "introducer" method can be used by either interventional radiologists or endoscopists to place a percutaneous gastric feeding tube. In this technique, the stomach is insufflated and anchored to the anterior abdominal wall with T-fasteners. Serial dilators are then used to enlarge the tract and the gastrostomy tube is introduced percutaneously. In this manner, the tube is not pulled through the cancerous region and risk for tumor seeding is decreased.[7]

Tube Selection

Physical Characteristics

Patient comfort and tube performance are the key criteria in choosing a feeding tube. Most commercially manufactured feeding tubes are made of polyurethane or silicone, each with its specific advantages and disadvantages (Table 12-1). Most nasogastric or nasoenteral tubes are constructed of polyurethane due to the ability to have a relatively larger inner tube diameter for a given outer diameter size. Most percutaneous tubes are constructed from silicone because of its inherent material longevity and comfort. Rubber tubes, used in Foley catheters and red rubber surgical jejunostomy tubes, are inferior due to their rapid degradation and lack of internal (red rubber) or external (Foley catheter) retaining devices.

Tube Types

Nasoenteric feeding tubes come in a wide array of diameters and lengths with an equally wide array of internal stylets, feeding and medication ports, weights, and tips (Table 12-2). Tubes are measured by their external diameter. However, flow through the tubes and susceptibility to clogging depend on a tube's inner diameter. The inner diameter may vary depending on the specific material used to construct the tube. In general, polyurethane tubes of the same outer diameter as a silicone tube will have a larger internal diameter.

Stylets or guidewires are provided with most nasoenteric feeding tubes to provide tube structure and/or guidance while passing these relatively floppy tubes. They are designed to be shorter than the length of the tube and to have a flexible distal tip to avoid perforation of the GI mucosa. A water-activated lubricant may be used to coat the tube's internal lumen to allow easier removal of these stylets or guidewires after the tube is in place. Commercially available nasoenteric feeding tubes

TABLE 12-1 Comparison of Polyurethane and Silicone Tube Characteristics

	Polyurethane	Silicone
Comfort	Lower	Higher
Stiffness	Higher	Lower
Wall width	Thinner	Thicker
Fungal degradation	More resistant	Less resistant
Common use	Nasoenteric feeding tubes	Percutaneous feeding tubes

TABLE 12-2 Nasoenteric and Enterostomy Tube Sizes

Tube Type	Size (French)	Length (cm)
Nasogastric	8–16	38–91
Nasoenteric	8–12	91–240
Gastrostomy	12–28	Not applicable
Gastrojejunal	6–12	
Jejunal extension tube through existing gastrostomy		15–95
Dual lumen tube (gastric and jejunal)	16–30	
Single lumen (jejunal only)	12–24	15–58
Low-profile gastrostomy (replacement)	12–24	0.8–6.5
Low-profile gastrojejunostomy	14–22	15–45

have either one port for feeding or two in a "Y" configuration: one for feeding and the other for medication and/or irrigation (Figure 12-1). These ports can accommodate either a feeding set or a syringe, or both. Dual ports allow concomitant feeding and medication administration and/or irrigation. However, to prevent clogging, medications should be administered through the tube only after enteral feedings are held and the feeding tube flushed. The Joint Commission has recognized that serious errors can occur when enteral feeding tubes are inadvertently connected to intravenous lines, and manufacturers have started to produce enteral feeding connectors that decrease this uncommon but catastrophic complication.[13]

Initially, weighted tube tips were thought to facilitate transpyloric passage. However, critical analysis of the literature does not demonstrate a clear advantage with the use of either weighted or unweighted tips.[14] Feeding tube tips come in a wide variety of sizes, number, and end versus side holes for feeding, although there is no specific data to favor any particular design. Therefore, the choice is left up to the personal preference of the individual clinician and mode of placement.

FIGURE 12-1 Nasoenteric Feeding Tube Ports

Y Port **Single Port**

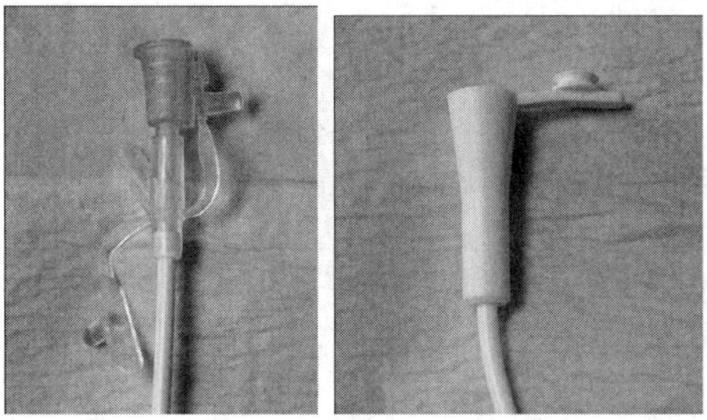

FIGURE 12-2 Percutaneous Endoscopic Gastrostomy Tube Internal Bolsters

Solid Type **Balloon Type**

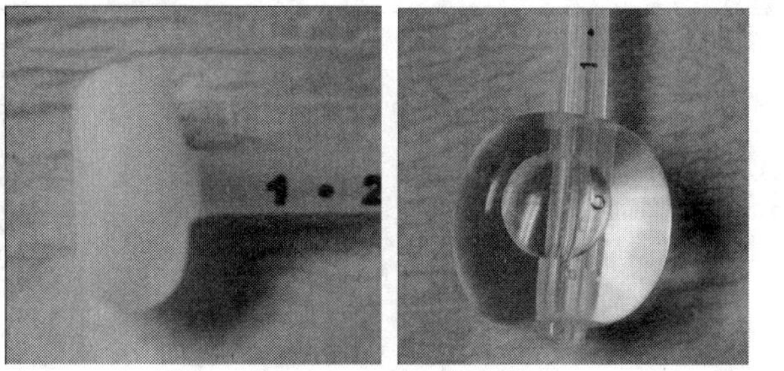

Enterostomy feeding tubes are available in a wide array of diameters and lengths (Table 12-2). The internal retention bolsters of percutaneous tubes are constructed of either solid material (silicone or polyurethane) or silicone balloons (Figure 12-2). Solid internal bolsters are more common with initial percutaneous enterostomy tube placement due to their greater longevity. Balloon-type internal bolsters are inserted more commonly with open and laparoscopic surgical tube placement and as replacement devices due to their ease in placement. These balloons generally only have a life span of 3 to 6 months.[15] If possible, use of a nonballoon tube is preferred for direct jejunal tube placement. Enterostomy feeding tubes may have multiple ports. Typically, separate ports are included for feeding and medication and/or irrigation. If the internal bolster is of the balloon type, an additional third port is present for balloon inflation or deflation.

Gastrojejunal feeding tubes are inserted using percutaneous, open, and laparoscopic techniques. These tubes are placed into the stomach with a smaller bore extension tube that passes through the pylorus into the jejunum. Some gastrojejunal tubes are specifically designed with separate gastric and jejunal lumens and ports, allowing for both jejunal feeding and gastric decompression (Figure 12-3). Jejunostomy tubes are placed directly into the jejunum without passage through the stomach. Low-profile tubes are skin-level devices that are used as replacement devices for gastrostomies, jejunostomies, and gastrojejunostomies (Figure 12-4). The length of the existing stoma tract is measured before choosing and placing the correct size of a low profile device.

Methods of Access

Nasal Tubes

Nasogastric and nasoenteric feeding tubes are inserted when short-term access is indicated. They can provide an opportunity to assess tolerance of enteral feedings before placement of a percutaneous enterostomy if longer-term access is required. They may be passed transorally or transnasally, although the nasal approach will be better tolerated in conscious patients. Contraindications to nasogastric or nasoenteric feeding tube placement are obstructing head, neck, and

FIGURE 12-3 Percutaneous Endoscopic Gastrojejunostomy Feeding Ports

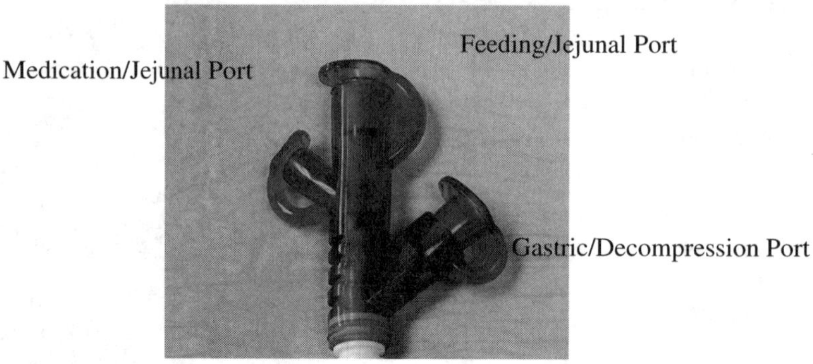

esophageal pathology, or injury preventing safe insertion. Nasogastric or nasoenteric feeding tubes should not be used until confirmation of proper position is obtained. Plain abdominal or chest radiography is the gold standard for confirmation of placement. However, recent studies suggest that radiographic confirmation may not be required when electromagnetic imaging technology is utilized for placement.[16,17] Other methods including auscultation, pH stepup, and capnography still require radiographic confirmation.[18–21]

Nasogastric tubes are the least difficult feeding tubes to insert. Placement may be performed by clinicians with all levels of training. Larger, stiffer tubes used for gastric decompression should be converted to a smaller bore feeding tube, if possible, for patient comfort and to decrease the risk of associated complications. The length of the tube necessary for gastric placement can be estimated by measuring the distance from the tip of the nose to the ear lobe and then to the xiphoid process. Placement of a nasogastric tube requires passage through a

FIGURE 12-4 Replacement Percutaneous Endoscopic Gastrostomy Tubes

Low-Profile Solid Internal Bolster

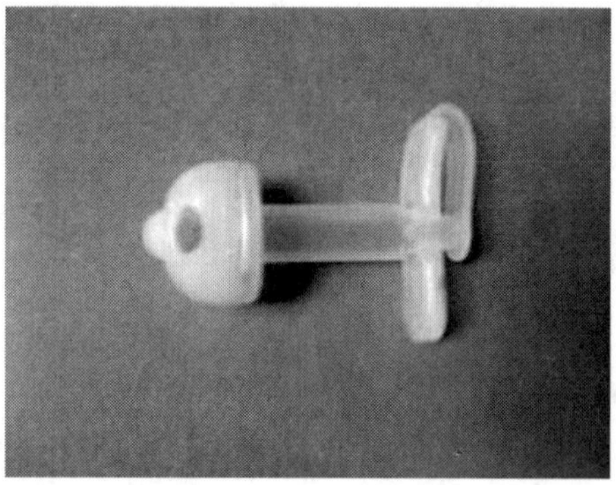

Low-Profile Balloon Internal Bolster

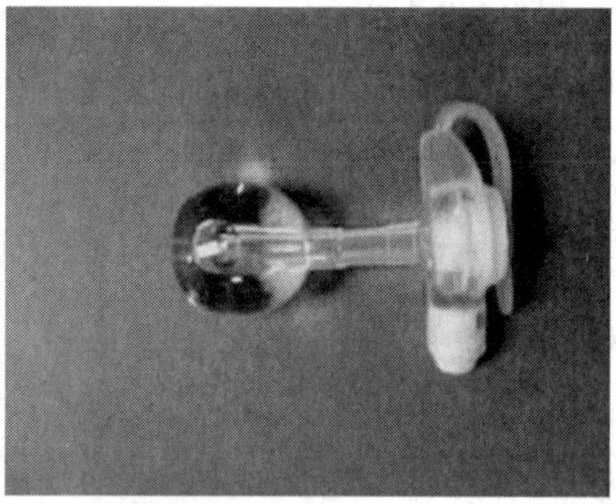

Standard-Profile Solid Internal Bolster

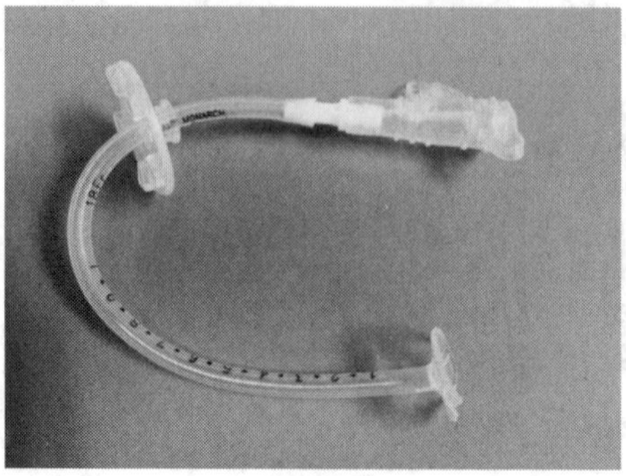

patent nare and may be facilitated by concurrent patient swallowing. Aspiration of gastric contents, auscultation of insufflated air over the stomach, and absence of patient coughing or choking suggests, but cannot ensure, correct tube placement. Again, correct position within the GI tract should be confirmed radiographically.

Nasoenteric feeding tubes are placed anywhere distal to the pylorus, whereas nasojejunal tubes are placed distal to the ligament of Treitz. Either is more difficult to place than nasogastric tubes. Nasoenteric tubes can be placed at the bedside, endoscopically, or fluoroscopically. Bedside placement usually requires experienced personnel with specialized training. The most common method uses the technique described by Zaloga.[22] This technique requires the patient to lie on the right side; the feeding tube tip is bent and advanced slowly with a combination of air insufflation, tube rotation, and auscultation. Prokinetics (erythromycin or metoclopramide) are often added to bedside techniques and may increase success rates.[23] Recently, devices have been developed to assist with nasoenteric tube placement including a bedside magnet and electromagnetic imaging system. Success rates > 90% have been reported using these systems.[17,20,21,24] Nasojejunal placement is most reliably achieved with endoscopic or fluoroscopic techniques, but are more costly, require advanced training, and are more invasive. The reported success rate for bedside nasoenteric tube placement ranges from 56% to 92% with > 90% success rates reported for endoscopic and fluoroscopic placement. However, success rates are lower for placement distal to the ligament of Treitz.[25]

Enterostomy Tubes

Enterostomy tubes are placed when long-term access (>4 weeks) is required. These tubes may be placed by endoscopic, fluoroscopic, or surgical methods. These methods have similar success rates, although there is less morbidity and cost with endoscopic or fluoroscopic techniques.[26–30] Routine preprocedural testing of coagulation parameters and platelets are no longer recommended, but they should be considered if there is concern for abnormal coagulation due to anticoagulant medication, medical history of excessive bleeding, or recent antibiotic use. Prophylactic antibiotics are administered as they have been shown to decrease peristomal infection rates when using endoscopic methods.[31,32]

Gastrostomy Tubes

Percutaneous endoscopic gastrostomy (PEG) is the most common technique for obtaining long-term gastric access, and it is generally performed under moderate sedation.[33] Specific contraindications for endoscopic placement include obstruction of the GI tract proximal to the stomach and the inability to transilluminate the abdominal wall for identification of a safe abdominal access site.[34] Additional relative contraindications include ascites, coagulopathy, gastric varices, active head and neck cancers, morbid obesity, and neoplastic, infiltrative, or inflammatory disease of the gastric or abdominal wall.[35]

The most common method of PEG insertion is the Ponsky (pull) technique.[36] Air is insufflated into the stomach via an endoscope. The optimal site for PEG placement is determined through simultaneous endoscopic transillumination noted on the abdominal wall and endoscopically visualized finger indentation at the site. A small incision is made at this site, and a needle/trocar is inserted through the abdominal wall and into the stomach. A guidewire is passed through the needle/trocar, and the snare is grasped endoscopically and withdrawn through the mouth. A gastrostomy tube is affixed to the guidewire and pulled through the esophagus into the stomach and out the abdominal wall. The gastrostomy tube is held in place by a solid mushroom-type internal retention device and an external bumper. Advantages of PEG placement include performance at bedside, lack of radiation, and ability to perform diagnostic and therapeutic endoscopic procedures simultaneously.

Percutaneous gastrostomy tubes can also be placed using fluoroscopic guidance using two general techniques. In the first, a nasogastric tube is placed to insufflate the stomach, a safe window is identified under fluoroscopy, and one to four T-fasteners are used to perform a gastropexy to secure the stomach wall to the abdominal wall. A needle is used to obtain gastric access, the guidewire is advanced through the needle, and the tract is dilated. Lastly, the gastrostomy tube is placed through the tract using a peel-away sheath.[37,38] A less commonly performed fluoroscopic method uses a slightly curved 18-gauge needle or vascular sheath; it is advanced into the stomach and pointed toward the gastroesophageal junction after gastric insufflation. The guidewire is then advanced with or without help of an angiographic catheter into the esophagus, the oropharynx, and out of the mouth. A gastrostomy tube is then threaded over the wire, advanced until it emerges from the abdominal wall, and then pulled into the desired position.[28,39] Advantages of fluoroscopic gastrostomy placement include lack of need for conscious sedation in some patients, ability to perform in patients with severe stenosis/trauma of the upper GI tract, and decreased risk of tumor seeding from upper aerodigestive tract cancers (Practice Scenario 12-1). Reported success rates for either fluoroscopic or endoscopic gastrostomies are greater than 95%.[40]

A gastrostomy tube inserted using the laparoscopic or open (laparotomy) method is performed in the operating room using general anesthesia. Surgical placement of feeding tubes is used when patients are undergoing another abdominal operation, when endoscopic and radiologic attempts fail, and/or in the presence of an aerodigestive tract obstruction or facial trauma. Direct jejunal tube placement is also done laparoscopically when there is not an endoscopy alternative available.

Laparoscopic techniques access the peritoneal cavity by way of small ports that enter through the abdominal wall.[36] A pneumoperitoneum is created through a port inserted just below the umbilicus through which a camera is passed. The stomach is accessed and manipulated through a second port entering in the left lower quadrant and a third port (if required) entering through the right upper quadrant. T-fasteners or laparoscopic sutures are placed to affix the stomach to the abdominal wall. The procedure then proceeds similar to fluoroscopic gastrostomy with a hollow needle advanced percutaneously into the stomach lumen followed by wire, dilators, peel-away sheath, and finally the gastrostomy tube.[41–44]

The Stamm technique is the most commonly used surgical placement of an open gastrostomy tube.[8,34] It requires a small laparotomy in the upper midline of the abdomen. The gastrostomy tube is brought into the stomach through a small stab wound in the upper abdominal wall. A small incision is made into the stomach through which the feeding tube enters and around which purse-string sutures are placed to secure the stomach around the gastrostomy tube. The stomach is then sutured to the anterior abdominal wall. This tube may be held in place with an inflated balloon or sutured to the abdominal wall to prevent tube migration.

Gastrojejunal Tubes

In the situation of impaired gastric motility, pancreatitis, pancreatic surgery, or any time that enteral feeding into the small bowel feeding with simultaneous stomach decompression is required, a gastrojejunal tube should be placed.[45,46]

Percutaneous endoscopic gastrojejunostomy may be performed immediately or any time after gastrostomy tube placement. Most commonly, a guidewire is placed through the existing gastrostomy. This is grasped endoscopically and carried into the jejunum. The endoscope is then withdrawn, leaving the guidewire in place. The jejunal extension tube is threaded over the guidewire into the small bowel.[34,47]

Fluoroscopic gastrojejunal access is becoming much more common. Initial steps are similar to fluoroscopic gastrostomy placement, as previously described. In addition, to facilitate placement of the gastrojejunostomy, puncture of the stomach is performed in the direction of the pylorus. A guidewire is advanced through the stomach to the ligament of Treitz, and the jejunal extension tube is advanced over the wire into the jejunum.[48,49] Fluoroscopic techniques can be used when the patient cannot undergo endoscopy; however, it does require transport to the radiology suite.

Gastrojejunal tubes can be placed during laparotomy or laparoscopy methods using any of the previously discussed methods. Using manual and/or endoscopic methods, the jejunal tube is positioned into the small bowel. The gastric component of the tube is left in the stomach. The patient benefits from gastric decompression while receiving enteral feeds into the small bowel, but there is greater risk of the jejunal tube piece migrating back into the stomach on a regular basis.

Jejunostomy Tubes

Direct percutaneous endoscopic jejunostomy is a modification of the pull PEG technique. A colonoscope or enteroscope is advanced into the small bowel. Transillumination and finger palpation is performed over the jejunum instead of the stomach. A sounding needle and/or trocar is passed through the anterior abdominal wall into the jejunum. An insertion wire is advanced through the trocar and grasped. The procedure is then completed as per the pull-type PEG.[49,50]

Fluoroscopic direct jejunostomy tube placement is performed a variety of different ways. In general, identification of the target bowel loop is performed by advancing an angiographic catheter into the proximal jejunum and insufflating it with air and contrast,[51] or by placing an angioplasty balloon[52] or snare loop[53] in the desired location to serve as a target. The jejunal loop is accessed with a needle, and a T-fastener device is then delivered to secure the jejunal loop against the abdominal wall. A guidewire is then advanced through the needle, the tract is dilated, and the jejunostomy tube is placed.

Direct percutaneous jejunostomy using either endoscopic or fluoroscopic guidance is considerably more difficult technically than percutaneous gastrostomy despite similar methods; it is not available in all institutions. Success rates for endoscopic jejunostomy range from 68% to 100% and from 87% to 100% for fluoroscopic jejunostomy.[54] Endoscopic jejunostomy tubes are more stable due to solid mushroom-type internal bolsters and larger tube diameters (18 to 20 vs. 10 to 14 French) than fluoroscopic tubes.

The technique of laparoscopic jejunostomy is similar to laparoscopic gastrostomy. Ports are placed in the left upper quadrant and lower abdominal midline. The jejunum is manipulated to affix it to the abdominal wall with T-fasteners. Then a guidewire is placed into the lumen of the jejunum, and a jejunostomy tube is advanced into the small bowel through a peel-away sheath.[36,42]

An open jejunostomy is placed using a Witzel technique. In this procedure, a submucosal tunnel is created in the small bowel through which the jejunostomy tube is threaded; this prevents leakage of small bowel contents onto the abdominal wall.[9] Less commonly, a needle catheter jejunostomy may be placed by laparotomy or laparoscopy.[9,55] In this procedure, a needle is threaded into the small bowel. A guidewire is passed into the jejunum. A small jejunostomy catheter (5 to 8 French) is passed over this guidewire into the jejunum. The small bore size of needle catheter jejunostomies make them prone to occlusion. Surgical jejunostomies are performed much more commonly due to the complexity of performing direct jejunostomies endoscopically or radiologically.

Skin-Level Devices

Skin-level devices are an excellent option for the patient who is concerned about cosmetic appearance. This device can also be more comfortable for the patient who is active, sleeps in the prone position, or who only needs intermittent therapy. Because of the need to attach a feeding connector to the skin-level device, adequate manual dexterity or caregiver assistance is needed. Skin-level devices are usually placed as an exchange tube for a preexisting gastrostomy or jejunostomy tube; however, they can also be inserted at the time of initial tube placement.[56] Newer skin-level device tubes are available for both gastric decompression and/or jejunal feeding. Skin-level tubes are held in place with an inflated internal balloon or a deformable solid silicone internal retention bolster.

Postinsertion Catheter Care

Skin Care

Regardless of the tube type or insertion technique, all patients require appropriate oral hygiene. This is often important for preventing aspiration pneumonia in ventilator-dependent patients or those with a depressed level of consciousness. Patients with nasal tubes benefit from skin care to the nasal area due to prolonged exposure to tape and adhesive products. Repositioning the nasal tube and avoiding pressure to the nares is important to prevent pressure necrosis. Patients and caregivers may use mild soap and water to cleanse the stoma site for percutaneous tubes. The area should be rinsed and dried thoroughly. Routine use of antibiotic ointments or hydrogen peroxide at the tube site is not recommended. Dressings can be applied if there is drainage from the stoma site; however, they should not be placed with excessive tension, which can promote infection and buried bumper syndrome.

Prevention of Clogging

All tubes are prone to clogging. Usual causes include suboptimal flushing, not flushing between each medication administration, accumulation of pill fragments, frequent checking of residuals, and administration of high-protein/-fiber formulas.[34,47] Compliance with intermittent flushing protocols is essential to prevent clogging. Water should be used as the flush fluid of choice. Two reports have demonstrated superiority of prophylactic use of pancreatic enzymes to prevent tube occlusion compared to standard water flushes.[57,58] Medications in liquid form are less likely to clog than crushed pills and should be used if available. Whether a medication is in pill or liquid form, each medication should be given separately with a water flush before and after each medication.[59]

Exchange and Removal of Enterostomy Tubes

Enterostomy tubes can be safely removed after the stoma tract has matured, usually > 2 weeks after insertion. In patients who are on steroids, immunosuppressed, obese, or otherwise suspected of poor wound healing, waiting 4 to 6 weeks is advised. Removal of enterostomy tubes before this time may result in the stomach falling away from the abdominal wall, allowing gastric contents to leak into the peritoneum. If this occurs, tube replacement with the assistance of endoscopy, interventional radiology, or surgery is required.

After stoma tract maturation, a replacement tube can be placed at the bedside without endoscopy or fluoroscopy. Removal of an endoscopically placed gastric tube with a mushroom internal bolster is accomplished at the bedside using the traction method. The patient is placed in the supine position with knees bent to relax the abdominal muscles. The exposed gastric tubing is firmly grasped and pulled forcefully. For devices held in place with an inflated balloon, the balloon is deflated and the tube is gently removed. Prior to removal using either technique, a surgical lubricant is placed at the tube site to thoroughly lubricate the stoma. When replacing a long-term enteral feeding device with a balloon replacement tube, follow the manufacturer's recommendations regarding balloon volume. Generally, 5 to 20 mL of sterile water should be used for gastric tubes and 3 mL for small bowel tubes. Standard and low-profile replacement tubes with solid internal bolsters are available as well (Figure 12-4). Correct tube position can be checked after replacement by aspiration of gastric contents or auscultation of insufflated air. However, these methods are not completely reliable, and if there is any concern for misplacement correct tube position should be confirmed with fluoroscopic or endoscopic imaging (Practice Scenario 12-2).

Practice Scenario 12-2

Question: What is the complication in a patient with percutaneous gastrostomy tube who develops abdominal pain after tube exchange?

Scenario: Patient is a 24-year-old female with a history of severe gastric and small bowel dysmotility. She has a 24 French gastric balloon decompression tube that was initially placed several years ago and is regularly changed by the patient at home. She most recently uneventfully changed her gastric tube the day prior. The next day she presented to the emergency room with severe abdominal pain. The patient awakened in the middle of the night with gastric leakage and intense pain around her feeding tube. She was unable to aspirate any gastric fluid from the feeding tube or move the tube within the tract. Her skin was very reddened and ulcerated from the leakage of gastric fluid.

Intervention: The patient had a radiologic evaluation of her feeding tube, and the tip was located within the gastric wall with leakage of the Gastrografin dye into the subcutaneous tissue. No peritoneal leakage was noted. The PEG was removed and a new PEG placed through the same tract. Proper position was confirmed by instillation of contrast through the tube with filling of the stomach with contrast noted.

Answer: Dislodgement of her abdominal feeding tube occurred after replacement. Health care providers should have an extremely low threshold for confirming tube position if there is any concern for tube malposition after replacement.

Rationale: If a patient develops abdominal pain after percutaneous feeding tube replacement, the concern is that the tube has not been placed back into the gastric lumen but was potentially placed within the stoma tract or has perforated into the peritoneal space. This most often occurs when there has been difficulty with tube replacement, but it can occur when replacement is reported to go smoothly as well. When this is suspected, the tube position should be evaluated fluoroscopically or endoscopically. Treatment of this problem depends on how severe the problem is and if there has been contamination of enteral feeds into the peritoneal cavity. For the patient in which significant peritoneal contamination has not occurred, the malpositioned tube can be removed and another tube placed using the same tract. If there is no further leakage into the peritoneal cavity, then the tube is safe to use. If more significant disruption of the tract occurs and a new tube cannot be placed at the existing site, the patient can be supported through a nasoenteric feeding tube while the stoma tract closes and any infection is treated.[60] If significant leakage has occurred and abdominal sepsis develops, the patient is supported with intravenous fluids and antibiotics, and a surgical consultation obtained. Necrotizing fasciitis has been reported in severe cases of untreated, uncontrolled infection. This is a surgical emergency with high morbidity and mortality. Emergency consultation for wide surgical debridement is indicated.

Complications of Enteral Access Devices

Nasal Tubes

Complications of nasogastric and nasoenteric feeding tubes can be divided into those occurring during the insertion procedure or those occurring in the postprocedure period. The overall procedure related complication rate is ~10% and includes epistaxis, aspiration, and circulatory or respiratory compromise. The most dreaded procedural complication is initial misplacement of the nasoenteric tube into the bronchopulmonary tree. This complication only occurs in 2% to 4% of nasoenteric tube placements. However, it is unsuspected in 80% of occurrences and results in pneumothorax up to 50% of the time it occurs.[18,61–63] Radiography is the gold standard for ensuring correct placement and should be performed before the feeding tube is used. Published data demonstrates that adopting radiographic confirmation protocols decreases inadvertent use of incorrectly placed feeding tubes.[19] As stated previously, use of a bedside electromagnetic imaging system may obviate need for radiographic confirmation.[16,17]

Postprocedural complications include inadvertent tube dislodgement, tube malfunction, tube occlusion, tube feeding aspiration, and intestinal ischemia. Dislodgement occurs in 25% to 41% of cases.[64–66] The use of a nasal bridle has clearly been shown to decrease tube dislodgment rate. A recent report decreased the incidence of accidental dislodgement from 36% to 10% by using a magnet-based system to place the nasal bridle.[67] Malfunction of the tube, including breaking, cracking, or kinking of the tube, occurs 11% to 20% of the time.[65,66] When accurately diagnosed by sinus needle puncture and aspiration, sinusitis occurs ~12% of the time.[68] This is believed secondary to obstruction of physiologic sinus drainage by the nasoenteric tube.

Tube occlusion is a frequent problem (20% to 45%) often requiring tube replacement.[66,69,70] Risk factors for tube occlusion include increasing tube length, decreasing tube caliber, inadequate water flushing, frequent medication delivery, and use of the tube to measure residual volumes.[70] When feeding tubes become clogged, simple flushing with water can relieve the obstruction in one-third of patients.[71] If this fails, the installation of pancreatic enzymes can reopen an additional 50% of the occluded tubes.[71,72] Mechanical dislodgement may also be achieved using a cytology brush, an endoscopic retrograde cholangiopancreatography catheter, or a commercial corkscrew device.[73] Finally, replacing the nasal feeding tube is the last resort.

Rarely, the provision of EN to a hypotensive, critically ill patient may be associated with intestinal ischemia. This is usually evidenced by increasing GI intolerance (increased tube output, abdominal pain and distension, ileus). This is best avoided by cessation of enteral feeding pending further evaluation in hypotensive patients requiring increasing doses of vasopressor agents with progressive GI intolerance.[25,74]

Enterostomy Tubes

Complications of enterostomy tubes can be divided into procedural and postprocedural events. Procedure-related complications and mortality are uncommon (1.5% to 4% and 0% to 2% of the time, respectively) and include intraprocedural aspiration, hemorrhage, perforation of the GI lumen, and prolonged ileus.[60] Risk factors for aspiration include the supine position, advanced age, need for sedation, and neurologic impairment.[75] Pneumoperitoneum as a result of the percutaneous procedure is common and in the absence of peritoneal signs is of no clinical consequence.[76] Infusion of water-soluble contrast with fluoroscopic imaging is the test of choice if peritonitis is suspected. The procedural and long-term mortality rate directly related to PEG placement is very low despite the up to 50% annual mortality in patients receiving gastrostomy tubes.[76] This very high rate is a function of the significant comorbidities of the patients rather than the procedure or the feeding tube itself.

The overall postprocedure complication rate of enterostomy tubes ranges from 4.8% to 10.8%.[60] Minor postprocedural complications are two to three times more common than major ones (Table 12-3). Peristomal infection is the most common complication of gastrostomy placement.[33,77] The majority of infections are mild. In rare cases, necrotizing fasciitis with high morbidity and mortality can develop. Prophylactic antibiotics before placement, early recognition of wound infections, treatment with antibiotics, local wound care, and debridement, if necessary, are the keys to successful management.[33,35,78]

Leakage around the gastrostomy site is a common and underrecognized problem facing nutrition support providers.[79] Risk factors include infection, excessive cleansing with irritant solutions (ie, H_2O_2, povidone-iodine), and excessive tension and side torsion on the external portion of the feeding tube. Prompt treatment of infection, good ostomy skin care, loosening of the outer bumper, and stabilizing the gastrostomy tube to prevent tension torsion on the tube will address these issues.[73]

Buried bumper syndrome results from growth of the gastric mucosa over the internal bumper. Risk factors include excessive tension between the internal and external bumpers, poor wound healing, and significant weight gain.[80–82] Treatment is based on maintaining the stoma tract while restoring the internal bumper entirely within the stomach lumen.[83,84]

TABLE 12-3 Major and Minor Complications of Enterostomy Tube Placement

	Reported Frequency (%)
Major Complications	
Aspiration	0.3–1.0
Hemorrhage	0–2.5
Peritonitis/necrotizing fasciitis	0.5–1.3
Death (related to percutaneous endoscopic gastrostomy placement)	0–2.1
Minor Complications	
Peristomal infection	5.4–30
Peristomal leakage	1–2
Buried bumper	0.3–2.4
Inadvertent removal	1.6–4.4
Fistulous tracts	0.3–6.7

As noted previously, accidental gastrostomy tube removal should be addressed urgently. If a standard tube is not promptly available, a suitably sized Foley catheter can be used to keep the tract open until a standard replacement tube can be placed. In patients prone to pulling tubes, the use of an abdominal binder, placing mittens on the patient's hands, cutting down the external tube length to 6 to 8 cm, or switching to a low-profile device can reduce the risk of future removal.[60]

Gastrojejunal and Jejunal Tubes

Complications of gastrojejunal tubes and jejunal tubes are similar to gastrostomy tubes described previously. Gastrojejunal feeding tubes are also complicated by frequent (up to 70%) malfunction, migration, and/or occlusion of the smaller jejunal extension tube.[85,86] Additional complications of direct jejunostomy tubes include jejunal volvulus and/or small bowel perforation.[87] Although often recommended by expert opinion, there is no clear evidence that more distal feeding with jejunal tubes markedly decreases a patient's aspiration risk. However, as stated previously, recent data suggests that jejunal feeding may be associated with decreased risk of aspiration pneumonia.[10–12]

Conclusion

Enteral feeding remains the feeding route of choice in the presence of a functional GI tract. Success depends on the placement of the appropriate access device in the correct location of the GI tract using the best insertion method available. Proper care and maintenance of these enteral access devices with early recognition and management of their complications is critical to successful EN therapy.

References

1. Vanek V. Ins and outs of enteral access. Part 1: short-term enteral access. *Nutr Clin Prac.* 2002;17:275–283.
2. Nguyen N, North D, Smith H, et al. Safety and effectiveness of prophylactic gastrostomy tubes for head and neck cancer patients undergoing chemoradiation. *Surg Oncol.* 2006;15:199–203.
3. Chang J, Gosling T, Larsen J, et al. Prophylactic gastrostomy tubes for patients receiving radical radiotherapy for head and neck cancers: a retrospective review. *J Med Imaging Radiation Oncology.* 2009;53:431–432.
4. Paleri V, Patterson J. Use of gastrostomy in head and neck cancer: a systematic review to identify areas for future research. *Clin Otolaryngology.* 2010;35:177–189.
5. Corry J. Feeding tubes and dysphagia: cause or effect in head and neck cancer patients. *J Med Imaging Radiat Oncol.* 2009;53:431–432.
6. Tsai J, Schattner M. Percutaneous endoscopic gastrostomy site metastasis. *Gastrointest Endosc Clin N Am.* 2007;17:777.
7. Foster J, Filocamo P, Nava H, et al. The introducer technique is the optimal method for placing percutaneous endoscopic gastrostomy tubes in head and neck cancer patients. *Surg Endosc.* 2007;6: 897–901.
8. Vanek V. Ins and outs of enteral access. Part 2: long-term access-esophagostomy and gastrostomy. *Nutr Clin Prac.* 2003;18:50–74.
9. Vanek V. Ins and outs of enteral access. Part 3: long-term access-jejunostomy. *Nutr Clin Prac.* 2003;18:201–220.
10. Metheny N, Stewart B, McClave S. Relationship between feeding tube site and respiratory outcomes. *J Parental Enteral Nutr.* 2011; 35:346–355.
11. Hsu C, Sun S, Lin S, et al. Duodenal versus gastric feeding in medical intensive care unit patients: a prospective, randomized, clinical study. *Crit Care Med.* 2009;37:1866–1872.
12. Panagiotakis P, DiSario J, Hilden K, et al. DPEJ prevents aspiration in high-risk patients. *Nutr Clin Prac.* 2008;23:172–175.
13. Joint Commission of Accreditation of Healthcare Organizations. Sentinel report on special events. *Jt Comm Perspect.* 1998;18: 19–33,36–42.
14. Levy H. Nasogastric and nasoenteric feeding tubes. *Gastrointest Endosc Clin N Am.* 1998;8:529–549.
15. Heiser M, Malaty H. Balloon-type versus non-balloon-type replacement percutaneous endoscopic gastrostomy: which is better? *Gastroenterol Nurs.* 2001;24:58–63.
16. Powers J, Luebbehusen M, Spitzer T, et al. Verification of an electromagnetic placement device compared with abdominal radiograph to predict accuracy of feeding tube placement. *Journal of Parenter and Enteral Nutr.* 2011;35:535–539.
17. Koopman M, Kudsk K, Szotkowski M, et al. A team-based protocol and electromagnetic technology eliminate feeding tube placement complications. *Ann Surg.* 2011;253:287–302.
18. Rassias A, Ball P, Corwin H. A prospective study of tracheopulmonary complications associated with the placement of narrow-bore enteral feeding tubes. *Crit Care.* 2009;2:25–28.
19. Marderstein E, Simmons R, Ochoa J. Patient safety: effect of institutional protocols on adverse events related to feeding tube placement in the critically ill. *J Am Coll Surg.* 2004;199:39–47.
20. Gray R, Tynan C, Reed L, et al. Bedside electromagnetic-guided feeding tube placement: an improvement over traditional placement technique? *Nutr Clin Prac.* 2007;22:436–444.
21. Stark S, Sharpe J, Larson G. Endoscopically placed nasoenteral feeding tubes. Indications and techniques. *Am Surg.* 1991;57:203–205.
22. Zaloga G. Bedside method for placing small bowel feeding tubes in critically ill patients. A prospective study. *Chest.* 1991;100: 1643–1646.
23. Booth C, Heyland D, Paterson W. Gastrointestinal promotility drugs in the critical care setting: a systematic review of the evidence. *Crit Care Med.* 2002;30:1429–1435.
24. Rivera R, Campana J, Seidner S, et al. Small bowel feeding tube placement using an electromagnetic tube placement device: accuracy of tip placement. *J Parental Enteral Nutr.* 2009;333:225.
25. McClave S, Chang W. Complications of enteral access. *Gastroentest Endosc.* 2003;58:739–751.
26. Cosentini E, Sauntner T, Gnant M, et al. Outcomes of surgical, percutaneous endoscopic, and percutaneous radiologic gastrostomies. *Arch Surg.* 1998;133:1076–1083.
27. Moller P, Lindberg C, Zilling T. Gastrostomy by various techniques: evaluation of indications, outcome, and complications. *Scand J Gastroenterol.* 1999;34:1050–1054.
28. Laasch H, Wilbraham L, Bullen K, et al. Gastrostomy insertion: comparing the options—PEG, RIG, or PIG? *Clin Radiol.* 2003;58: 398–405.
29. Stiegmann G, Goff J, Silas D, et al. Endoscopic versus operative gastrostomy: final results of a prospective randomized trial. *Gastrointest Endosc.* 1990;36:1–5.
30. Scott J, de la Torre RA, Unger S. Comparison of operative versus percutaneous endoscopic gastrostomy tube placement in the elderly. *Am Surg.* 1991;57:338–340.
31. Banerjee S, Shen B, Baron T, et al. Antibiotic prophylaxis for GI endoscopy. *Gastrointest Endosc.* 2008;67:791–798.

32. Lipp A, Lusardi G. Systemic antimicrobial prophylaxis for percutaneous endoscopic gastrostomy. *Coch Data System Rev*. 2006;4.
33. Gossner L, Keymling J, Hahn E, et al. Antibiotic prophylaxis in percutaneous endoscopic gastrostomy (PEG): a prospective randomized clinical trial. *Endoscopy*. 1999;31:119–124.
34. DiSario J, Baskin W, Brown R, et al. Endoscopic approaches to enteral nutritional support. *Gastrointest Endosc*. 2002;55:901–908.
35. Jain N, Larson D, Schroeder K, et al. Antibiotic prophylaxis for percutaneous endoscopic gastrostomy. A prospective, randomized, double-blind clinical trial. *Ann Intern Med*. 1987;107:824–828.
36. Ponsky J, Gauderer M. Percutaneous endoscopic gastrostomy: a non-operative technique for feeding gastrostomy. *Gastrointest Endosc*. 1981;27:9–11.
37. Cope C. Suture anchor for visceral drainage. *Am J Roentgenol*. 1986; 146:160–162.
38. Coleman C, Coons H, Cope C, et al. Percutaneous enterostomy with the Cope suture anchor. *Radiology*. 1990;174(3 Pt 1): 889–891.
39. Funaki B, Zaleski G, Lorenz J, et al. Radiologic gastrostomy placement: pigtail-placement versus mushroom-retained catheters. *Am J Roentgenol*. 2000;175:375–379.
40. Duszak R Jr, Mabry M. National trends in gastrointestinal access procedures: an analysis of Medicare services provided by radiologists and other specialists. *J Vasc Interv Radiol*. 2003;14: 1031–1036.
41. Lorentzen T, Skjoldbye B, Nolsoe C, et al. Percutaneous gastrostomy guided by ultrasound and fluoroscopy. *Acta Radiol*. 1995;36: 159–162.
42. Grant J. Comparison of percutaneous endoscopic gastrostomy with Stamm gastrostomy. *Ann Surg*. 1988;207:598–603.
43. Duh Q, Senokozlieff-Englehart A, Choe Y, et al. Laparoscopic gastrostomy and jejunostomy: safety and cost with local vs. general anesthesia. *Arch Surg*. 1999;134:151–156.
44. Lydiatt D, Murayama K, Hollins R, et al. Laparoscopic gastrostomy versus open gastrostomy in head and neck cancer patients. *Laryngoscope*. 1996;106:407–410.
45. Ho C. Radiologic placement of gastrostomy/jejunostomy tubes in high-risk patients. *Nutr Clin Prac*. 1997;12:S17–S19.
46. Ho C, Yeung E. Percutaneous gastrostomy and transgastric jejunostomy. *Am J Roentgenol*. 1992;158:251–257.
47. DeLegge M, Patrick P, Gibbs R. Percutaneous endoscopic gastrojejunostomy with a tapered tip, nonweighted jejunal feeding tube: improved placement success. *Am J Gastroenterol*. 1996;91: 1130–1134.
48. Peitgen K, Walz M, Krause U, et al. First results of laparoscopic gastroscopy. *Surg Endosc*. 1997;11:658–662.
49. Varadarajulu S, DeLegge M. Use of a 19-gauge injection needle as a guide for direct percutaneous endoscopic jejunostomy tube placement. *Gastrointest Endosc*. 2003;57:942–945.
50. Shike M, Latkany L, Gerdes H, et al. Direct percutaneous endoscopic jejunostomies for enteral feeding. *Gastrointest Endosc*. 1996; 44:536–540.
51. Yang Z, Shin J, Song H, et al. Fluoroscopically guided percutaneous jejunostomy: outcomes in 25 consecutive patients. *Clin Radiol*. 2007;62:1061–1065.
52. Szymski G, Albazzaz A, Funaki B, et al. Radiologically guided placement of pull-type gastrostomy tubes. *Radiology*. 1997;205: 669–673.
53. Richard H, Widlus D, Malloy P. Percutaneous fluoroscopically guided jejunostomy placement. *J Trauma*. 2008;65:1072–1077.
54. Itkin N, DeLegge M, Fang J, et al. Multidisciplinary practical guidelines for gastrointestinal access for enteral nutrition and decompression from the Society of Interventional Radiology and American Gastroenterological Association (AGA) Institute, with endorsement by Canadian Interventional Radiological Association (CIRA) and Cardiovascular and Interventional Radiological Society of Europe (CIRSE). *Gastroenterology*. 2011;141:742–765.
55. Hicks M, Surratt R, Picus D, et al. Fluoroscopically guided percutaneous gastrostomy and gastroenteroscopy: analysis of 158 consecutive cases. *Am J Roentgenol*. 1990;154:725–728.
56. Mack L, Kaklamanos I, Livingstone A, et al. Gastric decompression and enteral feeding through a double-lumen gastrojejunostomy tube improves outcomes after pancreaticoduodenectomy. *Ann Surg*. 2004;240:845–851.
57. Sriram K, VJayanthi, Lakshmi R, et al. Prophylactic locking of enteral feeding tubes with pancreatic enzymes. *J Parental Enteral Nutr*. 1997;21:353–356.
58. Bourgault A, Heyland D, Drover J, et al. Prophylactic pancreatic enzymes to reduce feeding tube occlusions. *Nutr Clin Prac*. 2003; 18:398–401.
59. Lord L. Restoring and maintaining patency of enteral feeding tubes. *Nutr Clin Prac*. 2003;18:422–426.
60. Lynch C, Fang J. Prevention and management of complications of PEG tubes. *Pract Gastroenterol*. 2004:66–76.
61. McWey R, Curry N, Schabel S, et al. Complications of nasoenteric feeding tubes. *Am J Surg*. 1988;155:253–257.
62. Odocha O, Lowery R, Mezghebe H, et al. Tracheopleuropulmonary injuries following enteral tube insertion. *J Natl Med Assoc*. 1989;81:275–281.
63. Roubenoff R, Ravich W. Pneumothorax due to nasogastric feeding tubes. Report of four cases, review of the literature, and recommendations for prevention. *Arch Intern Med*. 1989;149:184–188.
64. Damore LJ II, Andrus C, Herrmann V, et al. Prospective evaluation of a new through-the-scope nasoduodenal enteral feeding tube. *Surg Endosc*. 2002;11:460–463.
65. Lee S, Mathiasen R, Lipkin C, et al. Endoscopically placed nasogastrojejunal feeding tubes: a safe route for enteral nutrition in patients with hepatic encephalopathy. *Am Surg*. 2002;68:196–200.
66. McClave S, Sexton L, Spain D, et al. Enteral tube feeding in the intensive care unit: factors impeding adequate delivery. *Crit Care Med*. 1999;27:1252–1256.
67. Gunn S, Early B, Zenati M, et al. Use of a nasal bridle prevents accidental nasoenteral feeding tube removal. *J Parenter Enteral Nutr*. 2009;33:50–54.
68. Brandt C, Mittendorf E, Rassias A, et al. Endoscopic placement of nasojejunal feeding tubes in ICU patients. *Surg Endosc*. 1999;13: 1211–1214.
69. Patrick P, Marulendra S, Kirby D, et al. Endoscopic nasogastric-jejunal feeding tube placement in critically ill patients. *Gastrointest Endosc*. 1997;45:72–76.
70. Bosco J, Gordon F, Zelig M, et al. A reliable method for the endoscopic placement of a nasoenteric feeding tube. *Gastrointest Endosc*. 1994;40:740–743.
71. Marcuard S, Stegall K, Trogdon S. Clearing obstructed feeding tubes. *J Parental Enteral Nutr*. 1989;13:81–83.
72. Stahlfeld K, Hiltner L. Clogged feeding tube management now that Viokase is unavailable. *J Parental Enteral Nut*. 2011;35:11.
73. McClave S. Managing complications of percutaneous and nasoenteric feeding tubes. *Tech Gastrointest Endosc*. 2001;3:62–68.
74. Smith-Choban P, Max M. Feeding jejunostomy: a small bowel stress test? *Am J Surg*. 1988;155:112–117.
75. Safadi B, Marks J, Ponsky J. Percutaneous endoscopic gastrostomy. *Gastrointest Endosc Clin N Am*. 1998;8:551–568.
76. Wojtowycz M, Arata JA Jr, Micklos T, et al. CT findings after uncomplicated percutaneous gastrostomy. *Am J Roentgenol*. 1988; 151:307–309.

77. James A, Kapur K, Hawthorne A. Long-term outcome of percutaneous endoscopic gastrostomy feeding in patients with dysphagic stroke. *Age Ageing*. 1998;27:671–676.
78. Akkersdijk W, van Bergeijk JD, van Egmond T, et al. Percutaneous endoscopic gastrostomy (PEG): comparison of push and pull methods and evaluation of antibiotic prophylaxis. *Endoscopy*. 1995;27:313–316.
79. Lin H, Ibrahim H, Kheng J, et al. Percutaneous endoscopic gastrostomy: strategies for prevention and management of complications. *Laryngoscope*. 2001;111:1847–1852.
80. Segal D, Michaed L, Guimber D, et al. Late-onset complications of percutaneous endoscopic gastrostomy in children. *Pediatr Gastroenterol Nutr*. 2001;33:495–500.
81. Venu R, Brown R, Pastika B, et al. The buried bumper syndrome: a simple management approach in two patients. *Gastrointest Endosc*. 2002;56:582–584.
82. Walton G. Complications of percutaneous endoscopic gastrostomy in patients with head and neck cancer—an analysis of 42 consecutive patients. *Ann R Coll Surg Engl*. 1999;81: 272–276.
83. Ma M, Semlacher E, Fedorak R, et al. The buried gastrostomy bumper syndrome: prevention and endoscopic approaches to removal. *Gastrointest Endosc*. 1995;4:505–508.
84. Boyd J, DeLegge M, Shamburek R, et al. The buried bumper syndrome: a new technique for safe, endoscopic PEG removal. *Gastrointest Endosc*. 1995;41:508–511.
85. DiSario J, Foutch P, Sanowski R. Poor results with percutaneous endoscopic gastrojejunostomy. *Gastrointest Endosc*. 1990;36: 257–260.
86. DeLegge M, Duckworth PF Jr, McHenry L Jr, et al. Percutaneous endoscopic jejunostomy: a dual center safety and efficacy trial. *J Parental Enteral Nutr*. 1995;19:239–243.
87. Maple J, Baron T, Petersen B. The frequency, severity, and spectrum of adverse events associated with direct percutaneous endoscopic jejunostomy (DPEJ). *Gastrointest Endosc*. 2005; 61:AB80.

13 Complications of Enteral Nutrition

Ainsley Malone, MS, RD, LD, CNSC, David Seres, MD, ScM, PNS, and Linda Lord, NP, MSN, CNSN

CONTENTS

Background 219
Gastrointestinal Complications 220
Nausea and Vomiting 220
Abdominal Distention 220
Maldigestion/Malabsorption 220
Diarrhea 221
Etiologies 221
Drug-Induced Diarrhea 221
Infusion of Hypertonic Feeding Solutions 222
Lactose Intolerance 222
Management Strategies 222
Bacterial Overgrowth of the Intestinal Tract 222
Contamination of the Enteral Feeding Formula 222
Intestinal Ischemia 223
Gastrointestinal Diseases 223
Constipation 224
Aspiration 224
Definition 224
Incidence and Risk Factors 224
Methods of Detection 225
Strategies for Prevention 225
Metabolic Alterations 226
Electrolyte Imbalances 228
Hyperglycemia 229
Dehydration 229
Definition 229
Hospital-Acquired Dehydration 229
Risk Factors 229
Detecting Dehydration 229
Prevention of Dehydration 230
Determining Fluid Requirements 230
References 231

Objectives

1. Develop proficiency in preventing, recognizing, and treating gastrointestinal (GI) and metabolic complications of enteral nutrition (EN).
2. Outline strategies for minimizing and treating GI complications in patients receiving EN.
3. Understand the interactions between feeding formulation and patient tolerance.

Test Your Knowledge Questions

1. Which of the following actions is most appropriate for enhancing gastric emptying during EN?
   A. Keep the bed in Trendelenburg position.
   B. Decrease the rate of a continuous feeding infusion or changing from bolus to continuous feeding.
   C. Switch to an enteral formulation with a higher fat content.
   D. Switch to an enteral formulation with a higher protein content.
2. Which of the following is the most appropriate initial action for the management of tube feeding–associated diarrhea?
   A. Change to an enteral formulation with fiber.
   B. Review the patient's medication administration record to determine if hyperosmolar agents are being administered.
   C. Change to a peptide-based enteral formulation.
   D. Add an antimotility agent.
3. Which of the following methods is not recommended to minimize contamination of the enteral feeding formula?
   A. Preparation of enteral formulas following handwashing and with the use of sterile gloves.
   B. Immediate use of a newly opened enteral feeding formula container.
   C. Infusing reconstituted powered formulas or formulas with added modular components for more than 4 hours.
   D. Changing an "open" feeding container every 24 hours.

Test Your Knowledge Answers

1. The correct answer is **B**. Factors that delay gastric emptying include large boluses of fluid given at one time, increased rate of infusion, increased fat content of the solution, and infusion of solutions colder than room temperature. Elevation of the head of the bed and turning of the patient slightly to the right side allows gravity to help drain the stomach; however, such positions are often difficult to achieve in the hospital environment.
2. The correct answer is **B**. If clinically significant diarrhea develops during EN, the most appropriate initial action is to evaluate whether hyperosmolar medications are being administered that could result in liquid stooling. If none are in use, assessing for the presence of *Clostridium difficile*–induced diarrhea is suggested; if negative, the addition of fiber either by changing to a formulation that contains fiber or by providing supplemental fiber may be beneficial. Adding an antimotility agent or changing to a peptide-based formula should be considered if diarrhea continues despite these initial approaches. Parenteral nutrition (PN) should be initiated only if all treatment modalities fail (Figure 13-1).
3. The correct answer is **C**. Infusing a formula prepared from reconstituted powder or one in which modular components have been added should be infused for no more than 4 hours. Infusion times greater than this are associated with formula contamination. Other actions involved with the preparation and administration of enteral feedings including the use of good handwashing and sterile gloves along with immediately using a newly opened formula container will minimize contamination. In addition, changing an "open" feeding container every 24 hours will minimize the bacterial growth than can result in formula contamination.

FIGURE 13-1 Algorithm for Management of Diarrhea

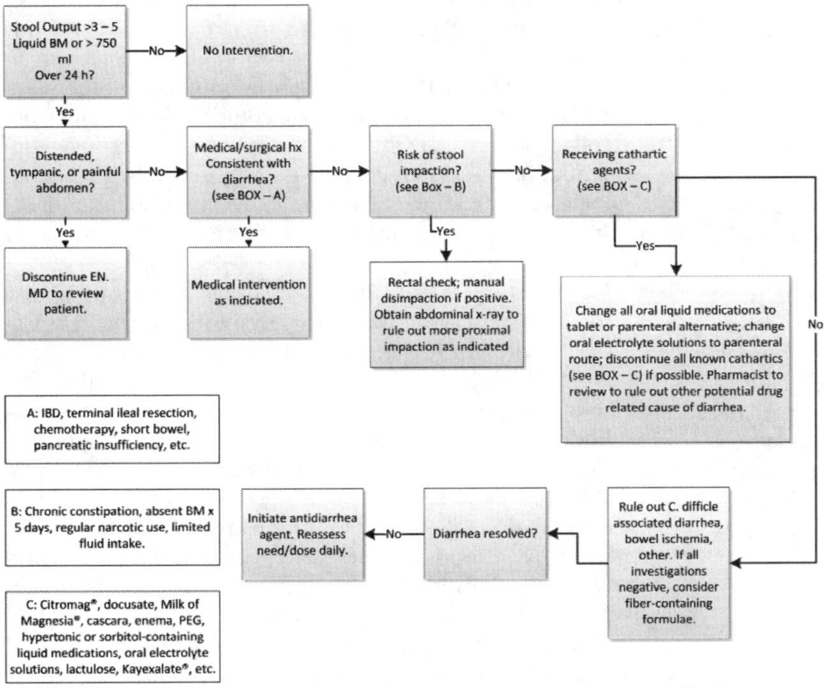

Reproduced with permission from Critical Care Nutrition. Greenwood J. Vancouver Coastal Health Authority. 2010. www.criticalcarenutrition.com/docs/tools/Diarrhea.pdf.

Background

Enteral tube feeding is the preferred feeding modality when the GI tract is functional and the patient is unable or unwilling to consume an oral diet adequately. The enteral route is promoted as an efficacious and cost-effective method of providing nutrients to patients. However, enteral tube feeding is not without its challenges. What may typically be considered "complications" are often a part of disease, illness, or trauma; treatment side effects; and iatrogenic conditions. Distinguishing potential causes is essential to controlling the complication. GI and metabolic complications that can contribute to a patient's morbidity and mortality are reviewed in this chapter. Chapter 12 examines complications specific to feeding tubes. A thorough evaluation of patients must take place before initiation of enteral tube feeding to identify and, when feasible, avoid or minimize potential problems. Ongoing monitoring and reassessment should be a standard component of follow-up care.

Gastrointestinal Complications

Nausea and Vomiting

Nausea and/or vomiting occur in approximately 7% to 26% of patients who receive EN support.[1-3] Vomiting, especially in minimally responsive patients, increases the risk of pulmonary aspiration, pneumonia, and sepsis. Multiple etiologies exist for nausea and vomiting with EN. Delayed gastric emptying is the most commonly identified problem.[4-6] Many potential causes of slowed emptying exist, including the following[7-13]:

- Hypotension
- Sepsis
- Stress
- Anesthesia and surgery
- Infiltrative gastric neoplasms
- Various autoimmune diseases
- Surgical vagotomy
- Pancreaticoduodenectomy
- Opiate analgesic medications (morphine sulfate, codeine, fentanyl)
- Anticholinergics (chlordiazepoxide hydrochloride and clidinium bromide)
- Excessively rapid infusion of formula
- Infusion of a very cold solution or one containing a large amount of fat

If delayed gastric emptying is suspected, appropriate interventions include reducing or discontinuing all narcotic medications, switching to a low-fat and/or isotonic formula, administering the feeding solution at room temperature, reducing the rate of infusion by 20 to 25 mL/h, changing infusion from bolus to continuous, and/or administering a prokinetic agent, such as metoclopramide or erythromycin.[5,6,10-12] Once tolerance is achieved, the rate or volume can be gradually increased every 8 to 24 hours until nutritional goals are met.[5,6] If nausea or vomiting occurs as the rate of administration or bolus volume of the EN increases, the rate or volume should be reduced to the highest tolerated amount, with an attempt to increase the rate again after symptoms abate.

The presence of abdominal distention in a patient with nausea indicates a need to monitor abdominal status closely—before the next bolus tube feeding or every 4 hours for continuous feeding.[14,15] A parameter often utilized in assessing enteral feeding tolerance is gastric residual volume (GRV). While elevated GRVs alone do not always correlate with intolerance,[16] the combination of an abnormal abdominal exam and an elevated GRV may be significant.[15] If GRVs are low, yet nausea persists, antiemetic medications may resolve the problem. Clinicians should also monitor stool frequency in patients who complain of nausea. Obstipation or fecal impaction may lead to distention and nausea, particularly in the institutionalized or chronically critically ill patient. Distention and vomiting may also occur as a result of diarrheal illness such as *C. difficile* colitis.

Abdominal Distention

Abdominal distention and increased GRV are two common reasons for interruption of EN.[1,2] Distention and its associated symptoms of bloating and cramping commonly occur as a result of GI ileus, obstruction, obstipation, ascites, and diarrheal illness. However, excessively rapid formula administration, infusion of very cold formula, or initial use of a fiber-supplemented formula may occasionally contribute to abdominal distention. Abdominal distention is diagnosed by visual inspection and palpation as well as from patient reports. Attempts have been made to define distention more objectively (eg, an increase of abdominal girth of more than 8 to 10 cm[17]), but careful clinical evaluation remains the most practical means of assessment. Distention due to ileus or mechanical bowel obstruction may often be diagnosed from a flat and upright abdominal x-ray; however, this method may miss fluid-filled loops of bowel and ascites. Injection of a small amount of contrast material into the feeding tube, with observation of intestinal anatomy and motility under fluoroscopy, can provide a clear picture of the clinical situation. If intestinal appearance and function are normal, EN may be continued, despite the distention. The discontinuation of feedings may be necessary, however, if motility is poor or if the bowel is markedly dilated.

Maldigestion/Malabsorption

Maldigestion refers to impaired breakdown of nutrients into absorbable forms, such as occurs in lactose intolerance. Clinical manifestations of maldigestion can include bloating, abdominal distention, and diarrhea, and may result in significant malabsorption, defined as defective mucosal uptake and transport of nutrients from the small intestine: fat, carbohydrate, protein, vitamins, electrolytes, minerals, or water. Clinical manifestations of malabsorption include unexplained weight loss, steatorrhea, diarrhea, anemia, tetany, bone pain, pathological fractures, bleeding, dermatitis, neuropathy, glossitis, and edema. Diagnostic studies for malabsorption include the following[18]:

- Screening: gross and microscopic examination of the stool, determination of fat and protein content of a random stool collection (qualitative), measurement of serum carotene concentration, measurement of d-xylose absorption, and radiological examination of intestinal transit time and motility
- Intake–output balance: stool collections for quantitative fecal fat study
- Maldigestion/malabsorption of specific nutrients: lactose tolerance test, Schilling test to screen for abnormal absorption of vitamin B_{12}, and various radioisotopic methodologies for identification of iron, calcium, various amino acids, folic acid, pyridoxine, and vitamin D malabsorption
- Endoscopic small bowel biopsy: helpful in diagnosing mucosal disorders such as celiac disease, tropical sprue, and Whipple disease

Causes of maldigestion/malabsorption include gluten-sensitive enteropathy, Crohn disease, diverticular disease, radiation enteritis, enteric fistulas, human immunodeficiency virus, pancreatic insufficiency, short gut syndrome, and numerous other syndromes. Knowledge of the patient's medical history and selection of an appropriate enteral product should help minimize the likelihood of malabsorption/maldigestion during enteral feeding. The use of an oligopeptide-based (whey protein hydrolysate, hydrolyzed sodium caseinate) formula with a greater percentage of medium-chain triglycerides or one with structured lipids may promote improved tolerance (see Chapter 11 for more information). However, depending upon the extent of disease, PN may be necessary in selected patients.[6,18,19]

Diarrhea

Diarrhea is the most commonly reported GI side effect in patients receiving EN (Practice Scenario 13-1).[20] No universally accepted definition of diarrhea exists.[21] However, a clinically useful definition is any abnormal volume or consistency of stool. Normal stool water content is 250 to 500 mL/d. Diarrhea has also been defined as > 500 mL stool output every 24 hours or more than three stools per day for at least 2 consecutive days.[22,23] Stool volume can be measured by placing a collection device in the toilet or by using a bedpan; in incontinent patients, this can be accomplished using a rectal tube or by placing a pad under the patient and weighing it after each stool (assuming 1 g/mL of stool).

Common causes of diarrhea in patients receiving EN include medications (liquid medications in a sorbitol base, antibiotics, etc.) and infection (*C. difficile* and nonclostridial bacteria). Intolerance due to characteristics of the formula (osmolality, fat content) or specific components in the formula (lactose) are less common. Because most standard 1 kcal/mL formulas are now lactose free, isotonic, and not excessively high in fat, a medical cause for diarrhea should be sought prior to initiating the nutritional maneuvers discussed below. See Practice Scenario 13-1 for the treatment of diarrhea in a tube-fed patient.

Practice Scenario 13-1

Question: How does one select an enteral formula in a tube-fed patient who experiences diarrhea?

Scenario: An isotonic, fiber-free nasogastric enteral feeding is initiated in a 78-year-old following surgical intervention for a perforated duodenal ulcer. His postoperative course is complicated by hospital-acquired pneumonia requiring ventilator support and the use of antibiotic therapy. His feeding is initiated and advanced over a 72-hour period. He has demonstrated good tolerance to his feeding with a slightly distended abdomen, hypoactive to active bowel sounds and one to two semiloose stools per day. After 5 days of feeding, he develops four to five watery stools/day requiring the use of a fecal management system.

Intervention: The nutrition support clinician reviewed the patient's medication profile and determined he was not receiving hypertonic or sorbitol-based medications nor was a prokinetic agent in use. The nutrition support clinician recommended use of a predominantly soluble-fiber EN formula to assist in controlling the patient's diarrhea.

Answer: Enteral formula modification for the patient experiencing diarrhea is one approach to assist in management. One modification is the inclusion of soluble fiber to the EN regimen. This can be done via an EN formula alone or in combination with a soluble fiber supplement.

Rationale: Multiple etiologies exist that can contribute to the development of diarrhea in patients receiving enteral feedings. In this patient, the use of antibiotics may be the contributing factor as a review of his medication record does not identify any motility agents, sorbitol based or hypertonic. Several management strategies can be employed to assist in controlling his diarrhea. One strategy is to add fiber to his enteral regimen. Several studies have demonstrated improvement in diarrhea with the addition of soluble fiber to an enteral feeding.[24–26] This can be achieved by using a fiber formula or by using a fiber modular supplement. If after initiation of a soluble fiber source, diarrhea continues, assessing for the presence of *C. difficile* in the stool culture is recommended followed by the initiation of antidiarrheal agents as appropriate.

Etiologies

Drug-Induced Diarrhea

Drugs may cause diarrhea because of hypertonicity (such as those that contain magnesium or sorbitol) or direct laxative action (such as occurs due to proton pump inhibitors or prokinetic medications). As little as 10 to 20 g of sorbitol can lead to GI side effects, including diarrhea.[6,27–30] Table 13-1 outlines the sorbitol content of selected liquid medications. Antibiotics commonly cause diarrhea without necessarily causing *C. difficile* overgrowth. Review medications and eliminate, if possible, those that might cause diarrhea. Table 13-2 provides a list of medications associated with an increased incidence of diarrhea. Any drug in a liquid vehicle given via a jejunal feeding tube should be diluted to avoid a hypertonic-induced dumping-like

TABLE 13-1 Sorbitol Content of Selected Medications

Generic	Trade Name	% Sorbitol (w/v)
Acetaminophen elixir	Tylenol	35.0
Amantadine	Symmetrel	72.0
Cimetidine	Tagamet	46.1
Doxycycline	Vibramycin	70.0
Furosemide	Lasix	35.0
Guafenesin/codeine	Robitussin AC	35.0
Hydroxyzine	Vistaril	116.0
Indomethacin	Indocin	35.0
Isoniazid	Generic	70.0
Metoclopramide	Reglan	28.0–42.0
Nortriptyline	Aventyl	64.0
Pseudoephedrine/ triprolidine	Actifed	49.0

w/v = weight per volume.
Adapted with permission from McCarthy MS, Fabling JC, Bell DE. Drug–nutrient interactions. In: Shikora SA, Martindale RG, Schwaitzberg SD, eds. *Nutritional Considerations in the Intensive Care Unit: Science, Rationale and Practice.* Dubuque, IA: Kendall-Hunt; 2002:153.

TABLE 13-2 Medications With Increased Incidence of Diarrhea

Ampicillin
Bisacodyl
Caffeine
Clindamycin
Colchicine
Digoxin
Erythromycin
Hydralazine
Lactulose
Magnesium-containing preparations
Metoclopramide
Methotrexate
Penicillamine
Procainamide
Neomycin
Quinidine
Theophylline

Reprinted with permission from Ratnaike RN, Jones TE. Mechanisms of drug–induced diarrhea in the elderly. *Drugs Aging*. 1998;13(3):245–253.

syndrome. Most drugs and electrolytes, for example, potassium, should be mixed with a minimum of 30 to 60 mL of water per 10 mEq dose to avoid direct irritation of the gut. Diarrhea may be inevitable due to the osmotic load. Medications administered via a feeding tube may not be compatible with EN formula and/or may cause feeding tube occlusion. Discussing drug delivery options with a pharmacist can assist in avoiding many problems related to medication administration in patients receiving EN (see Chapter 18).

Infusion of Hypertonic Feeding Solutions

Unless hypertonic enteral feeding products are infused at a very high rate, or by bolus into the small bowel, they rarely cause clinically significant diarrhea. If the enteral formula is thought to be causing diarrhea because of hypertonicity, changing to an isotonic formula may be beneficial. Diluting the formula with water, a measure that was once common for patients with diarrhea, may result in suboptimal nutrient provision, and formula dilution has not been shown to improve tolerance.[31,32] In addition, this practice may actually exacerbate symptoms by contaminating the formula and is discouraged.

Lactose Intolerance

Tube feeding product intolerance due to lactose intolerance is unlikely during EN because most formulas are lactose free, but may be observed during the transition from EN to an oral diet. Some patients are lactase deficient prior to the onset of illness, and others develop a transient lactase deficiency during their illness. A lactose-restricted diet may help reduce diarrhea in patients with lactase deficiency.

Management Strategies

If clinically significant diarrhea develops during EN, clinicians should consider the following options:

- Medical assessment of the patient to rule out infectious or inflammatory causes, fecal impaction, diarrheagenic medications, etc.
- Change of the formula type
- Addition of soluble fiber or insoluble fiber to the medication regimen, and/or changing to an enteral formula with added fiber, except in critically ill patients[16]
- Use of an antidiarrheal agent once *C. difficile* has been ruled out or is being treated (loperamide, diphenoxylate, paregoric, or octreotide).
- Continuation of EN as tolerated and initiation of PN to complete delivery of macro- and micronutrients if intolerance or malabsorption is prolonged

A systematic approach can be effective in the management of diarrhea. Figure 13-1 provides an algorithm for treatment of diarrhea in tube-fed patients.[33]

Bacterial Overgrowth of the Intestinal Tract

Bacterial overgrowth in the GI tract can cause severe enteritis with marked diarrhea, abdominal cramp pain, hypoalbuminemia and catabolism/cachexia, fever, and even sepsis. Increasingly, it is seen in patients after roux-en-Y gastric bypass for surgery.[34] Overgrowth is difficult to diagnose definitively without techniques such as hydrogen breath testing, but should be considered in the differential diagnosis when patients with altered GI anatomy or who have been treated with prolonged antibiotic therapy present with abdominal symptoms as previously discussed and/or catabolism/hypoalbuminemia. Prolonged use of broad-spectrum antibiotics increases the incidence of bacterial overgrowth.[35,36] Treatment is often empiric and includes antibiotics.

Contamination of the Enteral Feeding Formula

The enteral feeding formula can become contaminated with pathogenic microorganisms during formula preparation, storage, or administration. Enteral formulas that require minimal handling have a lower incidence of microbial contamination compared to those that require mixing, dilution, or transfer from the original container to a feeding bag for administration. Formulas that are provided in liquid form have undergone heat sterilization, whereas powdered formulas are not required to be sterile and may contain contaminants. Ideally, powdered formulas should be reconstituted with sterile water to minimize further contamination and prepared by trained personnel with aseptic technique in a clean environment.[37] Enteral formula preparation and administration should always involve good handwashing, clean gloves, and aseptic technique.

Formulas should be used immediately after being opened or after reconstitution with water, with strict adherence to the manufacturer-recommended formula hang times at room temperature. If there is excess formula left after the hang time volume is reached, then the excess amount can be refrigerated immediately and stored according to the manufacturer's recommendations.

For example, if the formula rate is 25 mL/hour and the formula hang time is 8 hours, then no more than 200 mL of formula should be administered at room temperature during that 8-hour period; the rest should be refrigerated for future use. Formula hang times at room temperature vary and are dependent on the formula composition and whether it is provided as an "open" versus "closed" delivery system.

Enteral open delivery systems are liquid formula delivered via syringe, or poured into a bag and delivered to the patient by gravity drip or pump. Reconstituted powered formulas or formulas with added modular components delivered by gravity drip or pump should hang no more than 4 hours at room temperature. Formulas poured into feeding bags from cans, screw top plastic bottles, and Brik Paks, have hang times from 4 to 12 hours, dependent on the feeding protocol at each facility and the manufacturer instructions. Lower levels of microbial growth have been shown with formulas poured from a screw top plastic bottles compared to flip top cans.[38] The lids of cans should be cleansed with isopropyl alcohol and allowed to dry before pouring the formula into the delivery receptacle.[39] The feeding bag itself should be changed every 24 hours.[40]

Enteral closed delivery systems are those that utilize prefilled, sterile bottles or non-air–dependent containers that are accessed with a spike or screw top tubing. These are administered by pump infusion and allowed longer hang times of 24 to 48 hours. There is reduced risk of contamination with the closed delivery system due to decreased exposure of the formula to outside contaminants.[41,42] However, prefilled containers require the attachment of tubing, so a contamination risk still remains. There is a reduction in contamination with delivery systems that have recessed spike sets and recessed nutrient container seals.[43] These features prevent inadvertent touching of the parts of the closed delivery system that come in contact with the formula.

Enteral formulas may also become contaminated in a retrograde manner with the patient's endogenous microorganisms (from stomach, throat, lungs) populating within the feeding tube and then migrating into the enteral delivery system.[44] These microorganisms would likely then proliferate within the feeding formula and then be reinfused to the patient in greater numbers. The majority of enteral delivery tubing systems contain a drip chamber that minimizes the occurrence of this during formula delivery.[45,46] However, if formula infusions are interrupted, the stagnant period could allow microorganisms to proliferate. Also, the procedure of checking for feeding residual volumes pulls potentially pathogenic microorganisms back up the feeding tube and can lead to a contaminated feeding tube hub and contaminated gloves.[47] The exposure of a patient's body fluids in this manner labels it a "dirty procedure." After the feeding residual volume check procedure, gloves must be removed and hands must be washed, or a U.S. Food and Drug Administration–approved[48] alcohol hand rub must be used, followed by donning of clean gloves prior to the administration of tube feeding formula, a "clean procedure."

The Y-ports of enteral delivery systems are used to deliver medications and water flushes to minimize disconnection of the tube feeding formula. In one investigation, contamination with ≥ 100 cfu/mL were cultured in 48.1% of the closed delivery systems at the Y-port compared to only 2.4% contamination in the formula container itself.[44] The investigators determined that this contamination was due to either administration of medications through the Y-port or retrograde movement of microorganisms from the feeding tube to the delivery system. Although this study looked at the results of cultures and not clinical outcomes of patients, they recommended that tube feedings not be allowed to remain within the delivery system without the infusion process occurring and that delivery sets be changed frequently.

Contamination of enteral formulas can lead to diarrhea, pneumonia, infectious enterocolitis, bacteremias, and septicemias.[49–52] Neonates, critically ill and immune-suppressed patients, as well as those with the loss of the gastric acid microbial barrier, may be predisposed to a greater risk of morbidity and mortality related to formula contamination. The implementation of enteral quality control programs have resulted in the reduction of enteral formula contamination to acceptable levels.[39]

Intestinal Ischemia

Multiple etiologies of intestinal ischemia exist and are often non-nutrition–related; however, ischemia in conjunction with EN resulting in nonocclusive bowel necrosis (NOBN) is associated with a high degree of morbidity and may result in a fatal outcome.[53] Neonates, critically ill and immune-suppressed patients, as well as those with the loss of the gastric acid microbial barrier may be predisposed to a greater risk of NOBN; the reported incidence is variable, ranging from 0.3% to 8.5%.[53] Underlying factors associated with the incidence of NOBN include the use of jejunal feedings and hyperosmolar formulas, feeding in the presence of hypotension, and disordered peristalsis.[54] Typical signs of enteral feeding intolerance, including abdominal distention and nausea and vomiting, are common with NOBN but are nonspecific and not uncommon in enterally fed patients in the intensive care unit without NOBN.[55] It is important to note that NOBN frequently presents later in the patient's clinical course rather than shortly after enteral feeding initiation. In a review of NOBN among surgical patients, the mean day of diagnosis after EN initiation was 6 days with a range of 4 to 18 days.[14]

While it is difficult to predict who may develop NOBN in conjunction with enteral feedings, there are practices that can be utilized as preventative measures. Of them, delaying EN until the patient is fully fluid-resuscitated is of greatest importance. In a review of case series reports of patients who developed NOBN, all cited the presence of hypotension and/or hypovolemia as precipitating factors.[53] Other considerations include the initial use of an isotonic and fiber-free enteral formula. Ongoing monitoring of EN is essential as acute changes in abdominal assessment can prompt early recognition and treatment of NOBN. A patient who previously demonstrated enteral feeding tolerance and then develops abdominal distention, abdominal pain, and an acute change in nasogastric tube output should be a cause of concern, and discontinuation of enteral feeding and further GI evaluation is advised.

Gastrointestinal Diseases

Many primary diseases of the intestine, including inflammatory bowel disease, short gut syndrome, gluten sensitive enteropathy, and acquired immunodeficiency syndrome, may result in

TABLE 13-3 Conditions Associated With Secretory Diarrhea

- Infection with enterotoxic organisms such as *Clostridium difficile*
- Abuse of stimulant laxatives
- Intestinal resection
- Inflammatory bowel disease
- Bile acid malabsorption
- Fatty acid malabsorption
- Chronic infections
- Celiac sprue
- Small intestinal lymphoma
- Villous adenoma of the rectum
- Zollinger–Ellison syndrome
- Collagen vascular diseases
- Congenital defects
- Malignant carcinoid syndrome

Reprinted with permission from Fine KD, Krejs GJ, Fordtran JS. Diarrhea. In: *Gastrointestinal Disease: Pathophysiology/Diagnosis/Management*, 5th ed. Philadelphia, PA: Saunders; 1995:1043.

malabsorption or secretory diarrhea. Table 13-3 outlines various disease states associated with secretory diarrhea. Recognition and treatment of these diseases can minimize diarrhea. In some disease states, PN may be required. In others, use of specialized enteral products are proposed to facilitate absorption.

Constipation

Defining constipation is difficult because normal defecation patterns may range from four stools each day to one stool every 4 or 5 days. With EN, this variation increases depending on the residue and extent of absorption of an enteral feeding product. The best clinical definition of constipation is the accumulation of excess waste in the colon, often up to the transverse colon or even the cecum. A rectal examination and plain abdominal x-ray are often effective for diagnosis and can differentiate constipation from small bowel obstruction or ileus. With uncomplicated constipation, there is rarely any small bowel dilatation.

Common causes of constipation include dehydration and either inadequate or excessive fiber in the diet.[7,20,56] To avoid dehydration, it is important to provide adequate fluid during EN. Hydration may be problematic when a concentrated formula is needed for fluid restriction. If usual hydration guidelines are contraindicated, consider a stool softener (docusate sodium or docusate calcium, or various emollients) and a laxative or cleansing enema. Chronic use of stimulants (eg, senna) often results in tachyphylaxis and is not indicated. Frequent rectal exams and abdominal radiographs may be required in patients with serious constipation.

Inadequate fiber intake can result in infrequent bowel movements without significant buildup of waste in the colon. Fiber helps propel waste through the colon. If fiber is added to the enteral regimen, patients must receive a minimum of 1 mL of fluid per kcal to prevent solidification of waste in the colon and constipation.[56] Additional fluid is often needed to facilitate regular stool output and minimize the chance of impaction. Inadequate physical activity can also contribute to constipation.[7,57] Patients should ambulate whenever possible.

A variant of constipation is impaction, a firm collection of stool in the distal colon (sigmoid colon or rectum). Liquid stool will seep around an impaction, occasionally at high volume. Impaction, if near to the rectum, can be diagnosed and may be treated by rectal exam. Impaction higher up in the sigmoid colon cannot be easily detected by examination, and a high level of clinical suspicion should be maintained in patients at risk. Impaction should be considered in patients, particularly the elderly and bed bound, when stool volumes have been small and then become liquid. Enemas, cathartics (sorbitol, lactulose), and even endoscopy may be required to treat severe impaction. Similarly, impaction may be the cause of delirium and agitation in the elderly.

Aspiration

Definition

Aspiration is defined as the inhalation of material into the airway. This is of concern in patients receiving EN when the inhalation of gastric contents and/or the tube feeding formula into the airway occurs. Clinical symptoms that can occur with aspiration include dyspnea, wheezing, frothy or purulent sputum, cyanosis, anxiety, and agitation. Patients can also develop a fever, tachycardia, tachypnea, rhonchi and rales, decreasing oxygenation, leukocytosis, leukopenia, and a new or progressing infiltrate on chest film. Pulmonary aspiration can also be asymptomatic (silent aspiration). In fact, aspiration of saliva is a normal phenomenon during sleep. Pneumonia can result from pulmonary aspiration of tube feeding formula; however, aspiration of very small amounts of fluid alone is insufficient to cause pneumonia. The progression of pulmonary aspiration of feeding formula to aspiration pneumonia is hard to predict and may depend on the quantity and acidity of the formula in addition to the particulates and contaminants in the formula. Age, immune status, and comorbidities also influence the tendency toward aspiration pneumonia development. When the quantity and acidity of the formula overwhelms either the patient's natural defense mechanisms or the patient's altered pulmonary defense mechanisms, pneumonia is more likely to occur.

Incidence and Risk Factors

Pulmonary aspiration of tube feeding formula is one of the most serious complications of EN support because it can lead to acute pulmonary pathology. Potential complications of aspiration include pneumonia, pneumonitis, atelectasis, empyema, bronchitis, acute lung injury, and acute respiratory distress syndrome. However, relating pathologic respiratory developments to the aspiration of tube feeding formula is difficult. Pulmonary aspiration can also occur with the inhaling of oropharyngeal secretions and gastric secretions, but it has not been consistently proven to be a consequence of high GRVs. Reported incidence in tube-fed patients varies depending on both the patient population studied and the technique used to identify aspiration. Recent investigations of critically ill, tube-fed patients utilizing advanced aspiration detection techniques report the presence of gastric contents in 22% to 31% of their tracheal secretions.[58,59] These research models have identified aspiration of gastric contents by detecting either pepsin (major enzyme in gastric fluid) or yellow microscopic beads (added to tube feeding formula) in tracheal aspirates. When pepsin positive secretions were used, Metheny et al. identified low head of the bed elevation, vomiting, gastric tube feedings (as opposed to small bowel feedings), a low Glasgow coma score, and GI reflux disease as risk factors for aspiration. Patients with a higher number of pepsin-positive secretions and those on paralytic agents and high sedation levels were at higher risk for pneumonia. Additional risk factors for aspiration include a malpositioned feeding tube, transportation within the hospital,[60] and inadequate nursing staff.[61]

Methods of Detection

No reliable method to detect pulmonary aspiration of tube feeding formula is currently available for routine clinical use. Radiographic findings are generally nonspecific and insensitive. However, if after an episode of emesis and regurgitation of tube feeding formula, a patient develops dyspnea, cyanosis, and agitation associated with a new infiltrate on chest film, then aspiration of feeding formula can be presumed. Patients with dysphagia may aspirate saliva and develop aspiration pneumonia independent of the presence of gastric contents. Regardless of the underlying cause, aspiration is a medical urgency. Emergency measures may include sitting the patient upright, orotracheal suctioning, oxygen, and antibiotics.

Methods historically used to predict pulmonary aspiration of formula, such as tinting enteral formula with blue dye or checking tracheal secretions with glucose oxidase strips, have proved unsatisfactory because neither method has ever been shown to be sensitive or specific.[59] Tinting enteral formulas with food coloring has been used as a method to reveal aspiration of feedings through the presence of the blue-tinted formula in tracheal aspirates. However, numerous problems surround this practice. The dose of food coloring has never been standardized, and bacterial contamination, allergic reactions, and false-positive guaiac testing have raised concerns about the use of this method. More important, a Public Health Advisory issued by the U.S. Food and Drug Administration on September 29, 2003, reported blue discoloration of body parts and fluids followed by refractory hypotension, metabolic acidosis, and death in patients receiving tube feedings containing Food Drug and Cosmetic Blue No. 1 dye.[48] Based on this report, the practice of tinting enteral formulas should be abandoned.

Glucose oxidase strips have been used to detect a high glucose reading in tracheal aspirates that contain feeding formula. However, high tracheal concentrations of glucose can also be found in aspirates of nonfed patients, those with elevated blood glucose levels, and in those aspirates that contain some blood.[62,63] A study using an animal model demonstrated a correlation between pepsin levels in tracheal aspirates and aspiration pneumonia, with a sensitivity of 90% and a specificity of 100%; however, this assay is not available for routine clinical use.[64]

Strategies for Prevention

The technique of withdrawing GRVs from enteral access devices, with a syringe, has been used to help determine the risk for aspiration. To prevent aspiration, tube feedings are held when the GRV is determined to be too high. But interpretation of GRVs is highly subjective (Practice Scenario 13-2). The accuracy of GRV measurements can be influenced by many factors, including the patient's position and type of access device. Metheny et al. reported that frequent aspirators, those with > 40% pepsin-positive secretions, had a significantly higher incidence of GRVs of at least 200 mL ×2 or 250 mL ×1.[65] They noted that aspiration can occur without high GRVs, but that it does occur more frequently when GRVs are high. Based on her research findings, Metheny encourages keeping GRV checks in nursing protocols.[66] Conversely, McClave et al. found no correlation between elevated GRVs of either > 200 mL or > 400 mL and aspiration in critically ill, mechanically ventilated patients receiving gastric tube feedings by either a nasogastric feeding tube or gastrostomy tube.[15] Aspiration was determined by the addition of yellow microscopic beads to the tube feeding formula and use of calorimetric fluoroscopy for detection in the tracheal aspirate. McClave and colleagues did note less aspiration with the gastrostomy tube feedings compared to the nasogastric tube feedings.

It is crucial to identify patients at high risk for aspiration and implement protocols aimed at risk reduction. Metheny designed an aspiration risk reduction protocol and studied critically ill, mechanically ventilated patients being fed through nasally inserted feeding tubes.[69] This protocol entailed head of bed (HOB) elevation at ≥ 30 degrees and GRV checks every 4 hours with an associated decision tree that directed actions depending on amount of GRV obtained. Raising the head of the bed to 45 degrees during gastric feedings is considered important because this simple measure has been associated with decreased esophageal and pharyngeal reflux of gastric contents and a lowered incidence of aspiration pneumonia.[70] In Metheny's study, a written doctor's orders for HOB elevation and the hourly recording of the bed angle on bedside flowsheets were recommended to improve compliance. When the GRV was ≥ 200 mL, a prokinetic agent was to be given once and repeated if still ≥ 200 mL. If the GRV continued to be ≥ 200 mL, then the feeding tube was converted to a small bowel feeding tube. With this protocol in place, the practice of HOB elevation increased from 38% to 88% and the conversion to small bowel feeding tubes increased from 39% to 68%. Aspiration incidence decreased from 88% to 39% and pneumonia decreased from 48% to 19%. Decreased delivery of nutrition and poorer achievement of nutritional goals have been shown to result when tube feeding infusions are held for GRVs < 200 mL.[71,72] Unless the patient is vomiting, GRVs should be reinstilled to replace fluid, electrolytes, and feeding formula. Newer techniques that strive to continually measure gastric pressure are being marketed but have not been studied for efficacy in improving delivery of calories or decreasing the incidence of pneumonia.

Different protocols should be followed for gastrostomy tubes as they are positioned in the anterior abdomen and as a result are unlikely to allow full withdrawal of stomach contents during GRV checks. A GRV of ≥ 100 mL with a gastrostomy tube has been suggested as a prudent trigger for careful evaluation of the patient for GI symptoms.[15] Neither the American Society for Parenteral and Enteral Nutrition (A.S.P.E.N.) critical care guidelines nor the A.S.P.E.N. enteral nutrition practice recommendations specifically address gastrostomy tubes and GRV checks.[16,37]

Tube-fed patients should be assessed continuously for tube feeding intolerance, such as abdominal distention, discomfort, or nausea, and measures should be implemented to reduce aspiration risk. Nutrition practice guidelines have been published for both EN[37] and critical care nutrition[16] that address the practice of GRV checks and HOB elevation. Continued study is required to delineate methods to assess risk of aspiration during tube feeding and to develop strategies to prevent this complication.

Practice Scenario 13-2

Question: How can GRV measurements best be used as a monitoring parameter to assess enteral feeding tolerance?

Scenario: A 53-year-old woman is admitted to the medical intensive care unit for sepsis and respiratory failure. Twenty-four hours following her admission, her hemodynamic status has stabilized and the medical intensive care unit team consults the dietitian to begin EN. A nasogastric feeding tube is placed, and an abdominal radiograph verifies the nasogastric tube position and also confirms absence of ileus. Based on the dietitian's recommendation, the nurse initiates an isotonic enteral formula at 20 mL/hour followed by an advancement of 10 mL every 6 hours until a goal rate of 55 mL/hour is achieved. The medical intensive care unit policy for monitoring enteral feeding tolerance includes checking GRVs every 4 hours.

GRV Data

1600 (start of enteral feeding)	GRV
2000	105 mL
0000	275 mL
0400	125 mL
0800	250 mL

At midnight and again at 8:00 am, the nurse holds the patient's enteral feeding due to elevated GRVs. As noted in the nursing flow record, the patient's abdominal assessment was negative with a soft abdomen and hypoactive bowel sounds.

Intervention: The dietitian speaks to the nurse as there is concern that this patient's nutrition needs are not being met. They review the medical intensive care unit policy for GRV monitoring with EN outlining that GRVs of < 500 mL without signs of intolerance (abdominal distention, nausea, vomiting, etc.) are acceptable. If the GRV is ≥ 250 mL, a stepwise approach is recommended to assess the aspiration risk. In addition to assessing for abdominal distention, the patient should be assessed for the following: nausea/emesis, the bowel pattern (to rule out constipation), abdominal discomfort, HOB elevation (should be 30 degrees or higher), the level of sedation, and the blood sugar control. The nurse notes that this patient is awake and alert, has been having regular bowel movements, has not reported any nausea or abdominal discomfort but is hyperglycemic, and the HOB is only at 20 degrees. The nurse resumes the tube feeding, but raises the HOB to 30 degrees and notifies the provider to manage the blood sugar more effectively.

Answer: GRV measurements are one of several parameters that can be used to monitor the patient's tolerance to EN. It is not meant to be used in isolation and therefore should not have resulted in cessation of EN unless other signs of intolerance were present. The EN policy in this medical intensive care unit indicates a maximal acceptable GRV of < 500 mL in the absence of overt intolerance, so this patient's EN should have continued after both the 275 mL and 250 mL GRV checks. The GRV of 275 mL should have initiated a stepwise approach that includes HOB elevation, GI assessment, and assessment of the level of sedation and glycemic control. Assessing GRVs at specific intervals in conjunction with maintaining HOB elevation between 30 and 45 degrees, ongoing GI assessment (degree, if any, of abdominal distention, abdominal pain, presence of nausea and/or vomiting), minimizing sedation, and assuring good glycemic control is the best approach to monitoring EN tolerance and lowering the aspiration risk in tube-fed patients. If GRV of ≥ 250 mL, a prokinetic agent can be recommended. Most clinicians agree that a GRV of ≥ 500 mL should warrant holding the EN and consideration of a small bowel feeding or a prokinetic agent, if not already initiated.

Rationale: The volume of fluid within the stomach at any given time during EN has historically been used as a measure to define tolerance to EN. However, other underlying conditions may cause slow gastric emptying and result in elevated and increasing GRVs. It is important to use GRV assessment in conjunction with other measures to assess EN tolerance including abdominal distention or discomfort, nausea and/or vomiting, etc. In addition, GRV checks do not always provide the full amount of fluid residing in the stomach and patients can still aspirate with low GRVs. Any patient receiving EN should have the HOB elevated 30 to 45 degrees if possible, be evaluated for GI tolerance, be minimally sedated, and have good glycemic control to minimize aspiration risk.

Using GRV measurements along with the patient's overall clinical assessment will lead to best practice decision making, ultimately resulting in achieving desired nutrition outcomes.[16,67,68]

Metabolic Alterations

With the exception of the refeeding syndrome, EN is, by itself, unlikely to be the cause of metabolic derangements or specific nutritional deficiencies. Rather, patients receiving EN support are more likely to have underlying conditions that predispose them to metabolic derangements. The nutrition support regimen may be the sole source of all nutrients, fluids, and electrolytes for the patient. Therefore, the nutrition support practitioner must be well schooled in the underlying medical issues that may affect formula selection, fluid and electrolyte prescription, and the response to feeding in previously starved or electrolyte-depleted patients. Nutrition support practitioners must work closely and as part of a team with the primary health care providers in setting therapeutic goals and in monitoring the patient's progress. Table 13-4 provides a summary

TABLE 13-4 Metabolic Complications of Enteral Nutrition

Problem	Possible Causes	Prevention or Therapy
Hypertonic dehydration	Excessive fluid loss Inadequate fluid intake Concentrated (energy, protein) formula administered to a patient who cannot express thirst	Monitor daily fluid intake and output (I/O) Monitor body weight daily Weight change of > 0.2 kg/d reflects change in ECF volume Estimate fluid losses: mild loss 3% decrease in body weight; moderate loss 6% decrease; severe loss 10% decrease Monitor serum electrolytes, urine specific gravity, BUN and Cr daily (BUN:Cr is usually 1:10 in state of normal hydration) Provide enteral or IV fluid as indicated
Overhydration	Excessive fluid intake Rapid refeeding Catabolism of lean body mass with potassium loss Refeeding syndrome Renal, hepatic, or cardiac insufficiency	Monitor I/O daily Assess fluid status daily Monitor body weight daily Weight change of > 0.2 kg/d reflects change in ECF volume Elevated aldosterone levels with sodium retention Consider use of less concentrated formula Diuretic therapy
Hypokalemia	Refeeding syndrome Catabolic stress Depleted body cell mass Supplement K and chloride Effect of ADH and aldosterone Diuretic therapy Excessive losses (diarrhea, nasogastric tube) Metabolic alkalosis (induce or result) Insulin therapy Dilution	Supplement K to normal before initiation of TF Monitor serum K daily until stable with patient at goal TF rate Consider supplementation protocol
Hyperkalemia	Metabolic acidosis Poor perfusion (eg, congestive heart failure) Renal failure Excessive potassium intake from TF, IV fluid, oral diet	Correct acidosis, if possible; recheck serum K Correct serum K before initiation of TF, if possible Monitor serum K daily Treat cause of poor perfusion Potassium binding resin, glucose, and/or insulin therapy Eliminate K from IV fluids; reduce K in TF and oral diet
Hyponatremia	Dilution, from elevated ADH levels Hepatic, cardiac, or renal insufficiency Reduced Na intake relative to output	Consider addition of table salt to TF Monitor Na level daily Assess fluid status Diuretic therapy, if indicated Fluid and/or sodium restriction
Hypernatremia	Inadequate fluid intake with increased fluid loss (sweating, osmotic diuresis) Increased Na intake (IV fluid) Depletion of total body Na, extracellular mass, ECF SIADH	Monitor daily I/O Monitor electrolytes, BUN:Cr daily Monitor body weight daily; weight change > 0.2 kg reflects change in ECF volume Estimate fluid loss: mild loss 3% weight decrease; moderate loss 6% weight decrease; severe loss 10% weight decrease; replace fluid loss via enteral or parenteral route to replete ECF
Hypophosphatemia	Refeeding syndrome Excessive calories Binding by epinephrine Sucralfate, antacids Insulin therapy	Supplement P to normal before initiation of TF Monitor serum P daily and replete as necessary with changing clinical course Supplement P as Na or K form, as clinically indicated, via enteral or parenteral route
Hyperphosphatemia	Renal insufficiency	Phosphate binder therapy Choose TF product with lower phosphorus content

(continued)

TABLE 13-4 Metabolic Complications of Enteral Nutrition ***(continued)***

Problem	Possible Causes	Prevention or Therapy
Hypercapnia	Overfeeding energy Excessive carbohydrate provision in patient with respiratory dysfunction	Measure energy requirement via IC if possible If IC not available, provide maintenance energy needs only until hypercapnia resolves Provide appropriate balance of carbohydrate, protein, and fat; consider fat as 30% to 50% of total energy
Hypozincemia	Excessive losses (nasogastric tube, protein-losing, enteropathy, ostomy, wound)	Supplement zinc via enteral or parenteral route
Vitamin K deficiency	Inadequate vitamin K intake Prolonged use of low-fat or low-vitamin K formula Antibiotic use, cirrhosis, malabsorption, pancreatic insufficiency	Supplement vitamin K Consider probiotic agents Measure prothrombin time and partial thromboplastin time or INR daily until stable
Thiamin deficiency	Chronic alcoholism Advanced age Long-term malnutrition Malabsorption Antacid therapy Dialysis	Thiamin supplementation for 3–7 days Consider addition of folate and multivitamin in cases of alcoholism or chronic disease
Essential fatty acid deficiency	Inadequate linoleic acid intake	Provide at least 4% of energy needs as linoleic acid Add modular fat component to TF if needed Provide 5 mL/d safflower oil via enteral route
Hyperglycemia	Refeeding syndrome Diabetes mellitus, sepsis, catabolism, trauma, or other disease states or conditions Insulin resistance Glucocorticoids Excessive carbohydrate	Correct serum glucose before initiation of TF, if possible Monitor serum glucose every 6 hours, or per protocol Treat underlying disease Maintain appropriate intervascular volume and hydration Provide oral hypoglycemic agent or insulin therapy as needed to maintain serum glucose as low as possible Consider providing 30% to 50% of total energy as fat Consider use of a product with fiber
Hypoglycemia	Abrupt cessation of EN in a patient receiving oral hypoglycemic agent or insulin	Monitor serum glucose every 6 hours, or per protocol Treat with IV or via tube glucose to increase serum level to > 100 mg/dL Taper TF gradually

ADH, antidiuretic hormone; BUN, blood urea nitrogen; Cr, creatinine; ECF, extracellular fluid; K, potassium; I/O, input/output; IC, indirect calorimetry; INR, international normalized ratio; IV, intravenous; Na, sodium; P, phosphorus; SIADH, syndrome of inappropriate secretion of antidiuretic hormone; TF, tube feeding. Adapted with permission from Ideno KT. Enteral nutrition. In: Gottschlich MM, Matarese LM, Shronts EP, eds. *Nutrition Support Dietetics Core Curriculum*. 2nd ed. Silver Spring, MD: American Society for Parenteral and Enteral Nutrition; 1193:98–99; Lord L, Trumbore L, Zaloga G. Enteral nutrition implementation and management. In: Merritt RM, Souba WW, Kohn-Keeth C, et al., eds. *The A.S.P.E.N. Nutrition Support Practice Manual*. Silver Spring, MD: American Society for Parenteral and Enteral Nutrition; 1998:5.10–5.14.

of the metabolic complications that can occur during enteral feeding.

A perception exists that there are fewer metabolic complications from EN when compared to PN (see Chapter 17). Certainly, PN carries greater potential for metabolic alterations considering the ability to manipulate the content of individual nutrients and the direct intravenous administration of the formulation. However, with the exception of hyperglycemia,[73] few controlled studies that randomize patients to receive either EN versus PN or EN versus no intervention have been done. Therefore, it is unclear whether enteral feedings may cause metabolic alterations or if there is an advantage of EN over PN in regards to metabolic complications. This by no means suggests that PN and EN are comparable therapies. EN is always preferred. It is more appropriate to discuss the following metabolic derangements that may be affected by enteral intake.

Electrolyte Imbalances

The frequency of refeeding syndrome has not been reported. The potential for the serious electrolyte decreases associated with refeeding syndrome should be anticipated in all malnourished patients, especially those with large electrolyte losses. Examples include those with diarrhea, high-output fistulae, or vomiting.

This syndrome, which has been reviewed extensively elsewhere,[74-76] typically occurs after nutritional formulas are started, but the problem may also arise in malnourished patients who are resuscitated with standard intravenous solutions containing dextrose. With refeeding syndrome, decrements in electrolyte levels may occur in a matter of hours and may lead to arrhythmias, respiratory and cardiac failure, aspiration, and death (see Chapters 7 and 17). While the occurrence of refeeding syndrome is more often thought of in association with the use of PN, its incidence has been well documented in those receiving EN support.[76-78] The nutrition support practitioner should examine the patient's chart for previous episodes of hypophosphatemia, hypomagnesemia, or hypokalemia because these abnormalities may suggest multiple unrecognized electrolyte deficiencies. Electrolyte deficiencies may occur in the presence of normal serum levels. A total body deficit of approximately 80 mEq of potassium is required before serum levels drop below normal. Clinicians should review the patient's history for evidence of prolonged starvation and chronic electrolyte-losing disease states, such as diarrhea or liquid stool from an ileostomy. Any patient thought to be at risk for refeeding syndrome requires frequent monitoring of electrolytes for the first few days of feeding and until stable. Furthermore, feedings should be advanced slowly to minimize the speed with which these abnormalities develop, perhaps not exceeding 15 to 20 kcal/kg/day in patients at high risk until electrolytes are stable.

Hyperglycemia

Hyperglycemia is reported in the literature to be more common with PN than with EN. The enteral products developed to improve glycemic control are typically higher in fat and contain fiber, both to slow gastric emptying and decrease the glycemic index. This may not be desirable in acutely ill patients in whom antropyloric dysfunction (poor gastric emptying, gastroparesis) commonly complicates gastric feeding. Further, absorption of glucose in continuous feeds is more affected by the rate of carbohydrate delivery than the glycemic index, because glycemic index refers to the rate of rise of glucose after a bolus. Slow advancement and close collaboration with the medical team should allow for adequate glucose control with standard feeding products. Glycemic control should be considered a primarily medical issue in the acutely ill patient. Diabetes-specific enteral products may help improve the ease of glycemic control in chronic care but has yet to be proven in the acutely ill.[79,80]

Dehydration

Definition

Dehydration is defined as a condition caused by the loss of too much water from the body. Dehydration can occur as a result of either inadequate fluid intake (orally, by tube, or intravenously) and/or excess fluid losses; it may be accompanied by sodium imbalance. Causes of dehydration are insufficient water intake, fever, diarrhea, vomiting, significant blood volume loss, chronic illnesses (eg, diabetes, kidney disease), overuse of diuretics, drainage tube or paracentesis losses, wound seepage, or high nasogastric, fistula, or ostomy outputs.

Hospital-Acquired Dehydration

Dehydration can also develop during hospitalization. One recent retrospective investigation compared hospitalized veterans between 1997 and 2000, with or without a diagnosis of one of three dehydration codes that developed during their hospital stay.[81] The overall development of dehydration in this group of patients was 3.5%. Overall mortality rates at 30 days and 6 months post discharge were significantly higher, about double, for those patients that developed dehydration during their hospital stay compared to those that did not. For the patients that developed volume-depleted dehydration, the 30 day mortality rate was 13.8% versus 6.0% (controls) and 29.3% versus 14.7% (controls) at 6 months.

Risk Factors

Patients who are tube fed are at risk for dehydration because enteral formulas alone typically do not meet total fluid needs and therefore additional water flushes need to be prescribed. The achievement of fluid balance in the tube-fed patient is dependent on the prescribers' and caregivers' knowledge base and the level of monitoring. The elderly patient population, in particular, has lower water reserves because of the decrease in lean body mass that occurs with aging. This puts the elderly tube-fed patient at higher risk for dehydration in addition to other age-related changes that include altered sense of thirst, diminished cognition, dysphagia, dysgeusia, hyposmia, reduced kidney function, impairment of hormonal modulators of sodium and water balance (lowered aldosterone secretion, vasopressin release and renin activity), and limitations in function.[82,83] Tube-fed patients with similar characteristics and those with chronic disease or at risk for adverse drug reactions are also at higher risk for dehydration.

Patients who become dehydrated are at increased risk for falls, pressure ulcers, constipation, urinary tract infections, respiratory infections, and medication toxicities. Persistent dehydration can lead to delirium, renal failure, coma, and death.

Detecting Dehydration

Clinicians need to assess for multiple signs and symptoms to determine dehydration. Early signs include dry mouth and eyes, thirst, light-headedness (especially when standing), headache, fatigue, loss of appetite, flushed skin, heat intolerance, and dark urine with a strong odor. Tongue dryness can be a simple, quick, reliable, cost-effective way to identify dehydration in the elderly, provided that other etiologies of dry mouth, such as diuretic and anticholinergic use, are ruled out.[84] Alternately, moist mucous membranes without tongue furrows can help rule out dehydration.[85] Dehydrated patients usually develop orthostatic hypotension, a drop in systolic blood pressure of 20 mm Hg or more on standing, and a rise in pulse rate by at least 10 beats/minute. Progressive dehydration can lead to dysphagia, clumsiness, poor skin turgor (sternum: more than 2 seconds), sunken eyes with dim vision, painful urination, muscle cramps, and delirium.

Laboratory results usually show an elevation in blood urea nitrogen (BUN), plasma osmolality, and hematocrit whereas serum sodium levels can be elevated, low, or normal, depending on the etiology of the dehydration. In dehydration, the BUN usually rises out of proportion to the usual BUN:creatinine ratio of 20:1. The BUN:creatinine ratio should be evaluated in the context of the patient's nutritional state, as well as underlying renal function. Patients with low muscle mass will have an artificially, and sometimes extremely, low creatinine. A rise in creatinine from 0.2 mg/dl to 0.4 mg/dl in a patient with severe muscle mass loss might signal a drop by 50% in glomerular filtration rate. BUN reflects protein intake as well as state of hydration and renal function. A patient with renal failure and no protein intake may have a normal or even low BUN. A severely cachectic patient with renal failure might have a creatinine significantly lower than 1 mg/dl, a BUN over 100 mg/dl, and a BUN:creatinine ratio > 100:1 and still be adequately hydrated.

An elevated urine specific gravity (> 1.028), paired with low urine output, usually reflects dehydration. Typical urine specific gravity measurements are 1.010 to 1.025. One report showed that urine color, using a standardized color reference chart, was comparable to urine specific gravity and osmolality results.[86,87] When greater precision and accuracy are not required, tube-fed patients can strive to achieve and maintain urine that is pale yellow or straw colored.

In hospitalized patients at risk for dehydration, fluid status can be tracked by strict intake and output measurements (including ostomy, fistula, liquid stool, drains, nasogastric tube, paracentesis outputs) and daily weights. The minimum urine output required to remove waste is 30 mL/hour or about 700 mL/day. The urine output range for adults is typically 0.5 to 2.0 mL/kg/hour,[17] and an output of >1 mL/kg/hour is useful as a guideline for adequate urine output. When viewing daily weight changes and intake/output volumes, comparisons can be made, noting that 1 kg weight change reflects 1 L of fluid. If total fluid output, in the euvolemic patient, begins to exceed total fluid intake by more than 800 mL to 1L daily (insensible losses from lungs, feces, and skin) with concurrent weight loss, dehydration can occur. Higher urine outputs with concurrent weight loss are expected when fluid overload is resolving.

Prevention of Dehydration

Clinicians need to be attuned to the fluid needs of their tube-fed patients to be sure they are providing maintenance fluid needs in addition to replacing any additional losses. Ongoing assessments need to be made and fluid intake increased with the development of fever (increase fluid intake by 12% per degree Celsius above 37.8°C),[88] emesis, diarrhea, high fistula and ostomy outputs, and hyperglycemia. If a patient misses a feeding, then the fluid content of that feeding should be replaced. At times, the replacement of large fluid losses cannot be accomplished via the GI tract. The clinician may then need to consider intravenous fluid therapy.

When a patient is being diuresed, the clinician needs to be watchful and determine when the patient achieves a euvolemic state (loss of edema) and then initiate adequate fluids to prevent dehydration. It should be noted that the presence of edema, indicating total body fluid and salt overload, does not guarantee intravascular volume adequacy. Aggressive diuresis of an acutely ill patient may lead to low vascular volume. This can lead to organ failure, particularly renal and cardiac, hypoperfusion, and hypotension, and may be difficult to detect, especially in the acutely ill. Some useful signs of intravascular volume depletion in these patients include an increase in heart rate, decreased or more concentrated urine, and an increase in oxygen extraction (an increase in the difference between arterial and venous oxygen concentration).

Determining Fluid Requirements

Formulas used to determine fluid requirements should account for weight and age differences. Water is needed to support an individual's lean body mass, but lean body mass fluctuates with body weight and decreases with age. A commonly used simplistic equation is 1 mL water per kcal required, but this has been shown to underestimate fluid needs.[89,90] The literature offers some equations that utilize body weight and age to determine fluid needs.[89–92] Some practitioners have found clinical success in determining and providing adequate fluid volume to adult tube-fed populations by calculating fluid needs using both of the following equations and then taking the average of the two. It is important to note that very muscular, active individuals likely require more water than what is provided in these equations. Conversely, the use of an obesity adjusted weight should be used to calculate the fluid needs of obese individuals.

Although there is a wide range, when an individual gains excess weight, about 75% is fat tissue and 25% is lean tissue. An obesity adjusted weight is often used when an individual is ≥ 125% ideal body weight (IBW), unless the excess weight is due to muscle mass. An obesity adjusted weight is obtained by subtracting the IBW from the actual weight and adding back one-quarter (25%) of the difference to the IBW. For obese and chronically inactive individuals, another approach is to calculate both calorie and fluid requirements using IBW alone and adjusting appropriately over time, based on response and observed needs.

- Ideal Body Weight Equation (± 10%):
  Female: 100 lbs for 5′; add 5 lbs for each inch over 5′
  Male: 106 lbs for 5′; add 6 lbs for each inch over 5′
- Obesity Adjusted Weight Equation:
  [(Actual Weight − IBW) × 0.25] + IBW = Adjusted Body Weight (for obesity)
  Example: 5′4″ 160-lb female:
  160 lb (actual weight) − 120 lbs (IBW) = 40
  40 × 0.25 = 10
  10 + 120 (IBW) = 130 lbs (adjusted body weight)
  2.2 lbs = 1 kg, therefore 130 lbs = 59 kg
  (Fifty-nine kilograms can then be used to calculate fluid requirements in the following equations.)
  Fluid Calculation Equations:

Equation 1:

- Adults age 18–55: 35 mL per kg body weight
- Adults age 55–75: 30 mL per kg body weight
- Adults age > 75 years: 25 mL per kg body weight
- Fluid restriction: ≤ 25 mL/kg body weight
  (renal and cardiac disease, fluid overload states)

Equation 2:

- 1500 mL for the first 20 kg
- + 20 mL per kg ≤ age 50
- + 15 mL per kg > age 50

Additional fluid must be provided for patients with severe diarrhea, large draining wounds, excessive diaphoresis, constant drooling, paracentesis losses, drains, high nasogastric fistula and ostomy outputs, and women who are lactating. Fluid losses should be measured when possible, but they are not always collectable. A clinician can be creative and weigh wound dressings before and after placement to determine the fluid loss from open wounds. Excessive diaphoresis that soaks bed linens enough to necessitate changing is usually equal to at least 1 L of fluid.[93] Some fluid losses contain significant amounts of electrolytes, minerals, or proteins that require replacement, along with water.

Some of the water requirements are provided in the tube feeding formula itself. Enteral formulas are 67% to 87% water (ranges from 161 to 208 mL water per 8 fl oz can). The remainder are solids consisting of macro- and micronutrients. The more calorically dense a formula is, the lower the percentage of water volume. The water content of formulas is provided in written materials distributed by the manufacturers, but is not usually listed on the formula label. After accounting for the water in the formula, the patient's remaining fluid needs are provided with water flushes, unless the patient can consume some oral fluids or is receiving intravenous fluids. Water flushes are administered with a large (50 to 60 mL) syringe or poured into a feeding bag either after feeding delivery or as a separate infusion. They are delivered every 4 to 6 hours during continuous feedings, before and after intermittent feedings, and around medication delivery. Automatic flush bags have been manufactured as part of some enteral delivery systems and are programmed to deliver a set amount of water at periodic intervals. These are purported to help maintain tube patency, lower contamination risk, and save nursing time. In addition to providing aliquots of water to maintain tube patency, some automatic flush bags can also be programmed to deliver larger quantities of water to meet patients' fluid requirements.

References

1. Poulard F, Dimet J, Martin-Lefevre L, et al. Impact of not measuring residual gastric volume in mechanically ventilated patients receiving early enteral feeding: a prospective before-after study. *J Parent Ent Nutr*. 2010;34:125–130.
2. Montejo JC, Grau T, Acosta J, et al. Multicenter, prospective, randomized, single-blind study comparing the efficacy and gastrointestinal complications of early jejeunal feeding with early gastric feeding in critically ill patients. *Crit Care Med*. 2002;30:796–800.
3. Heyland DK, Cahill NE, Dahliwal R, et al. Enhanced protein-energy provision via the enteral route in critically ill patients: a single center feasibility trial of the PEP uP protocol. *Crit Care*. 2010;14:R78.
4. Beyer PL. Complications of enteral nutrition. In: Matarese LE, Gottschlich MM, eds. *Contemporary Nutrition Support Practice; A Clinical Guide*. 2nd ed. Philadelphia, PA: Saunders; 1998:215–216.
5. Kozar RA, McQuiggan MM, Moore FA. Trauma. In: Merritt RM, ed. *The A.S.P.E.N. Nutrition Support Practice Manual*. Silver Spring, MD: American Society for Parenteral and Enteral Nutrition; 2005:271–276.
6. Malone AM, Brewer CK. Monitoring for efficacy, complications and toxicity. In: Rolandelli RH, ed. *Clinical Nutrition: Enteral and Tube Feeding*. 4th ed. Philadelphia, PA: Saunders; 2005:276–290.
7. Vickery G. Basics of constipation. *Gastroent Nurs*. 1997;20:125–128.
8. Davies A, Prentice W. Fentanyl, morphine, and constipation. *J Pain Sympt Manage*. 1998;16:141–144.
9. Ukleja A. Altered GI motility in critically Ill patients: current understanding of pathophysiology, clinical impact, and diagnostic approach. *Nutr Clin Pract*. 2010;25:16–25.
10. Ali T, Hasan M, Hamadani M, et al. Gastroparesis. *South Med J*. 2007;100:281–286.
11. Taylor SJ, Manara AR, Brown J. Treating delayed gastric emptying in critical illness: metoclopramide, erythromycin, and bedside (cortrak) nasointestinal tube placement. *J Parent Enteral Nutr*. 2010; 34:289–294.
12. Rhoney DH, Parker D Jr, Formea CM, et al. Tolerability of bolus versus continuous gastric feeding in brain-injured patients. *Neurol Res*. 2002;24:613–620.
13. Sidery MB, Macdonald IA, Blackshaw PE. Superior mesenteric artery blood flow and gastric emptying in humans and the differential effects of high fat and high carbohydrate meals. *Gut*. 1994; 35:186–190.
14. Spalding DR, Behranwala KA, Straker P, et al., Non-occlusive small bowel necrosis in association with feeding jejunostomy after elective upper gastrointestinal surgery. *Ann R Coll Surg Engl*. 2009;91: 477–482.
15. McClave SA, Snider HL, Lowen CC, et al. Use of residual volume as a marker for enteral feeding intolerance: prospective blinded comparison with physical examination and radiographic findings. *J Parenter Enteral Nutr*. 1992;16:99–105.
16. McClave SA, Martindale RW, McCarthy M, et al. Guidelines for the provision and assessment of nutrition therapy in the adult critically ill patient. *J Parent Ent Nutr*. 2009;33:277–316.
17. Ideno KT. Enteral nutrition. In: Gottschlich MM, Matarese LM, Shronts EP, eds. *Nutrition Support Dietetics Core Curriculum*. 2nd ed. Silver Spring, MD: American Society for Parenteral and Enteral Nutrition; 1993:98–99.
18. Wall-Alonso E, Sullivan MM, Byrne TA. Gastrointestinal and pancreatic disease. In: Matarese LE, Gottschlich MM, eds. *Contemporary Nutrition Support Practice: A Clinical Guide*. 2nd ed. Philadelphia, PA: Saunders; 2003:412–444.
19. Russell MK. Monitoring and complications. In: Charney P, Malone A, eds. *A Pocket Guide to Enteral Nutrition*. Chicago, IL: The American Dietetic Association, 2005:189–209.
20. Lefton J. Management of common gastrointestinal complications in tube-fed patients. *Support Line*. 2002;24:19–25.
21. Lebak KJ, Bliss DZ, Savik K, Patten-Marsh KM. What's new on defining diarrhea in tube feeding studies? *Clin Nurs Res*. 2003;12: 174–204.
22. Mobarhan S, DeMeo M. Diarrhea induced by enteral feeding. *Nutr Rev*. 1995;53:67–70.
23. Williams MS, Harper R, Magnuson B, et al. Diarrhea management in enterally fed patients. *Nutr Clin Pract*. 1998;13:225–229.
24. Spapen H, Diltoer M, Van Malderen C, et al. Soluble fiber reduces the incidence of diarrhea in septic patients receiving total enteral nutrition: a prospective, double-blind, randomized, and controlled trial. *Clinical Nutrition*. 2001;20(4):301–305.
25. Rushdi TA, Pichard C, Khater YH. Control of diarrhea by fiber-enriched diet in ICU patients on enteral nutrition: a prospective randomized controlled trial. *Clin Nutr*. 2004;23(6):1344–1352.
26. American Dietetic Association. Evidence Analysis Library. http://ada.portalxm.com/eal/conclusion.cfm?conclusion_statement_id=251597. Accessed July 28, 2011.

27. Reese JL, Means ME, Hanrahan K, et al. Diarrhea associated with nasogastric feedings. *Oncol Nurs Forum*. 1996;23:59–68.
28. Kely TW, Patrick MR, Kely TW, Patrick MR, Hillman KM. Study of diarrhea in critically ill patients. *Crit Care Med*. 1983;11:7–9.
29. Edes TE, Walk BE, Austin JL. Diarrhea in tube-fed patients: feeding formula is not necessarily the cause. *Am J Med*. 1990;88:91–93.
30. Monturo CA. Diarrhea in patients receiving enteral nutrition. *Oncol Nurs Forum*. 1995;22:1288.
31. Keohane PP, Attrill H, Love M, et al. Relationship between osmolality of diet and gastrointestinal side effects in enteral nutrition. *Br Med J*. 1984;288:678–680.
32. Gottschlich MM, Warden GD, Michel M, et al. Diarrhea in tube-fed burn patients: incidence, etiology, nutritional impact, and prevention. *J Parenter Enteral Nutr*. 1988;12:338–345.
33. Critical Care Nutrition. Tools. www.criticalcarenutrition.com/index.php?option=com_content&view=category&layout=blog&id=18&Itemid=19. Accessed July 26, 2011.
34. Marchado JD, Campos CS, Lopes Dah Silva C, et al. Intestinal bacterial overgrowth after Roux-en-Y gastric bypass. *Obes Surg*. 2008;18(1):139–143.
35. Fine KD, Krejs GJ, Fordtran JS. Diarrhea. In: Sleigenger MH, Fordtran JS, eds. *Gastrointestinal Disease: Pathophysiology/Diagnosis/Management*. 5th ed. Philadelphia, PA: Saunders; 1995:1043.
36. Powell DW. Approach to the patient with diarrhea. In: Yamada T, ed. *Textbook of Gastroenterology*. 2nd ed. Philadelphia, PA: Lippincott; 1995:830.
37. Bankhead R, Boullata J, Brantley S, et al. A.S.P.E.N. enteral nutrition practice recommendations. *J Parenter Enteral Nutr*. 2009;33(2):122–167.
38. Weenk GH, Kemen M, Wernert HP. Risks of microbiological contamination of enteral feeds during the set up of enteral feeding systems. *J Hum Nutr Diet*. 1993;6:307–316.
39. Fagerman KE. Limiting bacterial contamination of enteral nutrient solutions: 6-year history with reduction of contamination at two institutions. *Nutr Clin Practice*. 1992;7:31–36.
40. Kohn CL. The relationship between enteral formula contamination and length of enteral delivery set usage. *J Parenter Enteral Nutr*. 1991;15:567–571.
41. Vanek V. Closed versus open enteral delivery systems: a quality improvement study. *Nutr Clin Pract*. 2000;15:234–243.
42. Wagner DR, Elmore MF, Knoll DM. Evaluation of "closed" versus "open" systems for the delivery of peptide-based enteral diets. *J Parenter Enteral Nutr*. 1994;18:453–457.
43. Beattie TK, Anderton A. Microbiological evaluation of four enteral feeding systems which have been deliberately subjected to faulty handling procedures. *J Hosp Inf*. 1999;42:11–20.
44. Mathus-Vliegen EMH, Bredius WJ, Binnekade JM. Analysis of sites of bacterial contamination in an enteral feeding system. *J Parenter Enteral Nutr*. 2006;30(6):519–525.
45. Moffitt SK, Gohman SM, Sass KM, et al. Clinical and laboratory evaluation of a closed enteral feeding system under cyclic feeding conditions: a microbial and cost evaluation. *Appl Nutr Invest*. 1997;13:622–628.
46. Payne-James JJ, Rana SK, Bray MJ, et al. Retrograde (ascending) bacterial contamination of enteral diet administration systems. *J Parenter Enteral Nutr*. 1992;16(4):369–373.
47. Matlow A, Jacobson M, Wray R, et al. Enteral tube hub as a reservoir for transmissible enteric bacteria. *Am J Infect Control*. 2006;34:131–133.
48. U.S. Food and Drug Administration. FDA Public Health Advisory September 29, 2003: Reports of blue discoloration and death in patients receiving enteral feedings tinted with the dye, FD&C Blue No. 1.
49. Anderson KR, Norris DJ, Godfrey LB, et al. Bacterial contamination of tube-feeding formulas. *J Parenter Enteral Nutr*. 1984;8:673–678.
50. Anderton A. Bacterial contamination of enteral feeds and feeding systems. *Clin Nutr*. 1993;12(Suppl. 1):16–32.
51. Bliss DZ, Johnson S, Savik K, et al. Acquisition of *Clostridium difficile* and *Clostridium difficile*-associated diarrhea in hospitalized patients receiving tube feeding. *Ann Intern Med*. 1998;129:1012–1019.
52. Okuma T, Nakamura M, Totake H, et al. Microbial contamination of enteral feeding formulas and diarrhea. *Nutrition*. 2000;16:719–722.
53. Marvin RG, McKinley BA, McQuiggan M, et al., Nonocclusive bowel necrosis occurring in critically ill trauma patients receiving enteral nutrition manifests no reliable clinical signs for early detection. *Am J Surg*. 2000;179:7–12.
54. Sarap AN, Sarap MD, Childers J. Small bowel necrosis in association with jejunal tube feeding. *JAAPA*. 2010;23:28–32.
55. Munshi IA, Steingrub JS, Wolpert L. Small bowel necrosis associated with early postoperative jejunal feeding in a trauma patient. *J Trauma*. 2000;49:163–165.
56. Wong K. The role of fiber in diarrhea management. *Support Line*. 1998;20:16–20.
57. Metheny NM. Twenty ways to prevent tube feeding complications. *Nurs*. 1985;15:47–50.
58. McClave SA, Lukan JK, Stefater JA, et al. Poor validity of residual volumes as a marker for risk of aspiration in critically ill patients. *Crit Care Med*. 2005;33(2):324–330.
59. Metheny N, Clouse RE, Chang YH, et al. Tracheobronchial aspiration of gastric contents in critically ill tube-fed patients: frequency, outcomes and risk factors. *CCM*. 2006;34(4):1007–1015.
60. Kollef MH, Von Harz B, Prentice D, et al. Patient transport from intensive care increases the risk of developing ventilator-associated pneumonia. *Chest*. 1997;112:765–773.
61. Amaravadi RK, Dimick JB, Pronovost PJ, et al. IC nurse-to-patient ratio is associated with complications and resource use after esophagectomy. *Intens Care Med*. 2000;26:1857–1862.
62. Kinsey GC, Murray MJ, Swensen SJ, et al. Glucose content of tracheal aspirates: implications for the detection of tube feeding aspiration. *Crit Care Med*. 1994;22(10):1557–1562.
63. Metheny N, Dahms T, Stewart B, et al. Verification of inefficacy of the glucose method in detecting aspiration associated with tube feedings. *Medsurg Nurs*. 2005;14:112–121.
64. Metheny NA, Dahms TE, Chang YH, et al. Detection of pepsin intratracheal secretions after forced small-volume aspirations of gastric juice. *J Parenter Enteral Nutr*. 2004;28:79–84.
65. Metheny NA, Schallom L, Oliver DA, et al. Gastric residual volume and aspiration in critically ill patients receiving gastric feedings. *Am J Crit Care*. 2008;17(6):512–519.
66. Metheny NA. Residual volume measurement should be retained in enteral feeding protocols. *Am J Crit Care*. 2009;17(1):62–64.
67. Lin HC, Van Citters GW. Stopping enteral feeding for arbitrary gastric residual volume may not be physiologically sound: results of a computer simulation model. *J Parenter Enteral Nutr*. 1997;21:286–289.
68. McClave SA, Lukan JK, Stefater JA, et al. Poor validity of residual volumes as a marker for risk of aspiration in critically ill patients. *Crit Care Med*. 2005;33:324–330.
69. Metheny NA. Effectiveness of an aspiration risk-reduction protocol. *Nurs Research*. 2010;59(1):18–25.
70. Drakulovic MB, Torres A, Bauer TT, et al. Supine body position as a risk factor for nosocomial pneumonia in mechanically ventilated patients: a randomized trial. *Lancet*. 1999;354(9193):1851–1858.
71. Pinilla JC, Samphire J, Arnold C, et al. Comparison of gastrointestinal tolerance to two enteral feeding protocols in critically ill

patients: a prospective, randomized controlled trial. *J Parenter Enteral Nutr*. 2001;25:81–86.

72. Taylor SJ, Fettes SB, Jewkes C, Nelson RJ. Propective, randomized, controlled trial to determine the effect of early enhanced enteral nutrition on clinical outcome in mechanically ventilated patients suffering head injury. *Crit Care Med*. 1999;27:2525–2531.
73. Braunschweig CL, Levy P, Sheean PM, Wang X. Enteral compared with parenteral nutrition: a meta-analysis. *Am J Clin Nutr*. 2001; 74:534–542.
74. Crook MA, Hally V, Panteli JV, et al. The importance of the refeeding syndrome. *Nutrition*. 2001;17:632–637.
75. Brooks MJ, Melnik G. The refeeding syndrome: an approach to understanding its complications and preventing its occurrence. *Pharmacotherapy*. 1995;15:713–726.
76. Khan LU, Ahmed J, Khan S, Macfie J. Refeeding syndrome: a literature review. *Gastroenterol Res Pract*. 2011. doi:10.1155/2011/410971
77. Patel U, Sriram K. Acute respiratory failure due to refeeding syndrome and hypophosphatemia induced by hypocaloric enteral nutrition. *Nutrition*. 2009;25:364–367.
78. Lubart E, Leibovitz A, Dror Y, et al., Mortality after nasogastric tube feeding initiation in long-term care elderly with oropharyngeal dysphagia—the contribution of refeeding syndrome. *Gerontology*. 2009;55:393–397.
79. American Dietetic Association. Evidence Analysis Library; http://ada.portalxm.com/eal/topic.cfm?cat=1491. Accessed June 12, 2011.
80. Elia M, Ceriello A, Laube H, et al. Enteral nutritional support and use of diabetes-specific formulas for patients with diabetes: a systematic review and meta-analysis. *Diabetes Care*. 2005;28:2267–2279.
81. Wakefield BJ, Mentes J, Holman JE, et al. Postadmission dehydration: risk factors, indicators, and outcomes. *Rehabilitation Nursing*. 2009;34(5):209–216.
82. Feinsod F, Levenson M, Rapp SA, et al. Dehydration in frail, older residents in long-term care facilities. *J Am Med Dir Assoc*. 2004; 5(Suppl 2):S35–S41.
83. Xiao H, Barber J, Campbell ES. Economic burden of dehydration among hospitalized elderly patients. *Am J Health-Syst Pharm*. 2004;61:2534–2540.
84. Vivanti A, Harvey K, Ash S. Developing a quick and practical screen to improve the identification of poor hydration in geriatric and rehabilitative care. *Arch Gerontol Geriatr*. 2010;50:156–164.
85. McGee S, Abernethy WB III, Simel DL. The rational clinical examination: is this patient hypovolemic? *JAMA*. 1999;281:1022–1029.
86. Armstrong LE, Maresh CM, Castellani JW, et al. Urinary indices of hydration status. *Int J Sport Nutr*. 1994;4:265–279.
87. Wakefield B, Mentes J, Diggelmann L, et al. Monitoring hydration status in elderly veterans. *West J of Nurs Res*. 2002;24(2):132–142.
88. The Merck Manual. Dehydration in children. www.merckmanuals.com/professional/print/sec20/ch293/ch293b.html. Accessed July 4, 2011.
89. Chidester JC, Splanger AA. Fluid intake in the institutionalized elderly. *JADA*. 1997;97(1):23–28.
90. Kayser-Jones J, Schell ES, Porter C, et al. Factors contributing to dehydration in nursing homes: inadequate staffing and lack of professional supervision. *J Am Geriatr Soc*. 1999;47(10):1187–1194.
91. Holliday MA, Segar WE. The maintenance need for water in parenteral fluid therapy. *Pediatrics*. 1957;19:823–832.
92. Whitmire S. Fluid and electrolytes. In: Gottschlich MM, ed. *The A.S.P.E.N. Nutrition Support Core Curriculum*. Silver Spring, MD: The American Society for Parenteral and Enteral Nutrition; 2001:55–81.
93. Metheny NM. Nursing assessment. In: Metheny NM. *Fluid and Electrolyte Balance: Nursing Considerations*. Philadelphia, PA: JB Lippincott Publishers; 1987:11–35.

14 Overview of Parenteral Nutrition

Jay M. Mirtallo, MS, RPh, BCNSP, FASHP, and Meera Patel, PharmD, BCPS

CONTENTS

Background 235
Routes of Infusion 236
Central Parenteral Nutrition 236
Peripheral Parenteral Nutrition 236
Approaches to Parenteral Nutrition 237
Indications for Parenteral Nutrition 237
General Guidelines 237
Gastrointestinal Function 238
Clinical Status 238
Specific Guidelines 238
Gastrointestinal Disorders 238
Perioperative Nutrition 238
Critical Illness 240
Cancer 240
Home Parenteral Nutrition 240
The Parenteral Nutrition System 241
References 243

Objectives

1. Determine the appropriate indications for parenteral nutrition (PN).
2. Decide the best PN route based on the patient's nutritional, metabolic, and clinical status.
3. Initiate and manage PN therapy.
4. Describe the effects of PN on patient outcomes.

Test Your Knowledge Questions

1. What is the optimal nutritional support for a moderately malnourished patient with an ileus expected to resolve in 7 to 8 days?
   A. Central parenteral nutrition (CPN)
   B. Nasogastric enteral tube feedings
   C. Postpyloric enteral tube feedings
   D. Peripheral parenteral nutrition (PPN)
2. In which patient condition or treatment would PN elicit an improved patient outcome?
   A. Cancer chemotherapy
   B. Preoperative care of surgery patients with upper gastrointestinal (GI) cancer
   C. Allogeneic bone marrow transplantation
   D. Critical illness
3. CPN is contraindicated in which of the following conditions?
   A. Do Not Resuscitate (DNR) status
   B. Peritonitis
   C. Intestinal hemorrhage
   D. High-output fistulas

4. PN should be discontinued when which of the following criteria are met?
   A. A clear liquid diet is ordered.
   B. Tube feeding is initiated at 10% of goal rate.
   C. Solid food is well tolerated by mouth.
   D. Advancement to a regular diet is poorly tolerated.

Test Your Knowledge Answers

1. The correct answer is **D.** PPN may be used for short periods in patients who are not severely malnourished, have adequate peripheral venous access, and can tolerate large volumes of fluid. Although the most current American Society for Parenteral and Enteral Nutrition (A.S.P.E.N.) guidelines do not address appropriate PPN use, the previous A.S.P.E.N. guidelines indicated that PPN may be used in select patients to provide partial or total nutrition support for up to 2 weeks in patients who cannot ingest or absorb oral or enteral tube–delivered nutrients, or when central-vein PN is not feasible.[1] However, patients who are not severely malnourished may tolerate periods of no nutrition for varying periods (up to 7 to 10 days) without adversely affecting their outcome. Therefore, PPN is not the optimal choice for feeding patients with significant malnutrition, severe metabolic stress, large nutrient or electrolyte needs, fluid restriction, and/or the need for prolonged intravenous (IV) nutrition support.[2]
2. The correct answer is **B.** A review of PN literature has reported improved outcomes in patients with upper GI tract malignancies when PN is initiated 7 days before surgery.[3] An early report of a decrease in length of stay and infectious complications in allogeneic bone marrow transplant patients receiving PN has not been confirmed.[4] A review of published data on the use of PN in cancer chemotherapy, in the perioperative period, and during critical illness reports no positive effect of PN on the clinical outcome and a significant increase in infectious complications in patients randomized to PN therapy as compared to those receiving no nutritional support.[3]
3. The correct answer is **A.** Trujillo and colleagues[5] abstracted indications for PN from the 1993 A.S.P.E.N. guidelines as peritonitis, intestinal hemorrhage, intestinal obstruction, intractable vomiting, paralytic ileus, severe pancreatitis, stool output greater than 1 L/d, high-output fistulas, short bowel syndrome, and bone marrow recipients. Therapy was considered to be contraindicated if the patients were classified as well nourished and had inadequate enteral nutrition (EN) for less than 7 days; had a DNR status, and were deemed to warrant comfort measures only or terminally ill; or those receiving adequate EN.
4. The correct answer is **C.** The goal of PN therapy is to maintain the nutritional status of the patient until some form of EN is tolerated. The exception is the critically ill patient in whom therapy is withdrawn during the terminal stages of their disease process. In most other situations, GI function returns, or appropriate enteral access is obtained, and PN is tapered as the amount of reliable enteral intake increases. PN support may be discontinued when the patient is able to tolerate solid food by mouth unless they are elderly, debilitated, or there is a malignancy or ethnic food issue present. Then, a detailed transitional feeding plan should be established.[6]

Background

A successful infusion of hypertonic parenteral nutrients by Dudrick and colleagues[7] in the late 1960s was a major advancement in providing nutrition to patients with a nonfunctioning GI tract. Although IV nutrition has been of interest since the 1600s, Dudrick, Vars, and Rhoads' interest was in "patients seriously depleted of protein and in whom it was known that operation would carry an increased risk of various complications, both infectious and non-infectious."[8,9] Early problems with providing PN therapy included sources of safe IV nutrients and adequate venous access for hypertonic nutrient administration. Venous access problems were resolved by subclavian vein catheterization use, which minimized thrombotic complications associated with peripheral PN infusions (see Chapter 16). Early PN formulations consisted of dextrose and protein hydrolysates of either casein or fibrin. Protein hydrolysates were replaced by newer, crystalline amino acids, which are better used and lack preformed ammonia. Intravenous fat emulsions (IVFE) were not available in the United States until the 1970s and were used primarily as a source of essential fatty acids. It was not until the 1980s that IVFE were routinely used as a calorie source. This coincided with approval by the U.S. Food and Drug Administration (FDA) for fat emulsions to be compounded in the same container as other IV nutrients. Such a formulation is commonly referred to as a 3-in-1 admixture, or total nutrient admixture (TNA).

PN has been used in several clinical situations. Early use demonstrated a significant benefit to patients with GI fistulas who were unable to ingest nutrients by mouth.[9] Home PN has become a lifeline for patients with short bowel syndrome, allowing them to resume a nearly normal lifestyle (see Chapter 37). New knowledge and technology have improved patient selection, whereas individualized therapies and improved PN techniques have improved safety use. The refinement of PN will continue to make it a useful therapy for patients with complex diseases whose GI tract is nonfunctional.

The parenteral feeding formulation is a complex mixture containing up to 40 different chemical (nutrient) components that may cause problems with stability and compatibility (see Chapter 15). Serious harm and death have resulted from improperly compounded parenteral feeding formulations. Two deaths were attributed to the infusion of calcium phosphate precipitates, resulting from an improper admixture process.[10] Other complications, such as venous catheter infections, hepatobiliary disease, and glucose disorders, have contributed to patient morbidity (see Chapters 16 and 17).[11,12] The complication rate can be minimized through careful patient selection and by having knowledgeable clinicians oversee the specialized nutrition support program. Nehme[13] reported that the management of PN patients by an interdisciplinary team significantly reduced metabolic and fluid and electrolyte complications as compared to patients managed by individual clinicians. Eight of 11 patients with hyperglycemic, nonketotic dehydration and 2 of 7 patients with rebound hypoglycemia died in the group managed by individual clinicians, whereas no deaths occurred in the group managed by the interdisciplinary team. Interdisciplinary teams are also more likely to use PN according to A.S.P.E.N. guidelines.[5]

The benefit of PN in various conditions continues to be debated. Its use warrants a thorough evaluation of risk to benefit. The benefit is difficult to determine because it is influenced by the symptoms and nutritional effects of the patient's underlying disease process.

Routes of Infusion

The components of a parenteral feeding formulation will determine its osmolarity and infusion route. PN may be prepared for peripheral venous infusion or infusion through a central venous access device. PN may also be prepared as a TNA or a 2-in-1 solution. Two-in-1 solutions contain all necessary IV macronutrients and micronutrients in the same container except IVFE, which may be infused separately (see Chapter 15).

Parenteral feeding formulations are hypertonic to body fluids and, if administered inappropriately, may result in venous thrombosis, suppurative thrombophlebitis, and extravasation. Specifically, the osmolarity of a parenteral feeding formulation is dependent primarily on the dextrose, amino acid, and electrolyte content. Dextrose contributes approximately 5 mOsm/g, amino acids yield approximately 10 mOsm/g, and electrolytes provide approximately 1 mOsm/mEq of individual electrolyte additive. For example, the estimated osmolarity of a 1-L total volume parenteral feeding formulation providing 150 g of dextrose, 50 g of amino acids, and 150 mEq of electrolyte additives is 1400 mOsm/L. Central venous administration is preferred for this PN because the maximum osmolarity tolerated by a peripheral vein is 900 mOsm/L.[14]

Central Parenteral Nutrition

Central parenteral nutrition (CPN) is often referred to as total parenteral nutrition because the entire nutrient needs of the patient may be delivered by this route. A complete, balanced formulation includes dextrose; amino acids; IVFE; electrolytes such as potassium, magnesium, and phosphorus; vitamins; and multiple trace elements such as zinc, copper, manganese, chromium, and selenium. The glucose content (usually 150 to 600 g/d), along with amino acids and electrolytes, provides a hyperosmolar (1300 to 1800 mOsm/L) formulation that must be delivered into a large-diameter vein such as the superior vena cava adjacent to the right atrium. The rate of blood flow in these large vessels rapidly dilutes the hypertonic parenteral feeding formulation to that of body fluids, minimizing risk of complications associated with an IV infusion of hypertonic solutions. CPN provides complete nutrition in a reasonable fluid volume and may be concentrated to provide adequate calories and protein for those patients requiring a fluid restriction. Because central venous access can be maintained for prolonged periods (weeks to years), CPN is preferred for use in patients who will require PN support for longer than 7 to 14 days, including those patients receiving care at home or other extended health care environments, such as assisted living or extended care facilities and nursing homes (see Chapter 36).

Peripheral Parenteral Nutrition

Peripheral parenteral nutrition (PPN) has a similar composition as CPN, but lower concentrations of nutrient components are necessary to allow for peripheral venous administration. It has a lower dextrose dose of 150 to 300 g/d (5% to 10% final concentration) and amino acid content (50 to 100 g/d, or 3% final concentration) compared to CPN. Large fluid volumes must be administered to provide a comparable calorie and protein dose as CPN. PPN is usually an undesirable option for patients with fluid restriction because concentrating the solution frequently results in a hyperosmolar solution that is not suitable for peripheral administration. PPN may be used in patients with mild-to-moderate malnutrition to provide partial or total nutrition support when they are not able to ingest adequate calories orally or enterally, or when CPN is not feasible. However, this therapy is typically used for short periods (up to 2 weeks) because of limited tolerance and few suitable peripheral veins, so use in severely malnourished patients is generally not indicated.[2]

Patients considered for PPN must meet two criteria: (1) patients must have good peripheral venous access and (2) they must be able to tolerate large volumes (2.5 to 3 L) of fluid. They should require at least 5 days but no more than 2 weeks of partial or total PN. Contraindications to PPN are listed in Table 14-1. The use of PPN is controversial, with many believing that the risk of complications outweighs any potential benefit because candidates for this therapy have only minor, if any, nutritional deficits. The use of PPN to provide adequate doses of calories, protein, and other micronutrients in a limited fluid volume in critically ill patients is difficult. PPN formulations are hyperosmolar (600 to 900 mOsm/L) and may cause phlebitis and may require frequent peripheral IV site rotations (at least every 48 to 72 hours). IVFE may be used to increase the caloric density of the peripheral parenteral feeding formulation without increasing the osmolarity and has been reported to improve peripheral vein tolerance of PPN.[15] Although the use of midline catheters is recommended in patients needing PPN for more than 6 days due to their length and lower probability of dislodging compared to other peripheral cannulas, they do not eliminate the risk of thrombophlebitis.[16]

TABLE 14-1 Contraindications to Peripheral Parenteral Nutrition[16]

Significant malnutrition
Severe metabolic stress
Large nutrient or electrolyte needs (Potassium is a strong vascular irritant)
Fluid restriction
Need for prolonged parenteral nutrition (Greater than 2 weeks)
Renal or liver compromise

Approaches to Parenteral Nutrition

As practice has evolved, some new concepts or approaches to PN have surfaced in specific patient conditions such as the following: permissive underfeeding, hypocaloric feeding, and supplemental PN to avoid caloric deficits. Permissive underfeeding is a concept used in critically ill patients where nutrition and especially PN is not well tolerated. This approach is intended to minimize complications of PN delivery by providing only 80% of estimated caloric requirements until the patient's condition improves.[17] In contrast, hypocaloric feeding is used in both enteral and parenteral nutrition therapy for obese patients to provide adequate protein but lower than estimated needs of calories.[18] This approach is also designed to minimize the metabolic complications of PN while maintaining and improving protein stores. The approach is used for patients with a BMI >30 unless weight loss is not intended. It may be used in critically ill as well as other hospitalized patients. Very little data are available for long-term (>30 days) use of this approach. Lastly, supplemental PN is an approach designed to minimize the caloric deficit that accumulates during periods of no nutrition or undernutrition. It is used in those circumstances where EN is insufficient to meet energy needs.[17,19]

Indications for Parenteral Nutrition

General Guidelines

Malnutrition is associated with an increase in patient complications and mortality.[20] Although PN has been shown to improve several markers of nutritional status, prospective, randomized trials have rarely shown PN to improve patient outcomes.[3,21] However, many of these trials have been criticized for inadequate study designs, including inconsistent control for nutritional status, extent or type of underlying disease, or consistency in nutrient type and dose.[21,22] PN has been shown to be of benefit in the following circumstances: perioperative support of patients with moderate-to-severe malnutrition, acute exacerbations of Crohn's disease, GI fistulas, extreme short bowel syndrome, critical care patients who will be NPO for prolonged periods of time, and severe acute necrotizing pancreatitis.[3,21,23]

PN is costly and may result in serious complications when used inappropriately.[24] The costs of PN include not only the admixture but also costs, such as placing venous access, laboratory monitoring, and costs to treat complications.[24] As such, the use of PN is scrutinized.[3] The therapy should only be used in those patients who will demonstrably benefit.[25] Identifying these patients is not an easy task because the nutrition components of care may be confounded by the underlying disease process and its treatment. Specific guidelines for the implementation of PN have been developed by A.S.P.E.N.[1] Criteria that may be used in determining the appropriate application of PN are outlined in Table 14-2.[2,13] Considerations include the patient's nutritional status, GI function, and the extent and severity of the underlying disease. See Practice Scenario 14-1 for a discussion of indications for PN. Patients most likely to benefit from PN may be determined by evaluating the following criteria.

TABLE 14-2 Indications for Parenteral Nutrition[2,13]

Considerations for Parenteral Nutrition Use

1. Patients who are unable to meet nutrition requirements with EN. These patients are already or have the potential of becoming malnourished.
2. PPN may be used in selected patients to provide partial or total nutrition support for up to 2 weeks in patients who cannot ingest or absorb oral or enteral tube–delivered nutrients, or when central vein PN is not feasible.
3. CPN support is necessary when parenteral feeding is indicated for longer than 2 weeks, peripheral venous access is limited, nutrient needs are large, or fluid restriction is required, and the benefits of PN support outweigh the risks.

Use CPN when:

1. The patient has failed the EN trial with appropriate tube placement (postpyloric).
2. The EN is contraindicated or the intestinal tract has a severely diminished function due to the underlying disease or treatment. Specific applicable conditions are as follows:
   - Paralytic ileus
   - Mesenteric ischemia
   - Small bowel obstruction
   - GI fistula except when enteral access may be placed posterior to the fistula or volume of output (less than 200 mL/d) supports a trial of EN
3. As occurs in postoperative nutrition support, the exact duration of starvation that can be tolerated without increased morbidity is unknown. Expert opinion suggests that wound healing would be impaired if PN is not started within 5 to 10 days postoperatively for patients unable to eat or tolerate enteral feeding.[2]
4. The patient's clinical condition is considered in the decision to withhold or withdraw therapy. Conditions where nutrition support is poorly tolerated and should be withheld until the condition improves are severe hyperglycemia, azotemia, encephalopathy and hyperosmolality, and severe fluid and electrolyte disturbances.

PN, parenteral nutrition; CPN, central parenteral nutrition; PPN, peripheral parenteral nutrition; EN, enteral nutrition; GI, gastrointestinal.

Practice Scenario 14-1

Question: When is PN indicated?

Scenario: A 47-year-old female patient is admitted with recurring gastrointestinal problems. Nutritional parameters are listed as follows:

Weight loss, kg	8.4
Weight change, %	11
Time period of weight change, d	35
Intake history, % estimated nutritional needs	.25
Prealbumin, mg/dL	8

Abdominal scan findings demonstrated a partial/complete bowel obstruction with pockets of fluid collections consistent with an intra-abdominal abscess.

Intervention: At surgery, the patient was found to have a complete bowel obstruction, multiple adhesions, recurrence of Crohn's disease, and a large suprapubic abscess. The surgical procedure consisted of an exploratory laparotomy, lysis of adhesions, small bowel resection to remove the disease-affected bowel, and drainage of the abdominal abscess. A nasogastric tube was placed, which drained 1500 to 2000 mL on postoperative day 1.

Answer: The patient is at a high risk of developing postoperative complications such as wound dehiscence, wound infection, pneumonia, and renal failure. Because the problem with the GI tract is not expected to be resolved in 7 to 10 days, PN is indicated.[1]

Rationale: Whether PN is indicated is dependent on the severity of the patient's malnutrition, the period of time this patient will not be able to use the enteral route for nourishment, and the influence of the underlying clinical condition on the safety and efficacy of therapy. The Nutrition Consult Form in Figure 14-1 offers considerations for determining the appropriate indication for PN. The patient meets two criteria for severe malnutrition: more than 10% weight loss over a 2- to 3-month period and inadequate oral intake for more than 7 days before her surgery. Because of the severity of malnutrition in this patient, some form of nutrition support is indicated. At present, the problem with the GI tract precludes its use and is not expected to be resolved in 7 to 10 days. PN is indicated.[1]

Gastrointestinal Function

Symptoms such as nausea, vomiting, diarrhea, and abdominal distention or cramps may preclude the use of the GI tract for prolonged periods. The duration of inadequate oral nutrition and semi- or complete starvation that has an impact on patient outcomes is not known. Generally, treatment toxicities in cancer patients that preclude an adequate oral intake for more than a week are an indication for PN.[4] In critically ill patients, PN is indicated if EN is not possible, and hypermetabolism is expected to last more than 4 to 5 days.[21] For the severely malnourished patient, PN is indicated when an impairment of the GI tract occurs. PN is indicated in other conditions precluding the use of the GI tract for more than 7 to 10 days.[20] PN is often used when enteral tube feedings are unsuccessful as evidenced by high residuals or pulmonary aspiration. In some cases, enteral access is contraindicated or attempts at achieving enteral access may have failed. Finally, there are certain conditions where the GI tract should not be used until the underlying problem is treated (Table 14-2).

Clinical Status

PN should only be initiated in patients who are hemodynamically stable and who are able to tolerate the fluid volume, protein, carbohydrate, and IVFE doses necessary to provide adequate nutrient substrate. Examples of situations where PN warrants caution are found in Table 14-3.

These criteria can be easily adapted to a nutritional consultation form designed to educate the clinician requesting PN on the pertinent patient variables that identify a candidate for PN (Figure 14-1). By completing the nutrition consultation request section, the individual requesting PN addresses the previously mentioned criteria.

Specific Guidelines

Gastrointestinal Disorders

PN has not been shown to improve patient outcomes as the primary management of acute exacerbations of Crohn's disease or ulcerative colitis.[3,21] A retrospective analysis of data for PN use in patients with small bowel fistulas suggest an improvement in mortality rates and spontaneous and surgical closures except when the fistula arises from the bowel with active Crohn's disease (see Chapter 26).[3] Data suggest that bowel rest is not necessary to achieve remission in Crohn's disease.[21]

PN is unlikely to benefit patients with mild, acute, or chronic relapsing pancreatitis when the conditions last for less than 1 week.[1,3,26–28] A recent meta-analysis found that PN was not beneficial and was associated with net harm in patients with mild pancreatitis.[29] More recent reviews discuss the favorable response observed with EN in severe acute pancreatitis,[30,31] but evidence is lacking for those patients with more severe disease.[21] Patients who have a protracted course of pancreatitis or those with severe disease or complications often require PN (see Chapter 28); however, there is a paucity of clinical trials determining the optimal route, dose, or nutrient mix.[2]

Perioperative Malnutrition

The stress of surgical procedures produces an abundance of proinflammatory cytokines, which increase metabolic rate and cause catabolism, resulting in a depletion of lean body mass and aberrations in glycemic control. Studies have shown that patients at the highest risk of adverse outcomes postsurgery are those with low visceral protein stores at baseline, specifically, albumin.[17] The ratio of prealbumin to C-reactive protein may predict diminishing inflammation

FIGURE 14-1 Nutrition Assessment and Recommendation Form

Date: Time:	Consulting Service:		
IBW (Kg)	Actual Weight (Kg)	Dosing Weight (Kg)	Recent wt loss (Kg)

Indication
☐ Acute Pancreatitis ☐ SBO ☐ Ileus ☐ Fistula ☐ Short Bowel Syndrome ☐ Intractable Vomiting/Diarrhea
Other:

PMH
☐ DM1 ☐ DM2 ☐ CHF ☐ CRI ☐ ESRD- HD ☐ Liver Disease Other:

Current Medical Problems
☐ Hyperglycemia ☐ Sepsis ☐ Pregnancy ☐ Hyper TG ☐ ARF Other:

Current Medications

Glucose Control	Sedation	GI Meds
☐ Insulin drip: ☐ ICU- SSI every: ☐ SSI ( ) every: ☐ Oral Hypoglycemics: ☐ Octreotide: ☐ Steroids:	☐ Propofol drip:	☐ PPI (IV, po, tube) _____ ☐ H2 blocker: _____

Nutrient Access	Estimated Daily Needs
☐ PICC ☐ Central Line ☐ NG/OG-Tube	Calories:_____ Kcals / day Protein:_____ Grams / day

Baseline nutritional status
☐ Acute Malnutrition (acute injury/illness) ☐ Chronic disease related malnutrition
☐ Chronic Malnutrition (starvation) ☐ Well Nourished at baseline
☐ NPO for 24-72 hours ☐ NPO > 72 hours
☐ Currently receiving enteral nutrition meeting ___% goals

Refeeding risk ☐ Low ☐ Moderate ☐ High

Baseline Labs:

Na	K+	Cl	Bicarb	BUN	Crea	Gluc	Ca	Alb	Corr Ca
Mg	Phos	Chol	Trig	WBC	PLT	Hgb	HCT	PAB	ICa

CrCl: ml/min CBGs:

Impression			
Recommendation/ Formula	☐ Modified/Special Diet	☐ Enteral/Tube Feeding	☐ Parenteral Nutrition
Goals of Therapy	☐ ____ ☐ ____ ☐ ____		
Consult Completed By			

Sample/simulated form that may facilitate nutrition assessment including key components required to diagnose malnutrition, determine the indications for enteral or parenteral nutrition, and establish a nutrition care plan that is documented for the patient.

IBW, ideal body weight; SBO, small bowel obstruction; DM1, type-1 diabetes; DM2, type-2 diabetes; CHF, congestive heart failure; CRI, chronic renal insufficiency; ESRD-HD, end-stage renal disease on hemodialysis; Hyper TG, hypertriglyceridemia; ARF, acute renal failure; ICU, intensive care unit; SSI, sliding-scale insulin; PPI, proton-pump inhibitor; H2 blocker, H-2 receptor antagonist; PICC, peripherally-inserted central catheter; Kcals, kilocalories; Na, sodium; K+, potassium; Cl, chloride; Bicarb, bicarbonate; BUN, blood urea nitrogen; Crea, creatinine; Gluc, glucose; Ca, calcium; Alb, albumin; Corr Ca; corrected calcium; Mg, magnesium; Phos, phosphorus; Chol, cholesterol; Trig, triglycerides; WBC, white blood count; PLT, platelets; HCT, hematocrit; PAB, prealbumin, ICa, ionized calcium; CrCl, creatinine clearance; CBGs, complete blood gases.

TABLE 14-3 Clinical Conditions Warranting Cautious Use of Parenteral Nutrition

Condition	Suggested Criteria[a]
Hyperglycemia	Glucose >300 mg/dL
Azotemia	BUN >100 mg/dL
Hyperosmolality	Serum osmolality >350 mOsm/kg
Hypernatremia	Na >150 mEq/L
Hypokalemia	K <3 mEq/L
Hyperchloremic metabolic acidosis	Cl >115 mEq/L
Hypophosphatemia	Phosphorus <2 mg/dL
Hypochloremic metabolic alkalosis	Cl <85 mEq/L

BUN, blood urea nitrogen; Na, sodium; K, potassium; Cl, chloride.
[a]There is no evidence in the literature of the specific criteria noted in this column. These values are suggestions by the author(s) and should be modified based on the specific patient in question or the environment in which PN is being administered, such as intensive care, general medical ward, long-term care facility, or the home.

and therefore a patient's return to normal anabolic metabolism facilitated by feeding (PN) and subsequent repletion.[32] Well-designed and appropriately timed nutritional support in this population may help attenuate metabolic and oxidative stress and, as a result, improve postsurgical recovery in this patient population. Early nutrition in both the pre- and postoperative phases is associated with better patient outcomes. EN is the preferred form, mainly due to its protective effect on the gastrointestinal mucosal barrier. Parenteral nutrition is reserved for patients with severe malnutrition at baseline, in whom the risk of surgery would outweigh any benefit due to a high risk of postoperative complications, with maximal benefit derived in patients who receive PN for greater than 7 to 10 days.[32]

Critical Illness

Critical illness is characterized by a catabolic state that is generally the result of systemic inflammatory response to infectious or traumatic insult. In this state, gut failure is common due to preferential blood supply to vital organs. Additionally, mesenteric ischemia as a result of hemodynamic compromise and the use of vasopressors is a potential problem not usually seen in other conditions. These facts notwithstanding, the A.S.P.E.N./Society for Critical Care Medicine (SCCM) guidelines recommend the enteral route as the preferred means of nutrition support in this population, with the greatest benefit derived in patients started on enteral feedings within 24 to 48 hours of intensive care unit (ICU) admission. The benefit of EN is largely due to its positive impact on the immune barrier and decreasing the permeability of the GI tract to enteric organisms, which can contribute to the overall detrimental systemic inflammatory response, and due to the fact that the overall risk of causing mesenteric ischemia with introducing EN is, in fact, very low.[17] Expert recommendations place PN as a last line resort in this patient group for those who are unable to attain EN for greater than 7 days, if their baseline nutritional status was normal. Critically ill patients requiring PN are those who are malnourished at baseline and will not reliably ingest or absorb significant amounts of EN for a period of greater than 7 to 10 days, and have been adequately resuscitated from any hemodynamic compromise. Other scenarios where PN is indicated include patients who are hemodynamically stable and have a paralytic ileus, acute GI bleeding, or complete bowel obstruction (see Chapters 23 and 24).

Cancer

Routine PN use in patients receiving chemotherapy or radiation is associated with increased infectious complications and no improvement in clinical response, survival, or toxicity to chemotherapy. A.S.P.E.N. guidelines for the provision of nutritional support in adult patients receiving anticancer therapy recommend a thorough assessment of the patient's nutritional status and the use of PN only in those who are malnourished and are anticipated to be unable to ingest and absorb adequate nutrients for a period of 7 to 14 days.[33] EN is preferred in cancer patients with functional GI tracts. EN is also preferred in patients undergoing a hematopoietic cell transplant as a means to enhance glycemic control in comparison to PN.[33] There are data suggesting favorable outcomes in both of these patient groups with the use of immune-enhancing EN.[34] Until more specific data are available, indications for these patients are similar to those for other conditions (see Chapter 33).

Home Parenteral Nutrition

In general, indications for home PN are the same as for hospitalized patients but with careful consideration of the capabilities of the patient and family members as well as the safety of the home environment for PN. For home PN candidates (see Chapter 37), the duration of PN is prolonged (greater than 2 weeks), and hospitalization is no longer needed for medical reasons. However, federal (Medicare) and state (Medicaid) health care programs have developed criteria that must be met for reimbursement of home PN-associated costs that occur. Medicare requires documentation that the patient's GI tract is nonfunctional ("artificial gut"), and this condition is permanent (at least 90 days of therapy is needed). The patient must also have documented evidence of inability to tolerate enteral feeding (malabsorption, obstruction).

Outcomes of home PN patients vary depending on the underlying disease causing their nonfunctional GI tract. Cancer patients have more frequent PN complications, which are more likely to result in readmission to the hospital.[35] Also, the extent of the disease or its responsiveness to treatment is likely to influence the success of home PN in cancer patients with extensive disease.

Whether PN can be initiated in the home is controversial. Circumstances where the clinical risk warrants caution when considering the initiation of PN in the home are listed in Table 14-4.

TABLE 14-4 Conditions Warranting Caution When Initiating Parenteral Nutrition in the Home

Medical Condition	
	Diabetes mellitus
	Congestive heart failure
	Pulmonary disease
	Severe malnutrition
	Hyperemesis gravidarum
Electrolyte Disorder	
	Hypernatremia
	Hypokalemia
	Hyperchloremic metabolic acidosis
	Hypophosphatemia
	Hypochloremic metabolic alkalosis

The Parenteral Nutrition System

Outcomes from PN are dependent on the system by which it is managed within the health care system. A.S.P.E.N. guidelines provide practical advice for PN[1] use as well as safe practices.[14] As noted, PN is a therapy dependent on an adequate system to order, transcribe, prepare (compound), dispense, and administer.[14] It is a complex therapy requiring trained professionals to initiate and manage. Outcomes are optimized when interdisciplinary care or nutritional support teams manage PN.[36] Unfortunately, although the system is generally safe, when it fails, it is likely to cause patient harm.[36,37]

Pace and colleagues[38] used A.S.P.E.N. guidelines to assess the overuse of PN, the underuse of EN, and the need to update hospital policies and procedures to reflect recent advances and changes in nutrition support practice. A performance model was used to revise policies and procedures and to educate staff. This process resulted in a 52% decrease in PN use over a 4-year period, an increase in appropriate PN use from 74% to 95%, and an elimination of PPN use.

In a tertiary care teaching hospital, PN use was evaluated in 209 patients managed by either individual medical or surgical services or a metabolic support service.[5] Indications for PN were derived from A.S.P.E.N. guidelines.[1] PN therapy was considered to be preventable if there was a functional small bowel but there was no suitable enteral access. Therapy was considered to be contraindicated if the patients were classified as well nourished and had inadequate EN for fewer than 7 days, had a DNR status and were deemed to warrant comfort measures only or were terminally ill, or were receiving adequate EN. Of the PN regimens initiated, 62% were indicated, 23% were preventable, and 15% were not indicated. Compliance to established guidelines was improved when patients were managed by the metabolic support service.[5]

Parenteral nutrition therapy should be reserved for use in patients who are unable to tolerate enteral nutrients for prolonged periods of time due to physical or physiological impediments. PN has historically and again more recently been associated with complications and patient harm ranging from infections due to the introduction of IV catheters and their manipulations, the administration of essentially a viable growth medium, metabolic complications from overfeeding or refeeding, and simply errors that occur during prescription, transcription, or preparation.[14,39] In response to these errors, guidelines and expert recommendations have been developed in an attempt to curb harm resulting from PN use. Although the overall error rates may have decreased with the use of these recommendations, errors still occur and occasionally result in patient harm. This was recently shown by Sacks and colleagues[40] in a prospective observational study, where, in a cohort of 4730 prescriptions for PN, there were 74 (1.6%) errors, an overall error rate of 15.6/1000 PN prescriptions compounded. Of these errors, 67 (91%) were classified as nonharmful, whereas 6 (8%) resulted in temporary harm to a patient. Most errors occurred during the transcription and administration phase in this study. As suggested by the work of Sacks and colleagues, the incorporation of nutrition guidelines may help decrease error rates. In addition, the use of a multistep double check process that requires the verification of an electronically transcribed order against the actual written order may significantly decrease error rates.

In addition to incorporating systematic procedures for electronically transcribing and compounding PN accurately, the use of multidisciplinary teams in the ordering phase has been shown to be beneficial in ensuring the appropriate use of PN. See Practice Scenarios 14-2 through 14-5 for discussions of proper initiation, advancement, monitoring, and discontinuation of PN. In a recent study querying PN practices in statewide hospitals, results indicated that nutrition support teams and certified nutrition support clinicians can help cut down the inappropriate use of PN, and as a result, incur huge cost savings. In this particular study, of the 278 PN cases reviewed by registered dietitians, PN was inappropriately prescribed in 32% of cases, resulting in 552 days and $138,000 in preventable hospital costs.[41]

A recent review by Taylor and colleagues also suggests that the incorporation of a dietitian in the care of critically ill patients leads to a higher quality assessment of these patients' nutritional needs.[45] Dietitians are vital in thoroughly assessing patients' nutritional, fluid, and electrolyte needs as well as suggesting the appropriate route and timing of nutrition provision. Additionally, through the vast amount of research that dietitians have led, they have provided insight into the achievement of optimal blood glucose control and the use of specialized nutrition. They help adjust patients' nutrition plans according to changes in physiological status.[41]

A.S.P.E.N. guidelines are useful in identifying that the patient is likely to benefit from PN. CPN provides adequate nutrients to maintain and replete the patient's nutritional stores. PPN may be useful for limited periods in maintaining nutritional status until the GI tract is functional. Prospective randomized controlled studies have failed to provide significant evidence of PN benefits. Favorable physiological effects have been observed, but the impact on patient outcomes, such as the infection rate, the length of stay, and mortality, is not frequently reported. A meta-analysis of PN suggests that this route of nutrition support increases infection rates without measurable beneficial outcomes when compared with controls.[20,21] Still, malnutrition is a common comorbidity that influences a patient's response to treatment and outcomes.[27] Therefore, PN should be considered in those patients in whom the enteral route is contraindicated or in whom a trial of enteral feeding has failed.

TABLE 14-5 Suggested Monitoring for Parenteral Nutrition[6,44]

Parameter	Baseline	Initiation	Critically Ill Patients	Stable Patients
CBC with differential	Yes		Weekly	Weekly
INR, PT, PTT	Yes		Weekly	Weekly
Electrolytes: Na, K, Cl, CO_2 Mg, Ca, phosphorus, BUN, Cr	Yes	Daily × 3	Daily	1–2 × per week
Serum triglycerides	Yes	Day 1	Weekly	Weekly
Transferrin or prealbumin	Yes		Weekly	Weekly
Serum glucose	Yes	Daily × 3	Daily	1–2 × per week
Capillary glucose		As needed	At least 3 × day until consistent less than 150 mg/dL	As needed
Weight	Yes	Daily	Daily	2–3 × per week
Intake and output	Yes	Daily	Daily	Daily unless fluid status assessed by physical exam
ALT, AST, ALP, total bilirubin	Yes	Day 1	Weekly	Monthly
Nitrogen balance	As needed		As needed	As needed

ALP, alkaline phosphatase; ALT, alanine aminotransferase; AST, aspartate aminotransferase; BUN, blood urea nitrogen; CBC, complete blood cell count; Cl, chloride; CO_2, bicarbonate; Cr, serum creatinine; INR, International Normalized Ratio; K, potassium; Na, sodium; PT, prothrombin time; PTT, partial thromboplastin time.

Practice Scenario 14-2

Question: How should PN be initiated?

Scenario: PN is to be initiated in a 53-year-old male who has chronic disease-related malnutrition and a complete bowel obstruction. Nutritional and metabolic parameters in the patient are provided in table below.

Intervention: PN is initiated at a low rate (100 g dextrose per day) with a supplemental dose of phosphorus prior to start and an increased dose in PN.

Answer: A favorable clinical response to PN may be delayed by the patient's catabolic state. Glucose and phosphorus problems should be corrected prior to initiating PN. Then, PN should be initiated slowly beginning at a low caloric dose.

Rationale: The metabolic response to stress or injury (see Chapters 23 and 24) influences the efficiency by which nutrients are incorporated into the body. Also, the tolerance to nutrition support is influenced by abnormalities in carbohydrate, protein, and fat metabolism that are characterized in the stressed patient as hyperglycemia, insulin resistance, uremia, encephalopathy, hyperosmolality, and hypertriglyceridemia. Severe deficits in electrolytes (see Chapter 7) may be present and exacerbated by the initiation of a parenteral feeding formulation. Caution in initiating PN in some conditions is warranted (Table 14-3). The patient's laboratory data demonstrate an increased serum glucose and hypophosphatemia. Both of these conditions should be corrected before initiating PN and should be addressed in the PN formula. Answering the questions addressed on the Nutrition Consultation Form (Figure 14-1) not only assists with determining the appropriate indication for PN, but also establishes a framework by which PN may be safely initiated. This patient is severely malnourished and, as such, at significant risk of developing refeeding syndrome.[42] PN should be initiated slowly beginning at a low caloric dose. Electrolyte abnormalities should be corrected before initiating PN. Nutritional and metabolic parameters in the patient are provided below.

Practice Scenario 14-3

Question: When can PN be advanced to the goal infusion rate?

Scenario: PN is initiated in a 61-year-old female who has a history of type 2 diabetes.

Intervention: PN is initiated at a low caloric dose. The following morning, the patient's blood glucose concentration was in the range of 210 to 240 mg/dL. The patient's blood pressure and other vital signs are within acceptable parameters.

WBC 9.6 × 10^9/L	Na 135 mEq/L	K 4.1 mEq/L	Cl 103 mEq/L	CO_2 24 mmol/L
BUN 6 mg/dL	Cr 1.1 mg/dL	Gluc 234 mg/dL	Mg 1.8 mEq/L	Ca 9.8 mg/dL
Phosphorus 1.5 mg/dL	Prealbumin 2 mg/dL	Wt Loss 20 kg	% Wt loss 14%	Time of Wt change: 45 d

WBC, white blood cell; BUN, blood urea nitrogen; Na, sodium; Cr, creatinine; K, potassium; Gluc, glucose; Wt, weight; Cl, chloride; Mg, magnesium; CO_2, bicarbonate; Ca, calcium.

Answer: PN should be advanced only when the following criteria are met: stable blood pressure, pulse, and respiration rates; and normal serum phosphorus, potassium, and glucose concentrations. The best practice is to control the patient's blood glucose before advancing the rate of PN to its goal rate. A reasonable goal for blood glucose is 100 to 200 mg/dL.[12]

Rationale: PN contributes significantly to the fluid intake of the patient. Therefore, those with a limited cardiac function may not tolerate the PN infusion. The patient should be assessed for signs and symptoms of congestive heart failure and pulmonary edema. In addition, vital signs such as blood pressure and pulse may be adversely affected by PN. A useful guide would be not to advance the parenteral feeding formulation rate until the following criteria are met: stable blood pressure, pulse, and respiration rates; and normal serum phosphorus, potassium, and glucose concentrations. Hyperglycemia is frequently encountered in patients receiving PN (see Chapter 17).[43] The dextrose content of IV fluids and medications may contribute to excessive glucose administration in patients receiving PN.[12] The best practice is to control the patient's blood glucose before advancing the rate of PN to its goal rate.

Practice Scenario 14-4

Question: Once PN is infusing at its goal rate, what approach to monitoring should be taken?

Scenario: PN is advanced to the goal rate in a patient with normal renal function but a gastrointestinal fistula draining 800 mL per day. Laboratory values are normal after the acute replacement of potassium and magnesium and a correction of a metabolic acidosis.

Intervention: Follow-up labs are drawn on a daily/as needed basis, and capillary blood glucose checks continue four times a day with sliding scale insulin coverage.

Answer: Initially, fluid, electrolyte, and renal status should be monitored daily. Routinely, blood glucose monitoring should be conducted on a daily basis. Metabolic parameters (triglycerides and liver function tests) should be obtained periodically. The effectiveness of PN may be assessed, measuring serum visceral proteins on a weekly basis and determining nitrogen balance in patients with functioning kidneys and adequate urine output.

Rationale: Because PN may be a large source of fluid and electrolytes as well as other nutrients, serum levels of electrolytes, BUN, creatinine, and glucose should be assessed daily during the initial period of PN therapy. Patients receiving PN may be predisposed to fluid and electrolyte disturbances because of fluid losses from the GI tract, drug therapy such as diuretics, and electrolyte losses during periods of semi- or complete starvation. Other parameters of fluid and electrolyte status that are important to consider in monitoring the electrolyte content of PN are fluid intakes and outputs as well as daily weights in combination with physical assessment for signs and symptoms of dehydration or edema.

Metabolic disturbances are frequent in patients receiving PN. In addition to serum electrolytes and blood glucose monitoring, the periodic assessment of serum triglycerides is necessary if IVFE is administered. Abnormal hepatic function has also been associated with PN. Hepatic function should be assessed before initiating PN and then weekly.[11] Laboratory tests and a specific assessment along with the frequency of monitoring are outlined in Table 14-5.[44]

Practice Scenario 14-5

Question: When and how should PN therapy be discontinued?

Intervention: Following a surgical procedure for a bowel obstruction and the drainage of intra-abdominal abscess, PN is initiated in a 65-year-old woman. On postoperative day 8, nasogastric tube output dramatically declines, the patient is noted to have bowel sounds, and she has a bowel movement. The nasogastric tube was removed and orogastric tube feedings were initiated at this time.

Answer: PN may be discontinued when the patient is able to meet and tolerate an adequate percentage of their estimated energy and protein needs via the enteral route.

Rationale: The goal of PN therapy is to maintain the nutritional status of the patient until some form of EN is tolerated. The exception is the critically ill patient in whom therapy is withdrawn during the terminal stages of their disease process. In most other situations, the problem with the GI tract resolves or the appropriate enteral access is obtained. PN is tapered as the amount of reliable enteral intake increases. It may be discontinued when the patient is able to consume solid food or when an adequate percentage of his or her estimated energy and protein needs is tolerated.[4] In this patient, enteral tube feedings were initiated 8 days after the operation and was advanced to the goal infusion rate within 72 hours of initiation. PN therapy was decreased by 50% on postoperative day 9 and was discontinued on postoperative day 10.

To prevent rebound hypoglycemia, PN may be tapered over 1 to 2 hours. If PN needs to be stopped emergently, dextrose 10% in water should be infused at either the same rate as the PN or at 50 mL/h or more. When cyclic PN infusion is used in the home, some form of tapering is usually required during the last 2 hours of the cycle. Finally, PN may be rapidly discontinued if the patient is tolerating tube feeding in amounts adequate to maintain normal blood glucose levels.

References

1. A.S.P.E.N. Board of Directors and The Clinical Guidelines Task Force. Guidelines for the use of parenteral and enteral nutrition in adult and pediatric patients. *J Parenter Enteral Nutr.* 2002:26 (1 suppl):1SA–138SA.
2. A.S.P.E.N. Board of Directors. Guidelines for the use of parenteral and enteral nutrition in adult and pediatric patients. *J Parenter Enteral Nutr.* 1993;17(4):1SA–52SA.
3. Klein S, Kinney J, Jeejeebhoy K, et al. Nutrition support in clinical practice: review of published data and recommendations for future research directions. Summary of a conference sponsored by the National Institutes of Health, American Society for Parenteral and Enteral Nutrition, and American Society for Clinical Nutrition. *J Parenter Enteral Nutr.* 1997;2:133–156. Review.PMID:9168367
4. Weisdorf SA, Lysne J, Wind D, et al. Positive effect of prophylactic total parenteral nutrition on long-term outcome of bone marrow transplantation. *Transplantation.* 1987;43(6):833–838.

5. Trujillo EB, Young LS, Chertow GM, et al. Metabolic and monetary costs of avoidable parenteral nutrition use. *JPEN J Parenter Enteral Nutr.* 1999;23(2):109–113.
6. Sacks GS, Mayhew S, Johnson D. Parenteral nutrition implementation and management. In: Merritt R, et al. *The A.S.P.E.N. Nutrition Support Practice Manual.* 2nd ed. Silver Spring, MD: American Society for Parenteral and Enteral Nutrition; 2005:108–117.
7. Dudrick SJ, Wilmore DW, Vars HM, Rhoads JE. Long-term total parenteral nutrition with growth, development, and positive nitrogen balance. *Surgery.* 1968;64(1):134–142.
8. Dudrick SJ. Early developments and clinical applications of total parenteral nutrition. *JPEN J Parenter Enteral Nutr.* 2003;27(4): 291–299.
9. Rhoads JE, Dudrick SJ. History of intravenous nutrition. In: Rombeau JL, Caldwell MD, eds. *Clinical Nutrition, Parenteral Nutrition.* 2nd ed. Philadelphia, PA: Saunders; 1993:1–10.
10. Lumpkin MM. Safety alert: hazards of precipitation associated with parenteral nutrition. *Am J Hosp Pharm.* 1994;51(11): 1427–1428.
11. Btaiche IF, Khalidi N. Metabolic complications of parenteral nutrition in adults, Part 2. *Am J Health Syst Pharm.* 2004;61(19): 2050–2059.
12. Pleva M, Mirtallo JM, Steinberg SM. Hyperglycemic events in non-intensive care unit patients receiving parenteral nutrition. *Nutr Clin Pract.* 2009;24(5):626–634.
13. Nehme AE. Nutritional support of the hospitalized patient. *JAMA.* 1980;283(19):1906–1908.
14. Mirtallo J, Canada T, Johnson D, et al. Safe practices for parenteral nutrition. *JPEN J Parenter Enteral Nutr.* 2004;28(6):S39–S70.
15. Anderson ADG, Palmer D, MacFie J. Peripheral parenteral nutrition. *Br J Surg.* 2003; 90(9):1048–1054.
16. Pittiruti M, Hamilton H, Biffi R, et al. ESPEN Guidelines on Parenteral Nutrition: central venous catheters (access, care, diagnosis and therapy of complications. *Clin Nutr.* 2009;28(4): 365–377.
17. McClave SA, Martindale RG, Vanek VW, et al. Guideline for the provision and assessment of nutrition support therapy in the adult critically ill patient. Society for Critical Care Medicine (SCCM) and American Society for Parenteral and Enteral Nutrition (A.S.P.E.N.). *JPEN J Parenter Enter Nutr.* 2009;33(3):277–316.
18. Choban PS, Dickerson RN. Morbid obesity and nutrition support: Is bigger different? *Nutr Clin Pract.* 2005;20(4):480–487.
19. Heidegger CP, Romand JA, Treggiori MM, Pichard C. Is it now time to promote mixed enteral and parenteral nutrition for the critically ill? *Intensive Care Med.* 2007;33(6):963–969.
20. Dempsey DT, Mullen JL, Buzby GP. The link between nutritional status and clinical outcome. Can nutritional intervention modify it? *Am J Clin Nutr.* 1988;47(2 Suppl):352–356.
21. Koretz RL, Lipman TO, Klein S. AGA technical review: parenteral nutrition. *Gastroenterology.* 2001;121(4):970–1001.
22. Detsky AS, Baker JP, O'Rourke K, Goel V. Perioperative parenteral nutrition. A meta-analysis. *Ann Intern Med.* 1987;107(2):195–203.
23. Compher CW, Spencer C, Kinosian B. Perioperative parenteral nutrition: impact on morbidity and mortality in surgical patients. *Nutr Clin Pract.* 2005;20(4):460–467.
24. Twomey PL, Patching SC. Cost effectiveness of nutritional support. *JPEN J Parenter Enteral Nutr.* 1985;9(1):3–10.
25. Mullen JL, Buzby GP, Matthews DC, Smale BF, Rosato EF. Reduction of operative morbidity and mortality by combined preoperative and postoperative nutrition support. *Ann Surg.* 1980;192(5):604–613.
26. Kalfarentzos F, Kehagias J, Mead N, Kokkinis K, Gogos CA. Enteral nutrition is superior to parenteral nutrition in severe acute pancreatitis: results of a randomized prospective trial. *Br J Surg.* 1997; 84(12):1665–1669.
27. McClave SA, Greene LM, Snider HL, et al. Comparison of the safety of early enteral versus parenteral nutrition in mild acute pancreatitis. *JPEN J Parenter Enteral Nutr.* 1997;21(1):14–20.
28. Windsor AC, Kanwar S, Li AG, et al. Compared with parenteral nutrition, enteral feeding attenuates the acute phase response and improves disease severity in acute pancreatitis. *Gut.* 1998;42(3): 431–435.
29. Al-Omran M, Groof A, Wilke D. Enteral versus parenteral nutrition for acute pancreatitis. *Cochrane Database Syst Rev.* 2003;(1): CD002837.
30. Avgerinos C, Delis S, Rizos S, Dervenis C. Nutritional support in acute pancreatitis. *Dig Dis.* 2003;21(3):214–219.
31. Alsolaiman MM, Green JA, Barkin JS. Should enteral feeding be the standard of care for acute pancreatitis? *Am J Gastroenterol.* 2003;98(11):2565–2567.
32. Kudsk KA, Tolley EA, DeWitt RC, et al. Preoperative albumin and surgical site identify surgical risk for major postoperative complications. *JPEN J Parenter Enteral Nutr.* 2003;27(1):1–9.
33. August DA, Huhmann MB. A.S.P.E.N. Clinical Guidelines: Nutrition support therapy during adult anticancer treatment and in hematopoietic cell transplantation. *JPEN J Parenter Enteral Nutr.* 2009;33(5):472–500.
34. Braga M, Gianotti L, Vignali A, Carlo VD. Preoperative oral arginine and n-3 fatty acid supplementation improves the immunometabolic host response and outcome after colorectal resection for cancer. *Surgery.* 2002;132(5):805–814.
35. Hurley RS, Campbell SM, Mirtallo JM, Wade VR, Murphy C. Outcomes of cancer and non-cancer patients on HPN. *Nutr Clin Pract.* 1990;5(2):59–62.
36. A.S.P.E.N. Practice Management Task Force, DeLegge M, Wooley JA, Guenter P, et al. The state of nutrition support teams and update on current models for providing nutrition support therapy to patients. *Nutr Clin Pract.* 2010;25(1):76–84.
37. Seres D, Sacks GS, Pedersen CA, et al. Parenteral nutrition safe practices: results of the 2003 American Society for Parenteral and Enteral Nutrition survey. *JPEN J Parenter Enter Nutr.* 2006;30(3):259–265.
38. Pace NM, Long JB, Elerding S, et al. Performance model anchors successful nutrition support protocol. *Nutr Clin Pract.* 1997;12(6): 274–279.
39. Dimick JB, Swoboda S, Talamini MA, et al. Risk of colonization of central venous catheters: catheters for total parenteral nutrition vs catheters for other purposes. *Am J Crit Care.* 2003;12(4):328–335.
40. Sacks GS, Rough S, Kudsk KA. Frequency and severity of harm of medication errors related to the parenteral nutrition process in a large university teaching hospital. *Pharmacotherapy.* 2009;29(8): 966–974.
41. Martin K, DeLegge M, Nichols M, et al. Assessing appropriate nutrition ordering practices in tertiary care medical centers. *JPEN J Parenter Enter Nutr.* 2011;35(1):122–130.
42. Kraft MD, Btaiche IF, Sacks GS. Review of the refeeding syndrome. *Nutr Clin Pract.* 2005;20(6):625–633.
43. Rosemarin DK, Wardlaw GM, Mirtallo JM. Hyperglycemia associated with high, continuous infusion rates of total parenteral nutrition dextrose. *Nutr Clin Pract.* 1996;11(4):151–156.
44. A.S.P.E.N. Board of Directors. *A.S.P.E.N.'s Adult Parenteral Nutrition (PN) Support Pathway.* Silver Spring, MD: American Society for Parenteral and Enteral Nutrition; 1998.
45. Taylor B, Renfro A, Mehringer L. The role of the dietitian in the intensive care unit. *Curr Opin Clin Nutr Met Care.* 2005; Mar 8 (2): 211-216.

15 Parenteral Nutrition Formulations

Jacqueline R. Barber, PharmD, BCNSP, FASHP, and Gordon S. Sacks, PharmD, BCNSP, FCCP

CONTENTS

Formulation Components 246
Energy Substrates 247
Protein 247
Electrolytes 248
Vitamins 248
Trace Elements 248
Parenteral Nutrition Product Shortages 248
Disease-Specific Formulations/Special Nutrients 249
Modified Amino Acid Formulations 249
Glutamine 251
Omega-6 Fat Emulsions/Structured Lipids 251
Omega-3 and Omega-9 Fat Emulsions 251
Carnitine 252
Parenteral Nutrition Preparation 252
Admixtures: Dextrose-Amino Acids Versus Total Nutrient Admixtures 252
National Standards for Compounded Sterile Preparations 253
Automated Compounding Devices 254
Quality Control for the Preparation of Parenteral Nutrition Admixtures 255
Premixed Parenteral Nutrition Formulations 255
Stability/Compatibility of Parenteral Nutrition Formulations 256
Stability of Intravenous Fat Emulsion and Total Nutrient Admixture Formulations 256
Calcium and Phosphate 258
Medication Additives 259
Use of Filters 259
Control of Aluminum Contamination 259
Calculation of Parenteral Nutrient Formulations 262
References 262

Objectives

1. List 12 components typically incorporated into a parenteral nutrition (PN) formulation.
2. Summarize the major differences in commercially available crystalline amino acid formulations.
3. Compare and contrast the dextrose-amino acids (2-in-1) system for PN versus the total nutrient admixture (TNA) system in terms of convenience, stability and compatibility, and potential to support microbial growth if contaminated.
4. Describe the factors that influence the stability of PN formulations.
5. Explain the benefits of in-line filtration for PN formulations.
6. Perform calculations to construct a practical PN regimen given a patient's specific macrosubstrate needs.
7. List guidelines for "hang times" of various PN components.

Test Your Knowledge Questions

1. Which of the following may increase the risk of phlebitis with peripherally administered parenteral nutrition (PPN)?
   A. Osmolarity ≤900 mOsm/L
   B. Potassium 100 mEq/L
   C. Intravenous fat emulsion (IVFE) piggybacked with PPN
   D. Addition of heparin to the PPN
2. The smallest pore size filter that is recommended for TNA is
   A. 0.22 μm
   B. 0.5 μm
   C. 1.2 μm
   D. 5 μm
3. Which of the following will increase the solubility of calcium and phosphate in a PN formulation?
   A. Use of calcium as the chloride salt
   B. Use of phosphate as the sodium salt
   C. Increased amino acid concentration
   D. Increased temperature
4. According to recommendations by the National Advisory Group on Standards and Practice Guidelines for Parenteral Nutrition Formulations, the amount of dextrose used in preparation of a PN formulation is required to appear on the label as:
   A. The percent of original concentration and volume (eg, dextrose 50% water, 500 mL)
   B. The percent of final concentration after admixture (eg, dextrose 25%)
   C. Grams per liter of PN admixed (eg, dextrose 250 g per liter)
   D. Grams per day (eg, dextrose 250 g per day)
5. A patient requires approximately 70 g of protein and 1700 total kcal per day. Which of the following regimens would most closely supply this patient's needs?
   A. Manually compounded mix of equal volumes of dextrose 30% water and amino acids 8.5% (initial concentrations used in compounding) to infuse at 70 mL per hour with IVFE 10%, 500 mL per day, piggybacked in the PN line
   B. Manually compounded mix of equal volumes of dextrose 50% water and amino acids 10% (initial concentrations used in compounding) to infuse at 60 mL per hour with IVFE 20%, 300 mL per day, piggybacked in the PN line
   C. TNA containing amino acids 10%, 700 mL, dextrose 50% water, 650 mL, and IVFE 20%, 300 mL per daily bag
   D. TNA containing amino acids 8.5%, 850 mL, dextrose 30% water, 600 mL, and IVFE 10%, 500 mL per daily bag

Test Your Knowledge Answers

1. The correct answer is **B**. Potassium can be quite irritating to peripheral veins. Potassium in concentrations less than 60 mEq per liter and preferably less than 40 mEq per liter is generally suggested for fluids administered via the peripheral vein. All of the other choices may actually *decrease* the risk of phlebitis.[1–4]
2. The correct answer is **C**. The 1.2-μm filter is not a sterilizing filter, but it will remove large microorganisms such as *Candida albicans* and large particles that might otherwise lodge in pulmonary capillaries if allowed to pass through. A 0.22-μm filter is used for the 2-in-1 dextrose and amino acid type of PN, and this does qualify as a sterilizing filter. Because the size of fat particles is generally between 0.1 μm and 1 μm, IVFE could occlude 0.22-μm and 0.5-μm filters, or the emulsion could be destabilized if used with these filters. The 5-μm filter removes particulate matter but would allow many types of microbial contaminants to pass through.[5]
3. The correct answer is **C**. The higher the concentration of amino acids in the formulation, the less likely precipitation is to occur. Amino acids can form soluble complexes with calcium, which reduce the effective concentrations of free calcium available to form insoluble precipitates with phosphorus ions. Calcium chloride is more dissociated than calcium gluconate, making the risk of precipitation with phosphate higher. The salt form of phosphate does not affect calcium solubility if the phosphate amount remains constant; that is, 1 mmol of phosphate as the sodium salt has the same potential to precipitate with calcium as 1 mmol of phosphate as the potassium salt. However, there is more phosphate per milliequivalent of sodium as phosphate (4 mEq sodium to 3 mmol phosphorus) than per milliequivalent of potassium as phosphate (4.4 mEq potassium to 3 mmol phosphate). Precipitation is more likely to occur at warmer temperatures because the increased dissociation of calcium salts occurs as the temperature rises, promoting the availability of ions to form insoluble complexes with phosphate.[6]
4. The correct answer is **D**. Grams of dextrose per day is most consistent with that of a nutrient label, supports the use of the 24-hour nutrient infusion system, and requires the least number of calculations to determine the calories per day. Using the quantity per liter is an option that may appear on the label by adding a second column reflecting quantities per liter in parentheses.
5. The correct answer is **A**. At 70 mL per hour × 24 hour per day, a total of 1680 mL of dextrose/amino acids formulation will be infused each day, or dextrose 30% water, 840 mL, plus amino acids 8.5%, 840 mL. Dextrose 30% water, 840 mL, provides 30 g/100 mL = x g/840 mL; solving for x yields dextrose 252 g. This represents 252 g × 3.4 kcal per gram = 857 dextrose kcal. Amino acids 8.5%, 840 mL, provides 8.5 g/100 mL = x g/840 mL; solving for x yields amino acids 71 g, which supplies 284 kcal. IVFE 10%, 500 mL, supplies 500 mL × 1.1 kcal per milliliter or 550 kcal. Thus, the total kilocalories from this regimen is 857 + 284 + 550 = 1691 kcal. Answer B supplies 2112 kcal and amino acids 72 g. Answer C supplies 1985 kcal and amino acids 70 g. Answer D supplies 1451 kcal and amino acids 72 g.

Formulation Components

Components used in formulating PN typically include energy substrates such as carbohydrate, protein as amino acids and fat, as well as electrolytes, vitamins, and trace elements. Sterile water for injection may be added to provide necessary volume to the PN formulation. Various combinations of these components are incorporated into the regimen for intravenous (IV) administration based on the patient's individual requirements.

Energy Substrates

The most commonly used carbohydrate energy substrate is dextrose, which in its hydrated form, provides 3.4 kcal per gram. Dextrose is commercially available in multiple concentrations ranging from 2.5% to 70% as well as in combinations with other components of the PN formulation. According to the United States Pharmacopoeia (USP), dextrose solutions are acidic, with a pH ranging from 3.5 to 6.5, and vary in osmolarity depending on their concentration. Higher dextrose concentrations (greater than 10%) are generally reserved for central venous administration due to the propensity to cause thrombophlebitis in peripheral veins.[7]

Another carbohydrate energy substrate used less frequently is glycerol, a sugar alcohol that provides 4.3 kcal per gram. Glycerol, or glycerin, is contained in one premixed PN formulation marketed for peripheral administration. This formulation has been shown to be protein sparing and has been reported to induce less insulin response than dextrose-based regimens, although another study found the opposite to be true.[8–10] A brief discussion of rationales for the clinical use of this product is included in the section on peripheral PN (PPN) composition and preparation.

Lipids or intravenous fat emulsions (IVFEs) are used to provide energy as well as essential fatty acids for PN formulations. In the United States, IVFE components include 100% soybean oil or 50:50 mixes of soybean and safflower oils, egg yolk phospholipid as an emulsifier, glycerin to render the formulation isotonic, vitamin K, and sodium hydroxide to adjust the final pH (range 6 to 9).[11] IVFEs are commercially available in 10% (1.1 kcal per milliliter), 20% (2 kcal per milliliter), and 30% (2.9 to 3 kcal per milliliter, depending on the manufacturer) concentrations. Of these, the IVFE 30% formulation is only approved for the compounding of TNA, not for direct IV administration. Each gram of fat provides 9 kcal; however, the glycerol in IVFE adds calories such that each milliliter of fat in IVFE 10% is equivalent to 11 kcal, whereas each milliliter of fat in IVFE 20% and 30% is equivalent to 10 kcal.

Due to enhanced microbial growth potential with the infusion of IVFE separate from formulations that contain dextrose and amino acids, the Centers for Disease Control and Prevention (CDC) recommends a 12 hour hang-time limit for IVFE.[12] The USP has also endorsed using IVFE products within 12 hours of opening the original manufacturer's container if IVFEs are infused as separate preparations from dextrose and amino acids.[13] However, an admixture containing IVFE, dextrose, and amino acids in the same container may be administered over 24 hours. TNA, all-in-one (AIO), or 3-in-1 are terms used to describe this type of formulation in which all three base formula components (dextrose, amino acids, IVFEs) are combined together in one container. The hang time and infusion of this formulation is extended compared with an infusion of IVFEs alone because bacterial growth is inhibited due to reduced pH (pH approximately 5.6 to 6) and because of the increased total osmolarity with the combination of all three substrates in one container. Whether infused separately from amino acids and dextrose or as a TNA, the IVFE infusion rate should not exceed 0.11 g per kilogram per hour.[14] Greater infusion rates are associated with an increased risk of side effects such as hypertriglyceridemia and infectious complications.

Protein

Crystalline amino acids are used in PN formulations to provide protein and yield 4 kcal per gram if oxidized for energy. Nitrogen content varies depending on the concentration of the amino acid formulation and the mixture of individual amino acids; however, for nitrogen balance calculations, amino acid products are generally assumed to be 16% nitrogen (6.25 g protein = 1 g nitrogen). Standard or balanced amino acid products are mixtures of essential and nonessential amino acids. They are available from different manufacturers in stock solutions with concentrations ranging from 3% to 20%, although 8.5%, 10%, and 15% are most frequently used for PN compounding. Modified or specialty amino acid products are specifically formulated for certain disease states or special conditions (Table 15-1).[7] Commercially available amino acid formulations may also contain various concentrations and combinations of electrolytes and/or buffers, in addition to the inherent or endogenous electrolyte content of the individual amino acids.

Table 15-1 Commercially Available Crystalline Amino Acid Solutions

Brand Name	Type/Indication	Stock Concentrations
Travasol	Standard	3.5%, 4.25%, 5.5%, 8.5%, 10%
Clinisol	Standard/fluid restriction	15%
ProSol	Standard/fluid restriction	20%
Aminosyn II	Standard	3.5%, 4.25%, 5%, 7%, 8.5%, 10%, 15%
FreAmine III	Standard	8.5%, 10%
HepatAmine	Hepatic failure	8%
Hepatasol	Hepatic failure	8%
FreAmine HBC	Metabolic stress	6.9%
Aminosyn HBC	Metabolic stress	7%
BranchAmine[a]	Metabolic stress	4%
NephrAmine[b]	Renal failure	5.4%
Aminess[b]	Renal failure	5.2%
Aminosyn RF[c]	Renal failure	5.2%
RenAmin[d]	Renal failure	6.5%

[a]Contains branched chain amino acids only (leucine, isoleucine, and valine).
[b]Contains essential amino acids only.
[c]Contains essential amino acids plus arginine.
[d]Contains essential amino acids and some nonessential amino acids.

Table 15-2 Daily Electrolyte Requirements[5]

Electrolyte	Parenteral
Sodium	1–2 mEq/kg
Potassium	1–2 mEq/kg
Chloride	As needed to maintain acid–base balance
Acetate	As needed to maintain acid–base balance
Calcium	10–15 mEq
Magnesium	8–20 mEq
Phosphate	20–40 mmol

Electrolytes

Maintenance or therapeutic amounts of various electrolytes are added to PN formulations depending on the patient's requirements. Standard daily ranges for adults are listed in Table 15-2.[5] Acetate and chloride do not have specific ranges for intake; rather, they are adjusted as needed to maintain acid–base balance.[5] Electrolytes are also available in various salt forms (Table 15-3). Calcium gluconate and magnesium sulfate are the preferred forms of these cations for use in PN formulations because they are less likely to produce physicochemical incompatibilities compared to calcium chloride, calcium gluceptate, and magnesium chloride. Electrolytes are available commercially as individual salts and as "cocktails" (or combination products) for ease in admixing. They are also preadded in specified amounts to certain stock amino acid formulations or premixed PN formulations.

Vitamins

Commercially available vitamin products for PN supplementation include single vitamin products and multivitamin products that include both fat-soluble and water-soluble vitamins. Injectable multivitamin products for use in adults include ascorbic acid, retinol, ergocalciferol, thiamin, riboflavin, pyridoxine, niacinamide, dexpanthenol, dl-alpha tocopheryl acetate, folic acid, cyanocobalamin, biotin, and phylloquinone. However, parenteral formulations for single vitamins are not commercially available for biotin, pantothenic acid, riboflavin, vitamin A, vitamin D, and vitamin E. Table 15-4 lists the composition of adult parenteral multivitamin products available in the United Sates.[15,16] Micronutrient requirements and clinical indications are reviewed in Chapter 8.

Table 15-3 Commercially Available Parenteral Electrolyte Salts

Electrolyte	Salt Form
Sodium	Chloride, acetate, phosphate
Potassium	Chloride, acetate, phosphate
Chloride	Sodium, potassium
Acetate	Sodium, potassium
Calcium	Gluconate, gluceptate, chloride[a]
Magnesium	Sulfate, chloride[a]

[a]Preferred salt form for use in parenteral nutrition formulations.

Table 15-4 Composition of Adult Parenteral Multivitamin Products Available in the United States[a]

Component	Dose
Ascorbic acid	200 mg
Retinol	1 mg (3300 USP units)
Ergocalciferol	5 mcg (200 USP units)
Thiamin	6 mg
Riboflavin	3.6 mg
Pyridoxine	6 mg
Niacinamide	40 mg
Dexpanthenol	15 mg
dl-alpha Tocopheryl acetate	10 mg (10 USP units)
Biotin	60 mcg
Folic acid	600 mcg
Cyanocobalamin	5 mcg
Phylloquinone	150 mcg

[a]Note: One manufacturer provides a product that is phylloquinone free.
USP, United States Pharmacopeia.

Trace Elements

Commonly used trace elements in PN formulations include zinc, copper, chromium, manganese, and selenium. These are commercially available as single-entity products and in various multiple trace element combinations and concentrations for adults, pediatrics, and neonates. Other trace elements that may be supplemented in PN include molybdenum, iodine, and iron.[17] Four injectable iron products are available, all as single-entity products. Only iron dextran is approved for addition to PN, but this should only be considered for dextrose-amino acid formulations because IVFEs are disrupted by iron.[18]

Parenteral Nutrition Product Shortages

PN product shortages have occurred in the United States due to a variety of factors, including acquisition issues with raw materials, manufacturing/production interruptions, and consolidation of the market. The American Society for Parenteral and Enteral Nutrition (A.S.P.E.N.) assembled a group of experts to establish guidelines for managing shortages of IVFEs, amino acids, multivitamins, electrolyte/mineral injections, and trace element products (Tables 15-5 through 15-9).[19–23] Recommendations should only be used in the event of a national shortage of these products and should not be employed during routine (nonshortage) clinical practice. Although there are no substitutions for these products, dose conservation and alternate measures can be used during the shortage period. See Practice Scenario 15-1 for an example of dealing with a PN product shortage.

Table 15-5 Considerations for Use of Intravenous Fat Emulsions (IVFE) in Adults During a National Shortage[19]

- IVFEs should not be administered to adult, mild to moderately undernourished hospitalized patients on PN less than 2 weeks.
- Adult, hospitalized patients on PN longer than 2 weeks should receive a total of 100 g of fat per week in order to avoid essential fatty acid deficiency (EFAD).
- No additional IVFE is necessary in adult, hospitalized critically ill patients receiving propofol.
- Home or long-term care adult patients should receive a total of 100 g of fat per week to avoid EFAD.
- IVFEs should be included as a component of parenteral nutrition (PN) on a daily basis for special patient populations requiring PN (eg, patients with glucose intolerance, at risk for refeeding syndrome, during pregnancy).

Practice Scenario 15-1

Question: What is the most appropriate strategy to provide calcium to a PN-dependent patient in the event of an intravenous calcium gluconate shortage?

Scenario: AC, a surgical patient requiring central PN, has a single-lumen peripherally inserted central catheter (PICC). Pertinent laboratory and anthropometric data are as follows: weight = 40 kg; height = 170 cm; sodium (Na) = 145 mmol per liter (normal 135 to 145); potassium (K) = 3.5 mmol per liter (normal 3.5 to 5); chlorine (Cl) = 105 mmol per liter (normal 98 to 107); bicarbonate (HCO_3) = 21 mmol per liter (normal 22 to 30); blood urea nitrogen (BUN) = 37 mg per deciliter (normal 7 to 20); creatinine (Cr) = 0.8 mg per deciliter (normal 0.6 to 1.2); calcium (Ca) = 7.1 mg per deciliter (normal 8.5 to 10.2); magnesium (Mg) = 1.4 mEq per liter (normal 1.6 to 2.2); phosphate (PO_4) = 1.3 mg per deciliter (normal 2.5 to 4.5); albumin = 2.6 g per deciliter (normal 3.5 to 5); and ionized Ca = 2.25 mEq per liter (normal 2 to 2.5 mEq per liter).

The patient's energy and protein requirements are estimated to be 25 to 30 kcal per kilogram per day and 1.5 g protein per kilogram per day, respectively. A TNA formulation containing dextrose 175 g per day, amino acids 60 g per day, and IVFEs 37 g per day in a volume of 1200 mL per day to infuse at 50 mL per hour is prescribed to meet the patient's nutrition and fluid requirements. Additionally, IV fluids via a peripheral site are added to this regimen to correct dehydration. Due to a national shortage of intravenous concentrated calcium gluconate, the only salt form available for use is calcium chloride. The daily additives ordered for this 1200 mL per day PN formulation are:

Sodium acetate	40 mEq
Potassium chloride	80 mEq
Sodium phosphate	45 mmol
Calcium chloride	15 mEq
Magnesium sulfate	24 mEq
Multivitamins	10 mL
Multiple trace elements	5 mL

Intervention: Calcium is removed from the PN formulation and ionized calcium concentrations are monitored for evidence of calcium deficiency.

Answer: The patient is evaluated for signs related to low serum calcium concentrations, such as tetany, CNS, or cardiovascular symptoms. If calcium supplementation is necessary, administer calcium chloride separately from the PN formulation, taking care not to infuse intravenous calcium even through the same catheter as the PN formulation.

Rationale: Although AC's estimated total serum calcium concentration is 8.2 mg per deciliter (normal 8.5 to 10) (accounting for a decreased albumin concentration of 2.6 g per deciliter), the ionized calcium concentration is within the normal range. In this case, the dose of calcium in the PN can be removed to avoid precipitation from the addition of calcium chloride, a form of calcium that is less soluble than calcium gluconate, the preferred form of calcium for use in PN solutions. One of the most feared PN incompatibilities is the formation and infusion of calcium phosphate precipitates into the patient. The infusion of particulate matter, such as insoluble complexes of calcium phosphate, may block capillaries and have deleterious effects on vital organs such as the brain, lungs, kidneys, and liver. Case reports of pulmonary emboli and diffuse granulomatous interstitial pneumonitis have been attributed to calcium phosphate precipitates infused via PN formulations.[24,25]

Disease-Specific Formulations/Specific Nutrients

Modified Amino Acid Formulations

Specialty amino acid formulations are available for use in certain disease states or conditions (Table 15-1). These products are generally more expensive than standard formulations and should be reserved for patients meeting the intended indications who are expected to benefit clinically from their use.

Table 15-6 Considerations for Use of Intravenous Amino Acids in Adults During a National Shortage[20]

- Review all amino acid products currently available in the United States. Although there may be a limited supply in one concentration, availability may be present for a different concentration.
- Reserve high-concentration amino acid products (ie, > 10%) for use in fluid-restricted PN patients.
- Evaluate PN patient population to determine if a standardized, commercially available parenteral nutrition formulation (ie, premixed PN) is appropriate for use.
- Be aware that different brands of amino acids vary with respect to pH, electrolyte composition (eg, phosphorus), and calcium phosphorus solubility. As a result, compatibility and stability issues must be considered when substituting amino acid products.

PN, parenteral nutrition.

Table 15-7 Considerations for Use of Intravenous Multivitamins in Adults During a National Shortage[21]

- Substituting pediatric IV multivitamins for use in adults is not recommended because it may contribute to a shortage of pediatric products. The vitamin composition of pediatric products differs from adult products and may be inappropriate for use.
- Consider using oral or enterally administered multivitamin preparations whenever possible.
- When supplies of adult multivitamins are no longer available, reduce the daily dose by half or provide multivitamin doses three times a week.
- If supplies of adult multivitamins are exhausted, administer the following individual parenteral vitamins on a daily basis: thiamin 6 mg, ascorbic acid 200 mg, pyridoxine 6 mg, and folic acid 0.6 mg. Cyanocobalamin 100 mcg (vitamin B_{12}) should be administered at least once per month.
- Adult IV multivitamins should not be administered to neonates because these products contain propylene glycol and polysorbate, which may create toxic side effects.

IV, intravenous.

Table 15-8 Considerations for Use of Parenteral Electrolyte/Mineral Products in Adults During a National Shortage[22]

- Minimize the use of electrolyte/mineral additives to IV fluids and enteral nutrition products.
- Use oral or enteral electrolyte/mineral products for replacement therapy whenever possible.
- If appropriate for your PN patient population, consider using a standardized, commercially available multielectrolyte product or PN product with standard electrolytes.
- Consider compounding PN in a single, central location in order to decrease inventory waste.

IV, intravenous; PN, parenteral nutrition.

Table 15-9 Considerations for Use of Parenteral Trace Element Products in Adults During a National Shortage[23]

- Do not use pediatric/neonatal IV multitrace elements for adult populations because this may contribute to a shortage of pediatric products.
- The composition of pediatric multitrace element products differs from adult products and may be inappropriate for use.
- Use oral or enteral multitrace products whenever possible for replacement therapy.
- Consider decreasing or eliminating the daily amount of trace elements added to PN formulations.
- Consider using a different concentration or salt form if available.

IV, intravenous; PN, parenteral nutrition.

A.S.P.E.N. has published guidelines for the use of these products in clinical practice.[26]

Specialty formulations for use in renal failure are composed primarily of essential amino acids based upon the theory that nonessential amino acids can be physiologically recycled from urea, whereas essential amino acids must be provided from the diet. Despite the need for fluid restriction in many renal failure patients, these formulations are relatively dilute (5.2% to 6.5%) compared to commonly used standard amino acid formulations (8.5% and 10%). Essential amino acid formulas offer no significant advantage over the standard formulations and may result in metabolic complications; therefore, indications for these formulations are very limited.[27] Rather, standard formulations in reduced amounts are usually prescribed. Chapter 30 provides a discussion of nutrition in renal failure.

Modified amino acid formulations designed for use in hepatic encephalopathy contain increased amounts of branched-chain amino acids (BCAA) and decreased amounts of aromatic amino acids (AAA) compared to standard parenteral amino acid formulations.[27] An altered metabolism in patients with hepatic failure can result in a high serum ratio of AAA to BCAA. This imbalance is thought to cause increased transport of AAA into the brain, where they serve as precursors to neurotransmitters that may be responsible for altered mental status. As shown in Table 15-1, two therapeutically equivalent products are available. Indications for these formulations are very limited. See Chapter 28 for a discussion of nutrition in liver disease, including appropriate use and cost-effectiveness of specialized amino acid formulations.

Modified amino acid formulations are also available for use in metabolic stress, trauma, thermal injury, and/or hypercatabolic states. These products are formulated based on the theory that higher BCAA amounts are beneficial during severe metabolic stress because of increased skeletal muscle catabolism; therefore, significantly increased amounts of leucine, isoleucine, and valine are provided by all products. One product consists only of BCAAs, and is typically used to fortify a standard amino acid formulation to achieve the desired final BCAA concentration. The other products contain all the usual amino acids present in balanced amino acid formulations, with additional BCAA. Although the use of BCAA-enriched formulations slightly improves nitrogen balance in certain patient groups, clinical evidence does not support improved outcome.[26] Specialized nutrition support in trauma, critical care, and burns, including protein and amino acid requirements, is discussed in Chapter 23.

Concentrated amino acid formulations are available for use when fluid restriction is necessary. These are highly concentrated (15% and 20%), but are otherwise similar in composition to the standard amino acid formulations. Certain electrolytes such as chloride and acetate may be present in different amounts than in the standard formulations. Generally, the acetate content is higher in the more concentrated products compared to standard stock concentrations. However, chloride salts may be used to balance the chloride-to-acetate ratio in the final PN formulation to avoid iatrogenic acid–base disturbances.

Glutamine

Glutamine is an amino acid known to be conditionally essential during periods of metabolic stress. Crystalline amino acid formulations do not contain glutamine. As such, there has been considerable interest in adding glutamine to PN either as a separate entity, or as part of the amino acid stock formulations. However, due to stability and compatibility limitations, there is currently no IV form of glutamine commercially available in the United States for admixture in PN solutions. Studies of glutamine-supplemented PN have used extemporaneous preparations of powdered L-glutamine sterilized by filtration as well as commercially available products not available in the United States.[21,22] Parenteral glutamine supplementation in critically ill postoperative or ventilator-dependent patients requiring PN is associated with positive clinical outcomes such as reduced infectious complications and a shorter hospital length of stay.[28] Other patient populations, including adult surgical patients or those suffering thermal injuries and acute pancreatitis, may derive some benefit (Table 15-10).[28]

Omega-6 Fat Emulsions/Structured Lipids

IVFEs available in the United States are currently composed solely of long-chain triglycerides (LCTs; carbon chain length ≥ 14). Major fatty acid components in 100% soybean oil and 50% soybean/50% safflower oil mixtures include 51% to 63% linoleic, 18% to 23% oleic, 7% to 10% palmitic, 3.4% to 7% linolenic, and 2.9 to 4% stearic acid. Safflower oil contains only a trace of linolenic acid; thus, IVFEs using the 50:50 mix of soybean oil and safflower oil contains half as much omega-3 fatty acid (linolenic acid) as IVFEs using 100% soybean oil.[29]

Investigational IVFE products include physical mixtures of medium-chain triglycerides (MCTs; carbon chain length 6 to 12) and LCTs. Such formulations may be useful in patients intolerant to the currently available LCT products during critical illness and metabolic stress, and also in patients with carnitine deficiency because the transport of MCTs into mitochondria is carnitine independent.[32] Structured lipids containing laboratory-developed, chemically altered triglyceride molecules with specific fatty acids at the three binding sites of the glycerol backbone have also been investigated in various patient populations.[33,34] Specific fatty acids in structured lipids may include linoleic acid, a medium-chain fatty acid, and a very long chain omega-3 fatty acid, or various combinations of these or other fatty acids not found in nature. Because fatty acids at the 1 and 3 position of the glycerol backbone may be hydrolyzed more rapidly than those at the 2 position, the metabolism of structured lipids may be significantly different than that of typical LCT or MCT–LCT mixtures. Although currently under investigational study, neither MCT–LCT physical mixtures nor structured lipid products are commercially available for IV use in the United States.[35,36] Table 15-11 lists soybean, MCT, olive oil, and fish oil–based IVFEs currently available worldwide.

Table 15-10 Summary and Recommendations for Parenteral Nutrition Glutamine Supplementation in Adults[28]

- Parenteral glutamine administration is associated with a decrease in infectious complications, in hospital length of stay, and possibly in mortality in critically ill postoperative or ventilator-dependent patients requiring PN.
- Parenteral glutamine may be beneficial in certain other adult surgical patients, such as patients undergoing major abdominal surgery, or critically ill nonventilated patients requiring PN.
- There is a trend toward fewer positive blood cultures with the use of parenteral glutamine in adult hematopoietic stem cell transplant recipients receiving PN.
- Parenteral glutamine may be beneficial in adult burn patients or in acute pancreatitis patients who require PN.
- PN glutamine supplementation should probably be given early and in doses > 0.2 g/kg/day to be effective.
- To date, there is no evidence that parenteral glutamine is harmful. There are no absolute contraindications to the use of parenteral glutamine, but LFTs should be monitored in all patients, and it should be used with caution in end-stage hepatic failure patients and in patients with hepatic insufficiency.
- Parenteral free L-glutamine is available on an individual prescription, pharmacy-compounded basis in the United States. However, the practicality of compounding L-glutamine for use in or with PN should be weighed with the benefits that may be gained with its use.

PN, parenteral nutrition; LFT, liver function tests.

Omega-3 and Omega-9 Fat Emulsions

The incorporation of omega-3 fatty acids into IVFEs has been performed in an effort to produce less inflammatory and nonthrombogenic prostaglandins by the metabolic pathways responsible for lipoprotein breakdown. Studies indicating this effect have been performed in patients with sepsis,[37] atopic dermatitis,[38] severe ulcerative colitis,[39] and those undergoing elective surgery.[40] The most dramatic impact of IVFEs rich in omega-3 fatty acids has been demonstrated in the treatment of PN-associated liver disease (PNALD).[41] Omegaven (Fresenius Kabi AG, Bad Homburg VDH, Germany) is an IVFE that contains 100% fish oils with no oils from plant or vegetable sources. In murine models of PNALD, groups supplemented with fish oil failed to develop steatosis while on PN, in contrast to controls who developed severe macro- and microvesicular steatosis after receiving standard soybean-based IVFEs.[41] When used in a series of PN-dependent pediatric patients with cholestasis and compared to a group of historical controls who received conventional soybean oil–based lipid emulsions, patients receiving the fish oil–based IVFEs experienced reversal of cholestasis on the order of 7 times faster. Moreover, 2 of 18 infants receiving soybean-based IVFEs eventually required liver transplantation, whereas no liver transplants occurred in the 18 patients on Omegaven monotherapy.[42]

The substitution of olive oil for a portion of LCT in IVFEs has also been performed to reduce the risks of conventional LCT IVFE products in critically ill patients. Olive oil–based fat emulsions offer advantages over the current polyunsaturated LCT IVFEs, such as decreased peroxidation[43] and a lack of in vitro lymphocyte function inhibition.[44] Data from clinical

Table 15-11 Comparison of Parenteral Lipid Emulsions Per 10 g/100 mL

Oil source, %	Intralipid Fresenius Kabi	Liposyn II Hospira	Lipofundin MCT/LCT B. Braun	SMOF Lipid Fresenius Kabi	ClinOleic Baxter	Omegaven Fresenius Kabi
Soybean	100	50	50	30	20	0
Safflower	0	50	0	0	0	0
Coconut (MCT)	0	0	50	30	0	0
Olive	0	0	0	25	80	0
Fish	0	0	0	15	0	100
Phytosterols, mg/L	348±33	383	NP	47.6	327±8	0
α-Tocopherol, mg/L	38	NP	100	200	32	150–296
Fat composition, g						
Palmitic	1	0.88	0.55	0.9	0.65	0.25–1
Stearic	0.4	0.32	0.2	0.33	0.175	0.05–0.2
Oleic	2.6	1.82	1.16	2.8	2.83	0.6–1.3
Linoleic	5	6.54	2.66	2.85	0.86	0.1–0.7
α-Linolenic	0.9	0.39	0.1	0.275	0.115	< 0.2
EPA	0	0	0	0.25	0	1.28–2.82
Arachidonic	0	0	0	0.05	0.025	0.1–0.4
DHA	0	0	0	0.05	0	1.44–3.09

Data as provided by manufacturers. EPA, eicosapentaenoic acid; DHA, docosahexaenoic acid; LCT, long-chain triglyceride; MCT, medium-chain triglyceride; NP, not provided.

Reprinted from de Meijer VE, Gura KM, Le HD, Meisel JA, Puder M. Fish oil-based lipid emulsions prevent and reverse parenteral nutrition-associated liver disease: the Boston experience. *JPEN J Parenter Enteral Nutr.* 2009;33(5):541–547 with permission from the American Society for Parenteral and Enteral Nutrition (A.S.P.E.N.).

trials with olive oil–based IVFEs reveal these products to be clinically safe and well tolerated with a tendency to preserve hepatic function. Because olive oil contains approximately 20% omega-6 fatty acids, the supply of linoleic acid is enough to avoid the risk of essential fatty acid deficiency.

A combination IVFE product referred to as SMOF (Soy, MCT, Olive, Fish oil) capitalizes on the beneficial attributes of oils from non–soybean oil sources while reducing the amounts and detrimental effects of omega-6 fatty acids. Characterized as the "ideal" IVFE, it contains a mixture of 30% soybean oil, 30% MCTs, 25% olive oil, and 15% fish oil.[45] Clinical use of the product in comparison with soybean oil–based IVFE has shown reduced liver changes and the preservation of antioxidant capacity in critically ill patients.[46]

Carnitine

Carnitine is necessary for proper transport and metabolism of long chain fatty acids. Carnitine is not present in any component of PN formulations. An IV form of L-carnitine is commercially available for the treatment of carnitine deficiency, and is sometimes added to PN formulations for selected patients who have a documented deficiency or are susceptible to a deficiency.[47]

Parenteral Nutrient Preparation

Admixtures: Dextrose-Amino Acids Versus Total Nutrient Admixtures

PN admixtures may be prepared for the administration in either of two formats—the traditional or dextrose-amino acid (2-in-1) formulation, or the TNA system, which is also referred to as a 3-in-1 or all-in-one admixture. The dextrose-amino acid format incorporates the dextrose and amino acid–base solutions along with the prescribed electrolytes, minerals, vitamins, and trace elements in one or multiple containers each day. IVFE is administered separately as a piggyback infusion. In contrast, the TNA system incorporates dextrose, amino acids, and IVFEs along with the other prescribed micronutrients together in the same container for final administration.

Specific advantages and disadvantages are associated with the use of each PN formulation system.[48] Many institutions and home care providers have enthusiastically embraced the TNA system for overall convenience and cost advantages. Although these advantages are significant, especially in the home care setting, they must be weighed against the disadvantages, along with the particular circumstances of each situation.[49–51] A brief discussion of the major points follows.

Traditionally, the dextrose-amino acid format evolved as PN substrates were developed and refined, and standards of practice for specialized nutrition support matured. Concerns for the potential of IVFEs to support bacterial and fungal growth (if contaminated) led to CDC guidelines limiting the hang times of IVFE given in the piggyback fashion to a maximum of 12 hours.[12] At times, and with faster infusion rates (over 4 to 6 hours), this predisposed susceptible patients to hypertriglyceridemia that could be lessened by infusing IVFEs at a slower rate. Under these circumstances and in an effort to simplify administration procedures, the concept was developed to add the IVFEs directly to the PN admixture to provide the total daily infusion in one large container. This resulted in increased convenience for administration and a decreased risk for microbial contamination due to fewer manipulations or entries into the IV line. Initial concerns for increased risk of infection due to an IVFE hang time greater than 12 hours were not realized with adherence to proper sterile technique at all points in the preparation and administration process.[52] Table 15-12 presents the major advantages and disadvantages of the TNA system for PN.[50–53]

Either system may be infused via a central venous access device. If PN is to be administered via a true peripheral line (as opposed to a PICC), certain criteria are important to decrease risk of thrombophlebitis and damage to peripheral vein(s). Osmolarity should generally be kept below 900 mOsm per liter and calcium and potassium concentrations should be kept low (for some institutions, this may translate to calcium ≤ 5 mEq per liter and potassium ≤ 40mEq per liter whenever possible), and IVFE is generally given daily to provide adequate calories and decrease osmolarity.[1,5] In a dextrose-amino acid system for PPN, the IVFE is usually piggybacked into the same line and infused over 24 hours, replacing the IVFE bag at 12 hours to adhere to the 12 hour hang time limit. It has been speculated that this technique using daily IVFEs along with the dextrose-amino acid formulation may confer a modest protective effect on venous tolerance by the dilution of the PPN formulation and/or by some buffering action in the vein.[4] There has also been some success in reducing or preventing thrombophlebitis through the addition of heparin and/or small amounts of hydrocortisone to PPN, though this practice is variable.[1] Another technique to minimize thrombophlebitis includes the use of a nitroglycerin patch at the venous insertion site.

Table 15-12 Advantages and Disadvantages of the Total Nutrient Admixture System

Advantages

- All components aseptically compounded by the pharmacy
- Preparation is more efficient for pharmacy personnel, especially if automated
- Less manipulation of the system during administration
- Less risk of contamination during administration
- Inhibited or slower bacterial growth if contamination does occur compared to separate IVFE
- Less nursing time needed for one container/d and no piggyback IVFE to administer
- Less supply and equipment expense for only one infusion pump and IV tubing
- More convenient storage, fewer supplies, easier administration in home care settings
- Dextrose and venous access tolerance may be better in some situations
- Possible applications in fluid-restricted patients because IVFE 30% is restricted to use in TNA
- May be more cost-effective overall in certain settings
- Fat clearance may be better when IVFE is administered over more than 12 hours

Disadvantages

- Larger particle size of admixed IVFE precludes use of 0.22-μm (bacteria-eliminating) filter, and requires larger pore size filter of 1.2 μm
- Admixed IVFE less stable, more prone to separation of lipid components
- Formulations are more sensitive to destabilization with certain electrolyte concentrations
- Formulation more sensitive to destabilization with low concentrations of dextrose and amino acids
- Lower pH amino acid formulations may destabilize the IVFE portion of admixture
- Formulation may be unstable when the final concentration of IVFE is low
- Difficult to visualize precipitate or particulate material in the opaque admixture
- Certain medications are incompatible with the IVFE portion of admixture
- Catheter occlusion more common with daily IVFEs
- Less stable over time than dextrose–amino acid PN formulations with separate IVFE

IVFE, intravenous fat emulsions; IV, intravenous; TNA, total nutrient admixture; PN, parenteral nutrition.

National Standards for Compounded Sterile Preparations

A primary responsibility of the pharmacist is to ensure safe PN preparation. Compounding an accurate formulation free of microbial and particulate matter is an essential component of this process. A number of procedures have been developed by organizations, such as the USP and the American Society of Health-System Pharmacists (ASHP), to assist pharmacists in complying with sterile-product admixture guidelines. The USP is a private, nonprofit organization recognized by the federal government as the official group responsible for setting national standards for drug purity and safety. Most recently, the USP issued standards on the pharmaceutical compounding of sterile products. On January 1, 2004, the USP formally adopted Chapter {797}, the first official monograph enforceable by regulatory agencies concerning the procedures and requirements for compounded sterile preparations (CSPs). Much of the same information was previously published as recommendations in nonenforceable materials including USP Chapter {1206}, which focused on dispensing for home care and guidelines related to sterile product preparation published by ASHP.[54] Although Chapter {797} discusses the standards that apply to all sterile dosage forms that are compounded, only information pertinent to PN and its implications will be reviewed.

Chapter {797} identifies three different risk levels (low, medium, and high) for each CSP based on the potential for microbial contamination. The low-risk level typically involves a simple, closed-system aseptic transfer. A medium-risk level involves reconstitution of several sterile commercial products for transfer into several small-volume minibags or one large-volume parenteral preparation, such as PN. A high-risk compounding activity involves the preparation from bulk, nonsterile ingredients or the preparation from sterile ingredients but are exposed to less than the International Organization for Standardization (ISO) Class 5 standards. The ISO class used in USP Chapter {797} replaces previous terminology related to particle counts in the compounding area; ISO Class 5 is equivalent to Class 100 (ie, circulating particles 0.5 μm or larger do not exceed 100 particles per

Table 15-13 Risk Level Classification and Beyond-Use Dating Guidelines for Compounded Sterile Preparations

Risk Level	Example(s)	Beyond-Use Dating	
		Room (20°C–25°C)	Refrigeration (2°C–8°C)
Low	Reconstitution of a single dose vial of lyophilized powder with a sterile diluent for transfer into another container (eg, pediatric parenteral multivitamins)	48 hours	14 days
Medium	Mixing of multiple manufactured additives for transfer into a large-volume parenteral solution (eg, PN formulations)	30 hours	9 days
High	Preparation of nonsterile powder for intravenous infusion (eg, extemporaneously compounded L-glutamine for supplementation in PN formulation)	24 hours	3 days

PN, parenteral nutrition.

cubic foot). A low- or medium-risk product becomes high risk when any added component is high risk; thus, a PN formulation with L-glutamine compounded from nonsterile powder becomes a high-risk product. See Table 15-13 for further examples of risk level assessment and Practice Scenario 15-2 for more discussion of this topic.

Practice Scenario 15-2

Question: What is the most appropriate risk level and sterile environment for compounding a PN formulation from nonsterile powdered amino acids?

Scenario: An 82-year-old male is dependent on PN due to short bowel syndrome secondary to Crohn's disease and multiple bowel resections. There is currently a shortage of commercially available crystalline amino acids so the current PN formulation must be compounded with nonsterile powdered amino acids.

Intervention: The intravenous amino acid formulation is compounded from nonsterile powders as a result of a national shortage of commercially available crystalline amino acid formulations.

Answer: PN compounded from nonsterile powdered amino acids is classified as a high-risk level and must undergo terminal sterilization.

Rationale: Preparation of PN falls under the category of a CSP by the definition of USP Chapter {797}.[13] PN is classified as a medium-risk level CSP when it is prepared from crystalline amino acids and commercially available monohydrated dextrose, injectable lipid emulsions, electrolytes, multiple vitamins, trace elements, and sterile water. A medium-risk level procedure is characterized by the mixing of multiple small doses of different sterile products into one large bag. When PN is compounded using powdered amino acids as in this scenario, the procedure is elevated to a high-risk level because it involves the use of nonsterile ingredients and carries the highest risk for the contamination by microbial, chemical, or physical matter. High-risk level CSPs must undergo some type of terminal sterilization process prior to administration. All risk-level compounds should be prepared in an environment in which particulate matter and microorganisms are minimized, and the air quality must meet certain standards. Table 15-13 outlines the risk level classifications for all CSPs. To be compliant with USP Chapter {797}, institutions must show that all personnel are trained in garbing, aseptic work practices, and cleansing/disinfection procedures. Institutions must document that personnel complete didactic training, pass written competencies, and undergo skill assessment using observational audit tools and media-fill testing.

Risk level assessment is important because storage and expiration limits of CSPs are assigned based on the risk level. "Beyond-use dating" is the current terminology for what was formerly referred to as expiration dating. The difference is that an expiration date was based on drug stability, whereas the beyond-use date is defined as the date established by health care professionals from the published literature or manufacturer-specific recommendations beyond which the pharmacy-prepared product should not be used due to concerns of chemical instability and product sterility.[13] Sterility refers to the absence of viable microorganisms in a CSP. The beyond-use dating of individual CSPs cannot exceed the limits delineated in Chapter {797} unless formal sterility testing is performed. Beyond-use dating guidelines for CSPs based upon risk level are outlined in Table 15-13; these represent maximum beyond-use dating. For example, a pharmacy-prepared PN formulation stored at room temperature (20°C to 25°C) cannot be used after 30 hours, whereas a PN solution stored under refrigeration has a beyond-use date up to 9 days. However, certain PN formulations, particularly those mixed as a TNA and those with maximum calcium and phosphate concentrations, may require shorter beyond-use dating due to stability and/or compatibility issues.

Automated Compounding Devices

Automated compounding devices (ACDs) originally were developed to assist with streamlining the manufacturing sequence for PN formulations. The main advantage of ACDs is enhanced accuracy of the dosage form. Instead of trying to compound easily measured volumes (eg, 250- or 500-mL increments for amino acids or dextrose; refer to Figs. 15-1 and 15-2) any volume of a formulation can be programmed for pumping from large stock containers by ACDs. PN formulations can be more easily tailored to meet patient-specific needs and the process is more efficient. For institutions compounding more than a few PN formulations per day, ACDs are associated with decreased pharmacy labor and supply costs. This advancement in technology also reduces the risk of extrinsic contaminants that might be introduced with manually prepared formulations, such as "coring" of rubber vial tops and fibers from alcohol swabs. Ultimately, ACDs enable clinicians to provide more precise and safe preparations to patients.

ACDs are also available for the addition of the micronutrient components to PN formulations. Again, these may contribute to decreased labor and supply costs if an institution compounds many PN formulations daily. Some of these devices interface with bar code readers, which may help minimize compounding errors. However, ACDs may not be cost-effective for institutions making only a few PN formulations per day. The ACD uses a cassette with tubing that must be changed daily and represents a significant cost that may be more than offset by any savings in labor or supply costs. In pharmacies with limited space, there may simply not be enough space available for the ACD.

Quality Control for the Preparation of Parenteral Nutrition Admixtures

USP Chapter {797} describes the procedures for ensuring the accuracy and precision of the compounding process.[13] For conventional manual compounding of PN formulations, the additive vials and syringes must be inspected prior to dispensing the final product. A pharmacist other than the compounding personnel is preferred for confirming that the measured volumes in syringes correspond with the PN order. The two major methods used for verifying the accuracy of the compounding process by ACDs are either volumetric or gravimetric analysis. Each ACD has its own set of internal surveillance checks that assist the compounding pharmacist. These devices have the capability to measure each nutrient volume added to the final PN container. If the weight of the final PN container is different than the theoretical weight calculated by the automated system (the sum of the volume for each ingredient multiplied by its specific gravity), then the pharmacist is alerted to a possible error in the admixture process. Gravimetric analysis may also be used to assess the precision of the final PN admixture. Gravimetric analysis can be used as a quality control measure for manual or automated compounded systems, and is one method of quality assurance that can be applied independent of the ACD. Pharmacists can use an analytical balance to determine the weight of individual additive containers that have a narrow margin of safety. For example, if overfill for a final PN formulation was supplied solely from a potassium chloride container, the consequences of this error could be fatal. Thus, pharmacists can employ gravimetric techniques to assess the accuracy of individual additives delivered to the final PN formulation.

Refractometry also is used to determine if PN formulations have been compounded properly. The refractive index of dextrose and amino acids can be measured with a refractometer and compared to values established for known concentrations of dextrose and amino acids in PN base formulations. If the measured refractive indices differ substantially from predicted values, then the base formulation may have been improperly admixed. Refractometers cannot be used with IVFEs, so alternative methods must be used to assess the integrity of TNA systems. Research has shown that factors other than incorrect preparations can result in refractive indices deviating from predicted values. For example, Kitzen and colleagues[53] found that revised equations for predicting refractive indices may be needed when final dextrose concentrations exceed 15%. In contrast to indirectly measuring final dextrose concentrations with refractometric analysis, certain instruments use chemical analysis to directly measure final dextrose concentrations. Although dextrose concentrations of PN formulations administered in clinical practice may exceed the range of detection, samples can be diluted and compared against control solutions to determine if the formulation is within an acceptable margin of error.

Chapter {797} also addresses the responsibilities of the pharmacist for monitoring the quality of all CSPs after they leave the pharmacy for distribution.[13] This includes the processes for packaging, handling, and transport of the PN formulation to the patient or caregiver. For example, written procedures must be developed to ensure that the PN formulation is not exposed to extremes in temperature or light. The use of seals on all ports of PN containers can enhance product integrity during handling and transport. Particular attention to quality and control after dispensing is required for home care products because significant time and handling usually occur between the PN production in the pharmacy and delivery to the patient or caregiver.

Premixed Parenteral Nutrition Formulations

In addition to manual or automated methods for compounding PN formulations from the individual components, as discussed previously, there are two commercially available premixed dextrose-amino acid products (Nutrimix Labs, Hospira Inc., Lake Forest, IL and Clinimix, Baxter Healthcare Corporation, Deerfield, IL) for central and peripheral vein administration. The products for central vein infusion generally contain final concentrations of dextrose 15% to 25%, and amino acids 3.5%, 4.25%, or 5%, with or without a standard package of electrolytes. The products for peripheral vein infusion include those with final concentrations of dextrose 5% to 10%, and amino acids 2.75%, 3.5%, or 4.25% with or without electrolytes. These products require manipulation of the container to mix the dextrose and amino acid components just prior to use, because mixing prior to sterilization produces a chemical reaction that alters the integrity of the dextrose and amino acids (the Maillard reaction). Stacked chambers contain a separation strip that must be broken, causing the two chambers to form one large chamber containing both the dextrose and amino acids.

There is also a glycerol-based product containing final concentrations of amino acids 3%, glycerol 3%, and electrolytes (ProcalAmine, B. Braun) that is often used for short-term PPN administration.[56,57] Because glycerol is a sugar alcohol, this product can be premixed and sterilized in a single bag without undergoing the Maillard reaction that precludes the heat sterilization of mixed dextrose and amino acid solutions.

Premixed products may be preferred in settings where there is infrequent or irregular use of PN, such as in rural hospitals or long-term care facilities, because they have a reasonably stable shelf life and require minimal admixing. The usage of premixed products has recently increased in the setting of shortages of amino acid products for PN compounding. All premixed products require the addition of multiple vitamin injection shortly before administration because vitamins are essential components of PN that are not stable when added more than 24 hours in advance of use.

Stability/Compatibility of Parenteral Nutrition Formulations

Although stability and compatibility have been used interchangeably in the medical literature, a distinction exists between these two terms in reference to parenteral admixtures. The stability of PN formulations refers to the degradation of nutritional components that change their original characteristics. A classic example is the Maillard reaction, mentioned previously, that occurs between IV dextrose and certain amino acids such as lysine, resulting in a brownish discoloration of the final formulation. Stability may also refer to the ability of PN additives, including medications, to maintain their chemical integrity and pharmacologic activity. Photodegradation due to light exposure, particularly fluorescent light, results in a loss of some vitamins, including cyanocobalamin, folic acid, phylloquinone, pyridoxine, riboflavin, thiamin, and retinol.[58] In contrast, compatibility issues with PN formulations generally involve the formation of precipitates. These precipitates may be solid, such as crystalline matter, or liquid, such as phase separation of oil and water in a TNA. The distinction between stability and compatibility with IVFE can be difficult to discern, because all emulsions are inherently unstable systems that will return to their oil and water components over time, yet there are clearly compatibility issues that result in phase separation of the IVFE components. The majority of studies evaluating additive and Y-site compatibility with PN formulations evaluate only physical compatibility; a few include stability. For example, octreotide is listed as physically compatible when admixed in tested PN formulations but a study including stability data found highly variable drug activity.[59] Manufacturer information warns that the glycosylation of octreotide and the subsequent loss of activity may occur when the drug is added to PN formulations.[60] Unstable substances should not be added to PN regardless of physical compatibility.

When discussing medication incompatibilities, a distinction should be made between the use of dextrose-amino acids and TNA formulations. Presence of the IVFE in the same container and its chemical properties explain why some drugs are compatible in dextrose-amino acids but not in a TNA formulation. There are also a few medications, usually fat-soluble medications, that are compatible with TNA but not dextrose-amino acid formulations (Table 15-14).[59,61]

Table 15-14 Physical Compatibility of Parenteral Nutrition with Selected Medications via Y-site Administration[59,61]

Medication	Admixture Type: Dextrose–Amino Acids	Admixture Type: TNA
Acyclovir 7 mg/mL D5W	I	I
Amikacin 5 mg/mL D5W	C	C
Amphotericin B 0.6 mg/mL D5W	I	I
Ampicillin 20 mg/mL NaCl 0.9%	C	C
Butorphanol 0.04 mg/mL D5W	C	C
Cefazolin 20 mg/mL D5W	I	C
Ceftazidime 40 mg/mL D5W	C	C
Cimetidine 12 mg/mL D5W	C	C
Ciprofloxacin 1 mg/mL D5W	I	C
Cyclosporine 5 mg/mL D5W	I	I
Dopamine 3200 mcg/mL D5W	C	I
Dobutamine 4 mg/mL D5W	C	C
Famotidine 2 mg/mL D5W	C	C
Fentanyl 12.5 mcg/mL D5W	C	C
Fentanyl 50 mcg/mL undiluted	C	C
Ganciclovir 20 mg/mL D5W	I	I
Gentamicin 5 mg/mL D5W	C	C
Haloperidol 0.2 mg/mL D5W	C	I
Heparin 100 units/mL undiluted	C	I
Hydromorphone 0.5 mg/mL D5W	C	I
Insulin 1 U/mL D5W	C	C
Lorazepam 0.1 mg/mL D5W	C	I
Midazolam 2 mg/mL D5W	I	I
Morphine 1 mg/mL D5W	C	C
Morphine 15 mg/mL undiluted	NA	I
Ofloxacin 4 mg/mL D5W	C	C
Ondansetron 1 mg/mL D5W	C	I
Potassium phosphates 3 mmol/mL undiluted	I	I
Ranitidine 2 mg/mL D5W	C	C
Sodium bicarbonate 1 mEq/mL undiluted	I	C
Tacrolimus 1 mg/mL D5W	C	C
Ticarcillin/clavulanate 30/0.1 mg/mL D5W	C	C
Tobramycin 5 mg/mL D5W	C	C
Trimethoprim/sulfamethoxazole 0.8/4 mg/mL D5W	C	C
Vancomycin 10 mg/mL D5W	C	C
Zidovudine 4 mg/mL D5W	C	C

TNA, total nutrient admixture; C, compatible; I, incompatible; NA, not available.
Note: Certain medications may be physically compatible when coadministered with PN, but may not be suitable for coadministration due to loss of activity or inactivation of the medication.

Stability of Intravenous Fat Emulsion and Total Nutrient Admixture Formulations

The IVFE consists of an interior oil phase dispersed in an external water phase. Polar and nonpolar regions on the same fat droplet are responsible for maintaining stability. The polar regions create a negative charge, or zeta potential, on the surface of the fat droplet that promotes repulsion between neighboring lipid particles of the same charge.[24,51] When the surface charge becomes less negative, fat droplets begin to aggregate into larger fat globules ($> 1\ \mu m$ in diameter) and the emulsion becomes unstable. Clinically, the IVFE becomes unsafe for administration at this point, and fat globules may lodge in the pulmonary vasculature, compromising respiratory function.

Factors that may alter the electrical charge on the fat droplet surface include reductions in pH and the addition of electrolyte salts. A pH in the range of 6 to 9 is most favorable for IVFE stability, whereas additives lowering the pH below 5 or increasing the pH above 10 may irreversibly destabilize or "crack" the emulsion.[51] When a cracked IVFE occurs, the oil phase separates from the water phase and first appears as subtle changes in the uniformly white appearance of the emulsion, which may progress to yellow oil streaks throughout the bag or the development of an amber oil layer at the top of the admixture bag. A TNA with this appearance is unsafe for use. Low pH is especially damaging because, in addition to effects on the electrical charge, the egg phospholipid emulsifier begins to degrade. The single most critical factor influencing the pH of a PN formulation is the crystalline amino acid solution used for compounding. The final pH of a PN formulation is generally very near that of the amino acid solution unless the buffering capacity of the amino acids has been overwhelmed by other PN components. The pH of crystalline amino acid solutions varies by brand and ranges from about 5.2 to 7. Those with a pH of 5.3 or less, such as Aminosyn, Aminosyn-HBC, and Aminosyn RF, are not appropriate for use in a TNA preparation. Amino acid solutions with a pH in the range of 5.8 to 7, including Aminosyn II, FreAmine, Travasol, and Clinisol products, are generally acceptable for use in TNA compounding. Certain crystalline amino acid solutions used for pediatric patients and some concentrated solutions (15% and 20%) may be marginal for use in TNA formulations because the pH (5.4 to 5.7) is borderline for IVFE stability. Use of these amino acid formulations can be particularly problematic in home care where PN is made several days in advance of use and when other factors influencing TNA stability are marginal for IVFE stability. The addition of cysteine hydrochloride, as is routine with neonatal PN formulations and some pediatric PN formulations, renders the final admixture pH less than 5, promoting IVFE destabilization. However, some prescribers may request the use of pediatric amino acid products in adult PN patients because the pediatric amino acid formulations are the only products with taurine and, occasionally, pharmacists may add L-cysteine hydrochloride to an adult PN formulation in order to increase calcium phosphate solubility (eg, when a patient is eliminating high amounts of calcium in response to foscarnet therapy).

A concentrated dextrose solution should not be added directly to IVFE because of its acidic pH; rather, dextrose should be combined with the amino acid solution first during the compounding process. The amino acid solution serves as a buffer and low final concentrations of amino acids (less than 4%) may not provide adequate buffer capacity to prevent destabilization of a TNA. Low IVFE concentrations, especially below 2% or 2.5%, may also result in an unstable TNA.[62,63] When compounding PN for 3 to 7 days in advance of use, final IVFE concentrations may need to be higher for a stable TNA formulation, especially if other components contribute to destabilization. Stability studies should be reviewed carefully to ensure that the assigned beyond-use dating is reasonable for the final concentrations of base components and the combination of additives in the PN formulation. Manufacturers' data often list a range of dextrose, amino acids, and IVFE concentrations that have been evaluated for TNA stability but seldom include the specific combinations of base components, electrolytes, vitamins, and trace elements present in the PN formulations reported. Although this information provides some guidance to stability limits, it does not provide adequate practice guidelines. For instance, a range of final concentrations for each base component (dextrose, amino acids, and IVFE) is typically listed. If dextrose 10%, amino acids 1%, and IVFE 1% are each listed as within the range tested, there is no indication that this particular combination was tested. Although a final concentration of IVFE 1% may be stable with amino acids 5% or higher, this IVFE concentration is not likely to be compatible with the final concentration of amino acids 1%, but this is not stated. Home care practitioners must be particularly vigilant in assessing appropriate combinations of final concentrations and the beyond-use dating assigned. A PN formulation may be stable when used within 30 hours of compounding (in hospital) but may begin to destabilize before use when assigned a longer beyond-use date. Practice Scenario 15-3 further explores the topic of TNA stability.

Practice Scenario 15-3

Question: What are the limitations in compounding (ie, 3-in-1 versus 2-in-1) when compounding a peripheral parenteral nutrition formulation?

Scenario: SG is an 83-year-old male s/p fall from a stepladder at home who was admitted for repair of a hip fracture, mandibular fracture, and observation due to altered mental status. He has been NPO (nothing by mouth) for 5 days due to the mandibular fracture and impending surgery. On hospital day 7 (postoperative day 2), SG is advanced to full liquids but experiences abdominal pain and distention. A partial small bowel obstruction is confirmed upon abdominal X-ray. The Nutrition Support Team is consulted for the initiation of peripheral parenteral nutrition because long-term PN (> 10 days) is not anticipated and SG's primary physician does not want him to have a central venous line placed due to the risk for a central line infection.

Intervention: A 2-in-1 PN formulation with a separate infusion of IVFE is prepared for SG.

Answer: Three-in-one PN formulations or TNAs should be used with extreme caution or not at all as PPN formulations.

Rationale: Although published data are scarce, if final concentrations of amino acids are less than 4%, dextrose is less than 10%, or IVFE is less than 2%, TNA stability is compromised and coalescence of submicrometer droplets into large fat globules occurs often before the 30-hour beyond-use date assignment.[63] As a result, use of TNA for PPN formulations often does not meet stability requirements, and IVFEs should be infused separately in order to preserve a stable and safe formulation.

When reduced final concentrations of amino acids and glucose are used for compounding PN solutions, it has been difficult to accurately predict solubility limits between calcium (as the organic gluconate salt) and inorganic phosphate (as sodium or potassium salts) due to the lack of data. Low osmolarity PN formulations, such as PPNs, appear to pose a high threat for calcium–phosphorus precipitation.[64] Three different forms may arise from the interaction between these two ions: monobasic calcium phosphate [$Ca(H_2PO_4)_2$], dibasic calcium phosphate [$CaHPO_4$], and tribasic calcium phosphate [$Ca_3(PO_4)_2$]. Dibasic calcium phosphate (which is virtually insoluble in water) poses the greatest potential threat for lethal precipitants in the PN admixture and is commonly implicated in reports of significant morbidity and mortality among patients receiving incompatible mixtures. Comparatively, monobasic calcium phosphate is roughly 60 times more soluble.[65]

Excess cation amounts, especially divalent cations such as calcium (Ca^{++}) or magnesium (Mg^{++}), can reduce or neutralize the negative surface charge exerted by the emulsifier, thereby removing the repulsive force and allowing fat particles to combine.[51] Trivalent cations (ie, Fe^{+3}) have even greater destabilizing effects. There is no dosage of iron dextran that can be added to any TNA due to instability issues, nor are other parenteral iron products safe even if they were to be approved for addition to PN. As with base components, home care providers must be especially alert for inappropriate concentrations of electrolytes because the process of coalescence is not immediate, and formulations that are stable for 30 hours may not be stable for longer periods of time. Coalescence indicates that a fusion of fat droplets has occurred and the individual droplet size has increased. Formulations should no longer be infused after coalescence occurs because increased droplet sizes are capable of producing organ damage in experimental animal models.[66,67]

Calcium and Phosphate

The development of microprecipitates within PN formulations can occur as a result of incompatible combinations. In 1994, the U.S. Food and Drug Administration (FDA) released a safety alert in response to reports of two deaths and at least two cases of respiratory distress associated with the administration of PN formulations thought to contain an insoluble or unstable intermediate (ie, calcium phosphate crystals).[25,68] Diffuse microvascular pulmonary emboli containing calcium phosphate were confirmed upon patient autopsies.

Calcium phosphate solubility is a major compatibility concern with PN formulations. For patient safety, all health care professionals who prescribe PN formulations that deviate from preestablished standards should be familiar with limitations for addition of calcium and phosphate. This allows the compounding pharmacist to serve as a secondary check for calcium phosphate solubility rather than as a single evaluator.

Several factors can influence the calcium and phosphate solubility in a PN formulation (Table 15-15).[6] The pH of the final PN formulation plays a major role in dictating the solubility of calcium and phosphate. A low pH favors the presence of monobasic calcium phosphate, a relatively soluble salt form of calcium. Increasing the pH results in a greater availability of dibasic phosphate to bind with free calcium ions and increases the chance of precipitation. Thus, lowering the pH of the PN admixture lowers the likelihood that calcium and phosphate will precipitate. This concept has been used extensively in compounding pediatric PN formulations.[69] For example, relatively large doses of calcium and phosphorus are routinely required in neonatal PN formulations to optimize bone formation. Although pediatric amino acid products are formulated at a lower pH, L-cysteine hydrochloride can be added to further decrease pH and thereby increase calcium phosphorus solubility.[70] Because L-cysteine is considered a semiessential amino acid in premature infants, its addition to pediatric formulations serves a dual purpose. Yet, an acidic pH creates an unfavorable environment for IVFE, which may destabilize the final emulsion. As a result, TNA admixtures are discouraged for use in the neonatal and pediatric population where lowering the pH is an effective technique for increasing calcium phosphate solubility.

Table 15-15 Factors that Influence Calcium and Phosphorus Compatibility in Parenteral Nutrition Formulations

Amino acid concentration
Amino acid product composition (ie, pH or phosphorus content)
Calcium and phosphate concentration
Calcium salt form
Dextrose concentration
pH of formulation
Temperature of formulation
Order of mixing additives

Adapted from Trissel LA. *Trissel's Calcium and Phosphate Compatibility in Parenteral Nutrition.* Houston, TX: TriPharma Communications; 2001.

The concentration or amounts of calcium and phosphate ions are directly related to the risk of precipitation.[6] As the concentration of either micronutrient rises, precipitation is more likely to occur. A variety of resources are available to assist clinicians in determining appropriate calcium and phosphate concentrations to avoid precipitation. Product-specific solubility curves have been published that depict solubility limits for calcium and phosphate salts.[6,71] Unfortunately, most of these curves were developed using fixed concentrations of amino acids, dextrose, calcium, and phosphate and often omitted other components that might influence calcium–phosphate solubility. This makes use of such curves for determining solubility characteristics of patient-specific formulations difficult. When ACDs are used in the admixture process, the manufacturer's software may be helpful in predicting calcium and phosphate solubility for a given formulation.

The verification of large calcium doses (greater than 2 times the recommended daily allowance [RDA]) with the prescriber can help minimize the risk of precipitation. Low total serum calcium concentrations may arise from hypoalbuminemia, fluid retention, or acid–base disturbances, and supplemental calcium may be unnecessary. One practitioner has reported that reducing daily calcium doses from 13.5 mEq to 4.5 mEq in PN for stability reasons did not influence serum calcium concentrations.[71] However, because serum calcium is maintained at the expense of bone calcium when intake is inadequate, the risk of metabolic bone disease must be considered when calcium provision is below the recommended 10 to 15 mEq per day for adults.[5] If hypoalbuminemia is present, ionized calcium concentrations can be measured to verify the need for additional calcium.

The salt form of calcium added to the PN formulation can have a dramatic impact on the risk of precipitation. Calcium gluconate and calcium gluceptate are generally less dissociated salt forms of calcium than the chloride salts.[72] As a result, the amount of free calcium available to form insoluble complexes with phosphate is reduced. Solubility curves for calcium phosphate are specific for calcium salt and cannot be interchanged; most solubility curves are for calcium gluconate. High localized phosphate or calcium concentrations can occur if the final container is not sufficiently agitated or the contents are not sufficiently dispersed during the compounding process.

Medication Additives

Precipitates from medication incompatibilities or emulsion disruption from medication additives have also been reported. Studies of medications with dextrose-amino acids and TNA formulations during simulated Y-site administration have been performed, and incompatibilities ranged from the formation of precipitates to haziness, discoloration, and emulsion disruption with frank separation of oil and water phases. Table 15-14 summarizes the Y-site compatibility of selected medications with dextrose-amino acids and TNA formulations.[59,61] Compatibility by Y-site infusion (coinfusion) is not synonymous with admixture into the PN formulation because the time of exposure between the medication and PN components is greatly increased with admixture. In addition, pharmacokinetic variables must be considered with admixture of a medication into PN because the medication must be safe and effective when administered as a continuous infusion or over the cycle time of a PN formulation.

Use of Filters

The 1994 FDA safety alert on calcium phosphate precipitation highlighted the need for filtration of PN at the bedside. Relatively large-pore filters (5 μm) are adequate for the removal of precipitates (eg, calcium phosphate) and particulate matter (eg, plastic fragments from the bag) from a PN formulation. Filters, however, are not a substitute for good compounding practices intended to prevent precipitate formation.

The risk of infection associated with the preparation and administration of PN formulations further emphasizes the need for proper filtration techniques. In vitro studies have demonstrated that 0.22-μm filters are capable of removing pathogenic microorganisms, such as *Staphylococcus epidermidis*, *Escherichia coli*, and *Candida albicans*, from a PN administration line.[73] Yet the limitations of filters must also be recognized. Because fat particle sizes, even in the most stable formulations (including undiluted IVFEs from the manufacturer), contain fat droplets in excess of 5 μm, 0.22-μm filters are inappropriate for use with IVFEs.[74] Current recommendations include using 1.2-μm filters with IVFE-containing PN formulations to avoid particle shearing and instability that may occur with filters of smaller pore size. Despite the inability to remove bacterial contaminants such as *S. epidermidis* and *E. coli*, large organisms including *C. albicans* are trapped by a 1.2-μm filter.

In-line filters can increase the incidence of occlusion alarms during PN administration. Nursing interventions for frequent infusion pump alarms are often needed due to decreased flow rates or occlusions associated with filter use. However, these alarms should be recognized as a potential sign of a precipitate and should be investigated by a health care practitioner. An occluded filter should never be removed to allow a PN formulation to infuse freely without the use of any device to reduce the infusion of particulates and microprecipitates. Although filters may reduce the potential for patients to become infected due to contaminated PN formulations, they do not completely prevent this occurrence. As such, the CDC does not endorse the use of in-line filters solely for the purpose of infection control.

Control of Aluminum Contamination

On July 26, 2004, federal regulations regarding the labeling of aluminum content in large volume parenterals (LVPs), pharmacy bulk packaging (PBP), and small volume parenterals (SVPs) became effective.[75] Despite significant aluminum content in albumin, blood products, and certain medications, only products regulated by the Endocrine and Metabolic Products Division of the FDA, including products used in compounding PN formulations, are governed by the regulation.

The maximum aluminum load permitted in LVPs, including dextrose solutions, amino acid solutions with and without electrolytes, and premade PN solutions, is 25 mcg per liter. Labels on PBPs and SVPs must include the statement "not more than 25 mcg per liter of aluminum" or provide the aluminum content in micrograms per liter at product expiration. Thus, the label contains the potential *maximum* aluminum content, not the actual amount of aluminum at the time of use. Aluminum content increases over time and is influenced by the container material and closures. Products with an affinity for aluminum can leach aluminum from glass containers and elastomeric closures, causing a significant rise in aluminum contamination over the shelf life of the product. Specific amino acids, calcium salts, and phosphate salts have a high affinity for aluminum; therefore, storage of these products in plastic containers typically results in significantly less aluminum content at expiration than storage in glass containers.[76,77] Raw product contamination with aluminum also contributes to the aluminum load and may be responsible for some of the significant variability in aluminum content between different salt forms of products, such as calcium gluconate and calcium chloride.

Aluminum is widespread in the environment; however, under normal circumstances less than 1% of ingested aluminum is absorbed from the gastrointestinal tract.[77,78] The lungs also serve as an effective barrier. Unfortunately, the body has no effective barriers to aluminum contaminants in parenteral products and must rely on excretion to prevent toxicity. The kidneys are the primary route for the elimination of aluminum and remove unbound aluminum from the blood. The 95% of aluminum bound to protein, primarily transferrin, cannot be excreted; thus, elimination occurs slowly as equilibrium

FIGURE 15-1 Calculation of PN formulation

Clinical Presentation:

LT is a 45-year-old man hospitalized after a motor vehicle collision in which he suffered multiple injuries, including a liver laceration and several bone fractures. A feeding jejunostomy tube was placed during an emergent laparotomy. However, the patient develops abdominal distention following the initiation of enteral tube feedings; therefore, the feedings are discontinued and PN is initiated on day 2 of hospitalization. The patient is 72 in tall, with a precollision weight estimated at 74 kg. The nutrition support team determines that the patient should receive 1.5 g protein per kilogram day and between 25 to 30 total kcal per kilogram per day. The hospital pharmacy compounds PN formulations manually (ie, no ACD) and does not prepare TNA formulations.

Calculations:

Calculation of fluid requirements:

30 mL/kg/day × 74 kg = 2220 mL/day
Kcal: 25–30 kcal/kg/d × 74 kg = 1850–2220 total kcal/d

Usually start with ≤3 mg per kilogram per minute of dextrose so as to not exceed the maximum amount of dextrose the liver can oxidize (ie, 5 mg per kilogram per minute)

Dextrose: 74 kg × 3 mg/kg/min × 1440 min/day ÷1000 g/kg = 320 g dextrose

Protein: 1.5 g/kg/d × 74 kg = 111 g/d

Using amounts amenable to manual compounding:
Kcal to be supplied as dextrose = 300 g × 3.4 kcal/g = 1020 kcal/d
Kcal to be supplied by protein (amino acids) = 100 g/d × 4 kcal/g = 400 kcal/d

Therefore, kilocalories to be supplied by IVFE = 2220 kcal − 1020 kcal − 400 kcal = 800 kcal from IVFE to meet our maximum goal of 2220 kcal per day (or 1850 kcal − 1020 kcal − 400 kcal = 430 kcal from IVFEs to meet our minimum goal of 1850 kcal per day). Therefore, use IVFEs: 250 mL of IVFE 20% × 2 kcal/mL = 500 IVFE kcal

Therefore, the final prescription for the PN formulation is:
Dextrose: 300 g per day
Amino acids: 100 g per day
IVFEs: 250 mL of 20% IVFE infused per 12 hours = 21 mL per hour

Choosing amino acids 10% for compounding:
10 g/100 mL = 100 g/X mL; solving for *x* yields 1000 mL of amino acids 10%

Choosing dextrose 30% for compounding:
30 g/100 mL = 300 g/*x* mL; solving for *x* yields 1000 mL of dextrose 30%

Thus, 1000 mL amino acid + 1000 mL dextrose + 250 mL IVFE = 2250 mL. Estimate 30 mL per liter for additives:
30 mL/L × 2 L/d = 60 mL; 2250 mL/d + 60 mL/d = 2310 mL, which is close to the estimated fluid requirement of 2220 mL/day; 2310 mL/24 hrs = 96 mL/hr for PN infused continuously.

Discussion:

If 500 kcal are provided as IVFEs, approximately 1350 kcal remain to be provided as dextrose and protein (amino acids) for a goal of 1850 kcal per day. The patient requires about 110 g protein per day, but this is rounded down to 100 g due to the limitations of measurement with manual compounding. These 100 g of amino acids provide 400 kcal. Approximately 950 kcal remain to be provided as dextrose.

To provide 950 kcal of dextrose, a total of about 300 g of dextrose is necessary. A stock solution with a dextrose concentration that will provide close to 300 g is desirable. A stock solution of dextrose 30% can be used because 1000 mL provides 300 g. This relatively low dextrose concentration would not be a good option if the patient were fluid restricted. The total calories from IVFE 20%, 250 mL; amino acids 10%, 1000 mL; and dextrose 30%, 1000 mL is 1920 kcal per day.

The previous regimen is compounded as follows: amino acid 10%, 1000 mL is added to an empty 3 L ethylene vinyl acetate bag; then 1000 mL of dextrose 30% is added. Typical additives (electrolytes and multivitamins and trace elements) account for approximately 30 mL per liter. This bag will supply 24 hours of PN. The IVFE is administered separately, typically piggybacked over 12 hours onto the primary PN administration set at a port distal to the 0.22-μm filter.

FIGURE 15-2 Calculation for fluid-restricted PN formulation

Clinical Presentation:

A patient weighing 80 kg has estimated requirements of 30 kcal per kilogram per day, 1.5 g protein per kilogram per day. Twenty percent to 30% of total kilocalories will be provided as IVFEs. The PN formulation volume is restricted to 1.5 L per day.

Estimated Requirement Calculations:

Kcal: 30 kcal/kg/d × 80 kg = 2400 total kcal/d
Protein: 1.5 g/kg/d × 80 kg = 120 g/d
IVFE range: 2400 kcal/d × 0.2 – 0.3 = 480 kcal/d to 720 kcal/d

Example 1:

Stock solutions used by the pharmacy for compounding PN are amino acids 10%, dextrose 70%, and IVFE 20%. PN formulations are manually compounded without an ACD as dextrose –amino acid formulations.

Calculations: Using amounts amenable to manual compounding:

Amino acids 10%, 1000 mL yields 100 g; 100 g × 4 kcal/g yields 400 kcal/d
250 mL of 70% dextrose yields 175 g; 175 g × 3.4 kcal/g yields 595 kcal/d
250 mL of 20% lipid × 2 kcal/mL yields 500 kcal/d; the IVLE will be piggyback infused

Therefore, 400 + 500 + 595 = 1495 kcal/d in 1500 mL per day.

Discussion:

Meeting the caloric and protein needs of the fluid-restricted patient can be challenging and, in some cases, impossible. Amino acid stock solutions in 15% and 20% concentrations are available commercially. They are more expensive on a gram of protein basis compared to amino acid 8.5% or 10% formulations, especially if the pharmacy is purchasing 500 mL containers for manual compounding as opposed to larger stock bottles of amino acid 15% or 20% formulations for automated compounding. The 20% amino acid solution is available only as a 2-L volume unit for automated compounding. Dextrose 50% or 70% should be used for compounding PN in situations of fluid restriction.

If the pharmacy does not routinely use higher concentrated macronutrient stock solutions, the best plan would be to use amino acids 10%, dextrose 70%, and IVFE 20%, as outlined previously. Compounding this solution would require a special mix by the pharmacy because the volumes of dextrose and amino acids are not equal. The protein and calories provided by this regimen are significantly less than the patient's estimated requirements.

Example 2:

Stock solutions used by the pharmacy for compounding PN are amino acids 20%, dextrose 70%, and IVFE 30%. The pharmacy compounds TNA solutions with an ACD.

Calculations:

Protein: 20 g/100 mL = 120 g/x mL; solving for x yields 600 mL of amino acids 20%:
120 g amino acids × 4 kcal/g = 480 kcal/d from amino acids
IVFE: provide 20% to 30% of kcal as IVFE:
2400 kcal/d × 0.2–0.3 = 480 – 720 kcal/d

Because the PN formulation volume is restricted to 1.5 L per day, provide 30% or 720 kcal per day with IVFE 30%, which is more calorically dense (3 kcal per milliliter) than dextrose 70% (2.38 kcal per milliliter).

IVFE 30% provides 3 kcal/mL, therefore 720 kcal/d ÷ 3 kcal/mL = 240 mL
Dextrose: dextrose kcal needed = 2400 kcal – 480 kcal from amino acids – 720 kcal from IVFE = 1200 kcal/d
1200 kcal ÷ 3.4 kcal/g = 353 g dextrose
Dextrose 70% provides 70 g/100 mL = 353 g/x mL. Solving for x = 504 mL

Thus, the volume for the macronutrients is amino acids 20% 600 mL + IVFE 30% 240 mL + dextrose 70% 504 mL = 1344 mL per day. Additives, including electrolytes, parenteral multiple vitamins, and trace minerals, will provide an additional 100 to 120 mL per day. A final volume of 1500 mL per day or less can be achieved.

Discussion:

If the pharmacy does prepare TNA formulations and stocks amino acid 20% formulation and IVFE 30%, then the second scenario could be recommended. The goal protein of 120 g per day and kilocalories of 2400 kcal per day with 20% to 30% of kilocalories provided as IVFEs could be supplied in slightly less than 1500 mL.

between bound and unbound aluminum maintains about 5% of the aluminum available for filtration via the kidneys.[78,79] Eventually, about 60% of infused aluminum is eliminated in patients with adequate renal function.[77] The remaining aluminum is deposited in tissues, including the brain, bones, liver, and lungs.

Adult patients at risk of aluminum toxicity include those with significant renal dysfunction, with a high intake of parenteral products such as PN, or with iron deficiency.[75,78] These patients have either impaired excretion and/or excessive exposure such that aluminum accumulation is likely to occur. Progressive encephalopathy, patchy osteomalacia, reduced parathyroid hormone secretion, and erythropoietin (plus iron)-resistant microcytic anemia have been associated with aluminum toxicity. The final FDA ruling regarding the labeling of aluminum content selected 4 to 5 mcg per kilogram per day as the upper limit of acceptable aluminum exposure and requires a warning statement in the manufacturer's product information to this effect.[75] There is no mandate for the calculation of potential aluminum load or for inclusion of this information on compounded PN in the FDA ruling; however, minimizing aluminum exposure is an important clinical consideration for patients at risk of toxicity.

Calculation of Parenteral Nutrient Formulations

Common stock solutions of dextrose for use in manual PN compounding include 30%, 50%, and 70% concentrations. These are frequently supplied from the manufacturer in 500 mL partial-fill bags or bottles; that is, the bags or bottles in which they are supplied have a potential capacity of slightly more than a liter, allowing for the addition of amino acids and other additives to the formulation. Common stock solutions of amino acids for use in manual PN compounding include 8.5% and 10%. Manufacturers are transitioning from glass bottles to flexible plastic containers for IVFEs. These containers are non-phthalate (non-di-2-ethylhexyl phthalate [DEHP]) plastics, typically polypropylene or a copolymer of propylene, with an overwrap system that protects the IVFE from oxygen exposure.

The CDC recommends that IVFEs alone hang for no more than 12 hours; the CDC states that IVFEs incorporated into a TNA can hang for up to 24 hours.[12] The manufacturer may or may not specify a maximum hang time in their product information; however, since the release of USP Chapter {797}, which includes the CDC recommended times, this is considered the standard of practice. It is generally preferable to infuse an entire container of lipids over 12 hours to prevent wastage, although this must be balanced with adequate clearance of fats from the blood.

A variety of regimens can be constructed that will approximate the patient's predicted needs. If the PN formulation is going to be compounded manually, the pharmacy should be consulted before an order for a nonstandard formulation (ie, a formulation with different volumes of dextrose versus amino acids) is prescribed to determine the feasibility of mixing such a formulation and perhaps to explore alternative formulations that would be easier to compound.

Figure 15-1 illustrates one method of calculating the appropriate amounts of dextrose, amino acids, and IVFEs for the manual preparation of a PN formulation (ie, in an institution that does not use an ACD and does not prepare TNA formulations). Figure 15-2 (examples 1 and 2) depicts the calculations for a fluid-restricted PN formulation (ie, 1.5 L) with the same provision of calories and protein. The calculations are based on the use of commercially available products.

References

1. Isaacs JW, Millikan WJ, Stackhouse J, et al. Parenteral nutrition of adults with a 900 milliosmolar solution via peripheral veins. *Am J Clin Nutr.* 1977;30:552–559.
2. Hatton J, Cohen JL. Potassium. In: Baumgartner TG, ed. *Clinical Guide to Parenteral Micronutrition.* 3rd ed. Chicago, IL: Fujisawa USA; 1997: 239–254.
3. Gazitua R, Wilson K, Bistrian BR, et al. Factors determining peripheral vein tolerance to amino acid infusions. *Arch Surg.* 1979;114: 897–900.
4. Fujiwara T, Kawarasaki H, Fonkalsrud E. Reduction of post-infusion venous endothelial injury with Intralipid. *Surg Gynecol Obstet.* 1984;158:57–65.
5. Mirtallo JM, Canada TW, Johnson D, et al. Safe practices for parenteral nutrition. *JPEN J Parenter Enteral Nutr.* 2004;28: S39–S70.
6. Trissel LA. *Trissel's Calcium and Phosphate Compatibility in Parenteral Nutrition.* Houston, TX: TriPharma Communications; 2001.
7. Mirtallo JM. Parenteral formulas. In: Rombeau JL, Rolandelli RH, eds. *Parenteral Nutrition.* 3rd ed. Philadelphia, PA: WB Saunders; 2001:118–139.
8. Singer P, Bursztein S, Kirvela O, et al. Hypercaloric glycerol in injured patients. *Surgery.* 1992;112:509–514.
9. Lev-Ran A, Johnson M, Hwang DL, et al. Double-blind study of glycerol vs. glucose in parenteral nutrition of post-surgical insulin-treated diabetic patients. *JPEN J Parenter Enteral Nutr.* 1987;11: 271–274.
10. Fairfull-Smith RJ, Stoski D, Freeman JB. Use of glycerol in peripheral parenteral nutrition. *Surgery.* 1982;92:728–732.
11. Sacks GS, Driscoll DF. Does lipid hang time make a difference? Time is of the essence. *Nutr Clin Prac.* 2002;17:283–290.
12. Centers for Disease Control and Prevention. Guidelines for the prevention of intravascular catheter-related infections. *MMWR.* 2002;51(No. RR-10):1–28.
13. Chapter {797}. Pharmaceutical compounding—sterile preparations. Physical tests. In: *United States Pharmacopeia 28/National Formulary 23.* Rockville, MD: The United States Pharmacopeial Convention, Inc; 2005; 2461–2477.
14. Klein S, Miles JM. Metabolic effects of long-chain and medium-chain triglycerides in humans. *JPEN J Parent Enteral Nutr.* 1994;18: 396–397.
15. Food and Drug Administration. Notices/parenteral multivitamin products. *Federal Reg.* 2000;65:21200–21201.
16. American Medical Association Department of Foods and Nutrition. Multivitamin preparations for parenteral use: a statement by the Nutrition Advisory Group. *JPEN J Parenter Enteral Nutr.* 1979; 3:258–262.
17. American Medical Association Department of Foods and Nutrition. Guidelines for essential trace element preparations for parenteral use. A statement by an expert panel. *JAMA.* 1979;241: 2051–2054.

18. Kumpf VJ. Update on parenteral iron therapy. *Nutr Clin Prac.* 2003;18:318–326.
19. 2010 Information to Use in the Event of an Intravenous Fat Emulsion Shortage. American Society for Parenteral and Enteral Nutrition site. http://www.nutritioncare.org/Professional_Resources/Guidelines_and_Standards/Guidelines/Documents_Library_Table_of_Contents. Accessed June 1, 2011.
20. 2010 Information to Use in the Event of an Intravenous Amino Acids Shortage. American Society for Parenteral and Enteral Nutrition Web site. http://www.nutritioncare.org/Professional_Resources/Guidelines_and_Standards/Guidelines/Documents_Library_Table_of_Contents. Accessed June 1, 2011.
21. 2010 IV Multivitamin Shortage Information. American Society for Parenteral and Enteral Nutrition Web site. http://www.nutritioncare.org/Professional_Resources/Guidelines_and_Standards/Guidelines/Documents_Library_Table_of_Contents. Accessed June 1, 2011.
22. 2011 Parenteral Nutrition Electrolyte/Mineral Product Shortage Considerations. American Society for Parenteral and Enteral Nutrition Web site. http://www.nutritioncare.org/Professional_Resources/PN_Electrolyte_Shortage. Accessed June 1, 2011.
23. 2011 Parenteral Nutrition Trace Element Product Shortage Considerations. American Society for Parenteral and Enteral Nutrition Web site. http://www.nutritioncare.org/News/Parenteral_Nutrition_Trace_Element_Product_Shortage_Considerations. Accessed June 1, 2011.
24. Barnett MI. Physical stability of all-in-one admixtures: factors affecting fat droplets. *Nutrition.* 1989;5(5):348–349.
25. Food and Drug Administration. Safety alert: Hazards of precipitation associated with parenteral nutrition. *Am J Hosp Pharm.* 1994; 51:1427–1428.
26. A.S.P.E.N. Board of Directors and The Clinical Guidelines Task Force. Guidelines for the use of parenteral and enteral nutrition in adult and pediatric patients. *JPEN J Parenter Enteral Nutr.* 2002; 26(Suppl):1SA–138SA.
27. Melnick G. Value of specialty intravenous amino acid solutions. *Am J Health Syst Pharm.* 1996;53:671–674.
28. Vanek VW, Matarese LE, Robinson M, et al. A.S.P.E.N. position paper: parenteral nutrition glutamine supplementation. *Nutr Clin Pract.* 2011;26:479–494.
29. USDA National Nutrient Database for Standard Reference. USDA Web site. http://www.nal.usda.gov/fnic/foodcomp/search/index.html. Accessed June 1, 2011.
30. Schloerb PR, Skikne BS. Oral and parenteral glutamine in bone marrow transplantation: A randomized, double-blind study. *JPEN J Parenter Enteral Nutr.* 1999;23:117–122.
31. Ziegler TR, Benfell K, Smith RJ, et al. Safety and metabolic effects of L-glutamine administration in humans. *JPEN J Parenter Enteral Nutr.* 1990;14(suppl):137S–146S.
32. Ulrich H, Pastores SM, Katz DP, et al. Parenteral use of medium-chain triglycerides: A reappraisal. *Nutrition.* 1996;2:231–238.
33. Bellantone R, Bossola M, Carriero C, et al. Structured versus long-chain triglycerides: a safety, tolerance, and efficacy randomized study in colorectal surgical patients. *JPEN J Parenter Enteral Nutr.* 1999;23:123–127.
34. Nijveldt RJ, Tan AM, Prins HA, et al. Use of a mixture of medium-chain triglycerides and long chain triglycerides versus long-chain triglycerides in critically ill surgical patients: A randomized prospective double-blind study. *Clin Nutr.* 1998;17:23–29.
35. Gottschlich MM. Selection of optimal lipid sources in enteral and parenteral nutrition. *Nutr Clin Pract.* 1992;7:152–165.
36. Strausburg KM. Parenteral nutrition admixture. In: Merritt RJ, et al., eds. *A.S.P.E.N. Nutrition Support Practice Manual.* Silver Spring, MD: American Society for Parenteral and Enteral Nutrition; 1998:8.1–8.12.
37. Mayer K, Gokorsch S, Fegbeutel C, et al. Parenteral nutrition with fish oil modulates cytokine response in patients with sepsis. *Am J Respir Crit Care Med.* 2003;167:1321–1328.
38. Mayser P, Mayer K, Mahloudjian M, et al. A double-blind, randomized, placebo-controlled trial of n-3 vs. n-6 fatty acid based lipid infusion in atopic dermatitis. *JPEN J Parenter Enteral Nutr.* 2002;26:151–158.
39. Grimminger F, Führer D, Papavassilis C, et al. Influence of intravenous n-3 lipid supplementation on fatty acid profiles and lipid mediator generation in a patient with severe ulcerative colitis. *Eur J Clin Invest.* 1993;23:706–715.
40. Weiss G, Meyer F, Matthies B, et al. Immunomodulation by perioperative administration of n-3 fatty acids. *Br J Nutr.* 2002; 87:S89–S94.
41. De Meijer VE, Gura KM, Le HD, Meisel JA, Puder M. Fish oil-based lipid emulsions prevent and reverse parenteral nutrition-associated liver disease: The Boston Experience. *JPEN J Parenter Enteral Nutr.* 2009;33:541–547.
42. Gura KM, Lee S, Valim C, et al. Safety and efficacy of a fish-oil based fat emulsion in the treatment of parenteral nutrition-associated liver disease. *Pediatrics.* 2008;121(3):e678–686.
43. Goulet O, de Potter S, Antebi H, et al. Long-term efficacy and safety of a new olive-oil based intravenous fat emulsion in pediatric patients: a double-blind randomized study. *Am J Clin Nutr.* 1999;70:338–345.
44. Granot D, Blum S, Zbinden I, et al. Effect of ClinOleic®, an olive-oil based parenteral lipid emulsion on lymphocyte function in vitro. *Clin Nutr.* 1996;15:9(Suppl 1):3.
45. Waitzberg DL, Torrinhas RS, Jacintho TM. New parenteral emulsions for clinical use. *JPEN J Parenter Enteral Nutr.* 2006;30:351–367.
46. Antebi H, Mansoor O, Ferrier C, et al. Liver function and plasma antioxidant status in intensive care unit patients requiring total parenteral nutrition: comparison of 2 fat emulsions. *JPEN J Parenter Enteral Nutr.* 2004;28:142–148.
47. Borum PR. Is L-carnitine stable in parenteral nutrition solutions prepared for preterm neonates? *Neonatal Intensive Care.* 1993;6:30–32.
48. Mattox TW, Crill C. Parenteral nutrition. In: DiPiro JT, Talbert RL, Yee GC, et al., eds. *Pharmacotherapy.* 8th ed. Stamford, CT: McGraw-Hill; 2011:2505–2525.
49. Mirtallo JM. Should the use of total nutrient admixtures be limited? *Am J Hosp Pharm.* 1994;51:2831–2834.
50. Driscoll DF. Use of total nutrient admixtures should not be limited. *Am J Health Syst Pharm.* 1995;52:893–895.
51. Driscoll DF. Total nutrient admixtures: theory and practice. *Nutr Clin Pract.* 1995;10:114–119.
52. D'Angio RG, Reichers KC, Gilsdorf RB, Costantino JM. Effect of the mode of lipid administration on parenteral nutrition-related infections. *Ann Pharmacother.* 1992;26:14–17.
53. Erdman SH, McElwee CL, Kramer JM, et al. Central line occlusion with three-in-one nutrition admixtures administered at home. *JPEN J Parenter Enteral Nutr.* 1994;18:177–181.
54. American Society of Health-System Pharmacists. ASHP Guidelines on Quality Assurance for Pharmacy-Prepared Sterile Products. *Am J Health Syst Pharm.* 2000;57:1150–1169.
55. Kitzen JM, Halberstadt DJ, Nguyen H, et al. The effect of dextrose and amino acid composition on the refractive indices of parenteral nutrition solutions. *Hosp Pharm.* 1996;31:817–822.
56. Waxman K, Day AT, Stellin GP, et al. Safety and efficacy of glycerol and amino acids in combination with lipid emulsion for peripheral parenteral nutrition support. *JPEN J Parenter Enteral Nutr.* 1992;16:374–378.

57. Freeman JB, Fairfull-Smith R, Rodman GH, et al. Safety and efficacy of a new peripheral intravenously administered amino acid solution containing glycerol and electrolytes. *Surg Gyn Obstet.* 1983;156:625–631.
58. Smith JL, Canham JE, Wells PA. Effect of phototherapy light, sodium bisulfite, and pH on vitamin stability in total parenteral nutrition admixtures. *JPEN J Parent Enteral Nutr.* 1988;12(4):394–402.
59. Trissel LA, Gilbert DL, Martinez JF, et al. Compatibility of medications with 3-in-1 parenteral nutrition admixtures. *JPEN J Parenter Enteral Nutr.* 1999;23:67–74.
60. Octreotide acetate (Sandostatin) [package insert]. East Hanover, NJ: Novartis Pharmaceuticals Corporation; 2002.
61. Trissel LA, Gilbert DL, Martinez JF, et al. Compatibility of parenteral nutrient solutions with selected drugs during simulated Y-site administration. *Am J Health Syst Pharm.* 1997;54:1295–1300.
62. Driscoll DF. Physicochemical stability assessments of lipid emulsions of varying oil composition. *Clin Nutr.* 2001;20(Suppl 4):8–10.
63. Driscoll DF. Lipid injectable emulsions 2006. *Nutr Clin Prac.* 2006;21:381–386.
64. Joy J, Silvestri AP, Franke R, et al. Calcium and phosphate compatibility in low-osmolarity parenteral nutrition admixtures intended for peripheral vein administration. *JPEN J Parenter Enteral Nutr.* 2010;34:46–54.
65. Newton DW, Driscoll DF. Calcium and phosphate compatibility: revisited again. *Am J Health Syst Pharm.* 2008;65:73–80.
66. Brown R, Quercia RA, Sigman R. Total nutrient admixtures: a review. *JPEN J Parenter Enteral Nutr.* 1986;10:650–658.
67. Driscoll DF. Lipid injectable emulsions: pharmacopeial and safety issues. *Pharm Res.* 2006;23:1959–1969.
68. Knowles JB, Cusson G, Smith M, et al. Pulmonary deposition of calcium phosphate crystals as a complication of home parenteral nutrition. *JPEN J Parenter Enteral Nutr.* 1989;13:209–213.
69. Eggert LD, Rusho WJ, MacKay MW, et al. Calcium and phosphorus compatibility in parenteral nutrition solutions for neonates. *Am J Hosp Pharm.* 1982;39:49–53.
70. Schmidt GL, Baumgartner TG, Fischlschweiger W, et al. Cost containment using cysteine HCL acidification to increase calcium/phosphate solubility in hyperalimentation solutions. *JPEN J Parenter Enteral Nutr.* 1986;10:203–207.
71. Mirtallo JM. The complexity of mixing calcium and phosphate. *Am J Hosp Pharm.* 1994;51:1535–1536.
72. Driscoll DF, Newton DW, Bistrian BR. Precipitation of calcium phosphate from parenteral nutrition fluids. *Am J Hosp Pharm.* 1994;51:2834–2836.
73. Mershon J, Nogami W, Williams JM, et al. Bacterial/fungal growth in a combined parenteral nutrient solution. *JPEN J Parenter Enteral Nutr.* 1986;10:498–502.
74. McKinnon BT. FDA safety alert: hazards of precipitation associated with parenteral nutrition. *Nutr Clin Pract.* 1996;11:59–65.
75. Department of Health and Human Services, Food and Drug Administration. Aluminum in large and small volume parenterals used in total parenteral nutrition. *Federal Reg.* 2000;65(17): 4103–4111.
76. Bohrer D, do Nascimento PC, Binotto R, Carlesso R. Influence of the glass packing on the contamination of pharmaceutical products by aluminum. Part II: amino acids for parenteral nutrition. *J Trace Elem Med Biol.* 2001;15(2–3):103–108.
77. Bohrer D, do Nascimento PC, Binotto R, et al. Contribution of raw material to the aluminum contamination in parenterals. *JPEN J Parenter Enteral Nutr.* 2002;26(6):383–388.
78. Klein GL. Aluminum in parenteral solutions revisited—again. *Am J Clin Nutr.* 1995;61:449–456.
79. Yokel RA, McNamara PJ. Aluminum toxicokinetics: an updated minireview. *Pharmacol Toxicol.* 2001;88(4):159–167.

16 Parenteral Access Devices

Elizabeth A. Krzywda, APNP, MSN, Deborah A. Andris, APNP, MSN, and Charles E. Edmiston, Jr., PhD

CONTENTS

Introduction to Vascular Access . . . 266
Physiological Principles . . . 266
Vascular Anatomy . . . 267
Types of Access . . . 267
Peripheral Venous Access . . . 267
Central Versus Peripheral Access . . . 268
Central Venous Access . . . 268
Percutaneous Nontunneled Catheters . . . 268
Tunneled Catheters . . . 268
Implanted Catheters . . . 269
Device Selection and Patient Assessment . . . 270
Device Selection . . . 270
Patient Assessment . . . 270
Catheter Insertion and Maintenance . . . 272
Catheter Insertion . . . 272
Insertion Site Maintenance . . . 273
Hub Care . . . 274
Catheter Patency . . . 274
Device Stabilization . . . 275
Innovative Catheter Technology . . . 275
Central Venous Catheter Features . . . 275
Catheter Materials . . . 275
Antimicrobial Catheter Technology . . . 275
Device-Related Complications . . . 276
Infection – Central Line–Related Bloodstream Infections . . . 276
Microbial Etiology and Pathogenesis . . . 276
Risk Reduction Strategies – Care Bundles . . . 278
Device Occlusion . . . 279
Thrombotic Occlusion . . . 279
Nonthrombotic Occlusion . . . 280
Infusion Delivery Devices . . . 281
References . . . 281

Objectives

1. Identify the vascular anatomy pertinent to the placement of both peripheral and central venous catheters (CVCs).
2. Describe the key aspects of patient assessment and device selection.
3. Differentiate the key characteristics of various peripheral and central venous access devices (CVADs).
4. Discuss the plan of care for the maintenance of vascular access devices.
5. Identify patient risk factors, etiology, pathogenesis, and management of central line–associated bloodstream infections.
6. Define the appropriate approach to the clinical assessment of an occluded CVAD.

Test Your Knowledge Questions

1. Which of the following is the most appropriate vascular access device for a patient requiring long-term parenteral nutrition (PN) therapy?
   A. Use of a midclavicular catheter as a cost-effective measure
   B. Placing a percutaneous nontunneled catheter to initiate PN and then replacement with an implanted port
   C. Placement of a single-lumen tunneled cuffed catheter
   D. Placement of a triple-lumen antibiotic-coated catheter to ensure adequate access for future needs
2. Thrombotic occlusions are most commonly treated with which of the following?
   A. Thrombolytics
   B. Anticoagulants
   C. Ten percent hydrochloric acid
   D. Sodium bicarbonate
3. Which of the following practices has been shown to reduce the risk of central line–associated infections?
   A. Systemic use of antimicrobial prophylaxis at the time of insertion or access
   B. Routine replacement of central venous devices
   C. Use of the central line bundle for insertion and maintenance
   D. Selection of an internal jugular site as opposed to subclavian site
4. The National Healthcare Safety Network criteria for central line–associated bloodstream infection (CLABSI) includes all of the following except:
   A. The catheter must be in place for a minimum of 24 hours.
   B. The patient must have a recognized pathogen cultured from one or more blood cultures, which is not associated with any other site of infection.
   C. The patient exhibits one of the following: fever (>38 °C), chills, or hypotension.
   D. If the patient is <1 year of age and has at least one of the following signs or symptoms: fever, (>38 °C), hypothermia (<36 °C core), apnea or bradycardia, and a positive laboratory culture not related to another infected site.

Test Your Knowledge Answers

1. The correct answer is **C.** A single-lumen cuffed CVC would be the preferred device. The tunneled catheter was originally developed for patients with long-term PN.[1] Tunneled catheters have been demonstrated to be safe and effective in long-term therapies ranging from months to years.[2] A midclavicular catheter does not provide central access and, therefore, would not be an appropriate catheter choice. Percutaneous nontunneled catheters with additional features of multiple lumens and an antibiotic/antimicrobial coating provide PN access in the acute care setting for a shorter duration of time. It would be best to start with selection of the optimal device rather than a planned replacement. Ports are an alternative to external lumen catheters, and patients need to understand that repeated needle sticks will be required for daily therapy.
2. The correct answer is **A.** Catheter occlusions are commonly secondary to a thrombotic etiology. Thrombotic causes include an intraluminal thrombus, an extraluminal fibrin sleeve, and vessel thrombosis.[3] The successful use of thrombolytics to treat catheters occluded with a thrombus is well documented. Historically, streptokinase and urokinase have been used. These agents lyse thrombus by activating and converting plasminogen to plasmin. Plasmin degrades fibrin clots. More recently, tissue plasminogen activator (TPA) has also been used. Nonthrombogenic catheter occlusion includes intraluminal drug and lipid precipitates. Pharmacological agents that change the pH within the lumen increase the solubility of the precipitate.[3]
3. The correct answer is **C.** The central line bundle for insertion and maintenance includes: maximal barrier precautions; wearing a cap, masks, gown, and gloves; and skin antisepsis with chlorhexidine gluconate (CHG). The use of this bundle has been documented to decrease the incidence of catheter-associated infections. The systemic use of antimicrobial prophylaxis at the time of insertion or access is not recommended and may actually promote the resistance of microbial populations associated with catheter infections. The routine replacement of CVADs is not recommended, and catheters should only be removed when clinically indicated. Studies have shown a lower rate of catheter-associated infections in line placements via the subclavian site.[4]
4. The correct answer is **A.** CLABSI represents a new nomenclature that is slightly different from the previously used terminology, catheter-related bloodstream infection (CR-BSI).[4] CLABSI is primarily used for surveillance, whereas CR-BSI is designated as a clinical definition for practice and research. CR-BSI requires clear laboratory findings associating the catheter with infection, including a pathogen cultured with either a quantitative blood culture or a differential time to positivity laboratory testing and no other source of infection. CLABSI requires one of the following four criteria: the patient must have a recognized pathogen cultured from one or more blood cultures that is not associated with any other site of possible infection; symptoms of a fever; hypotension, or in the case of a patient <1 year of age, symptoms of fever, hypothermia, apnea, or bradycardia; and the catheter must have been in place for 48 hours.

Introduction to Vascular Access

Vascular access remains a key component of many medical therapies, including nutrition support. Maintaining vascular access can be as challenging as providing the primary therapy. Over the past 2 decades, complexities inherent in the use of vascular access devices have been recognized. This recognition has fueled scientific investigation and the development of innovative technologies, driving a change in clinical practice. The greatest benefit of success in maintaining vascular access is its translation to an improved quality of life for many patients.

Physiological Principles

Venous blood flow is influenced by several physiological principles promoting the return of blood to the heart and lungs.[5] Negative thoracic pressure occurs during inspiration; muscle contractions and valves within peripheral veins assist in blood return. In the upper and lower extremities, the system of paired valves prevents retrograde blood flow against gravity. In the large central veins, such as the inferior and superior vena cava SVC, blood flow is not dependent on valves but relies on negative intrathoracic pressure and abdominal and diaphragmatic muscle movement. Veins, as opposed to arteries, are able to compensate for occlusions via a rich collateral circulation.

Vascular Anatomy

The superficial veins of the upper extremity are visible and palpable because they lie in the superficial fascia. These vessels include the basilic, cephalic, and median antebrachial veins (Figure 16-1).

The SVC is the main vessel for venous return from the upper trunk emptying into the right atrium.[2] The subclavian vessels receive the external jugular veins and join with the internal jugular vein to form the brachiocephalic vein. The right brachiocephalic vein is directed vertically downward in the thorax. The left brachiocephalic vein crosses over to the right chest. The SVC is formed by the joining of the right and left brachiocephalic veins. The SVC is approximately 7 cm long and 20 to 30 mm in diameter. The estimated blood flow is 2000 mL per minute, making it the preferred vessel for central access and the infusion of vesicant and hyperosmolar fluids (Figure 16-1).[5]

Types of Access

Peripheral Venous Access

One of the easiest and safest ways to access the vascular system is to place a cannula into a peripheral vessel. Short-term peripheral devices are often placed in vessels that originate within the forearm. These devices provide access for a short duration—usually several days—in contrast to peripherally inserted central catheters that provide access for months.[6] The adequacy of the vein limits the use of the peripheral system for infusion. Catheter tips located in a peripheral vessel are not appropriate for the infusion of PN formulas ≥900 mOsm/L, small volume parenteral antibiotics, hypertonic solutions, or vesicants.[7,8] The indications for peripheral infusion are short-term access needs. Specially formulated PN solutions may be administered by peripheral access (see Chapters 14 and 15). These solutions are

FIGURE 16-1 Selected Vascular Anatomy

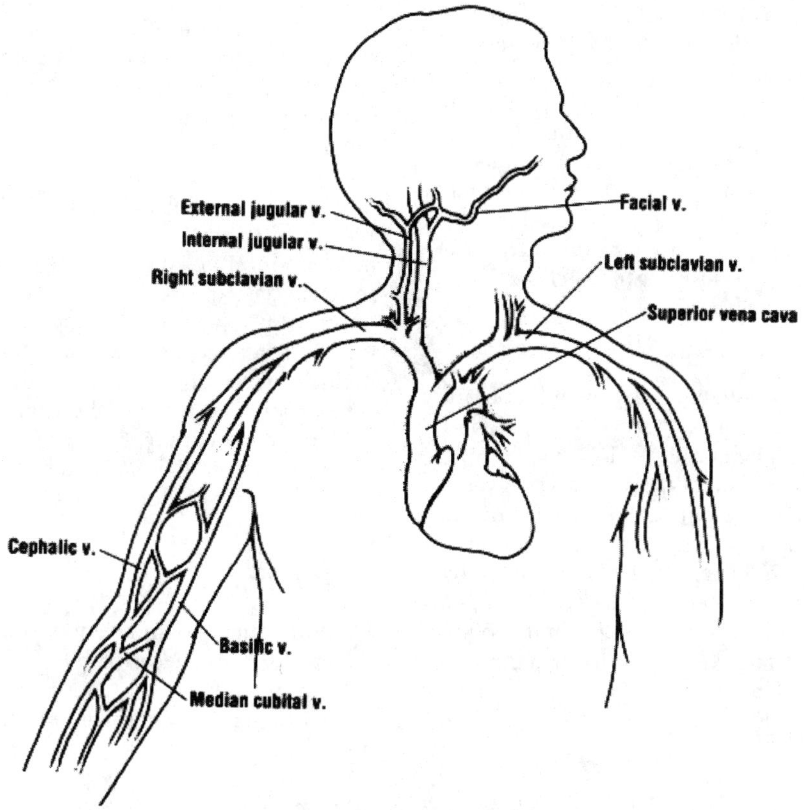

v, vein. Reprinted from Krzywda EA, Andris DA, Edmiston CE, Wallace JR. Parenteral access devices. In: Gottschlich M, ed. *The A.S.P.E.N. Nutrition Support Core Curriculum: A Case-Based Approach: The Adult Patient.* Silver Spring, MD: A.S.P.E.N.; 2007: 300–322, with permission from the American Society for Parenteral and Enteral Nutrition (A.S.P.E.N.).

based on a decreased dextrose concentration and osmolarity, and have been reported to be used for short-term therapies (≤10 to 14 days) when fluid restriction is not necessary.[8]

The leading complication associated with peripheral access is peripheral venous thrombophlebitis. The hallmark symptoms of infusion phlebitis (an inflammation of the cannulated vein) are pain, erythema, tenderness, or a palpable cord.[9] This phenomenon has been related to a number of risk factors including catheter material, size, operator skill, infusate, and duration of cannulation.[10] In one of the largest published studies of over 1000 peripheral cannulas, the risk for phlebitis exceeded 50% by the 4th day of catheterization.[11]

The duration of catheterization is the most common risk factor and in the past it was recommended that standard peripheral cannulas be rotated to a new site every 48 to 72 hours.[12] This concept has been challenged and a recent review found no conclusive benefit to routinely changing catheters every 72 or 96 hours.[13] Rather, it has been proposed that catheters should be changed when clinically indicated. The cannula should be removed as soon as thrombophlebitis develops. Replacement should be at some distance from the site of the phlebitis, preferably the other limb.

Various routines have been recommended as prophylaxis against peripheral vein thrombophlebitis. Heparin and hydrocortisone have been added to peripheral parenteral nutrition solutions resulting in extending the time of catheterization until the onset of thrombophlebitis.[14] However, the compatibility of these compounds in total nutrient admixtures is unknown. Although studied as a flush solution in neonates, there is insufficient data on the effectiveness of heparin flushes in decreasing the rate of phlebitis.[15]

Peripheral devices have the lowest risk of catheter-related infections. This may be related in part to the shortened dwell time, as well as a lack of adequate study and documentation. Peripheral catheters are the most commonly used vascular access devices; however, documented rates of infections are rarely reported and well-designed prospective studies are lacking to adequately support these commonly held beliefs.[16]

Central Versus Peripheral Access

Central or peripheral access is not defined by the initial point of entry into the vascular system but rather by the position of the distal catheter tip.[2] A peripheral catheter is defined as one in which the tip position is outside of the central vessels: the inferior or the superior vena cava. Peripheral catheters include standard peripheral cannulas and midline catheters. Midline catheters were initially introduced in 1950, temporarily removed from the market in the 1990s, and are now available as a redesigned catheter.[17] Catheters are 20 to 25 cm in length, inserted peripherally, and advanced to no further than the axillary vein. These catheters are suitable for all intravenous fluids and drugs that can be administered in a peripheral system. The average dwell time is 2 to 6 weeks.

Central Venous Access

Central venous access is defined as a catheter the distal tip of which lies in the distal vena cava or right atrium.[7] The most common sites of venipuncture for central access include the subclavian, jugular, femoral, cephalic, and basilic veins. CVCs provide access for infusion as well as blood aspiration for laboratory monitoring. The primary indications for central venous access are chemotherapy, antibiotics, and PN. Central venous access provides increased options for medications and infusions, which are not limited by drug pH, osmolarity, or volume. The risk of extravasation with vesicant drugs is reduced.

Conceptually, CVADs can be grouped into three broad categories: nontunneled, tunneled, and implanted.[2,7] This general classification provides a basis for catheter selection. Although no one catheter is ideal for all situations, catheter choice is guided by the advantages and drawbacks associated with these three general categories of devices (Table 16-1).

Percutaneous Nontunneled Catheters

Nontunneled CVADs are most commonly used in the acute care setting for therapies of short duration. Most often, access is obtained with a percutaneous venipuncture using a subclavian, jugular, femoral, or antecubital approach. To prevent dislodgment, sutures or a securement device are placed at the exit site, and a sterile dressing is used. Advantages to nontunneled catheters include decreased placement costs, ease of removal, and the ability to exchange these catheters over a guidewire (Figure 16-2).

Routinely scheduled catheter exchanges over a guidewire are no longer recommended as an effective means of preventing catheter-related infections.[4] Prospective studies have demonstrated a higher rate of infection when catheters are routinely exchanged over a guidewire.[18,19] The potential drawback associated with catheter guidewire exchanges is contamination of the new catheter.

A peripherally inserted CVC (PICC) is defined as a catheter inserted via a peripheral vein and the tip of which lies in the vena cava.[12] Therefore, by definition, these catheters are classified as nontunneled CVCs. PICCs are a common means for securing central vascular access in both acute care and home settings. PICC placement is accomplished using the antecubital vessels: basilic, cephalic, and brachial. This approach decreases the risks of a thoracic approach to catheter placement. Clinicians, mainly nurses and physicians with specialized training, place these catheters. The setting for PICC line placement varies and can occur in the patient's home, at the bedside, or in an interventional radiology suite (Figure 16-3).

Tunneled Catheters

The development of intravenous nutrition support served as an impetus for the technological development of long-term CVADs. Initially, central venous access was accomplished using surgically created arteriovenous fistulas. In an attempt to improve vascular access, a silicone elastomer catheter was inserted by subclavian venipuncture with the distal tip placed into the midatrium.[1] The Broviac catheter served as a model for the original tunneled catheter using an extravascular segment with an attached cuff that was brought through a subcutaneous tunnel on the anterior chest (Figure 16-4).

TABLE 16-1 Vascular Access Devices

Catheter Type	Access	Placement	Advantages	Disadvantages
Percutaneous nontunneled central catheter	Central	Jugular, femoral, subclavian vessels	Economical, easily removable, can be replaced over guidewire, useful in acute care and short duration therapies	Catheter breakage not repairable, patient self-care difficult, requires sutures to prevent dislodgment, high risk for catheter-related infections, not recommended for home care
Tunneled cuffed catheters	Central	Percutaneous placement via subclavian or jugular vessels; cephalic, jugular vein cutdown	Long-term usage, home care, dressings and sutures can be removed after 1 month, self-care easy, repair kit available	Operating room or specialized room for placement, requires small procedure for removal
Peripherally inserted central catheter (PICC)—nontunneled	Central	Percutaneous placement via a peripheral vein	Used in acute and home care for therapies ranging from several weeks to months, low risk of placement complications, placement occurs anywhere from radiology suite to patient bedside	Self-care may be difficult with antecubital placement because dressing changes require both hands, extended home care, repair kits may not be available
Implanted ports	Central	Percutaneous venous placement via subclavian, jugular, or peripheral vessels	Used for long-term therapies, site care only when accessed, monthly heparin flush, body image intact, no external segment for breakage	Needle access required, needle dislodgment can result in infiltration, placement in operating room or specialized room, surgical procedure for removal
Peripheral catheters	Peripheral	Percutaneous peripheral insertion	Least expensive, least risk for catheter-related infections, no special placement room, clinicians are easily trained in placement	Require site rotation 48–72 h, not appropriate to infuse solutions 400–600 mOsm/L, concentrated antibiotics, and vesicants
Midline catheters	Peripheral	Percutaneous peripheral insertion	Used for therapies lasting 2–4 weeks	Not appropriate for infusions requiring central access including PN
Midclavicular catheters	Peripheral	Percutaneous peripheral insertion	Used for therapies 2–3 months	Not appropriate for infusions requiring central access including PN

PN, parenteral nutrition.

Theoretically, catheter tunneling decreases the risk of catheter infection by separating the exit and venipuncture sites.[20,21] Catheter tunneling has, in general, been correlated with decreased rates of infection.[4] In one prospective study, catheter-related sepsis was confirmed in 28% of nontunneled catheters and 11.5% of tunneled catheters.[21] Recently, the benefit and cost-effectiveness of catheter tunneling has been debated.[22] Catheter-related infection rates for nontunneled catheters cared for meticulously by members of an infusion therapy team were comparable to infection rates of tunneled catheters (0.13 versus 0.14 of 100 catheter days).[23]

Tunneled catheters have been demonstrated to be safe and effective in long-term therapies ranging from months to years. Advantages to these catheters include ease of self-care by the patient, decreased risk of dislodgment, and the ability to repair the external lumen in the event of catheter breakage.

Implanted Catheters

Implanted catheters were introduced in 1982 as an alternative to external lumen catheters.[24] These devices consist of a silicone elastomer catheter attached to a plastic or titanium disk with a self-sealing silicone elastomer septum.[25] The port is placed into a subcutaneous pocket that is most often located in the anterior chest. Access is obtained by palpating the port and inserting a noncoring needle into the silicone septum. Ports can be accessed up to 1000 to 2000 times. Variations of the initial port design have included larger septums, double-lumen ports, side entry ports, power ports designed to be used for computed tomography (CT) contrast injection, and peripherally inserted ports, with port placement in the upper extremity.

Advantages to implanted catheters include minimal alteration in body image and ease of self-care. Implanted systems

FIGURE 16-2 A Percutaneous Nontunneled Catheter

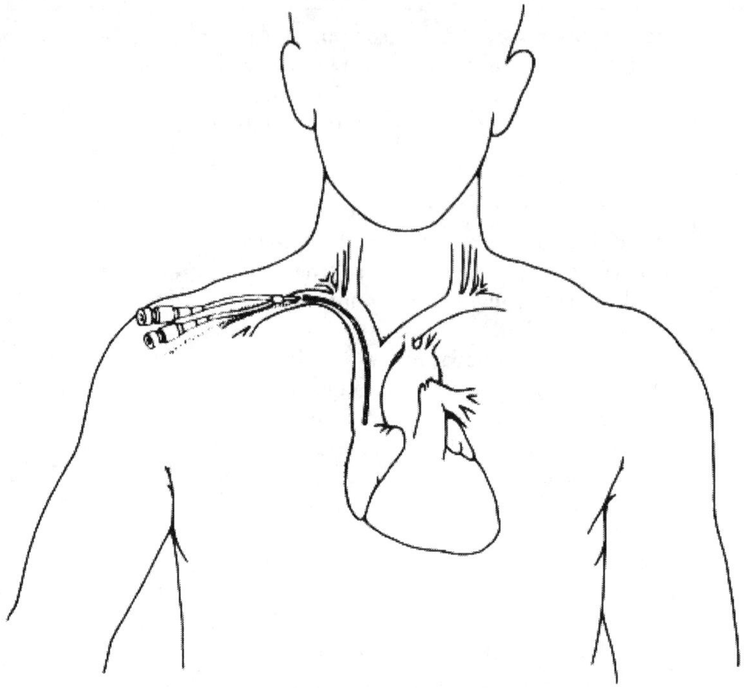

Reprinted from Krzywda EA, Andris DA, Edmiston CE, Wallace JR. Parenteral access devices. In: Gottschlich M, ed. *The A.S.P.E.N. Nutrition Support Core Curriculum: A Case-Based Approach: The Adult Patient.* Silver Spring, MD: A.S.P.E.N.; 2007: 300–322, with permission from the American Society for Parenteral and Enteral Nutrition (A.S.P.E.N.).

do not require routine site care when not in use and should be maintained with a monthly routine heparin flush. Ports are ideal for patients who require infrequent IV therapies, such as intermittent chemotherapy. Lower rates of infection and thrombosis have been demonstrated in a large group of patients (Figure 16-5).[26]

Device Selection and Patient Assessment

Device Selection

Few prospective randomized studies are available to compare various CVADs in terms of complications and outcome.[27] Overall, existing data do support the safety of either indwelling device. Early studies have demonstrated that implanted ports have the lowest rates of catheter-related bloodstream infections. These studies included a large prospective study, demonstrating significantly lower rates of infection in cancer patients with implanted ports as compared to tunneled catheters.[28] It is now recognized that the type of catheter is not the sole variable, but rather, multiple factors influence the potential for catheter complications and overall successful catheter outcomes. Selection of the vascular access device should address factors including the patient's needs, medical history, infusion needs, and device options.[2]

Patient Assessment

Device selection is an important consideration because it aligns the patient and his or her therapy with the appropriate catheter. The goal is to choose a device that is safe, meets the patient's access needs, and is cost-effective. Many factors play a role in the decision-making process, including the type of medication or solution to be delivered, overall therapeutic regimen, anticipated duration of therapy, the patient's lifestyle, the impact on body image, and activity level. The patient's cognitive ability and willingness to perform necessary tasks needs to be assessed because they will influence the degree of care and maintenance the patient will be able to provide. If the patient is unable to participate on a certain level, a device requiring less maintenance may be indicated. The need for and availability of an additional caregiver will impact on cost as well as the need for long-term home nursing assistance. The "ideal" goal of home therapy of a lifelong nature is to restore the patient to his or her prior level of function. When choosing a device, one must allow for an increasing level of activity as the patient recovers and even considers an eventual return to work (Table 16-1).

The educational needs of the patient must also need to be assessed. Patients not only have a need for knowledge that allows them to make an informed decision about device

FIGURE 16-3 A Peripherally Inserted Central Venous Catheter

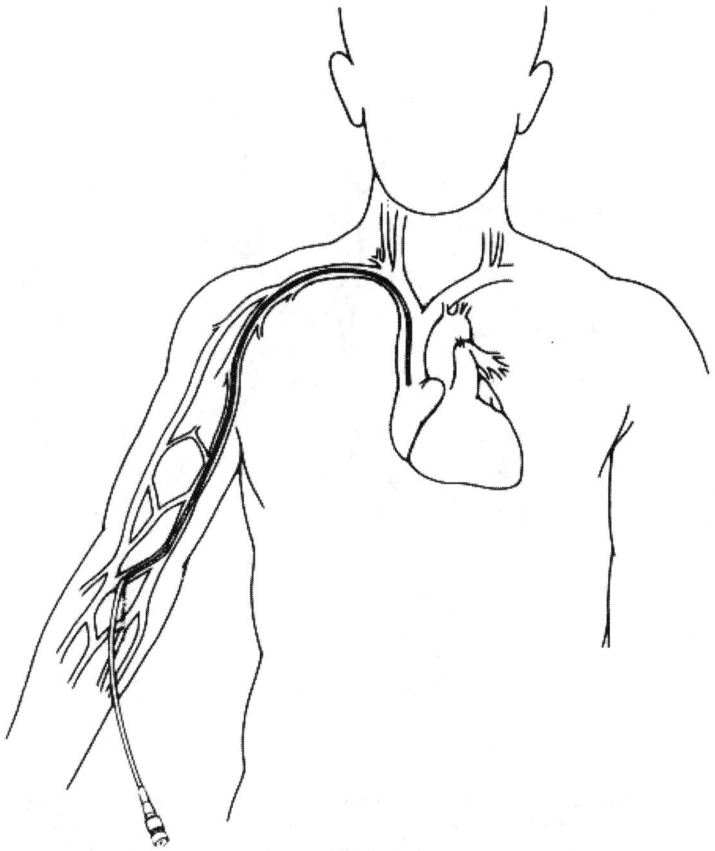

Reprinted from Krzywda EA, Andris DA, Edmiston CE, Wallace JR. Parenteral access devices. In: Gottschlich M, ed. *The A.S.P.E.N. Nutrition Support Core Curriculum: A Case-Based Approach: The Adult Patient.* Silver Spring, MD: A.S.P.E.N.; 2007: 300–322, with permission from the American Society for Parenteral and Enteral Nutrition (A.S.P.E.N.).

selection, but they also require information regarding ongoing care, potential complications, and how to respond appropriately to any problems that arise.

A vascular access history and a focused physical exam are components of the selection/preoperative assessment process. A comprehensive preoperative assessment may decrease the rate of insertion-related complications. In one randomized prospective study, three factors were associated with the failure of placement of a CVC in the subclavian vein: prior surgery or radiation in the region, body mass index >30 or <20, and previous catheterization.[29] A vascular access history identifies any previous devices, location, and length of time the device was in place. Prior device-associated complications such as thrombosis, infection, withdrawal occlusion, or difficult placements should be noted. Previous clavicular fracture, chest, neck, or breast surgery may alter normal anatomic landmarks used during insertion. The physical examination should focus on identifying any lesions, tumors, previous surgical procedures, venous abnormalities, or breaks in skin integrity near the intended placement site. The medication history screens for the use of drugs that could impact coagulation status such as aspirin, nonsteroidal anti-inflammatory agents, warfarin, or heparin. If the patient is on anticoagulants or antiplatelet medications, these medications should be held with a possible transition to low molecular weight heparin based on the individual's risk of thromboembolism.[30]

Venous duplex ultrasonography, or venous angiography, can be obtained when concerns regarding venous patency are present. Studies support the use of the subclavian approach and choosing a device with a minimal number or ports or lumens to minimize CVC-related infection and decrease placement complications.[4,31]

Contraindications to elective placement of a long-term CVC include sudden clinical deterioration with a change in the treatment plan; a new unexplained fever, or absolute neutropenia (white blood cell [WBC] <1000/mL). When platelet counts are less than 50,000, the efficacy of platelet administration within 2 hours of catheter insertion should be considered.

FIGURE 16-4 A Tunneled Central Venous Catheter

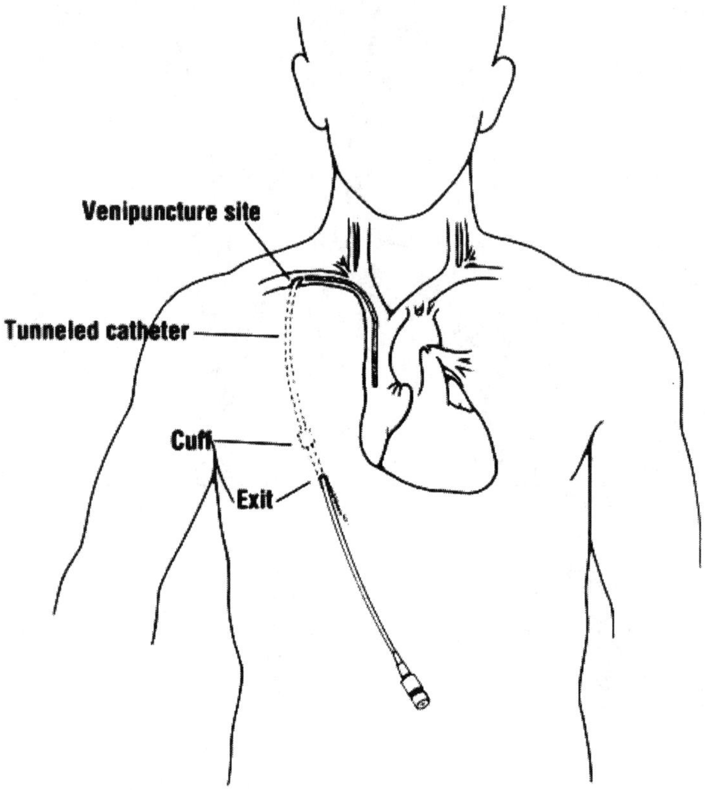

Reprinted from Krzywda EA, Andris DA, Edmiston CE, Wallace JR. Parenteral access devices. In: Gottschlich M, ed. *The A.S.P.E.N. Nutrition Support Core Curriculum: A Case-Based Approach: The Adult Patient.* Silver Spring, MD: A.S.P.E.N.; 2007: 300–322, with permission from the American Society for Parenteral and Enteral Nutrition (A.S.P.E.N.).

Catheter Insertion and Maintenance

The Centers for Disease Control and Prevention (CDC), Guidelines for the Prevention of Intravascular Catheter-Related Infections, 2011, recommends that an effective strategy should be in place to educate health care personnel regarding the indications for catheter use, proper procedures for insertion, and maintenance, which incorporates appropriate infection control measures to prevent intravascular catheter-related infections.[4,32]

Catheter Insertion

Catheters may be inserted at the patient's bedside, in the home, the procedure room, the operating room, or the interventional radiology suite. The setting may not be as critical a factor in minimizing infection risk as is the use of maximal barrier precautions such as the cap, mask, disposable gown, gloves, and large drape. Two landmark studies demonstrated a decrease in catheter colonization at the time of catheter insertion with use of these measures, thereby decreasing catheter-related sepsis risk.[33,34] The use of maximal barrier precautions during CVC insertion is given strong emphasis as a key recommended practice.[4]

Long-term CVADs are usually placed after the patient has received a local anesthetic with or without additional IV sedation. Catheter insertion is commonly performed by one of two techniques, either the percutaneous approach or venous cutdown. The percutaneous approach involves the following: (1) locating anatomic landmarks; (2) cannulating the vessel; (3) inserting a guidewire followed by an introducer; and (4) threading the catheter through the sheath of the introducer and advancing it into the central circulation.[35–37] Tunneled catheters are passed subcutaneously to a site 3 to 10 cm distal to the venotomy with the cuff 2 to 3 cm from the exit site. The percutaneous approach is associated with a risk of pneumothorax, arterial puncture, and catheter pinch-off. Pneumothorax is the most frequently observed complication with an incidence of 1% to 3%.[38]

A venous cutdown is performed using the cephalic, external jugular, or internal jugular vein. In this technique, the vein is dissected, and a venotomy allows for the direct visualization of the vessel while inserting the catheter. A cutdown approach virtually eliminates the risk of a pneumothorax.

The long-standing mandate to verify catheter placement and to detect a pneumothorax with a postprocedure chest X-ray has recently been challenged.[39,40] In a retrospective review of

FIGURE 16-5 An Implanted Port for Central Venous Access

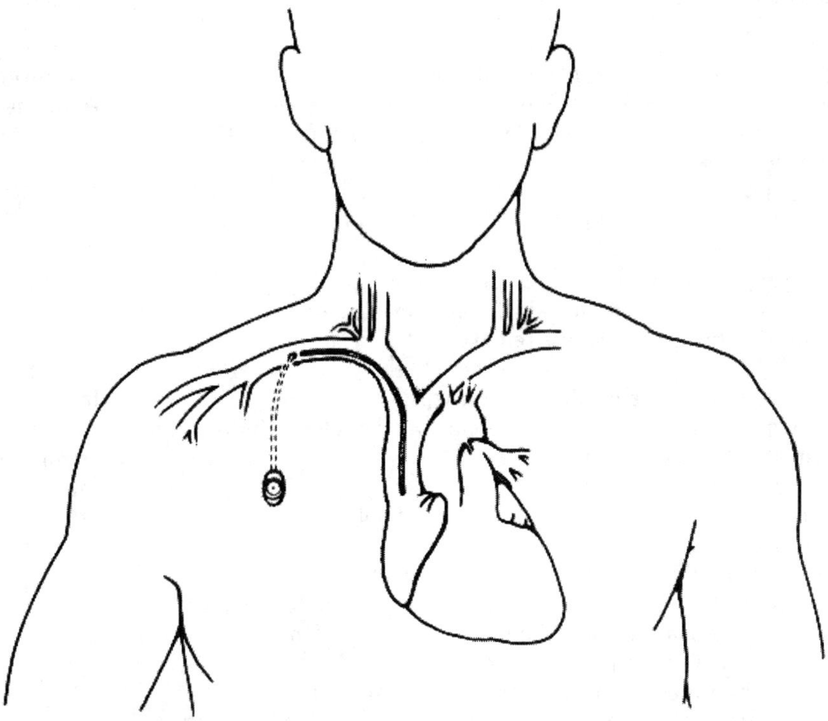

Reprinted from Krzywda EA, Andris DA, Edmiston CE, Wallace JR. Parenteral access devices. In: Gottschlich M, ed. *The A.S.P.E.N. Nutrition Support Core Curriculum: A Case-Based Approach: The Adult Patient.* Silver Spring, MD: A.S.P.E.N.; 2007: 300–322, with permission from the American Society for Parenteral and Enteral Nutrition (A.S.P.E.N.).

205 patients that underwent elective subclavian venous port placement, placement complications included pneumothorax (2%) and catheter malposition (2.4%).[39] A pneumothorax was not identified on the postprocedure chest X-ray, but only on a repeat chest X-ray when the patient was symptomatic. The catheter malpositions were recognized with intraoperative fluoroscopy and corrected.

The use of ultrasound as an adjunct to CVC placement has improved overall placement rates as well as decreased the complications associated with placement. In one of the largest published studies, Cavanna et al. prospectively monitored the safety of ultrasound-guided CVC placement. A total of 1,978 procedures were done with a single needle puncture in 98% of all procedures with a 0% pneumothorax.[40] Ultrasound guidance for central line placement should be used when the technology is available and clinicians are trained in the technique.[4]

Insertion Site Maintenance

Care of the catheter site and hub is considered to play a pivotal role in decreasing the risk for catheter-related sepsis.[41,42] General site care principles prevail regardless of the type of catheter (Table 16-2). The insertion site should be palpated daily for tenderness and, if present, visually inspected for signs of local infection. The catheter exit site should be cleansed with an appropriate antiseptic agent—either 70% alcohol, 10% povidone-iodine, or chlorhexidine. Maki and colleagues[40] pioneered research in this area by comparing these three agents and found 2% aqueous chlorhexidine to be significantly more effective in decreasing both local infection and catheter-related sepsis. In a similar vein, acetone was not found to have an effect on decreasing infection risk and is no longer recommended as a component of the site care regimen.[44]

Recent evidence shows significantly better immediate, persistent, and cumulative antimicrobial activity with products that combine 2% chlorhexidine gluconate (CHG) with 70% isopropyl alcohol.[45] The 2011 CDC guidelines recommend that the skin should be prepped with a >0.5% CHG preparation containing alcohol. In the event that the CHG is contraindicated, then tincture of iodine, an iodophor, or 70% alcohol can be used as an alternative.[4]

Routine use of antibiotic ointments at the catheter insertion site is not recommended due to the change in normal bacterial flora and the emergence of resistant bacteria or fungi.[46] However, recent studies have re-examined the use of antibiotic and antiseptic ointments to the catheter site in high risk patients such as the critically ill and those on hemodialysis.[4,47,48] These studies used either povidone-iodine or mupirocin ointments with a decrease in colonization and bloodstream infections. This decrease was seen primarily in nasal carriers of *Staphylococcus aureus*. However, concern for the emergence of resistant organisms is still a prime consideration.[4]

TABLE 16-2 Central Venous Catheter Maintenance

	Site Care	Flushing
Nontunneled CVC	Dressing: transparent or gauze Transparent enhances catheter stability Performed as a sterile dressing Skin antisepsis protocols include one or a combination of the following: 1. CHG 2. 10% povidone–iodine 3. 70% ethanol	Internal volume: 0.1–0.53 mL 1–2 mL flush is adequate Frequency: usually daily
Tunneled cuffed CVC	Dressing: transparent or gauze until incision healed Dressings often discontinued in double-valved catheters when incision healed and suture removed	Internal volume: 0.15–1.8 mL daily Groshong catheters: 5 mL 0.9% NS weekly
PICC	Performed as an aseptic dressing antisepsis (as previous) Dressing: transparent preferred to enhance catheter stability Preformed as a sterile procedure	Internal volume: 0.04–1.2 mL 2–3 mL flush is adequate Frequency: daily
Ports	Skin antisepsis (see previous) Dressings are required as long as catheter in place Securement devices are recommended Dressings until incision healed (several days post placement) Transparent dressing when port is accessed to stabilize needle Sterile gauze may be placed between needle and skin Huber needle change at least every 7 days Skin antisepsis as previous before needle placement Recommend sterile approach during needle insertion and dressing	Internal volume: 0.5–1.5 mL At least 3 mL adequate Frequency: every 4 weeks

CVC, central venous catheter; CHG, chlorhexidine gluconate; NS, normal saline; PICC, peripherally inserted central venous catheter. Reprinted from Krzywda EA, Edmiston CE. Parenteral access equipment. In: Crocker KS, Christensen ML, Gottschlich MM, et al., eds. *A.S.P.E.N. Nutrition Support Practice Manual.* Silver Spring, MD: The American Society for Parenteral and Enteral Nutrition; 1998.

Either sterile gauze or transparent dressings should be used to cover the catheter exit site. Results of studies comparing these two dressing types have yielded no difference in catheter site colonization rates.[4] Once the Dacron cuff has been incorporated into the subcutaneous tissue, some clinicians advocate cleansing the exit site with mild soap and water, and using no dressing.

Hub Care

Protocols focusing on care of the catheter hub are as critical as those emphasizing care of the site.[49] In most cases, a needleless connector is attached to the hub, which allows direct access to the catheter and obviates the use of needles.

Originally, these devices consisted of a simple split-septum design with no internal mechanism. Over the past 2 decades, connectors have become more sophisticated.[47] Connectors with a mechanical valve designed to control the flow within the system have been developed as well as devices that impact fluid displacement within the device. Microbial barriers are a new feature of some needleless connectors and incorporate the use of either silver or CHG. This development is in part due to studies in which the use of 70% alcohol to cleanse the connector did not reliably prevent entry of microorganisms into the catheter.[51] In an effort to reduce the risk of hub contamination an innovative silver nanohub technology has been developed that under in vitro conditions demonstrated a resistance to microbial contamination and biofilm formation involving selective microbial pathogens such as methicillin-resistant *S. aureus* (MRSA), vancomycin-resistant enterococci (VRE), *Pseudomonas aeruginosa*, coagulase negative staphylococci, and *Enterobacter cloacae*.[52,53]

The majority of new technology has not been analyzed in randomized studies. Jarvis et al.[51] noted an increase in bloodstream infections with the mechanical valve needleless connectors as compared to the split septum devices. The recent CDC guidelines recommend that, "when needleless systems are used, a split septum valve may be preferred over some mechanical valves due to an increase risk of infections with the mechanical values."[4]

Although disinfection of the hub is seen as an important step in preventing infection, there is a lack of consensus on the optimal agent. Available data suggest that vigorous scrubbing with an antiseptic such as CHG for 15 seconds may be preferable. There is no demonstrated benefit to changing connectors more frequently than every 72 hours.[4]

Catheter Patency

The role of routine anticoagulant flush solutions such as heparin to maintain catheter patency has been debated.[42] A recent study has shown that routine use of a heparin flush

(10 units/mL) decreased thrombotic occlusions.[55] Most institutional policies recommend flushing with a heparin flush solution at a regular interval. The volume of the solution should be twice the volume of the catheter and should not interfere with coagulation factors. New evidence suggests alternate anticoagulants such as ethylenediaminetetraacetate (EDTA) may be beneficial not only in maintaining patency but also providing anti-infective properties.[42] Split-valved catheters do not require a heparin flush secondary to their design (Table 16-2).

Device Stabilization

The venous access device must be anchored to prevent migration of the catheter and a loss of access. Effective catheter stabilization will help prevent subtle movement of the catheter tip against the wall of the blood vessel, which can create irritation and promote thrombosis formation. Methods commonly used to stabilize catheters include sutures, sterile tape, and surgical strips. Manufactured stabilization devices are available. Evidence suggests that the use of these products reduces the incidence of CR-BSI as well.[56] In recognition of these benefits, the most recent Infusion Nursing Standards of Practice as well as recent CDC guidelines recommend the use of manufactured securement devices to stabilize intravascular catheters whenever feasible.[4,57]

Innovative Catheter Technology

Central Venous Catheter Features

Catheter size is expressed as French size, diameter, and gauge. French size is the circumference of the outer diameter in millimeters. Diameter refers to both millimeter measurements of the internal and external diameters. The internal diameter may vary between catheters with similar external diameters based upon the catheter material. Gauge is an expression that is inversely proportional to the catheter's outer diameter. The total catheter length is dependent upon the site of insertion and any catheter trimming that is done at the time of insertion.

Most catheters are available in multilumen versions. This option provides for simultaneous infusion of multiple solutions or incompatible drugs. Design may vary among manufacturers in terms of both lumen size and distal tip configurations.

Cuffs attached to catheters are designed to serve as subcutaneous anchors and mechanical barriers. Dacron cuffs are most often attached to tunneled catheters. These cuffs are positioned in the subcutaneous tissue and serve to anchor the catheter by facilitating fibrous ingrowth. Collagen cuffs impregnated with silver ions can be attached to the catheter at insertion or are available preattached. The gradual release of the silver ion exerts short-term antimicrobial activity.[46] Specialized valves have been developed to help prevent retrograde blood flow, catheter occlusions, and air embolisms. A pressure sensitive three-way slit valve on the Groshong tunneled catheter eliminates the need for daily heparinized flushes and catheter clamping before disconnection at the catheter hub.

Catheter Materials

There are many inert biomaterials available for catheter construction. However, upon insertion into the patient, some materials may produce a variety of adverse effects. The ideal biomaterial is one that is nontoxic and nonpyrogenic, easily sterilized, biocompatible with host tissues, and durable. The compounds that most closely achieve these ideals include polyvinylchloride (PVC), polyethylene, polyurethane (PU), silicone elastomer, and hydrogels. PVC is a long-chain polymer that has seen many applications in the biomedical device field. Although this material is relatively inert, it is also quite rigid and demonstrates a high surface energy that is attractive to serum proteins. It has been shown that PVC catheters have been associated with an increase in thrombus formation and phlebitis compared with other polymeric catheters. There have also been reports in the literature suggesting that plasticizing substances added during manufacturing to confer catheter flexibility may leach out following placement and provoke an acute inflammatory reaction.[58]

PU catheters are characterized by a smooth surface, which demonstrates resistance to hydrolytic enzymes. PU offers tensile strength greater than silicone and evidence of lower degrees of microbial colonization.[59] It is felt that the properties of biocompatibility and versatility hold promise for upcoming catheter technology.[60]

The biomaterial most often used for long-term indwelling vascular access devices is silicone elastomer. Catheters constructed of silicone demonstrate excellent elasticity and softness; therefore, silicone catheters cause less damage to the vessel intima. In addition, silicone elastomer has a low inflammatory provoking potential in the tissues, whereas the surface is less attractive for adherence of microbial populations when compared to other biomaterials used in catheter construction. The material tends to be chemically inert to blood with reduced platelet adherence; however, serum protein will adsorb to the surface. Therefore, fibrin sleeve formation is seen as a common complication of these devices.[61]

A unique class of hydrophilic polymers has a cross-linked, three-dimensional structure, which allows water absorption—in some cases up to 90% of the catheter's dry weight. This polymer has been bonded to catheter surfaces. The polymer's negatively charged surface mimics the electrical characteristics of the host vessel wall, resulting in enhanced biocompatibility with a reduction in thrombogenicity. These specific catheters are stiffer for insertion and subsequently soften after placement in the vessel. Unfortunately, the hydrogels as a group lack the tensile strength and durability of other catheter materials, such as silicone elastomer. Acute hypersensitivity reactions have been associated with midline catheters composed of an elastomeric hydrogel material.[62]

Antimicrobial Catheter Technology

Initial trials of antiseptic- or antibiotic-impregnated catheters were noted to reduce the risk of microbial colonization and catheter-related bloodstream infection for short term access.[63,64] The 2011 CDC guidelines recommend that an antimicrobial-impregnated catheter be considered when other comprehensive strategies have failed to reduce the risk of CLABSIs. This technology alters the polymeric catheter surface to achieve increased resistance to microbial colonization.

In a prospective randomized trial, significantly decreased rates for both catheter colonization and CR-BSI were demonstrated with the use of a CHG and silver sulfadiazine coating on the external lumen of CVCs.[64] However, a recent investigation comparing a chlorhexidine/silver sulfadiazine-impregnated double-lumen CVC to a standard CVC found no difference in the colonization rate between both devices in ICU patients.[65] A recent economic analysis employing a Markov decision model has suggested that the cost-effectiveness of using an antimicrobial-impregnated CVC within the ICU patient population is "highly uncertain."[66] This uncertainty is often mirrored by the reticence of infection control personnel to universally adopt this technology as a risk-reducing strategy, thereby guiding the current CDC recommendation. However, the fear that the use of selective antimicrobial-impregnated catheters will promote antimicrobial resistance among hospital-acquired pathogens is currently unfounded based on recent clinical investigations.[67,68]

Limited reports in the literature address CHG hypersensitivities, especially with the use of CHG-impregnated CVC.[4] In Australia, a recent case report has been published noting an anaphylactic event following insertion for a CHG-impregnated CVC.[69]

Device-Related Complications

Complications associated with vascular access devices (VADs) have been divided into infectious and noninfectious complications. Infectious complications are the most frequently observed with intravascular devices. Noninfectious or mechanical complications include catheter occlusion, thrombosis, and breakage. Catheter occlusion is the most common noninfectious complication observed with the long-term use of VADs.

Infection – Central Line–Related Bloodstream Infections

Indwelling vascular access devices pose the greatest risk for the development of a bloodstream infection.[70] Nosocomial bloodstream infections associated with CVCs have an attributed mortality of 12% to 25%.[35] The key to decreasing CR-BSIs is prevention and, as such, is the main focus of the revised CDC report.[4] To give a rough estimate of potentially preventable nosocomial infections in health care, Harbarth et al.[69] conducted a systematic review of the literature assessing multimodal intervention studies and transmission studies published in the last decade. The most important reduction identified was the incidence of CR-BSI in CVADs with a crude reduction effect of 56% (from 8.7 episodes to 3.8 episodes/1000 catheter days).

Indwelling VADs pose the greatest risk for the development of a bloodstream infection. The CDC has published standardized definitions differentiating the types of catheter-related infections.[37] The use of consistent definitions will improve accuracy when comparing infection rates and treatments (Table 16-3).

Microbial Etiology and Pathogenesis

CVC-related infections can originate from one or more of the following pathways: endogenous skin flora, contamination of the catheter hub, hematogenous seeding of the device from a distant site, and contamination of infusate.[4] The two primary portals for the contamination of CVCs have been identified as the skin entrance site and the hub.[49] It is likely that hub contamination is the most frequent cause of intraluminal contamination in the long-term use of vascular access devices.[71] However, migration of endogenous skin flora from the insertion site results in extraluminal colonization of the catheter and is a more prevalent etiology in short-term catheters. Infusate contamination is rarely associated with catheter sepsis. Hematogenous seeding is an elusive mechanism requiring documentation of a primary infection at a distant site.

The microbial spectrum of CR-BSI has evolved over the past 30 years, with gram-positive isolates emerging as the predominant pathogens. Over 42% of catheter-associated bloodstream infections are caused by *Staphylococcus epidermidis*, an organism that, less than 20 years ago, would have been viewed primarily as a skin contaminant.[72] These organisms have emerged as a major nosocomial isolate and are the predominant pathogens associated with infections from biomedical devices.[4]

The coagulase-negative staphylococci are frequently capable of producing a biofilm composed of an exopolysaccharide (glycocalyx) that is also referred to as "slime." The exopolysaccharide allows the staphylococcal cells to cling tenaciously to the surface of a catheter or biomedical device (Figure 16-6). The staphylococcal cells embedded within this biofilm are protected from host phagocytic cells, antibodies, and antibiotic therapy.[70] In addition, selected strains of *S. epidermidis* that produce a biofilm often express phenotypic resistance to traditional antimicrobial agents.[73] The presence of a biofilm associated with a catheter-based infection increases the difficulty of successfully treating the infection without removing the catheter.[74]

S. aureus was at one time the most frequently reported pathogen associated with CR-BSI.[75] Adherence of *S. aureus* to a catheter surface is mediated by surface receptors that involve specific host protein interactions. Over the past 20 years, the importance of this microorganism has been compounded by the emergence of MRSA.[76] This resistance has contributed to an increase in the empiric use of vancomycin to treat nosocomial bloodstream infections. Hand contamination is viewed as the primary means of nosocomial acquisition for bloodstream infections. However, microbial aerosols produced during periods of rhinorrhea may also contribute to the distribution of these organisms, emphasizing the importance of maximal barrier precautions, including masks, while inserting central lines.

Enterococci currently account for 14.5% of nosocomial bloodstream infections.[71] Ninety percent of clinical enterococcal infections are caused by *Enterococcus faecalis*, whereas 5 % to 10% are associated with *Enterococcus faecium*. The emergence of VRE is associated with several sentinel risk factors, including: (1) previous antibiotic therapy involving third-generation cephalosporins and vancomycin use; (2) gastrointestinal colonization with VRE; (3) the severity of the underlying disease; (4) a prolonged hospital stay; and (5) the

TABLE 16-3 Catheter-Related Infections

	Infection Type			
	Exit Site	Tunnel	Pocket	Bloodstream
CDC definition	Erythema, tenderness, or purulence within 2 cm of site	Erythema, tenderness, or purulence >2 cm from site	Erythema and necrosis over port reservoir or purulent exudate in subcutaneous pocket	Same isolate on semiquantitative/quantitative catheter culture and blood; no other sign of infection, defervescence with catheter removal, paired blood samples: central five- to tenfold > than peripheral, or cultures are reported as positive from the central line 2 h sooner than the peripheral
Treatment options	Warm compresses, daily site care, oral antibiotics	Catheter removal	Port removal, antibiotic therapy	Antibiotic or antimicrobial lock, systemic antibiotics, catheter removal: yeast, *S. aureus*, polymicrobial, recurrent infection, persistent bacteremia

CDC, Centers for Disease Control.

use of indwelling VADs. Enterococcal bloodstream infections may arise from the patient's own endogenous flora or through nosocomial transmission involving the hands of health care workers and exposure to contaminated surfaces.[77] The increasing use of IV prophylactic vancomycin, especially in the neutropenic or high-risk population, is viewed as contributing to the emergence of VRE in the vascular access population.[78]

In general, *Candida* or yeast is associated with a 9% catheter-related sepsis rate.[79] The pathogenesis of these infections

FIGURE 16-6 The Role of Biofilm to Protect Bacteria on a Medical Device

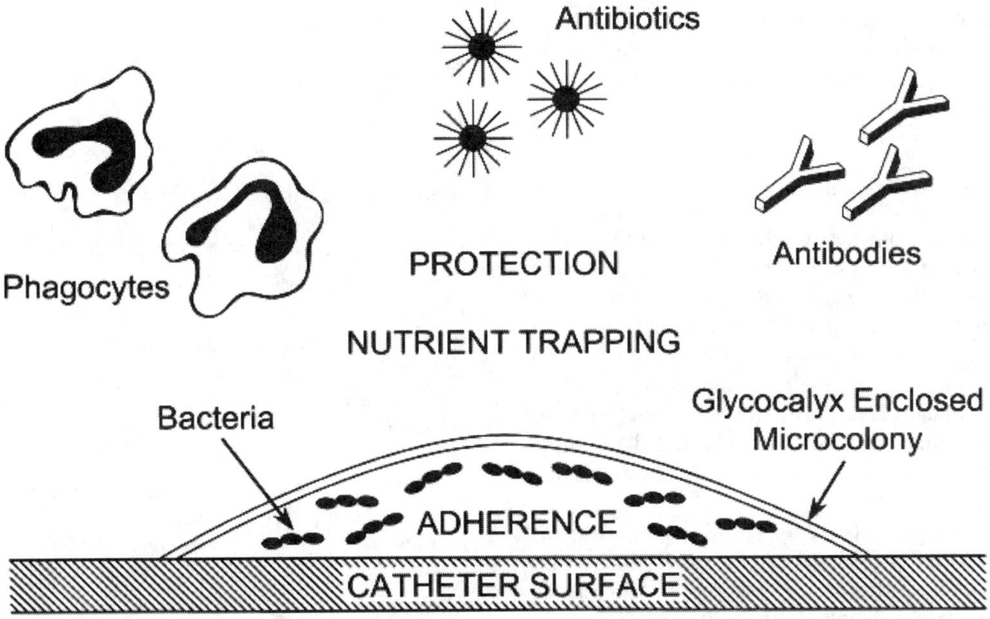

The exopolysaccharide (glycocalyx) substance elaborated by selected bacterial populations (staphylococci) facilitates microbial persistence and provides a protective environment on the catheter surface, preventing normal host defense mechanisms such as opsonizing antibodies and phagocytic cells from effectively dealing with the microbial pathogens. In addition, microbial populations enmeshed in glycocalyx are sequestered from the therapeutic activity of systemic antimicrobial agents. Reprinted from Krzywda EA, Andris DA, Edmiston CE, Wallace JR. Parenteral access devices. In: Gottschlich M, ed. *The A.S.P.E.N. Nutrition Support Core Curriculum: A Case-Based Approach: The Adult Patient.* Silver Spring, MD: A.S.P.E.N.; 2007: 300–322 with permission from the American Society for Parenteral and Enteral Nutrition (A.S.P.E.N.).

suggest that endogenous colonization is the principal mechanism of nosocomial acquisition.

Enterobacter spp., *Escherichia coli, Klebsiella pneumoniae,* and *Pseudomonas aeruginosa* are infrequent causes of CR-BSI. However, in the past, clusters of catheter infections associated with specific isolates such as *Enterobacter* or *Acinetobacter* may suggest the contamination of infusate solutions.[80] Infections involving *Pseudomonas* spp. and *Stenotrophomonas maltophilia* often require catheter removal because contamination with these specific pathogens is associated with a high rate of treatment failures.

Within the long-term PN patient population, many of the common microbial pathogens are similar to those seen within acute care patients. Specifically, coagulase-negative *Staphylococcus* occurs in approximately 60% of CVC infections followed by *Klebsiella pneumoniae, S. aureus,* and *Enterococcus.* However, *Candida* species, including *C. parapsilosis, C. glabrata,* and *C. albicans,* are often recovered from long-term CVCs used for PN.[81] Recurrent gram-negative infections of central lines have been observed in patients with short-gut syndrome receiving PN.[82]

Although antibiotic (or antimicrobial) lock has been validated as an effective strategy for the treatment of CR-BSIs and catheter salvage, the prophylactic use of antimicrobial lock to prevent CR-BSI is controversial. The CDC guidelines suggest that the practice should be limited to patients with long-term catheters who have a history of multiple CR-BSIs. Previous investigations have looked at the effectiveness of various antibiotic regimens; however, these studies have been fraught with flaws in both study design and implementation.[83] Several recent investigations have suggested that the use of 70% ethanol was effective at reducing the risk of primary CR-BSIs in high-risk patent populations.[84] Although these studies are intriguing, the CDC views the current evidence-based literature on this topic to be only category II.[4,83,84]

Risk Reduction Strategies – Care Bundles

The current focus on patient safety has brought the problem of CR-BSIs under closer scrutiny both by regulatory agencies and consumer groups. In a trend expected to become nationwide, several states have enacted laws mandating public disclosure of hospital-acquired infections, including central line infection rates. In response to this heightened awareness of the problem of CR-BSIs, the Institute for Healthcare Improvement (IHI) has proposed a set of evidence-based practices as a "Bundle," which has been designed to reduce the incidence of infections associated with central lines.

Based on CDC guidelines, the IHI Central Line Bundle has five components: (1) hand hygiene, (2) maximal barrier precautions, (3) CHG skin antisepsis, (4) optimal catheter site selection, and (5) daily review of line necessity, with the prompt removal of unnecessary lines. Maximal barrier precautions should be observed during the insertion of CVCs, PICCs, or guidewire exchange, which includes use of a cap, mask, sterile gown, sterile gloves, and a sterile full body drape (category 1B evidence-based practice).[4] Recent published studies have documented that the use of a catheter line care bundle incorporating maximal barrier precautions and CHG skin antisepsis is effective in reducing the incidence of CR-BSIs.[72,85–88]

According to the bundle concept, these measures are considered as a single intervention rather than as a set of individual processes. Failure to complete one aspect of the bundle is regarded as noncompliance with the entire protocol. Prospective clinical trials in which central line bundles have been rigorously implemented have yielded impressive reductions in the incidence of CR-BSIs. Some centers have virtually eliminated central line infections in intensive care units that employed the IHI bundle.[89,90]

An adjunctive interventional strategy that is supported by strong evidence-based data is the use of a CHG-impregnated sponge, which is affixed at the catheter exit site following line insertion. In a recent multicenter, randomized clinical study involving over 1600 ICU patients and >28,000 catheter days, the use of the CHG-impregnated sponges was effective at significantly reducing the rate of CR-BSIs from 1.1 per 1000 catheter days to 0.6 per 1000 catheter days ($p<.03$).[91] The use of this innovative technology resulted in a 60% reduction in the risk of catheter-related infections within a patient population with a low background rate of CR-BSIs.

Although implementation of the catheter care bundle has resulted in a significant reduction in the global rate of CR-BSIs (CLABSI), the adjunctive addition of selective evidence-based interventions has allowed many institutions to essentially eliminate line-associated infections within selective critical care patient populations.[91] These results underscore the importance of evidence-based practice and how strict adherence to standards of care can improve patient outcomes (Practice Scenario 16-1).

Practice Scenario 16-1

Question: What is the appropriate treatment of CR-BSI in a patient with a tunneled cuffed vascular access catheter?

Scenario: A 55-year-old woman on long-term home PN presents to the clinic with a fever of 102°F and shaking chills that started 2 hours after beginning her PN infusion. The patient had been on home PN for 8 months after a complicated surgical history resulting in stenosis of the superior mesenteric artery as well as celiac artery, bowel ischemia, small bowel resection, and short-gut syndrome. A single-lumen, tunneled, cuffed silicone elastomer catheter is in place.

The physical exam reveals a middle-aged woman who appears ill. Her skin was warm and dry. Vital signs were as follows: temperature, 101.8°F; blood pressure 130/80; pulse, 100; respiratory rate, 18. The catheter site was clean, nontender, and nonreddened. Laboratory testing is significant for a white blood cell count of 15,000 (5,000 to 10,000) and an elevated blood glucose level of 160 mg/dL (70 to 120). CR-BSI is suspected and blood cultures are obtained both through the catheter and via a peripheral blood sample. Results indicate *S. epidermidis* from the catheter specimen within 4 hours, and the same organism is identified in the peripheral sample in 10 hours.

Intervention: Treatment included both systemic antibiotic therapy as well as locking the catheter with a 70% ethanol lock of 2 mL daily with a 6-hour dwell time. She was discharged home with treatment planned for 7 days. Home PN was also continued.

Answer: Although the gold standard for the diagnosis of a CR-BSI requires catheter removal, in patients that require long-term IV therapies, catheter salvage rather than removal is desirable. Blood cultures are obtained using a method of "differential time to positivity." CVC blood cultures that become positive ≥2 hours earlier than the peripheral culture are considered predictive for CR-BSIs, with 85% sensitivity and 81% specificity. Blood cultures confirmed a CR-BSI. Catheter salvage using both an ethanol lock as well as systemic antibiotic therapy is often successful in treating a CR-BSI.

Rationale: The decision to remove an infected CVC depends, in part, on the virulence of the microorganism.[92] Removal of the catheter is recommended for documented fungal infections and *S. aureus*. Ethanol is an antiseptic that provides bactericidal activity against a broad range of organisms and is less likely to promote resistance.[84] A growing number of studies have documented the efficacy of locking catheters as both a treatment option as well as a method of prevention in patients with recurrent CR-BSIs.[4]

Device Occlusion

Catheter occlusion is the most common noninfectious complication. Depending upon the series, occlusion has been identified in up to 50% of CVCs.[93] Occlusion can be secondary to thrombotic as well as nonthrombotic causes. Catheter patency is defined by two criteria—the ability to infuse without resistance and the ability to aspirate blood without resistance. When either of these criteria are not met, the catheter is occluded (Table 16-4).

Thrombotic Occlusion

Thrombotic causes are the primary source of catheter dysfunction.[93] In the early 19th century, Virchow proposed a triad of key factors resulting in the development of vessel thrombosis. These three causative factors are (1) vessel wall damage, (2) blood flow changes, and (3) a systemic alteration in coagulation.[82] Today, these factors continue to form a physiological explanation for catheter-related thrombosis. Vessel wall injury occurs with catheter placement. Venous thrombi are composed of fibrin, and trauma induced by the catheter tip against the vessel wall binds platelets and blood cells. In response to this injury, coagulation factors are activated. Fibrin becomes cross-linked and erythrocytes interweave with platelets and leukocytes. In addition, blood flow dynamics are altered by the presence of a catheter in a vessel. Malignancy and certain other diseases can produce procoagulants that alter the physiological equilibrium and predispose the patient to thrombotic phenomena.

The initiation of a thrombotic process on a catheter surface occurs minutes after vascular catheter insertion. In a landmark study, Horshal et al.[94] described the presence of fibrin sleeves surrounding subclavian CVCs. Upon autopsy inspection, all catheters were noted to have circumferential fibrin sleeves. The origin of these collections seemed to occur at two points. The most common point was where the catheter entered the vessel. The second point identified was at the intima adjacent to the distal catheter tip. Risk factors for thrombus formation include: catheter tip position, catheter material, type of infusate, and length of catheter duration. A prospective study of 444 patients with indwelling CVCs identified three significant baseline factors associated with the incidence of catheter-related thrombosis: more than one insertion attempt, ovarian cancer, and previous CVC insertion.[95] The incidence of symptomatic catheter-related thrombosis varies from 0.3% to 28.3%; when assessed by venography, it is reported to range from 27% to 66%.[96] The thrombotic complications associated with PICCs are fewer, but not infrequent, ranging from 1% to 4% (based on symptoms alone) to 23% (based on radiographic findings).[97,98]

Catheter-related thrombosis has been differentiated according to the location and extent of the thrombus.[3] Distinct thrombotic occlusions include an intraluminal clot, a fibrin sleeve formation, a mural thrombus, or thrombosis of the vessel.

Intraluminal clotting as a result of inadequate flushing or blood reflux can result in sluggish catheter function as well as catheter occlusion. Inadequate saline flushing following blood aspiration and the administration of blood products can lead to intraluminal clotting. The volume of flush solution is recommended to be at least twice the volume of the catheter.[42] Fibrin sleeves can encase the catheter and distal catheter tip. Venous thrombosis refers to a thrombus in the vessel that may partially or totally occlude the vessel. This mural thrombus may initially present as a venous obstruction.

TABLE 16-4 Catheter Occlusions

Etiology	Symptoms	Treatment
Intraluminal occlusion	Resistance to infusion/aspiration	a. Blood clotting—use thrombolytic in volume to fill catheter lumen b. Drug/lipid precipitate—use appropriate pharmacologic agent: (0.1 N HCl, sodium bicarbonate, ethyl alcohol)
Fibrin sleeve—distal catheter tip	Inability to aspirate blood sample	a. Thrombolytic agents given as catheter infusion or overfill method b. Endovascular catheter stripping
Vessel thrombosis/ pericatheter thrombosis	Resistance to infusion and aspiration	a. Thrombolytic agents given as systemic infusion and/or catheter directed b. Endovascular stenting
Mechanical occlusion	Resistance to infusion and aspiration	a. Rectify closed clamp/tight suture/catheter malposition b. Pinch-off syndrome—remove catheter

The primary symptom suggesting a catheter-related thrombosis is a loss of catheter patency. Fibrin sleeve formation at the distal catheter tips often presents as a withdrawal occlusion. Catheters remain fully functional for infusion; however, blood cannot be aspirated from the lumen. Physiologically, the fibrin sleeve acts as a one-way valve. As negative pressure is applied, the sleeve is pulled over the open catheter tip and prevents blood aspiration. Catheter phlebography has demonstrated the presence of presumed fibrin collections encasing the distal catheter tips. In some cases, the sleeve may extend to the venous entry site and result in extravasation of infusate into the surrounding tissues. Overall, the exact incidence of fibrin sleeve formation resulting in withdrawal occlusion is not clearly determined but may be evident in 47% of CVCs.[96]

Catheter-related venous thrombosis may present as a catheter occlusion, with clinical symptoms of vascular obstruction. These symptoms include neck vein distension, edema, tingling or pain over the ipsilateral arm and neck, a tight feeling in the throat, and a prominent venous pattern over the anterior chest.[99] SVC thrombosis can result in a permanent vascular obstruction, chronic venous insufficiency, and loss of future access.[95]

Treatment will depend on the extent of the thrombus, severity of symptoms, and the need to reestablish access and available alternatives. Treatment is most successful when the cause of the catheter occlusion is correctly identified. The effectiveness and safety of the use of thrombolytics in the treatment of intraluminal clot and fibrin sleeve formation has been documented.[3,100] Thrombolytics such as alteplase 2 mg in a 2 ml volume are injected into the catheter and allowed to dwell for 30 minutes to 4 hours. If patency is not reestablished, the dose may be repeated.

In patients with catheter-associated mural or venous thrombosis, catheter removal is not recommended as the first treatment.[99] In one pilot study,[99] the use of standard dalteparin/warfarin in patients with upper extremity deep vein thrombosis (DVT) secondary to central catheters resulted in the ability to maintain access without the risk of recurrence or extension of the DVT. Catheter-directed thrombolysis has typically been used in cases with a recent onset of symptoms, extensive edema, and an impairment of function. To date there is a lack of randomized studies addressing the optimal time of anticoagulation for catheter-related thrombosis.[99]

In terms of thrombosis prophylaxis, early evidence had suggested a benefit of low dose anticoagulation. This practice is no longer supported; an analysis of randomized studies found no significant effect for either vitamin K antagonists or heparin on symptomatic DVT.[101] One prognostic factor that has been identified is that of catheter tip placement. Catheter tips that are positioned during placement in the lower vena cava have a decreased rate of thrombosis as compared to those with tips more proximal in the vena cava.[98]

Thrombosis has been linked to an increased risk of infection.[102] Fibrin sheaths, rich in fibrin and fibronectin, promote bacterial adherence. In a study of 72 postmortem examinations, catheter-related septicemia was only demonstrated in patients with underlying mural thrombosis.[102] van Rooden et al.,[103] in a prospective study, evaluated 105 patients for catheter-related infections and thrombosis. In patients with two or more positive cultures, 71.4% developed thrombosis; the incidence of thrombosis was 3.3% in patients with a negative or a single positive culture. These results highlight the potential benefit of using thrombolytics in the treatment and prevention of catheter-related bloodstream infections.

Nonthrombotic Occlusion

The leading causes of intraluminal occlusions are drug/heparin interactions, parenteral nutrition formulations with inappropriate calcium/phosphate ratios, and lipid residue.[3] Lipid occlusions may slowly accumulate within the catheter lumen, resulting in sluggish catheter flow before a complete occlusion. The compounding of total nutrient admixtures requires close attention to prevent the precipitation of components. The use of a 0.9% normal saline flush between all intravenous medications, infusions, and heparin is the key to prevention.

Various factors can lead to a nonthrombotic or mechanical catheter occlusion. Mechanical occlusions can be caused by external clamps, kinking of the catheter, occluded port needles, and constricting sutures (Practice Scenario 16-2).

Practice Scenario 16-2

Question: How do you successfully establish catheter patency in an occluded central catheter?

Scenario: A 70-year-old man with a pseudo-obstruction has a single-lumen tunneled catheter for administration of PN. After his hospital discharge, he is transferred to an intermediate skilled nursing facility. Within the first week at this facility, the nurse began the nightly PN infusion; 3 hours after PN infusion, the pump alarms occlusion. The following assessment is completed: (1) no extrinsic compression from clamps, sutures, or kinked catheter tubing is noted; (2) the occlusion is relieved by postural changes, such as raising the ipsilateral arm and shrugging the shoulders forward; (3) recent infusion history includes only PN with no recent blood draws or medications; and (4) there are no physical signs of edema, redness, pain, or dilated vessels.

Intervention: In view of the assessment of an occlusion that resolves with postural changes, catheter pinch-off syndrome is suspected. The physician is contacted and arrangements are made for a chest X-ray and possible catheter replacement.

Answer: An often unrecognized cause of catheter occlusion is catheter pinch-off syndrome. A pinch-off presents as an intermittent mechanical obstruction related to postural changes caused by catheter compression between the clavicle and the first rib.[104] In select patients, an anatomic narrow triangle exists at the junction of the axillary vein and the subclavian vein. This junction is in the lateral aspect of the clavicle, and pinch-off may occur with medial placement of a percutaneous CVC in this area. Changing the patient's position by raising the ipsilateral arm, and thereby opening this angle, relieves the occlusion. In 1400 patients, pinch-off syndrome was identified in 1.1%.[104] Chest X-rays will demonstrate a luminal narrowing of the catheter.

Rationale: Pinch-off syndrome can lead to catheter transection and embolus; therefore, removal is recommended.[105]

Infusion Delivery Devices

Infusion delivery devices are an integral component of parenteral therapy. These devices add a level of safety and ensure accuracy to IV infusions. Significant advances in device design have led to the availability of a variety of infusion pumps on the market. Ease of operation, mobility, and acquisition cost have been major incentives for technological advances. In addition to the cost of the infusion device, one must consider the cost of the tubing. The advantage of low cost-per-use standard PVC IV administration sets have promoted the use of stationary pumps. New technology that will allow this tubing to be used with ambulatory electronic devices may shift the market toward these infusion devices. However, a calculation of the total cost of a specific infusion device includes more than the actual equipment needs. Factored into this cost are the ease of training for staff and patients, device complications, waste and disposal, availability, down time, inventory costs, and overall product reliability.

References

1. Broviac JW, Cole JJ, Scribner BH. A silicone rubber atrial catheter for prolonged parenteral alimentation. *Surg Gynecol Obstet.* Apr 1973;136(4):602–606.
2. Sansivero GE. Features and selection of vascular access devices. *Semin Oncol Nurs.* May 2010;26(2):88–101.
3. Baskin JL, Pui CH, Reiss U, et al. Management of occlusion and thrombosis associated with long-term indwelling central venous catheters. *Lancet.* Jul 11 2009;374(9684):159–169.
4. O'Grady NP, Alexander M, Burns LA, et al. Guidelines for the prevention of intravascular catheter-related infections. *Am J Infect Control.* May 2011;39(4 Suppl 1):S1–34.
5. Sansivero GE. Venous anatomy and physiology. Considerations for vascular access device placement and function. *J Intraven Nurs.* 1998;21(5 Suppl):S107–114.
6. Amerasekera SS, Jones CM, Patel R, Cleasby MJ. Imaging of the complications of peripherally inserted central venous catheters. *Clin Radiol.* 2009;64(8):832–840.
7. Mirtallo J, Canada T, Johnson D, et al. Safe practices for parenteral nutrition. *JPEN J Parenter Enteral Nutr.* 2004;28(6):S39–70.
8. Gura KM. Is there still a role for peripheral parenteral nutrition? *Nutr Clin Pract.* Dec 2009;24(6):709–717.
9. Uslusoy E, Mete S. Predisposing factors to phlebitis in patients with peripheral intravenous catheters: a descriptive study. *J Am Acad Nurse Pract.* 2008;20(4):172–180.
10. Tagalakis V, Kahn SR, Libman M, Blostein M. The epidemiology of peripheral vein infusion thrombophlebitis: a critical review. *Am J Med.* 2002;113(2):146–151.
11. Maki DG, Ringer M. Risk factors for infusion-related phlebitis with small peripheral venous catheters. A randomized controlled trial. *Ann Intern Med.* 1991;114(10):845–854.
12. Pearson ML. Guideline for prevention of intravascular device-related infections. Part I. Intravascular device-related infections: an overview. The Hospital Infection Control Practices Advisory Committee. *Am J Infect Control.* 1996;24(4):262–277.
13. Webster J, Osborne S, Rickard C, Hall J. Clinically-indicated replacement versus routine replacement of peripheral venous catheters. *Cochrane Database Syst Rev.* 2010(3):CD007798.
14. Catton JA, Davies J, Dobbins BM, et al. The effect of heparin in peripheral intravenous nutrition via a fine-bore midline: a randomised double-blind controlled trial. *Clin Nutr.* Jun 2006;25(3): 394–399.
15. Shah PS, Ng E, Sinha AK. Heparin for prolonging peripheral intravenous catheter use in neonates. *Cochrane Database Syst Rev.* 2005(4):CD002774.
16. Zingg W, Pittet D. Peripheral venous catheters: an under-evaluated problem. *Int J Antimicrob Agents.* 2009;34(Suppl 4):S38–42.
17. Griffiths V. Midline catheters: indications, complications and maintenance. *Nurs Stand.* 2007;22(11):48–57.
18. Cobb DK, High KP, Sawyer RG, et al. A controlled trial of scheduled replacement of central venous and pulmonary-artery catheters. *N Engl J Med.* 1992;327(15):1062–1068.
19. Marschall J, Mermel LA, Classen D, et al. Strategies to prevent central line-associated bloodstream infections in acute care hospitals. *Infect Control Hosp Epidemiol.* 2008;29(Suppl 1):S22–30.
20. de Cicco M, Panarello G, Chiaradia V, et al. Source and route of microbial colonisation of parenteral nutrition catheters. *Lancet.* 1989;2(8674):1258–1261.
21. Keohane PP, Jones BJ, Attrill H, et al. Effect of catheter tunnelling and a nutrition nurse on catheter sepsis during parenteral nutrition. A controlled trial. *Lancet.* 1983;2(8364):1388–1390.
22. Darouiche RO, Berger DH, Khardori N, et al. Comparison of antimicrobial impregnation with tunneling of long-term central venous catheters: a randomized controlled trial. *Ann Surg.* 2005;242(2):193–200.
23. Raad I, Davis S, Becker M, et al. Low infection rate and long durability of nontunneled silastic catheters. A safe and cost-effective alternative for long-term venous access. *Arch Intern Med.* 1993;153 (15):1791–1796.
24. Niederhuber JE, Ensminger W, Gyves JW, et al. Totally implanted venous and arterial access system to replace external catheters in cancer treatment. *Surgery.* 1982;92(4):706–712.
25. Gullo SM. Implanted ports. Technologic advances and nursing care issues. *Nurs Clin North Am.* 1993;28(4):859–871.
26. Maki DG, Kluger DM, Crnich CJ. The risk of bloodstream infection in adults with different intravascular devices: a systematic review of 200 published prospective studies. *Mayo Clin Proc.* 2006;81(9): 1159–1171.
27. Bouza E, Guembe M, Munoz P. Selection of the vascular catheter: can it minimise the risk of infection? *Int J Antimicrob Agents.* 2010;36 Suppl 2:S22–25.
28. Groeger JS, Lucas AB, Thaler HT, et al. Infectious morbidity associated with long-term use of venous access devices in patients with cancer. *Ann Intern Med.* 1993;119(12):1168–1174.
29. Mansfield PF, Hohn DC, Fornage BD, Gregurich MA, Ota DM. Complications and failures of subclavian-vein catheterization. *N Engl J Med.* 1994;331(26):1735–1738.
30. Nagelhout J, Elisha S, Waters E. Should I continue or discontinue that medication? *AANA J.* 2009;77(1):59–73.
31. Lorente L, Henry C, Martin MM, Jimenez A, Mora ML. Central venous catheter-related infection in a prospective and observational study of 2,595 catheters. *Crit Care.* 2005;9(6):R631–635.
32. Aarons L, Schulman J, Masserman JH, Zimmar GP. Behavioral adaptations after parietal cortex ablation in the neonate macaque. *Recent Adv Biol Psychiatry.* 1961;4:347–361.
33. Mermel LA, McCormick RD, Springman SR, Maki DG. The pathogenesis and epidemiology of catheter-related infection with pulmonary artery Swan-Ganz catheters: a prospective study utilizing molecular subtyping. *Am J Med.* 1991;91(3B):197S–205S.
34. Raad, II, Hohn DC, Gilbreath BJ, et al. Prevention of central venous catheter-related infections by using maximal sterile barrier precautions during insertion. *Infect Control Hosp Epidemiol.* 1994;15(4 Pt 1):231–238.

35. Safdar N, Fine JP, Maki DG. Meta-analysis: methods for diagnosing intravascular device-related bloodstream infection. *Ann Intern Med.* 2005;142(6):451–466.
36. Harbarth S, Sax H, Gastmeier P. The preventable proportion of nosocomial infections: an overview of published reports. *J Hosp Infect.* 2003;54(4):258–266.
37. O'Grady NP, Alexander M, Dellinger EP, et al. Guidelines for the prevention of intravascular catheter-related infections. *Am J Infect Control.* 2002;30(8):476–489.
38. Thompson EC, Calver LE. Safe subclavian vein cannulation. *Am Surg.* 2005;71(2):180–183.
39. Brown JR, Slomski C, Saxe AW. Is routine postoperative chest x-ray necessary after fluoroscopic-guided subclavian central venous port placement? *J Am Coll Surg.* 2009;208(4):517–519.
40. Cavanna L, Civardi G, Vallisa D, et al. Ultrasound-guided central venous catheterization in cancer patients improves the success rate of cannulation and reduces mechanical complications: a prospective observational study of 1,978 consecutive catheterizations. *World J Surg Oncol* 2010 Oct 19;8:91.
41. Krzywda EA, Andris DA. Twenty-five years of advances in vascular access: bridging research to clinical practice. *Nutr Clin Pract.* 2005;20(6):597–606.
42. Ryder M. Evidence-based practice in the management of vascular access devices for home parenteral nutrition therapy. *JPEN J Parenter Enteral Nutr.* 2006;30(1 Suppl):S82–93.
43. Maki DG, Ringer M, Alvarado CJ. Prospective randomised trial of povidone-iodine, alcohol, and chlorhexidine for prevention of infection associated with central venous and arterial catheters. *Lancet.* 1991;338(8763):339–343.
44. Maki DG, McCormack KN. Defatting catheter insertion sites in total parenteral nutrition is of no value as an infection control measure. Controlled clinical trial. *Am J Med.* Nov 1987;83(5):833–840.
45. Hibbard JS. Analyses comparing the antimicrobial activity and safety of current antiseptic agents: a review. *J Infus Nurs.* 2005; 28(3):194–207.
46. Crnich CJ, Maki DG. The promise of novel technology for the prevention of intravascular device-related bloodstream infection. II. Long-term devices. *Clin Infect Dis.* 2002;34(10): 1362–1368.
47. Fukunaga A, Naritaka H, Fukaya R, Tabuse M, Nakamura T. Povidone-iodine ointment and gauze dressings associated with reduced catheter-related infection in seriously ill neurosurgical patients. *Infect Control Hosp Epidemiol.* 2004;25(8):696–698.
48. Johnson DW, MacGinley R, Kay TD, et al. A randomized controlled trial of topical exit site mupirocin application in patients with tunnelled, cuffed haemodialysis catheters. *Nephrol Dial Transplant.* 2002;17(10):1802–1807.
49. Mermel LA. What is the predominant source of intravascular catheter infections? *Clin Infect Dis.* 2011;52(2):211–212.
50. Hadaway L, Richardson D. Needleless connectors: a primer on terminology. *J Infus Nurs.* 2010;33(1):22–31.
51. Menyhay SZ, Maki DG. Disinfection of needleless catheter connectors and access ports with alcohol may not prevent microbial entry: the promise of a novel antiseptic-barrier cap. *Infect Control Hosp Epidemiol.* 2006;27(1):23–27.
52. Maki DG. In vitro studies of a novel antimicrobial luer-activated needleless connector for prevention of catheter-related bloodstream infection. *Clin Infect Dis.* 2010;50(12):1580–1587.
53. Edmiston CE Jr, Markina V. Reducing the risk of infection in vascular access patients: an in vitro evaluation of an antimicrobial silver nanotechnology luer activated device. *Am J Infect Control.* 2010;38(6):421–423.
54. Jarvis WR, Murphy C, Hall KK, et al. Health care-associated bloodstream infections associated with negative- or positive-pressure or displacement mechanical valve needleless connectors. *Clin Infect Dis.* 2009;49(12):1821–1827.
55. Jonker MA, Osterby KR, Vermeulen LC, Kleppin SM, Kudsk KA. Does low-dose heparin maintain central venous access device patency?: a comparison of heparin versus saline during a period of heparin shortage. *JPEN J Parenter Enteral Nutr.* 2010;34(4):444–449.
56. Yamamoto AJ, Solomon JA, Soulen MC, et al. Sutureless securement device reduces complications of peripherally inserted central venous catheters. *J Vasc Interv Radiol.* 2002;13(1):77–81.
57. Infusion Nursing Standards of Practice. *J Infus Nurs.* 2006;29(1 Suppl):S1–92.
58. Kim SW, Petersen RV, Lee ES. Effect of phthalate plasticizer on blood compatibility of polyvinyl chloride. *J Pharm Sci.* 1976; 65(5):670–673.
59. Zdrahala RJ, Zdrahala IJ. Biomedical applications of polyurethanes: a review of past promises, present realities, and a vibrant future. *J Biomater Appl.* 1999;14(1):67–90.
60. Brown JM. Polyurethane and silicone: myths and misconceptions. *J Intraven Nurs.* 1995;18(3):120–122.
61. Larsson N, Stenberg K, Linder LE, Curelaru I. Cannula thrombophlebitis: a study in volunteers comparing polytetrafluoroethylene, polyurethane, and polyamide-ether-elastomer cannulae. *Acta Anaesthesiol Scand.* 1989;33(3):223–231.
62. Adverse reactions associated with midline catheters—United States, 1992–1995. From the Centers for Disease Control and Prevention. *JAMA.* 1996;275(10):749–750.
63. Darouiche RO, Raad II, Heard SO, et al. A comparison of two antimicrobial-impregnated central venous catheters. Catheter Study Group. *N Engl J Med.* 1999;340(1):1–8.
64. Maki DG, Stolz SM, Wheeler S, Mermel LA. Prevention of central venous catheter-related bloodstream infection by use of an antiseptic-impregnated catheter. A randomized, controlled trial. *Ann Intern Med.* 1997;127(4):257–266.
65. Camargo LF, Marra AR, Buchele GL, et al. Double-lumen central venous catheters impregnated with chlorhexidine and silver sulfadiazine to prevent catheter colonisation in the intensive care unit setting: a prospective randomised study. *J Hosp Infect.* 2009;72(3): 227–233.
66. Halton KA, Cook DA, Whitby M, Paterson DL, Graves N. Cost effectiveness of antimicrobial catheters in the intensive care unit: addressing uncertainty in the decision. *Crit Care.* 2009;13(2):R35.
67. Aslam S, Darouiche RO. Prolonged bacterial exposure to minocycline/rifampicin-impregnated vascular catheters does not affect antimicrobial activity of catheters. *J Antimicrob Chemother.* 2007; 60(1):148–151.
68. Ramos ER, Reitzel R, Jiang Y, et al. Clinical effectiveness and risk of emerging resistance associated with prolonged use of antibiotic-impregnated catheters: more than 0.5 million catheter days and 7 years of clinical experience. *Crit Care Med.* 2011;39(2): 245–251.
69. Kluger M. Anaphylaxis to chlorhexidine-impregnated central venous catheter. *Anaesth Intensive Care.* 2003;31(6):697–698.
70. Trautner BW, Darouiche RO. Catheter-associated infections: pathogenesis affects prevention. *Arch Intern Med.* 2004;164(8): 842–850.
71. Gaynes R, Edwards JR. Overview of nosocomial infections caused by gram-negative bacilli. *Clin Infect Dis.* 2005;41(6):848–854.
72. Schulman J, Stricof R, Stevens TP, et al. Statewide NICU central-line-associated bloodstream infection rates decline after bundles and checklists. *Pediatrics.* 2011;127(3):436–444.

73. Mehall JR, Saltzman DA, Jackson RJ, Smith SD. Fibrin sheath enhances central venous catheter infection. *Crit Care Med.* 2002;30(4):908–912.
74. Costerton W, Veeh R, Shirtliff M, et al. The application of biofilm science to the study and control of chronic bacterial infections. *J Clin Invest.* 2003;112(10):1466–1477.
75. Schaberg DR, Culver DH, Gaynes RP. Major trends in the microbial etiology of nosocomial infection. *Am J Med.* 1991;91(3B):72S–75S.
76. Klevens RM, Edwards JR, Tenover FC, et al. Changes in the epidemiology of methicillin-resistant Staphylococcus aureus in intensive care units in US hospitals, 1992-2003. *Clin Infect Dis.* 2006;42(3):389–391.
77. Boyce JM, Opal SM, Chow JW, et al. Outbreak of multidrug-resistant Enterococcus faecium with transferable vanB class vancomycin resistance. *J Clin Microbiol.* 1994;32(5):1148–1153.
78. Ena J, Dick RW, Jones RN, Wenzel RP. The epidemiology of intravenous vancomycin usage in a university hospital. A 10-year study. *JAMA.* 1993;269(5):598–602.
79. Wisplinghoff H, Bischoff T, Tallent SM, et al. Nosocomial bloodstream infections in US hospitals: analysis of 24,179 cases from a prospective nationwide surveillance study. *Clin Infect Dis.* 2004;39(3):309–317.
80. Maki DG, Rhame FS, Mackel DC, Bennett JV. Nationwide epidemic of septicemia caused by contaminated intravenous products. I. Epidemiologic and clinical features. *Am J Med.* 1976; 60(4):471–485.
81. Marra AR, Opilla M, Edmond MB, Kirby DF. Epidemiology of bloodstream infections in patients receiving long-term total parenteral nutrition. *J Clin Gastroenterol.* 2007;41(1):19–28.
82. Mammen EF. Pathogenesis of venous thrombosis. *Chest.* 1992;102(6 Suppl):640S–644S.
83. Snaterse M, Ruger W, Scholte OP, Reimer WJ, Lucas C. Antibiotic-based catheter lock solutions for prevention of catheter-related bloodstream infection: a systematic review of randomised controlled trials. *J Hosp Infect.* 2010;75(1):1–11.
84. Maiefski M, Rupp ME, Hermsen ED. Ethanol lock technique: review of the literature. *Infect Control Hosp Epidemiol.* 2009;30(11): 1096–1108.
85. Koll BS, Straub TA, Jalon HS, et al. The CLABs collaborative: a regionwide effort to improve the quality of care in hospitals. *Jt Comm J Qual Patient Saf.* 2008;34(12):713–723.
86. Galpern D, Guerrero A, Tu A, Fahoum B, Wise L. Effectiveness of a central line bundle campaign on line-associated infections in the intensive care unit. *Surgery.* 2008;144(4):492–495.
87. Marra AR, Cal RG, Durao MS, et al. Impact of a program to prevent central line-associated bloodstream infection in the zero tolerance era. *Am J Infect Control.* 2010;38(6):434–439.
88. Furuya EY, Dick A, Perencevich EN, et al. Central line bundle implementation in US intensive care units and impact on bloodstream infections. *PLoS One.* 2011;6(1):e15452.
89. Reduction in central line-associated bloodstream infections among patients in intensive care units—Pennsylvania, April 2001–March 2005. *MMWR Morb Mortal Wkly Rep.* 2005;54(40): 1013–1016.
90. Berenholtz SM, Pronovost PJ, Lipsett PA, et al. Eliminating catheter-related bloodstream infections in the intensive care unit. *Crit Care Med.* Oct 2004;32(10):2014–2020.
91. Timsit JF, Schwebel C, Bouadma L, et al. Chlorhexidine-impregnated sponges and less frequent dressing changes for prevention of catheter-related infections in critically ill adults: a randomized controlled trial. *JAMA.* 2009;301(12):1231–1241.
92. Raad, II, Hanna HA. Intravascular catheter-related infections: new horizons and recent advances. *Arch Intern Med.* 2002;162(8): 871–878.
93. Moureau N, Poole S, Murdock MA, Gray SM, Semba CP. Central venous catheters in home infusion care: outcomes analysis in 50,470 patients. *J Vasc Interv Radiol.* 2002;13(10):1009–1016.
94. Hoshal VL Jr, Ause RG, Hoskins PA. Fibrin sleeve formation on indwelling subclavian central venous catheters. *Arch Surg.* 1971;102(4):353–358.
95. Lee AY, Levine MN, Butler G, et al. Incidence, risk factors, and outcomes of catheter-related thrombosis in adult patients with cancer. *J Clin Oncol.* 2006;24(9):1404–1408.
96. Verso M, Agnelli G. Venous thromboembolism associated with long-term use of central venous catheters in cancer patients. *J Clin Oncol.* 2003;21(19):3665–3675.
97. Kovacs MJ, Kahn SR, Rodger M, et al. A pilot study of central venous catheter survival in cancer patients using low-molecular-weight heparin (dalteparin) and warfarin without catheter removal for the treatment of upper extremity deep vein thrombosis (The Catheter Study). *J Thromb Haemost.* 2007;5(8): 1650–1653.
98. Cadman A, Lawrance JA, Fitzsimmons L, Spencer-Shaw A, Swindell R. To clot or not to clot? That is the question in central venous catheters. *Clin Radiol.* 2004;59(4):349–355.
99. Kucher N. Clinical practice. Deep-vein thrombosis of the upper extremities. *N Engl J Med.* 2011;364(9):861–869.
100. Ponec D, Irwin D, Haire WD, et al. Recombinant tissue plasminogen activator (alteplase) for restoration of flow in occluded central venous access devices: a double-blind placebo-controlled trial—the Cardiovascular Thrombolytic to Open Occluded Lines (COOL) efficacy trial. *J Vasc Interv Radiol.* 2001;12(8):951–955.
101. Akl EA, Vasireddi SR, Gunukula S, et al. Anticoagulation for patients with cancer and central venous catheters. *Cochrane Database Syst Rev.* 2011;4:CD006468.
102. Raad II, Luna M, Khalil SA, et al. The relationship between the thrombotic and infectious complications of central venous catheters. *JAMA.* 1994;271(13):1014–1016.
103. van Rooden CJ, Schippers EF, Barge RM, et al. Infectious complications of central venous catheters increase the risk of catheter-related thrombosis in hematology patients: a prospective study. *J Clin Oncol.* 2005;23(12):2655–2660.
104. Andris DA, Krzywda EA, Schulte W, Ausman R, Quebbeman EJ. Pinch-off syndrome: a rare etiology for central venous catheter occlusion. *JPEN J Parenter Enteral Nutr.* 1994;18(6):531–533.
105. Mirza B, Vanek VW, Kupensky DT. Pinch-off syndrome: case report and collective review of the literature. *Am Surg.* Jul 2004; 70(7):635–644.

17 Complications of Parenteral Nutrition

Vanessa J. Kumpf, PharmD, BCNSP, and Jane Gervasio, PharmD, BCNSP

CONTENTS

Background 285
Macronutrient-Related Complications 285
Hyperglycemia 285
Hypoglycemia 286
Essential Fatty Acid Deficiency 286
Hypertriglyceridemia 286
Azotemia 287
Micronutrient-Related Complications 287
Fluid and Electrolytes 287
Vitamins 288
Trace Elements 288
Refeeding Syndrome 288
Hepatobiliary Complications 289
Types of Hepatobiliary Disorders 289
Prevalence of Hepatobiliary Complications 289
Parenteral Nutrition–Related Risk Factors 290
Energy 290
Carbohydrate 290
Protein 290
Intravenous Fat Emulsion 290
Carnitine 291
Choline 291
Strategies to Manage Parenteral Nutrition–Associated Hepatobiliary Complications 291
Oral and Enteral Nutrition 292
Cyclic Infusion 292
Pharmacotherapeutic Options 292
Transplantation 292
Metabolic Bone Disease 292
Prevalence of Metabolic Bone Disease 293
Parenteral Nutrition–Related Factors 293
Calcium 293
Vitamin D 293
Aluminum Toxicity 294
Magnesium Deficiency 294
Copper Deficiency 294
Prevention and Management 294
Summary 295
References 295

Objectives

1. Identify potential acute and long-term metabolic complications associated with parenteral nutrition (PN).
2. Describe the laboratory and clinical monitoring parameters required to identify metabolic complications associated with PN.
3. List clinically relevant metabolic complications that develop from administration of inadequate or excessive nutrients.
4. Develop strategies to avoid and treat metabolic complications associated with PN.

Test Your Knowledge Questions

1. Which of the following is the most common metabolic complication associated with PN?
   A. Hyperglycemia
   B. Essential fatty acid deficiency (EFAD)
   C. Azotemia
   D. Hyperammonemia
2. After periods of prolonged uncomplicated starvation, which of the following metabolic and physiologic changes occur as a patient begins PN therapy?
   A. Anabolism begins almost immediately.
   B. Basal metabolic rate decreases to conserve energy.
   C. Insulin levels decrease.
   D. Liver gluconeogenesis decreases.
3. Which of the following measures would be considered most beneficial in a patient receiving long-term PN that is infused over 12 hours nightly who develops cholestasis?
   A. Stop all oral or enteral intake.
   B. Switch from a cyclic to continuous method of PN administration.
   C. Decrease intravenous fat emulsion (IVFE) dose from 1.5 g/kg daily to 1 g/kg twice weekly.
   D. Increase protein dose from 1 to 2 g/kg/d.
4. Which of the following PN modifications is recommended in the prevention and/or treatment of osteoporosis in a long-term PN patient?
   A. Maintain protein intake at least 2 g/kg/d.
   B. Provide calcium > 20 mEq/d.
   C. Add injectable vitamin D to the PN formulation.
   D. Provide phosphorus 20 to 40 mmol/d.

Test Your Knowledge Answers

1. The correct answer is **A**. Hyperglycemia is the most common metabolic complication that occurs with PN. Hyperglycemia is associated with overfeeding but occurs frequently in appropriately fed patients. This is attributed to insulin suppression, resistance, and gluconeogenesis from stress and infection. Nondiabetic hospitalized patients receiving intravenous (IV) dextrose infusions at rates > 4 mg/kg/min have a 50% chance of developing hyperglycemia.[1] EFAD is associated with fat-free PN and can be avoided by administering minimal amounts of IVFE. Azotemia may occur but is usually associated with renal or hepatic dysfunction or protein overfeeding. Hyperammonemia rarely occurs because of the implementation of crystalline amino acids.
2. The correct answer is **A**. During starvation, the body adapts by decreasing gluconeogenesis and increasing use of ketones and fatty acids that do not require phosphate to produce energy.[2] When refeeding occurs, there is a sudden shift to glucose as the primary fuel.[3] Basal metabolic rate increases when nutrition support is initiated after starvation. Anabolism begins almost immediately. There is a rapid alteration in hormone levels, primarily insulin as glucose becomes the dominant fuel. A rapid alteration in calories, fluid, and particularly sodium intake may cause fluid shifts and intravascular volume overload, which may increase risk for developing congestive heart failure.[4] Management and prevention of refeeding syndrome involves identifying patients at risk, serum electrolyte monitoring, restoring circulatory volume, and increasing calories slowly.[5]
3. The correct answer is **C**. Cholestasis has been associated with IVFE doses > 1 g/kg/d in adult patients receiving long-term PN,[6] and a trial of lowering the IVFE dose may, therefore, be beneficial. Cyclic infusion has been shown to reduce serum liver enzyme and conjugated bilirubin concentrations when compared to continuous infusion.[7] Enteral feeding should be attempted to promote enterohepatic circulation of bile acids. Protein dose does not appear to play a role in the development of cholestasis in adults.
4. The correct answer is **D**. An inadequate phosphorus dose may increase urinary calcium excretion; therefore, doses of 20 to 40 mmol/d added to the PN formulation have been recommended.[8] Although patients receiving PN are vulnerable to a negative calcium balance, calcium supplementation in the PN formulation is limited by physical compatibility with phosphorus, and higher doses are offset by higher urinary losses. The recommended dose of calcium gluconate to be added to the PN formulation is 10 to 15 mEq per day.[8] High protein doses (2 g/kg/d compared to 1 g/kg/d) in PN formulations have been associated with increased urinary calcium excretion in adult patients. Excessive vitamin D doses can be detrimental to the bone because they can suppress parathyroid hormone and promote bone resorption.

Background

PN-associated complications can be categorized as mechanical, metabolic, and infectious. Metabolic complications are more commonly associated with PN rather than enteral nutrition. Therefore, patients receiving PN require close monitoring for prevention and early detection of complications. Mechanical complications related to the venous access device and infectious complications will be presented elsewhere (see Chapter 16). This chapter will focus on the recognition, prevention, and treatment of metabolic complications associated with PN in the adult patient.

Macronutrient-Related Complications

Hyperglycemia

Hyperglycemia is the most common complication associated with PN administration and can be caused by various factors.

Stress-associated hyperglycemia in acutely ill and septic patients often develops as a result of insulin resistance, increased gluconeogenesis and glycogenolysis, and suppressed insulin secretion.[1] Excess carbohydrate administration has been associated with hyperglycemia, hepatic steatosis, and increased carbon dioxide production. Maintaining blood glucose concentrations between 80 to 110 mg/dL in patients in the surgical intensive care unit and < 180 mg/dL in patients in the medical (nonsurgical) intensive care unit and non-critically ill patients has been associated with decreased morbidity and mortality.[1,8,9] PN should be initiated at half of the estimated energy needs or approximately 150 to 200 grams dextrose for the first 24 hours. Lesser dextrose delivery (approximately 100 grams) is warranted in the hyperglycemic patient requiring insulin therapy or a hypoglycemic agent. Carbohydrate administration should not exceed a rate of 4 to 5 mg/kg/min or 20 to 25 kcal/kg/d.[10] Capillary blood glucose concentrations should be monitored every 6 hours and more frequently in hyperglycemic patients.

Blood glucose concentrations can be controlled with insulin therapy, which may be administered subcutaneously, intravenously via an insulin infusion, or directly to the PN solution. An initial regimen of 0.05 to 0.1 units of insulin per gram of dextrose in the PN solution is common, or 0.15 to 0.2 units of insulin per gram of dextrose in patients already hyperglycemic. Supplemental subcutaneous regular insulin may be administered if needed, utilizing a sliding scale regimen. Two-thirds of the total amount of sliding scale insulin required over 24 hours may then be added to the next day's PN formulation. Increases in dextrose concentrations in PN should not be implemented until glucose concentrations are controlled. Insulin should be proportionally increased and decreased with respect to the PN glucose concentration. Alternatively, an insulin infusion may be instituted and provides a more consistent and safe glucose control. A proportional increase of fat may be necessary to increase calories. Rarely, hyperglycemia may be due to chromium deficiency. Insulin is ineffective in patients with chromium deficiency. Increasing the chromium dose in the PN formulation beyond the standard amount in commercially prepared multiple trace element injections may be necessary.[11,12] Uncontrolled hyperglycemia may result in hyperosmolar hyperglycemia, nonketotic dehydration, coma, and death secondary to osmotic diuresis.[13]

Hypoglycemia

PN-associated hypoglycemia can occur from excess insulin administration via the PN solution, IV infusion, or subcutaneous injection. Excessive or erroneous administration of insulin is a severe medication error, and resulting hypoglycemia may be life-threatening. Treatment includes initiation of a 10% dextrose infusion, administration of an ampule of 50% dextrose, and/or stopping any source of insulin administration. Abrupt discontinuation of PN solutions has been associated with rebound hypoglycemia.[14] Studies have reported no symptomatic hypoglycemia after abruptly stopping PN infusions given over 16 to 24 hours.[15,16] However, nonsymptomatic hypoglycemia did occur in some patients. Patients requiring large doses of insulin have a greater propensity for rebound hypoglycemia, but predetermining which patients will experience rebound hypoglycemia is difficult. Therefore, to reduce the risk of rebound hypoglycemia in susceptible patients, a 1- to 2-hour taper down of the infusion, or half the infusion rate, may be necessary. If a PN solution must be discontinued quickly, a dextrose-containing fluid should be infused for 1 or 2 hours following PN discontinuation to avoid a possible rebound hypoglycemia. Obtaining a capillary blood glucose concentration 30 minutes to 1 hour after the PN solution is discontinued will help identify rebound hypoglycemia.

Essential Fatty Acid Deficiency

IVFE is generally provided as a source of essential fatty acids and as a nonprotein caloric source (see Chapters 5 and 15). Although the incidence is low, there are several potential complications associated with IVFE use, such as infusion-related adverse reactions and allergy to the IVFE components. Depending on the length of the PN therapy and the nutrition status of the patient, IVFE-free PN may result in EFAD. Two polyunsaturated fatty acids, linoleic and alpha-linolenic, cannot be synthesized by the body and are considered essential. Clinical manifestations of EFAD include scaly dermatitis, alopecia, hepatomegaly, thrombocytopenia, fatty liver, and anemia.[17] Biochemical evidence of EFAD is determined by a triene:tetraene ratio of more than 0.2 and can occur within 1 to 3 weeks in adults receiving IVFE-free PN.[18] The adult requirements for linoleic acid are met through exogenous sources or endogenously through the lipolysis of adipose tissue. However, when hypertonic dextrose is infused, insulin is secreted and lipolysis is reduced. Thus, an exogenous source of fat must be provided. To prevent EFAD, 1% to 2% of daily energy requirements should be derived from linoleic acid and about 0.5% of energy from linolenic acid.[19] This translates into approximately 250 mL of 20% IVFE or 500 mL of 10% IVFE administered over 8 to 10 hours, twice a week. Alternately, 500 mL of a 20% IVFE can be given once a week. In patients who are intolerant to IVFE, a trial of topical skin application or oral ingestion of oils to alleviate biochemical deficiency of EFAD may be given.[20,21]

Hypertriglyceridemia

Hypertriglyceridemia can occur with dextrose overfeeding or with rapid administration rates of IVFE (> 110 mg/kg/hr). Hyperlipidemia may impair immune response, alter pulmonary hemodynamics, and increase the risk of pancreatitis.[22,23] Reducing the dose and/or lengthening the infusion time of IVFE will help minimize these effects. IVFE intake should be restricted to less than 30% of total calories or 1 g/kg/d and be provided slowly over no less than 8 to 10 hours if administered separately.[22] Serum triglyceride concentrations should be checked in any patient with a known history of hyperlipidemia prior to IVFE administration. Acceptable serum triglyceride concentrations are < 400 mg/dL.[8,19] Occasionally, serum triglyceride concentrations will rise in a patient who is fat-intolerant. In such patients, IVFE infusions should be reduced or discontinued. Pancreatitis due to IVFE-induced hyperlipidemia is rare unless serum triglyceride concentrations exceed 1000 mg/dL. IVFE is considered safe for use in patients with pancreatitis without hypertriglyceridemia.[24] However, IVFE should be withheld from the PN regimen if serum triglyceride concentrations exceed 400 mg/dL (see Chapter 28 for more details).

Although rare, allergic reactions to IVFE can occur, especially in patients with history of egg allergy. This is most likely a result of the egg phospholipid that is used as an emulsifier. Other acute infusion-related adverse reactions include hyperlipidemia, dyspnea, cyanosis, flushing, sweating, dizziness, headache, back or chest pain, nausea, and vomiting.

Azotemia

Excessive protein administration results in an increased metabolic demand on the body for disposing of the byproducts of protein metabolism. Prerenal azotemia can result from dehydration, excess protein, and/or inadequate nonprotein calories. Intolerance to the protein load will be exhibited by an increase in blood urea nitrogen. Patients with hepatic or renal disease are prone to developing azotemia due to the impaired ability to metabolize and eliminate urea. When urea clearance is impaired, dialysis may be required in order to assist with the elimination of urea and allow for the adequate intake of protein.

The incidence of hyperammonemia has been a rare occurrence since the advent of crystalline amino acid solutions. The early protein hydrolysates contained excessive amounts of ammonia and insufficient arginine for urea cycle metabolism. However, hyperammonemia has been observed with the new crystalline amino acid solutions in patients with urea cycle defects, such as ornithine transcarbamylase deficiency.[25,26]

Patients who develop amino acid intolerance such as prerenal azotemia, hepatic encephalopathy, or hyperammonemia may benefit from a reduction in the amount of amino acids provided. In patients with hepatic failure and hepatic encephalopathy, the use of high branched chain, low aromatic amino acid formulations has provided inconsistent results (see Chapter 27 for appropriate usage of these specialized amino acid formulations).

Micronutrient-Related Complications

Fluid and Electrolytes

Once macronutrient tolerance has been established, the routine management of the patient receiving PN centers on fluid and electrolytes (see Chapter 7). The requirements vary depending on the patient's renal, fluid, and electrolyte status when starting PN, as well as his or her underlying disease process and any losses they may incur.[27,28] Daily fluid and electrolyte shifts between the intracellular and extracellular space or changes in total body water or electrolyte content will require changes in the PN solution composition and volume.

Evaluation of concurrent IV fluids and medications provided during PN therapy is necessary when determining the fluid and electrolyte status. PN formulations should be prescribed with consideration of all fluids being infused. Fluid and electrolyte replacement with separate IV fluids outside of the PN formulation may be necessary when the patient has excessive losses. Treatment involves replacing the lost fluids with IV fluid of similar electrolyte composition. Accurate intake and output records are necessary to show the amount of loss from various body fluids. See Chapter 7 for a complete review of fluid and electrolytes and Practice Scenario 17-1 for a discussion of metabolic monitoring during PN.

Practice Scenario 17-1

Question: What parameters should be monitored and with what frequency to help identify and prevent metabolic complications in a patient initiating PN?

Scenario: A 52-year-old female, postoperative day 7, presents with a small bowel obstruction. She is experiencing elevated gastric residuals, abdominal distention, and hypogastric bowel sounds. Her nutritional status is as follows: height 165 cm, weight 63 kg with no muscle or adipose tissue wasting noted. Signs of edema are not present. Serum laboratory values include albumin 3.7 g/dL; prealbumin 16 mg/dL; sodium 139 mmol/L; potassium 3.9 mmol/L; chlorine 101 mmol/L; carbon dioxide 25 mmol/L; blood urea nitrogen 10 mg/dL; creatinine 0.7 mg/dL; glucose 112 mg/dL; ionized calcium 4.7 mg/dL; phosphate 3.3 mg/dL; magnesium 1.9 mg/dL. Vital signs include heart rate 74; blood pressure 118/70; input 2400 mL; output 2370 mL.

Intervention: The patient's IV solution has been discontinued and PN has been initiated.

Answer: The patient's fluid status as well as a complete metabolic panel including a phosphate, magnesium, and ionized calcium level should be obtained and assessed before PN is initiated. If depleted, electrolytes, specifically potassium, phosphate, magnesium, and calcium, should be repleted before PN is administered. After PN is initiated, electrolytes should be evaluated daily until stable in part to assess for potential refeeding syndrome. PN may be administered slowly and titrated to goal over a period of days to prevent hyperglycemia. Glucose levels should be monitored at least every 6 hours until the patient is euglycemic. More frequent monitoring may be necessary if insulin administration is begun and consideration for resulting hypoglycemia is imperative. Triglyceride levels should also be evaluated before the initiation of PN, then once weekly to prevent hypertriglyceridemia. Supplementation or elimination of specific vitamins or trace elements may be necessary depending on the patient's medical condition and presentation. Prealbumin can be evaluated initially and serially during PN administration. Prealbumin can be a useful indicator of inflammatory metabolism when levels are below normal as well as an indication that normal postprandial metabolism (and anabolism) is possible when levels are normal (see Chapter 9 for further discussion).

Rationale: Initial presentation of the patient does not warrant any additional concerns except the standard considerations of fluid status, electrolytes, and glucose levels. Her electrolytes are within normal values, her vital signs and fluid status are appropriate, and she has no signs of wasting. She is being initiated on PN so the complication of hyperglycemia must be considered. Additionally, until she is stable, daily electrolyte monitoring is necessary.

Vitamins

Vitamins are essential for effective nutrient utilization (see Chapter 8). A sustained exogenous intake of vitamins is essential to avoid deficiency. However, excessive intake of lipid-soluble vitamins A, D, E, and K has the potential for accumulation and, therefore, the potential for toxicity. Provision of adequate vitamin intake in the PN patient may be complicated by conditions that increase requirements, such as sepsis, trauma, or following surgery. Identifying vitamin deficiency or toxicity states can be difficult due to limitations in correlating serum vitamin concentrations with body stores and often because of vague clinical symptoms. Therefore, adult patients receiving PN should receive a standard daily dose of parenteral multivitamins.[8] Delaying IV multivitamin therapy until development of clinical signs of vitamin deficiency is inappropriate.

Certain clinical situations warrant special attention. Patients receiving both PN and warfarin therapy require close monitoring of the desired anticoagulation level because of the inclusion of vitamin K in the multivitamin preparation. PN supplementation with additional thiamin (25 to 100 mg/d) is reasonable in PN patients with a history of alcohol abuse, especially if the patient did not receive thiamin upon hospital admission. Thiamin supplementation is also recommended upon initiation of specialized nutrition support in patients with a prolonged history of poor dietary intake. During the period of parenteral vitamin shortages in the United States in the late 1980s and 1990s, several cases of lactic acidosis due to thiamin deficiency were reported, including three deaths.[29] The American Society for Parenteral and Enteral Nutrition (A.S.P.E.N.) recommends that the following practices be implemented during periods of short supply: (1) use oral or enterally administered multivitamins whenever possible, especially liquid multivitamins of defined content; (2) when all options to obtain IV multivitamins have been exhausted, ration use by reducing the dose by 50% or giving one dose three times a week; (3) if IV multivitamins are no longer available, administer thiamin, ascorbic acid, pyridoxine, and folic acid daily as individual entities and vitamin B_{12} at least once per month.[30] Vitamin toxicity, particularly of the fat-soluble vitamins, is also a potential complication of PN. Vitamin A toxicity has been reported in patients with chronic renal failure receiving PN. Therefore, some clinicians have recommended reducing the frequency of fat-soluble vitamin administration to twice per week in renal failure patients. However, because there are no injectable multivitamin preparations available without fat-soluble vitamins, the potential for developing water-soluble vitamin deficiency exists with restricted dosing. In addition, because some water-soluble vitamins may be lost with hemodialysis, provision of water-soluble vitamins to patients receiving dialysis has been recommended.[19] This requires use of an oral vitamin B complex supplement or individual parenteral vitamin B supplementation, as available.

Several vitamins are known to undergo substantial degradation after addition to the PN formulation. This is not considered a significant problem in the acute care setting because of the relatively short time period between compounding and administration. However, when PN formulations are compounded in a batch fashion for patients in the home setting, this degradation must be considered. The degradation was clearly demonstrated in a home PN patient who developed night blindness within 6 months of receiving PN that was prepared on a weekly basis with the vitamins added to the PN formulation by the pharmacy before delivery.[31] Although night blindness resolved after a therapeutic dose of vitamin A, symptoms returned 6 months later before the source of the problem was identified. Substantial amounts of vitamin A were likely lost to degradation and adsorption to the plastic matrix of the bag because the vitamins were added to the PN formulation up to a week before administration. Therefore, daily addition of vitamins to the PN formulation before infusion has been recommended.[8]

Trace Elements

Trace element deficiency states are relatively uncommon in patients receiving PN, but they can occur when there is insufficient intake or increased utilization or excretion over a prolonged period of time. For example, zinc deficiency may occur in the patient with high intestinal losses due to increased loss of zinc. Cardiomyopathy caused by selenium deficiency has been reported in patients receiving long-term PN without selenium supplementation. The development of trace element excess is also a potential complication in the long-term PN patient and in the patient with hepatobiliary disease. Available parenteral multitrace preparations may exceed actual requirements in many patients receiving PN. In addition, many of the components of the PN formulation have been shown to be contaminated with trace elements such as zinc, copper, manganese, chromium, selenium, and aluminum.[32] Tissue elevations of copper, manganese, and chromium have been noted on autopsy in patients receiving long-term PN.[33] Although serum trace element monitoring at baseline and routine follow-up is recommended in patients receiving long-term PN, it is an unreliable measure of total body balance.[34] Empiric adjustments in trace element intake may be warranted. Reductions in manganese and copper dosing should be considered in patients with hepatobiliary disease due to impaired excretion. Removal of supplemental manganese from the PN formulation and reduction in the copper dose may be necessary in long-term PN patients.

Iron is not a component of the PN formulation, primarily due to compatibility limitations. Parenteral iron supplementation at repletion doses is warranted in conditions of iron deficiency when the oral route is ineffective or not tolerated and can be provided as an infusion separate from the PN formulation. Delivery of maintenance iron (around 1 mg of elemental iron per day in adult men and menstruating women) in patients receiving PN has been suggested and may be given on an intermittent (eg, monthly) basis.[35] When parenteral iron is provided, especially as chronic supplementation, monitoring of iron status (eg, serum ferritin every 1 to 3 months) is necessary to prevent iron overload[36] (see Chapter 8 for more details about trace elements).

Refeeding Syndrome

The delivery of calories, particularly in the form of carbohydrate, may induce refeeding syndrome in a malnourished patient. Refeeding syndrome (see Chapters 7 and 13) refers to the metabolic and physiologic shifts of fluid, electrolytes, and minerals (eg, phosphorus, magnesium, and potassium) that occur as a result of aggressive nutrition support or nutritional repletion of a malnourished patient.[37] Carbohydrate delivery stimulates insulin secretion, which causes an intracellular shift of these electrolytes and minerals with the potential for severe hypophosphatemia, hypomagnesemia, and hypokalemia. Refeeding syndrome is characterized by symptoms of generalized fatigue, lethargy, muscle weakness, edema, cardiac arrhythmia, and hemolysis. Thus, for patients who are at risk for refeeding, calories should be initiated and advanced slowly[37] (Practice Scenario 17-2).

Practice Scenario 17-2

Question: How can the complications of refeeding syndrome be minimized when providing PN to a nutritionally depleted patient?

Scenario: A 54-year-old male with a history of gastric cancer was status post partial gastrectomy and small bowel resection. Nasogastric output equals 1250 mL per day with absent bowel sounds. A kidney, ureter, and bladder x-ray is consistent with a small bowel ileus. His nutritional status is as follows: height 180 cm; weight 66 kg; usual body weight 75 kg; malnourished, with lean muscle and adipose stores slightly wasted; slight edema post surgery; prealbumin 10 mg/dL; albumin 3.1 g/dL.

Intervention: IV fluids are tapered as PN is initiated on postoperative day 8.

Answer: Start nutrition slowly by providing half of the energy requirements, or approximately 15 kcal/kg/d, on the first day of PN. The first bag should contain about 1000 total calories. Recommendations differ with regard to initial protein dosing. The effect of protein on glycolysis is not as concerning as dextrose, so some have recommended starting at the goal dose for amounts less than or equal to 1.5 g/kg/d. Dextrose and fat should comprise the rest of the formulation, although dextrose should not exceed approximately 200 g/d. Nutrition should be slowly increased to full nutritional goal over the next few days. Monitor electrolytes daily, paying particular attention to sodium, potassium, phosphorous, and magnesium. Daily intake and output, as well as the patient's weight, must be assessed. Administer vitamins and trace elements daily.

Rationale: The patient is at risk for refeeding syndrome complications because he is malnourished; his lean muscle and adipose stores are slightly wasted. He should be monitored closely for electrolyte abnormalities and volume overload.

Hepatobiliary Complications

Disorders of the liver and biliary system are complications commonly reported in patients receiving PN. These complications may be life-threatening and are particularly concerning for patients dependent on long-term support. Mechanisms explaining the influence of PN on the development of liver disease are lacking. Historically, it was thought that some existing component of the PN formulation or nutrient not provided by the PN formulation caused the liver disease. However, that simplistic concept has been replaced with the realization that liver dysfunction can result from a complex set of risk factors present in patients receiving PN. The term PN-induced liver disease has therefore been replaced with the term PN-associated liver disease (PNALD).[38] Intestinal failure is a primary risk factor; therefore, the term intestinal failure–associated liver disease has also been used.[39] The terms PNALD and intestinal failure–associated liver disease have been used interchangeably to refer to hepatic dysfunction secondary to intestinal failure that occurs in the setting of parenteral nutrition.

Types of Hepatobiliary Disorders

The types of hepatobiliary disorders associated with PN differ among adult and pediatric patients, although the distinction becomes less evident in the long-term PN patient. There are three types of hepatobiliary disorders associated with PN therapy: steatosis, cholestasis, and gallbladder sludge/stones; however, these disorders may coexist.[40] Steatosis, or hepatic fat accumulation, is predominant in adults and is generally benign. It typically presents as modest elevations of serum aminotransferase concentrations that occur within 2 weeks of PN therapy and may return to normal, even when PN is continued. Most patients are asymptomatic. Steatosis appears to be a complication of overfeeding and has probably decreased in prevalence over the years with the decrease in estimates of PN calorie requirements. Although steatosis is generally thought to be a nonprogressive lesion, progression to fibrosis or cirrhosis may become an issue in patients receiving long-term PN.[6]

PN-associated cholestasis (PNAC) is a condition of impaired secretion of bile or frank biliary obstruction that occurs predominantly in children, but may also occur in adult patients receiving long-term PN. PNAC typically presents as an elevation of alkaline phosphatase, gamma-glutamyl transpeptidase, and conjugated (direct) bilirubin concentrations with or without jaundice. Although both gamma-glutamyl transpeptidase and alkaline phosphatase are sensitive markers for hepatobiliary disease, they lack specificity because levels may be elevated in other diseases as well. An elevated serum conjugated bilirubin is considered the prime indicator for cholestasis, typically defined as a concentration > 2 mg/dL. PNAC is a serious complication because it may progress to cirrhosis and liver failure.

Last, gallbladder stasis during PN therapy may lead to the development of gallstones or gallbladder sludge with subsequent cholecystitis. It is related more to the lack of enteral stimulation than the PN infusion itself. The lack of oral intake results in decreased cholecystokinin (CCK) release and impaired bile flow and gallbladder contractility. The duration of PN therapy appears to correlate with the development of biliary sludge.[41] Biliary sludge may progress to acute cholecystitis in the absence of gallstones. This condition is also referred to as acalculous cholecystitis.

Prevalence of Hepatobiliary Complications

Reported prevalence rates of PNALD vary greatly. In adult patients receiving PN, the reported incidence of abnormal enzyme elevations has varied from 25% to 100%.[40] However, few studies have correlated enzyme changes to permanent hepatic function or histological damage. Development of liver disease in patients receiving long-term PN is particularly concerning because its occurrence and severity appear to increase with longer duration of PN usage. The prevalence of chronic cholestasis in a group of 90 patients receiving home PN for permanent intestinal failure was 55% at 2 years, 64% at 4 years, and 72% at 6 years.[6]

Many of the studies evaluating prevalence of PNALD also attempted to identify risk factors unrelated to the PN therapy. Bacterial and fungal infections have been documented to be associated with cholestasis. Sepsis likely causes liver inflammation because of the release of proinflammatory cytokines that are activated by endotoxins. This is especially relevant in the long-term PN patient who may suffer from recurrent central line–associated bloodstream infections. Many patients receiving PN have disorders that predispose them to developing small intestinal bacterial overgrowth, which is considered another risk factor for liver disease. Bacterial overgrowth occurs when large amounts of bacteria normally confined to the colon and lower small bowel populate the upper small intestine. It has been postulated that these anaerobic bacteria in the small intestine may produce hepatotoxins. Massive intestinal resection has also been identified as a risk factor for PNALD.[6,42] A small bowel remnant < 50 cm in length has been significantly associated with chronic cholestasis.[6]

Parenteral Nutrition–Related Risk Factors

Although supporting data are limited, various factors related to the nutrient composition of the PN formulation have been suggested to contribute to the development of liver complications. Therefore, it is important to evaluate the merits of these potential risk factors in order to design a PN formulation that minimizes risk of PNALD.

Energy

Clinical studies suggest that the development of steatosis during PN administration is primarily due to excessive energy intake.[40] Overfeeding either combined or individual energy substrates (carbohydrate, fat, protein) can contribute to liver complications. The administration of excessive energy is thought to promote hepatic fat deposition by stimulating insulin release, which, in turn, promotes lipogenesis and inhibits fatty acid oxidation.[40]

Carbohydrate

Dextrose-based PN formulations that contain little or no fat have been implicated in the development of steatosis. Not only do excess carbohydrates deposit in the liver as fat, but a dextrose-based PN formulation may result in EFAD. EFAD may lead to impaired lipoprotein formation and triglyceride secretion, resulting in steatosis. Providing balanced dextrose and fat calories seems to decrease the incidence of steatosis, possibly by decreasing hepatic triglyceride uptake and promoting fatty acid oxidation. A balanced PN formulation should provide 70% to 85% of nonprotein calories as carbohydrate and 15% to 30% as fat.[8] In addition, carbohydrate content should not exceed 7 g/kg/d in adults.

Protein

Early sources of amino acids for parenteral use included protein hydrolysates that had significant amounts of aluminum contamination. Animal studies suggest that high levels of aluminum contamination may lead to the development of cholestasis. However, the replacement of protein hydrolysates with crystalline amino acids has significantly reduced the overall aluminum contamination in PN formulations. Amino acid–associated aluminum toxicity is not considered a risk factor for the development of liver complications.[43] Although the role amino acids play in the development of cholestasis in adults is unclear, it does not appear to be as significant as it is in infants.

Intravenous Fat Emulsion

There are various concerns regarding the role of IVFE in the development of liver complications, including fat source, the phytosterol content, and the dose. In the United States, the available IVFE is soybean oil–based and contains high concentrations of ω-6 fatty acids and significant quantities of phytosterols. Phytosterols are inefficiently metabolized to bile acids by the liver, and it has been postulated that they may impair bile flow and cause biliary sludge and stones. Adult patients with short bowel syndrome receiving IVFE-containing PN have been shown to have much higher serum phytosterol levels than other patients with short bowel syndrome or healthy controls.[44] Case reports of children with PN-related cholestasis have documented high serum phytosterol levels.[45] In addition, there is concern that the high ω-6 fatty acids content of soybean-based IVFE may initiate or worsen inflammatory states and has been shown to have immunosuppressive effects.[46] The presence of phytosterols and proinflammatory ω-6 fatty acids may contribute to the hepatotoxic effects seen in patients receiving long-term PN with a soybean oil–based IVFE. The use of a fish oil–based fat emulsion, primarily composed of ω-3 fatty acids and containing no phytosterols, has shown promising results in reversing PNALD in pediatric patients when used in place of conventional IVFE.[47] Further study evaluating safety and efficacy of fish oil–based IVFE for prevention and treatment of PNALD is under way. The IVFE dose is another concern. Although liver complications have been associated with EFAD, they can also occur when the IVFE dose is excessive. Steatosis can occur when the IVFE infusion rate exceeds the liver's ability to clear the phospholipids and fatty acids, leading to direct deposition in the liver. Cholestasis may also be associated with high IVFE doses, especially with long-term use. Multivariate analysis demonstrated that chronic cholestasis and severe PNALD was strongly associated with IVFE intake > 1 g/kg/d in patients receiving long-term PN.[6] The results demonstrated no association between dextrose intake or nonprotein calorie intake and PNALD.

Carnitine

Carnitine plays an important role in fat metabolism (see Chapters 5 and 15). Primary carnitine deficiency has been associated with the development of steatosis. Because carnitine is not routinely added to PN, plasma carnitine concentrations may decrease below the reference range within a few weeks of starting PN therapy. Carnitine supplementation has been shown to help mobilize hepatic fat stores and prevent steatosis in neonates receiving PN.[45] However, low serum carnitine concentrations do not necessarily correlate with hepatic dysfunction in adults. In adult home PN patients with abnormal serum liver enzymes and low serum carnitine concentrations, no improvement was shown in liver enzymes after carnitine was supplemented for 1 month, despite normalization of serum carnitine concentrations.[48] The role of carnitine in the prevention and treatment of PN-associated liver complications in adults remains to be established.

TABLE 17-1 Strategies to Manage Parenteral Nutrition–Associated Liver Complications

1. Rule out non-PN factors	Hepatotoxic medications Herbal supplements Biliary obstruction Hepatitis Sepsis
2. Consider PN modifications	Decrease dextrose Decrease IVFE (less than 1g/kg/d) Provide a balance of dextrose and IVFE Cyclic PN infusion
3. Maximize enteral intake	Encourage oral diet Tube feeding, even at slow rate
4. Prevent/treat bacterial overgrowth	Enteral antibiotics, such as: • Metronidazole • Neomycin • Doxycycline • Ciprofloxacin • Rifaximin In CIPO patients, consider agents to enhance motility: • Metoclopramide • Erythromycin • Tegaserod • Octreotide[a]
5. Pharmacotherapy	Aggressive treatment of infection Ursodeoxycholic acid (ursodiol) Treatment of pruritus: • Cholestyramine • Rifampin • Phenobarbital
6. Intestinal transplantation	Consider for patients with PN failure

CIPO, chronic intestinal pseudo-obstruction; IVFE, intravenous fat emulsion; PN, parenteral nutrition.
[a]Octreotide delays gastric emptying, but stimulates small intestinal motility.

Choline

Choline is a nutrient found in many foods that is essential for normal function of all cells and required for lipid transport and metabolism (see Chapter 8). It is not a component of PN formulations because it is assumed that endogenous synthesis is possible from methionine contained in the crystalline amino acid solution. However, the conversion of methionine to choline may be less efficient when methionine is given parenterally than when given orally.[49] Low plasma-free choline concentrations have been reported in patients receiving long-term PN and have been associated with elevated serum hepatic aminotransferase concentrations. Steatosis reportedly resolved following choline supplementation.[50] Additional studies are needed to further evaluate the role of choline supplementation in the prevention and treatment of PNALD. At present, there is no commercially available injectable choline preparation.

Strategies to Manage Parenteral Nutrition–Associated Hepatobiliary Complications

When a patient receiving PN develops liver complications, a review of all aspects of care is necessary to identify and eliminate or treat other contributing factors. Table 17-1 outlines strategies to consider when a patient receiving PN develops liver complications (see Practice Scenario 17-3 for a discussion of management of cholestasis in an adult patient on long-term PN).

Practice Scenario 17-3

Question: What modifications can be made to the PN formulation to minimize and manage the development of cholestasis in an adult patient requiring long-term PN?

Scenario: A 72-year-old female with a history of ovarian cancer and short bowel syndrome due to intestinal ischemia presents to the intestinal failure clinic for home PN management. She has been receiving home PN for the past year. She has approximately 120 cm of small bowel and partial colon remaining, and an end jejunostomy. A recent liver biopsy shows cholestasis and steatosis, and laboratory studies show elevated serum transaminase levels, alkaline phosphatase, and conjugated/direct bilirubin (8 mg/dL). She is eating a regular diet and empties the ostomy appliance 10 times daily. Weight is 50 kg and has been stable; body mass index is 18.9. Home PN regimen provides protein 60 g, dextrose 275 g, standard electrolytes, vitamins, and trace elements, and volume 2000 mL cycled over 15 hours nightly through a single lumen tunneled catheter. IVFE 50 g is coinfused via Y-site over 15 hours three times weekly.

Intervention: Modifications made to the PN formulation include a reduction in frequency of IVFE from three to one times weekly, a proportional increase in dextrose to account for the decrease in IVFE, and conversion from separate IVFE infusion to total nutrient admixture on the day she receives it each week. The infusion cycle is shortened from 15 to 12 hours. Trace element levels are obtained and supplemental copper and manganese are removed from the PN formulation.

Answer: The PN formulation does not appear excessive in dextrose or overall calories based on a stable weight and a total calorie dose of 28 kcal/kg/d. Although the dose of IVFE does not exceed 1 g/kg/d, a trial to decrease the dose may be beneficial. Providing IVFE via a total nutrient admixture is preferable to a separate coinfusion in the home setting due to less manipulation required for administration and therefore potentially less risk of infection. Infusing PN over a cyclic period rather than a continuous, 24-hour infusion rate may be beneficial in reducing risk of PNALD. Even though the impact in changing from her current 15- to a 12-hour cycle may be minimal, all efforts to minimize risk are warranted as long as it is otherwise tolerated. Finally, the dose of copper and manganese should be reduced or eliminated and levels monitored in this patient due to impaired excretion.

Rationale: A critical review of the PN formulation should be undertaken whenever liver complications develop. Although the PN therapy may not be implicated as the cause of the complication, it may contribute to or exacerbate the problem. Overfeeding should be avoided, and a trial of decreasing calories may be warranted. Infection risk should be minimized because it has been identified as a risk factor for development of PNALD. In the long-term patient who develops cholestasis, specifically limiting IVFE dose may be beneficial.

Oral and Enteral Nutrition

Oral and enteral nutrition should be optimized whenever feasible in the patient on long-term PN because even small amounts of dietary or enteral intake may be beneficial in promoting enterohepatic circulation of bile acids. Oral nutrition is generally preferable to tube feeding for obvious reasons, but tube feeding may offer certain advantages in select patients. For example, a trial of jejunal feeding at a slow rate may be tolerated during a portion of the day or night in the patient with chronic intestinal pseudo-obstruction who is dependent on PN and requires gastric decompression. Medications to enhance motility may be necessary to aid success, and multiple attempts may be required before feeding tolerance is achieved. During periods of acute illness, enteral tolerance may be more difficult to achieve, and setbacks can be expected, but attempts should be made to restart enteral feeding as soon as possible once the condition has stabilized. Patients with short bowel syndrome should be encouraged to maximize oral intake because at least some of their intake will be absorbed. Depending on the severity of the short bowel syndrome, a reduction in PN calories may be necessary to prevent unwanted weight gain. However, fluid requirements generally remain high because stool output tends to increase when oral intake increases.

Cyclic Infusion

Cyclic PN infusion refers to the infusion of a PN formulation over less than a 24-hour period (generally 8 to 12 hours), allowing a period of time off PN. Continuous PN infusion can result in hyperinsulinemia and fat deposition in the liver, thereby potentially increasing the risk of liver complications. Cyclic PN infusion has been shown to reduce serum liver enzyme and conjugated bilirubin concentrations when compared to continuous PN infusion.[7] Allowing a period of time each day off PN may reduce the risk of PNALD, especially in long-term PN-dependent patients.

Pharmacotherapeutic Options

In addition to enteral intake, medications can also be used to help stimulate bile flow and maintain gallbladder contractility. Ursodiol (ursodeoxycholic acid) is a form of bile acid that has been widely used in the treatment of various chronic cholestatic liver diseases and has been shown to improve biochemical markers of cholestasis. When given orally at therapeutic doses, it becomes the predominant biliary bile acid and is thought to displace potentially hepatotoxic bile salts. Experience using ursodiol to treat PNAC is limited, but it may improve biochemical markers and symptoms of pruritis.[51] However, there is no evidence that the progression of disease is delayed. In addition, ursodiol has limited use in patients who cannot absorb oral medications because no IV form is available. CCK-octapeptide is a synthetic fragment of CCK that produces the biologic activities of CCK and is available in an injectable form. However, there is not enough evidence at this time to support its use in the prevention or treatment of PNAC. Phenobarbital has been used in relieving pruritus in patients with cholestasis and has been used in the treatment of other types of cholestatic liver disease. However, evidence supporting use for treating PNAC remains lacking.

Transplantation

In the long-term PN patient with significant or progressive liver disease, an isolated intestinal or combined liver/intestinal transplant may be the only remaining treatment option.[52,53] Medicare has approved payment for intestinal transplantation in patients who fail PN therapy. One of the criteria used by Medicare to define PN failure is the development of impending or overt liver failure. The choice of isolated small bowel versus combined small bowel and liver transplantation depends on the extent of liver disease. Although many patients are able to stop PN after receiving intestinal transplantation, there are other life-threatening complications and quality-of-life issues that must be considered before deciding on this option (see Chapter 31).

Metabolic Bone Disease

Osteoporosis and osteomalacia have been associated with long-term PN use. Osteoporosis is the most common form of metabolic bone disease and is defined as a loss of bone mass and microarchitectural deterioration of the skeleton leading to increased risk of fractures.[54] According to World Health

Organization criteria, the diagnosis of osteoporosis is based on a bone mineral density measurement that is more than 2.5 standard deviations below the mean score of young adult ethnicity and sex-matched controls. It is reported as a T-score below −2.5. A T-score that ranges between −1 and −2.5 is considered low bone mass, or osteopenia. Osteomalacia is characterized as softening and bending of the bones that occurs because the bones contain osteoid tissue that has failed to calcify. This generally occurs because of vitamin D deficiency. Bone biopsy for histologic examination of bone tissue is necessary for the diagnosis of osteomalacia and is, therefore, more difficult to identify. A combination of osteoporosis and osteomalacia may also occur.

Prevalence of Metabolic Bone Disease

The prevalence of PN-associated metabolic bone disease is unknown, but it is of concern in all patients requiring long-term PN. Osteoporosis was reported in 41% of patients after at least 6 months of home PN in one group,[55] and in 67% of patients on long-term PN because of intestinal failure in another group.[56] There are many diseases, conditions, and medications that have been associated with bone loss (Table 17-2). Because essentially all patients receiving long-term PN manifest at least one of these risk factors, it is unclear whether or not PN actually contributes to accelerated bone loss. A follow-up study in a relatively large patient group receiving long-term PN according to more current protocols showed moderate bone loss that was not statistically larger than in age- and sex-matched healthy subjects.[57]

TABLE 17-2 Diseases or Conditions Associated With Bone Loss

Postmenopausal osteoporosis
Long-term PN
Endocrine disease
Cushing's syndrome
Hypogonadism
Amenorrhea
Hyperthyroidism
Hyperparathyroidism
Gastrointestinal disease
Crohn's disease
Short bowel syndrome
Malabsorption
Malignancy
Multiple myeloma
Leukemia
Medications
Corticosteroids
Heparin
Warfarin
Levothyroxine overreplacement
Phenytoin
Phenobarbital
Leuprolide
Methotrexate
Genetic disease
Osteogenesis imperfecta
Immobilization
Spinal cord injury
Prolonged bed rest
Other
Alcohol abuse
Anorexia nervosa

PN, parenteral nutrition.

Parenteral Nutrition–Related Factors

Various factors related to the nutrient composition of the PN formulation have been suggested to interfere with bone metabolism.[58,59] Therefore, designing a PN formulation that minimizes the risk is important.

Calcium

Calcium plays a vital role in maintaining bone integrity by decreasing bone turnover and slowing bone loss. Patients receiving PN are particularly vulnerable to negative calcium balance because of limited intake and increased urinary calcium loss. Not only is calcium supplementation in the PN formulation limited by physical compatibility with phosphorus, but there also seems to be a threshold for calcium uptake when given parenterally. Higher calcium doses provided in the PN formulation are offset by higher urinary calcium losses. Therefore, the recommended daily intake of calcium gluconate added to the PN formulation is 10 to 15 mEq.[8] An inadequate phosphorus dose may also increase urinary calcium excretion. Phosphorus seems to enhance calcium reabsorption by the renal tubules and thereby promote a positive calcium balance. The recommended daily intake of phosphorus added to the PN formulation is 20 to 40 mmol.[8] Higher protein doses (2 g/kg/d as compared to 1 g/kg/d) in PN formulations have been associated with increased urinary calcium excretion, so reducing protein intake to maintenance doses whenever possible has been recommended. Chronic metabolic acidosis has also been associated with hypercalciuria and metabolic bone disease. Correction of the acidosis with acetate in the PN formulation has been shown to reduce urinary calcium excretion, so adequate acetate amounts should be added to the PN formulation to avoid metabolic acidosis. Finally, cyclic PN infusion has been shown to result in higher urinary calcium losses when compared to continuous infusion. However, this potential disadvantage associated with cyclic infusion should be weighed against its potential benefits to the liver and quality of life in long-term PN patients when compared to continuous infusion.

Vitamin D

Data regarding vitamin D requirements in patients receiving PN is controversial. Both vitamin D deficiency and vitamin D toxicity can result in bone disease. The adult multivitamin preparation used for PN formulations contains 200 IU of vitamin D (ergocalciferol or cholecalciferol). Vitamin D can be detrimental to the bone when excessive doses are given because it can suppress parathyroid hormone (PTH) secretion and directly promote bone resorption. There are reports that short-term removal of vitamin D from the PN formulation resulted in decreased hypercalciuria and an improvement in osteomalacia, although the results may have been influenced by the presence of significant aluminum contamination. Long-term (average of 4.5 years) removal of vitamin D in nine long-term PN patients with low serum PTH and low 1,25-hydroxyvitamin D resulted in normal PTH and 1,25-hydroxyvitamin D concentrations and improvement in bone mineral density of the spine.[60] Although vitamin D removal may be beneficial in certain patients, such as those with a low serum PTH concentration, it is impractical because there are no commercially available injectable multivitamin preparations without vitamin D. Because vitamin D deficiency can also result in bone disease, it seems reasonable to provide PN patients with the maintenance vitamin D dose contained in the injectable multivitamin preparation. Excessive supplementation should be avoided.

Aluminum Toxicity

Osteomalacia had been associated with PN formulations that once contained significant aluminum contamination because of protein hydrolysates. A low turnover bone disease and decreased bone formation was described in patients with elevated plasma, urine, and bone aluminum concentrations. Aluminum contamination of PN formulations is significantly lower now that crystalline amino acids have replaced protein hydrolysates. However, aluminum contamination is still a concern and has prompted the U.S. Food and Drug Administration to establish labeling requirements. Manufacturers of large-volume parenterals, small-volume parenterals, and pharmacy bulk packages used in PN compounding are required to measure the aluminum content of their product and disclose the concentration on the label.[61] Large-volume parenterals, including amino acid and concentrated dextrose solutions, IVFE, and sterile water for injection, are required to contain no more than 25 mcg/L of aluminum. There is no limit for the aluminum content in small-volume parenterals (ie, electrolyte salts) and pharmacy bulk packages (ie, parenteral multivitamins and trace element solutions), but manufacturers are required to provide the maximum aluminum level at expiry in the products' labeling.

Magnesium Deficiency

Hypocalcemia is a prominent manifestation of magnesium deficiency. Magnesium deficiency results in decreased mobilization of calcium from bone through several mechanisms. Hypomagnesemia causes an increased release of magnesium ions at the bone surface in exchange for increased bone uptake of calcium ions from the serum. In addition, chronic severe hypomagnesemia inhibits PTH release, resulting in inappropriately low PTH levels for the degree of hypocalcemia. The response of bone to PTH can also be diminished, resulting in functional hypoparathyroidism. Hypomagnesemic hypocalcemia should be treated with magnesium supplementation because it is often refractory to calcium therapy alone. Magnesium deficiency can also lead to hypophosphatemia because of increased phosphorus excretion.

Copper Deficiency

Copper deficiency impairs bone formation and can cause osteoporosis. Bone disease has been reported in infants receiving a copper-free PN formulation.

Prevention and Management

Because most patients with osteoporosis are asymptomatic, a screening process is important to identify patients at risk. A thorough history, physical examination, and laboratory assessment should be performed to identify risk factors. Decreased height may occur as a result of compression fractures of the vertebral bodies in patients receiving long-term PN. A baseline dual energy X-ray absorptiometry scan is recommended for all patients who require long-term PN therapy. If results are normal, then follow-up bone mineral density measurements may be considered in 2 to 3 years.[58] If osteopenia or osteoporosis is present, repeat measurement should be considered in 1 to 2 years. In addition to routine laboratory monitoring, patients with low bone mineral density may require further diagnostic testing, including measurement of thyroid-stimulating hormone, intact parathyroid hormone, 25-hydoxyvitamin D, 24-hour urine calcium and magnesium, urine markers of bone turnover (such as N-telopeptide collagen), and serum markers of bone turnover (such as osteocalcin and C-telopeptide collagen).

Strategies to prevent and treat osteoporosis should be considered in all patients who require long-term PN therapy, as outlined in Table 17-3. The PN formulation should be designed to minimize hypercalciuria; provide adequate magnesium, calcium, and phosphorus; avoid metabolic acidosis; provide vitamins and trace elements; and minimize aluminum contamination.[53] Selection of individual products with the lowest reported maximal aluminum content should be utilized in PN compounding whenever possible, such as use of sodium phosphate instead of potassium phosphate.[62] Patients with osteoporosis should be educated on lifestyle modifications, low intensity exercises, and fall prevention measures to minimize risk. Medications are available that have shown safety and efficacy in improving bone mineral density and decreasing fracture risk in patients with osteoporosis. Medications used for the prevention or treatment of osteoporosis that decrease bone resorption include bisphosphonates, raloxifene (a selective estrogen-receptor modulator), calcitonin, estrogen, and the newly approved monoclonal antibody denosumab. Teriparatide is the only approved medication that stimulates bone formation.

Special considerations are required in the pharmacologic approach to the treatment of osteoporosis in PN-dependent patients because of impaired gastrointestinal (GI) absorption of oral medications. Oral bisphosphonate therapy, including alendronate and risedronate, are considered first-line treatment options in the general population but are problematic in patients on PN. Oral bioavailability of these agents is less than 1% in the fasting state of normal subjects and requires special

TABLE 17-3 Strategies to Prevent and Treat Osteoporosis in Long-Term Parenteral Nutrition Patients

Strategy	Considerations
PN modifications	Avoid high doses of protein Avoid excessive doses of sodium Calcium 10 to 15 mEq/d Phosphorus 20 to 40 mmol/d Treat metabolic acidosis Maintain adequate magnesium intake Maintain adequate copper intake Minimize aluminum contamination Avoid adding heparin
Lifestyle modification	Weightbearing exercise Stop smoking Reduce caffeine Reduce alcohol
Fall prevention measures	Home safety Discontinue medications that may increase risk of falls, if possible
Calcium	Consider oral supplementation
Antiresorptive agents	Avoid oral route due to malabsorption and tolerance issues Consider IV bisphosphonate (ie, zoledronic acid 5 mg IV once yearly)
Estrogen	Estrogen approved for prevention of postmenopausal osteoporosis, but may not be safest option Raloxifene, a selective estrogen-receptor modulator, is approved for prevention and treatment of postmenopausal osteoporosis
Nasal calcitonin	Shown to reduce risk of vertebral fractures, but not hip fractures
Teriparatide	Recombinant human parathyroid hormone Stimulates bone formation Dose approved for osteoporosis is 20 mcg subcutaneously daily for up to 2 years

IV, intravenous; PN, parenteral nutrition.

measures to ensure adequate absorption even when GI anatomy and function are normal. The ability to achieve adequate absorption in patients with impaired absorptive capacity is questionable. In addition, oral bisphosphonates can cause mucosal inflammation and ulceration, which may lead to GI intolerance. IV bisphosphonate therapy provides a therapeutic option for patients on PN. Zoledronic acid is approved for the treatment of postmenopausal osteoporosis, and pamidronate has been effectively used off-label for the treatment of postmenopausal osteoporosis.[63–65] Teriparatide, a recombinant human parathyroid hormone, is approved for treatment of glucocorticoid-induced osteoporosis, postmenopausal osteoporosis, and osteoporosis in men. Its subcutaneous route of administration offers a therapeutic option for patients unable to take oral medications. Although IV bisphosphonate agents and teriparatide may provide a safe and effective therapeutic option for the treatment of PN-associated metabolic bone disease, further study is warranted. To date, only a single randomized controlled study has evaluated the use of bisphosphonate therapy in patients on home PN.[66]

Summary

Patients receiving PN therapy are at risk of developing metabolic complications and therefore require close monitoring. Refeeding syndrome and hyperglycemia are of particular concern in patients receiving PN in the acute care setting. In patients receiving long-term PN, the development of micronutrient abnormalities, hepatobiliary complications, and metabolic bone disease are of concern. Even though the PN itself may not be the sole cause of these complications, efforts to minimize contributing risk factors from the PN formula should be taken. A thorough monitoring plan is required to identify and prevent the development of both short- and long-term metabolic complications in all patients receiving PN.

References

1. Lewis KS, Kane-Gill SL, Bobek MB, et al. Intensive insulin therapy for critically ill patients. *Ann Pharmacother*. 2004;38:1243–1251.
2. Mehanna HM, Moledina J, Travis J. Refeeding syndrome: what it is, and how to prevent and treat it. *BMJ*. 2008;336:1495–1498.
3. Byrnes MC, Stangenes J. Refeeding in the ICU: an adult and pediatric problem. *Curr Opin Clin Nutr Metab Care*. 2011;14:186–192.
4. Weinsier RL, Krumdieck CL. Death resulting from overzealous total parenteral nutrition: the refeeding syndrome revisited. *Am J Clin Nutr*. 1981;34:393–399.
5. Brown KA, Dickerson RN, Morgan LM, et al. A new graduated dosing regimen for phosphorus replacement in patients receiving nutrition support. *J Parenter Enteral Nutr*. 2006;30:209–214.
6. Cavicchi M, Beau P, Crenn P, et al. Prevalence of liver disease and contributing factors in patients receiving home parenteral nutrition for permanent intestinal failure. *Ann Intern Med*. 2000;132:525–532.
7. Hwang TL, Lue MC, Chen LL. Early use of cyclic TPN prevents further deterioration of liver functions for the TPN patients with impaired liver function. *Hepatogastroenterology*. 2000;47:1347–1350.
8. Task Force for the Revision of Safe Practices for Parenteral Nutrition. Safe practices for parenteral nutrition. *J Parenter Enteral Nutr*. 2004;28(6 suppl):S39–S70.
9. Griesdale DE, de Souza RJ, van Dam RM, et al. Intensive insulin therapy and mortality among critically ill patients: a meta-analysis including NICE-SUGAR study data. *CMAJ*. 2009;180:821–827.
10. McMahon MM. Management of parenteral nutrition in acutely ill patients with hyperglycemia. *Nutr Clin Pract*. 2004;19:120–128.
11. Hopkins LL Jr, Ransome-Kuti O, Majaj AS. Improvement of impaired carbohydrate metabolism by chromium (III) in malnourished infants. *Am J Clin Nutr*. 1968;21;203–211.
12. Jeejeebhoy KN, Chu RC, Marliss EB, et al. Chromium deficiency, glucose intolerance, and neuropathy reversed by chromium supplementation, in a patient receiving long-term total parenteral nutrition. *Am J Clin Nutr*. 1977;30:531–538.
13. McCurdy DK. Hyperosmolar hyperglycemia non-ketotic diabetic coma. *Med Clin No Am*. 1970;54:683–699.

14. Stout SM, Cober MP. Metabolic effects of cyclic parenteral nutrition infusion in adults and children. *Nutr Clin Pract.* 2010;25:277–281.
15. Krzywda EA, Andris DA, Whipple JK, et al. Glucose response to abrupt initiation and discontinuation of total parenteral nutrition. *J Parenter Enteral Nutr.* 1993;17:64–67.
16. Eisenberg PG, Gianino S, Clutter WE, et al. Abrupt discontinuation of cycled parenteral nutrition is safe. *Dis Colon Rectum.* 1995;38:933–939.
17. Hamilton C, Austin T, Seidner DL. Essential fatty acid deficiency in human adults during parenteral nutrition. *Nutr Clin Pract.* 2006;21:387–394.
18. Holman RT, Smythe L, Johnson S. Effect of sex and age on fatty acid composition of human serum lipids. *Am J Clin Nutr.* 1979;32:2390–2399.
19. American Society for Parenteral and Enteral Nutrition Board of Directors and The Clinical Guidelines Task Force. Guidelines for the use of parenteral and enteral nutrition in adult and pediatric patients. *J Parenter Enteral Nutr.* 2002;26(1 Suppl):1SA–138SA.
20. Miller DG, Williams SK, Palombo JD, et al. Cutaneous application of safflower oil in preventing essential fatty acid deficiency in patients on home parenteral nutrition. *Am J Clin Nutr.* 1987;46:419–423.
21. Friedman Z, Shochat SJ, Maisels MJ, et al. Correction of essential fatty acid deficiency in newborn infants by cutaneous application of sunflower-seed oil. *Pediatrics.* 1976;58:650–654.
22. Seidner DL, Mascioli EA, Istfan NW, et al. Effects of long-chain triglyceride emulsions on reticuloendothelial system function in humans. *J Parenter Enteral Nutr.* 1989;13:614–619.
23. Carpentier YA, Kinney JM, Sidedrova VS, et al. Hypertriglyceridemia clamp: a new model for studying lipid metabolism. *Clin Nutr.* 1990:9(Suppl 1):1–9.
24. Adamkin DH, Gelke KN, Andrews BF. Fat emulsions and hypertriglyceridemia. *J Parenter Enteral Nutr.* 1984;8:563–567.
25. Kapila S, Saba M, Lin CH, Bawle EV. Arginine deficiency-induced hyperammonemia in a home total parenteral nutrition-dependent patient: a case report. *J Parenter Enteral Nutr.* 2001;25:286–288.
26. Felig DM, Brusilow SW, Boyer JL. Hyperammonemic coma due to parenteral nutrition in a woman with heterozygous ornithine transcarbamylase deficiency. *Gastroenterology.* 1995;109:282–284.
27. Sacks GS, Mayhew S, Johnson D. Parenteral nutrition implementation and management. In: Merritt RM (ed). *The A.S.P.E.N. Nutrition Support Practice Manual.* 2nd ed. Silver Spring, MD: American Society for Parenteral and Enteral Nutrition; 2005:108–117.
28. Kraft MD, Btaiche IF, Sacks GS, et al. Treatment of electrolyte disorders in adult patients in the intensive care unit. *Am J Health Syst Pharm.* 2005;62:1663–1682.
29. Centers for Disease Control and Prevention. Lactic acidosis traced to thiamin deficiency related to nationwide shortage of multivitamins for total parenteral nutrition – United States, 1997. *JAMA.* 1997;278:109–111.
30. American Society for Parenteral and Enteral Nutrition. *Product Shortages Recommendations: 2010 IV Multivitamin Shortage Information.* www.nutritioncare.org/lcontent.aspx?id=5346. Accessed August 20, 2011.
31. Howard L, Chu R, Feman S, et al. Vitamin A deficiency from long-term parenteral nutrition. *Ann Intern Med.* 1980;93:576–577.
32. Pluhator-Murton MM, Fedorak RN, Audette RJ, et al. Trace element contamination of total parenteral nutrition.1. Contribution of component solutions. *J Parenter Enteral Nutr.* 1999;23:222–227.
33. Howard L, Ashley C, Lyon D, et al. Autopsy tissue trace elements in 8 long-term parenteral nutrition patients who received the current U.S. Food and Drug Administration formulation. *J Parenter Enteral Nutr.* 2007;31:388–396.
34. Buchman AL, Howard LJ, Guenter P, et al. Micronutrients in parenteral nutrition: too little or too much? The past, present, and recommendations for the future. *Gastroenterology.* 2009;137:S1–S6.
35. Forbes A. Iron and parenteral nutrition. *Gastroenterology.* 2009; 137:S47–S54.
36. Kumpf VJ. Update on parenteral iron therapy. *Nutr Clin Pract.* 2003;18:318–326.
37. Solomon SM, Kirby DF. The refeeding syndrome: a review. *J Parenter Enteral Nutr.* 1990;14:90–97.
38. Kumpf VJ. Parenteral nutrition-associated liver disease in adult and pediatric patients. *Nutr Clin Pract.* 2006;21:279–290.
39. Kelly DA. Intestinal failure-associated liver disease: what do we know today? *Gastroenterology.* 2006;130:S70–S77.
40. Quigley EMM, Marsh MN, Shaffer JL, et al. Hepatobiliary complications of total parenteral nutrition. *Gastroenterology.* 1993;104:286–301.
41. Messing B, Bories C, Kunstlinger F, et al. Does total parenteral nutrition induce gallbladder sludge formation and lithiasis? *Gastroenterology.* 1983;84:1012–1019.
42. Luman W, Shaffer JL. Prevalence, outcome and associated factors of deranged liver function tests in patients on home parenteral nutrition. *Clin Nutr.* 2002;21:337–343.
43. Buchman A. Total parenteral nutrition-associated liver disease. *J Parenter Enteral Nutr.* 2002;26(5 suppl):S43–S48.
44. Ellegard L, Sunesson A, Bosaeus I. High serum phytosterol levels in short bowel patients on parenteral nutrition support. *Clin Nutr.* 2005;24:415–420.
45. Btaiche IF, Khalidi N. Parenteral nutrition-associated liver complications in children. *Pharmacotherapy.* 2002;22:188–211.
46. Calder PC. Hot topics in parenteral nutrition: rationale for using new lipid emulsions in parenteral nutrition and a review of the trials performed in adults. *Proc Nutr Soc.* 2009;68:252–260.
47. de Meijer VE, Gura KM, Meisel JA, et al. Parenteral fish oil monotherapy in the management of patients with parenteral nutrition-associated liver disease. *Arch Surg.* 2010;145:547–551.
48. Bowyer BA, Miles JM, Haymond MW, et al. L-carnitine therapy in home parenteral nutrition patients with abnormal liver tests and low plasma carnitine concentrations. *Gastroenterology.* 1988;94:434–438.
49. Chawla RK, Berry CJ, Kutner MH, et al. Plasma concentrations of transsulfuration pathway products during nasoenteral and intravenous hyperalimentation of malnourished patients. *Am J Clin Nutr.* 1985;42:577–584.
50. Buchman AL. The addition of choline to parenteral nutrition. *Gastroenterology.* 2009;137:S119–S128.
51. San Luis VA, Btaiche IF. Ursodiol in patients with parenteral nutrition-associated cholestasis. *Ann Pharmacother.* 2007;41:1867–1872.
52. American Gastroenterological Association Clinical Practice Committee. AGA technical review on short bowel syndrome and intestinal transplantation. *Gastroenterology.* 2003;124:1111–1134.
53. Staun M, Pironi L, Bozzetti F, et al. ESPEN guidelines on parenteral nutrition: home parenteral nutrition (HPN) in adult patients. *Clin Nutr.* 2009;28:467–479.
54. Consensus development conference: Diagnosis, prophylaxis and treatment of osteoporosis. *Am J Med.* 1994;94:646–650.
55. Pironi L, Labate AM, Pertkiewicz M, et al. Prevalence of bone disease in patients on home parenteral nutrition. *Clin Nutr.* 2002;21:289–296.
56. Cohen-Solal M, Baudoin C, Joly F, et al. Osteoporosis in patients on long-term home parenteral nutrition: a longitudinal study. *J Bone Miner Res.* 2003;18:1989–1994.
57. Haderslev KV, Tjellesen L, Haderslev PH, et al. Assessment of the longitudinal changes in bone mineral density in patients receiving home parenteral nutrition. *J Parenter Enteral Nutr.* 2004;28:289–294.

58. Seidner DL. Parenteral nutrition-associated metabolic bone disease. *J Parenter Enteral Nutr*. 2002;26(5 suppl):S37–S42.
59. Buchman AL, Moukarzel A. Metabolic bone disease associated with total parenteral nutrition. *Clin Nutr*. 2000;19:217–231.
60. Verhage AH, Cheong WK, Allard JP, et al. Increase in lumbar spine bone mineral content in patients on long-term parenteral nutrition without vitamin D supplementation. *J Parenter Enteral Nutr*. 1995;19:431–436.
61. Department of Health and Human Services (HHS), Food and Drug Administration (FDA). Amendment of regulations on parenteral nutrition; delay of effective date. *Federal Register*. 2003; 68:32979–32981.
62. Smith BS, Kothari H, Hayes BD, et al. Effect of additive selection on calculated aluminum content of parenteral nutrient solutions. *Am J Health-Syst Pharm*. 2007;64:730–739.
63. Reid IR, Brown JP, Burckhardt P, et al. Intravenous zoledronic acid in postmenopausal women with low bone mineral density. *N Engl J Med*. 2002;346:653–661.
64. Miller RG, Chreitien KC, Meoni LA, et al. Comparison of intravenous pamidronate to standard therapy for osteoporosis. Use in patients unable to take oral bisphosphonates. *J Clin Rheumatol*. 2005;11:2–7.
65. Vis M, Bultink IEM, Dijkmans BAC. The effect of intravenous pamidronate versus oral alendronate on bone mineral density in patients with osteoporosis. *Osteoporos Int*. 2005;16: 1432–1435.
66. Haderslev KV, Tjellesen L, Sorensen HA, et al. Effect of cyclical intravenous clodronate therapy on bone mineral density and markers of bone turnover in patients receiving home parenteral nutrition. *Am J Clin Nutr*. 2002;76:482–488.

18 Drug–Nutrient Interactions

Carol J. Rollins, MS, RD, CNSD, PharmD, BCNSP

CONTENTS

Background 299
Types of Interactions 300
Physical Interactions 300
Parenteral Nutrition 301
Enteral Nutrition 301
Preventing or Mitigating Physical Interactions 302
Pharmaceutical Interactions 303
Dosage Forms 303
Preventing or Mitigating Pharmaceutical Interactions 304
Pharmacokinetic Interactions 305
Definition 305
Apparent Absorption and Metabolism 305
Administration-Related Factors 305
Tubing and Bag Characteristics 305
Site of Delivery 305
Delivery Environment 306
Administration Regimen 307
Drug-Related Factors 307
Presystemic Metabolism 308
Therapeutic Index 308
Formula-Related Factors 308
Macronutrients 308
Micronutrients 308
Disease-Related Factors 308
Specific Drugs—Enteral Nutrition Interactions 309
Phenytoin 309
Carbamazepine 309
Fluoroquinolones 309
Warfarin 310
Summary 311
References 311

Objectives

1. Describe three different types of drug–nutrient interactions (DNIs) related to parenteral nutrition (PN) or enteral nutrition (EN), and give an example of each.
2. List two drug- or formula-related factors that may contribute to DNIs with PN formulations and EN formulations.
3. Determine when intermittently stopping enteral feeding or changing the EN formulation is more likely to result in successful management or prevention of a DNI.
4. List the usual steps for administering a drug via the feeding tube or when PN is also being administered, and explain why these steps are more appropriate than other methods including admixture of a drug with parenteral or enteral feeding formulations.

Test Your Knowledge Questions

1. An alert and oriented patient is receiving a continuous infusion of a standard, fiber-containing enteral feeding formulation through an 8 Fr nasogastric (NG) tube. Drugs administered by bolus administration through the side port of the tube are phenytoin suspension 400 mg daily and nizatidine 150 mg every 12 hours. The feeding tube becomes occluded and must be removed. Which of the following measures is most appropriate for preventing occlusion of the new tube?
   A. Replace the 8 Fr tube with a 16 Fr NG tube.
   B. Flush the feeding tube with 15 mL of water before and after administering each medication.
   C. Discontinue the fiber-containing enteral feeding formulation, and initiate feeding with a fiber-free formulation.
   D. Hold the feeding infusion for 2 hours before and after administering phenytoin.
2. The EN formulation for a home patient receiving EN through a percutaneous gastrostomy was recently changed from a high-protein, fiber-containing, 1 kcal/mL formulation to the only 1.5 kcal/mL formulation available in the local store. The new product is marketed for use in patients with compromised pulmonary function and contains low amounts of carbohydrate, 55% of calories from fat, about 15% less protein per day than the 1 kcal/mL formulation, and no fiber. What component of the new formulation is most likely to contribute to interactions resulting from slow gastric emptying?
   A. Lower fiber content
   B. Lower protein content
   C. Higher fat content
   D. Higher caloric density
3. Which of the following is the preferred method of administering a hospitalized patient's antihypertensive medication when tube feeding is started due to poor oral intake?
   A. By the oral route
   B. As an oral liquid via the feeding tube
   C. As a crushed tablet via the feeding tube
   D. By the intravenous (IV) route
4. A medication that is ordered as a liquid to be administered via the feeding tube is available in the pharmacy in the IV form, as a capsule (powdered drug in a hard gelatin capsule), and as a film-coated tablet. What is the most appropriate and cost-effective choice for administration of this medication?
   A. Administer the IV form via the IV route.
   B. Administer the IV form via the feeding tube.
   C. Make a slurry of the capsule's powder and administer via the feeding tube.
   D. Crush the tablet to a fine powder and administer via the feeding tube.

Test Your Knowledge Answers

1. The correct answer is **B**. The most likely cause of the feeding tube occlusion is improper flushing technique (see Chapters 12 and 13). The tube should be flushed with a minimum of 15 mL of water before and after each medication, but 30 mL is commonly recommended and may be required to properly flush longer or larger tubes.[1,2] Although the risk of occlusion is potentially greater with an 8 Fr small-bore tube than with a 16 Fr tube, the discomfort associated with such a large-bore tube would make it a poor choice for enteral access in an alert patient, especially for more than a day or two. Switching from a fiber-containing to a fiber-free enteral feeding formulation would have little influence on risk of tube occlusion. The fiber used in enteral feeding formulations has been processed to a degree that makes its viscosity similar to that of polymeric fiber-free formulations.[3] Holding the feeding infusion for 2 hours before and after phenytoin administration has been recommended as a method to enhance drug absorption; it would not be expected to influence tube occlusion.
2. The correct answer is **C**. High fat intake slows gastric emptying. High protein intake and high caloric density can also slow gastric emptying but have less effect than high fat. In addition, protein intake will be lower with the new formulation. Low fiber intake has been associated with slow colonic transit and constipation rather than altered gastric emptying.
3. The correct answer is **A**. The oral route is preferred whenever possible because this is the route by which oral medications were designed to be administered. If the patient is allowed to take adequate water to swallow the medication, the oral route should be considered. For medications to be taken with food, the patient should have either food from oral ingestion or enteral formulation in the stomach before medication administration by mouth. Medications that are not administered via the feeding tube will not cause tube occlusion, making this a very effective method of preventing tube occlusion caused by medications.
4. The correct answer is **C**. IV administration is generally the most expensive and requires IV access. Use of IV dosage forms via the gastrointestinal (GI) tract is not usually recommended because these dosage forms are not designed to withstand the environment of the GI tract (gastric acid), and adequate amounts may not reach the bloodstream after presystemic metabolism in the GI tract mucosa (eg, cytochrome P450 [CYP450] metabolism) and first pass metabolism in the liver. Crushing a film-coated tablet can be difficult because the film coating tends to remain intact and can become sticky when wetted with water. This makes administration via a feeding tube difficult. Most hard gelatin capsules can be opened and the powder inside combined with water to make a slurry for administration via a feeding tube.

Background

Interactions between medications (ie, drugs) and PN or EN have the potential to affect patient outcomes adversely because of loss of feeding access, loss of access for drug administration, or inappropriate response to drugs and/or altered absorption of nutrients. Numerous factors must be considered to prevent or mitigate DNIs including the route and method of drug administration, the dosage form, and pharmacokinetic properties (primarily absorption and metabolism), as well as stability and compatibility characteristics. Factors related to nutrition support that may influence DNIs include the type and site of access, method of administration, and content of the PN or EN formulation.

Unfortunately, the U.S. Food and Drug Administration does not require manufacturers to evaluate drugs for altered pharmacokinetic parameters or potential DNIs when administered via tube into the stomach, duodenum, or jejunum. Few DNIs are well studied in patients receiving PN and EN therapy, and studies that do exist often focus on in vitro physical interactions or use small numbers of healthy volunteers with simulated feeding access (eg, ingesting an EN formulation by mouth rather than by feeding tube). Studies in patients are typically not blinded, lack placebo control, and are retrospective in nature. Observational studies and case reports from very small numbers of patients are often the only data available. Thus, understanding of the mechanism of interaction is often poor, and the strength of evidence supporting methods to prevent or mitigate interactions in patients receiving PN and EN therapy is seldom strong. Even the limited data available in the literature are sometimes conflicting, leading to multiple approaches to manage an interaction. Despite these limited and conflicting data, it is often possible to identify general principles that apply to management of DNIs. This chapter presents general principles to consider with DNIs and discusses specific issues related to the concurrent administration of drugs with PN or EN therapy. The chapter is not intended to be inclusive of all potential DNIs that the clinician may encounter; it is intended to illustrate certain common clinical dilemmas.

Types of Interactions

The American Society for Parenteral and Enteral Nutrition (A.S.P.E.N.) has defined a DNI as "an event that occurs when nutrient availability is altered by a medication, or when a drug effect is altered or an adverse reaction is caused by the intake of nutrients."[4] This is a broad definition that encompasses many types and potential mechanisms of interaction between drugs and nutrients. Table 18-1 illustrates one system for classifying DNIs; other systems using somewhat different categories and terminology are also in use.[5] The focus of this chapter is primarily on the physical, pharmaceutical, and pharmacokinetic interactions because these are the types most likely to present problems specific to PN or EN therapy, although they can occur in patients receiving an oral diet as well. Other types of interactions, such as electrolyte alterations related to specific medications, also occur in patients receiving nutrition support, but they tend to be independent of the route of nutrition and will occur whether the patient receives PN, EN, or an oral diet.

Physical Interactions

Interactions that result in altered physical characteristics of the nutrition formulation or the drug occur with both PN and EN therapy. Occlusion of the feeding access device is frequently the outcome from physical interactions. Other outcomes can include reduced bioavailability of the drug or nutrients, although studies seldom address effects of DNIs on the nutrients. Physical interactions typically occur in the delivery device before the drug or nutrients reach the patient; therefore, this type of interaction can be referred to as an ex vivo interaction.[5] Variables that are important to consider when assessing the risk of physical interactions include the pH at which the drug and the PN or EN formulation are most stable; presence of cations and anions known to react chemically; concentration and chemical complexity of nutrients; and time, temperature, and duration of exposure to one another. This latter factor is one reason admixture of drugs with a PN or EN formulation is very different than y-site or coadministration.

TABLE 18-1 Classification of Drug–Nutrient Interactions

Type of Interaction	Effect of Interaction	Associated Factors
Physical	Precipitation in PN or EN formulations; disruption of emulsion for IVFE or EN formulation; altered viscosity,change in consistency, clumping, or curdling of EN formulation	Drug and formulation pH; reactive chemical moieties; protein complexity; time; temperature; duration of exposure
Pharmaceutical	Loss of drug activity; toxicity	Alteration of a specialized dosage form or administration by a different route than that for which it was designed
Pharmacokinetic	Loss of drug activity; toxicity	Occurs before the drug or nutrient reaches the site of action; altered absorption, presystemic metabolism, hepatic metabolism
Pharmacodynamic	Loss of drug activity; toxicity	Occurs at the site of action; binding sites or receptors usually involved
Pharmacological	Inability to provide PN or EN therapy because of adverse effects	Extension of a drug's normal pharmacological actions

EN, enteral nutrition; IVFE, intravenous fat emulsion; PN, parenteral nutrition.

Parenteral Nutrition

Many studies evaluating compatibility between drugs and PN rely on visual inspection, measured turbidity, or increased particle count. Visually evident physical changes, such as turbidity, haziness, cloudiness, color changes, or precipitate formation in PN formulations, indicate incompatibility, as does emulsion disruption in fat-containing PN. Drugs that show no evidence of physical interaction with PN are generally classified as compatible. However, some interactions result in loss of drug or nutrient activity that requires chemical or molecular analysis for detection; no visible changes occur in the product(s). For example, injectable multivitamin preparations are compatible with PN formulations, although some vitamins, such as thiamin, have limited stability and begin to lose their activity very quickly once added to the PN formulation because of hydrolysis, photodegradation, or other forms of chemical degradation (see Chapter 15).

Safety guidelines that address the stability and compatibility of PN formulations have been developed.[6] When drugs are administered with PN, either by admixture or coinfusion, the method of administration should assure that both the drug and the PN formulation are stable and free from incompatibility. General principles for evaluating compatibility of drugs with a PN formulation include obtaining data for both physical compatibility and chemical stability of the drug and PN components whenever possible.

Both physical compatibility and chemical stability are influenced by pH. Because most PN formulations have a slightly acidic pH (5 to 6.5), drugs requiring a high pH or low pH for best solubility are typically incompatible with PN (see Practice Scenario 18-1 for a discussion of drug compatibility with PN). Increasing time of exposure between the PN and drug increases the risk of interactions; therefore, admixture of a drug into a PN formulation poses greater risk of interaction than coinfusion. Details related to the specific drug formulation (eg, with or without preservative, salt form) and drug concentrations evaluated, specific components in the PN formulation, and environmental conditions during evaluation (temperature[s] in particular) should be considered. Dextrose and amino acid concentration, specific brand of amino acids used for compounding, inclusion of intravenous fat emulsion (IVFE), electrolyte concentrations and specific electrolytes added, and addition of trace elements, heparin, insulin, and other components can all influence compatibility and stability of PN formulations. Efficacy and toxicity profiles must be acceptable with administration by continuous infusion rather than intermittent infusion when admixing drug with PN. Clinical application of principles of drug compatibility and PN formulations is discussed in Chapter 15.

Practice Scenario 18-1

Question: What factor(s) is most likely to result in occlusion of the vascular access device (VAD) when a patient is receiving several drugs and PN through the VAD?

Scenario: A 57-year-old man who underwent hematopoietic cell transplant 2 months ago is currently receiving PN with separate fat emulsion, patient-controlled analgesia with morphine sulfate (1 mg/mL concentration), ceftazidime, fluconazole, and foscarnet through his tunneled VAD. Calcium chloride, 1 g every 8 hours, is ordered due to a shortage of calcium gluconate for adding to PN and the patient's increased calcium requirements. He receives platelet and red blood cell transfusions a minimum of twice weekly. The VAD is double lumen; however, the patient's nurse states that one lumen is occluded. Two attempts to clear the catheter with a thrombolytic agent failed. The morphine has continued through the patent line. Foscarnet, ceftazidime, fluconazole, and PN are on hold until access can be obtained.

Intervention: A 0.1 N hydrochloric acid solution is instilled in the occluded lumen and allowed to dwell for 30 minutes before attempting to withdraw the solution. The procedure is repeated once because the catheter was still "sluggish" after the first attempt.

Answer: Several factors, including pH, time, administration method, and PN composition can contribute to physical interactions resulting in VAD occlusion. When the pH of PN and the pH at which a drug is most soluble differ significantly, there is a high risk of the drug precipitating when coinfused with PN. The administration regimen should be reviewed. Precipitation of calcium phosphate is the most likely cause of VAD occlusion if calcium is coinfused with PN.

Rationale: Evidence supports most antibiotics in the cephalosporin class, including ceftazidime, as compatible with PN; therefore, ceftazidime is unlikely to have caused the occlusion.[7] Data also support fluconazole compatibility with PN. Limited evidence suggests foscarnet is compatible for coinfusion with PN; however, other data indicate incompatibility with calcium-containing solutions. Given this mixed picture of compatibility, foscarnet may cause problems if coinfused with PN containing calcium. In this case, the patient is receiving calcium chloride outside the PN. Calcium is known to precipitate with phosphate when the solubility product of calcium phosphate is exceeded, which is likely to occur if calcium chloride is coinfused with PN containing phosphate. Thrombolytic agents are not effective in clearing drug precipitate. Altering the pH within the VAD lumen to make the drug more soluble can often clear the occlusion. However, the risk versus benefit of attempting line salvage should be considered. Generally, salvage is more likely to be attempted with a long-term tunneled or implanted VAD. With calcium phosphate precipitate, decreasing the pH by instilling 0.1 N hydrochloric acid will increase calcium phosphate solubility and may be effective in clearing the occlusion. Discussion with the nurse reveals the infusion arrangement changed last evening. The patient was receiving a blood transfusion when his calcium dose was due, and he was to receive platelets once the red cell transfusion was completed. Therefore, the nurse coinfused calcium chloride with the PN, which contained above standard amounts of potassium phosphate due to effects of foscarnet.

Enteral Nutrition

Use of enteral feeding tubes as a drug delivery device increases the risk of various interactions between the drug, the EN formulation, and the feeding tube. Physical interactions can be a significant problem when drugs are allowed to mix with EN formulations. Several studies have evaluated physical compatibility between various drugs in liquid form (elixirs, solutions, suspensions) and EN formulations. All of these studies were performed more than

20 years ago, generally did not use a rigorous study design, and tested relatively few drugs and even fewer EN formulations.[8–13] Direct application of these results to current clinical practice is difficult because drug and EN formulations may have been altered by the manufacturer while maintaining the same product name. Nevertheless, principles of compatibility can be gleaned from these studies.

Both the drug and the EN formulation affect the risk of physical interactions. The presence of complex protein (ie, intact or whole protein, not hydrolyzed protein or free amino acids) seems to be a critical property for determining risk of developing a physical interaction. Protein source (caseinates, soy, whey) may have some effect on interactions; however, fiber content, nitrogen content, and dilution of the EN formulation have not been shown to affect the risk of physical interactions with drugs in studies reported in the literature.[8–12,14] Theoretically, dilution of the EN formula is expected to improve drug dissolution and reduce interactions; however, formula dilution is not recommended due to increased risk of microbial contamination.[2] Two factors are of particular importance with drugs in liquid form: (a) acidic pH, and (b) base components, especially sugar-water syrups, alcohol-containing elixirs, or oil-based products.[8–10] These factors are probably more important than the drug per se in most cases; however, it is important to recognize that pH and base components are selected to optimize solubility of a particular drug.

Overall, approximately one-third of drugs in liquid dosage forms evaluated for physical interactions with EN formulations have demonstrated undesirable effects (precipitation, curdling, clumping) with at least one EN formulation.[8–11] Of 25 drugs reported to be incompatible with intact protein formulations in these studies, only 3 (one potassium chloride liquid and two oil-based products—medium chain triglyceride oil and methenamine suspension) were incompatible with a hydrolyzed EN formulation. One drug (Reglan syrup, Baxter Healthcare Corporation, Deerfield, IL) of the twelve tested with both fiber-free and fiber-containing EN formulations was reported as incompatible with fiber and compatible without fiber. The formulation tested contained soy polysaccharide as the fiber source. There are no data for EN formulations containing soluble fiber (guar gum, acacia, gum arabic, pectin) or fructo-oligosaccharides. Soluble fibers have a propensity to form gels. Therefore, the risk of undesirable interactions between drugs and EN formulations containing these fiber sources may be greater than with soy polysaccharide. An acidic pH was reported for all except two of the incompatible drugs, the exceptions being antacids (Mylanta II, McNeil Consumer Pharmaceuticals Co., Fort Washington, PA; Riopan, Takeda Pharmaceuticals International, Inc., Deerfield, Il.), both with pH 7.5.

The protein source for all of the intact protein EN formulations in these studies included caseinates.[8–11] There is limited evidence that soy protein results in finer precipitate than caseinates, and whey-based formulations are unlikely to curdle and clump when mixed with acidic drug products because of the acid-stable characteristics of whey protein.[14] However, these are primarily observations that should be confirmed in scientifically rigorous studies with current EN and drug formulations. The data suggest protein denaturation, especially for caseinates, may be responsible for much of the physical incompatibility when drugs in liquid dosage form and EN formulations interact.

Preventing or Mitigating Physical Interactions

Physical interactions are best avoided by not allowing drugs to mix with either PN or EN formulations. Ideally, drugs should be administered via a route other than the feeding administration device (VAD or feeding tube), although this is not always possible. There are a few exceptions where products are added directly to the PN or EN formulation, including drugs such as insulin in PN and electrolytes such as sodium chloride in EN formulations. For patients who are allowed oral intake, the best route for administration of oral drugs is by mouth (see Practice Scenario 18-2 for a discussion of oral vs. tube administration of medications). Routes such as rectal, transdermal, sublingual, intramuscular, and subcutaneous can be considered when drugs are available in these forms.

When a drug must be administered through the same device as the PN or EN formulation, feeding should be stopped, and the access device should be flushed with fluid that is compatible with the PN or EN formulation as well as the drug. The access device should be flushed before and after drug administration and between drugs if more than one drug is administered. The "flush" volume must be adequate to clear the administration device of the feeding formulation or the drug. Sodium chloride 0.9% is the usual fluid of choice for flushing VADs, but 5% dextrose solution is sometimes required. Minimum flush volume for VADs is typically specified by the manufacturer based on catheter size and type. Water is the fluid of choice for enteral feeding tubes. Other fluids should generally be avoided to reduce the risk of interactions with the EN formulation. Acidic products, such as carbonated beverages and cranberry juice, may be particularly problematic.[15,16] The volume used to flush enteral feeding tubes is often more than the minimum for clearing the tube, and 15 mL is the minimum recommended volume for flushing feeding tubes in adults.[2]

Other potential methods of preventing physical interactions with PN and EN formulations include altering the infusion time, the nutrition formulation, or the drug. For PN, a cyclic regimen might allow an incompatible drug to infuse during the off time, although this is rarely an effective approach for drugs administered more than once daily. Ideally, a therapeutically equivalent drug with evidence of compatibility for coadministration with the PN formulation could be used if changing administration schedules is not possible. Altering the PN formulation to omit the interacting component may be possible in limited circumstances and for a limited duration. For example, omitting fat emulsion for a few days while other vascular access is obtained may be possible when the emulsion is known to be the incompatible component and the patient's clinical condition is acceptable for this approach.

Changing to a hydrolyzed or free amino acid EN formulation rather than an intact protein source could be considered, although these formulas tend to be considerably more expensive and this is not typically a preferred approach to preventing interactions. Alternative dosage forms (eg, powder from a capsule can be made into a slurry rather than using an elixir) or drugs that are therapeutic equivalents (different drug with the same therapeutic effect) but with different potential to interact may be viable options in some cases.

Practice Scenario 18-2

Question: What is the most effective method for preventing feeding tube occlusion related to medication administration in a patient receiving jejunal feedings to supplement inadequate oral intake associated with gastroparesis?

Scenario: A 63-year-old woman was admitted to the hospital due to nausea and weight loss. The GI workup, including small bowel follow through, indicates gastroparesis, likely secondary to type 2 diabetes mellitus. Thin liquids empty from the stomach with only slight delay; however, progression of thick liquids and solids into the duodenum is severely delayed. A percutaneous gastrojejunostomy tube is placed by interventional radiology, and the patient is started on tube feeding in addition to a modified consistency (thin liquid) diet. Although the patient's chart from another hospital indicates poor response to prokinetic agents, metoclopramide is ordered and home medications are restarted, including levothyroxine, lovastatin, amlodipine, calcium citrate, and fluoxetine.

Intervention: Medications are ordered for administration through the feeding tube. After reviewing the chart, the nutrition support clinician recommends changing to oral administration of medications.

Rationale: Medication administration through a feeding tube is a contributing factor to tube occlusion. Medications administered by mouth do not cause tube occlusion. In this case, the patient is allowed an oral diet with thin liquids to reduce gastric stasis. Medications taken with water should have minimal effect on gastric emptying compared to water alone, and thin liquids empty with only slight delay per the GI evaluation.

Pharmaceutical Interactions

Dosage Forms

Interactions that occur because a drug dosage form is altered are more likely to occur with EN therapy and are seldom necessary for consideration with PN therapy. Drug dosage forms include the drug itself and other nonmedicinal components (excipients) necessary to make a stable and efficacious product that has suitable administration characteristics (eg, palatable for oral administration, nonirritating for dermal administration). Some dosage forms are designed for specific applications, such as enteric-coated tablets to protect drugs from gastric acid or the stomach from an irritating drug, long-acting products to reduce the number of daily doses, and sublingual or rectal products that avoid first pass metabolism in the liver. Altering certain dosage forms can dramatically increase or decrease drug bioavailability and trigger adverse effects, or conversely, destroy the active ingredient. Thus, pharmaceutical interactions can also be classified as pharmacokinetic interactions.

The most common method of altering a dosage form is to crush or dissolve solid dosage forms to create a liquid for administration via the feeding tube. When a solid dosage form is to be administered via a feeding tube, it must first be determined that crushing or dissolving will not disrupt the drug's pharmaceutical activity. Solid dosage forms that are appropriate to crush should be prepared as a very fine powder and mixed with warm water before administering through the tube. In addition, many capsules may be opened and the contents administered after forming a slurry with water from the powder or finely crushed solids. Consult manufacturers' product information and the medical literature for information regarding crushing tablets or capsules. A list of dosage forms that should not be crushed is published periodically.[17]

As a general rule, special dosage forms such as long-acting, sustained-release, slow-release, or delayed-release forms containing several doses in one tablet or capsule should not be crushed or dissolved. These dosage forms are designed to slowly release the drug in the GI tract, often over 12 to 24 hours. Crushing may cause immediate release of the total drug dose, increasing the risk of toxicity and reducing efficacy. For example, a 200-mg extended-release morphine capsule is designed to gradually release drug over 24 hours. When crushed or dissolved before administration, the full 200-mg dose is immediately released, resulting in increased risk of respiratory depression and potentially respiratory arrest. However, conventional (non-extended–release) morphine is usually dosed every 4 to 6 hours so the patient is likely to experience pain, and potentially withdrawal symptoms, if the conventional dosage form is given according to the schedule intended for the extended-release formulation. The risk of toxicity from crushing an extended-release formulation is exacerbated when bioavailability is increased disproportionately as the drug dose increases, as it does with diltiazem.[18] The metabolic effects of the immediate release of large drug doses intended for extended delivery, such as nifedipine from crushing an extended-release tablet, can be life-threatening.[19] Drugs that contain initials such as CD, CR, ER, LA, SA, SR, TR, XL, and XR following the name generally need to be taken intact and should not be crushed or dissolved for administration.

Enteric-coated products, often denoted by EC after the name, are another special dosage form that generally should not be altered for administration. The coating is intended to protect a drug from destruction by gastric acid or to protect the stomach from irritation caused by the drug. When the coating is disrupted by crushing or dissolving the tablet, adverse effects are likely to occur. In one case, the drug is destroyed by exposure to gastric acid, and the patient receives less than the desired dose, thereby placing the patient at risk of treatment failure. Gastric irritation from removal of a protective tablet coating may also result in treatment failure if the patient experiences emesis from the drug.

Enteric coatings should be distinguished from film coatings on tablets. Film coatings are used to make tablets easier to swallow or to mask unpleasant taste, but do not impart special characteristics such as those associated with enteric coatings. Crushed film-coated tablets should not result in altered drug activity or increased risk of adverse effects. However, film coatings can be problematic because they often remain as undissolved pieces that become sticky in water and can occlude the feeding tube. Sublingual dosage forms are designed to dissolve under the tongue for absorption via oral mucosa. Enteric mucosal and endoplasmic reticulum enzymes (eg, CYP450) and transporters (eg, p-glycoprotein and anion-transporting polypeptides) are bypassed with this route, thereby eliminating presystemic metabolism. In addition, blood flow is not routed to the liver, so first pass effects from hepatic enzymes, including hepatic CYP450 enzymes, are eliminated. Sublingual doses are typically small compared to oral doses, and sublingual doses administered via a feeding tube are unlikely to provide an appropriate treatment dose of the drug.

Dosage forms designed to disintegrate rapidly in the mouth before swallowing (solutabs) avoid the need for crushing and administering through the feeding tube when the patient is able to take such products. Pellets contained inside microencapsulated dosage forms should generally not be crushed. Intact pellets may be administered through the feeding tube, provided the pellets are small enough to completely pass through the tube. Usually, a larger tube such as a 16 Fr gastrostomy tube is necessary for successful administration of these dosage forms. Suggestions for administering the microencapsulated beads or pellets include pouring them down the tube or suspending them in an acidic juice before administering through the tube.[20] Using an acidic juice as the vehicle for microencapsulated pieces should reduce the risk of the beads or pellets sticking to the tube. However, water should be used to clear the tube of the EN formulation before and after administration of the acidic juice–drug mixture to avoid physical DNIs between the EN formulation and an acidic product (see Practice Scenario 18-3 for an example of such a drug administration situation).

Administration of IV dosage forms via the GI tract is similar to altering a dosage form. In general, IV dosage forms are poorly suited to withstand gastric acidity and enzyme activity within the GI tract. Substantial drug loss can occur, resulting in poor drug absorption and delivery to the site of activity. IV electrolyte preparations are an exception and seem to be effective when administered via the GI tract. However, the osmolality of such preparations can be very high and potentially result in GI intolerance, including osmotic diarrhea. Oral liquid dosage forms can also have a high osmolality and result in diarrhea or cramping. Osmolality of oral liquids and IV drugs often exceeds 1000 mOsm/kg and may be several thousand mOsm/kg.[21,22] The effect of high osmolality is most pronounced when a large volume is needed for each dose of drug. Diluting hyperosmolar products with water before administration reduces the osmolality and may reduce the risk of GI intolerance.

Sweetening agents such as mannitol, sucrose, and sorbitol are used in many oral liquid dosage forms and contribute to increased osmolality. Sorbitol is particularly troublesome because the cumulative daily dose from oral liquid drugs can reach 20 to 50 g, an amount commonly used as an osmotic laxative.[23,24] With only 5 to 10 g daily of sorbitol, a considerable portion of people experience bloating and flatulence.[25] An important factor in promoting EN tolerance is identification, prevention, and management of diarrhea due to the sorbitol content or hypertonicity of concurrent liquid medications.

Practice Scenario 18-3

Question: Which of the available dosage forms of lansoprazole should be ordered, and how should it be administered through a nasal-jejunal feeding tube?

Scenario: A 49-year-old man is receiving lansoprazole due to a GI bleed. He is being fed via a small bore nasal-jejunal tube because of poor nutritional status, inability to take an oral diet, and aspiration risk while on mechanical ventilation. He was taken off mechanical ventilation yesterday and is transferring from the intensive care unit (ICU) to a medicine unit today. His continuous IV infusion of lansoprazole was stopped today and administration via the feeding tube is ordered.

Intervention: The ICU pharmacist discusses the options for acid suppression with the physician and obtains an order to change to famotidine.

Answer: Lansoprazole is problematic for administration through a small-bore feeding tube using commercially available dosage forms. Either an extemporaneously prepared oral suspension or therapeutic alternatives should be considered to avoid occlusion of the feeding tube. In addition, the continued need for acid suppression once the patient is off mechanical ventilation, especially after he leaves the ICU, should be addressed. If acid suppression is to continue, the histamine-2 receptor antagonist on the hospital's formulary may be adequate. Otherwise, extemporaneous preparation of a suspension will be required.

Rationale: Lansoprazole is available as a delayed-release capsule and as a delayed-release orally disintegrating tablet (ODT). These dosage forms should not be crushed because of the delayed-release characteristics. The capsule can be opened and intact granules administered with apple juice via feeding tube.[26] However, the tube must be of adequate size to allow intact granules to pass through the tube without causing occlusion. The ODT was previously recommended for small bore tubes (≥ 8 French); however, due to the risk of tube occlusion, one manufacturer's ODT is no longer recommended, and caution must be used with any ODT.[26,27] A histamine-2 receptor antagonist available in a liquid dosage form or crushable tablet, such as famotidine, can be considered if acid suppression is still necessary once the patient leaves the ICU. Recipes are available for preparation of an oral lansoprazole liquid dosage form; however, this requires preparation from the available delayed-release capsule.[28]

Preventing or Mitigating Pharmaceutical Interactions

Methods of preventing or mitigating pharmaceutical interactions include using immediate-release dosage forms rather than long-acting forms and avoiding special dosage forms, such as enteric-coated or sublingual, when they must be crushed or dissolved for administration through the feeding tube. Proper tube flushing cannot prevent pharmaceutical interactions. However, flushing with adequate quantities of water remains an important technique to prevent concomitant physical interactions. Pharmaceutical interactions may also be minimized by using alternate routes of administration or by using a therapeutic alternative that is available in a form conducive to administration via the feeding tube. Exposure to sorbitol may be controlled by use of alternate administration routes or by use of therapeutic alternatives. Unfortunately, current information on the sorbitol content of a drug is often unavailable, so selecting a therapeutic alternative with less sorbitol may not be easy. The drug manufacturer is generally the best source of information for current sorbitol content. Published information may not reflect current content, and wide variation in sorbitol content can be found between manufacturers of a given product. Many pediatric drugs in liquid form, such as antibiotics, are now formulated without sorbitol.[29]

Pharmacokinetic Interactions

Definition

The term "pharmacokinetics" refers to studies of the time course for drug absorption, distribution, metabolism, and excretion.[30] However, the term can also be applied to nutrients because these same processes occur with nutrients. Pharmacokinetic DNIs are characterized by alterations in one or more pharmacokinetic parameters of a drug or nutrient due to an interaction between them. Changes in drug absorption and metabolism are most often reported. The effects of drugs on nutrient pharmacokinetics are rarely evaluated. Pharmacokinetic DNIs occur as the result of multiple factors, including those related to administration of EN or PN, the drug, and the PN or EN formulation. The disease process resulting in a requirement for EN or PN can also contribute to pharmacokinetic DNIs, especially as it affects protein status, organ perfusion, and GI motility.

Apparent Absorption and Metabolism

Bioavailability describes the amount of drug reaching systemic circulation after administration. Drug or nutrient loss during administration, adverse pH effects, complex formation between nutrient(s) and drug, presystemic metabolism in the gut mucosa (eg, CYP450 metabolism), and hepatic first pass metabolism can cause product losses that decrease bioavailability. Product loss during administration may reflect a chemical interaction that results in deterioration of the drug or nutrient without causing a change in the physical appearance of the PN or EN formulation or the drug product. A change in product color without precipitate formation or changes in viscosity may also indicate an interaction. Photodegradation, oxidation, and hydrolysis are typical chemical reactions resulting in stability problems. These chemical reactions tend to be exacerbated by pH changes, increased time of exposure (eg, admixture in a PN formulation rather than coinfusion), and increased temperature. Photodegradation requires light exposure and tends to be limited by opaque formulations, including IVFE and most EN formulations.

Amino acids are frequently associated with chemical reactions in PN and EN formulations. The Maillard reaction occurs between the amine group of amino acids, including those in proteins, and the carbonyl moiety of certain carbohydrates, resulting in a browning reaction that alters taste, appearance, and potentially, nutritional value. The carbohydrates involved are reducing sugars (eg, glucose, lactose). Sucrose and complex carbohydrates commonly found in EN formulations do not react unless hydrolyzed to monosaccharides. Heat (eg, heat sterilization) and water accelerate the reaction.

The potential for chemical reactions and stability issues exists whenever a solid dosage form of drug is made into a liquid form. Water tends to accelerate chemical reactions that result in loss of drug activity. Solid dosage forms (tablets, capsules) may not contain protective additives or stabilizers needed for liquid dosage forms of the same drug. For example, aspirin is very unstable in water, and an aspirin tablet dissolved in water quickly loses most of its pharmacological activity. Solid drug dosage forms should, therefore, be prepared as a slurry with water just before administration through the feeding tube. Occasionally, extended stability data for an extemporaneous liquid preparation is available, and the pharmacist can make the liquid product a few days in advance.[7,28]

Administration-Related Factors

Tubing and Bag Characteristics

Adsorption of a drug or nutrient into a container or administration tubing results in product loss without changes in the physical appearance of the products and is difficult to separate from chemical instability without sophisticated analysis. Specific chemical characteristics of the container or administration set must be considered before extrapolating data from a study to the practice site. Results of studies conducted in foreign markets relative to the clinician's practice may be especially problematic for extrapolation as differences in container and tubing characteristics, as well as medication formulation, may influence results.

Products with high fat solubility are more likely to undergo adsorption with plastics, but other drugs (eg, insulin) can also be adsorbed. The classic example of nutrient loss to the container is vitamin A loss into diethylhexylphthalate (DEHP)-containing plastics.[31] IVFE actually leaches DEHP from the bags into the emulsion, as does the castor oil emulsion used in formulating certain fat-soluble drugs, such as cyclosporine A. Although not DNIs in the usual sense, these interactions are concerning because the solubilized DEHP may pose a health risk.

Loss of certain drugs into feeding tubes has been suggested.[32,33] However, it is likely that most, if not all, of the loss was caused by adherence to the intraluminal surface of the tube because diluting phenytoin and carbamazepine suspensions before administration reduced drug losses during in vitro studies. Irrigating the feeding tubes after drug administration also reduced drug loss. Thus, suspensions, especially viscous suspensions, are best diluted to a relatively thin consistency before administration through a feeding tube. Slurries made from powdered or crushed drug should also be a thin consistency to avoid drug loss in the feeding tube. In addition, the tube must be adequately flushed to remove residual drug. Failure to do so may result in physical DNIs between drug retained in the feeding tube and the EN formulation, resulting in a high likelihood of feeding tube occlusion.

Site of Delivery

The site of drug delivery has minimal effect on PN-associated DNIs but can be a major administration-related factor for EN therapy. For PN therapy, the delivery sites are peripheral vein or central venous circulation, and the primary difference in PN formulations is the lower osmolarity of peripheral PN. On the other hand, efficacy and bioavailability of EN therapy may be greatly altered by site of delivery. Drugs with a "local" effect must be delivered to that locale. For example, antacids and sucralfate have no therapeutic effect with postpyloric delivery because they act locally in the stomach. Drug or nutrient absorption from the GI tract requires that the product be in a ready state for absorption. Nutrients must be released from the food matrix and specific complexes (eg, vitamin B_{12} and intrinsic factor) or valences (eg, ferric vs. ferrous iron) may be needed. Drugs generally must be dissolved and have some portion in the nonionized (noncharged) state. The site of feeding and drug delivery determines the environment to which a product is exposed, thereby affecting readiness for absorption. The location of the tube's distal tip determines the delivery environment for products administered through a feeding tube.

Delivery Environment

Feeding tubes can deliver drugs and nutrients to the stomach, duodenum, or jejunum (see Chapter 12). The environment changes from highly acidic to moderate acidity to near neutrality as the tip of the feeding tube moves deeper into the GI tract. These environmental changes in pH influence degree of absorption. Feeding and drug delivery into the stomach allow most of the normal physiological functions associated with digestion to be utilized. The stomach serves as a mixing chamber, helping release nutrients from the food matrix and mixing foods and drugs with gastric acid. Drugs soluble in acid generally complete the dissolution process in the stomach. Drugs that are not soluble in acid dissolve once they reach the small bowel.

Little absorption actually occurs in the stomach; rather, the vast majority of absorption occurs in the small bowel because of the enormous surface area. Thus, gastric emptying is a rate-controlling step for absorption, and any nutrient or drug that alters gastric emptying rate will affect pharmacokinetic parameters. Table 18-2 lists several EN formulation characteristics and drug examples that may be associated with altered gastric emptying. The rate of nutrient and drug absorption typically follows the direction of change in gastric emptying. Slow gastric emptying slows absorption and rapid gastric emptying increases the absorption rate.

Effects of altered gastric emptying on bioavailability, or extent of absorption, can be difficult to predict and are dependent on chemical characteristics and mechanisms of absorption for a particular drug or nutrient. Rapid gastric emptying accompanied by rapid GI transit can result in poor absorption because there is too little contact time between the drug or nutrient and the absorptive surface of the small bowel. Rapid gastric emptying in the presence of normal small bowel motility is expected to reduce the extent of absorption for nutrients and drugs requiring an acidic environment in order to create readiness for absorption. Slow gastric emptying allows increased release of nutrients from the food matrix, increased exposure to acid, and slower presentation of chyme to the small bowel. This translates into an increased extent of absorption for nutrients such as iron, calcium, and magnesium that benefit from acid exposure and for nutrients such as riboflavin that undergo active absorption by a saturable mechanism in the upper small bowel. Dissolution of acid soluble (eg, tetracycline) and poorly soluble (eg, carbamazepine, digoxin) drugs is improved with slow gastric emptying; however, bioavailability depends on stability in an

TABLE 18-2 Factors Associated with Delayed Gastric Emptying

Factors	Amount/ Characteristics	Concomitant Effect on Intestinal Motility
Formulation-related:		
Long-chain fats[a]	High concentration	Decrease (gastric)
Protein	High concentration	Decrease (gastric)
pH	Low	Decrease (gastric) Increase (small bowel)
Osmolarity (mOsm/L)	< 250 and > 800	Decrease (gastric) Increase (small bowel)
Viscosity	High	Decrease (gastric)
Volume	Large	Decrease (gastric) Increase (small bowel)
Drugs[b]/Drug-related:		
Particle size	Large or tablets	Decrease (gastric)
Anticholinergic agents		Decrease (gastric and small bowel)
Narcotic agents		Decrease (gastric and small bowel)
Octreotide		Decrease (gastric and small bowel)

[a]Greatest effect of formulation-related factors.
[b]This list of drugs is not all-inclusive.
Sources: Cullen J, Kelly K. Gastric motor physiology and pathophysiology. *Surg Clin North Am.* 1993;73:1145–1160; Fleischer D, Li C, Zhou Y. Drug, meal and formulation interactions influencing drug absorption after oral administration. *Clin Pharmacokinet.*1999;36:233–254; Singh BN. Effects of food on clinical pharmacokinetics. *Clin Pharmacokinet.* 1999;37:213–255.

acid environment. For example, bioavailability increases for carbamazepine, an acid stable drug, but decreases for digoxin, which is hydrolyzed in the presence of acid.

Delivery of the EN formulation and drugs into the small bowel bypasses problems with gastric emptying. Experience with use of short- and long-term jejunal feeding using both hydrolyzed and intact protein formulations suggests that delivery beyond the duodenum has negligible effects on overall nutrient absorption. The effect on drugs is largely dependent on their solubility and need for acid exposure for absorption. For example, poorly soluble drugs that benefit from an increased time for dissolution and drugs that require exposure to acid are expected to exhibit reduced bioavailability with administration into the small bowel. Thus, drugs such as carbamazepine, itraconazole, and tetracycline are likely to have reduced bioavailability with postpyloric administration. Limited data support poor itraconazole absorption with jejunal administration.[34]

The balance between reduced dissolution and less acid destruction with postpyloric administration of poorly soluble but acid-labile drugs, such as digoxin, is difficult to predict. Reduced hydrolytic products (0.6% vs. 2.9%) and greater nonmetabolized digoxin recovery (96.3% vs. 90.8%) were reported with jejunal administration compared to oral intake in a small study, suggesting the balance may be in favor of reduced destruction.[35] Because serum digoxin levels were not reported in this study, it is unclear if more nonmetabolized digoxin in the jejunum results in greater drug absorption. However, evaluation of serum digoxin levels within a few days of changing between oral or gastric administration and jejunal administration is recommended.

The site of drug absorption is an important consideration when administering drugs into the jejunum. Although most drugs are absorbed throughout the small bowel, a few are best absorbed in the duodenum and are likely to exhibit a significant decrease in bioavailability when administered into the jejunum compared to the duodenum. Ciprofloxacin serves as an example for duodenal absorption because up to 40% of an oral dose is absorbed in the duodenum.[36] Duodenal administration results in greater absorption than gastric administration in both healthy subjects and patients in the ICU, reflecting the acid labile nature of ciprofloxacin.[37] In addition, duodenal administration results in higher serum concentrations compared to jejunal administration.[38] Gastric versus jejunal administration of ciprofloxacin has produced mixed results relative to serum concentrations of drug.[38,39] One study reported higher ciprofloxacin serum concentrations with jejunal compared to gastric administration of drug with water, and equivalent concentrations between jejunal and gastric administration in the presence of enteral feeding.[38] However, compared to gastric administration in normal volunteers, a case report found the peak serum concentration to be lower with jejunal administration despite no feeding or other medications for 2 hours after drug administration.[39]

It is unclear if the absorption characteristics demonstrated by ciprofloxacin are applicable to other drugs in the fluoroquinolone class because similar studies are not available for the other drugs. Lack of data concerning potential pharmacokinetic problems with postpyloric administration of drugs is the norm rather than the exception. This situation is further confounded by published data, including the manufacturers' "package insert," that rarely provides information on the proportion of a drug absorbed in specific segments of the small bowel. Fortunately, most drugs have a wide therapeutic range and seem to be efficacious and nontoxic, despite potential changes in bioavailability related to the delivery site and environment. For drugs with a narrow therapeutic index, it is advisable to monitor for changes in the serum drug level whenever administration occurs through a feeding tube.

Administration Regimen

Food is known to interact with many drugs and alter pharmacokinetic profiles, particularly absorption and metabolism.[40] Recommendations for oral administration of many drugs commonly includes directions for taking the drug with or without food. Logic suggests that an EN formulation is equivalent to oral food ingestion; however, limited data suggest the method of EN administration influences GI tract response. Particular patterns of GI motility and secretions are associated with the "fed" state, including slowed gastric emptying and increased release of digestive enzymes and GI tract secretions. The "nonfed" state is associated with more rapid gastric emptying and fewer digestive enzymes and secretions.

One study of hydralazine pharmacokinetics in eight healthy volunteers receiving an EN formulation via NG tube reported similar results with fasting and continuous infusion of the EN formulation.[41] Hydralazine parameters with bolus administration of the EN formulation were similar to those with a standard breakfast (controlled for effects of nutrient content, such as fat) and differed from fasted parameters. These results suggest that holding continuous EN administration for drugs to be taken on an empty stomach (1 hour before or 2 hours after a meal) is not necessary. However, extrapolating results from a single investigation of one drug in healthy subjects to other patient populations and other medications is difficult. There is little evidence of therapeutic failure in most cases (a few notable exceptions are discussed later in the chapter) when continuous EN administration is stopped only during the short time needed to properly flush the tube and administer the drug. Clinical experience does, however, suggest that holding EN administration for approximately 1 to 2 hours every 6 to 8 hours for drug administration is likely to result in inadequate nutritional support and deterioration in nutritional status.

Drug-Related Factors

Factors associated with the drug itself can result in pharmacokinetic DNIs. These factors include the dosage form, chemical characteristics, and susceptibility to presystemic enzymatic degradation, cellular transport, and hepatic metabolism. For PN formulations, drug-related factors are largely associated with stability of the IV dosage form and the potential for loss of drug activity due to chemical reactions (photodegradation, oxidation, hydrolysis). Alteration of dosage forms and chemical characteristics relative to the delivery environment are important drug-related factors pertinent to EN therapy that have been discussed previously in this chapter. Susceptibility of drugs to presystemic enzymatic degradation, cellular transport, and hepatic metabolism can play a major role in apparent absorption for drugs administered into the GI tract; however, these processes are not specific to EN therapy and are reviewed only briefly here.

Presystemic Metabolism

Metabolism that occurs before reaching systemic circulation is known as presystemic metabolism and occurs in both the gut mucosa and liver. The CYP450 enzyme system includes many isoenzymes involved in drug metabolism and is a major component of presystemic metabolism. It is estimated that about 60% of drugs currently available are metabolized by CYP450 isoenzymes, specifically CYP3A4.[42] Drug interactions with grapefruit juice are the classic example of CYP450-mediated DNIs. Grapefruit juice inhibits the isoenzyme CYP3A4, thereby increasing serum levels of drugs normally metabolized by this isoenzyme.[43] Considerable research has been devoted to understanding effects of the CYP450 system on drug metabolism and DNIs because these enzymes can dramatically alter bioavailability, and, in some cases, this can result in life-threatening DNIs. In addition, drug transporters have increasingly been recognized for their importance in drug metabolism and disposition.

The best known transporter is P-glycoprotein, which serves as an efflux mechanism to pump xenobiotics, such as drugs, out of cells and prevent entry to the compartment the cells protect. P-glycoprotein is located on the luminal surface of cells lining the small bowel and prevents systemic absorption of certain drugs. The bile canalicular membrane in the liver and cells in the renal proximal tubule also contain p-glycoprotein. Organic anion-transporting polypeptides serve as uptake transporters in the intestine, opposing the efflux effect of P-glycoprotein.[44] The net effect of inhibition, induction, and interaction between CYP450 enzymes, uptake transporters, and efflux transporters can be complex and requires continued research to understand. To date, there are no data to sugget that any component of EN formulations significantly inhibits or induces these enzymes and transporters.

Therapeutic Index

Drugs with a narrow therapeutic index require serum drug concentrations within a small range to avoid therapeutic failure or toxicity. Any alteration in absorption of these drugs can be problematic; thus routine monitoring of serum drug levels or surrogate markers (eg, prothrombin time [PT]/International Normalized Ratio [INR] for warfarin) is generally conducted. Monitoring of narrow therapeutic index drugs is also advised with initiation and changes in an EN regimen.

Formula-Related Factors

Macronutrients

The association of complex proteins and fiber with physical DNIs was discussed previously in this chapter. Protein may also influence drug metabolism through effects on enzymes of the mixed function oxidase system in the liver.[40,45] Activity of the mixed function oxidase system seems to be stimulated with high protein intake and with riboflavin, niacin, and large ascorbic acid doses, thereby increasing clearance of drugs metabolized by these enzymes. Protein intake may also influence blood flow, with low intake reducing flow to the kidney and lowering renal elimination of some drugs. However, most data on protein effects come from animal studies, and more research is required before any definitive statement or recommendations can be made regarding the effect of protein on DNIs in the clinical setting. Nutrients that alter gastric emptying and GI motility can alter the rate and extent of drug absorption, thereby contributing to DNIs. The effects of macronutrients on gastric emptying and GI motility are included in Table 18-2.

Micronutrients

Micronutrients in EN formulations have the potential to cause DNIs. For example, divalent and trivalent minerals (calcium, magnesium, and iron) are known to form complexes with certain drugs, such as tetracycline and ciprofloxacin, which results in poor absorption of the drugs. Degradation products from micronutrients have also been reported to cause physical interactions. For example, oxalate from ascorbic acid degradation has been reported to interact with calcium in PN formulations forming an insoluble precipitate.[46]

The vitamin K content of EN formulations is a concern because of potential DNIs with warfarin. Formation of vitamin K–dependent blood clotting factors in the liver (Factors II, VII, IX, X) is inhibited by warfarin resulting in an anticoagulation effect. Significant vitamin K intake from an EN formulation can antagonize this anticoagulant effect and result in treatment failure. Most EN formulations marketed today contain modest amounts of vitamin K and provide daily vitamin K intake similar to average dietary intake from foods (90 to 120 mcg/d in adults).[47] Consistent intake of an EN formulation containing under 100 mcg of vitamin K per 1000 calories is not expected to cause warfarin resistance. Nonetheless, warfarin resistance has been reported in EN patients with relatively low vitamin K intake and seems to respond to changes in the warfarin administration schedule.[48,49] This suggests a mechanism other than vitamin K antagonism of warfarin activity, because the duration of warfarin antagonism is several days, not hours. Further discussion of this interaction occurs under the "Specific Drugs–Enteral Nutrition Interactions" section.

Disease-Related Factors

Malnutrition is a disease associated with alterations in body composition that may affect the risk of pharmacokinetic DNIs. Pharmacokinetic parameters can be affected by decreased serum concentrations of visceral proteins, especially albumin, which binds many drugs (eg, phenytoin, valproic acid, warfarin). Edema, increased body water, and decreased lean muscle mass may also affect pharmacokinetic parameters. Other disease-related factors include alterations in organ function and perfusion, as well as effects on GI motility. A full discussion of disease-related factors is beyond the scope of this chapter.

Specific Drugs—Enteral Nutrition Interactions

There are many potential DNIs involving EN therapy; however, a few drugs are particularly troublesome and have generated more discussion than most. Four of these drugs are discussed in this section.

Phenytoin

Phenytoin is a notorious drug for interaction with EN therapy. Many studies and case reports have been published but few are prospective, randomized, controlled trials. There are multiple theories regarding the interaction and many proposed solutions. Four prospective, randomized, controlled trials of phenytoin and EN in healthy volunteers have been reviewed.[50,51] Only one study investigated the effect of the EN formulation delivered through a feeding tube while the others investigated the effect of oral EN on serum phenytoin concentrations. None of these studies found an interaction between phenytoin and EN formulations. Countering these results were 25 reports and studies with less rigorous designs (no randomization or placebo control) that supported an interaction in patients.[50] Theories regarding the mechanism of interaction focus on issues related to pH[52–55] and phenytoin binding, either to tubing[32] or to an EN component.[56] Dosage form issues (eg, suspension, chewable tablets, capsule, IV formulation), chemical form (phenytoin acid vs. phenytoin sodium), and solubility are encompassed in the discussion of pH.

Of the various methods proposed to manage the phenytoin–EN interaction, none is completely reliable, and monitoring of serum phenytoin concentrations is highly recommended. Holding administration of the EN formulation for at least 1 hour, and possibly 2 hours, before and after phenytoin administration seems to produce the most consistent results.[56,57] However, some practitioners choose to continue adjusting the phenytoin dose to achieve therapeutic serum concentrations because adjustment of the EN infusion schedule can create problems related to inadequate EN delivery. Relatively high phenytoin doses are typically required to achieve therapeutic levels with this approach, and close monitoring of serum concentrations is required when the EN is discontinued. Dilution of phenytoin suspension is also recommended when the suspension is administered through a feeding tube.[32] Regardless of the method used, consistency of administration is important in order to control one of the variables influencing the phenytoin concentration.

Carbamazepine

Carbamazepine is a relatively insoluble drug and is acid stable; thus, slow gastric emptying improves bioavailability. Limited data suggest EN therapy reduces bioavailability, possibly by altering solubility. Relative bioavailability of 90% was reported in a randomized, crossover study comparing administration of carbamazepine suspension via NG tube with continuous EN and oral intake after an overnight fast in seven healthy males.[58] Serum carbamazepine concentrations with tube feeding were significantly lower at 8 hours and the lower maximum concentration approached statistical significance, although the small study size limited ability to show significance. In vitro recovery of carbamazepine also seems to be reduced after mixing with an intact protein EN formulation (58% recovery) compared to recovery after mixture with a simulated gastric juice (79% recovery).[59] Recovery was similar for the EN formulation and simulated intestinal juice (59% recovery). This suggests that postpyloric administration of carbamazepine may result in poor bioavailability.

Binding of carbamazepine to a component of EN formulations has not been demonstrated; thus, it is unclear if holding administration of the EN formulation for 2 hours before and after the drug dose, as has been recommended, is the best method of mitigating this potential interaction.[60,61] Adequate dilution of the suspension (or slurry from a crushed tablet) prior to administration and adequate flushing after the dose should be the first choice of methods to mitigate the EN–carbamazepine interaction because this does not impact delivery of adequate nutrition. When adequate dilution and flushing fail in patients with postpyloric administration, it would be reasonable to hold feedings before and after drug administration in this population. Gastric administration could be cautiously monitored without routinely holding the EN formulation unless there is evidence of an interaction. Carbamazepine suspension should be diluted at least 1:1 with water if administered via a feeding tube because drug loss in the feeding tube seems to be reduced with dilution.[33]

Fluoroquinolones

Bioavailability of fluoroquinolone antibiotics seems to be reduced by EN formulations. Studies in healthy volunteers have reported a 25% to 28% decrease in ciprofloxacin bioavailability when administered with an EN formulation, and decreases of 27% to 67% have been reported in hospitalized patients.[38,62,63] Reduced bioavailability is also reported with repeated doses of ciprofloxacin via NG tube in critically ill patients receiving continuous infusion of an EN formulation.[64,65] Jejunal feeding has the greatest potential of reducing ciprofloxacin bioavailability; however, the limited data available do not provide clear evidence of clinically significant differences in absorption based on the site of administration.[38,39] It is unclear whether reduced bioavailability with gastric or jejunal feeding is clinically significant because serum drug concentrations above the minimum inhibitory concentration have been reported for many pathogenic microorganisms.[39,66]

Complex formation of ciprofloxacin with divalent cations in the EN formulation was initially thought to be responsible for reduced bioavailability of ciprofloxacin with EN therapy. Fluoroquinolones are known to bind with divalent cations, and manufacturers' instructions advise separating drug administration from intake of foods, dietary supplements, or other drugs containing calcium, magnesium (eg, antacids), or iron. However, one in vitro study failed to find a correlation between cation content of the EN formulation and loss of different fluoroquinolones mixed directly into the formulation.[67] Ciprofloxacin loss was greatest (82.5%), followed by levofloxacin (61%) and ofloxacin (46%). The amount of loss seemed to increase with the degree of hydrophilicity of the individual drug. Limited in vivo data support this finding. Better bioavailability of ofloxacin (90%) compared to ciprofloxacin (72%) has been reported in healthy volunteers receiving the antibiotics with an EN formulation.[62]

The current recommendation is to hold administration of the EN formulation for at least 1 hour before a fluoroquinolone dose and 2 hours after the dose.[61] This approach seems to minimize effects of the DNI on ciprofloxacin and norfloxacin; however, data supporting holding EN are very limited, especially in patients actually receiving tube feedings. Well-designed studies comparing proper drug dilution and adequate flush volumes with holding of EN therapy with each of the fluoroquinolones are necessary to confirm the validity of holding feedings. Nonetheless, in the absence of such a study or drug-specific data clearly showing lack of a DNI, holding feedings remains a potential method of mitigating the fluoroquinolone–EN interaction.

Warfarin

One proposed mechanism for warfarin resistance with low vitamin K intake is binding of warfarin to a component of the EN formulation, most likely protein.[68] Warfarin resistance due to protein binding has not been adequately studied to confirm this as an in vivo mechanism of DNI. The study used to promote protein binding as a mechanism of interaction was conducted in vitro at a pH outside the physiologic range.[68] Use of a free amino acid (elemental) EN formulation is expected to prevent the interaction if protein binding actually causes the DNI; however, this premise has not been tested. Practitioners may elect to manage the interaction by methods other than using an elemental formula (ie, increase the warfarin dose or change to an alternative anticoagulant therapy) given the higher cost, potential for the high osmolality to cause GI intolerance, and greater difficulty in justifying use of these formulas. Many questions remain relative to the theory of warfarin–EN protein binding, including the reversibility of such binding during or after absorption, and potential for release of warfarin from protein during protein metabolism. Binding of warfarin to the protein component of EN remains a theory with limited data supporting this mechanism of interaction.

A recent in vitro study presents data supporting another potential mechanism for the warfarin–EN interaction.[69] Loss of warfarin was demonstrated when drug was infused through a polyurethane feeding tube under defined laboratory conditions and when weighed amounts of sliced feeding tube were added to beakers containing three different concentrations of warfarin. Binding of warfarin to the polyurethane feeding tube material did not appear to be a saturable process in this study. The authors concluded that holding EN around administration of warfarin through a feeding tube should not affect bioavailability of warfarin, and they did not recommend holding feedings to mitigate the warfarin–EN interaction. This study only evaluated warfarin binding to polyurethane feeding tube material under simulated gastric conditions. Further studies are needed to determine if other feeding tube materials or small bowel conditions would produce the same effects.

The mechanism of interaction between warfarin and EN has not been clearly delineated, and no definitive recommendation can be provided for mitigating warfarin resistance associated with relatively low vitamin K intake. Nonetheless, interactions involving warfarin can be life-threatening. Response to warfarin therapy must be closely monitored when EN therapy is started, stopped, or altered (see Practice Scenario 18-4 for a discussion of this interaction).

Potential methods of mitigating the warfarin–EN interaction include using concentrated drug administered rapidly to minimize contact with the feeding tube, separating warfarin administration from EN administration, increasing the warfarin dose until a therapeutic PT/INR is achieved, or changing to an alternative anticoagulation therapy that does not interact with EN therapy. Minimizing contact with the feeding tube has a low potential to cause unintended consequences and is a reasonable first approach. If this fails to resolve warfarin resistance, separating the warfarin dose from EN by holding EN for at least 1 hour before and after the warfarin dose is a likely next step. Increases in PT/INR should be evident within a few days if the warfarin resistance is resolved. Increasing the warfarin dose periodically until a therapeutic INR is achieved can result in high drug doses that may place the patient at risk of bleeding should EN administration be reduced for any reason. In addition to routine monitoring, the PT/INR should be re-evaluated with any change in the EN regimen.

Practice Scenario 18-4

Question: Should tube feeding be held when a therapeutic INR is not achieved with the home dose of warfarin after tube feeding starts?

Scenario: A 68-year-old man was admitted to the hospital with suspected sepsis and required mechanical ventilation. Broad-spectrum antibiotic coverage was initiated immediately after admission. Antibiotics changed to high-dose IV nafcillin on hospital day 3, based on blood culture results. Tube feeding started on hospital day 5 through a small-bore NG tube and reached goal rate within 48 hours. Mechanical ventilation stopped on day 10, and the patient was transferred to a medical floor. Tube feeding continued due to possible esophageal damage. IV nafcillin and the heparin infusion continued. Lisinopril and warfarin were initiated through the feeding tube at home dosages. Morphine liquid was ordered via NG tube, with 1 mg IV morphine allowed every 4 hours, as needed for pain.

After 2 weeks of gradually increasing the daily warfarin dose from 5 mg (home dose) to 12 mg, the INR remained subtherapeutic at 1.4.

Past medical history: Hypertension, recurrent deep vein thrombosis, and osteoarthritis with left knee replacement 2 months ago. Medications before admission included lisinopril 20 mg tablet daily, acetaminophen/hydrocodone 500/5 mg 1 tablet every 6 hours and up to two additional tablets daily as needed for pain, paroxetine 20 mg tablet daily, and warfarin 5 mg tablet daily.

Answer: The pharmacist recommends restarting paroxetine and changing to acetaminophen/hydrocodone (home medication) for pain management, rather than holding tube feedings around warfarin administration.

Rationale: Assessing drug interactions with warfarin before altering the tube feeding regimen is important. Paroxetine increases INR.

The patient received paroxetine at home and will likely be discharged on this medication. Acetaminophen interrupts the vitamin K cycle through effects of the *N*-acetyl (p)-benzoquinoneimine metabolite on vitamin K-dependent carboxylase, an enzyme in the vitamin K cycle.[70] Standard doses of acetaminophen increase INR significantly in some patients. Nafcillin decreases INR and could contribute to warfarin "resistance." Keeping the warfarin concentration relatively high in the slurry prepared for administration through the feeding tube and administering it rapidly would be an appropriate administration technique. Holding tube feedings for 1 to 2 hours on each side of the warfarin dose may be reasonable if the INR does not increase within a few days of restarting acetaminophen/hydrocodone and paroxetine at the home doses; however, data supporting this action are limited. Binding of warfarin with a component of the EN formulation has been proposed to explain warfarin resistance with modest vitamin K intake.[68] The feeding rate will need to be increased to make up for the hours feedings are held. Assuming protein is the component that binds warfarin, changing to a hydrolyzed formulation would be expected to resolve the warfarin resistance because hydrolyzed protein lacks the complex structure to form binding sites. However, there are no data to confirm this hypothesis, and a hydrolyzed formulation would be much more expensive. Changing to IV warfarin administration would also be expected to resolve the problem of warfarin resistance but is more expensive and complicated than changing the administration schedule of the EN formulation. A low-molecular-weight heparin or one of the new oral anticoagulants could also be used for anticoagulation but cost is higher than warfarin therapy.

Summary

DNIs are an important consideration with both PN and EN therapy. The consequences of such interactions range from relatively benign to life-threatening. All nutrition support clinicians should be involved in establishing safe practices that minimize the risk of various types of DNIs occurring and mitigate adverse effects associated with such interactions.

References

1. Rollins CJ. General pharmacologic issues. In: Matarese LE, Gottschlich MM, eds. *Contemporary Nutrition Support Practice*. 2nd ed. Philadelphia, PA: Saunders; 2003:315–335.
2. Bankhead R, Boullata J, Brantley S, et al. A.S.P.E.N. Enteral Nutrition Practice Recommendations. *J Parenter Enteral Nutr*. 2009; 33:122–167.
3. Scheppach W, Burghardt W, Bartram P, et al. Addition of dietary fiber to liquid formula diets: the pros and cons. *J Parenter Enteral Nutr*. 1990;14:204–209.
4. American Society for Parenteral and Enteral Nutrition. Definition of terms, style, and conventions used in A.S.P.E.N. guidelines and standards. *Nutr Clin Pract*. 2005;20:281–285.
5. Chan LN. Drug-nutrient interaction in clinical nutrition. *Curr Opin Clin Nutr Metab Care*. 2002;5:327–332.
6. Task Force for the Revision of Safe Practices for Parenteral Nutrition. Safe practice for parenteral nutrition formulations. *J Parenter Enteral Nutr*. 2004;28(6 suppl):S39–S70.
7. Trissel LA. *Handbook on Injectable Drugs*. 16th ed. Bethesda, MD: American Society of Health-System Pharmacists; 2011.
8. Fagerman KE, Ballou AE. Drug compatibilities with enteral feeding solutions co-administered by tube. *Nutr Support Serv*. 1988; 8:31–32.
9. Altman E, Cutie AJ. Compatibility of enteral products with commonly employed drug additives. *Nutr Support Serv*. 1984;4:8–17.
10. Cutie AJ, Altman E, Lenkel L. Compatibility of enteral products with commonly employed drug additives. *J Parenter Enteral Nutr*. 1983;7:186–191.
11. Burns PE, McCall L, Wirsching R. Physical compatibility of enteral formulas with various common medications. *J Am Diet Assoc*. 1988;88:1094–1096.
12. Holtz L, Milton J, Sturek JK. Compatibility of medications with enteral feedings. *J Parenter Enteral Nutr*. 1987; 11:183–186.
13. Strom JG, Miller SW. Stability of drugs with enteral nutrient formulas. *Drug Intell Clin Pharm*. 1990;24:130–134.
14. Rollins CJ. Tube feeding formula and medication characteristics contributing to undesirable interactions. *J Parenter Enteral Nutr*. 1999;23:S13 (abstract).
15. Nicolau DP, Davis SK. Carbonated beverages as irrigants for feeding tubes. *Ann Pharmacother*. 1990;24:840.
16. Metheny N, Eisenberg P, McSweeney M. Effect of feeding tube properties and three irrigants on clogging rates. *Nurs Res*. 1988;37: 165–169.
17. Mitchell JF. Oral dosage forms that should not be crushed. Do not crush list. www.ismp.org/Tools/DoNotCrush.pdf. Accessed July 2, 2011.
18. Höglund P, Nilsson LG. Pharmacokinetics of diltiazem and its metabolites after repeated multiple-dose treatments in healthy volunteers. *Therapeutic Drug Monitoring*. 1989;11:551–557.
19. Schier JG, Howland MA, Hoffman RS, et al. Fatality from administration of labetalol and crushed extended-release nifedipine. *Ann Pharmacother*. 2003;37:1420–1423.
20. Beckwith MC, Barton RG, Graves C. A guide to drug therapy in patients with enteral feeding tubes: dosage form selection and administration methods. *Hosp Pharm*. 1997;32:57–64.
21. Niemiec PW, Vanderveen TW, Morrison JI, et al. Gastrointestinal disorders caused by medication and electrolyte solution osmolality during enteral nutrition. *J Parenter Enteral Nutr*. 1983;7: 387–389.
22. Dickerson RN, Melnik G. Osmolality of oral drug solutions and suspensions. *Am J Hosp Pharm*. 1988;45: 832–834.
23. Lutomski DM, Gora ML, Wright SM, et al. Sorbitol content of selected oral liquids. *Ann Pharmacother*. 1993;27:269–274.
24. Johnston KR, Govel LA, Andritz MH. Gastrointestinal effects of sorbitol as an additive in liquid medications. *Am J Med*. 1994;97: 185–191.
25. Hyams JS. Sorbitol intolerance: an unappreciated cause of functional gastrointestinal complaints. *Gastroenterology*. 1983;84:30–33.
26. Wensel TM. Administration of proton pump inhibitors in patients requiring enteral nutrition. *P&T*. March 2009;34:143–160.
27. U.S. Food and Drug Administration. Letter to healthcare professionals: communication on lansoprazole delayed-release orally disintegrating tablets manufactured by Teva Pharmaceuticals. April 15, 2011. www.fda.gov/Drugs/DrugSafety/ucm251485.htm. Accessed July 3, 2011.
28. Rollins CJ, Thomson CA, Crane T. Pharmacotherapeutic issues. In: Rolandelli RH, Bankhead R, Boullata JI, et al., eds. *Clinical Nutrition: Enteral and Tube Feeding*. 4th ed. Philadelphia, PA: Elsevier Saunders; 2005:291–305.
29. Introduction to pharmacokinetics and pharmacodynamics. In: DiPiro JT, Spruill WJ, Blouin RA, et al., eds. *Concepts in Clinical Pharmacokinetics*. 3rd ed. Bethesda, MD: American Society of Health-System Pharmacists, 2002:1–17.

30. Jew RK, Soo-Hoo W, Erush S. *Extemporaneous Formulations for Pediatric, Geriatric, and Special Needs Patients.* 2nd ed. Bethesda, MD: American Society of Health-System Pharmacists; 2010.
31. Howard L, Chu R, Feman S, et al. Vitamin A deficiency from long-term parenteral nutrition. *Ann Intern Med.* 1980;93:576–577.
32. Cacek AT, DeVito JM, Koonce JR. In vitro evaluation of nasogastric administration methods for phenytoin. *Am J Hosp Pharm.* 1986;43:689–692.
33. Clark-Schmidt AL, Garnett WR, Lowe DR, et al. Loss of carbamazepine suspension through nasogastric feeding tubes. *Am J Hosp Pharm.* 1990;47:2034–2037.
34. Kintzel PE, Rollins CJ, Yee WJ, et al. Low itraconazole serum levels following administration of itraconazole suspension to critically ill allogeneic bone marrow transplant recipients. *Ann Pharmacother.* 1995;29:140–143.
35. Magnusson JO. Metabolism of digoxin after oral and jejunal administration. *Br J Clin Pharmacol.* 1983;16:741–742.
36. Staib AH, Beerman D, Harder S, et al. Absorption differences of ciprofloxacin along the human gastrointestinal tract determined using remote-control drug delivery device. *Am J Med.* 1989;97 (suppl 5A):66S–69S.
37. Yuk JH, Nightingale CH, Quintiliani R, et al. Absorption of ciprofloxacin administered through a nasogastric or a nasoduodenal tube in volunteers and patients receiving enteral nutrition. *Diag Microbiol Infect Dis.* 1990;13: 99–102.
38. Healy DP, Brodbeck MC, Clendening CE. Ciprofloxacin absorption is impaired in patients given enteral feedings orally and via gastrostomy and jejunal tubes. *Antimicrob Agents Chemother.* 1996;40:6–10.
39. Sahai J, Memish Z, Conway B. Ciprofloxacin pharmacokinetics after administration via a jejunostomy tube. *J Antimicrob Chemother.* 1991;28:936–937.
40. Singh BN. Effects of food on clinical pharmacokinetics. *Clin Pharmacokinet.* 1999;37:213–255.
41. Semple HA, Koo W, Tam YK, et al. Interactions between hydralazine and oral nutrients in humans. *Ther Drug Monit.* 1991; 13:304–308.
42. Zhou S, Chan SY, Goh BC, et al. Mechanism-based inhibition of cytochrome P450 3A4 by therapeutic drugs. *Clin Pharmacokinet.* 2005;44:279–304.
43. Dresser GK, Bailey DG. The effects of fruit juices on drug disposition: a new model for drug interactions. *Eur J Clin Invest.* 2003;33 (suppl 2):10–16.
44. Cvetkovic M, Leake B, Fromm MF, et al. OATP and P-glycoprotein transporters mediate the cellular uptake and excretion of fexofenadine. *Drug Metab Dispos.* 1999; 27:866–871.
45. Williams L, Davis JA, Lowenthal DT. The influence of food on the absorption and metabolism of drugs. *Med Clin North Am.* 1993; 77:815–829.
46. Gupta DV. Stability of vitamins in total parenteral nutrient solutions. *Am J Hosp Pharm.* 1986;43:2132.
47. Food and Nutrition Board, Institute of Medicine. Vitamin K. In: Dietary Reference Intakes for Vitamin A, Vitamin K, Arsenic, Boron, Chromium, Copper, Iodine, Iron, Manganese, Molybdenum, Nickel, Silicon, Vanadium, and Zinc. *The National Academies Press.* 2001:162–196. Available at http://www.nap.edu/openbook.php?record_id=10026&page=162#. Accessed April 12, 2012.
48. Petretich DA. Reversal of Osmolite–warfarin interaction by changing warfarin administration time [letter]. *Clin Pharm.* 1990;9:93.
49. Dickerson RN, Garman WM, Kuhl DA, et al. Vitamin K-independent warfarin resistance after concurrent administration of warfarin and continuous enteral nutrition. *Pharmacotherapy.* 2008;28:308–313.
50. Au Yeung SC, Ensom MHH. Phenytoin and enteral feedings: does evidence support an interaction? *Ann Pharmacother.* 2000;34: 896–905.
51. Doak KK, Curtis EH, Dunnigan KJ, et al. Bioavailability of phenytoin acid and phenytoin sodium with enteral feedings. *Pharmacotherapy.* 1998;18:637–645.
52. Splinter MY, Seifert CF, Bradberry JC, et al. Recovery of phenytoin suspension after in vitro administration through percutaneous endoscopic gastrostomy Pezzer catheters. *Am J Hosp Pharm.* 1990; 47:373–377.
53. Fleisher D, Sheth N, Kou JH. Phenytoin interaction with enteral feedings administered through nasogastric tubes. *J Parenter Enteral Nutr.* 1990;14:513–516.
54. Hooks MA, Longe RL, Taylor AT, Francisco GE. Recovery of phenytoin from an enteral nutrient formula. *Am J Hosp Pharm.* 1986; 43:685–688.
55. Guidry JR, Eastwood TF, Curry SC. Phenytoin absorption on volunteers receiving selected enteral feedings. *West J Med.* 1989;150: 659–661.
56. Gilbert S, Hatton J, Magnuson B. How to minimize interaction between phenytoin and enteral feedings: two approaches—therapeutic options. *Nutr Clin Pract.* 1996;11:28–31.
57. Bauer LA. Interference of oral phenytoin absorption by continuous nasogastric feedings. *Neurology.* 1982;32:570–572.
58. Bass J, Miles MV, Tennison MB, et al. Effects of enteral tube feeding on the absorption and pharmacokinetic profile of carbamazepine. *Epilepsia.* 1989;30:364–369.
59. Kassam RM, Friesen E, Locock RA. In vitro recovery of carbamazepine from Ensure. *J Parenter Enteral Nutr.* 1989;13:272–276.
60. Estoup M. Approaches and limitations of medication delivery in patients with enteral feeding tubes. *Crit Care Nurse.* 1994;14:68–79.
61. Engle KK, Hannawa TE. Techniques for administering oral medications to critical care patients receiving continuous enteral nutrition. *Am Society Health-Syst Pharm.* 1999;56:1441–1444.
62. Mueller BA, Brierton DG, Abel SR, et al. Effect of enteral feeding with Ensure on oral bioavailabilities of ofloxacin and ciprofloxacin. *Antimicrob Agents Chemother.* 1994;38:2101–2105.
63. Piccolo ML, Toossi Z, Goldman M. Effect of coadministration of a nutritional supplement on ciprofloxacin absorption. *Am J Hosp Pharm.* 1994;51:2697–2699.
64. Mimoz O, Binter V, Jacolot A, et al. Pharmacokinetics and absolute bioavailability of ciprofloxacin administered through a nasogastric tube with continuous enteral feeding to critically ill patients. *Intensive Care Med.* 1998;24:1047–1051.
65. de Marie S, VandenBergh MFQ, Buijk SL, et al. Bioavailability of ciprofloxacin after multiple enteral and intravenous doses in ICU patients with severe Gram-negative intra-abdominal infections. *Intensive Care Med.* 1998;24:343–346.
66. Cohn SM, Sawyer MD, Burns GA, et al. Enteric absorption of ciprofloxacin during tube feeding in the critically ill. *J Antimicrob Chemother.* 1996;38:871–876.
67. Wright DH, Pietz SL, Konstantinides FN, et al. Decreased in vitro fluoroquinolone concentrations after admixture with an enteral feeding formulation. *J Parenter Enteral Nutr.* 2000;24:42–48.
68. Penrod LE, Allen JB, Cabacungan LR. Warfarin resistance and enteral feedings: two case reports and a supporting in vitro study. *Arch Phys Med Rehabil.* 2001;82:1270–1273.
69. Klang M, Graham D, McLymont V. Warfarin bioavailability with feeding tubes and enteral formula. *J Parenter Enteral Nutr.* 2010;34:300–304.
70. Thijssen HH, Soute BA, Vervoort LM, et al. Paracetamol (acetaminophen) warfarin interaction: NAPQI, the toxic metabolite of paracetamol, is an inhibitor of enzymes in the vitamin K cycle. *Thromb Haemost.* 2004;92:797–802.

19 Dietary Supplements

Joseph I. Boullata, PharmD, RPh, BCNSP, Michele Nicolo, MS, RD, CDE, CNSD, LDN, and Kathleen W. Stratton, JD, MA, RD, LDN

CONTENTS

Introduction 314
Current Use in Adults 314
Definitions 314
Regulatory Issues 319
The U.S Food and Drug Administration's General Authority 319
History of Dietary Supplement Regulation 319
Labeling Requirements and Claims 319
Labeling 319
Claims 320
Nutrient Content Claims 320
Structure/Function Claims (Statements of Nutritional Support) 320
Health Claims 320
Advertising and Promotion 320
Product Quality 321
Adverse Event Reporting 321
Efficacy of Dietary Supplements 322
Safety of Dietary Supplements 322
Clinician's Role and Implications for Nutrition Support Practice 324
Summary 325
References 325

Learning Objectives

1. Define various terms utilized in relation to dietary supplements and complementary and alternative medicine.
2. Describe regulatory issues relating to dietary supplements, including labeling requirements, advertising, product quality, and adverse event reporting.
3. Identify potential safety problems with dietary supplements including issues involving either intrinsic or extrinsic ingredients.

Test Your Knowledge Questions

1. Which one of the following claims for a dietary supplement would most likely cause the FDA to consider that the supplement should be regulated as a drug rather than as a dietary supplement?
   A. Supports strong bones and teeth
   B. Treats influenza
   C. Promotes urinary health
   D. Improves immune function
2. Which of the following best describes dietary supplements in the United States?
   A. Only a minority of the population uses dietary supplements.
   B. Most patients report their dietary supplement use to their primary care providers.
   C. Most patients think that their health care providers are knowledgeable about dietary supplements.
   D. Many patients using prescription medicines concomitantly use dietary supplements.

3. Even if current Good Manufacturing Practices (cGMPs) promulgated by the DSHEA are being properly implemented, which of the following would still be likely to occur?
   A. A dietary supplement product adulterated with a prescription drug such as sibutramine is being marketed and sold.
   B. A dietary supplement product is analyzed and found to have much less of the active ingredient than what is indicated on the label.
   C. A dietary supplement product is analyzed and found to have much more of the active ingredient than what is indicated on the label.
   D. A dietary supplement product is marketed and sold, but there are no studies to confirm its efficacy for any condition.

Test Your Knowledge Answers

1. The correct answer is **B.** Under DSHEA, manufacturers of dietary supplements may make statements regarding product ability to affect structure or function of the body. Any claim regarding diagnosis, treatment, cure, or prevention of a disease is disallowed. Therefore, a claim to support strong bones and teeth would be allowed as a structure claim. The claims to promote urinary health and support the immune system would be function claims. The claim that a product treats influenza is an obvious claim regarding treatment of disease and would thus be disallowed.
2. The correct answer is **D.** Surveys have shown varying percentages of the U.S. population using dietary supplements. Data from a large nationwide survey published in 2011 indicated that about 53% of adults use them. Many persons using dietary supplements do not report this use to their allopathic health providers. This lack of disclosure could be due to the patient's not thinking of these supplements as medications or their believing that the health provider will be judgmental about their use. Although most patients think that their health care provider should be knowledgeable regarding dietary supplements, only about half of patients in a recent survey felt that these providers actually were knowledgeable. Many patients using dietary supplements also use prescription medications; this concomitant use could result in supplement interactions with medication or increased incidence of adverse events.
3. The correct answer is **D.** The DSHEA mandated that cGMPs be set up for the dietary supplement industry. Under these cGMPs, which were supposed to be fully implemented by 2010, process controls are to be in place at each step of manufacturing. Thus, the dietary supplements arriving on the shelf should contain the correct ingredients in the correct amounts and should be free of adulterants. There should be consistency between lots in terms of content. Unfortunately, the FDA does not have the manpower to do extensive inspection of manufacturing plants and final products. The cGMPs do not address whether there are any data supporting the efficacy of dietary supplements.

Introduction

Dietary supplements are widely used by consumers and likely to be used by some patients receiving nutrition support. Nutrition support clinicians are in an important position to not only identify patient use, but to provide information to patients and other health care providers about dietary supplement indications, efficacy, safety and governing regulations. This chapter will provide an overview of the subject that involves tens of thousands of dietary supplements on the market. More complete information on specific dietary supplement ingredients is available from specialized resources (Table 19-1). A relatively small number of ingredients account for a large portion of the most popular dietary supplement products.

Current Use in Adults

Sales of dietary supplement products in the United States exceed 26 billion dollars annually when accounting for traditional retail markets as well as direct marketing methods that include the Internet.[1] The prevalence of dietary supplement use varies by the population evaluated and the products included in the survey. The most recent National Health and Nutrition Examination Survey data, published in 2011, suggests that approximately 53% of adults use dietary supplements—an increase from previous years.[2] Other surveys confirm similar rates of dietary supplement use among older adults.[3] The results of a 2002 study in a community hospital indicate that of the patients taking dietary supplements, less than half reported this to their primary providers. Documentation of dietary supplement use in the medical record was found to be insufficient in a prospective study of interviewed patients.[4] Product description, product name, and frequency of use were often missing. Reported use of a supplement 2 to 3 days prior to surgery was also not recorded in the medical record.[5] Dietary supplements are used regularly by 37% to 59% of physicians and 59% of nurses, with a majority of those surveyed also recommending dietary supplements to their patients.[6,7]

Definitions

For purposes of this chapter, the ingredients that can be found in dietary supplements are divided into one of three groups based in part on raw material sources. The first group is comprised of ingredients accepted as nutrients that have been recognized with dietary reference intake values (Table 19-2). The second group is herbal ingredients that contain parts or extracts of medicinal plants (Table 19-3). Lastly, are the other dietary supplement ingredients that are not officially recognized as nutrients and are not of botanical origin (Table 19-4). The official regulatory framework surrounding dietary supplements, including definitions, is important for better appreciating their role in patient care.

The controlling legal definition of a "dietary supplement" is that which the U.S. Congress included in the Dietary Supplement Health and Education Act of 1994 (DSHEA),[8] which amended the U.S. Food and Drug Administration (FDA) authority under the Federal Food, Drug, and Cosmetic Act

TABLE 19-1 Select Resources on Dietary Supplements

Publication

Reference Books

- Barnes J, Anderson LA, Phillipson JD (eds). *Herbal Medicines.* 3rd ed. London, UK: Pharmaceutical Press; 2007.
- Batz F, Hitchens K, Jellin JM. Pharmacist's Letter/Prescriber's Letter: Natural Medicines Comprehensive Database. Stockton, CA: Therapeutic Research Faculty; 2006.
- Coates PM, Betz JM, Blackman MR, et al (eds). *Encyclopedia of Dietary Supplements.* 2nd ed. London, UK: Informa Healthcare; 2010.
- Cupp MJ, Tracy TS (eds). *Dietary Supplements: Toxicology and Clinical Pharmacology.* Totowa, NJ: Humana Press; 2003.
- Dasgupta A, Hammett-Stabler C (eds). *Herbal Supplements.* Hoboken, NJ: John Wiley & Sons, Inc.; 2011.
- Mason P. *Dietary Supplements.* 3rd ed. London, UK: Pharmaceutical Press; 2007.
- Pathak Y (ed). *Handbook of Nutraceuticals.* Boca Raton, FL: CRC Press; 2010.
- Stargrove MB, Treasure J, McKee DL. *Herb, Nutrient, and Drug Interactions.* St. Louis, MO: Mosby Elsevier; 2008.
- Tracy TS, Kingston RL (eds). *Herbal Products: Toxicology and Clinical Pharmacology.* 2nd ed. Totowa, NJ: Humana Press; 2010.
- Ulbricht CE. *Natural Standard Herb and Supplement Guide.* St. Louis, MO: CV Mosby; 2010.

Online

Organization	Website
American Botanical Council	www.herbalgram.org and www.herbmed.org
ConsumerLab	www.ConsumerLab.com
Federal Trade Commission	www.ftc.gov
Food and Drug Administration	www.fda.gov/Food/DietarySupplements/default.htm
National Sanitation Foundation	www.nsf.org/certified/dietary/
Natural Products Association	www.npainfo.org
Natural Standard	www.naturalstandard.com
Natural Medicine Comprehensive Database	www.naturaldatabase.com
NIH Office of Dietary Supplements	http://ods.od.nih.gov/
QuackWatch	www.quackwatch.org
U.S. Pharmacopeia	www.usp.org

(FDCA).[9] The legal definition of a "dietary supplement" is broad and includes products taken by mouth that contain one or more of the following "dietary ingredients": a vitamin; a mineral; a herb or other botanical; an amino acid; a dietary substance for use by man to supplement the diet by increasing the total dietary intake; or a concentrate, metabolite, constituent, extract, or combination of any ingredient previously described. A dietary supplement must be labeled as such and may be in tablet, capsule, powder, softgel, gelcap, or liquid form. It is "supplementary" in that it is not represented for use as a conventional food or as a sole item of a meal or the diet.[10]

In addition to defining the term, Congress included dietary supplements under the general category of "foods" for purposes of the FDCA.[10] Hence, dietary supplements do not undergo the stringent premarket approval process required for prescription or over-the-counter drugs. Congress also excluded dietary supplements from the definition of "food additives"[11] so that manufacturers are exempt from the food additive premarket approval provisions of the FDCA as well.

It is informative to visit some other terms that exist outside of the legal definition that come up in a discussion of dietary supplements to put them into perspective.

The National Institutes of Health defines "complementary and alternative medicine" (CAM) as a group of diverse medical and health care systems, practices, and products that are not generally considered part of conventional medicine (also called allopathic medicine).[12] Complementary medicine refers to practices/products used together with conventional medicine, whereas alternative medicine refers to systems/practices/products as a substitute for conventional medicine. Integrative medicine (also called integrated medicine) refers to a practice that combines both conventional and CAM approaches for which there is evidence of safety and effectiveness.[12] It is important to note that both conventional and CAM practitioners may use dietary supplements as part of a patient's biologically based treatment. What defines a dietary supplement product is the legal definition (as previously described) rather than who recommends it. "Naturopathy" is a medical system that aims to support the body's ability to heal itself through dietary and lifestyle changes with therapies including the use of herbal supplements, massage, and joint manipulation.[12] The term phytotherapy is the science of using plant-based medicines to prevent or treat illness.[13]

The terms "nutraceutical" and "functional food" may be used frequently in the context of dietary supplements. The term nutraceutical can refer to nutrients or other active food ingredients delivered in a pharmaceutical dosage form. By contrast, an active ingredient delivered within a food matrix, whether added or natural, may be considered a functional food whether those ingredients are nutrients, herbals, or other compounds.[14] For example, vitamin C tablets might be described as a nutraceutical, whereas orange juice might be

TABLE 19-2 Common Nutrient Supplement Ingredients

			Major Adverse Effects		
Ingredient Name	**Common Uses[a]**	**Daily Dose[b]**	**Side Effects**	**Interactions**	**Comments**
Arginine	Athletic performance, wound healing	2–3 g	GI discomfort, headache	Antihypertensives, blood thinners	Avoid use status post myocardial infarction; caution in hepatic/renal impairment
Ascorbic acid	Wound healing	100–1000 mg	GI discomfort, hemolysis	Aspirin, estradiol, iron, indinavir	Dose cautiously in glucose-6-phosphate dehydrogenase deficiency; caution in renal impairment
Biotin	Alopecia, brittle nails	300 μg	NK	Antiepileptics	High dose pantothenic acid reduces biotin absorption
Calcium	Osteoporosis	400–2000 mg	Hypercalcemia, constipation	Bisphosphonates, digoxin, fluoroquinolones, levothyroxine	Caution in those at risk of Ca-oxalate stones
Cholecalciferol	Osteoporosis	10–25 μg	Hypercalcemia	Antiepileptics	1 μg = 40 IU
Choline	Athletic performance, dementia	250–500 mg	GI discomfort	NK	Lecithin (phosphatidyl-choline) has a less fishy odor
Chromium	Diabetes, depression	200–500 μg	Hypoglycemia	Insulin	Trivalent form and chloride salt preferred
Copper	Hypercholesterolemia	1–2 mg	GI discomfort	Penicillamine, iron, zinc	Chloride, acetate, or sulfate salt
Folic acid	NTD prevention	400–1000 μg	NK	Phenytoin, methotrexate	Assess vitamin B_{12} status
Iron	Fatigue	60–180 mg	GI discomfort	ACE inhibitors	Fumarate or sulfate if inorganic; RDA 8 mg (men and post-menopausal women), 18 mg (nonpregnant women)
Pyridoxine	PMS, depression	50–150 mg	Neuropathy	Isoniazid, hydralazine	Allergic reaction and photosensitivity is rare
Selenium	CVD, rheumatoid arthritis, cancer	50–100 μg	Hair loss	Clozapine	Sodium selenite or selenomethionine preferred
Taurine	Athletic performance, CVD	0.5–2 g	NK	NK	Nonprotein amino acid
Zinc	Diarrhea, wound healing	25–100 mg	Immunosuppression, anemia	Fluoroquinolones	Sulfate or chloride preferred; RDA 11 mg (men), 8 mg (women)

ACE, angiotensin-converting-enzyme; CVD, cardiovascular disease; GI, gastrointestinal; NK, none known or not known; NTD, neural tube defects; PMS, premenstrual syndrome; RDA, recommended dietary allowance.
[a]In addition to prevention/treatment of nutrient deficits.
[b]Elemental doses listed for minerals.

TABLE 19-3 Popular Herbal Supplement Ingredients

Ingredient Name				Major Adverse Effects	
Familiar	**Botanical**	**Common Use**	**Daily Dose**	**Side Effects**	**Interactions**
Black cohosh	*Cimicifuga racemosa*	Menopausal symptoms	40–80 mg	Headache, GI discomfort	Tamoxifen
Chamomile	*Matricaria recutita*	Indigestion; insomnia	400–1600 mg	Allergic reactions, drowsiness	Benzodiazepines
Echinacea	*Echinacea purpurea* *Echinacea pallida* *Echinacea angustifolia*	Upper respiratory infection	600–1600 mg	Allergic reactions, headache, GI discomfort	Acetaminophen, steroids, and other immunosuppressants
Feverfew	*Tanacetum parthenium*	Migraine prevention	125 mg	Allergic reactions, joint pain, mucositis, photosensitivity	NK
Garlic	*Allium sativum*	Hyperlipidemia	600–900 mg	Bleeding, body odor, GI discomfort	Blood thinners, saquinavir
Ginger	*Zingiber officinale*	Nausea, vomiting	1000 mg	Heartburn	Blood thinners
Ginkgo	*Ginkgo biloba*	Vascular insufficiency	80–240 mg	Allergic reactions, bleeding, GI discomfort	Blood thinners
Ginseng	*Panax ginseng* *Panax quinquefolius*	Panacea	100–200 mg	Headache, insomnia, GI discomfort	Antihypertensives
Goldenseal	*Hydrastis canadensis*	Dyspepsia, diarrhea	400–800 mg	GI discomfort, hypoglycemia, mucositis, photosensitivity	Blood thinners
Green tea	*Camellia sinensis*	Weight loss	100–750 mg	Stimulant	Warfarin
Hawthorn	*Crataegus monogyna*	Heart failure	160–900 mg	GI discomfort, headache, insomnia	Antihypertensives, digoxin
Milk thistle	*Silybum marianum*	Liver disease	200–400 mg	Anaphylaxis, GI discomfort	NK
Saw palmetto	*Serenoa repens*	Benign prostatic hyperplasia	320 mg	Dry mouth, GI discomfort, headache	NK
St. John's wort	*Hypericum perforatum*	Depression	240–1800 mg	Dry mouth, GI discomfort, confusion, hypomania, photosensitivity	Antiepileptics, cyclosporine, digoxin, indinavir, oral contraceptives, triptans,warfarin
Valerian	*Valeriana officinalis*	Anxiety; insomnia	400–1200 mg	Drowsiness	Benzodiazepines

GI, gastrointestinal; NK, none known or not known.

considered a functional food because it is high in vitamin C. However, the terms nutraceutical and functional food have no legal meaning under the FDCA, and the FDA has regulatory authority over them either as dietary supplements or as foods, depending on the product.[15] The American Dietetic Association (ADA) defines functional foods as foods that "move beyond necessity to provide additional health benefits that may reduce disease risk and/or promote optimal health." According to the ADA, this would include conventional foods, modified foods (fortified, enriched, or enhanced), medical foods, and foods for special dietary use, such as infant foods and weight loss foods.[16]

Dietary supplements are also distinguished from medical foods, such as enteral nutrition formulas. The legal definition of a medical food comes from the Orphan Drug Act and is a "food which is formulated to be consumed or administered enterally under the supervision of a physician and which is intended for the specific dietary management of a disease or condition for

TABLE 19-4 Other Popular Supplement Ingredients[a]

			Major Adverse Effects		
Ingredient Name	**Common Uses**	**Daily Dose**	**Side Effects**	**Interactions**	**Comments**
Beta carotene	Cardiovascular disease	5–15 mg	Diarrhea, joint pain	Colestipol, ethanol, orlistat	Avoid in smokers (increased risk of lung cancer and cardiovascular mortality)
Chitosan	Hypercholesterolemia	1.3 g	Bleeding, GI discomfort, hypoglycemia	Antiplatelets	Avoid in persons with shellfish allergy; may interfere with vitamin absorption
Chondroitin	Osteoarthritis	800–1200 mg	GI complaints	Warfarin	May be natural (cartilage, trachea) or synthetic
Coenzyme Q	Hypertension, heart failure	100–600 mg	Headache, fatigue	Warfarin	Synthesized by body; decreases with age
Creatine	Muscle mass/ strength	2–5 g	GI complaints, muscle cramps	Caffeine	Synthesized by body; influences creatinine
Curcumin	Wound healing, inflammation	NK	NK	NK	A component of turmeric
Fish oils	Cardiovascular disease	1–4 g	Anticoagulant	Antiplatelets	Contents may vary with fish sources used
Glucosamine	Osteoarthritis	1500 mg	GI complaints, proteinuria	Antiplatelets, diuretics	Source may be natural (shellfish)
Lutein	Ocular disorders	2–20 mg	NK	NK	Carotenoid found in a variety of foods
Lycopene	Cancer, cardiovascular disease	2–30 mg	GI discomfort	Antiplatelets	Carotenoid found in tomato products
Melatonin	Sleep disturbances	0.5–5 mg	Dysphoria, headache, infertility	Antiepileptics, sedatives, warfarin	Pineal gland hormone
MSM	Allergic rhinitis, osteoarthritis	0.5–2.5 g	GI discomfort	NK	MSM is an oxidation product of dimethyl sulfoxide
Resveratrol	Cancer, cardiovascular disease	NK	NK	Antiplatelets	Oral bioavailability unclear

GI, gastrointestinal; MSM, methylsulfonylmethane; NK, None known or not known.
[a]Data on adverse effects and interactions are limited for this category of dietary supplements.

which distinctive nutritional requirements, based on recognized scientific principles, are established by medical evaluation."[17] The original reasoning behind orphan drugs and this subcategory of orphan foods was to ease premarket development costs for those products not anticipated to recoup costs due to minimal need.[18] Examples include liquid protein and other modular components used in enteral nutrition, some oral nutritional drinks, and a few vitamin products approved for use as medical foods. Medical foods are exempt from both food labeling[19] and dietary supplement labeling requirements, so even though a product might look like a dietary supplement in terms of content, if it is labeled as a medical food, different regulations apply.

Homeopathy is a system of medicine that originated in Europe over 200 years ago. It is based on the "principle of similars," or "like cures like," which is described by practitioners of homeopathy as the observation that while high doses of pharmacologically active substances cause symptoms when administered to healthy people, those same substances when prepared in very dilute form may relieve similar symptoms in conditions resulting from different etiologies.[20] Homeopathic remedies are not dietary supplements within the meaning of the FDCA. Although two products may contain similar ingredients, they may also be subject to different regulations depending on whether the product is officially recognized as a homeopathic medicine or a dietary supplement. Articles listed in the official Homœopathic Pharmacopœia of the United States are categorized as drugs by the FDCA.[21] These are products that have official monographs that provide drug information in the Homœopathic Pharmacopœia of the United States.[20] However, whereas the premarket approval process for most new drugs is governed by the FDA, the homeopathic products' premarket approval process is controlled by the Homœopathic Pharmacopœia Convention of the United States, which is comprised of scientists and clinicians trained in homeopathy.[20]

Regulatory Issues

The U.S. Food and Drug Administration's General Authority

Under DSHEA, the manufacturer is responsible for ensuring that a dietary supplement is safe before it is marketed. The FDA is responsible for taking action against an unsafe product and its manufacturer after it reaches the market. Generally, manufacturers do not need to register their products with the FDA nor obtain FDA approval before producing or selling dietary supplements unless the product contains a new dietary ingredient (NDI).[22] This refers to any ingredient not previously marketed in the United States before the enactment of DSHEA (October 15, 1994).[23] A dietary supplement product on the market is considered adulterated if it contains an ingredient that was not present in the food supply prior to DSHEA or a known ingredient that has been chemically altered, if it is marketed without prior notification to the FDA.[24] If a product includes an ingredient formerly unknown to the food supply, the manufacturer must make an NDI submission to the FDA that includes premarket safety data. The agency has rejected some for failure to adequately identify the ingredient or for failure to provide sufficient safety information.[25] For more information on premarket notification requirements for NDIs, see the FDA's guidance available on their website.[26] In addition, a number of compilations of dietary supplement regulations exist, which can make referring to them easier.[27,28]

History of Dietary Supplement Regulation

The Pure Food and Drug Act of 1906 prohibited "adulterated or misbranded" products from reaching consumers. The FDCA (1938) required products to be safe and subsequent amendments created the requirement of efficacy.[14] In the 1960s and early 1970s, the FDA attempted to increase regulation of vitamin and mineral formulations under its authority to regulate special dietary foods.[29] In 1966, the FDA issued regulations that created several new requirements for vitamins and mineral formulations including the requirement that products carry a statement that "there is no scientific basis for recommending the routine use of dietary supplements."[29] Due to strenuous objection, regulations were stayed and the agency eventually revoked them. In response to the FDA's attempts to assert its control over the dietary supplement industry, critics supported legislation that would severely limit the FDA's role in regulating dietary supplements. In 1976, amendments to the FDCA substantially limited the agency's authority to regulate the composition of dietary supplements.[29]

The FDA again attempted to increase regulation of dietary supplements in the 1990s. The Nutritional Labeling and Education Act (NLEA) of 1990 contained legislation governing labeling and claims of food and food products, including dietary supplements. At that time, a review of over-the-counter products revealed a lack of safety and efficacy documentation, which meant that many dietary supplement products would have to be pulled from store shelves.[14] The dietary supplement industry also argued that herbs, botanicals, and their components would not have been adequately quantified on labels under the nutrition labeling rules of the NLEA.[30] Further debate resulted in the Dietary Supplement Act of 1992, which delayed the NLEA and exempted dietary supplements from the purview of the legislation.

This is the backdrop for the U.S. Congress passing the DSHEA in 1994 despite strong objection from the FDA. Passage of DSHEA meant an inclusive definition of dietary supplements, which covers a wide range of products. Dietary supplements were relegated to the category of "foods," not drugs or food additives, both of which require submission of premarket safety data to the FDA. Congress specifically allowed structure/function claims that prior to this time would have made the product a drug for regulatory purposes. This allowance placed the burden on the FDA to show that a product is unsafe after it is already being sold instead of requiring the manufacturer to demonstrate safety prior to a product's sale.[29] While the legislative intent was to improve access to dietary supplements for consumers and prevent burdensome and time-consuming premarket requirements, a consequence has been reduced regulation of dietary supplements in comparison with medications and food additives. Despite the length of time that DSHEA has been in place, several studies demonstrate that the public does not understand how dietary supplements are regulated; in particular, they believe that the FDA or another government agency approves dietary supplements prior to their sale.[31] Safety considerations have led to recommending a return to more stringent regulation.[32]

Labeling Requirements and Claims

Labeling

The DSHEA amended the FDCA to add specific requirements for dietary supplement labels and ingredient declarations.[33] The FDA has jurisdiction to promulgate rules to prevent the misbranding of dietary supplements. These rules, which have been in effect since 1999, require dietary supplements to carry a supplement facts label that meets specific requirements.[34] Among other requirements, daily values must be listed for dietary ingredients present in a significant amount and for which a daily consumption value has been established. This daily reference value (ie, the daily values) does not necessarily reflect the nutrient recommended dietary allowance (RDA) or adequate intake levels. If no daily value has been established, the ingredient must still be listed but identified as having no such recommendation.[33] The label must also contain contact information identifying a "responsible person" who can receive serious adverse event reports.[35] Manufacturers must ensure that product label information is truthful and not misleading.[22] For a complete description of labeling and claims requirements, see the FDA's *Dietary Supplement Labeling Guide* intended for industry.[15]

Scientific literature from a peer-reviewed publication that is used in connection with the sale of a dietary supplement is exempt from labeling requirements if it is reprinted in its entirety; is not false or misleading; does not promote a particular manufacturer or brand; is presented with other items on the same subject matter to give a balanced view of available scientific information; if displayed in an establishment, is physically separate from the dietary supplements; and does not have appended to it any other information.[36] This provision is referred to as the third party literature exemption, but there is no requirement that the publication be prepared by an independent party with no financial interest in the successful marketing and sale of the product.[29]

Claims

Dietary supplements may carry a variety of different types of claims. Some require approval by the FDA prior to use and some do not. All must comply with pertinent statutes and regulations. Three types of claims—nutrient content, structure/function, and health—are described subsequently but many more exist and a complete description may be found on the FDA's website in its *Guidance for Industry*.[15]

Nutrient Content Claims

Manufacturers are required to accurately describe nutrient content of a dietary supplement; if claims regarding the content do not meet statutory requirements, the product may be deemed misbranded within the meaning of the FDCA.[37] A product is misbranded if it:

- Fails to list (1) the name of each ingredient in the supplement and (2) the quantity of each ingredient or, if it contains a proprietary blend, the total quantity of all the ingredients in the blend
- Is a botanical product and fails to identify the part of the plant from which the ingredient is derived
- Purports to conform to the specifications of an official compendium but fails to do so
- Fails to have the identity and strength that the supplement is represented to have or fails to meet the quality, purity, or compositional specifications based on the assay or method the supplement purports to meet.

Structure/Function Claims (Statements of Nutritional Support)

Under the FDCA, articles intended for use in the diagnosis, cure, mitigation, treatment, or prevention of a disease and articles (other than food) intended to affect the structure or any function of the body are drugs.[21] However, the DSHEA specifically allows dietary supplements to make structure/function claims if they meet the statutory criteria described in the following, including a disclaimer statement that the product is not intended to prevent or cure a disease. Before DSHEA, herbal supplements (but not vitamin/mineral supplements) were classified as drugs if they made structure/function claims.[29]

These statements of nutritional support tend to be nonspecific (eg, "helps support the immune system"). Premarket notification or approval by the FDA is not required. The label can include one of these claims if:

- The benefit is related to a classical nutrient deficiency disease, describes the role of the ingredient in affecting structure or function in humans, and characterizes the mechanism by which the ingredient acts to maintain such structure or function
- Describes general well-being from consumption of a nutrient or dietary ingredient and the statement is truthful and not misleading; and contains the following disclaimer in full: "This statement has not been evaluated by the FDA. This product is not intended to diagnose, treat, cure, or prevent any disease."[38]

Health Claims

A health claim is an explicit or implied characterization of a relationship between a substance and a disease or a health-related condition. This type of claim requires significant scientific agreement and must be authorized by the FDA. A health claim describes the effect a substance has on reducing the risk of or preventing a disease (eg, "calcium may reduce the risk of osteoporosis"). By contrast, a structure/function claim describes the role of a substance intended to maintain the structure or function of the body (eg, "calcium for bone and colon health") and does not require approval by the FDA before use.[39,40] It is important to note that although homeopathic remedies may contain the same ingredients as a dietary supplement (eg, cold remedies), they are not recognized legally as dietary supplements and therefore can make more specific claims about treating or curing illness without having to demonstrate scientific evidence to the FDA.[41]

Advertising and Promotion

The Federal Trade Commission (FTC) is responsible for ensuring that dietary supplement advertising is truthful, not misleading, and based on sound scientific evidence. The FTC publishes an *Advertising Guide for Industry* to assist those who sell or market dietary supplements with compliance.[42] The FTC can send warning letters to companies making potentially misleading statements in their advertisements. If a clinician believes advertising is false, misleading, or without scientific proof, complaints can be filed with the FTC (www.ftc.gov/complaint). The FTC has brought more than 100 law enforcement actions over the past decade challenging claims about the effectiveness of a wide variety of supplements, including cold and flu products, weight loss products, and supplements that claim to treat serious diseases, including cancer and acquired immunodeficiency syndrome.[43] The advertising and sale of dietary supplements on the Internet is common in today's economy and estimated to account for at least 4% of total dietary supplement sales.[44] It can be difficult for consumers and health professionals to find sites that provide reliable information. Several sources are available (Table 19-1), and some perform better than others.[45] For a discussion of current actions brought by the FTC against Internet supplement advertisers, see the FTC press releases found on the FTC website.

Despite the FTC's role in preventing deceptive advertising, the public is inundated with marketing about dietary supplements that may not be accurate or based in science. Adolescents have been identified as a group at risk for susceptibility to questionable advertising in fashion, sports, and lifestyle magazines because of a reported desire to improve the body's appearance or performance and because of an observation that teenagers identify with celebrities and sports figures.[46] One study of advertising in magazines with a high adolescent readership showed problems with the accuracy of information about dietary supplements in these publications.[46]

Product Quality

The quality of dietary supplement products has long been an area of concern given the minimal regulation involved since the passage of DSHEA in 1994. DSHEA gave the FDA the authority to promulgate rules to prevent dietary supplement products of poor quality.[47] However, rules relating to current good manufacturing practices (cGMPs) for dietary supplements took time to develop. The final rule governing cGMPs was published in June of 2007, but compliance dates exempted smaller manufacturers until June 2010.[48,49] For a complete history of dietary supplement cGMPs, see the FDA's *Compliance Guide* found on their website.[50] Prior to adoption of the final rule, general food good manufacturing practices applied to dietary supplements but, unlike foods, most dietary supplements are packaged into tablets, gelcaps, and capsules with concerns very different from foods.

The cGMPs require process controls to be in place at each step of the manufacturing process, regardless if one or multiple firms are involved, to ensure that the product contains what it purports to contain. These controls include establishing and meeting specifications to ensure the finished supplement contains the correct ingredient, purity, strength, and composition intended consistently and reliably each time.[49] While establishing standardized cGMPs for dietary supplements is an important step in promoting product quality, the onus remains on the manufacturer to ensure that these processes are established and being followed. The FDA has limited resources to inspect manufacturing plants and products for compliance with cGMPs, but if a violation is found, the agency can take steps to remove the offending product from the market (see Practice Scenario 19-1 for discussion of an adulterated dietary supplement).

Practice Scenario 19-1

Question: What steps would you take in the case of a woman who is admitted to the hospital with unexplained rapid heartbeat and high blood pressure who admits to using weight loss supplements in the recent past?

Scenario: A 45-year-old woman with a history of obesity and fluctuating weight is admitted for unexplained hypertension and tachycardia. She admits to using a weight loss product but states that the label says it is "100% natural." The dietitian reviews the label and confirms the "100% natural" label but notes that it does not list any ingredients known to cause these symptoms. A call to the hospital pharmacist identifies the product as a dietary supplement and not a drug. After searching the Internet for further product information, the dietitian locates the FDA website and discovers that the FDA has warned consumers about tainted weight loss products containing sibutramine, a prescription medication that was taken off the market in 2010. The particular supplement used by this patient is one of the products identified as containing sibutramine.

Intervention: Inform the patient to stop taking the supplement and explain the rationale. Discuss with the medical team the results of the search and the advice given to the patient. This adverse event should then be reported using the FDA's MedWatch Safety Information and adverse event reporting program (www.fda.gov/medwatch/report.htm).

Answer: (1) Discuss the supplement with the pharmacist. (2) Investigate supplement on the FDA's website and other reliable sites (refer to Table 19-1). (3) Communicate all information to the patient and medical team. (4) Report the adverse event on MedWatch.

The FDA has reported incidents of weight loss products marketed as "100% natural" being adulterated with prescription medications including sibutramine, which was removed from the market in 2010 for safety reasons. Sibutramine is known to substantially increase blood pressure and/or pulse rate in some patients and may present a significant risk for patients with a history of coronary artery disease, congestive heart failure, arrhythmias, and stroke. Sibutramine may also interact with medications in a life-threatening way.

Adverse Event Reporting

In 2006, Congress amended the FDCA to require dietary supplement manufacturers to report any serious adverse events that they learn of to the FDA.[51,52] A serious adverse event is defined as an event that either results in death, a life-threatening experience, inpatient hospitalization, a persistent or significant disability or incapacity, or a congenital anomaly or birth defect, or any event that requires a medical or surgical intervention to prevent one of these outcomes.[52] If a consumer or clinician reports such an event to the manufacturer identified on the label of the suspect product, the manufacturer is bound by law to file a report of the event to the FDA through the agency's MedWatch reporting system.[52] At this point, the agency can take appropriate steps to investigate the product and consider requiring the manufacturer to remove it from store shelves, if appropriate. However, submission of a serious adverse event report by a manufacturer does not constitute an admission that the product caused the event.[52]

Only serious events, as defined by law, require this type of reporting to the FDA. While manufacturers do have to keep records of both serious and nonserious events for 6 years and make them available to the FDA if the plant is inspected, nonserious events are not presently reported publicly for health care professionals to review. So, for example, if a product causes mild rash in many people but no hospital admissions or other serious event criteria apply, the general public will not have access to this information. Due to the lack of premarket testing data in addition to this reporting system, availability of minor adverse reaction data is limited with dietary supplements. Clinicians who believe a patient's illness or injury might be related to the use of a dietary supplement should report the event directly to the FDA. Previously reported adverse events are also published on the FDA's website for review by clinicians.[53]

In February 2010, U.S. Senators McCain and Dorgan introduced a bill that proposed to amend the FDCA to tighten regulation of dietary supplements on the basis that these products may pose safety risks unknown to consumers.[54] While this bill has not been signed into law, it reflects the efforts of those who believe increased regulation of dietary supplements would benefit the public. The bill proposed requires dietary supplement facilities to register with the FDA and requires manufacturers to submit a compilation of all nonserious adverse events to the FDA.

Efficacy of Dietary Supplements

Given the diversity of dietary supplement ingredients, it is not possible to generalize about the clinical efficacy of all dietary supplements as a group. Thousands of marketed products contain countless ingredients often in a variety of combinations. Data on efficacy will vary with the individual ingredient(s) in a product. As with any therapeutic intervention, the value of a dietary supplement ingredient or a specific combination of ingredients in a dietary supplement product is based on an evaluation of known benefits and risk.

For the patients' benefit, a thorough and critical evaluation of the data precedes any consideration for incorporating a dietary supplement into clinical practice. The trials used to evaluate clinical efficacy should meet accepted criteria for a well-designed study. Well-designed clinical intervention studies provide the highest level of data to support the effectiveness of therapeutic interventions. Once published, such studies can provide information on indications, contraindications, dosing, and monitoring of a dietary supplement. As the regulatory framework for dietary supplements varies between countries, it is important to pay particular attention to the description of the pharmaceutical quality of the product used in each study.

Epidemiologic data and case reports on the use of a dietary supplement ingredient are less valuable in making clinical decisions about efficacy. Information on traditional use—including dietary patterns that include a given component—cannot necessarily be extrapolated to the use of dietary supplement ingredients in a pharmaceutical regimen. Common uses of popular dietary supplement ingredients (Tables 19-2 to 19-4) are supported by widely varying levels of evidence. Although there is a growing body of peer-reviewed literature studying the use of individual dietary supplement ingredients or specific combinations of ingredients, many marketed products are not yet supported by the data. Differentiating the available evidence from the marketing hype is important for consumers and clinicians alike.[55] Although having adequate efficacy data would be ideal to evaluate a dietary supplement, a patient could choose to use a product even in the absence of any supporting data once it is in the marketplace. In such a case, it would be valuable to know that the product is at least reasonably safe and of high quality (see Practice Scenario 19-2 for an example of questionable use of a dietary supplement).

Practice Scenario 19-2

Question: What advice would you give to the medical team treating a young woman admitted with a severe Crohn's disease flare who refuses conventional medications in favor of using aloe vera?

Scenario: A 25-year-old woman with an established history of Crohn's disease, a body mass index of 17.5 kg/m^2, and a weight loss of 10 pounds over the last 3 months is admitted to the hospital with an acute Crohn's disease flare and iron deficiency anemia. In taking her history, she tells you she is refusing anti-inflammatory medications in favor of natural dietary supplements because of potential side effects of the medications. She is taking aloe vera on the advice of a natural medicine practitioner. The medical team assumes taking aloe vera orally is not harmful and agrees to allow the patient a trial period of treatment with the aloe vera. They mutually agree that if there is no improvement, the patient will try conventional medications used for treating Crohn's disease. The team asks you for information on appropriate dosage of oral aloe vera.

Intervention: Tell the team that oral aloe vera is relatively contraindicated given the patient's current presentation.

Answer: (1) Research information on oral aloe vera use. (2) Communicate results of search to patient and team. (3) Recommend against its use in this patient.

Aloe vera is used in its topical form to treat wounds, minor burns, and other dermatological conditions. Its traditional use in oral form is for managing constipation, for which there is supporting scientific evidence. For inflammatory bowel disease, there is no convincing evidence of any benefit nor has it been compared to conventional treatments for Crohn's disease. Risks include exacerbating abdominal pain, cramping, diarrhea, and significant electrolyte imbalances. The risk of harm outweighs any potential benefit, and the medical team should be advised that oral aloe vera is not safe for this patient.

Safety of Dietary Supplements

Given the presence of biologically active ingredients, dietary supplement product safety shares many similarities with the more closely regulated pharmaceutical products, but also has a few more unique concerns. As with other pharmaceutical products, adverse effects resulting from the intrinsic (ie, labeled) ingredients may occur. These may be predictable and dose-related, or unexpected allergic or idiosyncratic reactions, as well as interactions with prescribed medication. The risk to the patient may vary by age, sex, genetics, nutrition status, conditions or disorders, and treatments. Adverse effects may influence any organ system; for example, the influence on the liver may be mild transient transaminitis to fulminant hepatic failure (eg, kava), or influence on the skin may be a self-limited rash to exfoliative dermatitis (eg, ginkgo).

Safety evaluation based on epidemiologic data or traditional use data may fall short of identifying or predicting potential adverse effects. The doses, matrixes, and chronicity of exposure using pharmaceutical dosage forms may all present unique features for these products compared to traditional use or findings from epidemiologic data or even short-term clinical intervention trials. Unfortunately, clinical trials that are designed specifically to evaluate adverse effects are not common.[56] In part, this is due to the large number of subjects—and the associated cost—needed to detect less common harmful events. As a result adverse effects of dietary supplements are not as well characterized, recognized, or reported as they are with medications. When adverse effects are identified, reported, and documented, it is not always clear whether the findings can be attributed to the labeled ingredients or to poor product quality. In either case, potential harm to a patient is critical to know, allowing informed decision making about the use of a dietary supplement. Some ingredients are recognized to have risks that outweigh benefits (Table 19-5).

The safety of multi-ingredient products in particular is not always known given limited study.[57] Determining the maximum safe levels of dietary supplement ingredients needs to account for the interindividual variability of intake of foods fortified with nutrients or other ingredients.[58] This risk assessment approach can be most easily conducted for nutrient ingredients. Toxicological data on many of the plant sources of herbal ingredients are still lacking.[59]

The incidence of adverse effects with a dietary supplement product or ingredient is therefore difficult to ascertain given a voluntary system of reporting that captures very few events in combination with little valuable denominator data on overall use.[60] Some of the best data come from poison control centers with estimates of about 30% to 40% of referred dietary supplement exposures being associated with adverse effects.[60] About one half of calls to poison control centers concerning dietary supplement exposures described symptoms, with 62% of these considered "probably" associated with the supplement.[61] Dietary supplements ranked second behind only antidepressants in adverse reaction hospitalizations following exposures as evaluated by poison control centers.[62] Adverse effects related to dietary supplement interactions with medications are not always delineated, but they need to be taken into account.

At least 43% of ambulatory adults regularly use dietary supplements concurrently with prescription medicine.[63] Among adults using prescription drugs, 32% to 39% are also taking a dietary supplement.[64,65] Forty-four percent of patients with two or more chronic medications reported use of herbal dietary supplements.[65] Among women 75 years and older using prescription medication, 60% combined them with dietary supplements.[3] An estimated 12% to 45% of individuals using dietary supplement products with prescription drugs are at risk for an interaction, with 6% to 29% considered potentially serious or clinically significant.[66–69]

Approximately 90% of dietary supplement users thought that pharmacists should routinely be checking for interactions.[63] The information on documented interactions or potential interactions is limited but continues to grow.[68,70] These may occur within the gastrointestinal lumen, but more likely occur at the level of transporters and metabolizing enzymes found in the intestinal epithelium and the liver. Many of the dietary polyphenols as well as botanicals found in dietary supplement products are substrates for—or influence expression and activity of—drug transporters and drug metabolizing enzymes.[71–77] For example, soy isoflavones (eg, daidzein, genistein) can significantly upregulate two drug transporters and five enzymes.[78,79] Also, catechins found in green tea can significantly influence drug transporters in enterocytes and hepatocytes.[80] Nutrient transporters (eg, thiamin, folic acid) can also be reduced by polyphenols.[81] Even specific probiotic strains may play a role in altering transporter function responsible for drug and nutrient absorption.[82] Cautious interpretation and extrapolation from in vitro and in vivo data is necessary until more human data become available.

In contrast to prescription and nonprescription medication, dietary supplements may also be associated with adverse effects that are extrinsic to the labeled ingredients. This relates to the quality of the product and may be caused by misidentification of the raw material or ingredients, as well as the presence of impurities whether by adulteration (eg, prescription drugs), substitution (eg, different plant), or contamination (eg, heavy metals, pesticides). The full implementation of cGMPs is intended to reduce the likelihood of this group of adverse effects.

Plant-derived (ie, botanical) ingredients in particular may vary widely in their chemical content, depending in part on soil and environmental conditions. This emphasizes the value of adhering to Good Agricultural Practices. Quality assurance of dietary supplement products containing botanical ingredients should take this into account, with manufacturers requiring an independent certificate of analysis for all raw materials purchased (botanical or otherwise) that provide thorough documentation of composition including concentrations of

TABLE 19-5 Dietary Supplement Ingredients Where Risk Outweighs Benefit

Ingredient Name	Potential Danger
Androstenedione	Carcinogenic
Bitter orange (*Citrus aurantium*)	Cardiotoxic, hypertension
Blue-green algae	Hepatotoxic, neurotoxic
Blue cohosh (*Caulophyllum thalictroides*)	Cardiotoxic, hypertension
Calamus (*Acorus calamus*)	Carcinogenic, nephrotoxic
Chaparral (*Larrea tridentata*)	Hepatotoxic
Coltsfoot (*Tussilago farfara*)	Carcinogenic, hepatotoxic
Comfrey (*Symphytum spp.*)	Carcinogenic, hepatotoxic
Dong quai (*Angelica sinensis*)	Anticoagulant, carcinogenic
Ephedra [aka ma huang] (*Ephedra sinica*)	Cardiotoxic, hepatotoxic
Germander (*Teucrium chamaedrys*)	Hepatotoxic
Germanium	Nephrotoxic
Kava (*Piper methysticum*)	Hepatotoxic
Lobelia (*Lobelia inflata*)	Coma, hepatotoxic, neurotoxic
Pennyroyal (*Hedeoma pulegioides; Mentha pulegium*)	Multiorgan dysfunction, neurotoxic, abortifacient
Sassafras (*Sassafras albidum*)	Genotoxic, hepatocarcinogenic, abortifacient
Skullcap (*Scutellaria spp.*)	Hepatotoxic
Snakeroot or boneset (*Eupatorium perfoliatum*)	Carcinogenic, hepatotoxic, nephrotoxic
Wormwood (*Artemisia absinthium*)	Neurotoxic
Yohimbe (*Pausinystalia yohimbe*)	Cardiotoxic

any contaminants.[83] The ability to analyze dietary supplement ingredients containing or extracted from plant sources is improving. To monitor the quality of these herbal ingredients requires validated and adopted standard assays for chemical constituents (ie, marker compounds) but also evaluation of contaminants.[84–86]

Ideally, quality control methods would occur with raw material as well as finished products.[83] Any manufacturing practice that cannot confirm the identity, purity, strength, and quality of a dietary supplement product falls short of maximizing patient safety. There are a number of independent testing programs accessible to the public that provide data on quality of dietary supplements. Manufacturers may choose to submit their products for independent testing, and the results are published in reports available to consumers. Only a small proportion of products on the market are independently tested. These programs include the U.S. Pharmacopeia Dietary Supplement Verification Program, ConsumerLab.com, the National Sanitation Foundation, and the Natural Products Association (formerly the National Nutritional Foods Association), which offers a third-party cGMP certification program specific to dietary supplements that includes the FDA cGMP requirements. Aside from general tests and assays, many dietary supplement ingredients have officially recognized monographs in the U.S. Pharmacopeia that can be used to better identify high-quality products.[87]

Clinician's Role and Implications for Nutrition Support Practice

Open dialogue between clinicians and patients is vital in communicating health-related information. This includes regular discussions with patients about their medications and dietary supplements. It is recommended that clinicians have a good working knowledge of common dietary supplements based on validated sources of information.[88] One goal is to support informed decision making by the patient. Another goal is to prevent adverse outcomes associated with dietary supplement use, keeping in mind that the risk for adverse reactions is increased for individuals receiving concurrent drug therapy or undergoing surgery. The involved clinician should be willing to evaluate the dietary supplement literature and report any observed adverse effects including interactions when needed.[88] Of patients regularly using dietary supplements, 93% think it is important for their health care provider to be knowledgeable about them but only about half felt that they actually were.[63]

For a practitioner to be able to counsel patients on the use of dietary supplements, he or she first needs to be familiar with common ingredients, their safety and efficacy, and any potential interactions between the supplements and medications. It is important for health care providers to inquire about supplement use often and to collect data on the current or proposed use of vitamins, minerals, herbals, and other dietary supplements, including the specific regimen and the reason/indication for each. This allows an evaluation of indications and dosing, as well as safety and efficacy data. Knowing the patient's intended or current use of supplements provides an opportunity for counseling on safety of supplement use. Clinicians should approach the subject of supplement use with a "buyers beware" perspective. Having documented the use of supplements allows the practitioner to continually monitor for potential adverse reactions. For patients who have taken their supplements consistently with other medications, it is important they are counseled on checking with a provider prior to making any changes in dose or discontinuing the product. One study demonstrated that certain ethnic groups (eg, Asian Americans and Hispanics) may be less likely to disclose dietary supplement use to health care providers.[65] The authors suggest that this is associated with decreased language ability and socioeconomic level, which may inhibit seeking medical attention. Other potential influences on patient disclosure include avoiding negative responses from their health care provider.[65] Significant deficits do exist in consumer knowledge about dietary supplement safety, efficacy, and regulation that can be significantly improved through education by clinicians.[29]

Given the limited evidence on safety and efficacy, clinicians have had little guidance in directing patient use of dietary supplements. Weiger et al. developed a systems approach to guiding clinicians to "recommend," to "accept," or to "discourage" dietary supplement use.[89] Recommendation for a specific dietary supplement should be based on evidence that supports its efficacy and safety. Supplement acceptance can be considered if evidence for efficacy is questionable but safety has been established. Clinicians should discourage use of supplements in which lack of efficacy and potential harm has been established.

Among the oncology populations, patients may opt for alternative treatments instead of conventional therapy. Michaud et al. present an algorithm for evaluating dietary supplement use in oncology patients; however, it may be applied to other medical situations.[90] Oral supplement products increase potential risk for interaction between drug and nondrug therapies for oncology patients. Under safety review, the supplement should be evaluated according to several characteristics. Identify dietary supplement ingredients that may have antioxidant, anticoagulant, procoagulant, immune modulator, or hormonal properties, particularly if there are established safety concerns or known drug interactions. If any of these characteristics apply, patient risk level should be addressed. Even if it is only a hypothetical concern or questionable data exist, individuals at risk should be discouraged from using the product. If patient risk level is absent, clinicians should proceed to evaluate the efficacy of the product. If there is decisive evidence for lack of efficacy, use of the product should be discouraged. If convincing evidence exists to support efficacy, use of the product may be recommended. For supplements in which evidence is lacking or questionable, it is up to clinical judgment on whether to accept use of the supplement. Supplements falling into this category may warrant continued follow-up and close monitoring.[90]

The ADA recommends that any dietetics professional considering being engaged in the sale of supplements should consider several factors.[91] Providers should avoid selling products that are beyond their scope of practice or are not compliant with institutional policies regarding sales and distribution of dietary supplements. They should acknowledge the patient's choice and avoid any potential preference in persuading patients to choose specific dietary supplements. Accurate and relevant education information should be included when providing/selling dietary supplements. If the providers gain financial revenue from the sale of the product(s), they need to disclose this to their patients via face-to-face interaction or in writing that is easily understood and readily available. Information for comparable products on the market should also be presented. Legal issues including malpractice is a concern for providers who choose to sell dietary supplements. It is further recommended that providers have a grasp of federal and state regulations pertaining to licensure and business practices.

Recommendations for individual patients do not preclude setting institutional protocols or policies that address dietary supplements. The Joint Commission has set forth recommendations for health system formulary implementation on the use of dietary supplements, but otherwise is silent on specifics.

The American Society of Health-System Pharmacists (ASHP) issued clinical practice recommendations on the use of dietary supplements because of the increased frequency of use.[92] Because of safety concerns, ASHP discouraged use of supplements in situations where irrevocable consequences may occur such as use in conjunction with immune suppression, chemotherapy, human immunodeficiency virus infection, anticoagulation therapy, or for those on hormonal contraceptives. Health-system formularies should have established criteria for inclusion of dietary supplements. Dietary supplements should undergo the same scrutiny as prescription and nonprescription medications in order to decrease institutional liability. ASHP suggests discontinuing use of patient self-administered dietary supplement use upon admission especially as diagnostic workup continues. Allowing patient dietary supplement use during hospital admission should require documentation in the medical record, include a physician order, and include the supplement name. In addition, a pharmacist should review and verify the ordered supplement prior to dispensing.[92] The safety of hospitalized patients may be compromised if written policies about dietary supplements are inadequate[93] (see Practice Scenario 19-3 for an example of dealing with dietary supplements in an inpatient setting).

Practice Scenario 19-3

Question: What dietary supplement would you recommend for a patient with heart failure and with history of gastric bypass surgery 5 years earlier?

Scenario: A 57-year-old man presented with new onset mild heart failure, leukopenia, and peripheral neuropathy. He reported that he had never been fully compliant with advice to take a multivitamin with minerals and a calcium supplement following his gastric bypass procedure. The team immediately ordered the oral multivitamin supplement on the hospital formulary and ordered a laboratory micronutrient panel for bariatric patients to check for a number of deficiencies (ie, thiamin, vitamin B_{12}, vitamin C, vitamin D, iron, copper, selenium, and zinc). The results of the panel revealed deficiencies of thiamin, copper, zinc, and vitamin D. The neurology team, concerned with the patient's neuropathy, calls you to ask whether the formulary micronutrient product contains the necessary amount of copper for repletion. As the nutrition support clinician, you check with the pharmacy for the supplement label information. You learn that the current formulary product supplied by the wholesaler to the pharmacy and dispensed contains the following:

Vitamin A (no β-carotene)	5000 IU
Thiamin mononitrate	1.5 mg
Riboflavin	2 mg
Niacinamide	20 mg
Pyridoxine	0.1 mg
Calcium pantothenate	1 mg
Vitamin C	37.5 mg
Vitamin D	400 IU

You quickly realize that this is not a multivitamin/mineral product, but only a multivitamin product, and incomplete at that. The content of vitamin A (salt not described) exceeds the RDA of 900 μg (5000 IU = 1500 μg), while the content of pyridoxine, pantothenic acid, and vitamin C are below the RDA; the form of vitamin D is not described for the dose (400 IU = 10 μg).

Interventions: Initially recommend a complete therapeutic multivitamin/mineral preparation. Investigate the product on formulary to determine the product composition and identify whether it contains adequate amounts and forms of the nutrients to replete the identified deficiencies. Additionally, consider repleting individual deficiencies using single ingredient products of appropriate dose and salt.

Answer: (1) Identify a therapeutic multivitamin/mineral product containing adequate amounts to meet the patient's specific needs. (2) Communicate the information to the patient and the team.

The composition of the formulary oral micronutrient supplement did not meet the patient's needs. The patient was deficient in copper, and the supplement available on formulary did not contain any minerals including trace elements. An individual oral copper supplement containing 2 to 8 mg of copper that is not the sulfide or oxide forms would be most appropriate. A set of criteria for selecting an appropriate multivitamin/mineral product should be determined and shared with the purchasing officer.

Summary

The popularity of dietary supplement products containing nutrient, herbal, and/or other ingredients remains unabated. The well-informed nutrition support clinician understands what constitutes a dietary supplement and how these products are regulated. Whenever required to do so, the responsible clinician will determine clinical effectiveness and safety of specific dietary supplement ingredients through a careful review of evidence-based compilations and the primary literature. Patients should be supported in making fully informed decisions about dietary supplements.

References

1. Council for Responsible Nutrition. Fact sheet, Mar 2011. www.crnusa.org/pdfs/DSSafeRegulatedBeneficial_rev031411.pdf. Accessed September 2011.
2. Gahche J, Bailey R, Burt V, et al. *Dietary Supplement Use Among U.S. Adults has Increased Since NHANES III (1988-1994)*. NCHS data brief no 61. Hyattsville, MD: National Center for Health Statistics, 2011.

3. Qato DM, Alexander GC, Conti RM, et al. Use of prescription and over-the-counter medications and dietary supplements among older adults in the United States. *JAMA*. 2008;300:2867–2878.
4. Chhay C, Rynes R, Kajimura-Beck M, et al. Alternative medicine use in a community hospital. *Am J Health-Syst Pharm*. 2002;59: 2452–2453.
5. Cockayne NL, Duguid M, Shenfield GM. Health professionals rarely record history of complementary and alternative medicines. *Br J Clin Pharmacol*. 2004;59:254–258.
6. Dickinson A, Boyon N, Shao A. Physicians and nurses use and recommend dietary supplements: report of a survey. *Nutr J*. 2009;8:29.
7. Dickinson A, Shao A, Boyon N, et al. Use of dietary supplements by cardiologists, dermatologists and orthopedists: report of a survey. *Nutr J*. 2011;10:20.
8. Pub Law No. 103-417, 108 Stat 4325 (1994).
9. 21 USC 321 et seq.
10. 21 USC 321(ff).
11. 21 USC 321(s).
12. National Center for Complementary and Alternative Medicine. What is complementary and alternative medicine? Publ No D347, updated November 2010. http://nccam.nih.gov/health/whatiscam/#definingcam. Accessed September 2011.
13. Thompson CA. Intervention: dietary supplementation and integrative care. In: Escott-Stump S, Mahan LK (eds). *Krause's Food, Nutrition, & Diet Therapy*. 12th ed. St. Louis, MO: Saunders Elsevier, 2008:470–488.
14. Boullata JI. Dietary supplements. In: Rolandelli RH, Bankhead R, Boullata J, et al (eds). *Clinical Nutrition: Enteral and Tube Feeding*. 4th ed. Philadelphia, PA: Elsevier Saunders, 2005:248–264.
15. U.S. Food and Drug Administration. Dietary supplement labeling guide, April 2005. Updated April 2011. www.fda.gov/Food/GuidanceComplianceRegulatoryInformation/Guidance Documents/DietarySupplements/DietarySupplementlabeling-guide/default.htm. Accessed September 2011.
16. Position of the ADA. Functional foods. *J Am Diet Assoc*. 2009;109: 735–746.
17. 21 USC 360ee.
18. Bankhead R, Boullata J, Brantley S, et al., A.S.P.E.N. Board of Directors. Enteral nutrition practice recommendations. *J Parenter Enteral Nutr*. 2009;33:122–167.
19. 21 CFR 101.9.
20. Borneman JP, Field RI. Regulation of homeopathic drug products. *Am J Health-Syst Pharm*. 2006;63:86–91.
21. 21 USC 321(g).
22. U.S. Food and Drug Administration. Dietary supplements. Updated December 2010. www.fda.gov/Food/DietarySupplements/default.htm. Accessed September 2011.
23. 21 USC 350b.
24. 21 CFR 190.6.
25. McGuffin M, Young AL. Premarket notifications of new dietary ingredients: a ten-year review. *Food Drug Law J*. 2004;59:229.
26. U.S. Food and Drug Administration. Chapter VII. Premarket notification of new dietary ingredients, April 2005. Updated April 2011. www.fda.gov/Food/GuidanceComplianceRegulatoryInformation/GuidanceDocuments/DietarySupplements/DietarySupplement labelingguide/ucm070614.htm. Accessed September 2011.
27. Allport-Settle MJ. *Dietary Supplements: Current Good Manufacturing Practice, Labeling and Pre-market Notification*. Willow Springs, NC: PharmaLogika, 2010.
28. U.S. Pharmacopeia. *USP Dietary Supplements Compendium: The Authoritative Reference*. Rockville, MD: U.S. Pharmacopeial Convention, 2012.
29. Hutt PB, Merrill RA, Grossman LA (eds.). *Food and Drug Law: Cases and Materials*. 3rd ed. New York, NY: Foundation Press, 2007: 246–268.
30. Dickinson A. History and overview of DSHEA. *Fitoterapia*. 2011;82:5–10.
31. Dodge T, Litt D, Kaufman A. Influence of the Dietary Supplement Health and Education Act on consumer beliefs about the safety and effectiveness of dietary supplements. *J Health Communic*. 2011;16:230–244.
32. Rogovik AL, Vohra S, Goldman RD. Safety considerations and potential interactions of vitamins: should vitamins be considered drugs? *Ann Pharmacother*. 2010;44:311–324.
33. 21 USC 343(q)(5)(F).
34. Federal Register 1997;62(184):49825-49858.
35. 21 USC 343(y).
36. 21 USC 343-2.
37. 21 USC 343(s).
38. 21 USC 343(r).
39. 21 USC 101.14.
40. 21 CFR 101.93.
41. Anonymous. In from the cold. *Nutr Action Health Letter*. 2011:10–11.
42. Federal Trade Commission. Dietary supplements: an advertising guide for industry, April 2001. http://business.ftc.gov/documents/bus09-dietary-supplements-advertising-guide-industry. Accessed September 2011.
43. Federal Trade Commission. FTC submits statement to Congress on deceptive marketing of dietary supplements, May 2010. www.ftc.gov/opa/2010/05/supplement.shtm. Accessed September 2011.
44. Saldanha LG, Dwyer JT, Andrews KW, et al. Online dietary supplement resources. *J Am Diet Assoc*. 2010;110:1427–1431.
45. Clauson KA, Polen HH, Peak AS, et al. Clinical decision support tools: personal digital assistant versus online dietary supplement databases. *Ann Pharmacother*. 2008;42:1592–1599.
46. Shaw P, Zhang V, Metalinos-Katsaras E. A content analysis of the quantity and accuracy of dietary supplement information found in magazines with high adolescent readership. *J Alternat Complement Med*. 2009;15:159–164.
47. 21 USC 342(g).
48. 21 CFR 111.1.
49. Federal Register 2007;72(121):34752-34800.
50. U.S. Food and Drug Administration. Guidance for industry: current good manufacturing practice for dietary supplements, Dec 2010. Updated May 2011. www.fda.gov/Food/Guidance ComplianceRegulatoryInformation/GuidanceDocuments/SmallBusinessesSmallEntityComplianceGuides/ucm238182.htm. Accessed September 2011.
51. 120 Stat 3469 2006.
52. 21 USC 379aa-1.
53. U.S. Food and Drug Administration. Dietary supplement alerts and safety information, Oct 2009. www.fda.gov/Food/Dietary Supplements/Alerts/default.htm. Accessed September 2011.
54. The Library of Congress. Bill summary & status, 111th Congress (2009–2010), S.3002, Feb 2010. http://thomas.loc.gov/cgi-bin/bdquery/z?d111:S.3002. Accessed September 2011.
55. Temple NJ. The marketing of dietary supplements in North America. *J Alt Complem Med*. 2010;16:803–806.
56. Lobb A. Science of weight loss supplements: compromised by conflicts of interest? *World J Gastroenterol*. 2010;16(38):4880–4882.
57. Higgins JP, Tuttle TD, Higgins CL. Energy beverages: content and safety. *Mayo Clin Proc*. 2010;85(11):1033–1041.
58. Dufour A, Wetzler S, Touvier M, et al. Comparison of different maximum safe levels in fortified foods and supplements using a

probabilistic risk assessment approach. *Br J Nutr*. 2010;104: 1848–1857.

59. Fu PP, Chiang H-M, Xia Q, et al. Quality assurance and safety of herbal dietary supplements. *J Environ Sci Health Part C*. 2009;27: 91–119.
60. Gardiner P, Sarma DN, Dog TL, et al. The state of dietary supplement adverse event reporting in the United States. *Pharmacoepidemiol Drug Saf*. 2008;17:962–970.
61. Palmer M, Haller C, McKinney P, et al. Adverse events associated with dietary supplements: an observational study. *Lancet*. 2003;361:101–106.
62. Vassilev ZP, Chu AF, Ruck B, et al. Evaluation of adverse drug reactions reported to a poison control center between 2000 and 2007. *Am J Health-Syst Pharm*. 2009;66:481–487.
63. Braun LA, Tiralongo E, Wilkinson JM, et al. Perceptions, use and attitudes of pharmacy customers on complementary medicines and pharmacy practice. *BMC Complement Altern Med*. 2010;10: 38.1–38.7.
64. Slone Epidemiology Center at Boston University. Patterns of medication use in the United States, 2006. www.bu.edu/slone/SloneSurvey/AnnualRpt/SloneSurveyWebReport2006.pdf. Accessed September 2011.
65. Mehta DH, Gardiner PM, Phillips RS, et al. Herbal and dietary supplement disclosure to health care providers by individuals with chronic conditions. *J Alt Complem Med*. 2008;14:1263–1269.
66. Peng CC, Glassman PA, Trilli LE, et al. Incidence and severity of potential drug-dietary supplement interactions in primary care patients: an exploratory study of 2 outpatient practices. *Arch Intern Med*. 2004;164:630–636.
67. Lee AH, Ingraham SE, Kopp M, et al. The incidence of potential interactions between dietary supplements and prescription medications in cancer patients at a Veterans Administration hospital. *Am J Clin Oncol*. 2006;29:178–182.
68. Sood A, Sood R, Brinker FJ, et al. Potential for interactions between dietary supplements and prescription medications. *Am J Med*. 2008;121:207–211.
69. Loya AM, González-Stuart A, Rivera JO. Prevalence of polypharmacy, polyherbacy, nutritional supplement use and potential product interactions among older adults living on the United States-Mexico border: a descriptive, questionnaire-based study. *Drugs Aging*. 2009;26:423–436.
70. Chan L-N. Interaction of natural products with medication and nutrients. In: Boullata JI, Armenti VT (eds). *Handbook of Drug-Nutrient Interactions*. 2nd ed. New York, NY: Humana Press, 2010: 341–366.
71. Nabekura T, Kamiyama S, Kitagawa S. Effect of dietary chemopreventive phytochemicals on P-glycoprotein function. *BiochemBiophys Res Comm*. 2004;327:866–870.
72. Morris ME, Zhang S. Flavonoid-drug interactions: effects of flavonoids on ABC transporters. *Life Sci*. 2006;78:2116–2130.
73. Shim C-K, Cheon E-P, Kang KW, et al. Inhibition effect of flavonoids on monocarboxylate transporter 1 (MCT1) in Caco-2 cells. *J Pharm Pharmacol*. 2007;59:1515–1519.
74. Cermak R. Effect of dietary flavanoids on pathways involved in drug metabolism. *Expert Opin Drug MetabToxicol*. 2008;4:17–35.
75. Volak LP, Ghirmai S, Cashman JR, et al. Curcuminoids inhibit multiple human cytochromes P450, UDP-glucuronosyltransferase, and sulfotransferase enzymes, whereas piperine is a relatively selective CYP3A4 inhibitor. *Drug Metab Disp*. 2008;36:1594–1605.
76. Sergent T, Dupont I, Van Der Heiden E, et al. CYP1A1 and CYP3A4 modulation by dietary flavonoids in human intestinal Caco-2 cells. *Toxicol Lett*. 2009;191:216–222.
77. Chen Y, Liu W-H, Chen B-L, et al. Plant polyphenol curcumin significantly affects CYP1A2 and CYP2A6 activity in healthy, male Chinese volunteers. *Ann Pharmacother*. 2010;44:1038–1045.
78. Peng WX, Li HD, Zhou HH. Effect of daidzein on CYP1A2 activity and pharmacokinetics of theophylline in healthy volunteers. *Eur J Clin Pharmacol*. 2003;58:237–241.
79. Li Y, Mezei O, Shay NF. Human and murine hepatic sterol-12-α-hydroxylase and other xenobiotic metabolism mRNA are upregulated by soy isoflavones. *J Nutr*. 2007;137:1705–1712.
80. Roth M, Timmermann BN, Hagenbuch B. Interactions of green tea catechins with organic anion-transporting polypeptides. *Drug Metab Disp*. 2011;39:920–926.
81. Martel F, Monteiro R, Calhau C. Effect of polyphenols on the intestinal and placental transport of some bioactive compounds. *Nutr Res Rev*. 2010;23:47–64.
82. Chen H-Q, Shen T-Y, Zhou Y-K, et al. *Lactobacillus plantarum* consumption increases PepT1-mediated amino acid absorption by enhancing protein kinase C activity in spontaneously colitic mice. *J Nutr*. 2010;140:2201–2206.
83. Singh SK, Jha SK, Chaudhary A, et al. Quality control of herbal medicines by using spectroscopic techniques and multivariate statistical analysis. *Pharm Biol*. 2010;48(2): 134–141.
84. Waksmundzka-Hajnos M. Modern high performance liquid chromatography in the analysis of phytochemicals. *J AOAC Internat*. 2011;94:1–3.
85. Chen P, Harnly JM. Flow injection mass spectroscopic fingerprinting and multivariate analysis for differentiation of three *Panax* species. *J AOAC Internat*. 2011;94:90–99.
86. Zhou L, Duan C, Wang M, et al. Analysis of residues of 81 pesticides on Ginkgo leaves using QuEChERS sample preparation and gas chromatography/mass spectrometry. *J AOAC Internat*. 2011; 94:313–321.
87. U.S. Pharmacopeia Convention. *United States Pharmacopeia/National Formulary, Edition 34/29*. Rockville, MD: United States Pharmacopeia Convention, Inc.; 2011.
88. Glisson JK, Walker LA. How physicians should evaluate dietary supplements. *Am J Med*. 2010;123:577–582.
89. Weiger WA, Smith M, Boon H, et al. Advising patients who seek complementary and alternative medical therapies for cancer. *Ann Intern Med*. 2002;137:889–903.
90. Michaud LB, Phillps-Karpinski J, Jones KL, et al. Dietary supplements in patients with cancer: risks and key concepts, part 1. *Am J Health-Syst Pharm*. 2007;64:369–381.
91. Thompson C, Diekman C, Saurubin-Fragakis A, et al. Guidelines regarding the recommendation and sale of dietary supplements. *J Am Diet Assoc*. 2002;102:1158–1164.
92. American Society of Health-System Pharmacists. ASHP statement on the use of dietary supplements. *Am J Health-Syst Pharm*. 2004; 61:1707–1711.
93. Gardiner P, Phillips RS, Kemper KJ, et al. Dietary supplements: inpatient policies in US children's hospitals. *Pediatrics*. 2008;121: e775–e781.

PART III

NUTRITION SUPPORT OF SPECIFIC STATES

20. **Pregnancy and Lactation** 331
Catherine Cimbalik, RN, RD, CNSC
James D. Paauw, MD, PhD

21. **Wound Healing** 348
Joyce K. Stechmiller, PhD, ACNP-BC, FAAN

22. **Nutrition in Neurologic Impairment** 363
Kathryn Ruf, PharmD
Barbara Magnuson, PharmD, BCNSP
Jimmi Hatton, PharmD
Aaron M. Cook, PharmD, BCPS

23. **Critical Care Sepsis** 377
Keith Miller, MD
Laszlo Kiraly, MD
Robert G. Martindale, MD, PhD

24. **Trauma, Surgery, and Burns** 392
Bryan R. Collier, DO, FACS, CNSC
Jill R. Cherry-Bukowiec, MD, MS, FACS
Mary E. (Beth) Mills, MS, RD, CNSC, LDN

25. **Pulmonary Failure** 412
Krista L. Turner, MD, FACS

26. **Gastrointestinal Disease** 426
David Frantz, MD, MS
Craig Munroe, MD
Carol Rees Parrish, MS, RD
Joseph Krenitsky, MS, RD
Kate Willcutts, MS, RD, CNSC
Amy Fortune, RD, PA-C

27. **Liver Disease** 454
Thomas H. Frazier, MD
Craig J. McClain, MD
Benjamin E. Wheeler, MD
Matthew Cave, MD

28. **Pancreatitis** 472
Carol Rees Parrish, MS, RD
Joseph Krenitsky, MS, RD
Stephen A. McClave, MD

29. **Renal Disease** 491
Robert Wolk, PharmD
Charles J. Foulks, MD, FACP, FACN

30. **Short Bowel Syndrome** 511
Sherry Tarleton, RD, CNSC
John K. DiBaise, MD, FACG

31. **Solid Organ Transplantation** 523
Jeanette M. Hasse, PhD, RD, LD, FADA, CNSC
Laura E. Matarese, PhD, RD, LDN, FADA, CNSC

32. **Human Immunodeficiency Virus (HIV) Infection** 536
Peter J. Wasserman, RD, MA
Sorana Segal-Maurer, MD
David S. Rubin, MD

33. **Cancer** 563
Robin B. Mendelsohn, MD
Mark A. Schattner, MD

34. **Nutritional and Medical Management of Diabetes Mellitus in Hospitalized Patients** 580
Laura Newton, MA, RD
W. Timothy Garvey, MD

35. **Obesity** 603
Ryan T. Hurt, MD, PhD
Thomas H. Frazier, MD

36. **Nutrition Support for Older Adults** 620
Charles Mueller, PhD, RD, CNSD
Rena Zelig, MS, RD, CSG

37. **Chylothorax and Chylous Ascites** 630
Thomas H. Frazier, MD
David A. Spain, MD, FACS
Stephen A. McClave, MD

20 Pregnancy and Lactation

Catherine Cimbalik, RN, RD, CNSC, and James D. Paauw, MD, PhD

CONTENTS

Background 332
Multiple Gestation 332
Maternal Weight Gain 333
Fetal Growth 333
Macronutrients 333
  Calories 333
  Carbohydrate 334
  Protein 335
  Fat 335
Micronutrients 335
  Deficiency 336
  Toxicity 336
Enteral Nutrition 336
  Indications/Contraindications 336
  Formula Composition 336
  Access 337
  Complications 337
Parenteral Nutrition 337
  Indications/Contraindications 337
  Formula Composition 338
  Access 338
  Complications 338
Monitoring Nutrition Support 338
  Serum Analysis 338
  Urinalysis 340
  Acid-Base 340
  Transitional Feeds 340
Lactation 341
Special Consideration: Hyperemesis Gravidarum 341
Trauma 342
Other Considerations 343
References 344

Objectives

1. Describe the changes in requirements for macronutrients and micronutrients that occur with pregnancy and lactation.
2. Summarize modifications to a nutrition support regimen that are indicated to ensure optimal maternal and fetal outcomes during pregnancy.
3. Discuss selection, placement, and maintenance of enteral and parenteral access devices during pregnancy.
4. Identify nutrition monitoring parameters that are altered by pregnancy.

Test Your Knowledge Questions

1. Which of the following parameters is appropriate for monitoring glycemic control of pregnant women receiving nutrition support?
   A. Urine glucose
   B. Serum glucose
   C. Serum insulin
   D. Urine lactic acid
2. Which of the following statements is true regarding the nutrition management of pregnant women receiving nutrition support?
   A. Hyperlipidemia is a normal occurrence of pregnancy.
   B. Women with hyperemesis gravidarum (HG) should not be fed via feeding tube.
   C. Placement of percutaneous endoscopic gastrostomy (PEG) tubes is contraindicated in pregnancy.
   D. Administration of parenteral lipid emulsions is associated with preterm labor in humans.
3. Which of the following statements about maternal energy needs in pregnancy is accurate?
   A. Five hundred kcals/d to support pregnancy should be added to calculated energy needs derived from traditional energy predictive formulas used in potentially hypermetabolic conditions.
   B. Providing 36 to 40 kcals/kg of pregravid weight is acceptable to support pregnancy in most women.
   C. Estimated daily energy requirement in pregnancy increases above nonpregnant values by about 180 to 340 kcals/d.
   D. An extra 5 kcals/kg of pregravid weight should be added to daily energy calculations during the first trimester of pregnancy.

Test Your Knowledge Answers

1. The correct answer is **B**. Serum glucose levels must be strictly monitored during pregnancy to avoid the possible detrimental effects of neonatal hyperglycemia and hyperinsulinemia. The presence of glucose in a pregnant woman's urine is not abnormal and therefore does not necessarily indicate the presence of maternal diabetes.[1] The presence of lactic acid in the urine is typically observed during strenuous exercise and has no value in terms of monitoring glycemic control.
2. The correct answer is **A**. Hyperlipidemia is a common occurrence during pregnancy. Serum triglyceride and cholesterol may rise to 150% and to 125% to 150%, respectively, of nonpregnant levels. This is the result of enhanced adipose tissue lipolysis, increased triglyceride synthesis, increased chylomicron production from dietary lipids, and reduced lipoprotein lipase activity in extrahepatic tissues.[2,3] Women with HG may be successfully fed via an enteral feeding tube.[4,5] There are no reports of aspiration of enteral feeding. PEG feeding in conscious pregnant women has been reported,[6] and PEG feedings may be a possible feeding alternative. At this time, parenteral lipids in reasonable amounts are considered safe for pregnant women.[7]
3. The correct answer is **C**. The Food and Nutrition Board has determined that the daily estimated energy requirement in pregnancy should be increased by 8 kcals per each second or third trimester week plus 180 kcals/d energy deposition.[8] Formulas used to calculate energy needs in potentially hypermetabolic conditions should be adjusted by 200 to 300 kcals/d to support pregnancy. While 36 to 40 kcals/kg is recommended for women whose pregravid weight was less than desirable, lower energy provisions are recommended for other pregnant women.[9] No increase in energy needs are indicated during the first trimester.

Background

Overwhelming evidence links maternal nutrition during pregnancy with fetal outcome.[10] In particular, poor maternal weight gain increases the risk for delivery of a low-birth-weight infant (< 2500 g), thus increasing the risk for neonatal death or long-term medical and developmental sequelae.[10] Prolonged nutrient deprivation is likely to result in an exacerbation of the fasting state of pregnancy, known as "accelerated starvation," in which there is an increased rate of turnover of maternal metabolic fuels. This state is associated with higher fasting plasma concentrations of free fatty acids, triglycerides, and an increased predisposition for fasting ketosis.[11,12] Significant nutritional deficits may occur in pregnant women with preexisting or intercurrent illnesses that affect nutrient intake or absorption (eg, inflammatory bowel disease, bowel obstruction, cancer, coma associated with head injury or intracranial hemorrhage, anorexia nervosa, diabetic gastroparesis, pancreatitis, or previous surgery for obesity), or in women with conditions such as HG with intractable nausea and vomiting.[4,5,13–16]

Both parenteral nutrition (PN) and enteral nutrition (EN) have been used during pregnancy and have been associated with adequate maternal nutrition and promotion of fetal growth.[4,5,13–16] The potential for additional benefit with optimal timing for initiation of "early" nutrition support in the pregnant population as compared to the nonpregnant population has yet to be determined. Ultrasonography to monitor fetal growth is a valuable tool for assessing the adequacy of PN or EN during pregnancy.[17] Preterm delivery is usually the consequence of medical or obstetric rather than nutrition-related complications.[10]

Multiple Gestation

Multiple gestations would be expected to require additional nutritional support for the patient. Casele et al. has shown that twin gestation has dramatic effects upon glucose and fat metabolism, particularly during the second half of pregnancy.[18] Luke,

TABLE 20-1 Recommended Weight Gain Based on Prepregnancy Body Mass Index[22]

Prepregnancy BMI	Total Weight Gain (in kg)	Rate of gain/ week	Second and Third Trimester Range in kg/week[a]
Underweight (BMI < 18.5)	12.5–18	0.51	(0.44–0.58)
Normal weight (BMI 18.5–24.9)	11.5–16	0.42	(0.35–0.50)
Overweight (BMI 25–29.9)	7–11.5	0.28	(0.23–0.33)
Obese (BMI > 30.0)	5–9	0.22	(0.17–0.27)

BMI, body mass index.
[a]Weight gain recommendations based on pregravid weight status.

in her excellent review of nutrition and multiple gestation, recommended a diet composed of 20% of calories from protein, 40% of calories from fat, and 40% of calories from carbohydrate for pregnant women carrying twins or triplets.[19] The recommendation is based on a diabetic regimen for better glycemic control and less bulk in an oral diet. Iron deficiency, a concern in single gestation, is thought to pose an even greater risk in mothers with multiple gestation.[20] There are no published reports of EN or PN in multiple gestation.

Maternal Weight Gain

Maternal weight gain is strongly correlated with infant birth weight.[21] Recently, the Institute of Medicine reexamined the guidelines for weight gain during pregnancy in response to the changing demographic of women of childbearing age. It is recommended that an underweight woman (body mass index [BMI] < 18.5) gain 12.5 to 18 kg, compared with 11.5 to 16 kg for a normal weight woman (BMI 18.5 to 24.9), 7 to 11.5 kg for an overweight woman (BMI 25 to 29.9), and 5 to 9 kg for an obese woman (BMI ≥ 30) (Table 20-1).[22] Lack of weight gain throughout pregnancy in women with low or average pregravid weight may be associated with fetal growth restriction.[21] Lack of weight gain in the second trimester is strongly correlated with decreased birth weight, and supplementary feedings have been shown to increase maternal weight gain, birth weight, length, and head and chest circumference of newborns of women with low socioeconomic status.[23,24] On the other hand, if the mother is significantly overweight but otherwise healthy, below average weight gain is unlikely to be associated with appreciable fetal growth restriction.[25] Other factors besides maternal weight gain and poor nutrition that may decrease fetal birth weight include chromosomal abnormalities, substance abuse, fetal infections, congenital malformations, constitutionally small mothers, chemical teratogens, and maternal disease.[26]

Weight gain in multiple gestations has been reported and is described by Luke (Table 20-2). The intrauterine growth of multiples peaks earlier than that in single pregnancies. With each additional fetus, the chance of intrauterine growth restriction rises with length of gestation. [27] In twin pregnancies, the pattern of weight gain has been related to outcome. Poor weight gain (≤ 0.85 lb/week before 24 weeks of gestation) is associated with decreased intrauterine growth and higher morbidity with twins regardless of late weight gain after 24 weeks.[28] The Institute of Medicine provided the following provisional guidelines for weight gain in twin pregnancies: normal weight women should gain 17 to 25 kg, overweight women 14 to 23 kg, and obese women 11 to 19 kg total.[22] There is insufficient information to provide guidelines for underweight women with multiple gestations.

Fetal Growth

Fetal growth should be regularly monitored by fundal height measurements and/or serial ultrasound measurements to ensure adequate nutrition support of the pregnancy. However, clinicians should be aware that fundal height is only an estimate of gestational age and fetal growth. Deviations occur in women who are short or tall, underweight or overweight, and have a dull bladder, and in multiples. Fundal height that measures smaller or larger than expected, or increases more or less quickly than expected, could indicate intrauterine growth restriction or macrosomia but also polyhydramnios, uterine fibroids, or premature descending into the pelvis or settling into a breech or other unusual position.

Macronutrients

Refer to prior segments of this text for more information pertaining to general nutrient guidelines: Chapters 2, 3, 5, and 6.

Calories

Additional calories are required in order to support the normal processes during pregnancy: maternal fat deposition and the development of fetal, uterine, and mammary tissue, and an

TABLE 20-2 Summary of Multiple Gestations and Maternal Gain

Plurality	No. of Infants	% LBW (< 2500 g)	% VLBW (< 1500 g)	To 24 Weeks (lb)	Total (lb)	Range of Gestation (weeks)	Average Weight (g)
Singletons	3,851,109	6	1	12	25–35	38–41	3700–4000
Twins	97,064	50	10	24	40–45	36–38	2500–3800
Triplets	4,233	90	32	36	50–60	34–35	1900–2200
Quadruplets	360	98	75	50	65–80	31–33	1500–1800

LBW, low birth weight; VLBW, very low birth weight.
Adapted from Luke B. What is the Influence of maternal weight gain on the fetal growth of twins? *Clinical Obstetrics and Gynecology.* March 1998;41(1):57–64.

TABLE 20-3 Estimated Energy Requirements for Adolescent and Adult Females[8]

EER for women 19 years and older
$EER = 354 - 6.91 \times age\ (y) + PA \times (9.36 \times weight\ [kg] + 726 \times height\ [m])$

Where PA is the physical activity coefficient:
PA = 1.00 if PAL is estimated to be ≥ 1.0 < 1.4 (sedentary)
PA = 1.12 if PAL is estimated to be ≥ 1.4 < 1.6 (low active)
PA = 1.27 if PAL is estimated to be ≥ 1.6 < 1.9 (active)
PA = 1.45 if PAL is estimated to be ≥ 1.9 < 2.5 (very active)

EER for girls 9 through 18 years
$EER = 135.3 - 30.8 \times age\ (y) + PA \times (10.0 \times weight\ [kg] + 934 \times height\ [m] + 25\ [kcal\ for\ energy\ deposition])$

Where PA is the physical activity coefficient:
PA = 1.00 if PAL is estimated to be ≥ 1.0 < 1.4 (sedentary)
PA = 1.16 if PAL is estimated to be ≥ 1.4 < 1.6 (low active)
PA = 1.31 if PAL is estimated to be ≥ 1.6 < 1.9 (active)
PA = 1.56 if PAL is estimated to be ≥ 1.9 < 2.5 (very active)

EER, estimated energy requirements; PA, physical activity.

increased basal metabolism associated with these newly synthesized tissues. The Dietary Reference Intakes (DRIs) for energy use the term "estimated energy requirement" (EER). EER is defined as "the dietary energy intake that is predicted to maintain energy balance in healthy normal weight individuals of a defined age, gender, weight, height and level of physical activity consistent with good health."[8] Energy requirements for females (adolescent and adult) can be calculated using Table 20-3. EERs for pregnancy in adolescents and adults are shown in Table 20-4. These EER formulas are typically not used for overweight or obese persons, and there is little data published regarding formulas for energy needs in this pregnant population.[9] Close monitoring of weight trends is encouraged, and adjustments can be made for inadequate or excessive weight gains. During the first trimester, energy needs are not significantly increased. Extra energy intake is needed only in the second and third trimesters.

When various hypermetabolic conditions (ie, trauma, sepsis, burns; see Chapters 23 and 24) are superimposed on pregnancy, basal caloric requirements may be increased from normal pregnancy. In this situation, indirect calorimetry (see Chapter 2), if available to the clinician, is probably the most accurate method for estimating maternal caloric requirements for supporting adequate fetal growth. If indirect calorimetry is not available, traditional formulas that estimate needs for these potentially hypermetabolic conditions may initially be used with 200 to 300 kcal/d added to support pregnancy. Caloric delivery should then be adjusted as needed based on frequent monitoring of maternal metabolic parameters, weight gain, and fetal growth using ultrasonography exams.

Carbohydrate

Compared with protein and fat, carbohydrates have the greatest effect on blood glucose levels (see Chapter 3). In normal pregnancy, the consumption of a high carbohydrate meal results in postprandial hyperglycemia and hyperinsulinemia.[29] This suggests that the hyperglycemic response to meals ensures a constant supply of glucose to the fetus.[29] However, pregnant women tend to have lower premeal and fasting blood glucose levels. This is probably due to a constant uptake of glucose by the placenta along with altered hepatic gluconeogenesis. Overall, the mean 24-hour blood glucose level of pregnant women is comparable to that of nonpregnant women.

Prolonged elevated maternal blood glucose concentrations, as occurs in conditions such as diabetes mellitus (see Chapter 34) or metabolic stress (see Chapters 23 and 24), causes an excess transfer of glucose across the placenta. In the second trimester of pregnancy, several hormone concentrations rise (progesterone, estrogen, human placental lactogen, growth hormone, cortisol) and can promote an increase in insulin resistance as well as a decrease in insulin sensitivity, which are associated with the development of gestational diabetes.[30] In particular, human placental lactogen is a major contributor to this impaired glucose tolerance state.[31] This, in turn, results in fetal hyperglycemia and hyperinsulinemia, both of which are detrimental to the fetus at any stage of pregnancy. During early pregnancy, chronically elevated fetal blood glucose levels are associated with fetal anomalies and increased risk of miscarriages. Later in pregnancy, poor maternal glycemic control is associated with increased risk of stillbirth and fetal macrosomia, which may result in birth trauma and shoulder dystocia, and increased rates of cesarean deliveries.[32–35] Therefore, when pregnancy is complicated by diabetes, fasting blood glucose levels should be ≤ 90 mg/dL and 2-hour postprandial values should be kept at ≤ 120 mg/dL.[36–38]

Inadequate amounts of carbohydrate in the maternal diet can exacerbate the underlying ketonemia and ketonuria of pregnancy. Studies have shown deleterious effects of ketone bodies on embryogenesis[39] and behavioral and intellectual development in childhood.[40] Given these deleterious effects, it is essential to provide sufficient dietary carbohydrate to prevent ketonemia. The current DRI for carbohydrate consumption in pregnancy, required to provide energy for both mother and fetus, is 175 g/day, but this may not prevent ketonemia in all

TABLE 20-4 Estimated Energy Requirements for Pregnancy in Adolescent and Adult Females[8]

14–18 Years	EER = adolescent EER + pregnancy energy deposition
First trimester	Adolescent EER + 0 (pregnancy energy deposition)
Second trimester	Adolescent EER + 160 kcal (8 kcal/wk × 20 wks) + 180 kcal
Third trimester	Adolescent EER + 272 kcal (8 kcal/wk × 34 wks) + 180 kcal
19–50 Years	EER = adult EER + pregnancy energy deposition
First trimester	Adult EER + 0 (pregnancy energy deposition)
Second trimester	Adult EER + 160 kcal (8 kcal/wk × 20 wks) + 180 kcal
Third trimester	Adult EER + 272 kcal (8 kcal/wk × 34 wks) + 180 kcal

EER, estimated energy requirements.

individuals.[8] Catabolic illness and hyperglycemia superimposed on pregnancy may further increase the risk for ketonemia despite the level of carbohydrate in the diet.

Oral ingestion of fructose-oligosaccharide has been shown to enhance the growth of bifidobacteria in the gut, a beneficial strain.[41] Fructose-oligosaccharide, one of a general group of compounds known as prebiotics, has also been hypothesized to enhance gastrointestinal (GI) immunity, as well as have a inhibitory effect in the development of colon cancer.[42] The current recommendation is that pregnant and lactating women should only take prebiotic supplements if prescribed by their physician.[42]

Protein

Additional protein intake is required during pregnancy to support increased maternal protein synthesis for expansion of the blood volume, uterus, and mammary tissue, and to supply selected amino acids for synthesis of fetal and placental proteins.[32] Inadequate protein supply in humans is believed to result in reduced growth during blastogenesis and small for gestational age babies.[43,44] Also, observations in animals indicate that reduced nonprotein energy supply results in increased fetal protein catabolism at the expense of fetal growth. Historically, excessive protein amounts have been suggested not to be well tolerated by the fetus.[45,46] However, no recent study has shown that high protein intakes are necessarily detrimental to the fetus.

The DRI for protein during the second and third trimesters of a normal pregnancy is about 1.1 g/kg/d body weight, or +25 g/day additional protein above the DRI for a nonpregnant female.[8] Protein deposition for the second and third trimesters is estimated to be 3.66 and 7.2 g/d, respectively.[8] As with nonpregnant patients (see Chapters 5 and 24), up to 2 g/kg of total protein may be required for pregnant patients with moderate or severe stress.[29] Recent American Society for Parenteral and Enteral Nutrition (A.S.P.E.N.) guidelines further specify protein requirements in the critically ill obese patient as follows: > 2.0 g/kg ideal body weight/day for BMI of 30 to 40, and > 2.5 g/kg ideal body weight/day for BMI > 40.[47]

Fat

Lipid metabolism is significantly altered by pregnancy. Transient maternal hyperlipidemia is common during pregnancy; free fatty acids, triglycerides, and cholesterol tend to be significantly higher in pregnancy than in nonpregnancy, especially during the late stages of gestation.[32,48] Triglyceride levels may rise 150% and cholesterol to 125% to 150% of prepregnancy levels without adverse sequelae.[2] Maternal hypertriglyceridemia results from several factors: enhanced adipose tissue lipolysis, which increases the amount of substrate available to the liver for triglyceride synthesis, reduced lipoprotein lipase activity in extrahepatic tissues, and increased chylomicron formation from dietary lipid.[3] In terms of fetal metabolism, fat deposition increases markedly in the second half of gestation. At term, lipid stores account for about 16% of the fetus' body weight.[49] Maternal intake of essential fatty acids (EFAs) has been associated with fetal growth and lung maturation. EFAs are necessary for the production of fetal phosphatidylglycerol, pulmonary surfactant, and myelin. An adequate intake for α-linolenic acid and linoleic acid are 1.4 g/d and 13 g/d, respectively (see Chapter 5).[8] There is increasing evidence that the long chain n-3 fatty acid docosahexaenoic acid (DHA) is required for optimal fetal growth and cognitive development and to promote optimal maternal stores to support lactation.[50] Fetal accretion rates in the third trimester cannot be met by conversion from α-linoleic acid alone.[51] Conversion of α-linoleic acid to DHA is slightly higher in pregnancy than in nonpregnant women[52] but overall less than 1% of intake.[53] Many groups such as the Perinatal Lipid Nutrition Project and Great Britain recommend 200 to 300 mg DHA/day during pregnancy and lactation.[50]

Micronutrients

According to the DRIs, there is an increased requirement for vitamins and minerals during pregnancy relative to the nonpregnant state (Tables 20-5 and 20-6).[54,59] (See Chapters 7 and 8 for a discussion of general electrolyte and micronutrient requirements.)

TABLE 20-5 Daily Requirements in Normal Pregnancy Compared with a Standard Intravenous Vitamin Preparation[54–56,58,59]

Vitamins	*RDI*	MVI-12
A	≤18y 750 μg retinol equivalent 19–30 y 770 μg retinol equivalent 31–50 y 700 μg retinol equivalent	3300 USP units (retinol)
D	600 IU (15 μg cholecalciferol)	200 USP units
E (ditocopheryl acetate)	10 mg-tocopherol equivalents	10 USP units
Ascorbic acid	≤18y 80 mg 19–30 y 85 mg 31–50 y 85 mg	200 mg
Thiamin (B_1)	1.4 mg	6.0 mg
Riboflavin (B_2)	1.4 mg	3.6 mg
Pyridoxine (B_6)	1.9 mg	6.0 mg
Niacin	18 mg	40.0 mg
Pantothenic acid	6 mg	15.0 mg
Biotin	30 μg	60 μg
Folic acid	600 μg	600 μg[a]
B_{12}	2.6 μg	5 μg
K	≤18y 75 μg[b] 19–30y 90 μg[b] 31–50y 90 μg[b]	

RDI, recommended daily intake; MVI, multivitamin; USP, U.S. Pharmacopeia.
[a]Requires additional supplementation.
[b]Must be added to the standard vitamin regimens.

TABLE 20-6 Recommended Daily Intakes for Minerals for Enteral and Parenteral Nutrition Support during Pregnancy[58,59]

RDI	Mineral
Calcium	
18 yr	1300 mg
19–30 yr	1000 mg
31–50 yr	1000 mg
Phosphorus	
18 yr	1250 mg
19–30 yr	700 mg
31–50 yr	700 mg
Magnesium	
18 yr	400 mg
19–30 yr	350 mg
31–50 yr	360 mg
Zinc	12 mg
Copper	1 mg
Manganese	2 mg
Iodine	22 μg
Selenium	60 μg
Iron	27 mg
Chromium	
≤ 18 yr	29 μg
19–30 yr	30 μg
31–50 yr	30 μg

RDI, recommended daily intake.

Deficiency

Maternal intake of certain vitamins and minerals affects fetal growth or length of gestation, and deficiencies have been linked with maternal complications and teratogenesis. Specifically, low maternal and newborn levels of vitamin A have been strongly associated with growth restriction, eye abnormalities, and impaired vision in children.[60] Zinc deficiencies are suspected to result in central nervous system malformations, and low red cell folate levels have been correlated with increased neural tube defects, malformations, small for gestational age infants, and third-trimester bleeding.[54,55] Studies of supplementation with calcium and magnesium have shown a substantial increase in length of gestation and reduction in prematurity.[57,58] Maternal calcium and vitamin D deficiency may be related to neonatal hypocalcemia and rickets.[60] Mild iron deficiency, resulting in microcytic anemia, is probably one of the most common mineral deficiencies of pregnancy.[61] Very low levels of hematological values (eg, hemoglobin) have been associated with increased incidences of growth retardation, prematurity, and fetal death.[62]

Toxicity

Vitamin A and zinc are nutrients that may have toxic effects on the fetus if consumed during pregnancy in quantities that are several times that of the DRIs. During pregnancy, excess intake of vitamin A of greater than 10,000 IU daily[63] or in the amount of 0.5 to 1.5 mg/kg of 13-cis retinoic acid (isotretinoin) has been associated with a high incidence of spontaneous abortions and birth defects.[64] Large daily doses of retinyl esters or retinol in amounts ≥ 6000 RE or 20,000 IU may cause similar abnormalities.[60,65,66] Excessive zinc supplementation may also be harmful during pregnancy. In one study, three out of four pregnant women to whom zinc sulfate supplements were given in amounts of 300 mg daily, which is significantly above the DRI of 15 mg/d, delivered prematurely; the fourth woman gave birth to a stillborn infant.[60,67]

Application of the normal pregnancy DRIs to pregnant patients who have acute or chronic disease and/or are receiving artificial nutrition support is problematic for several reasons. First, alterations in the metabolism of nutrients are suspected to occur during metabolic stress of acute and chronic disease; requirements for vitamins and minerals for individual disease states either in the nonpregnant or pregnant population are not completely known at this time. Second, artificial nutrition formulations may not contain the same sources or combinations of vitamins and minerals as naturally occurring foods. Therefore, absorption or requirements for these nutrients may not be comparable. Third, DRIs are based on nutrient balances from normal oral intake. When providing nutrients via the parenteral route, the gut, which normally regulates nutrient entry into the bloodstream, is bypassed and requirements may be entirely different than when administered via the enteral route. These concerns apply to all patients, but have a special importance when pregnancy is involved. Ideally, micronutrient intake should be monitored in pregnant women receiving long-term EN or PN in order to avoid the possible ill effects of deficiency or toxicity of individual nutrients (see Chapters 13 and 17) on fetal growth and maturation.

Enteral Nutrition

Enteral tube feedings (see Chapters 10 to 13) may be useful for preventing nutritional deficits and promoting adequate weight gain in pregnant women with impaired intake resulting from complications of pregnancy (eg, HG) or from illnesses unrelated to pregnancy (eg, trauma, diabetic gastroparesis).[10]

Indications/Contraindications

Enteral intake is the preferred route for nutrient intake when the GI tract is intact.[10] Enteral feeding supports the integrity of the GI tract and prevents mucosal atrophy. Enteral feeding is associated with fewer complications when compared to parenteral feeding. Also, enteral formula, feeding equipment, and placement procedures are generally less costly when compared to parenteral support (see Chapter 12). Common conditions during pregnancy that may warrant feeding by tube include gastroparesis, HG, and trauma.

Formula Composition

The macronutrient composition of most enteral products seems to be adequate for support of most pregnant patients when estimated total calorie and nitrogen requirements are provided (see Chapter 11). The clinician should evaluate the micronutrient composition of standard formulae because formulae vary in vitamin, mineral, and trace element composition. If evaluation of a particular formula indicates that certain vitamins or minerals may be inadequate in the context of the DRIs, the clinician should consider supplementation of those nutrients.

Access

Nasoenteric feeding tube placement is less invasive than other routes for placement such as surgical or percutaneously placed gastrostomy or jejunostomy (see Chapter 12). A potential disadvantage of nasogastric placement is the increased risk of aspiration of the enteral feeding in pregnant women. During pregnancy, there is delayed gastric emptying and decreased gastroesophageal sphincter tone.[68] Additionally, because the nasogastric feeding tube keeps the gastroesophageal sphincter from closing completely, there is an increased risk of reflux of stomach contents into the esophagus.

Enteral feeding via percutaneously placed gastrostomy[69] or gastrojejunostomy[70,71] in pregnant women has been reported in the literature. As noted by Koh and Lipkin,[72] this type of access for feeding may have some advantages over nasogastric access. Percutaneous gastrostomy can be placed endoscopically without need for radiologic confirmation of position and may reduce the potential for gastroesophageal reflux, esophagitis, and aspiration pneumonia. Percutaneous fluoroscopic gastrostomy placement by a radiologist is considered to be a safe and effective alternative to endoscopic placement. The risk of fetal radiation exposure is discussed in the Practice Scenario 20–1.

Practice Scenario 20-1

Question: How do you prevent adverse neurologic outcome when initiating nutrition support in a patient with severe intractable hyperemesis gravidarum?

Scenario: A 23-year-old woman presents in her 11th week of pregnancy with persistent nausea and emesis of 7 weeks' duration. She reports vomiting between two and eight times daily over that time period, over which she lost 12 pounds, or 10% of her body weight. Rehydration is started with a dextrose solution. A nasogastric feeding tube is placed and feeding of a standard 1 kcal/mL formula is advanced over a 2-day period to her goal, providing 2000 kcals and 84 g protein daily. On the second hospital day, she became confused and began to exhibit short-term memory loss. Physical examination revealed nystagmus that was not present on her admitting examination, as well as gait ataxia.

Intervention: The patient is given 100 mg thiamin intravenously immediately, and again over the next 2 days. Her symptoms rapidly resolve.

Answer: Do not proceed with dextrose or other carbohydrate repletion without first providing supplemental thiamin. Prompt thiamin replacement should be given if neurologic symptoms develop in patients with HG. Confusion, opthalmoplegia, and ataxia represent the classic triad of Wernicke encephalopathy caused by thiamin deficiency.

Rationale: Any patient with repetitive vomiting, such as this patient, is at significant risk for development of Wernicke encephalopathy. This is usually precipitated by provision of glucose without prior or concurrent thiamin supplementation.

Complications

Diarrhea often occurs in patients requiring tube feedings for nutrition support for a variety of reasons (ie, gut flora alteration caused by antibiotic therapy, the administration of hypertonic medications via the feeding tube, bowel edema caused by severe hypoalbuminemia) (see Chapter 13). Once the contributing factor to the diarrhea is identified, steps can be taken to provide the appropriate treatment. Use of antidiarrheal drugs containing narcotics (ie, paregoric or diphenoxylate/atropine) should be reconsidered in pregnant women because of potential adverse effects on the fetus. Adding psyllium to the enteral program may be a more appropriate therapy instead of using these types of medications.

Conversely, constipation is common during pregnancy. As much as 40% of women complain of constipation at various gestational stages,[73] most commonly in the third trimester. Adequate fiber (see Chapter 3) and fluid intake (see Chapter 7) are usually all that are needed to prevent constipation in normally active pregnant women. For pregnant women receiving nutrition support, prophylactic treatment with bulk-forming laxatives and fiber-containing formulae may be beneficial, especially if the patient is confined to bed. Stool softeners may be needed on an individual basis.

Parenteral Nutrition

Indications/Contraindications

The preferred route for provision of nutrition support is via the GI tract. In situations where this is not possible, PN (see Chapters 14 to 17) has been used successfully during pregnancy to support fetal and maternal growth.[13,74,75] One of the more common GI conditions necessitating PN support during pregnancy is inflammatory bowel disease. HG refractory to attempts at EN is another. Pancreatitis and diabetic gastroparesis, formerly thought to be initially appropriate for PN, are now considered to be better and more safely managed by jejunal tube feeding. As with any use of PN, fastidious care must be afforded to central venous catheter use and maintenance to avoid septic complications.[76,77]

Peripheral PN (PPN) is usually reserved for patients who meet several conditions: those who have a nonfunctioning GI tract, do not have a severely catabolic illness, have reasonably good venous integrity, can tolerate a more aggressive fluid load, and are anticipated to need support for only 5 to 7 days. Providing adequate nutrition support with PPN is more challenging than with central PN because of the limited ability of peripheral veins to tolerate higher calorie hypertonic formulations. Consequently, PPN usually serves as a temporary measure of nutrition support. Use of small amounts of hydrocortisone (5 mg/mL) and heparin (1 U/ml) in the PPN solution to minimize phlebitis, as well as achievement of target solution osmolarity by addition of calculated amounts of free water, enhances the success of PPN.[78] PPN may also serve as an adjunct to tube feeding for patients who experience GI intolerance when high enteral infusion rates are required to meet total caloric needs. The higher volume required to provide a more limited amount of calories may limit the benefit of PPN for patients in whom fluid overload is a concern (see Chapters 14 to 17). PPN as a sole source of nutrition may not provide pregnant women with 100% of their estimated calorie requirements. PPN is a more appropriate method to provide PN support in women who are unable to ingest adequate calories either orally or enterally, and in whom central venous PN is not feasible or desirable.

Formula Composition

The macronutrient composition of the PN formulation required to meet the needs for pregnancy is similar to the standard composition routinely provided for nonpregnant patients (see Chapters 14 and 15). The percentage of total calories provided as carbohydrate should range from 40% to 50%, as fat from 20% to 30%, and as protein from 15% to 20%. A relative limitation of carbohydrate in PN for pregnancy is based on concern for the diabetogenic effect of placental hormones on insulin resistance. While carbohydrate in the form of intravenous (IV) dextrose should not be provided in excessive amounts likely to predispose to hyperglycemia, care also should be taken to avoid ketonemia from inadequate carbohydrate provision. Insulin may be added to PN if glucose intolerance develops, although limiting the dextrose load to 5 mg/kg/min should help avoid the need for insulin. Standard parenteral amino acid solutions provide an appropriate balance of amino acids to support pregnancy adequately when total estimated or measured protein requirements are met. Standard commercially available parenteral lipid solutions derived from vegetable oils contain adequate amounts of linoleic and linolenic acid.

Providing 4% of calories as EFAs is necessary to satisfy requirements for these nutrients. Practically, this can be achieved by giving as little as 10% to 15% of total calories from a commercially prepared lipid emulsion.[79] Although concerns have been expressed relative to the possible deleterious effect of administering higher amounts of triglycerides containing long-chain fatty acids on the immune system (see Chapter 5), current understanding is that these triglycerides can be used safely in PN when limiting the provision of lipids to less than 30% of total calories.[80,81]

PPN admixtures contain dextrose in a final concentration ≤ 10%. Lower dextrose concentrations are necessary to keep the osmolarity of the solution within a range that can be tolerated by peripheral veins (850 mOsm/kg, with an upper limit of 900 mOsm/kg).[82] The addition of lipid increases caloric delivery to the patient while diluting the final osmolarity of the PPN admixture (see Chapters 14 and 15). Nitrogen requirements can usually be met with amino acids at a final concentration of 3.5% to 5.0%.

Standard multivitamin and trace element packets may not meet the DRIs of pregnancy for all nutrients. The composition of these preparations should be examined to ensure adequacy of intake (Table 20-5). Specifically, magnesium, vitamin D, folic acid, vitamin K, iron, iodine, and selenium may need to be supplemented on an individual basis. The mineral requirements of pregnancy usually can be met by providing the amounts suggested by the DRIs (Table 20-6).

Access

Catheter selection for PN administration is based on the anticipated duration of need for nutrition support (see Chapter 16). Short-term nutrition support is usually defined as < 30 days for which temporary percutaneously placed central venous catheters or peripherally inserted central catheters (PICCs) are used. While PICCs have been proposed as a means to eliminate risks associated with placement of central venous access devices,[13] the significant risk of venothrombotic events associated with PICCs may outweigh any advantages with the use of PICCs. When PICCs are used, placement in the right arm may be preferable because patients are instructed to rest in the left lateral decubitus position later in pregnancy.[83] Long-term PN (30 days or more) is usually administered via a subcutaneous port or a tunneled catheter because these access devices are thought to reduce the risk of catheter-associated infection over time. The procedure for obtaining access for PPN and the complications thereof are no different in pregnant women than with nonpregnant individuals (see Chapter 16).

Complications

Although PN has been used with successful outcomes in pregnancy for many years, it has been associated with a variety of maternal complications.[13,84] Many of the risks associated with PN are similar in nonpregnant and pregnant patients (see Chapter 17). However, pregnant women are at higher risk for hyperglycemic complications.[85] At least one study suggests that they may be at higher risk for sepsis.[13] The incidence of catheter-related sepsis, which is generally independent of type (not site) of central venous catheter used, is approximately 25%.[13,84] In nonpregnant adult patients, the incidence of PICC-related upper extremity venous thrombosis detected by Doppler ultrasound is 62% in patients not on prophylactic anticoagulants and still 23% in those who are on such therapy.[86] Venous thromboembolism, which occurs in 2% of all patients receiving long-term PN, is estimated to be up to five times as likely to occur in pregnant women than in nonpregnant women of similar age.[85,87,88] Routine use of anticoagulant chemoprophylactic agents is recommended in all patients with PICCs.

Monitoring Nutrition Support

Serum Analysis

In normal pregnancy, many serum proteins, electrolytes, vitamins, and minerals are altered compared to the nonpregnant state. An increase in the blood volume by as much as 50% results in lower concentrations of a number of nutrients (although total circulating levels may actually be higher), and many components exhibit changes independent of blood volume. Normal values for pregnancy are represented in Table 20-7.[89] Hyperglycemia is one of the most common metabolic complications associated with PN. Accordingly, it is critical to monitor glucose concentration closely, particularly during the first 72 hours, in order to provide adjustments to the dextrose or insulin administration to the patient. The serum glucose should initially be checked every 6 hours. In cases where the patient has known glucose intolerance, more frequent assessments may be required, even on an hourly basis if deemed necessary.

TABLE 20-7 Laboratory Values in Pregnancy

	Value	
	Nonpregnant	**Pregnant**
Electrolytes and acid-base values		
Sodium (mEq/L)	135–145	132–140
Potassium (mEq/L)	3.5–5.0	3.5–4.5
Chloride (mEq/L)	100–106	90–105
Bicarbonate (mEq/L)	24–30	17–22
Pco_2 (mm Hg)	35–50	25–30
Po_2 (mm Hg)	98–100	101–104
Base excess	0.7	3–4
Arterial pH	7.36–7.44	7.40–7.45
BUN (mg/dL)	10–18	4–12
Creatinine (mg/dL)	0.6–1.2	0.4–0.9
Creatinine clearance (mL/min)	3.5–5.0	2.0–3.7
Osmolality (mOsm/kg)	275–295	275–285
Lipids and liver function tests		
Total bilirubin (mg/dL)	1.0	1.0
Direct bilirubin (mg/dL)	0.4	0.4
Alkaline phosphatase (IU/mL)	13–35	25–80
SGOT/AST (IU/mL)	10–40	10–40
Total protein (g/dL)	6.0–8.4	5.5–7.5
Albumin (g/dL)	3.5–5.0	3.0–4.5
Globulin (g/dL)	2.3–3.5	3.0–4.0
Total lipids (mg/dL)	460–1000	1040
Total cholesterol (mg/dL)	120–200	250
Triglycerides (mg/dL)	45–150	230
Free fatty acid (mcg/L)	770	1226
Phospholipids (mg/dL)	256	350
Hematologic laboratory values		
CBC		
Hematocrit (%)	37–48	32–42
Hemoglobin (g/dL)	12–16	10–14
Lymphocytes (%)	38–46	15–40
Platelets	150,000–350,000	Normal or slightly decreased
Serum iron (μg)	75–150	62–130
Iron binding capacity (μg)	250–410	300–500
Iron saturation (%)	30–40	15–30
Ferritin (ng/mL)	35	10–12

AST, aspartate aminotransferase; BUN, blood urea nitrogen; CBC, complete blood count; SGOT, serum glutamic-oxaloacetic transaminase.
Gleicher N, ed. *Principles of Medical Therapy in Pregnancy*. New York: Plenum Publishing Group; 1985 with kind permission from Springer Science+Business Media B.V.

Serum albumin has historically been used to assess hepatic protein synthesis and nutriture of patients. However, its long half-life and large circulating pool size make it insensitive to detecting consequences of short-term alterations to calorie intake. During the latter stages of pregnancy, the concentration of albumin decreases due to a shift in gamma-globulin to alpha- and beta-globulins. Also, a dilutional effect from normal plasma expansion occurs.[90] This results in reduced plasma oncotic pressure and increases the tendency to develop edema. In critically ill patients (see Chapter 24), rapid decreases in albumin may be more reflective of inflammation and extravasation rather than the result of true nutritional deficits.

Prealbumin and retinol-binding protein (RBP) have considerably shorter half-lives than albumin and have been used to assess protein nutriture in relatively stable patients. Normal values for prealbumin have not yet been established for pregnancy. RBP concentrations in pregnant women have been demonstrated to be similar to those seen in a nonpregnant control group.[91] In any case, newer publications question the validity of using prealbumin and RBP as indicators of protein or calorie adequacy.[92] Creatinine levels generally are lower in pregnancy than in the average population because of increased renal clearance. Pregnant women with a creatinine level ≥ 0.9 mg/dL should be evaluated for possible developing renal insufficiency,[93] and protein intake may need to be adjusted based on the clinical situation. In pregnant women who receive nutrition support, a baseline triglyceride level should be evaluated with respect to subsequent values to ensure adequate utilization of lipids. If subsequent measurements of triglyceride levels are significantly increased from baseline, lipid intolerance may be present, and the enteral or parenteral formulation should be modified to decrease the provision of lipids. When intake of fat from enteral or parenteral feedings approaches an amount that meets only the minimum estimated needs for pregnancy, patients should be monitored closely for developing signs of EFA deficiency. Although deficiency symptoms may be visually apparent within 1 to 3 weeks,[94] it is not known whether compromise of fetal development occurs before the observance of maternal physical signs. Therefore, practitioners should be encouraged to provide adequate EFAs to avoid the possibility of deficiency.

Total iron-binding capacity (TIBC), serum iron, hemoglobin, and hematocrit levels may be used to assess iron status. A transferring saturation of 16% or a serum iron level of < 60 to 70 mcg/dL may indicate iron deficiency during pregnancy.[54] The National Research Council recommends that transferrin saturation in pregnancy be maintained above 20%.[95] TIBC and iron levels may be affected by factors other than nutrition during illness; for example, TIBC, which normally increases in iron deficiency, may function as a metabolic fuel during acute or chronic illness, creating difficulties in using it solely for evaluating iron status. Also, iron tends to be acutely sequestered during infection, rendering serum levels an inadequate marker for existing stores. Because serum ferritin concentration more accurately reflects the body's iron stores, it may help differentiate iron deficiency from dilutional changes in pregnancy. A serum ferritin concentration of 12 mcg/L is classified as iron deficiency; however, concentrations < 35 mcg/L may indicate deficiency during pregnancy. In the face of a depressed serum hemoglobin concentration, with low mean corpuscular volume and mean corpuscular hemoglobin concentration, assaying serum ferritin should be considered in order to confirm iron deficiency. Generally, serum hemoglobin and hematocrit levels < 11.0 mg/dL and 33.0%, respectively, in the first trimester, 10.5 mg/dL and 32.0% in the second trimester, or 11.0 mg/dL and 33.0% in the third trimester indicate possible iron deficiency anemia.[61] In this regard, a test dose of 1 g using either iron sucrose or iron gluconate over divided daily doses is recommended. Measures of iron deficiency can then be evaluated to determine when iron status achieves normal range.

Urinalysis

Glomerular filtration increases significantly in pregnancy beginning in the first trimester. This may result in glucosuria, which may be present in more than 50% of pregnant women.[1] Glucosuria is not necessarily related to maternal hyperglycemia, and urine glucose levels should not be used to diagnose diabetes or for monitoring glycemic status in pregnant women. The presence of ketones in the urine can be caused by inadequate hydration, hyperglycemia, or inadequate calorie intake. Catabolic illness during pregnancy may also increase the risk of ketonuria. Monitoring urine ketones during the provision of artificial nutrition support is advisable for every patient so that calorie and fluid intake from enteral and parenteral formulations may be adjusted appropriately. The presence of ketones should initially be checked daily, and then as needed, if weight loss, hyperglycemia, or change in maternal status (eg, fever) occurs that might affect fluid requirements. Nitrogen balance studies may be helpful to the clinician when evaluating individual total nitrogen requirements (see Chapter 9). It is desirable to maintain a positive nitrogen balance during pregnancy to ensure adequate protein intake for fetal growth. A positive balance of 4 to 6 g of nitrogen per day is ideal. Positive nitrogen balance may not be obtainable during the immediate period following acute illness (ie, trauma, sepsis) (see Chapters 23 and 24). However, every effort should be made to minimize net nitrogen losses to avoid possible detriment to fetal protein status. Balance studies should initially be obtained at least weekly until positive balance is achieved, and then should be repeated as needed when changes in the formula type or amounts delivered are deemed necessary.

Acid-Base

Clinicians monitoring tolerance to EN and PN support should be familiar with normal changes in acid-base status (see Chapter 7) associated with pregnancy. During pregnancy, a chronic state of compensated respiratory alkalosis exists, and buffering capacity is decreased. The alteration is mostly due to an increase in maternal respiratory rate and increased excretion of bicarbonate by the maternal kidneys; the result is that the maternal pH is maintained within normal limits. These changes facilitate the transfer of carbon dioxide from the fetus to the mother.

Transitional Feeds

The transition to enteral or oral support should be initiated and tolerated before the discontinuation of parenteral or enteral therapies, similar to the nonpregnant state (see Chapters 10 and 14).

TABLE 20-8 Daily Recommended Intakes for Vitamins and Minerals during Lactation[54–56,58,59]

Mineral	DRI
Minerals and Trace Elements	
Calcium	
18 yr	1300 mg
19–30 yr	1000 mg
31–50 yr	1000 mg
Phosphorus	
18 yr	1250 mg
19–30 yr	700 mg
31–50 yr	700 mg
Magnesium	
18 yr	360 mg
19–30 yr	310 mg
31–50 yr	320 mg
Zinc	
≤18 yr	13 mg
19–50 yr	12 mg
Copper	1300 μg
Manganese	2.6 mg
Iodine	290 μg
Selenium	70 μg
Iron	15 mg
Chromium	
≤ 18 yr	44 μg
19–50 yr	45 μg
Vitamins	
Vitamin A	
18 yr	1200 μg retinol equivalent
31–50 yr	1300 μg retinol equivalent
Thiamin (B_1)	1.4 mg
Riboflavin (B_2)	1.6 mg
Pyridoxine (B_6)	2.0 mg
Vitamin B_{12}	2.8 μg
Ascorbic acid	
18 yr	115 mg
31–50 yr	120 mg
Vitamin D	600 IU (15 μg cholecalciferol)
Vitamin E	19 mg–tocopherol equivalents
Vitamin K	
18 yr	75 μg
31–50 yr	90 μg
Folic acid	500 μg
Niacin	17 mg
Biotin	35 μg
Pantothenic acid	7 mg

DRI, daily recommended intake.

Lactation

Table 20-8 outlines the vitamin and mineral DRIs for lactation. EERs for lactation in females (adolescent and adult) can be determined using Table 20-8. No known reports or specific guidelines exist regarding breastfeeding during PN or EN therapy. The item "milk energy output" in Table 20-9 is computed from production and energy density of human milk. The value for the first 6 months of lactation is 500 kcal/d and 400 kcal/d for the second six months of lactation.

Special Consideration: Hyperemesis Gravidarum

Typical morning sickness of pregnancy involves occasional vomiting and does not cause significant weight loss. It has been estimated to occur in 45% to 90% of all pregnancies.[96–100] One study indicated that nausea and vomiting of pregnancy was associated with a normal pregnancy outcome with regard to fetal weight, and some even suggest a decreased risk of spontaneous abortion.[101–103] However, many of these studies did not stratify the outcome data with regard to the severity of nausea and vomiting. HG is a more severe form of this condition, which results in dehydration, electrolyte imbalance, and a loss of > 5% of body weight.[98] When severe, this condition may be characterized by ketonuria, abnormal liver enzyme profile, and vitamin deficiencies.[104–106] One such deficiency, Wernicke encephalopathy, characteristically develops when dextrose is started without first replacing thiamin (Practice Scenario 20-1). A recent study of over 500,000 births identified by California birth certificate date linked with hospital discharge data found a prevalence of HG of about 0.5% of all pregnancies resulting in live births.[107] HG typically begins between the 6th and 12th week and resolves by the 20th week of pregnancy.[100,101] Singleton infants of hyperemetic mothers tend to be smaller,[107,108] small for gestational age,[107] and have shorter gestations.[108] HG is associated with additional maternal hospitalizations averaging 2.6 days in length and an estimated $5,932 increase in the cost of pregnancy.[107]

Initial support for HG usually involves supplemental thiamin followed by IV fluids to treat ketonuria, dehydration, and electrolyte and acid-base imbalances; avoiding oral intake; and the administration of antiemetics. A multivitamin may be added to the IV fluid because the patient's intake likely had been poor for the past several weeks, and she probably had suboptimal vitamin status. Van Stuijvenberg and colleagues documented that the intake of most nutrients by women with HG fell below the 50% of the DRI, and 60% of patients had suboptimal levels of thiamin, riboflavin, vitamin B_6, and vitamin A.[109] The consequences of a mild, transient depletion of maternal stores of most vitamins are unknown and are probably of little significance. However, the administration of glucose-based IV fluids may exacerbate an existing mild thiamin deficiency, and cases of Wernicke encephalopathy occurring in women with HG have been reported.[107,110] The inclusion of a multivitamin in the IV fluids is a simple and inexpensive therapy that may be beneficial. While promethazine and pyridoxine are considered to be first-line therapies,[111] women taking pyridoxine-metoclopramide reported improved subjective response and fewer emeses than those receiving monotherapy with either promethazine or prochlorperazine.[112] Continuous subcutaneous metoclopramide has been reported to give complete symptom resolution in more than 60% of cases, with only mild side effects.[113] Subcutaneous metoclopramide should be considered, and if successful, can be converted to home use, with a possible significant reduction in costly hospitalization. Several randomized, double blind, placebo-controlled trials of corticosteroid use have been done, supporting a beneficial role in the relief of symptoms.[114,115] However, corticosteroid use did not prevent future hospitalizations, nor did it offer rapid and complete remission of symptoms.[114,115] Pulsed high-dose IV hydrocortisone is significantly more effective at reducing episodes of vomiting and preventing hospital readmission in women with intractable HG than regularly scheduled IV metoclopramide.[116] The presence of weight loss may be predictive of successful response to corticosteroids in that women who lost more than 5% of prepregnant weight uniformly improved with corticosteroids.[117] In pregnant women receiving corticosteroids, the rate of fetal malformations is 3.5%, very similar to the rate seen for the general population.[118] Although ondansetron is frequently used in refractory HG, it is not thought to be more effective than promethazine.[119] In addition, ginger has been shown to be effective in reducing the nausea and vomiting of pregnancy in patients not responding to first-line therapies.[120,121]

Failure of attempts to stop the vomiting and continued weight loss with a 48-hour trial of IV fluids and antiemetics indicate that a patient is unable to support her nutritional needs on her own. At this point, nutrition support should be considered to avoid further deterioration of the mother's nutriture and possible deleterious effects of continued inadequate nutrient intake on the fetus.

As in many disease states, EN, associated with lower risk than PN, should be considered as the first choice for nutrition intervention in HG. EN has been successfully used as a source of nutrition but also as a means to improve the nausea and vomiting of HG, especially when these symptoms are associated with the consumption of food.[5,122] In HG, initial patient stabilization with appropriate hydration and electrolyte balance is essential to successful EN, which should not be started until after electrolyte imbalances have been corrected and the acute phase of vomiting has subsided, even if nausea has not resolved.[4] At that time, a small bore feeding tube may be passed. Continuous gastric feedings with an

TABLE 20-9 Estimated Energy Requirements for Lactation in Adolescent and Adult Females[8]

14–18 Years	EER = adolescent EER + milk energy output − weight loss
First 6 mo	Adolescent EER + 500 − 170 (milk energy output − weight loss)
Second 6 mo	Adolescent EER + 400 − 0 (milk energy output − weight loss)
19–50 Years	EER = adult EER + milk energy output − weight loss
First 6 mo	Adult EER + 500 − 170 (milk energy output − weight loss)
Second 6 mo	Adult EER + 400 − 0 (milk energy output − weight loss)

EER, estimated energy requirements.

iso-osmotic solution should be initiated at a low rate and increased slowly at regular intervals; this should continue as long as the nausea is not exacerbated and if no diarrhea or gastric residuals occur.[123] In intractable cases necessitating long-term gastric tube feedings, a gastrostomy tube, such as a PEG, can be safely placed.[6] Antiemetics are often used in conjunction with enteral tube feedings so that continued retching, which increases risk of aspiration and tube dislodgement, can be minimized. When patients with HG manifest intolerance to gastric feeding, jejunal feeding may be necessary. Nasojejunal tubes can be placed either endoscopically or fluoroscopically with appropriate shielding.[124] With placement of a nasojejunal feeding tube after failure of hydration and hyperemetic therapy, reduced vomiting occurred within 48 hours, with complete cessation after an average of 5 days.[124] For jejunally fed patients with severe refractory HG, the use of a PEG with a jejunal limb has been shown to be a safe, effective, and relatively cost-effective modality in several case reports.[15,70] Because use of a jejunal feeding tube necessitates feedings in a continuous or cyclic fashion to avoid the usual jejunal intolerance of bolus feedings, in refractory HG a trial of nasogastric feeding should be attempted before moving to a jejunal tube. A PEG should be considered if gastric feedings are tolerated but become prolonged. If a patient fails gastric feeding, a trial of nasojejunal feeding should be undertaken before placement of a PEG with a jejunal limb. Only when a patient experiences complete failure of enteral nutrition should PN be considered (Figure 20-1).

Although PN has been used to achieve successful outcomes in pregnancy for many years, it has been associated with a variety of maternal complications.[13,84] As noted previously, PN entails significant risk of infection and, if a PICC is used, PICC-related upper extremity venous thrombosis. Moreover, venous stasis related to dehydration places the patient with HG at above-average risk for central catheter-related thromboembolic phenomena. PN should only be initiated in those meeting the criteria of weight loss over a period of at least 4 weeks, failed conservative therapy, failed attempts at enteral feeding (Figure 20-1), and persistent laboratory findings such as serum electrolyte abnormalities and progressive hypoalbuminemia.[84]

Trauma

Medical and nutrition support of pregnant trauma patients are especially challenging because of catecholamines released in response to stress causing increased nutrient catabolism and vasoconstriction of the placental vasculature, reducing the nutrient and oxygen supplies to the fetus. The nutritional needs to support maternal illness together with demands of the growing fetus are difficult to estimate. Requirements for nutrients are likely to be altered by trauma, but the degree of alteration is dependent on the nature and extent of the injury. In the few published case reports of pregnant trauma patients receiving nutrition support,[72,125–128] various methods for estimating caloric requirements in the absence of indirect calorimetry were used. In these cases, caloric support ranged from 2000 to 3000 kcal/d. Indirect calorimetry is a valuable tool for determining the resting energy expenditure of the maternal–fetal unit so that under- or overfeeding can be prevented. If indirect calorimetry is not available, traditional formulas that estimate the needs of critically ill patients can be used with 200 to 300 kcal/day added for pregnancy. Weight gain goals are as described previously in the chapter (Table 20-1). The initial estimation for protein requirements can be calculated by using the same methods for nonpregnant patients, beginning with 1.5 to 2.0 g/kg body weight.

Low protein markers in the pregnant trauma patient most likely reflect a colloid shift from the intravascular to the extravascular space as an acute response to trauma and dilution from volume support. The normal physiology of pregnancy may also

FIGURE 20-1 Algorithm for preference of route of nutrition support in hyperemesis gravidarum

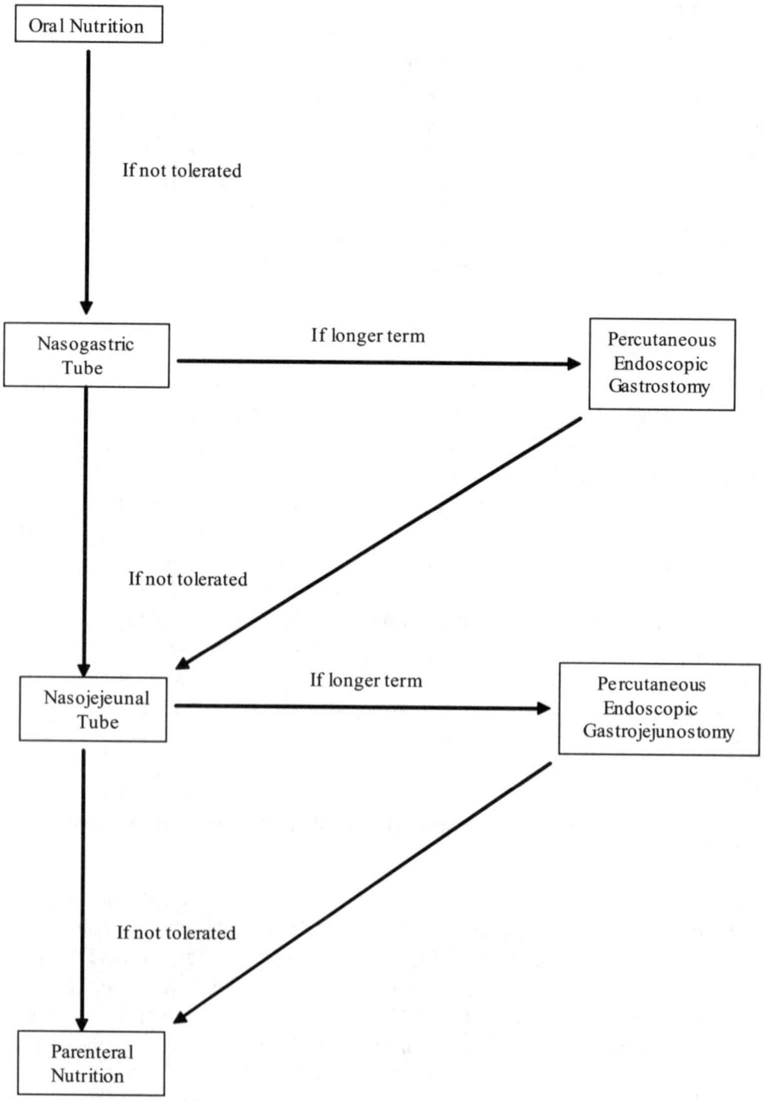

account for a portion of the decreased albumin and total protein. During pregnancy, a greater shift in gamma-globulin to alpha- and beta-globulin and a dilutional effect from normal plasma expansion occurs, especially during the latter stages of pregnancy. This effect levels off around the 28th week of gestation.

Fluoroscopic nasoenteric feeding tube placement is a successful, safer, and more cost-effective approach than endoscopic placement.[129] Endoscopic placement should be reserved for cases of failed fluoroscopic placement. Although no reports on fetal radiation exposure in fluoroscopic feeding tube placement exist, safe use of fluoroscopy in pregnant patients has been reported for other fluoroscopic procedures such as endoscopic retrograde cholangiopancreatography[130] and cardiac catheter ablation procedures.[131]

Although some controversy exists, a systematic review and consensus statement of immune-enhancing diets in critically ill patients concluded that these products resulted in reductions of infection rate, time on mechanical ventilation, and hospital length of stay.[132] Given beneficial effects, immune-enhancing formulas are recommended in critically ill patients requiring enteral feeding. Because no firm data exist as to the ideal duration of use of immune-enhancing formula, a consensus is developing to limit use of these products to 5 to 7 days. Additional information on these enteral formulations is available in Chapter 11. A review of enteral feeding patients advanced to goal rate by 18 hours, on average, showed no negative clinical effects despite some evidence of refeeding syndrome, when an electrolyte replacement protocol was in effect.[133] Additional iron may need to be added to the enteral regimen to provide the DRI of pregnancy of 27 mg of iron per day, but not in the first trimester.

Guidelines for blood glucose management in pregnant women, as well as in critically ill patients, are more rigorous than in nonpregnant patients. The insulin resistance that typically accompanies critical illness may result in hyperglycemia that is difficult to control in the pregnant woman, and elevated blood glucose levels can harm the fetus. The clear benefit of intensive glycemic management has made it the standard of care in both pregnant and critically ill patients.[134-137] Unfortunately, specific guidelines for blood glucose management in pregnant women receiving continuous enteral or parenteral nutrient infusions do not exist at this time. Jovanovic-Peterson and Peterson recommended that women whose pregnancies are complicated by diabetes maintain fasting blood glucose levels < 90 mg/dL and 2-hour postprandial blood glucose values < 120 mg/dL.[36] However, because these guidelines were designed for meal-eating women who also experience a fasting period, they are impractical and may possibly be inappropriate for those patients receiving continuous feedings. Mean 24-hour blood glucose levels, in which the postprandial states and fasting states are averaged, may have more practical application in this situation. Of particular interest is a study by Kitzmiller[138] in which pregnancy outcome was associated with mean 24-hour maternal blood glucose levels (average of fasting and postprandial blood glucose values). In this study, it was observed that keeping mean blood glucose levels < 100 mg/dL was also associated with good pregnancy outcome (ie, reduced incidence of macrosomia, neonatal hypoglycemia). This type of protocol may be a more practical application of blood glucose management for women who are receiving continuous enteral or parenteral feedings.

Ordering a 24-hour urine nitrogen study is helpful in assessing the protein needs of both pregnant and nonpregnant trauma patients. A positive nitrogen balance is difficult to obtain in the early posttrauma period, but efforts to minimize net nitrogen losses should be made. A modular protein may need to be added to the tube feeding formulation to increase protein intake to 2.0 g/kg body weight, close to the presumed maximal amount thought to be beneficial. Another option is to increase the nonprotein calorie to nitrogen ratio in order to minimize nitrogen losses.

In pregnant patients receiving nutrition support, prophylactic treatment with bulk-forming laxatives and use of fiber-containing formulas may be beneficial, especially if the patient is confined to bed (Practice Scenario 20-2). Adding free-water flushes as appropriate may also be helpful. Constipation in a patient who is inactive could easily develop into an impaction, which increases the risk of preterm labor or toxic megacolon.

Practice Scenario 20-2

Question: What measures should be taken to minimize the incidence of constipation and impaction in an immobilized pregnant patient receiving nutrition support?

Scenario: A 39-year-old woman in the 34th week of pregnancy is involved in a motor vehicle collision in which she strikes her head on the windshield. She has loss of consciousness at the scene, where she is orotracheally intubated before being transported to the emergency department. Computed tomography scan reveals an intraparenchymal hemorrhage, and her Glascow Coma Scale measure of 6 requires her to be mechanically ventilated. A nasojejunal feeding tube is placed under fluoroscopic guidance with appropriate shielding, and the patient is advanced to goal tube feedings using a high-protein 1 kcal/mL solution and water flushes of 30 mL every 6 hours. On the seventh hospital day, the patient's abdomen becomes more firm, and her bowel sounds become hyperactive. Nursing notes reveal no bowel movement for the past 3 days.

Intervention: The patient is started on bulk-forming laxatives, and the feeding formula is switched to one that contains fiber. The water flushes are increased to 60 ml every 4 hours. The patient has three bowel movements the next day, and her abdominal exam normalizes.

Answer: Prophylactic measures should be undertaken at the outset of enterally feeding an immobilized pregnant patient, including use of bulk-forming laxatives such as psyllium seed and the use of fiber-containing enteral formulas. In addition, water flushes more generous than standard amounts should be given.

Rationale: The patient was at increased risk to experience constipation and impaction by virtue of both her late-stage pregnancy and her immobility. This complication is aggravated by insufficient dietary fiber and water.

Other Considerations

In regards to eating disorders, two studies revealed that pregnant women with active eating disorders are at high risk for delivering by cesarean section[139] and also at high risk for delivering infants with lower birth weights, smaller head circumference, microcephaly, and small for gestational age.[140] No other studies were found that specifically linked pregnant eating disorder patients and nutritional support.

Gestational diabetes and pregnancy that requires nutritional support may be best managed with the avoidance of overfeeding and adequate glycemic control. There are commercially available enteral formulas for diabetic patients that contain less carbohydrate (40% of total kcals compared to a standard formula that provides 55% carbohydrate). For further discussion on the use of diabetic formulas, see Chapter 34.

As far as nutritional support and inflammatory bowel diseases, no published studies specific to this subject were found.

References

1. Davison JM, Hytten FE. The effect of pregnancy on the renal handling of glucose. *Br J Obstet Gynecol.* 1975;82:374–381.
2. Everson GT. Liver problems in pregnancy: distinguishing normal from abnormal hepatic changes. *Medscape Women's Health.* 1998;3:3.
3. Herrera E, Gomez-Coronado D, Lasuncion MA. Lipid metabolism in pregnancy. *Biol Neonate.* 1987;51:70–77.
4. Gulley RM, Pleog NV, Gulley JM. Treatment of hyperemesis gravidarum with nasogastric feeding. *Nutr Clin Pract.* 1993;8:33–35.
5. Hsu JJ, Clark-Glena R, Nelson DK, Kim CH. Nasogastric enteral feeding in the management of hyperemesis gravidarum. *Obstet Gynecol.* 1996;88:343–346.
6. Godil A, Chen YK. Percutaneous endoscopic gastrostomy for nutrition support in pregnancy associated with hyperemesis gravidarum and anorexia nervosa. *J Parenter Enter Nutr.* 1998;22:238–241.
7. Amato P, Quercia RA. A historical perspective and review of the safety of lipid emulsion in pregnancy. *Nutr Clin Pract.* 1991;6:189–192.
8. Institute of Medicine, Food and Nutrition Board. *Dietary Reference Intakes for Energy, Carbohydrate, Fiber, Fat, Fatty Acids, Cholesterol, Protein and Amino Acids.* Washington, DC: National Academies Press; 2002.
9. Thomas AM, Gutierrez YM. *American Dietetic Association Guide to Gestational Diabetes Mellitus.* Washington, DC: American Dietetic Association; 2005:49–52.
10. A.S.P.E.N. Board of Directors. Clinical guidelines for the use of parenteral and enteral nutrition in adults and pediatric patients. *J Parenter Enteral Nutr.* 2002;17:1SA–52SA.
11. Metzger BE, Freinkel N. Accelerated starvation in pregnancy: implications for dietary treatment of obesity and gestational diabetes mellitus. *Biol Neonate.* 1987;51:78–85.
12. Carpenter MW. Metabolic changes in gestational diabetes. *Clin Perinatol.* 1993;20:583–591.
13. Russo-Stieglitz KE, Levine AB, Wagner BA, Armenti TV. Pregnancy outcomes in patients requiring parenteral nutrition. *J Maternal–Fetal Med.* 1999;8:164–167.
14. Campo M, Albinana S, Garcia-Burguillo A, et al. Pregnancy in a patient with chronic intestinal pseudoobstruction on long term parenteral nutrition. *Clin Nutr.* 2000;19:455–457.
15. Irving PM, Howell RJ, Shidrawi RG. Percutaneous endoscopic gastrostomy with a jejunal port for severe hyperemesis gravidarum. *Eur J Gastroenterol Hepatol.* 2004;16:937–939.
16. Pendlebury J, Phillips F, Ferguson A, Ghosh S. Successful pregnancy in a patient with chronic intestinal pseudo-obstruction while on ambulatory percutaneous endoscopic gastrostomy feeding. *Eur J Gastroenterol Hepatol.* 1997;9:711–713.
17. Merialdi M, Caulfield LE, Zavaleta N, et al. Randomized controlled trial of prenatal zinc supplementation and fetal bone growth. *Am J Clin Nutr.* 2004;79:826–830.
18. Casele HL, Dooley SL, Metzger BE. Metabolic response to meal eating and extended overnight fast in twin gestation. *Am J Obstet Gynecol* 1996;175:917–921.
19. Luke B. Nutrition and multiple gestation. *Semin Perinatol.* 2005;29:349–354.
20. Blickstein I, Goldschmit R, Lurie S. Hemoglobin levels during twin vs. singleton pregnancies: parity makes the difference. *J Reprod Med.* 1995;40:47–50.
21. Ehrenberg HM, Dierker L, Milluzzi C, Mercer BM. Low maternal weight, failure to thrive in pregnancy, and adverse outcomes. *Am J Obstet Gynecol.* 2003;189:1726–1730.
22. Institute of Medicine and National Research Council. *Weight Gain During Pregnancy: Reexamining the Guidelines.* Washington, DC: The National Academies Press; 2009.
23. Abrams B, Selvin S. Maternal weight gain pattern and birth weight. *Obstet Gynecol.* 1995;86:163–169.
24. Begum N, Hussain T, Afridi B, Hamid A. Effect of supplementary feeding of pregnant women on birth weight of the newborn. *Plant Foods Hum Nutr.* 1991;41:329–336.
25. Hise, M. Metabolism and life cycle: pregnancy and lactation. In: Rolandelli RH, Bankhead R, Boulata JI, Compher CW, eds. *Clinical Nutrition: Enteral and Tube Feeding.* 4th ed. Philadelphia, PA: Elsevier Saunders; 2005:58.
26. Cunningham GF, Gant NF, Leveno KJ, et al. Fetal growth restriction. In: *Williams Obstetrics.* 21st ed. New York, NY: McGraw-Hill; 2001:745–757.
27. Luke B. Reducing fetal deaths in multiple births: optimal birth weights and gestational ages for infants of twin and triplet births. *Acta Genet Med Gemellol.* 1996;45:333–348.
28. Luke B, Minogue J, Witter FR, et al. The ideal twin pregnancy: patterns of weight gain, discordancy, and length of gestation. *Am J Obstet Gynecol.* 1993;169:588–597.
29. MacBurney M, Matarese LE. Pregnancy. In: Matarese L, Gottschlich MM, eds. *Contemporary Nutrition Support Practice.* 2nd ed. Philadelphia, PA: Saunders; 2003:337–343.
30. Catalano PM, Kirwan JP, de Mouzon SH, King J. Gestational diabetes and insulin resistance: role in short- and long-term implications for mother and fetus. *J Nutr.* 2003;133:1674S–1683S.
31. Thomas AM, Gutierrez YM. *American Dietetic Association Guide to Gestational Diabetes.* Washington, DC: American Dietetic Association; 2005:11–12.
32. Butte NF. Carbohydrate and lipid metabolism in pregnancy: normal compared with gestational diabetes mellitus. *Am J Clin Nutr.* 2000;71:1256S–1261S.
33. Turok DK, Ratcliffe SD, Baxley EG. Management of gestational diabetes mellitus. *Am Fam Physician.* 2003;68:1767–1772.
34. Christoffersson M, Rydhstroem H. Shoulder dystocia and brachial plexus injury: a population-based study. *Gynecol Obstet Invest.* 2002;53:42–47.
35. Hod M, Bar K, Peled Y, et al. Antepartum management protocol. Timing and mode of delivery in gestational diabetes. *Diabetes Care.* 1998;21(suppl 2):B113–117.
36. Jovanovic-Peterson L, Peterson CM. Dietary manipulation as a primary treatment strategy for pregnancies complicated by diabetes. *J Am Coll Nutr.* 1990;9:320–325.
37. American Diabetes Association. Preconception care of women with diabetes. *Diabetes Care.* 2001;24(suppl):66S–68S.

38. American Diabetes Association. Gestational diabetes mellitus. *Diabetes Care.* 2004;27(suppl 1):88S–90S.
39. Weigensberg M, Sobel R, Garcia-Palmer F, Freinkel N. Temporal differences in vulnerability to fuel mediated teratogenesis. *Diabetes.* 1988;37(suppl 1):85A.
40. Rizzo T, Metzger BE, Burns WJ, Burns K. Correlations between antepartum maternal metabolism and child intelligence. *N Engl J Med.* 1991;325:911–916.
41. Gibson GR. Dietary modulation of the human gut microflora using the prebiotics oligofructose and inulin. *J Nutr.* 1999;129: 1438S–1441S.
42. PDR Health. Prebiotics. www.pdrhealth.com/drug_info/nmdrug-profiles/nutsupdrugs/pre_0326.shtml. Accessed April 26, 2006.
43. Khoushabi F, Saraswathi G. Impact of nutritional status on birth weight of neonates in Zahedan City, Iran. *Nutr Res Pract.* 2010; 4(4):339–344.
44. Moore VM, Davies MJ, Willson KJ, Worsley A. Dietary composition of pregnant women is related to size of the baby at birth. *J Nutr.* 2004;134:1820–1826.
45. Landon MB, Gabbe SG, Mullen JL. Total parenteral nutrition during pregnancy. *Clin Perinatol.* 1986;13:57–72.
46. Rush D. *The National WIC Evaluation: An Evaluation of the Special Supplemental Food Program for Women, Infants, and Children.* Vols. I, II. New York, NY: Research Triangle Institute and New York State Research Foundation for Mental Hygiene; 1986.
47. McClave SA, Martindale RG, Vanek VW, et al. Guidelines for the provision and assessment of nutrition support therapy in the adult critically ill patient. Society of Critical Care Medicine (SCCM) and American Society for Parenteral and Enteral Nutrition (A.S.P.E.N.). *J Parenter Enteral Nutr.* 2009;33:277–316.
48. Hachey DL. Benefits and risks of modifying maternal fat intake in pregnancy and lactation. *Am J Clin Nutr.* 1994;59(2 suppl): 454S–464S.
49. Kimura RE. Lipid metabolism in the fetal–placental unit. In: Cowett RM, ed. *Principles of Perinatal–Neonatal Metabolism.* 2nd ed. New York, NY: Springer-Verlag; 1998:389.
50. Koletzko B, Lien E, Agostoni C, et al. The roles of long-chain polyunsaturated fatty acids in pregnancy, lactation and infancy: review of current knowledge and consensus recommendations. *J Perinatal Med.* 2008;36(1):5–14.
51. Makrides M, Gibson RA. Long-chain polyunsaturated fatty acid requirements during pregnancy and lactation. *Am J Clin Nutr.* 2000;71(suppl):307S–311S.
52. Welch AA, Shakya-Shrestha S, Lentjes MAH, Wareham NJ, Khaw K-T. Dietary intake and status of n-3 polyunsaturated fatty acids in a population of fish-eating and non-fish eating meat-eaters, vegetarians and vegans and the precursor-product ratio of α-linolenic acid to long chain n-3 polyunsaturated fatty acids: results from the EPIC-Norfolk cohort. *Am J Clin Nutr.* 2010:92:1040–1051.
53. Brenna JT, Salem N, Sinclair AJ, Cunnane SC. Alpha-linolenic acid supplementation and conversion of n-03 long chain polyunsaturated fatty acids in humans. *Prostaglandins Leukot Essent Fatty Acids.* 2009:80:85–91.
54. Institute of Medicine, Food and Nutrition Board. *Dietary Reference Intakes. Vitamin A, Vitamin K, Arsenic, Boron, Chromium, Copper, Iodine, Iron, Manganese, Molybdenum, Nickel, Silicon, Vanadium, and Zinc.* Washington, DC: National Academies Press; 2001.
55. Institute of Medicine, Food and Nutrition Board. *Dietary Reference Intakes. Thiamin, Riboflavin, Niacin,Vitamin B6, Folate, Pantothenic Acid, Biotin, and Choline.* Washington, DC: National Academies Press; 1998:233–238.
56. Institute of Medicine, Food and Nutrition Board. *Dietary Reference Intakes. Vitamin C, Vitamin E, Selenium, and Carotenoids.* Washington, DC: National Academies Press; 2000.
57. Pathak P, Kapil U. Role of trace elements zinc, copper and magnesium during pregnancy and its outcome. *Indian J Pediatr.* 2004;71:1003–1005.
58. Institute of Medicine, Food and Nutrition Board. *Dietary Reference Intakes. Calcium, Phosphorus, Magnesium, Vitamin D, and Fluoride.* Washington, DC: National Academies Press; 1997.
59. Institute of Medicine, Food and Nutrition Board. *Dietary Reference Intakes. Calcium and Vitamin D.* Washington, DC: National Academies Press; 2011.
60. Worthington-Roberts B, Williams SR. Appendix A. Vitamins and minerals and pregnancy outcome. In: Worthington-Roberts BS, Williams SR, eds. *Nutrition in Pregnancy and Lactation.* 6th ed. St. Louis, MO: Times Mirror/Mosby; 1997:480–486.
61. Centers for Disease Control and Prevention. Recommendations to prevent and control iron deficiency in the United States. *MMWR Morb Mortal Wkly Rep.* 1998;47:1–36.
62. Yip R. Significance of an abnormally low or high hemoglobin concentration during pregnancy: special consideration of iron nutrition. *Am J Clin Nutr.* 2000;72(suppl):272S–279S.
63. Rothman KJ, Moore LL, Singer MR, et al. Teratogenecity of high vitamin A intake. *N Engl J Med.* 1995;333:1369–1373.
64. Lammer EJ, Chen DT, Hoar RM, et al. Retinoic acid embryopathy. *N Engl J Med.* 1985;313:837–841.
65. Costas K, Davis R, Kim N, et al. Use of supplements containing high-dose vitamin A—New York state, 1983–1984. *JAMA.* 1987; 257:1292–1297.
66. Bernhart IB, Dorsey DJ. Hypervitaminosis A and congenital renal anomalies in a human infant. *Obstet Gynecol.* 1974;43:750–755.
67. Kumar S. Effect of zinc supplementation on rats during pregnancy. *Nutr Rpts Intl.* 1976;13:33–36.
68. Cunningham GF, Gant NF, Leveno KJ, et al. Gastrointestinal disorders. In: *Williams Obstetrics.* 21st ed. New York, NY: McGraw-Hill; 2001:1273–1306.
69. Shaheen NJ, Crosby MA, Grimm IS, Isaacs K. The use of percutaneous endoscopic gastrostomy in pregnancy. *Gastrointest Endosc.* 1997;46:564–565.
70. Serrano P, Velloso A, Garcia-Luna PP, et al. Enteral nutrition by percutaneous endoscopic gastrojejunostomy in severe hyperemesis gravidarum: a report of two cases. *Clin Nutr.* 1998;17:135–139.
71. Wejda BU, Soennichsen B, Huchzermeyer H, et al. Successful jejunal nutrition therapy in a pregnant patient with apallic syndrome. *Clin Nutr.* 2003;22:209–211.
72. Koh ML, Lipkin EW. Nutrition support of a pregnant comatose patient via percutaneous endoscopic gastrostomy. *J Parenter Enteral Nutr.* 1993;17:384–387.
73. Everson GT. Gastrointestinal motility in pregnancy. *Gastroenterol Clin North Am.* 1992;21:751–776.
74. Badgett T, Feingold M. Total parenteral nutrition in pregnancy: case review and guidelines for calculating requirements. *J Maternal–Fetal Med.* 1997;6:215–217.
75. Caruso A, De Carolis S, Ferrazzani S, et al. Pregnancy outcome and total parenteral nutrition in malnourished pregnant women. *Fetal Diagn Ther.* 1998;13:136–140.
76. Folk JJ, Leslie-Brown HFM, Nosovitch JT, et al. Hyperemesis gravidarum. Outcomes and complications with and without total parenteral nutrition. *J Repro Med.* 2004;49:497–502.
77. Yousuf F. Comment. *Nutr Clin Pract.* 2005;20:364–365.
78. Tighe MJ, Wong C, Martin IG, McMahon MJ. Do heparin, hydrocortisone, and glyceryl trinitrate influence thrombophlebitis during full intravenous nutrition via a peripheral vein? *J Parenter Enteral Nutr.* 1995;19:507–509.
79. Martindale RG, Cresci GA, Leibach FH. Nutrition and metabolism. In: JP O'Leary, ed. *The Physiologic Basis of Surgery.* 3rd ed. Philadelphia, PA: Lippincott Williams & Wilkins; 2002:133–167.

80. Waitzberg DL, Lotierzo PH, Logullo AF, et al. Parenteral lipid emulsions and phagocytic systems. *Br J Nutr.* 2002;87(suppl 1): S49–S57.
81. MacMahon MM, Driscoll DF, Bistrian BR. Design of nutritional therapy for the fluid-restricted patient. In: Kinner JM, Borum PR, eds. *Perspectives in Clinical Nutrition.* Baltimore, MD: Urban & Schwarzenberg; 1989:169–180.
82. Task Force for the Revision of Safe Practices for Parenteral Nutrition. Safe practices for parenteral nutrition. *J Parenter Enteral Nutr.* 2004;28:S39–S70.
83. Levine MG, Esser D. Total parenteral nutrition for the treatment of severe hyperemesis gravidarum: maternal nutritional effects and fetal outcome. *Obstet Gynecol.* 1988;72:102–107.
84. Folk JJ, Leslie-Brown HFM, Nosovitch JT, Silverman RK, Aubry RH. Hyperemesis gravidarum. Outcomes and complications with and without total parenteral nutrition. *J Reprod Med.* 2004; 49:497–502.
85. National Institutes of Health Consensus Development Conference. Prevention of venous thrombosis and pulmonary embolism. *JAMA.* 1986;256:744–749.
86. Paauw JD, Borders H, Ingalls N, et al. The incidence of PICC line associated thrombosis with and without the use of prophylactic anticoagulants. *J Parenter Enter Nutr.* 2008;32(4):443–447.
87. Greenspoon JS, Rosen DJ, Ault M. Use of the parenterally inserted central catheter for parenteral nutrition during pregnancy. *Obstet Gynecol.* 1993;81:831–834.
88. Fabri PJ, Mirtallo JM, Ruberg RI, et al. Incidence and prevention of thrombosis of the subclavian vein during total parenteral nutrition. *Surg Gynecol Obstet.* 1982;115:238–242.
89. Aubry RH, Roberts A, Quencs VG. The assessment of maternal nutrition. *Clin Perinatol.* 1975;2:207–219.
90. Mendenhall HW. Serum protein concentrations in pregnancy. *Am J Obstet Gynecol.* 1970;106:388–399.
91. Sapin V, Alexandre MC, Chaib S, et al. Effect of vitamin A status at the end of term pregnancy on the saturation of retinol binding protein with retinol. *Am J Clin Nutr.* 2000;71:537–543.
92. Jensen GL, Bistrian B, Roubenoff R, Heimburger DC. Malnutrition syndromes: a conundrum vs continuum. *J Parenter Enter Nutr.* 2009;33:710–716.
93. Cunningham GF, Gant NF, Leveno KJ, et al. Assessment of renal disease during pregnancy. In: *Williams Obstetrics.* 21st ed. New York, NY: McGraw-Hill; 2001:1252–1253.
94. Goodgame JT, Lowry SF, Brennan MF. Essential fatty acid deficiency in total parenteral nutrition: time course of development and suggestions for therapy. *Surgery.* 1978;84:271–277.
95. National Research Council. *Laboratory Indices of Nutritional Status in Pregnancy.* Washington, DC: National Academy of Science; 1978.
96. Brandes JM. First trimester nausea and vomiting as related to outcome of pregnancy. *Obstet Gynecol.* 1967;30:427–431.
97. Fairweather DV. Nausea and vomiting in pregnancy. *Am J Obstet Gynecol.* 1968;102:135–175.
98. Biggs JS. Vomiting in pregnancy: causes and management. *Drugs.* 1975;9:299–306.
99. Jarnfelt-Samsioe A. Nausea and vomiting in pregnancy: a review. *Obstet Gynecol Surg.* 1987;42:422–427.
100. Walters WA. The management of nausea and vomiting during pregnancy. *Med J Aust.* 1987;147:290–291.
101. Schulman PK. Hyperemesis gravidarum: an approach to the nutritional aspects of care. *J Am Diet Assoc.* 1982;80:577–578.
102. Gross S, Librach C, Cecutti A. Maternal weight loss associated with hyperemesis gravidarum: a predictor of fetal outcome. *Am J Obstet Gynecol.* 1989;160:906–909.
103. Weigel RM, Weigel MM. Nausea and vomiting of early pregnancy and pregnancy outcome. A meta-analytical review. *Br J Obstet Gynaecol.* 1989;96:1312–1318.
104. Chatwani A, Schwartz R. A severe case of hyperemesis gravidarum. *Am J Obstet Gynecol.* 1982;143:964–965.
105. Morali GA, Braverman DZ. Abnormal liver enzymes and ketonuria in hyperemesis gravidarum. A retrospective review of 80 patients. *J Clin Gastroenterol.* 1990;12:303–305.
106. Lavin PJM, Smith D, Kori SH, Ellenberger CJ. Wernicke's encephalopathy: a predictable complication of hyperemesis gravidarum. *Obstet Gynecol.* 1983;62(suppl):13S–15S.
107. Bailit JL. Hyperemesis gravidarum: epidemiological findings from a large cohort. *Am J Obstet Gynecol.* 2005;193:811–814.
108. Paauw JD, Bierling S, Cook C, Davis AT. Hyperemesis gravidarum and fetal outcome. *J Parenter Enteral Nutr.* 2005;29: 93–96.
109. Van Stuijvenberg ME, Schabort I, Labadarios D, Nel JT. The nutritional status and treatment of patients with hyperemesis gravidarum. *Am J Obstet Gynecol.* 1995;172:1585–1591.
110. Wood P, Murray A, Sinha B, et al. Wernicke's encephalopathy induced by hyperemesis gravidarum. Case reports. *Br J Obstet Gyneacol.* 1983;90:583–586.
111. Paauw JD, Davis AT. Specialized requirements: Hyperemesis in pregnancy. In: Symonds ME, Ramsay MM, eds. *Maternal-Fetal Nutrition During Pregnancy and Lactation.* Cambridge, UK: Cambridge University Press; 2010:138–146.
112. Bsat FA, Hoffman DE, Seubert DE. Comparison of three outpatient regimens in the management of nausea and vomiting in pregnancy. *J Perinatol.* 2003;23:531–535.
113. Buttino L, Coleman SK, Bergauer NK, et al. Home subcutaneous metoclopramide therapy for hyperemesis gravidarum. *J Perinatol.* 2000;20:359–362.
114. Nelson-Piercy C, Fayers P, de Swiet M. Randomized, double-blind, placebo-controlled trial of corticosteroids for the treatment of hyperemesis gravidarum. *Br J Obstet Gynecol.* 2001;108:9–15.
115. Yost NP, McIntire DD, Wians FH Jr, et al. A randomized, placebo-controlled trial of corticosteroids for hyperemesis due to pregnancy. *Obstet Gynecol.* 2003;102:1250–1254.
116. Bondok RS, El Sharnouby NM, Eid HE, Abd Elmaksoud AM. Pulsed steroid therapy is an effective treatment for intractable hyperemesis gravidarum. *Crit Care Med.* 2006;34:2781–2783.
117. Moran P, Taylor R. Management of hyperemesis gravidarum: the importance of weight loss as a criterion for steroid therapy. *Q J Med.* 2002;95:153–158.
118. Danesi R, Del Tacca M. Teratogenesis and immunosuppressive treatment. *Transplant Proc.* 2004;36:705–707.
119. Sullivan CA, Johnson CA, Roach H, et al. A pilot study of intravenous odansetron for hyperemesis gravidarum. *Am J Obstet Gynecol.* 1996;174:1565–1568.
120. Boone SA, Shields KM. Treating pregnancy-related nausea and vomiting with ginger. *Ann Pharmaco.* 2005;39:1710–1713.
121. Borrelli F, Capasso R, Aviello G, et al. Effectiveness and safety of ginger in the treatment of pregnancy-induced nausea and vomiting. *Obstet Gynecol.* 2005;105:849–856.
122. Boyce RA. Enteral nutrition in hyperemesis gravidarum: a new development. *J Am Diet Assoc.* 1992;92(6):733–736.
123. van de Ven CJM. Nasogastric enteral feeding in the management of hyperemesis gravidarum. *Lancet.* 1997;349:445–446.
124. Vaisman N, Kaidar R, Levin I, Lessing JB. Nasojejunal feeding in hyperemesis gravidarum—a preliminary study. *Clin Nutr.* 2004; 23:53–57.
125. Landye ST. Successful enteral nutrition support of a pregnant, comatose patient: a case study. *J Am Diet Assoc.* 1988;88:718–720.

126. Smith BK, Rayburn WF, Feller I. Burns and pregnancy. *Clin Perinatol.* 1983;10:383–398.
127. Wong M, Apodaca CC, Markenson MG, Yancey M. Nutrition management in a pregnant comatose patient. *Nutr Clin Pract.* 1997;12:63–67.
128. Aderet NB, Cohen I, Abramowicz JB, et al. Traumatic coma during pregnancy with persistent vegetative state. Case report. *Br J Obstet Gynaecol.* 1984;91:939–941.
129. Foote JA, Kemmeter PR, Prichard PA, et al. A randomized trial of endoscopic vs. fluoroscopic placement of post pyloric feeding tubes in critically ill patients: a randomized trial. *J Parenter Enteral Nutr.* 2004;28:154–157.
130. Kahaleh M, Hartwell GD, Arseneau KO, et al. Safety and efficacy of ERCP in pregnancy. *Gastrointest Endoscopy.* 2004;60:287–292.
131. Damilakis J, Theocharopoulos N, Perisinakis K, et al. Conceptus radiation dose and risk from cardiac catheter ablation procedures. *Circulation.* 2001;104:893–897.
132. Montejo JC, Zarazaga A, Lopez-Martinez J, et al. Immunonutrition in the intensive care unit. A systematic review and consensus statement. *Clin Nutr.* 2003;22;221–233.
133. Flesher ME, Archer KA, Leslie BD, et al. Assessing the metabolic and clinical consequences of early enteral feeding in the malnourished patient. *J Parenter Enteral Nutr.* 2005;29: 108–117.
134. McMahon MM, Rizza RA. Nutrition support of hospitalized patients with diabetes mellitus. *Mayo Clin Proc.* 1996;71: 587–594.
135. Krinsley J, Grissler B. Intensive glycemic management in critically ill patients. *Joint Commission J Quality Patient Safety.* 2005; 31:308–312.
136. Digman C, Borto D, Nasraway SA. Hyperglycemia in the critically ill. *Nutr Clin Care.* 2005;8:93–101.
137. Christiansen C, Toft P, Jorgensen HS, et al. Hyperglycemia and mortality in critically ill patients. A prospective study. *Intensive Care Med.* 2004;30:1685–1688.
138. Kitzmiller JL. Intensified glucose monitoring in gestational diabetes. *Clin Diabetes.* 1995;6:110–111.
139. Franko DL, Blais MA, Becker AE, Delinsky SS, Greenwood DN, Flores AT, Ekeblad ER, Eddy KT, Herzog DB. Pregnancy complications and neonatal outcomes in women with eating disorders. *Am J Psychiatry.* 2001 Sep;158(9):1461–1466.
140. Koubaa S, Hallstrom T, Lindholm C, Hirschberg AL. Pregnancy and neonatal outcomes in women with eating disorders. *Obstet Gynecol.* 2005;105(2):255–260.

21 Wound Healing

Joyce K. Stechmiller, PhD, ACNP-BC, FAAN

CONTENTS

Introduction ... 349
Wound Healing Process ... 349
Skin as an Organ ... 349
Phases of Acute Wound Healing ... 350
Chronic Wounds ... 351
Incidence or Prevalence Data on Pressure Ulcers ... 351
Diabetic Ulcers, Venous Ulcers, and Other Chronic Wounds ... 352
Etiology of Delayed Healing ... 352
Nutrition Screening and Assessment ... 353
Nutrition Requirements ... 353
Energy Requirements ... 353
Protein Requirements ... 353
Arginine ... 353
Other Amino Acid Supplements ... 356
Fatty Acids ... 356
Hydration ... 356
Vitamins, Minerals and Other Micronutrients ... 356
Vitamin A ... 356
Vitamin C ... 357
Vitamin E ... 357
Zinc ... 357
Other Micronutrients ... 357
Nutrition Support ... 357
Monitoring of Wound Healing and Outcomes ... 358
References ... 359

Objectives

1. Describe the process of wound healing with specific focus on the requirements of macro- and micronutrients.
2. Describe the incidence and etiology of chronic wounds.
3. Discuss nutrition screening approaches of individuals at risk and in the presence of chronic wounds.
4. Specify nutrition support interventions to augment healing of chronic wounds.

Test Your Knowledge Questions

1. What are the goals for protein support for adults with delayed healing of pressure ulcers?
   A. Provide adequate protein: 0.8 g protein/kg per day
   B. Provide adequate protein: 1.2 to 2.1 g protein/kg with recommended evening supplements (protein and energy) for depletion
   C. Ensure adequate protein: 1.25 to 1.5 g protein/kg per day
   D. All of the above

2. Zinc is necessary for which of the following processes?
   A. Cell replication and growth
   B. Muscle contraction
   C. Red cell formation
   D. All of the above
3. What factors differentiate patients experiencing a chronic wound from an acute wound?
   A. No differences in baseline demands for protein and energy metabolism
   B. Endogenous arginine stores meet the needs of both groups
   C. Adequate protein and energy has been shown to enhance healing in both groups
   D. None of the above

Test Your Knowledge Answers

1. The correct answer is **C**. The goal for protein support for patients with pressure ulcers is to ensure 1.25 to 1.5 g/kg body weight per day.[1–5]
2. The correct answer is **A**. Zinc is an essential trace mineral necessary for cell replication and growth. Zinc supplementation is recommended only for patients with zinc deficiencies. For patients with normal levels of zinc, supplementation offers no benefit and may result in zinc toxicity.[6,7]
3. The correct answer is **C**. Although there are distinct differences from acute wounds that should be taken into account when considering the nutritional requirements in an individual with a chronic wound, adequate protein and energy has been shown to enhance healing in both groups. These differences may be due to a number of factors including chronic stress state, greater than baseline demands for protein metabolism, protein calorie malnutrition, hypercatabolism, comorbidities, and/or dehydration. Chronic wounds are characterized by a disruption in the sequence of expected healing events or prolonged inflammatory metabolism.[8–13] There are also distinct differences at the molecular level of chronic wounds; increased levels of inflammatory cytokines such as tumor necrosis factor alpha, interleukin-1 and -6, and proteases such as matrix metalloproteinases, particularly matrix metalloproteinase-2 and matrix metalloproteinase-9, are evident in chronic wound fluid. This results in an inhibition of fibroblast and endothelial cell proliferation and function, as well as decreased levels of tissue inhibitors of metalloproteinases. Increased bacterial burden (tissue bacterial levels exceed 100,000 colony forming units per gram of tissue) and altered keratinocyte function as well as extracellular matrix degradation have also been implicated in chronic wounds.[8–13] Endogenous sources of arginine stores are compromised and may not adequately meet the needs for adequate wound healing of complex acute and chronic wounds.

Introduction

Nutrition is a key factor that impacts wound healing.[1–5] Dietary protein, energy, and certain key nutrients such as vitamins (A, B, and C) and trace elements (selenium, zinc, copper, and manganese) are necessary for optimal wound healing.[1–5] Individuals who experience involuntary weight loss and protein calorie malnutrition (PCM) are at risk for delayed wound healing. Although PCM is implicated as a factor in impaired wound healing, it is also related to susceptibility to infection and increased risk of developing chronic wounds including pressure ulcers, diabetic ulcers, venous ulcers, and dehisced surgical wounds.[4,5]

Nutrition regimens for preventing skin breakdown and enhancing wound healing are controversial because of a lack of randomized clinical trials and outcomes data to support treatment. This demonstrates the need for further research and emphasizes the importance of individualized nutrition care plans for high-risk patients. This chapter presents an overview of literature on the role of nutrition support in the healing of wounds to help guide clinical practice and identify implications for further research. There is also a section on monitoring wound healing. Finally, the chapter concludes with practice scenarios that illustrate common practice problems associated with wound healing and nutrition support.

Wound Healing Process

Skin as an Organ

The skin is the largest organ of the human body. The skin functions as a protective barrier from external environmental factors while attempting to maintain homeostasis internally.[12] The layers of the skin include the epidermis, or outermost layer; the dermis, which is the thickest tissue layer of the skin; the basement membrane that separates the epidermis from the dermis; and the hypodermis, or the superficial fascia, which rests beneath the dermis but covers the muscle, ligaments, tendon, and bone that reside beneath these layers of skin.[12] The epidermis is comprised mostly of keratinocytes in several stratums of various stages of maturation. This layer of skin does not contain nerve endings or blood vessels, but is responsible for epithelialization (skin closure) of wounds. The dermis provides the supportive matrix upon which the epidermis sits and is composed of various connective tissue elements such as collagen fibers, elastic fibers, ground substance, mast cells, macrophages, lymphocytes, fat cells, fibroblasts, hair follicles, nerve endings, sweat glands, and blood vessels.[12] Ground substance, a gelatinous material composed largely of water, glycoproteins, glycosaminoglycans, and proteoglycans, plays a role in connective tissue similar to that of plasma in blood. The fibroblast, the most common cell found in connective tissue, is responsible for secreting the essential elements of the extracellular matrix such as collagen. The various types of collagen and other components of the extracellular matrix secreted by the fibroblasts are necessary for wound bed epithelialization or granulation of full thickness or partial thickness wounds that extend past the epidermal layer. Thus, the role of the dermis is providing critical components of the immune response for the complex processes of wound healing.[12]

An alteration in the skin's integrity is considered a wound and may be caused by injury (including pressure), disease, surgery, or environmental factors.[13] Chronic, recalcitrant or nonhealing wounds represent a significant health, economic, and quality of life burden to individuals as well as to society in general. To review how wounds typically heal, one must examine basic wound and tissue physiology. Partial thickness wounds are shallow wounds involving full or partial epidermal loss and partial loss of the dermal layer. Full thickness wounds involve total loss of both epidermal and dermal layers, extending to at least the subcutaneous tissue layer and possibly as deep as the fascia, muscle layer, and the bone.[12,13]

Phases of Acute Wound Healing

Wound healing, or tissue repair, has been well documented to occur in a sequence of specific events. Inflammation, proliferation, reconstruction, granulation, wound contraction, epithelialization, remodeling, and scar maturation are several generally accepted terms used to describe the phases of acute wound healing.[12,13] The following describes these phases further, and Figure 21-1 illustrates the phases of wound healing.

Injury is when wounding initially occurs, resulting in the stimulation of the inflammatory response. This leads to platelet aggregation and initiation of the coagulation at the wound site. Hemostasis usually takes place very quickly (within minutes) unless damage has occurred to large blood vessels or the individual's clotting mechanisms are impaired. The process of hemostasis includes the breakdown of platelets and release of platelet derived growth factors and proinflammatory cytokines. The commencement of the inflammatory response consequently spurs the aggregations of neutrophils, macrophages, prostaglandins, lymphocytes, cytokines, various enzymes and histamines at the area of injury, and in some cases systemic generation of the same.[11-14] The classic signs of inflammation include rubor, swelling, increase in local temperature, and pain.[15] Rubor is a response of body tissues to injury or irritation that is characterized by pain, swelling, redness, and heat inflammation. The inflammatory phase typically lasts about 4 to 5 days but may be prolonged due to infection, foreign bodies, additional trauma to the wound, chronic comorbid conditions, or other unknown reasons.[10,13] The inflammatory phase leads to tissue reconstruction and the proliferative phase in which fibroblast formation, angiogenesis (growing new capillaries), and the development of granulation tissue occur. This phase also includes wound

FIGURE 21-1 Phases of Wound Healing

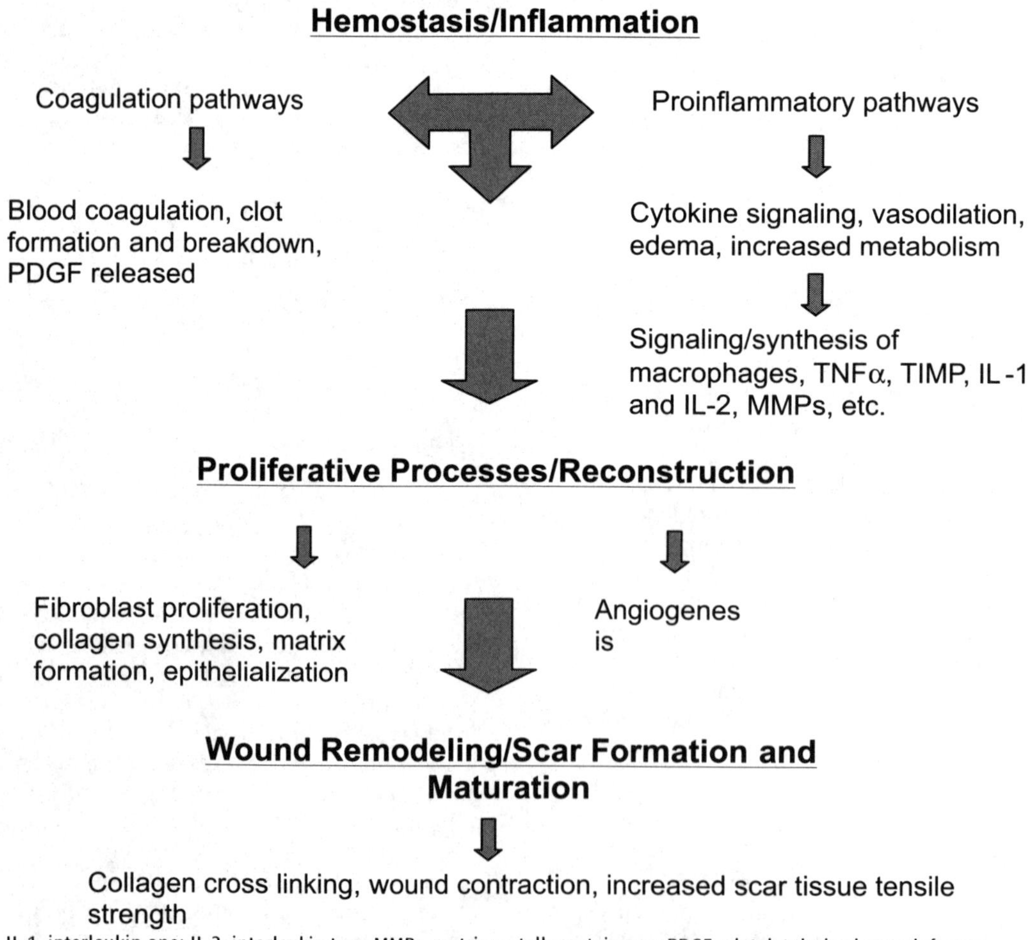

IL-1, interleukin one; IL-2. interleukin two; MMPs, matrix metalloproteinases; PDGF, platelet derived growth factor; TIMP, tissue inhibitors of metalloproteinases; TNFα, tumor necrosis factor alpha.

FIGURE 21-2 Wound Categories

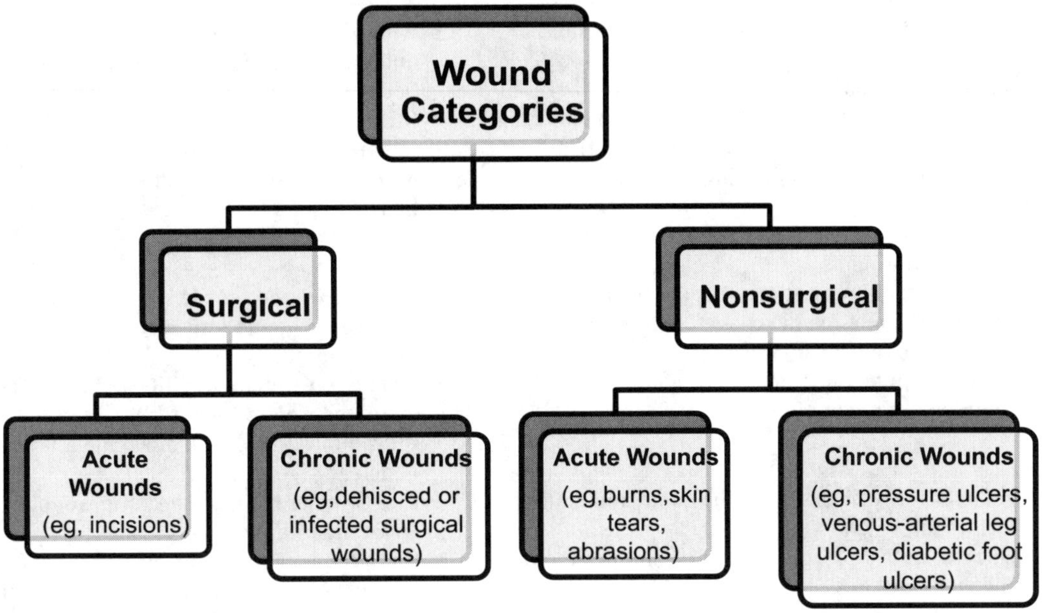

contraction, in which the volume of the wound (wound size in length, width, and depth) decreases. Epithelialization occurs when surface epithelial cells cover the wound and eventually close it. Keratinocytes in various stages of maturity are the key cells in this process. Macrophages release epidermal growth factors, which stimulate the proliferation and migration of these epithelial cells. Remodeling, or scar maturation, is the final stage of wound healing during which collagen fibril cross-linking and scar tissue tensile strength is maximized. Wound contraction continues from the reconstruction phase into the remodeling phase. Maturation may begin approximately 21 days after wounding and may take up to a year to reach maximum potential tensile strength of 80% normal, uninjured tissue.[10–14] Examples of acute and chronic wounds include surgical incision wounds, traumatic burns, and skin tear wounds (Figure 21-2).

At every phase of acute wound healing, nutrients play a critical role.[1–5,16] Research suggests that the body's endogenous supply of amino acids is seldom sufficient to meet the demands that occur in response to injury or metabolic stress.[17] Arginine and glutamine are nitrogen-rich endogenous amino acids that have been shown to play a vital role in normal wound healing.[16–18] Arginine is a precursor for proline, a building block of collagen, as well as a precursor for nitric oxide, and stimulates release of insulin, human growth factor, anabolic hormones, and insulin-like growth factor.[18] Glutamine improves the killing ability of neutrophils, stimulates the release of growth hormone, and provides fuel for lymphocytes, epithelial cells, fibroblasts, and macrophages.[19,20] In addition, glutamine may also play a role in preserving lean muscle mass as an anticatabolic agent.[19,20] Carbohydrates are a major energy source for wound healing. Collagen synthesis uses glucose stores in various ways, and the extracellular matrix is comprised of scaffolding (proteoglycans and glycosaminoglycans) made from polysaccharide chains linked to protein.[13] Macrophages appear to produce lactate as a byproduct of glucose metabolism. Lactate stimulates fibroblast synthesis of collagen, as well as activates specific cellular genetic expression responsible for stimulating factors in vital healing pathways, such as angiogenesis and mitogenesis. Zinc is known to play a role in immune function, but it is also critical for protein synthesis, cell proliferation, cell membrane stabilization, and the production and regulation of matrix metalloproteinases. Copper is a micromineral necessary for erythropoiesis and plays an important role in the hydroxylation of proline and hydroxyproline, which is involved in collagen cross-linking, especially crucial during remodeling, wound contraction, and scar maturation when the tensile strength of the scar tissue will achieve its maximum potential. Table 21-1 reviews the role of micronutrients in wound healing.[21]

Chronic Wounds

Incidence or Prevalence Data on Pressure Ulcers

There are approximately 6 million chronic wounds in the United States annually and 37 million globally.[1,22] The most common chronic wounds include pressure ulcers and lower extremity ulcers including diabetic ulcers, venous ulcers, and arterial ulcers. Additional types of chronic wounds include burns, skin cancers, fistulae, nonhealing surgical wounds, radiation wounds, and dermatitis or vasculitis wounds (Figure 21-2). Chronic wounds may persist for months or years.

Most chronic wounds are pressure ulcers with an estimated 2.5 million cases each year in the United States and 9 million per year worldwide.[1,17] There is a high prevalence of pressure ulcers in hospitals (3% to 14%) and nursing homes (20% to

TABLE 21-1 Role of Micronutrients in Wound Healing

	Function in Wound Healing	Effects of Deficiency
Vitamin A	• Maintains integrity of epithelial and mucosal surfaces • Stimulates fibroblasts, which increases collagen synthesis; cross-linking and remodeling of collagen • Antagonizes inhibitory effects of glucocorticoids	• Widespread alterations in immune function (altered and mucosal surfaces, T and B cell function and antibody response) • Increased risk of infection (diarrheal and respiratory) • Impaired collagen synthesis with delayed wound healing
Vitamin E	• No clear role in wound healing • Antioxidant • Inhibits collagen synthesis, decreases tensile strength of wounds	• No clinically significant effects on wound healing known
Vitamin C	• Required for fibroblast maturation; hydroxylation of proline and lysine in collagen synthesis • Required for angiogenesis • Affects immune function (leukocyte function and complement production)	• Reduced wound tensile strength and increased wound dehiscence due to impaired fibroblast and collagen maturation • Increased capillary fragility and angiogenesis; with increased wound hemorrhage • Old wounds may break down in very severe vitamin C deficiency
Vitamin K	• Cofactor for synthesis of prothrombin and clotting factors VII, IX, and X	• Excessive bleeding can occur in wounds and predispose to wound infection
Iron	• Cofactor in hydroxylation of lysine and proline for collagen synthesis • Oxygen transport to wounded tissue • Component of many enzymes (eg, required in oxidative burst of phagocytosis)	• If low hemoglobin concentration is due to iron deficiency anemia, it may be a factor in tissue hypoxia and impair wound healing if compensatory mechanisms cannot maintain adequate tissue perfusion • Impaired hydroxylation of collagen due to iron deficiency is rarely seen in clinical practice • Impairment of immune response (T cell and phagocytic function)
Zinc	• Component of many enzyme systems (eg, various growth factors, synthesis of fibroblasts, deoxyribonucleic acid and ribonucleic acid) • Affects multiple aspects of immune function • Production of metalloproteinases are zinc dependent	• Impaired wound strength (decreased fibroblast proliferation, collagen synthesis, and rate of epithelialization) • Depressed immunity even in mild deficiency; increased susceptibility to a variety of pathogens

33%) and also a high prevalence of malnutrition (30% to 50% and 19% to 59%, respectively).[1] Pressure ulcer risk factors include malnutrition, weightbearing pressure, shear, friction, old age, immobility, incontinence, and comorbidities including catabolic injury and illness.[1,2,23-27] One longitudinal study found that higher body mass index was associated with lower risk for the development of pressure ulcers.[26] Poor appetite, low intake of protein and calories, or the need for nutrition support (enteral or parenteral) increases the risk for pressure ulcer formation.[24-26] Cost estimates for treating pressure ulcers range from $5000 per year for Stage I to $60,000 or more for Stage IV ulcers.[1]

Diabetic Ulcers, Venous Ulcers, and Other Chronic Wounds

Diabetes affects millions of people around the world. Healing of wounds is impaired in individuals with diabetes. Patients with diabetes are at risk for developing nonhealing diabetic foot ulcers, which are a significant complication of diabetes and can result in lower leg amputations. The treatment of diabetic foot ulcers requires adequate nutrition to stabilize blood sugar levels, proper wound care, prevention and treatment of inflammation and infection, and off loading pressure.[27]

Venous ulcers are common lower limb ulcerations in older adults with a history of deep vein thrombosis and previous surgery for varicose veins. The ulcerations drain moderate amounts of protein-rich exudate and are painful and debilitating. Improved patient outcomes have been achieved by the use of interdisciplinary teams, surgical interventions, compression systems, and adequate nutrition.[10,13]

Etiology of Delayed Healing

Chronic wounds exhibit distinct differences from acute wounds that should be taken into account when considering the nutrition requirements in an individual with a chronic wound.[1,2,4,5,15,23-26] Factors that may contribute to these differences include the presence of a chronic inflammatory state causing catabolic metabolism, frequent protein calorie malnutrition, and dehydration. Increased bioburden and altered keratinocyte function, as well as extracellular matrix degradation, have also been implicated in chronic wounds.[10–13] Bioburden refers to the number of microorganisms present on a contaminated object or in this case in a wound.[13] In addition, the production (or overproduction) of enzymes in the wound fluid of chronic wounds further complicates this process by breaking down the protein-rich collagen and matrix materials that are attempting to close the wound.[8,9]

Nutrition Screening and Assessment

Nutrition screening and assessment should be conducted for individuals at risk or in the presence of a wound.[1,28–30] Initial screening identifies an individual at nutritional risk who may require a referral for a comprehensive nutrition assessment (see Chapter 9). Patients must be screened for pressure ulcer risk on admission to any health care agency and reassessed periodically as their condition changes. The Braden Pressure ulcer risk assessment scale is widely used to screen for pressure ulcer risk in adults in all settings and includes a subscale for nutrition risk.[30]

Once identified, the individual at nutritional risk or with malnutrition is referred to a registered dietitian (RD) to perform a comprehensive nutrition assessment (see Chapter 9) to develop nutrition interventions that are appropriate for each individual's nutrition-related care. The comprehensive nutrition assessment provides a review of all pertinent data including, but not limited to, anthropometric measurements, biochemical data, nitrogen balance, physical examination, and diet history. From this information, nutrition diagnoses or problems are identified, nutrient requirement estimated, and nutrition intervention(s) planned and implemented.

Nutrition Requirements

As previously stated, wound healing is a complex process requiring adequate nutrition for healing to occur.[31–36] The following will address the best clinical advice on the nutritional requirements of those with acute and chronic wounds and also roles of specific nutrient and adequate hydration in the healing of wounds. Table 21-2 presents nutritional requirements recommended for pressure ulcers based on ulcer stage.

Energy Requirements

Adequate energy is essential for optimal wound healing, specifically for cell metabolism, anabolism, collagen formation, nitrogen retention, and angiogenesis.[1,2,4,5,15] Estimated energy needs should be individualized based on age, comorbidities, body weight, activity level, severity and number of wounds, size of the wound(s), stage in the healing process, nutritional state, basal metabolic rate, and level of physiologic stress.[31–39] For example, as one ages, basal energy requirements decrease over time.[37–39] Obesity also requires an individualized nutritional approach because it is an important factor in delayed wound healing.[40,41] Obese patients are at risk for immune incompetence, wound infections, and delayed wound healing. Adipose tissue is associated with poor vascularity to tissues, which can impair blood flow and delivery of essential nutrients to the wound.[40] In critically ill adults, providing adequate energy in hypermetabolic states is often problematic and may require indirect calorimetry for more accurate determination of energy needs.[41]

A common energy prescription guideline for optimal wound healing is 30 to 35 kcal/kg body weight.[42] The National Pressure Ulcer Advisory Panel recommends individuals who are underweight or losing weight to increase their energy goals to 35 to 40 kcal/kg/day to enhance wound healing.[1] Blood glucose control should be maximized for patients with diabetes mellitus or corticosteroid-induced hyperglycemia. Uncontrolled blood glucose is associated with impairment of the production of leukocytes. This has implications for the healing process, risk for infection, and impaired wound healing.[27]

Protein Requirements

Protein is a required structural component for skin integrity, for growth and maintenance of cells, and for fluid and electrolyte balance. Protein plays an essential role in immune system cells responsible for the inflammatory response, fibroblast proliferation, collagen production, and angiogenesis, all of which are necessary for wound healing. Studies indicate that protein deficiency results in delayed wound healing.[43–46] Protein loss associated with acute soft-tissue wounds have been studied and estimations have been determined in practice to plan replacement.[47] For example, the relative loss of nutrients from a Stage I pressure ulcer versus a Stage IV ulcer should be taken into consideration; restoring protein losses that occur in draining wound fluids should be accounted for according to the number, size, and depth of the wound.[48]

The recommended daily allowance (RDA) for protein in healthy adults is 0.8g/kg body weight/day.[49] Older adults ($\geq$ 65 years of age) have an increased protein requirement of 1.0 g/kg body weight/day to maintain a positive nitrogen balance.[50] For individuals with pressure ulcers, the National Pressure Ulcer Advisory Panel recommends 1.25 to 1.5 g/kg body weight per day.[1] Research has shown that increasing protein intakes above RDA enhances pressure ulcer wound healing.[43,44]

Arginine

Arginine is a conditionally essential amino acid produced in the body for cellular metabolism and has been studied extensively as a factor in enhancing wound healing.[17,18] During stress, endogenous stores may be depleted and supplemental sources of arginine may be given.[51] Arginine has been used for protein synthesis, cell signaling through nitric oxide production, stimulation of immune function, and cell proliferation through metabolism to ornithine and polyamines.[52–54] Arginine is also obtained from the diet and enteral tube feeding formulas. In healthy volunteers and rodents, studies have shown that arginine supplementation will enhance wound strength and collagen deposition in artificial incisional wounds.[17,18] However, few studies have focused on chronic wounds and arginine's effectiveness to enhance healing of delayed chronic wounds has not been determined.[52–54]

Recommendations for a safe regimen of arginine supplementation in humans with wounds have not been determined.[55]

TABLE 21-2 Oral/Enteral Nutrition Therapy for Adult Patients with Pressure Ulcers

Stage	Total Calories[a]	Protein[b]	Fluid	RDA/DRI	Vitamin C[c]	Zinc[d]	Vitamin A[e]
STAGE I–II	**Stage I** Maintenance: ≥25 calories/kg **Stage II** Slightly above maintenance: Approximately 28–30 calories/kg	**Stage I** 1–1.2 gm/kg **Stage II** 1.25–1.4 gm/kg	≥ 30 mL/kg with a minimum of 1 mL/kcal or 1500 mL (unless medical limitations [eg, renal or cardiac disease])	If oral/enteral intake inadequate to achieve 100% of RDA/DRI, give multivitamin/mineral supplement daily; all stages: evaluate for deficiency of zinc, and vitamins C and A; replete as needed	100–200 mg vitamin C per day	RDA (8 mg female, 11 mg male) or 15 mg elemental zinc per day; if deficiency is suspected, give up to 220 mg zinc sulfate (50 mg elemental zinc) twice daily for 10–14 days	RDA/DRI daily 700 mcg/d (2310 units) females, 900 mcg/d (3333 units) males; if deficiency is suspected, replete with 10,000–50,000 units daily × 10 days
STAGE III–IV Small, nondraining pressure ulcer	30 calories/kg	1.5 gm/kg	30–40 mL/kg or 1–1.5 mL/kcal with a minimum of 1 mL/kcal or 1500 mL per day; consider fluid losses (eg, fever, draining wounds, stool/ostomy output, air-fluidized beds)	Add multivitamin mineral supplement at RDA/DRI level	Up to 1000–2000 mg/d in divided doses for stressed patients or those at risk of deficiency; reassess after 10–14 days	25–40 mg elemental zinc per day; same as previous if deficiency is suspected	Same as previous; or, if concomitant use of glucocorticoids, consider supplement with 10,000–15,000 units/day × 7 days
STAGE III–IV Large, multiple, and/or draining pressure ulcer(s)	33–35 calories/kg	1.5–2.0 gm/kg					
MAXIMUM	40 calories/kg (eg, patient in anabolic phase with minimal risk of complications from overfeeding)	2.2 gm protein/kg; consider need to replace protein from wound losses or malabsorption	As tolerated to maintain adequate hydration	Multivitamin/mineral supplement twice daily	2000 mg vitamin C per day	If severe deficiency or significant wound/GI losses, give up to 150 mg elemental zinc per day × 2 weeks	25,000–50,000 units vitamin A per day × 10–14 days

The previous guidelines were developed to standardize practice at one facility and have not been validated. Clinical judgment is required to develop a nutrition regimen appropriate for individual patients. Consider the quantity of calories; protein; and vitamins A, C, and zinc provided from **all** sources; and evaluate actual (versus prescribed) intake. The progress of wound healing must be evaluated on a regular/timely basis and consideration should be given to the nutrition regimen to determine if/when changes are appropriate.

[a]**CALORIES** – Conduct indirect calorimetry if feasible or use the most reliable energy equation considering weight (obese, nonobese), severity of illness/comorbid conditions, activity level, and stage in the healing process. "Individuals who are underweight or who have had significant unintentional weight loss may need additional calories to cease weight loss and/or regain lost weight. (Strength of Evidence = C) ERUAP/NPUAP, 2009)."

Maintaining tight glucose control is paramount, given the increased susceptibility to infection associated with hyperglycemia. Consider calories from all sources including dextrose from intravenous fluids and lipid-based medications (eg, propofol).

[b]**PROTEIN** – Use a higher protein enteral formula (24%–25%) or a modular protein supplementation to meet needs. Consider protein losses from draining wounds (eg, negative pressure wound therapy devices). Although nitrogen losses from an open abdominal wound are estimated to be approximately 12.5 g protein per liter of wound drainage (Cheatham, 2007), losses from pressure ulcers may be relatively low (Iizaka, 2010).

ARGININE – There are no evidence-based recommendations to guide the use of arginine supplementation for chronic wounds. Improved markers of collagen synthesis were observed after volunteers received oral arginine supplementation at doses of 17–24.8 g free arginine/day for 2 weeks (Kirk, 1993; Barbul 1990). Preliminary studies using a high-protein oral supplement with arginine and antioxidants show some promise. In addition, enhanced nitrogen retention and immune function have been reported in several but not all studies (Thompson, 2005). Arginine supplementation should be used with caution in patients with severe sepsis (McClave, 2009).

GLUTAMINE – Glutamine appears to play an indirect role in wound healing (eg, fuel source for fibroblasts, epithelial cells, enterocytes, lymphocytes, and macrophages). Supplementation can improve nitrogen balance and attenuate immunosuppression in times of relative deficiency such as catabolic states and elective surgery (Wilmore, 2001). However, glutamine supplementation has not been proven to have a noticeable effect on wound healing (Arnold, 2006). The safe maximum supplemental glutamine dosage for adults is 0.57 gm/kg/day (Ziegler, 1990).

FATS – In one study using an animal model, high-dose supplementation with omega-3 fatty acids delayed wound healing (Albina,1993). The clinical effect of omega-3 fatty acids on human wound healing has not been adequately studied; and their potentially beneficial effects to support immune function and decrease infection rates should also be considered.

[c]**VITAMIN C** – Vitamin C deficiency is known to impair wound healing; however, supplementation of nondeficient patients is unlikely to accelerate wound healing. The current RDA is 75 mg women, 90 mg men with an additional 35 mg/day recommended for smokers; the tolerable upper intake level is 2,000 mg/day. In patients with renal failure, some authorities recommend no more than 100–500 mg/d due to the increased risk of oxalate stone formation and soft tissue damage (Winkler, 2000). Additional research is required to confirm the optimal dosage and populations that would achieve a clinical benefit from vitamin C supplementation.

[d]**ZINC** – Zinc supplementation can enhance wound healing; however, only in those patients who are zinc deficient. Plasma zinc concentrations do not accurately reflect tissue stores during acute injury/illness. Low dose zinc supplementation (15–25 mg elemental zinc/d) is frequently given to patients with pressure ulcers because zinc intakes below the RDA are frequently seen in elderly patients; increased losses can occur from large skin wounds, the GI tract (eg, diarrhea, fistulae output), or urine (after trauma, closed head injury, etc); and a potential for decreased bioavailability. The tolerable upper limit is 40 mg/d. Guidelines for replacement therapy have not been well defined. To treat zinc deficiency in adults, 220 mg zinc sulfate twice daily is often recommended because it is rather insoluble and poorly absorbed from the intestine. Some authors suggest limiting high-dose supplementation to as brief as 2–3 weeks to minimize the risk of adverse effects. Prolonged high-dose zinc supplementation can adversely affect copper status, immune response, and lipid profiles. Note: Parenteral requirements are significantly less than oral/enteral dosage due to differing rates of absorption; and the oral supplement of 220 mg zinc sulfate provides 50 mg elemental zinc.

[e]**VITAMIN A** – Vitamin A supplementation is warranted to help restore wound healing that has been retarded by vitamin A deficiency; and in some patients with diabetes or who receive glucocorticoids, radiation, or chemotherapy (Thompson, 2005; Arnold, 2006). In patients with chronic renal failure, vitamin A supplementation is frequently contraindicated because vitamin A levels are typically high in this population and there is an increased risk of hypercalcemia. The recommended level of supplementation/repletion may exceed the tolerable upper intake limit of 3000 mcg (or ~10,000 units/d) if medically indicated. For patients with fat malabsorption, such as those with advanced liver failure or cystic fibrosis, a water miscible form may be appropriate.

OTHER VITAMINS AND MINERALS – Many nutrients are involved in the wound healing process. Thiamin, riboflavin, and pantothenic acid are involved in collagen production; copper and manganese are required for tissue regeneration; and vitamin K is essential for the synthesis of prothrombin and other clotting factors (Thompson, 2005). However, verification is lacking that a deficiency state would result in a clinically significant effect on wound healing (Albina, 1994). The impact of vitamin E supplementation on wound healing appears to vary with the type of wound. A few studies have shown a possible benefit of vitamin E supplementation in situations such as hyperbaric oxygen therapy, after irradiation, or to minimize ischemia-reperfusion tissue damage. However, supplementation with vitamin E appears to have either no benefit or even a detrimental effect on healing other types of wounds, such as surgical wounds. In animal studies, supplementation with vitamin E delayed wound healing by retarding collagen synthesis and decreasing wound tensile strength. Further research is needed to address the potential risks and benefits of vitamin E and other antioxidants in wound healing.

Selected References:

- Academy of Nutrition and Dietetics. Nutrition for spinal cord injured patients with pressure ulcers. http://adaevidencelibrary.com http://www.adaevidencelibrary.com/template.cfm?template=guide_summary&key=2378.
- Albina JE. Nutrition and wound healing. *JPEN J Parenter Enteral Nutr.* 1994;18:367–376.
- Albina JE, Gladden P, Walsh WR. Detrimental effects of an omega-3 fatty acid-enriched diet on wound healing. *JPEN J Parenter Enteral Nutr.* 1993;17:519–521.
- Arnold M, Barbul A. Nutrition and wound healing. *Plast Reconstr Surg.* 2006;117(Suppl):425.
- Barbul A, Lazarou S, Efron DT, et al. Arginine enhances wound healing and lymphocyte immune responses in humans. *Surgery.* 1990;108(2):331–337.
- Cheatham ML, Safcsak K, Brzezinski SJ, Lube MW. Nitrogen balance, protein loss and the open abdomen. *Crit Care Med.* 2007;35:127–131.
- Dorner B, Posthauer ME, Thomas D, National Pressure Ulcer Advisory Panel. The role of nutrition in pressure ulcer prevention and treatment: National Pressure Ulcer Advisory Panel White Paper 2009. http://www.npuap.org/Nutrition%20White%20Paper%20Website%20Version.pdf.
- Ellinger S, Stehle P. Efficacy of vitamin supplementation in situations with wound healing disorders: results from clinical intervention studies. *Curr Opin Clin Nutr Metab Care.* 2009;12:588–595.
- European Pressure Ulcer Advisory Panel and National Pressure Ulcer Advisory Panel. *Treatment of Pressure Ulcers: Quick Reference Guide.* Washington, DC: National Pressure Ulcer Advisory Panel; 2009. http://www.epuap.org
- Hunt TK, Hopf HW. Wound healing and wound infection: what surgeons and anesthesiologists can do. *Surg Clin North Am.* 1997;77:587–606.
- Iizaka S, Sanada H, Nakagami G, et al. Estimation of protein loss from wound fluid in older patients with severe pressure ulcers. *Nutrition.* 2010;16:890–895.
- Kirk SJ, Hurson M, Regan MC, et al. Arginine stimulates wound healing and immune function in elderly human beings. *Surgery.* 1993;114(2):155–160.
- McClave SA, Martindale RG, Vanek VW, et al. Guidelines for the provision and assessment of nutrition support therapy in the adult critically ill patient: Society of Critical Care Medicine (SCCM) and American Society for Parenteral and Enteral Nutrition (A.S.P.E.N.) *JPEN J Parenter Enteral Nutr.* 2009; 33(3):277–316.
- National Academy of Sciences. Institute of Medicine. Food and Nutrition Board. Dietary Reference Intakes: Recommended Intakes for Individuals http://www.iom.*edu*/Activities/Nutrition/SummaryDRIs/~/media/Files/Activity%20Files/Nutrition/DRIs/5_Summary%20Table%20Tables%201-4.pdf.
- Stechmiller JK. Understanding the role of nutrition and wound healing. *Nutr Clin Pract.* 2010;25:61–68.
- Thompson CW, Fuhrman MP. Nutrients and wound healing – still searching for the magic bullet. *Nutr Clin Pract.* 2005;20:331–347.
- Wilmore DW. The effect of glutamine supplementation in patients following elective surgery and accidental injury. *J Nutr.* 2001;131(suppl):2543S–2549S.
- Winkler MR. Inquire here. *Support Line.* 2000;22:20–21.
- Zielger TR, Benfell K, Smith RJ, et al. Safety and metabolic effects of L-glutamine administration in humans. *JPEN J Parenter Enteral Nutr.* 1990;14(suppl 4):137S–146S.

Adapted with permission from the Intermountain Medical Center's Nutrition Support Service, Murray UT. The above guidelines have not been validated but were compiled from a literature review to assist with standardizing clinical practice. They are to be used along with the text information provided to develop a nutrition regimen appropriate for individual patients.

The use of oral arginine supplementation in elderly with pressure ulcers has been evaluated using 17 g free arginine as an intervention.[53,54]

Other Amino Acid Supplements

One study has examined the effect of B-hydroxy B-methylbutyrate (HMB), a metabolite of leucine, on wound healing, based on the theory that HMB may increase collagen formation, modulate protein utilization, and inhibit muscle breakdown.[56] In a study of two groups of healthy elderly humans, one group was given an oral supplement consisting of 3 g HMB, 14 g arginine, and 14 g glutamine, and the other an isonitrogenous control diet. After 14 days, an increase in collagen deposition was found in the supplemented group.[56]

Several additional amino acids may enhance wound healing. Cysteine is a cofactor for enzyme systems involved in collagen formation. Methionine is necessary for collagen formation and fibroblast proliferation. Lysine and proline are precursors of collagen.[31] However, no randomized clinical trials have examined the effect of dietary supplementation of these amino acids on wound healing.

Glutamine serves as a fuel source for enterocytes, lymphocytes, fibroblasts, epithelial cells, and macrophages. As such, it plays an important role in wound healing.[31] Research indicates, but does not confirm, that supplementation can enhance immune function in elective surgery and in catabolic states.[19] The current maximum recommended dosage of supplemental glutamine for adults is 0.57g/kg/day.[20]

Fatty Acids

Lipid is an essential nutrient that is a dense source of energy, provides essential fatty acids, and acts as a carrier for fat-soluble vitamins (vitamins A, D, E, and K). However, the role of essential fatty acids in wound healing has not received sufficient study to yield definitive recommendations.[57,58] Omega-3 fatty acids have been shown to affect proinflammatory cytokine production, gene expression, cell metabolism, and angiogenesis in the wound bed.[59,60] Albina et al. supplemented rats with omega-3 fatty acids for 3 weeks prior to wounding and 10 to 30 days post wounding and found that excessive supplementation of omega-3 fatty acids impairs wound healing.[61] Recommendations for the use of specific fatty acids for the healing of wounds remain obscure given the inconsistencies reported in the literature.

Hydration

Adequate hydration contributes to good skin turgor, perfusion, and oxygenation of healthy and wounded tissues.[1,4,5] Furthermore, maintaining normal fluid status is an important factor in prevention and treatment of skin breakdown.[1,4,5] Dehydration, on the other hand, impairs oxygen delivery to wounded tissues.[1,4,5] Oxygen is necessary for hydroxylation of lysine and proline during the formation of collagen.[57] Research indicates that in a state of hypoxia, the healing of acute wounds is impaired.[58]

Two general guidelines for daily fluid intake are (1) 30mL/kg body weight or (2) 1.0 to 1.5 mL/kcal consumed.[32] Patients experiencing increased fluid losses due to evaporation of fluids from severe pressure ulcers, draining wounds, open wounds, persistent diarrhea and/or vomiting, diuresis, fever, sweating, mechanical ventilation, and other causes of fluid losses require judicious monitoring of fluid status.

Vitamins, Minerals, and Other Micronutrients

Vitamin A

Vitamin A acts as a stimulant of the immune system and may be important during the inflammatory phase of wound healing by increasing the number of macrophages and monocytes in the wound environment.[62–65] In addition, vitamin A maintains the integrity of mucosal and epithelial surfaces, enhances epithelization, increases collagen formation, and inhibits the detrimental effects of glucosteroids, chemotherapy, radiation, diabetes, and excessive vitamin E supplementation on wound healing.[63–72] Deficiency results in impaired wound healing and alterations in immune function that may increase the likelihood of wound infections.[32,72–78]

The recommendation for vitamin A is 900 retinol activity equivalents for men and 700 for women per day.[75] In international units, this is approximately 3000 IU and 2300 IU, respectively.[75] The recommended amount of vitamin A for enhanced wound healing in injured patients is 25,000 to 50,000 IU per day orally.[74] For individuals receiving steroids, vitamin A doses of 10,000 to 15,000 IU/day for 1 week are recommended prophylactically to counteract the anti-inflammatory effects of steroid therapy and immune suppression.[78,79] Animal studies have shown that high doses of vitamin A increase the tensile strength of wound tissue and reverse the anti-inflammatory effect of steroids.[80] Studies have also shown that vitamin A supplementation in combination with glucocorticoid administration in immunosuppressed animals with renal or skin allografts did not affect the graft healing outcomes.[81–83] Beta carotene is a precursor of vitamin A and is found in some dietary supplements. Animal research has implicated the efficacy of beta carotene in restoring wound strength in rats also given steroids. However, effectiveness of beta carotene in human wound healing and recommended dosage has not been established.

Symptoms of vitamin A toxicity include dryness of the mucous membranes, vomiting, headache, liver damage, alopecia, muscle or bone pain, bleeding, and coma.[84,85] Patients with abnormal liver function or malnutrition need special attention because toxicity may occur in this group; vitamin A is stored in the liver and its transport is protein dependent.[21] Renal failure also places patients at high risk for vitamin A toxicity, and levels and supplementation measures should be monitored closely.[32] Infections, malnutrition, and other metabolic conditions may alter plasma vitamin A concentrations. The best evaluation of retinol status is a liver biopsy, which is not realistic in the majority of cases. Vitamin A supplementation should be done cautiously and judiciously (Table 21-1).[32]

Vitamin C

Vitamin C is an essential water-soluble nutrient known to enhance normal wound healing. Vitamin C functions as a cofactor in the hydroxylation of proline and lysine in collagen formation. Vitamin C is also required for angiogenesis and fibroblast formation and acts on immune function, specifically neutrophil activity, which aids in preventing wound infections.[86,87] Vitamin C deficiency has been associated with delayed wound healing. The recommendation to prevent scurvy is 10 to 20 mg/day; for nonsmokers, the recommendation is 75 mg/day for women and 90 mg/day for men.[88,89] In patients with vitamin C deficiency, supplementation has been shown to enhance wound healing. However, vitamin C supplementation in nondeficient individuals has not been proven to enhance wound healing. High doses of vitamin C supplementation for wound healing of chronic wounds may be problematic in patients at risk for kidney stones. Current guidelines for patients with renal failure recommend giving no more than 60 to 100 mg vitamin C per day due to the risk of renal oxalate stone formation.[90–92]

Vitamin E

Vitamin E is an antioxidant that has no clear role in healing of acute or chronic wounds. However, some speculation suggests that the antioxidant properties of vitamin E may play a role during the inflammatory phase of wound healing. Some research has determined that vitamin E supplementation, given in conjunction with hyperbaric oxygen therapy, improves skin flap survival.[93] Vitamin E supplementation also appears to limit the degree of impairment in wound breaking strength that occurs following irradiation therapy.[94,95] In addition, vitamin E supplementation may also minimize ischemia-reperfusion tissue damage, which may have implications for pressure ulcer healing.[96] Many individuals take supplemental vitamin E above the dietary reference intake (DRI) for presumed antioxidant benefits. However, supplementation has been shown to inhibit collagen formation and to decrease the tensile strength of acute surgical wounds resulting in delayed wound healing.[95] Further research is needed in humans using controlled randomized trials to determine the risks and benefits of various doses of vitamin E and the effect on wound healing.

Zinc

Zinc is an essential trace mineral necessary for cell replication and growth; it is a cofactor for collagen and other wound protein synthesis.[6,7] Zinc supplementation is recommended only for patients with zinc deficiencies.[68] Serum concentration of zinc may not be a reliable indicator to reflect total body status. For patients with normal levels of zinc, supplementation offers no benefit and may result in zinc toxicity.[76] Zinc toxicity can have adverse effects on wound healing and the immune system. Impaired neutrophil and lymphocyte function has been observed in men receiving 150 mg of oral, elemental zinc twice a day for 6 weeks.[6] Excess zinc is associated with copper and calcium-binding interactions that reduce availability of these nutrients for wound healing.[7] Excess zinc supplementation can lead to gastrointestinal tract irritation resulting in nausea, vomiting, and diarrhea.[76]

Zinc deficiencies are associated with delayed wound healing due to decreased collagen and protein synthesis, and impaired immune competence.[97,98] Zinc deficiencies are commonly seen in patients with diarrhea, malabsorption, or in hypermetabolic states (stressed, sepsis, burns, venous ulcers, or seriously injured).[99–102] The DRI for zinc is 11 mg/day for men and 8 mg/day for women.[75] However, zinc sulfate 220 mg daily has been used as a standard adult oral replacement dose because zinc is rather insoluble and difficult to absorb. It should be noted that guidelines for replacement therapy have not been well defined in the literature. For patients receiving parenteral nutrition, the recommended dose is 2.5 to 4 mg zinc/day for noncatabolic states and 4.5 to 6.0 mg zinc/day for severely injured patients. For individuals with small intestinal fluid loss, an additional 12.2 mg zinc per liter of fluid loss and 17.1 mg zinc per kilogram of stool output or ileostomy drainage is recommended.[76,102] In severe deficiency states, zinc supplements can be continuously infused over 24 hours at 50 to 100 mg per day if well tolerated; close monitoring of response is recommended.

Other Micronutrients

There is limited information regarding deficiency of other vitamins and minerals required for wound healing (Table 21-2). Adequate levels of copper and manganese are required for tissue regeneration.[103–105] Adequate levels of manganese are responsible for collagen and ground substance synthesis. Adequate levels of iron, riboflavin, thiamin, and pantothenic acid contribute to the formation of collagen.[104,105]

Nutrition Support

The goals for nutritional support for individuals with chronic wounds are to restore and/or maintain adequate nutritional status, enhance wound healing and immune function, and reduce susceptibility to wound infection.[1–5] Nutritional interventions are based on a thorough nutritional assessment in concert with a skin risk assessment that includes determining the severity of the wounds, and the size and staging of any pressure ulcers that may be present.

Early recognition of a depleted nutritional state and an aggressive nutritional regimen may help prevent delays in pressure ulcer wound healing.[1,106–112] Strategies to increase oral intake are of paramount importance. This includes giving protein and energy dense nutritional supplements to provide energy at 35 kcal/kg/day and 1.5 g/kg/day protein with DRI of micronutrients.[1] One study showed that giving an oral supplement of 254 kcal and 20 g of protein in the evening may reduce nutritional risk, prevent pressure ulcers, and provide significantly better clinical outcomes in older patients.[107] Other evidence suggests that nutritional interventions can have a positive effect on chronic pressure ulcer healing.[1,3,4,36] Increasing protein intake either through protein supplements, sip feedings, or conventional food showed a beneficial effect on the healing rate.[36] Research suggests that nutritional interventions show little effect in preventing pressure ulcer formation

FIGURE 21-3 Process of Care for Patient and Wound Healing Assessment

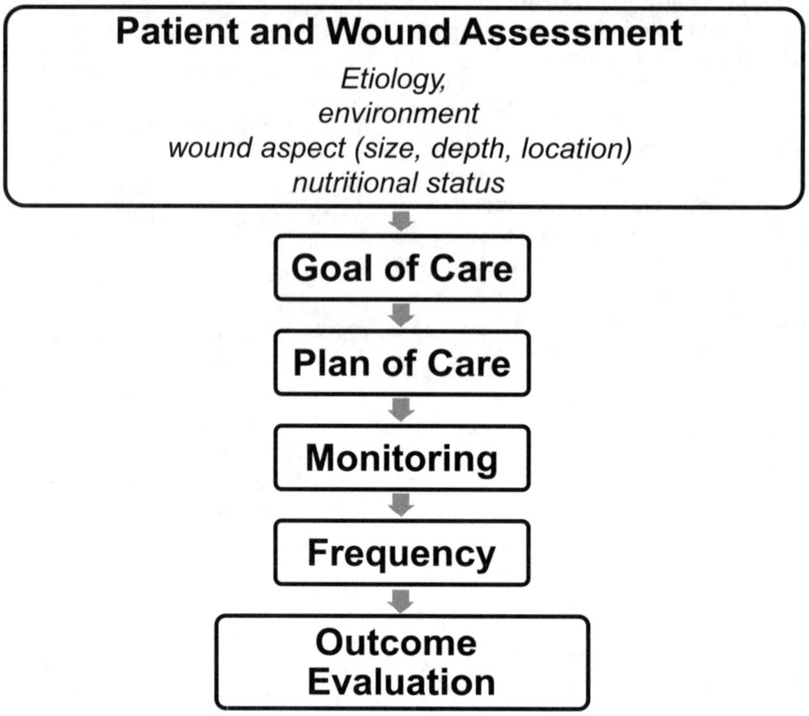

in individuals with cachexia when compared to an underfed state.[108–113] In acutely ill older patients, adding two oral supplements of 200 kcal each to an 1800 kcal hospital diet resulted in a tendency for fewer pressure ulcers to occur.[113]

Enteral nutrition formulas that are recommended for promoting wound healing are energy dense, are high in protein, and provide DRI levels of micronutrients. Formulas fortified with arginine, glutamine, vitamins A and C, zinc, and omega-3 fatty acids are also available, but their efficacy is somewhat controversial, as previously discussed. Enteral feedings should be considered for those individuals who cannot meet their nutritional goals orally.[111] Further research using randomized trials is needed to determine nutritional needs of patients with specific types of chronic wounds.

Monitoring of Wound Healing and Outcomes

Regular assessment of the wound (ie, monitoring) is necessary to determine the effectiveness of care and clinical outcomes including the progression of tissue granulation formation, changes in wound size and depth, and eventual wound closure and healing. Outcomes of care are based on a complete patient history, assessment, and regular follow-up assessments.[13] The patient and wound should be monitored for signs of improvement, infection, or complications, and a complete wound assessment should be performed to determine progress. Realistic and clearly defined goals of care help achieve the desired outcome. Figure 21-3 outlines the process of patient and wound assessment, development of goals, plan of care, and monitoring with outcomes and evaluation.[114]

The first step in the assessment process is to classify the wound (Figure 21-2). Two categories of wounds are commonly used related to the cause: surgical or nonsurgical, and whether the wound is chronic or acute. The goals of therapy are different for these two types of wounds. Superficial or partial thickness wounds are expected to heal in less time when compared to deeper full thickness wounds that are associated with complications. There are wound classification systems for lower limb chronic wounds. For example, diabetic and venous ulcers are graded according to clinical signs, etiologic classification, anatomic distribution, and depth. A wound assessment and monitoring model considers close evaluation of the wound bed, size, wound edges, and surrounding skin.[14] A recommended approach for wound bed assessment is the TIME acronym: *tissue* characteristics, *i*nfection, *m*oisture, and *e*dges of the wound described elsewhere.[14] This approach is widely used in the clinical setting as a helpful guide for including all aspects of the wound bed in monitoring wound healing.

Throughout the process and progress of wound healing, nutritional adequacy as previously described is requisite for tissue granulation, reduction in wound size and depth, and wound closure. Practice Scenarios 21-1 and 21-2 discuss the approach to nutrition support in the healing of chronic wounds (pressure ulcers) and acute wounds (surgical wound).

Practice Scenario 21-1

Question: What are the protein and energy recommendations for Stage II and Stage III pressure ulcers in a nutritionally depleted elderly patient?

Scenario: A 72-year-old female is admitted to the hospital with a history of hypertension, decompensated congestive heart failure, and dysphagia due to a stroke. On admission her height was 5′3″ and weight was 104 lbs with a Braden scale score of 14. A swallow evaluation by the speech pathologist was completed on day 2 and tube feeding was initiated the same day. Based on the hospital tube feeding protocol, the tube feeding was progressed to goal rate as designated by the RD. On day 3, a Stage II pressure ulcer was observed on her coccyx. On day 5, a Stage III coccyx pressure ulcer (4 cm × 5 cm × 6 cm) was observed with exudates consisting of moderate amounts of serous drainage from the wound. The wound bed was covered with yellow slough, and a tissue culture revealed a wound infection with gram-negative organisms.

Intervention: The RD determined that the tube feeding order met the estimated needs for the patient, but the tube feeding was held for presumed elevated gastric residuals, when these residuals were below the hospital threshold of 250 mL. This resulted in inadequate nutrient infusion based on the recommended amounts for wound healing indicated in this chapter and the following. The RD reviewed this finding with the physician and nursing staff and completed a 2-day calorie count to determine the adequacy of the actual nutrient infusion. Nursing was reminded that the tube feeding need not be held for gastric residuals less than 250 mL (see Chapter 13).

Answer: A chronic wound with an active infection results in increased physiological stress that would increase dietary protein needs.[10–13] Age, immobility, and chronic disease states such as congestive heart failure and diabetes are all risk factors for protein calorie malnutrition. In the older adult with a traumatic injury this is a challenge, particularly because it is difficult to orally deliver the amount of calories and nutrients needed to promote nutritional well-being and to prevent and treat pressure ulcers. This will be accomplished by the following:

- Provide 30 kcal/kg/day
- Provide 1.2 to 1.5 g protein/kg/day
- Ensure 100% of the RDA of vitamins and minerals; supplementation of micronutrients and other amino acids not known to accelerate healing of pressure ulcers
- Provide adequate hydration (30 mL/kg)
- Monitor nutritional status and individualize nutritional care plan as appropriate (Table 21-2)[1]

The goals for nutritional support for individuals with pressure ulcers are to restore and/or maintain adequate nutritional status, enhance wound healing and immune function, and reduce susceptibility to wound infection.[1,28–30]

Practice Scenario 21-2

Question: What are the recommendations for micronutrients in a patient with an acute surgical wound?

Scenario: A 78-year-old male with chronic obstructive pulmonary disease was admitted to the surgical intensive care unit following prostate surgery. Despite spontaneous breathing trials each morning, the patient was unable to be weaned from the ventilator. Enteral nutrition was initiated on day 3 due to the concern for prolonged inability to resume oral feedings, with patient failing weaning trials and the need for adequate nutrients for surgical wound healing.

Intervention: The patient was started on enteral nutrition based on the nutrition assessment, including a multivitamin once daily. The RDA for protein in healthy adults is 0.8g/kg body weight/day.[49] The RD determined the additional nutrient needs for wound healing, documented the information in the medical record, and obtained the order from the physician.

Answer: A surgical patient intubated postoperatively with acute wounds and comorbidities has increased requirements for protein and calories.

Rationale: A common energy prescription guideline for optimal wound healing is 30 to 35 kcal/kg body weight.[42] Older adults (≥ 65 years of age) have an increased protein requirement of 1.0 g/kg body weight/day to maintain a positive nitrogen balance.[50] The optimal micronutrient intake to promote wound healing is unknown. What is known is that all nutrients potentially are important to wound healing; energy, protein, arginine, water, and vitamins A, C, and E and minerals play a critical role in the process of wound healing, as discussed in the chapter.

References

1. National Pressure Ulcer Advisory Panel. www.npuap.org. Accessed June 5, 2011.
2. Horn SD, Bender SA, Ferguson ML, et al. The national pressure ulcer long-term care study: pressure ulcer development in long-term care residents. *J Am Geriatr Soc.* 2004;52:359–367.
3. Stratton RJ, Ek AC, Engfer M, et al. Enteral nutritional support in prevention and treatment of pressure ulcers: a systematic review and meta-analysis. *Ageing Res Rev.* 2005;4:422–450.
4. Posthauer ME, Dorner B, Collins N. Nutrition: a critical component of wound healing. *Adv Skin Wound Care.* 2010;23(12):560–572.
5. Stechmiller JK. Understanding the role of nutrition and wound healing. *Nutr Clin Pract.* 2010;25(1):61–68.
6. Chandra RK. Excessive intake of zinc impairs immune responses. *JAMA.* 1984;252:1443–1446.
7. Lansdown AB. Zinc in the healing wound. *Lancet.* 1996;347:706–707.
8. Stechmiller JK, Kilpadi D, Childress B, et al. Effect of vacuum-assisted closure therapy on the expression of cytokines and proteases in wound fluid of adults with pressure ulcers. *Wound Repair Regen.* 2006;14(3):371–374.
9. Trengove NJ, Stacey MC, MacAuley S, et al. Analysis of the acute and chronic wound environments: the role of proteases and their inhibitors. *Wound Repair Regen.* 1999;7(6):442–452.
10. Jones V, Harding K, Stechmiller JK, et al. Acute and chronic wound healing. In: Baranoski S, Ayello E, eds. *Wound Care Essentials: Practice Principles.* 3rd ed. Baltimore, MD: Wolters Kluwer, Lippincott Williams & Wilkins; 2012:83–100.
11. Schultz GS, Sibbald RG, Falanga V, et al. Wound bed preparation: a systematic approach to wound management. *Wound Repair Regen.* 2003;11(suppl 1):S1–28.
12. Wysocki AB. Skin anatomy, physiology, and pathophysiology. *Nurs Clin North Am.* 1999; 34(4):777–797.
13. Cowan L, Stechmiller JK, Phillips P, et al. Science of wound healing: translation of bench science into advances for chronic wound care. In Krasner D, Sibbald G, Rodeheaver G, eds. *Chronic Wound Care: A Clinical Source Book for Healthcare Professionals.*

5th ed. King of Prussia, PA: Health Management Publications; In Press.
14. Chin GA, Diegelmann RF, Schultz GS. Cellular and molecular regulation of wound healing. *Wound Heal.* 2005;14:17–39.
15. Wild T, Rahbarnia A, Kellner M, et al. Basics in nutrition and wound healing. *Nutrition.* 2010;26:862–866.
16. Stechmiller JK, Childress B, Cowan L. Arginine supplementation and wound healing. *Nutr Clin Pract.* 2005;20:52–61.
17. Barbul A, Lazarou S, Efron DT, et al. Arginine enhances wound healing and lymphocyte immune responses in humans. *Surgery.* 1990;108:331–337.
18. Kavalukas S, Barbul A. Nutrition and wound healing: an update. *Plast Reconstr Surg.* 2010;38S–43S.
19. Wilmore DW. The effect of glutamine supplementation in patients following elective surgery and accidental injury. *J Nutr.* 2001; 131(suppl):S2543–S2549.
20. Ziegler TR, Benfell K, Smith RJ, et al. Safety and metabolic effects of L-glutamine administration in humans. *J Parenter Enteral Nutr.* 1990;14(suppl 4):137S–146S.
21. Doley J. Nutrition management of pressure ulcers. *Nutr Clin Pract.* 2010;25:50–57.
22. *World Wound Care Markets 2008*. New York: Kalorama Information; 2008.
23. Mathus-Vliegen EH. Old age, malnutrition, and pressure sores: an ill-fated alliance. *J Gerontol.* 2004;4:355–360.
24. Mathus-Vliegen EM. Nutrition status, nutrition and pressure ulcers. *Nutr Clin Pract.* 2001;16:286–291.
25. Thomas DR. Improving outcome of pressure ulcers with nutrition interventions: a review of the evidence. *Nutrition.* 2001;17: 121–125.
26. Berlowitz DR, Brandeis GH, Morris JN, et al. Deriving a risk-adjustment model for pressure ulcer development using the Minimum Data Set. *J Am Geriatr Soc.* 2001;49:866–871.
27. Guo S, DiPietro LA. Factors affecting wound healing. *J Dental Res.* 2010;89:223–229.
28. Stechmiller JK, Cowan L, Whitney JD, et al. Guidelines for pressure ulcer prevention. *Wound Repair Regen.* 2008;151–168.
29. Thomas DR. Nutritional assessment in long-term care. *Nutr Clin Pract.* 2008;23:383–387.
30. Braden B. The Braden scale for predicting pressure sore risk. www.bradenscale.com/images/bradenscale.pdf. Accessed October 17, 2011.
31. Gordon MD, Gottschlich M, Helvig EI, et al. Review of evidence-based practice for the prevention of pressure sores in burn patients. *J Burn Care Rehabil.* 2004;25:388–410.
32. Thompson C, Fuhrman M. Nutrients and wound healing: still searching for the magic bullet. *Nutr Clin Pract.* 2005;20:331–347.
33. Langer G, Schloemer G, Knerr A, et al. Nutritional interventions for preventing and treating pressure ulcers. *Cochrane Database Syst Rev.* 2003;(4):CD003216.
34. van Anholt RD, Sobotka L, Meijer EP, et al. Specific nutritional support accelerates pressure ulcer healing and reduces wound care intensity in non-malnourished patients. *Nutrition.* 2010;26: 867–872.
35. Fuhrman MP. Wound healing and nutrition. *Top Clin Nutr.* 2003; 18:100–110.
36. Schols JM, Jager de-van den Ende MA. Nutrition intervention in pressure ulcer guidelines: an inventory. *Nutrition.* 2004;20:548–553.
37. Chernoff R. Normal aging, nutritional assessment, and clinical practice. *Nutr Clin Pract.* 2003;18:12–20.
38. Shock NW, Greulich RC, Andres R, et al. *Normal Human Aging: The Baltimore Longitudinal Study of Aging.* NIH publication 82-2450. Baltimore, MD: USDHHS Public Health Service; 1984.
39. McGandy R, Barrows CH, Spanias A, et al. Nutrient intakes and energy expenditures in men of different ages. *J Gerontol.* 1966;21: 581–587.
40. Gottschlich MM, Mayes T, Khoury JC, et al. Significance of obesity on nutritional, immunologic, hormonal and clinical outcome parameters in burns. *J Am Diet Assoc.* 1993;93:1261–1268.
41. Frankenfield D, Roth-Yousey L, Compher C. Comparison of predictive equations for resting metabolic rate in healthy nonobese and obese adults: a systematic review. *J Am Dietetic Assoc.* 2005; 105(5):775–789.
42. Bergstrom N, Bennett MA, Carlson CE, et al. *Treatment of Pressure Ulcers: Clinical Practice Guideline,* No. 15. Rockville, MD: US Department of Health and Human Services, Public Health Service, Agency for Health Care Policy and Research; 1994.
43. Chernoff RS, Milton KY, Lipschitz DA. The effect of a very high-protein liquid formula (Replete) on decubitus ulcer healing in long-term tube fed institutionalized patients [abstract]. *J Am Diet Assoc.* 1990;90:A-130.
44. Breslow RA, Hallfrisch J, Guy DG, et al. The importance of dietary protein in healing pressure ulcers. *J Am Geriatr Soc.* 1993;41: 357–362.
45. Mora RJ. Malnutrition: organic and functional consequences. *World J Surg.* 1999;23:530–535.
46. Doweiko JP, Nompleggi DJ. The role of albumin in human physiology and pathophysiology. Part III: albumin and disease states. *J Parenter Enteral Nutr.* 1991;15:476–483.
47. Waxman K, Rebello T, Pinderski L, et al. Protein loss across burn wounds and for acute soft tissue wounds. *J Trauma.* 1987;27: 136–140.
48. Hourigan LA, Hourigan L, Linfoot JA, et al. Loss of protein, immunoglobulins, and electrolytes in exudates from negative pressure wound therapy. *Nutr Clin Pract.* 2010;25(5):510–516.
49. National Research Council. *Recommended Dietary Allowances.* 10th ed. Washington, DC: The National Academies Press; 1989.
50. Goldberg JP, Smith JA, Economos C. Dietary management of the "old-old": an individualized approach. *Nutr Clin Care.* 1998;1: 126–137.
51. Heyland DK, Dhaliwal R, Drover JW, et al., Canadian Critical Care Practice Guidelines Committee. Canadian clinical practice guidelines for nutrition support in mechanically ventilated, critically ill adult patients. *J Parenter Enteral Nutr.* 2003;27:355–373.
52. Desneves KJ, Todorovic BE, Cassar A, et al. Treatment with supplementary arginine, vitamin C and zinc in patients with pressure ulcers: a randomized controlled trial. *Nutr Clin Care.* 2005;24: 979–987.
53. Langkamp-Henken B, Herrlinger-Garcia KA, Stechmiller JK, et al. Arginine supplementation is well tolerated but does not enhance mitogen-induced lymphocyte proliferation in elderly nursing home residents with pressure ulcers. *J Parenter Enteral Nutr.* 2000; 24:280–287.
54. Stechmiller JK, Langkamp-Henken B, Childress B, et al. Arginine supplementation does not enhance serum nitric oxide levels in elderly nursing home residents with pressure ulcers. *Biol Res Nurs.* 2005;6(4):289–299.
55. Langer G, Schloemer G, Knerr A, et al. Nutritional interventions for preventing and treating pressure ulcers. *Cochrane Database of Syst Rev.* 2007;(1).
56. Williams JZ, Abumrad N, Barbul A. Effect of specialized amino acid mixture on human collagen deposition. *Ann Surg.* 2002;236: 369–375.
57. Ahn C, Mulligan P, Salcido RS. Smoking—the bane of wound healing: biomedical interventions and social influences. *Adv Skin Wound Care.* 2008;21:227–238.

58. Pai MP, Hunt TK. Effect of varying oxygen tensions on healing of open wounds. *Surg Gyecol Obstet.* 1972;135:756–758.
59. McDaniel JC, Belury M, Ahijevych K, et al. Omega-3 fatty acids effect on wound healing. *Wound Repair Regen.* 2008;16:337–345.
60. Shingel KI, Faure MP, Azoulay L, et al. Solid emulsion gel as a vehicle for delivery of polyunsaturated fatty acids: implications for tissue repair, dermal angiogenesis and wound healing. *J Tissue Eng Regen Med.* 2008;2:383–393.
61. Albina JE, Gladden P, Walsh WR. Detrimental effects of an omega-3 fatty acid-enriched diet on wound healing. *J Parenter Enteral Nutr.* 1993;17:519–521.
62. Burgess C. Topical vitamins. *J Drugs Dermatol.* 2008;7(suppl 7):S2–6.
63. Conner MJ. Retinoid stimulation of epidermal differentiation in vivo. *Life Sci.* 1986;38:1807–1812.
64. Demetriou AA, Levenson SM, Rettura G, et al. Vitamin A and retinoic acid: induced fibroblast differentiation in vitro. *Surgery.* 1985;98:931–934.
65. Niu XT, Cushin B, Reisner A, et al. Effect of dietary supplementation with vitamin A on arterial healing in rats. *J Surg Res.* 1987;42:61–65.
66. Wicke C, Halliday B, Allen D, et al. Effects of steroids and retinoids on wound healing. *Arch Surg.* 2000;135:1265–1270.
67. Ulland AE, Shearer JD, Coulter C, et al. Altered wound arginine metabolism by corticosterone and retinoic acid. *J Surg Res.* 1997; 70:84–88.
68. Levenson SM, Gruber CA, Rettura G, et al. Supplemental vitamin A prevents the acute radiation-induced defect in wound healing. *Ann Surg.* 1984;200:494–512.
69. Weinzweig J, Levenson SM, Rettura G, et al. Supplemental vitamin A prevents the tumor-induced defect in wound healing. *Ann Surg.* 1990;211:269–276.
70. Seifter E, Rettura G, Padawer J, et al. Impaired wound healing in streptozotocin diabetes: prevention by supplemental vitamin A. *Ann Surg.* 1981;194:42–49.
71. Anstead GM. Steroids, retinoids, and wound healing. *Adv Wound Care.* 1998;11:277–285.
72. Gerber LE, Erdman JW. Effect of dietary retinyl acetate, β-carotene and retinoic acid on wound healing in rats. *J Nutr.* 1982;112: 1555–1564.
73. The National Academies Press. Dietary reference intakes. http://nap.edu. Accessed June 8, 2011.
74. Gottschlich MM. Fat soluble vitamins in wound healing. In: Molnar JA, ed. *Nutrition and Wound Healing.* Boca Raton, FL: CRC Press; 2007:149–171.
75. Standing Committee on the Scientific Evaluation of Dietary Reference Intakes, Food and Nutrition Board. *Dietary Reference Intakes for Vitamin A, Vitamin K, Arsenic, Boron, Chromium, Copper, Iodine, Iron, Manganese, Molybdenum, Nickel, Silicon, Vanadium, and Zinc.* Washington, DC: The National Academies Press; 2001.
76. Levenson SM, Demetrious AA. Metabolic factors. In: Cohen IK, Diegelmann RF, Lindblad WJ, eds. *Wound Healing Biochemical and Clinical Aspects.* Philadelphia, PA: Saunders; 1992:248–273.
77. Pollack SV. Wound healing: a review. III: nutritional factors affecting wound healing. *J Derm Surg Oncol.* 1979;5:615–619.
78. Lown D. Wound healing. In: Matarese LE, Gottschlich MM, eds. *Contemporary Nutrition Support Practice: A Clinical Guide.* Philadelphia, PA: Saunders; 1998.
79. Hunt TK. Vitamin A and wound healing. *J Am Acad Dermatol.* 1986;15:817–821.
80. Phillips JD, Kim CS, Fonkalsrud EW, et al. Effects of chronic corticosteroids and vitamin A on the healing of intestinal anastomoses. *Am J Surg.* 1992;163:71–77.
81. Schweizer RT, Bartus SA. Vitamin A and immunosuppression of allografts in dogs and rabbits. *J Surg Res.* 1975;19:229–232.
82. Neifeld JP, Lee HM, Hutcher NE. Lack of effect of vitamin A on corticosteroid-induced immunosuppression. *J Surg Res.* 1975;19: 225–228.
83. Haick A, Johnson D, Raju S. Vitamin A does not alter immunosuppressive properties of simultaneously administered steroids. *Am Surg.* 1981;47(12):533–537.
84. Ross AC. Vitamin A and retinoids. In: Shils ME, Olson JA, Shike M, et al., eds. *Modern Nutrition in Health and Disease.* 9th ed. Baltimore, MD: Williams & Wilkins; 1999:305–307.
85. Underwood BA. Methods for assessment of vitamin A status. *J Nutr.* 1990;120(suppl 12):S1459–S1463.
86. Goetzl EJ, Wasserman SI, Gigli I, et al. Enhancement of random migration and chemotactic response of human leukocytes by ascorbic acid. *J Clin Invest.* 1974;53:813–818.
87. Nicosia RF, Belser P, Bonanno E, et al. Regulation of angiogenesis in vitro by collagen metabolism. *In Vitro Cell Dev Biol.* 1991; 27A:961–966.
88. ter Riet G, Kessels AG, Knipschild PG. Randomized clinical trial of ascorbic acid in the treatment of pressure ulcers. *J Clin Epidemiol.* 1995;48:1453–1460.
89. Standing Committee on the Scientific Evaluation of Dietary Reference Intakes, Food and Nutrition Board. *Dietary Reference Intakes of Vitamin C, Vitamin E, Selenium, and Beta-Carotene, and other Carotenoids.* Washington, DC: The National Academies Press; 2000.
90. American Dietetic Association and Morrison Health Care, Inc. Pressure ulcer (Stage I–IV) medical nutrition therapy protocol. In: *Medical Nutrition Therapy across the Continuum of Care.* Chicago, IL: The American Dietetic Association; 1997 (suppl 1:Older Adult Section).
91. Jacob RA. Vitamin C. In: Shils ME, Olson JA, Shike M, et al., eds. *Modern Nutrition in Health and Disease.* 9th ed. Baltimore, MD: Williams & Wilkins; 1999:131–132.
92. Vilter RW. Nutritional aspects of ascorbic acid: uses and abuses. *West J Med.* 1980;133:485–492.
93. Stewart RJ, Moore T, Bennett B, et al. Effect of free radical scavengers and skin hyperbaric oxygen on random pattern flaps. *Arch Surg.* 1994;129:982–988.
94. Taren DL, Chvapil M, Weber CW. Increasing the breaking strength of wounds exposed to preoperative irradiation using vitamin E supplementation. *Int J Vitamin Nutr Res.* 1987;57:133–137.
95. Havlik RJ. Vitamin E and wound healing: Plastic Surgery Educational Foundation DATA Committee. *Plast Reconstr Surg.* 1997;100:1901–1902.
96. Houwing R, Overgoor M, Kon M, et al. Pressure-induced skin lesions in pigs: reperfusion injury and the effects of vitamin E. *J Wound Care.* 2000;9:36–40.
97. Williams JZ, Barbul A. Nutrition and wound healing. *Surg Clin North Am.* 2003;83:571–596.
98. Gray M. Does oral zinc supplementation promote healing of chronic wounds? *J Wound Ostomy Continence Nurs.* 2003;30: 295–299.
99. Selmanpakoglu AN, Cetin C, Sayal A, et al. Trace element (Al, Se, Zn, Cu) levels in serum, urine, and tissues of burn patients. *Burns.* 1994;20:99–103.
100. King JC, Keen DL. Zinc. In: Shils ME, Olson JA, Shike M, et al., eds. *Modern Nutrition in Health and Disease.* 9th ed. Baltimore, MD: Williams & Wilkins; 1999:223–239.
101. Pennington JA, Young BE, Wilson DB. Mineral content of foods and total diets: the selected minerals in foods survey, 1982 to 1984. *J Am Diet Assoc.* 1986;86:876–891.
102. Wolman SL, Anderson GH, Marliss EB, et al. Zinc in total parenteral nutrition: requirements and metabolic effects. *Gastroenterology.* 1979;76(3):458–467.

103. Baumgartner TG, ed. *Clinical Guide to Parenteral Micronutrition.* 3rd ed. Chicago, IL: Fujisawa USA, Inc.; 1997.
104. Albina JE. Nutrition and wound healing. *J Parenter Enteral Nutr.* 1994;18:367–376.
105. Berger MM, Cavadini C, Bart A, et al. Cutaneous copper and zinc losses in burn. *Burns.* 1992;18(5)373–380.
106. Reddy M. Pressure ulcers. *Clin Evid (Online).* 2011;1901.
107. Delmi M, Rapin C-H, Bengoa JM, et al. Dietary supplementation in elderly patients with fractured neck of the femur. *Lancet.* 1990;335:1013–1016.
108. Gilmore SA, Robinson G, Posthauer ME, et al. Clinical indicators associated with unintentional weight loss and pressure ulcers in elderly residents of nursing facilities. *J Am Diet Assoc.* 1995;95: 984–992.
109. Bourdel-Marchasson I, Barateau M, Rondeau V, et al. A multicenter trial of the effects of nutritional supplementation in critically ill older inpatients. GAGE Group. *Nutrition.* 2000;16:1–5.
110. Thomas DR. The role of nutrition in prevention and healing of pressure ulcers. *Clin Geriatr Med.* 1997;13:497–511.
111. Stratton RJ, Ek A-C, Engfer M, et al. Enteral nutritional support in prevention and treatment of pressure ulcers: a systematic review and meta-analysis. *Ageing Res Rev.*2005;4:422–450.
112. Dorner B, Posthauer ME, Thomas D. National Pressure Ulcer Advisory Panel: the role of nutrition in pressure ulcer prevention and treatment: National Pressure Ulcer Advisory Panel white paper. *Adv Skin Wound Care.* 2009;22(5): 212–221.
113. Henderson CT, Trumbore LS, Mobarhan S, et al. Prolonged tube feeding in long-term care: nutritional status and clinical outcomes. *J Am Coll Nutr.* 1992;11:309–325.
114. van Rijswijk L, Catanzaro J. Wound assessment and documentation. In: Krasner D, Rodeheaver G, Sibbald RG, eds. *Chronic Wound Care.* 4th ed. Malvern, PA: HMP Publishers; 2007:113–126.

22 Nutrition in Neurologic Impairment

Kathryn Ruf, PharmD, Barbara Magnuson, PharmD, BCNSP, Jimmi Hatton, PharmD, and Aaron M. Cook, PharmD, BCPS

CONTENTS

Introduction and Background 364
Metabolism 364
Complications of Neurologic Illness Affecting Nutrition Support 365
Nutrition Assessment and Requirements 366
Route of Nutrition Support 369
Complications and Monitoring 370
Emerging Nutritional Interventions 371
References 373

Objectives

1. Compare and contrast options for fluid resuscitation in neurologic injury.
2. Discuss appropriate assessment of caloric need in patients with traumatic brain injury, spinal cord injury, stroke, or cerebral palsy.
3. Describe common challenges inherent in the neurologically injured population related to provision of nutrition.
4. Explain the rationale and current clinical status of immunonutrients such as L-arginine and glutamine in acute neurologic injury.

Test Your Knowledge Questions

1. Fluid resuscitation is a key component in the management of traumatic brain injury (TBI). Which of the following statements is true?
   A. Immediately following a TBI, large volumes of free water supplements should be added to the enteral nutrition regimen to prevent frequent hypernatremia.
   B. High dextrose-containing parenteral solutions are beneficial following TBI.
   C. Advantages of using normal saline (0.9% sodium chloride [normal saline (NS)]) in fluid resuscitation include isotonicity, the lack of salt-free water, and diminished likelihood of cerebral edema.
   D. Glucose administration rates should exceed 5.3 g/kg/day.
2. An accurate assessment for both calories and protein is critical for the neurologically injured patient. Which of the following statement is false?
   A. Patients with TBI exhibit a definite hypermetabolic and hypercatabolic phase that can last for weeks to months following injury.
   B. Delaying nutrition support results in negative outcomes and denies the patient of the benefits of early enteral nutrition.
   C. Indirect calorimetry remains the current "gold standard" for best accuracy of determining the caloric requirements.
   D. Barbiturate-induced coma to control refractory intracranial hypertension following TBI increases energy expenditure by up to 40%.
3. Metabolic changes following spinal cord injuries (SCIs) depend on the level of cord injury and the extent of injuries. Which of the following statements is true?
   A. The energy expenditure following a SCI is approximately 48% higher than patients with TBI.
   B. To accurately assess the caloric requirements for a patient with SCI, multiply the Harris-Benedict equation (HBE) by 1.6 for an injury factor and then again by 1.2 for an activity factor.
   C. A modified body mass index (BMI) scale has been proposed for individuals with SCI, with healthy normal as 18 to 22 kg/m^2.
   D. Patients with chronic SCI require approximately 30 to 33 kcal/kg/day, depending on their physical activity.

Test Your Knowledge Answers

1. The correct answer is **C**. Aggressive fluid resuscitation is critical following TBI to maintain adequate cerebral perfusion pressure. Large volumes of salt-free water can be deleterious and contribute to cerebral edema. Dextrose solutions and hyperglycemia may increase brain injury severity and may be associated with worsened neurologic outcomes and increased mortality. Glucose administration rates should not exceed 3.5 g/kg/day.
2. The correct answer is **D**. A, B, and C are true statements. Barbiturate-induced coma to control refractory intracranial hypertension following traumatic brain injury also drastically decreases energy expenditure by up to 40%. Calorie provision should be decreased during the barbiturate-induced coma to avoid potentially detrimental hyperglycemia and other adverse events associated with overfeeding.
3. The correct answer is **C**. Energy expenditure following SCI has been repeatedly reported to be almost 48% lower than TBI. Most patients with SCI will expend 5–15% more than the HBE, and therefore no extreme injury or activity factors should be multiplied to the equation. In the chronic phase, patients with SCI are at risk for obesity and related disorders such as diabetes and cardiovascular disease. Generally, these patients require approximately 20 to 23 kcal/kg/day depending on their physical activity. A modified proposed BMI scaled suggests a normal healthy BMI be 18 to 22 kg/m^2.

Introduction and Background

The central nervous system (CNS) acts as a regulator of nutrient intake. This is accomplished by internal signaling mechanisms that maintain homeostasis of blood glucose and electrolytes along with triggering the consciousness of hunger and thirst. In CNS injury, these normal physiologic functions become disrupted, the severity of which depends on the acuity and magnitude of the brain insult. Acute brain trauma and stroke generate immediate consequences on nutritional intake and metabolic parameters. More chronic, degenerative diseases of the brain can also cause significant nutritional complications, which present gradually as the disease progresses. Residual neurologic function often changes over time, generating different nutritional concerns depending on the stage of CNS recovery.

Trauma is often the cause of neurologic injury. Traumatic brain injury (TBI) accounts for approximately 33% of injury-related deaths.[1] Nearly 1.4 million individuals suffer from TBI each year.[2] A number of these patients survive but are left with significant cognitive or physical disabilities that require extensive rehabilitation.[3] Early and adequate nutrition support is challenging to provide in the complex TBI population, but may improve the overall clinical course of this population.[4] SCI is less common than TBI (there are approximately 14,000 SCIs in North America annually), but no less devastating.[5] Patients with SCI often have varying degrees of permanent neurologic dysfunction resulting in lack of movement and/or sensation.[6]

Other causes of neurologic injury may present in an acute or chronic fashion such as stroke or Parkinson disease (PD). In the United States, it is estimated that 700,000 new or recurrent strokes occur annually with estimated costs in 2005 of $57 billion for medical costs and disability.[7] Stroke is a medical emergency requiring immediate intervention to restore blood and oxygen to the injured brain. Precipitating causes are vascular or thrombotic changes associated most commonly with underlying cardiovascular disease or diabetes. The area of brain and extent of tissue loss will dictate signs and symptoms associated with the acute event and the subsequent complications.[8] Conversely, cerebral palsy (CP) and PD affect 764,000 and 1 million Americans, respectively.[9,10] Nutritional needs are rarely acute as in trauma or stroke, but symptoms associated with these diseases make self-feeding progressively difficult such that baseline malnutrition is common.

Numerous considerations are pertinent when evaluating nutrition support in a neurologically injured patient. Nutritional assessment provides the basis for nutritional interventions, especially in acute care settings. CNS trauma often affects young, healthy, adult males in contrast to acute stroke patients and those with CP or PD where malnutrition and concomitant disease are more common. The extent of neurologic recovery following CNS injury will be a common, primary factor determining nutrition recommendations, independent of the initial diagnosis. Safe and effective enteral access can be a challenge in the CNS-injured patient. Bedside placement of a postpyloric feeding may be difficult due to facial or sinus fracture sustained during the trauma, and endoscopic placement of postpyloric feeding tubes may be challenging in patients with intracranial pressure problems or cervical spine instability. The presence of neurotransmitters and inflammatory mediators, along with other factors such as fluid/electrolyte balance and CNS-specific medications each should be considered when providing nutritional support in this fragile patient population. Other important considerations include preventing dramatic shifts in glucose (hyperglycemia/hypoglycemia) and acid-base abnormalities related to the use of mechanical ventilation, nasogastric suctioning, and certain intravenous fluids.

Nutrition support interventions can have significant CNS effects. Excessive protein can lead to azotemia or hyperammonemia, aromatic amino acids can affect neurotransmitter production, the effect of glutamine on glutamate production is unknown, and finally, providing excessive "free water" can significantly affect sodium balance in the CNS-injured patient, a population already predisposed to sodium abnormalities. Reduced muscle mass may lower serum creatinine, masking compromised renal function. These conditions can predispose the patient to complications from his or her nutritional support regimens. Micronutrients are important in acute and chronic neurologic disease. Antioxidants, B vitamins, selenium, and zinc each have been used in different phases of CNS illness.

Metabolism

TBI and SCI are typified by a vigorous hypermetabolic, catabolic stress response that is proportional to the severity of injury and motor dysfunction.[11] Numerous abnormalities in the neuroendocrine axis, acute phase reactants, electrolytes,

Table 22-1 Metabolic Alterations after Central Nervous System Injury[115–118]

Diminished Concentrations in CNS Injury	Elevated Concentrations in CNS Injury
• Albumin	• Alpha-1 acid glycoprotein
• Insulin-like growth factor-1	• C-reactive protein
• Iron	• Ceruloplasmin
• Prealbumin	• Interleukin-1
• Thyroxine	• Interleukin-6
• Thyroid stimulating hormone	• Vasopressin (in SIADH)
• Transferrin	• Cortisol (acute)
• Vasopressin (in diabetes insipidus)	• Growth hormone (acute)
• Zinc	
• Cortisol (chronic)	
• Growth hormone (chronic)	

CNS, central nervous system; SIADH, syndrome of inappropriate antidiuretic hormone.

and peripheral amino acid concentrations may occur after neurotrauma (Table 22-1). These problems may lead to increased morbidity and mortality related to hyperglycemia, protein wasting, increased energy demand, and altered neurotransmitter function. Often, the patient with SCI loses weight during his or her acute rehabilitation phase due to obligatory nitrogen losses and mismatched nutrition intake and expenditure. Following an SCI, a resultant change in the body composition develops with reduction in lean body mass, reduction in bone mineral density, and an increase in fat mass.[12,13] Effective nutrition support can play a major role in attenuating the catabolic response and avoiding the potentially harmful effects of prolonged hypermetabolism (Table 22-2).

Table 22-2 Nutritional Consequences of Central Nervous System Injuries[1,7–10]

- Difficulty chewing/swallowing
- Dysphagia
- Muscle catabolism
- Muscle denervation
- Severe hand tremors
- Delayed gastric emptying
- Dehydration
- Decreased salivation
- Weight loss
- Aspiration pneumonia
- Taste, smell, and appetite abnormalities
- Glucose intolerance
- Negative nitrogen balance
- Osteoporosis
- Depression
- Anemia

The metabolic phase following TBI is vastly different than the metabolic response after a stroke. In contrast to the severe hypermetabolic response seen following TBI, the acute stroke patient dose not experience the initial severe increase in energy expenditure as previously assumed. The small landmark study by Weekes and Elia reported the stroke patient did not experience a severe hypermetabolic phase. [14] Several larger, more recent studies have validated this finding, suggesting that basal energy needs vary as little as 7% to 14% from baseline.[15,16]

Complications of Neurologic Illness Affecting Nutrition Support

Fluid resuscitation is a key component in the management of traumatic brain injury. Aggressive fluid resuscitation to maintain adequate cerebral perfusion pressure may prevent hypotension, which has a negative correlation with patient outcomes.[1] An understanding of its potential to cause iatrogenic sodium disturbances is critical. However, the Brain Trauma Foundation guideline does not make a specific recommendation about the type of fluid used for resuscitation and generally, the optimal fluid used during TBI fluid resuscitation is not well defined. When providing fluid replacement for patients with TBIs, considerations include crystalloid versus colloid solution, glucose content, free water content, and serum sodium level abnormalities. The goal of fluid resuscitation should be to provide adequate intravascular volume and optimal hemodynamics without worsening hyponatremia and cerebral edema.

Crystalloids and colloids both have distinct advantages and disadvantages in the setting of TBI. There is no supporting evidence that the use of albumin (colloid) solutions instead of crystalloid solutions is beneficial in the setting of TBI. To the contrary, the Saline versus Albumin Evaluation trial revealed a small mortality increase in trauma patients receiving albumin (relative risk of death 1.36 [0.99 to 1.86]) that appeared to be driven by those patients with TBI.[17] Formal subgroup analysis of the TBI population in this trial was described in Saline versus Albumin Evaluation-TBI.[18] The authors noted that albumin-resuscitated patients with TBI had significantly higher mortality (relative risk 1.8 [1.31 to 2.71]). Advantages of using normal saline (0.9% sodium chloride, NS) in fluid resuscitation include isotonicity and the lack of salt-free water. These characteristics diminish the likelihood that NS would have deleterious effects on plasma osmolarity or cerebral edema.[19] For this reason, solutions containing dextrose only (sodium-free water) are generally avoided. Even "balanced" salt solutions, like Ringer lactate, provide 114 mL of free water per liter and may also contribute to cerebral edema.[20–22]

In addition to the potential to exacerbate cerebral edema, solutions containing dextrose contribute to hyperglycemia. Hyperglycemia may increase brain injury severity and may be associated with worsened neurologic outcomes and increased mortality. [23–29] It is postulated that glucose may increase secondary to a stress-induced cortisol response.[30] Hyperglycemia may be further magnified by a dysfunction in glucose utilization and a shift to anaerobic metabolism and cellular destruction.[20,31–33] Hyperglycemia may also independently worsen cerebral edema and cause direct insulin-independent cell toxicity.[34,35] Thus, careful use of dextrose, or other hypotonic solutions, is paramount. Glucose administration rates should not exceed 3.5 g/kg/day to avoid complications associated with hyperglycemia and impaired glucose utilization.[36] Generally, fluid management should include an iso-osmotic, isotonic salt solution that does not contain free water and will not contribute to cerebral edema. Judicious use of NS seems to be the safest option at this time. Diligent monitoring of sodium concentration is often necessary because wide perturbations in serum sodium may affect brain tissue volume.

Dysphagia is prevalent in patients with neurologic impairment. Sixty-one percent of patients with TBI and 43% of patients on first episode of stroke will experience swallowing difficulty.[37] Negative sequelae have been associated with dysphagia. In stroke patients, dysphagia has been associated with longer hospital length of stay and increased need for institutionalized care.[38] Thus, evaluation for and treatment of dysphagia should be addressed in all patients with neurologic impairment.

Evaluation of dysphagia is multimodal. An initial bedside swallow examination may be performed to screen patients, but it may not be a sufficient method for identifying aspiration or the degree of laryngeal dysfunction.[39] A modified barium swallow can be performed to radiographically assess a patient's risk of aspiration. Evaluation for dysphagia should be ongoing, and patients should be continually evaluated for swallowing difficulty.[40] For example, in patients after stroke, it has been noted that 86% will recover swallowing function in 2 weeks.[41]

Treatment of dysphagia should focus on the etiology of the condition and may include modifications of swallowing technique and selecting an appropriate diet. Recommendations for a diet based on the severity of the patient's dysphagia were developed in 2002 by the American Dietetic Association. The National Dysphagia Dietary Task Force published the National Dysphagia Diet (NDD).[42] The NDD is a hierarchy of dietary recommendations divided into three distinct food levels based on food consistency, viscosity, and texture. Subjective evaluation of the patient's degree of swallowing impairment (mild to moderate-severe) drives the selection of the appropriate food level. The hierarchy progresses from level 1, a pureed diet, through level 3, an advanced diet (Table 22-3). Patients with severe dysphagia are at high risk for aspiration and may require percutaneous endoscopic gastrostomy (PEG) or nasogastric (NG) feedings instead of or in addition to the oral feedings recommended in the NDD. Such methods of enteral feeding may provide for the provision of early enteral nutrition in this patient population.[40] However, enteral nutrition therapy, amongst other issues, carries special considerations for the administration of medications that must be addressed.

Swallowing difficulties must be considered in all neurologically impaired patients. The management of dysphagia is a critical consideration in the care of these patients. Accurate diagnosis, selection of optimal nutritional support strategies, and frequent care plan modifications are keys to successful management of this patient population.

Table 22-3 National Dysphagia Diet[42,119–122]

Dysphagia Level	Description	Degree of Dysphagia
Level 1: Dysphagia pureed	Cohesive and pudding-like texture; little chewing required	Moderate to severe
Level 2: Dysphagia mechanically altered	Semisolid and moist texture; easily form bolus; some chewing required	Mild to moderate
Level 3: Dysphagia advanced	Soft-solid regular texture (no hard, sticky, or crunchy foods); more chewing required; provides a transition to a regular diet	Mild dysphagia

Nutrition Assessment and Requirements

An accurate assessment for both calories and protein is critical for the neurologically injured patient. Increases in metabolic activity and demand are common during the acute phase of illness. The increased metabolic need may persist for weeks to months after injury, depending on severity and recovery. There is a marked hypermetabolic and hypercatabolic phase following TBI.

Precise estimation of metabolic needs in the patient with TBI is difficult (Practice Scenario 22-1). Indirect calorimetry remains the current "gold standard" for best accuracy of determining the caloric requirements. However, the results from a metabolic cart study may be imprecise due to numerous factors such as paroxysmal sympathetic storming, muscle contractions, seizure, and fever. Studies in the 1980s estimated the energy expenditure to be much higher than is currently used in practice today. Early studies predicted energy expenditure using the Harris-Benedict equation (HBE) with a 1.6 stress/injury factor and then multiplied again by 1.2 for an activity factor.[43,44] However, recent evidence suggests the needs for nutrition are lower. American Society for Parenteral and Enteral Nutrition (A.S.P.E.N.) guidelines currently recommend the use of the Mifflin-St. Jeor equation for basal energy expenditure. However, the equation has not been validated for use in the TBI population.[45] As consistent with the Brain Trauma Foundation guidelines, aiming for estimated calorie provision between 120% to 160% of estimated basal needs (as determined by the HBE) and 1.5 to 2 gm/kg/day of protein, while also monitoring for signs of overfeeding such as an elevated respiratory quotient and hyperglycemia, is sufficient.[1,30]

McCall and colleagues evaluated the effect of neuromuscular blockade on the energy expenditure with severe head injury.[46] They reported the measured energy expenditure by indirect calorimetry to be 120% above the HBE (using actual weight) without blockade and a 4% to 5% decrease of below the HBE with blockade that nearly eliminated any hypermetabolic response due to TBI. Ignoring the significant changes in metabolism from continuous neuromuscular blockade can result in excessive caloric intake and negative consequences of hyperglycemia, refeeding syndrome, and hypercarbia.

Barbiturate-induced coma to control refractory intracranial hypertension following TBI also decreases energy expenditure. Dempsey and colleagues measured energy expenditure in 10 patients with TBI within 2 weeks of injury.[47] They demonstrated a change of nearly 40% when barbiturates were administered. Dempsey reported brain-injured patients averaged 26% above predicted energy expenditure using the HBE without barbiturates to a decrease of nearly 14% below the predicted energy expenditure. These are consistent with results reported from other studies. Fried and colleagues also evaluated energy expenditure and nitrogen elimination of patients with TBI within the first week of injury.[48] They demonstrated a 42% decrease of measured energy expenditure by indirect calorimetry during barbiturate therapy (132% plus 28% without barbiturate versus 76% plus 23% with barbiturate, $p < 0.01$) and nitrogen elimination decreased by approximately 40%. Even though these therapies are clearly not intended for long-term use, the energy prescription should be adjusted accordingly.

Metabolic changes following SCI depend on the level of cord injury and the extent of injuries (Practice Scenario 22-2). A landmark study published in 1979 by Long and colleagues attempted to predict energy expenditure for injured patients by multiplying the basal energy expenditure as determined from the HBE by a 1.6 injury factor and then multiplied again by 1.2 for an activity factor.[43] Several studies have since refuted the philosophy that SCI elicits a severe hypermetabolic phenomenon as seen in multiple trauma or TBI. Kolpek et al. reported a decrease in measured energy expenditure (MEE) compared to predicted energy expenditure (PEE). During the first week after SCI, the ratio of MEE/PEE was a mean of 0.56. Overall, during the 3 weeks after SCI, patients exhibited a MEE/PEE ratio of 0.94, indicating a lower metabolic need than normal.[44] The MEE was determined by indirect calorimetry, and the PEE was estimated as the HBE multiplied by 1.2 to 1.6. These energy expenditure values were approximately 48% lower for patients with SCI than for patients with TBI. In contrast to quadriplegic patients, the paraplegic patient expends more energy initially and throughout rehabilitation. Cox et al. reported the MEE of 5 paraplegic patients to be 27.9 kcal/kg/day during the early rehabilitation phase compared to 15 quadriplegic patients who required only 22.7 kcal/kg/day.[49] While others have confirmed these figures as estimates for nutritional need, patients with SCI are also known to have persistent negative nitrogen balance despite aggressive calorie provision and providing 2 g/kg/day of protein.[50]

Patients with SCI appear to have lower metabolic needs than one would predict well after the acute stages of injury. Bauman and colleagues studied energy expenditure in adult twins with one having an SCI and the other as a control.[51] All SCIs were from 3 to 26 years previous to the study. They reported that the energy expenditure remained low for years following injury. The MEE was an average 15% less than the PEE using the HBE, and their mean caloric requirement was approximately 20.4 kcal/kg. Monroe and colleagues evaluated 10 males with SCI beyond 2 years following injury. They concluded the individuals with SCI expended significantly lower daily energy than the control subjects. The lower energy expenditure in those with SCI were explained by lower levels of physical activity, lower resting metabolic rate, and the thermogenic effect of food.[52]

Clearly, there is a legitimate risk for obesity-related disorders such as diabetes and cardiovascular disease in the long-term SCI population. A modified BMI scale has been proposed for individuals with SCI, with healthy normal as a BMI of 18 to 22kg/m^2, overweight as a BMI of 22 to 25 kg/m^2, and obese as a BMI of over 25 kg/m^2.[53] Groah reported nearly 70% overweight individuals with SCI in his study of 73 persons with over 1 year from cord injury (along with deficient intake of some vitamins, minerals, and macronutrients).[54] Another study evaluated 7,959 veterans with SCI and reported that almost 53% were obese or overweight using the standard BMI scale of $\geq$ 25kg/m^2.[55] When the BMI scale was adjusted for overweight at 23 kg/m^2 and obese at 28 kg/m^2, then 68% were then classified as overweight or obese. The quadriplegic and chronic SCI individual requires 20 to 23 kcal/kg/day, depending on his or her physical activity. Alternatively, the calories can be estimated by the HBE adjusted to 85% to 100% of the result (basal energy expenditure).[49,51,56] As suggested by Rodriquez's study, protein requirements immediately following SCI are 1.5 to 2 g/kg/day. In the long-term setting, persons with SCI will only require typical protein needs from 0.8 to 1 gm/kg/day of ideal (or adjusted if obese) body weight, adjusting the range up if decubitus ulcers are present.

Preexisting malnutrition prior to an ischemic stroke may worsen complications and outcome. Yoo and colleagues reviewed 113 ischemic stroke patients and reported a 12% prevalence of undernutrition upon admission and nearly 20% undernutrition at 1 week. The 1-week undernutrition assessment statistically predicted poor 3-month outcomes.[57] The multicenter comprehensive trial Feed or Ordinary Diet enrolled 5,033 patients admitted to a hospital following a recent stroke. This study had three trial arms to determine whether routine oral nutritional supplementation of the hospital diet improved outcome after the stroke (Trial 1); whether early tube feeding improved outcomes of dysphagic stroke patients (Trial 2); and if enteral feeding via a PEG tube resulted in better outcomes than with an NG tube (Trial 3). Trial 1 showed there was no benefit for routine supplementation of hospital diet for unselected stroke patients who are predominantly well nourished on admission in providing nutritional supplementing. In Trial 2, 859 dysphagic patients were allocated to early enteral nutrition or avoiding enteral nutrition for 1 week. Early enteral nutrition was associated with an absolute reduction in risk of death. Throughout the first 5 days of study, the energy expenditure did not vary greatly from 19.2 $\pm$ 2 kcal/kg (with protein needs ranging from 1 to 1.2 gm/kg/day).[58] Trial 3 included dysphagic patients who received enteral nutrition via either PEG or NG tube. Trial 3 data suggested best outcomes from feeding with the NG tube and does not support a policy of early initiation of PEG feedings. Foley also confirmed that patients fed with enteral feeding tubes following a stroke received significantly more calories and protein than those eating a regular hospital or dysphagia diet.[59]

Patients with CP pose a continuing challenge to clinicians regarding their nutritional assessment. The usual anthropometric measurements are not reliable in assessing the nutritional status of patients with moderate to severe CP nor are the traditional estimated energy equations. The person with CP typically has very low lean body mass. Many do not bear weight, and their neurologic insult is often associated with endocrine dysfunction. Nutrition support recommendations in CP populations have focused on pediatric populations. Extrapolating to adults with CP is somewhat speculative. Several studies have documented the resting energy expenditure (REE) of nonambulatory spastic quadriplegic children with CP is much lower than their developed counterparts. The REE in these studies were generally about 75% of predicted requirements. The energy expenditure likely remains lower throughout their adulthood due to lower fat-free mass and less physical activity.[60-62] Children with mild CP appear to expend significantly more energy during walking than do developing peers. Conversely, adolescents with mild CP often exhibit lower physical activities and overall also have lower energy expenditures.[63]

Dickerson and colleagues have reported the most extensive studies evaluating and validating energy expenditure estimations for adults with CP or other severe neurodevelopment disabilities.[64] They reported the Arlington Developmental Center equation as the most precise and unbiased estimate for adult patients with severe neurodevelopment disabilities and fixed upper extremity contractures, while the HBE remained precise and unbiased for adults with CP who have preserved upper body movements.[65-67]

Arlington Developmental Center equation: REE (kcal/day) = (22.3 * FFM in kg) – (9.4 * age in yrs) + 557

Adults with CP and athetosis, a continuous involuntary movement that is a slow and worm-like motion involving extremities, neck, face, and trunk, also have an increase in REE by almost 14% when adjusted for fat-free mass.[69] Indirect calorimetry is perhaps the most valid tool for determining energy requirements in adults with CP.

Practice Scenario 22-1

Question: How do you estimate the energy and protein requirements of a patient in the acute phase of a TBI?

Scenario: A 22-year-old male was admitted with a severe TBI after falling from a roof while at work and required intubation on the scene. His presenting Glasgow Coma Score was 8T. He suffered only minor other injuries and had no other significant medical history. He remained intubated secondary to neurologic status. You were asked to evaluate his current tube feeding regimen and recommend changes if necessary. The patient was receiving a calorically dense enteral formula (2 kcal/mL) that was advanced to a goal of 50 mL/hr through a postpyloric small bore feeding tube without any noted NG residuals. His latest serum chemistries were all within normal limits.

Height: 177 cm; weight: 72 kg

Enteral formula: 2 kcal/mL and 83.5 g/L of protein and 725 mL/L free water at 50 mL/hr

Medications: Phenytoin suspension 150 mg per tube every 8 hours for 7 days holding tube feeds 1 hour before and 1 hour after each dose, docusate sodium 100 mg per tube twice a day, enoxaparin 30 mg subcutaneously every 12 hours, and insulin drip (added this morning during rounds)

Intervention: Tube feedings were increased to a goal of 75 mL/hr for 18 hours daily to provide 2700 kcals and 113 g of protein. Phenytoin administration was changed to 200 mg twice a day (or appropriate dose per levels) so the enteral nutrition will only be interrupted for 4 hours/day. Tube feeding goal at 65 mL/hr for 20 hr/day provides 2600 kcal and 109 g/day protein.

Answer: Current nutritional goals with the selected enteral formula at goal of 50 mL/hr (over 18 hours daily due to phenytoin therapy) would provide only 900 mL for 1800 kcal and 75.15 grams of protein. Acutely, patients after TBI are hypermetabolic and hypercatabolic and require an estimated 120% to 160% of their basal energy expenditure and 1.5 to 2 g/kg/day of protein. Indirect calorimetry is considered to be the "gold standard" for estimating their metabolic needs. The ideal equation to estimate basal energy expenditure in the setting of TBI has not been established. The Mifflin-St. Jeor equation, recommended by the A.S.P.E.N. guidelines, has not been validated for use in the TBI population. The HBE can be used to estimate the caloric requirements.[1] The current regimen of calorically dense tube feeding at a goal of 50 mL/hr to run over 18 hours daily did not meet the estimated needs of the patient. Using the HBE, the patient's basal needs are 1972 kcal, with a stress/injury factor of 120% to 160%; the estimated needs are 2152 to 2870 kcals/day. Protein need is estimated at 108 to 144 g/day, and free water requirement is estimated at 2 to 2.5 L/day. Increasing the tube feed goal to 75 mL/hr over 18 hours per day will provide 2700 kcals, 112 g of protein, and 979 mL of free water, which is within target range. By adding 250 mL of free water every 6 hours to provide 1973 mL daily, this would include his medication flushes and meet his daily requirements.

Rationale: Adequate nutrition support is critical in the setting of TBI, and the benefits of early enteral nutrition in TBI have been established. Patients with TBI may also require medications that will affect their nutrition support regimen. Phenytoin suspension, an antiepileptic medication used to treat or prevent seizures after TBI, combined with enteral nutrition results in decreased levels compared to patients that swallow it. The exact cause of interaction and decreased absorption is unknown. It may bind with the tube feeding and thereby become ineffective or due to an overall decreased absorption in the acute critical illness state. Thus, enteral feeds can be held 1 hour before and 1 hour after administration to circumvent the drug-nutrient interaction. Also, some patients with TBI may be receiving neuromuscular blocking agents or barbiturates to induce a coma or reduce intracranial pressure, which may slow their metabolism and decrease their metabolic needs. Propofol, also a commonly administered sedative in this population, is prepared as a 10% lipid emulsion.

*FFM = fat free mass was determined by skinfold thickness measurements and technique as described by Slaughter et al.[68]

The caloric content, 1.1 kcal/mL, of the propofol emulsifier must be considered when selecting a nutrition regimen to avoid overfeeding.

Practice Scenario 22-2

Question: What is the initial nutritional support regimen for a patient with an SCI?

Scenario: A 23-year-old male was admitted to the intensive care unit with acute SCI following a diving accident 3 hours earlier. He was intubated for ventilator support, and an NG tube was placed. He is presently unable to move any of his extremities. The working diagnosis is a complete SCI in his cervical spine. His prior medical history is insignificant, and his current laboratory values are within normal limits.

Height: 183 cm; weight: 75 kg

Answer: Calories and protein were calculated by the use of the HBE minus 6% (1800 kcals) and protein at 114 g/day when at goal rate. Tube feedings were initiated via the NG tube.

Rationale: In acute injury, stress factors are not recommended for patients with SCI. Studies have shown the metabolic rate to be 6% to 10% lower than predicted using the HBE.[44,49] Obtaining accurate weight may be very difficult in patients with SCI. The best estimation of the weight of a patient with SCI can be provided by family, as often patients are intubated, combined with current weights from nursing records. Obese patients with acute SCI should initially be prescribed calories and protein based on ideal body weight. A high protein prescription (1.5 to 2 g/kg/day) was implemented due to accelerated muscle catabolism, which cannot be completely corrected but may assist immune function. Most trauma patients will have a NG tube in place for decompression purposes initially. Using this access port for enteral nutrition is acceptable for the first few days until a percutaneous feeding tube can be safely inserted, but should be used with caution due to the risk of gastroparesis. The NG tube should be removed as soon as possible to limit nasal trauma and sinusitis risk. Small-bowel access should be obtained for tube feeding intolerance. The enteral formula should provide between 114 and 150 g of protein and between 1800 to 1900 kcals/day. Consideration of the volume required is important because gastric motility and paralytic ileus are common.

Route of Nutrition Support

As mentioned previously, swallowing dysfunction, or dysphagia, is a common problem following a cerebral vascular accident and can result in malnutrition, aspiration pneumonia, and other complications.[70,71] Dysphagia has been reported in 64% of patients with stroke upon initial presentation utilizing video fluoroscopy.[72] Up to 20% of patients with stroke are not formally evaluated for swallowing function within the first 48 hours of their admission,[58] and aspiration has been detected in nearly 40% of the patients following an acute stroke.[71,73] The presence of dysphagia significantly increases the odds of developing malnutrition, especially in the rehabilitation stage. Efforts to regain swallowing function should be implemented early, as nearly 70% of patients may have improvements in swallowing function during hospitalization.[58,74,75] Dysphagia following the first stroke episode has been reported in up to 43% of cases with the majority of these (86%) recovering swallowing function within 2 weeks.[57] Patients with dysphagia tend to have a prolonged length of hospital stay (up to three times longer) and higher associated complications and need for institutionalized care compared to patients without dysphagia.

Proactive initiation of oral nutrition is likely to benefit patients with stroke, even if oral intake is less than optimal. In one study of 21 patients with acute stroke able to swallow, the combination of enteral sip feedings with hospital food resulted in more favorable clinical outcomes and lower death rates compared to patients with acute stroke who received only hospital food. [59] The average daily intake was approximately 1800 kcal/day and approximately 64 g/day protein for the supplemented group compared to approximately 1200 kcal/day and approximately 43 g/day protein for hospital food–only patients. Improved outcome at hospital discharge has been reported even when only 60% of estimated energy requirements were met.

Benefits of early enteral nutrition that apply to patients with multitrauma patients also apply to patients with TBI.[76] Delaying nutrition support results in negative outcomes and denies the patient of the benefits of early enteral nutrition.[77] Early enteral nutrition in the intensive care unit results in downregulation of the systemic immune response, a reduction in oxidative stress, and overall improved outcome.[4] The use of enteral nutrition is contingent upon having access to the stomach or small bowel. In patients who cannot swallow adequately or who have diminished consciousness, placement of a nasoduodenal or nasojejunal feeding tube would be preferred largely because many critically ill individuals exhibit gastroparesis. This is often due to neurologic failure, administration of vasoactive agents, or opioid pain medications. Patients typically tolerate continuous enteral nutrition early in injury (particularly in TBI), but as the stress response wanes, gastric motility typically returns, making gastric feeding more feasible. The placement of a gastrostomy tube allows a more permanent feeding access, but it should first include an open discussion with the patient, family, caregiver, and referring physician.

If patients are dysphagic, oral administration of medications can be difficult. Guidelines for crushing oral tablets or using a liquid dosage form for delivery through an enteral access device should be followed. Unless otherwise directed, enteral feedings should be held for at least 30 minutes prior to and following administration of most medications. The tube should be flushed before and after the drug is administered. Other special considerations for many commonly used medications are summarized in Table 22-4.

The advantages and disadvantages of parenteral nutrition are well documented.[78] Currently, the routine use of parenteral nutrition is not preferable for neurologically injured patients. Some clinical scenarios exist where parenteral nutrition may be preferable including the use of high-dose vasopressor agents in

Table 22-4 Medication Considerations in Neurologic Disease[123–127]

Medication	Nutritional Implications
Barbiturates	• Infusion rate or as needed use should be monitored closely (may cause constipation) • Should be combined with bowel regimen • May diminish caloric requirements
Carbamazepine	• Avoid combining suspension with water or other medication diluents (forms an orange, rubbery precipitate) • Monitor for hyponatremia (may cause SIADH)
Corticosteroids	• Monitor for hyperglycemia • May increase risk for osteoporosis, gastric ulcers (chronic use)
Cyclosporine	• Monitor for hyperkalemia, hyperlipidemia, hypomagnesemia
Demeclocycline	• Monitor sodium concentrations/free water provision (used for SIADH) • Avoid combining with polyvalent cations or enteral nutrition (chelation/diminished absorption)
Desmopressin/ vasopressin	• Monitor sodium concentrations/free-water provision (used for diabetes insipidus)
Levodopa	• Individual meals high in protein may delay levodopa absorption (should encourage consistent levodopa dosing with food or meals) • Pyridoxine (vitamin B_6) reduces levodopa efficacy (unless combined with carbidopa) • Use caution combining with herbal preparations such as kava (may cause diminished efficacy)
Loop diuretics	• Monitor for hypokalemia, hypomagnesemia, hypocalcemia, decreased zinc
Mannitol	• Monitor for hypokalemia, hypomagnesemia, hypovolemia
Narcotic analgesics	• Infusion rate or as needed use should be monitored closely (may cause constipation) • Should be combined with bowel regimen
Penicillin G	• Monitor for hyperkalemia
Phenytoin	• Caution combining suspension with enteral nutrition (diminished/delayed absorption—consider holding enteral nutrition for 1 to 2 hours before and after administration) • Decreased folate, vitamin D (with chronic use)
Potassium	• Caution when repleting potassium with concentrated solutions or powders (may cause diarrhea)
Propofol	• Infusion rate should be monitored to determine the number of lipid calories provided by the phospholipid vehicle
Sorbitol (some liquid medications)	• May cause diarrhea
Ticarcillin/Piperacillin	• Monitor for hypernatremia
Monoamine oxidase inhibitors	• Hypertensive crisis when combined with wine, aged cheeses (tyramine-containing foods)

SIADH, syndrome of inappropriate antidiuretic hormone.

the setting of hypotension in SCI or TBI, enteral nutrition failure during pentobarbital coma, or polytrauma situations where bowel integrity may be compromised.[79] Parenteral nutrition can be used relatively safely in most patients, but neurologically injured patients require special care to avoid hyponatremia and hyperglycemia (among other complications), as these may directly exacerbate acute neurologic illness.

Complications and Monitoring

Hyponatremia (serum sodium < 135 mEq/L) is common in neurosurgical intensive care unit populations and may be manifest as focal neurologic deficits, altered mental status, and even seizure.[80] Further, hyponatremia may contribute to worsening cerebral edema, intracranial pressure elevations, and death from herniation.[20] Thus, the management of sodium may become challenging. Careful attention to serum sodium concentrations becomes fundamental in the management of neurologic illness. Sodium abnormalities can occur quickly in neurologically injured patients, particularly those with TBI or stroke and in those receiving enteral or parenteral nutrition. TBI and stroke are common causes of syndrome of inappropriate antidiuretic hormone (SIADH), particularly early after the event. Patients are usually euvolemic but have a low serum sodium concentration. The urine output is usually appropriately concentrated and of a normal volume, so SIADH is often difficult to detect before clinical symptoms begin unless serum sodium is monitored. In most patients, the SIADH is transient and related to the acute event. Fluid restriction is the primary method of treatment, though caution should be used in the acute phases of illness, as fluid restriction may be inappropriate in many patients with severe neurologic insult. Other treatments such as demeclocycline, sodium supplementation, or vasopressin-receptor antagonists should be reserved for patients with refractory cases that do not resolve as the acute phase of illness subsides.

Cerebral salt wasting (CSW) syndrome is another potential cause of hyponatremia, which, like SIADH, is also usually transient and related to early phases of illness after TBI.[81] The typical characteristic of CSW syndrome that distinguishes it from SIADH is the tendency for the patient to be volume depleted, due to natriuresis. Response to treatment may also provide clues to the etiology of the hyponatremia. CSW syndrome is usually best addressed by close monitoring of serum sodium concentrations and urine output, while also carefully supplementing sodium intravenously to restore sodium concentrations back to normal (whereas patients with SIADH tend not to have as robust response to sodium supplementation). Very low sodium values should be carefully returned to values nearer to normal at a rate no greater than 12 mEq/L/day in order to prevent central pontine myelinolysis.[80]

Diabetes insipidus, on the other hand, is related to a deficiency in vasopressin, resulting in hypernatremia. Diabetes insipidus may be nephrogenic or neurogenic in origin. Neurogenic diabetes insipidus is usually associated with pituitary dysfunction or a devastating neurologic event. Supplementation of salt-free water and use of vasopressin or analogs can reduce serum sodium concentrations to normal levels. Overly enthusiastic correction of hypernatremia can result in exacerbation of cerebral edema, so great care in supplementation and monitoring should be taken to avoid harm. As in hyponatremia, correction of serum sodium concentration back to a more normal range should occur slowly (no greater than 12 mEq/L/day serum sodium level).

Emerging Nutritional Interventions

Advancement in the understanding of neurologic illness has created a special niche for the nutrition support of these patients (Table 22-5). Supplementation of branched-chained amino acids (BCAAs), glutamine, L-arginine, omega-3 fatty acids (eicosapentaenoic acid [EPA]), gamma-linolenic acid (GLA), and supraphysiologic replacement of micronutrients have emerged as potential therapies for the neurologically impaired patient. Leucine, valine, isoleucine, or BCAAs are considered essential and must come from dietary sources. These amino acids have an important role in increasing hepatic and muscle synthesis as well as inhibiting protein muscle breakdown.[82] For this reason, they have been studied in critical illness, including patients with severe TBI. A small study of 40 patients with TBI and 20 healthy volunteers who received 15 days of intravenous BCAA supplementation revealed a significant improvement in the Disability Rating Score.[83] The difference was noted both within each group and between both the healthy volunteers and patients with TBI.

L-arginine is of particular interest and is a component of many immune-enhancing enteral formulations. L-arginine functions to upregulate the immune system via conversion into nitric oxide and has been shown to modulate the immune system by improving Th1/Th2 neutrophil response.[84] L-arginine also augments both phagocytosis and neutrophil generation of reactive oxygen species.[85,86] In sepsis, L-arginine has been shown to decrease blood pressure via a reduction in systemic vascular resistance. Cytokine-induced L-arginine oxidation and depletion has also been described.[87,88] Therefore, the clinical significance of arginine as an immune-enhancing supplement in sepsis remains a matter of debate.[89] Similarly, in severe neurologic illness, the effects of L-arginine supplementation and the associated nitric oxide generation are complex and difficult to predict. Nitric oxide in both the right amount and clinical conditions facilitates adequate brain perfusion. This may be a particular advantage in the setting of ischemia as is common in TBI and stroke. However, combination of nitric oxide with

Table 22-5 Immunonutrients in Neurologic Injury[87,93,94,104,108,113]

Immunonutrient	Potential Mechanism	Neurologic Impact	Recommendation
Branched-chain amino acids	Reduced skeletal muscle catabolism	Possible improved muscle mass retention after illness	Omit from nutrition supplementation plan until more evidence is available to support use
Docosahexaenoic acid	Anti-inflammatory	Possible prevention or reduction of traumatic axonal injury	Omit from nutrition supplementation plan until more evidence is available to support use
Eicosapentaenoic acid/glutamine	Reduced proinflammatory cytokines	Possible improved immune function, blunted inflammatory response	Omit from nutrition supplementation plan until more evidence is available to support use Potential harm has been noted in acute lung injury
Glutamine	Improved enterocyte and immune function	Possible improved immune function Possible conversion to damaging neurotransmitter (glutamate)	Omit from nutrition supplementation plan until more evidence is available to support use
L-arginine	Substrate for producing nitric oxide	Possible increase in perfusion Possible increase in damaging reactive nitrogen species	Omit from nutrition supplementation plan until more evidence is available to support use
Selenium	Antioxidant	Possible reduction in oxidative stress in acute injury	Supplement recommended daily allowance Supranormal doses should be avoided until more evidence is available to support use
Zinc	Cofactor for normal enzymatic activity	Zinc loss may be associated with poor outcome in traumatic brain injury	Supplement recommended daily allowance Supranormal doses should be avoided until more evidence is available to support use

local reactive oxygen species may produce peroxynitrite, a particularly nefarious mediator of neurologic harm in acute injury.[90] Also, a significant amount of arginine metabolism results in the synthesis of glutamate, an excitatory neurotransmitter.[91] Thus, more supportive data and understanding of the dynamics of nitric oxide in acute neurologic injury is needed before L-arginine can be recommended.

Glutamine, while not traditionally considered an essential amino acid, may be conditionally essential during critical illness. Glutamine deficiency may result in immune dysfunction, impaired organ integrity, and decreased energy availability.[92] Glutamine stores become rapidly depleted during inflammatory catabolic states and its biosynthesis is upregulated. This may result in muscle wasting because BCAAs are released from lean muscle tissues to serve as nitrogen donors for this process. Thus, glutamine supplementation has been evaluated in critical illness. Limited clinical evidence suggests a potential reduction in infectious morbidity with glutamine supplementation.[92–96] However, no mortality benefit has been noted with enteral glutamine supplementation. Glutamine may increase glutathione production and also has a role in anabolism, increasing growth hormone and insulin-like growth factor-1, which may be advantageous in acute neurologic injury.[97]

Extrapolation of data supporting glutamine in other areas of critical illness should be done with caution in acute neurologic illness such as TBI. It is evident that astrocytes and other brain cells have the ability to convert glutamine to glutamate via the enzyme glutaminase.[91,98] Glutamate is a well-known agonist for the N-methyl-D-aspartic acid receptor, which is one of the primary mechanisms for secondary injury and cytotoxic edema after TBI. Inhibition of glutamate and the N-methyl-D-aspartic acid receptor is a common target for neuroprotective therapies. Several small studies have been reported that may indicate that generation of significant amounts of glutamate from exogenous glutamine does not occur, though data is conflicting as to whether glutamine is actually helpful for patients with TBI.[92,99–101] However, given the physiologic potential for this process to occur and the deleterious impact it may have, more adequately powered trials are probably warranted to ensure that the findings of these smaller trials are correct. Routine supplementation in neurologic injury is not supported by current evidence nor Brain Trauma Foundation guidelines.[1]

Overall, the delicate balance of glutamine and arginine metabolism is poorly defined in acute neurologic illness. The precise impact of these amino acids on cerebral blood flow, metabolism, and excitotoxicity in TBI, as well as the dynamic process of amino acid shuttling during physiologic stress, needs to be defined in order to make a reasonable assessment of the potential for benefit or harm in this population. Clinicians should use these nutrients with caution in patients with acute neurologic injury until more information is available.

Omega-3 fatty acid, EPA, and docahexaenoic acid supplementation is another area of interest in neurologic illness. Omega-3 fatty acids, unlike long-chain polyunsaturated fatty acids, omega-6 fatty acids, have been shown to improve some cognitive and physiologic functions in a healthy patient population.[102] Animal studies have also revealed that omega-3 fatty acid supplementation may increase the seizure threshold, although human study has revealed only a transient decrease in seizure incidence during the first 6 weeks of supplementation.[103] Further, an omega-3 fatty acid-rich diet may reduce the prostaglandin E2 production and decrease the production of inflammatory cytokines.[104] Experimental animal data has highlighted the potential role of docosahexaenoic acid to both prevent and reverse traumatic axonal injury.[105,106]

GLA has also been evaluated for its potential anti-inflammatory effects. GLA, lengthened to dihomo-γ-linolenic acid in vivo, has been shown to reduce leukotriene biosynthesis.[107] Thus, both EPA and GLA have a potential role in the setting of many proinflammatory states, though few studies exist in the neurologically injured population. The use of enteral formulas rich in EPA, GLA, and antioxidants has been more rigorously evaluated in the setting of severe sepsis and acute lung injury. Previous studies have suggested that supplementation with EPA-/GLA-rich nutrition appears to result in improvement in oxygen status, more ventilator-free days, and decreased new organ dysfunction for those patients who received the study formula, as well as a possible decrease in mortality.[108,109] However, a recent placebo controlled trial evaluating EPA/GLA supplementation in patients with acute lung injury was stopped early for futility.[110] Patients in the EPA/GLA group had significantly less ventilator-free days and a trend toward increased 60-day mortality. Clinical data are lacking in neurologic illness, despite the plausible mechanism of EPA/GLA supplementation to counter the proinflammatory response typified by severe neurologic events. No definitive recommendations can be made regarding routine EPA/GLA supplementation at this time for this patient population. Clinicians should carefully weigh the risks and benefits of EPA/GLA supplementation in patients with acute lung injury.

Immune-enhancing enteral formulas (those rich in omega-3 fatty acids, L-arginine, nucleotides, and nucleic acids) have also been studied in critical illness as well as neurologic injury, though with only a modicum of success. While some studies suggest benefit in critically ill populations such as trauma, current data in patients with severe TBI do not reveal any difference in hospital length of stay or infectious complications compared with traditional enteral formulations.[111] However, because of the strong theoretical basis for benefit, immune-enhancing enteral formulas continue to be an area of research.[112]

Micronutrient supplementation has also been evaluated in neurologic illness. Antioxidants, B vitamins, selenium, and zinc each have been used in different phases of CNS illness, and supplementation is supported with various levels of evidence. Zinc is of particular interest in TBI. It was included for discussion in the TBI guidelines after a nonsignificant trend toward decreased mortality was noted in a small prospective trial.[113] Vitamin E has been evaluated in Alzheimer disease. Supplementation with 2000 IU vitamin E per day resulted in a significant delay in median time to death, institutionalization, loss of ability to perform two of three activities of daily living, or progression to severe dementia compared to placebo.[114] Micronutrient supplementation will undoubtedly continue to be an area of continued evaluation in neurologic illness.

References

1. Brain Trauma Foundation. Management of severe traumatic brain injury. *J Neurotrauma*. 2007;24(Suppl 1):S1–S95.
2. Langlois JA, Rutland-Brown W, Thomas KE. *Traumatic Brain Injury in the United States: Emergency Department Visits, Hospitalizations, and Deaths*. Atlanta, GA: Centers for Disease Control and Prevention, National Center for Injury Prevention and Control; 2006.
3. Centre for Neuro Skills. Centre for neuro skills Bakersfield, CA Tbi resource guide [online]. www.neuroskills.com. Accessed June 6, 2011.
4. Taylor SJ, Fettes SB, Jewkes C, et al. Prospective, randomized, controlled trial to determine the effect of early enhanced enteral nutrition on clinical outcome in mechanically ventilated patients suffering head injury. *Crit Care Med*. 1999;27(11):2525–2531.
5. Section on Disorders of the Spine and Peripheral Nerves. The American Association of Neurological Surgeons. Introduction. *Neurosurgery*. 2002;50(3):S1.
6. The National Spinal Cord Injury Association. Resource center: A-z index by subject [online]. www.spinalcord.org/resources. Accessed June 6, 2011.
7. Gariballa S. *Nutrition and Stroke: Prevention and Treatment*. Oxford, UK: Blackwell Publishing; 2004.
8. American Heart Association, American Stroke Association. American Heart Association, [online]. www.strokeassociation.org. Accessed June 6, 2011.
9. National Parkinson Foundation. National Parkinson Foundation, [online]. www.parkinson.org. Accessed June 6, 2011.
10. United Cerebral Palsy. United Cerebral Palsy, [online]. http://www.ucp.org/. Accessed June 6, 2011.
11. Fruin AH, Taylor C, Pettis MS. Caloric requirements in patients with severe head injuries. *Surg Neurol*. 1986;25(1):25–28.
12. Zehnder Y, Luthi M, Michel D, et al. Long-term changes in bone metabolism, bone mineral density, quantitative ultrasound parameters, and fracture incidence after spinal cord injury: a cross-sectional observational study in 100 paraplegic men. *Osteoporos Int*. 2004;15(3):180–189.
13. Spungen AM, Adkins RH, Stewart CA, et al. Factors influencing body composition in persons with spinal cord injury: a cross-sectional study. *J Appl Physiol*. 2003;95(6):2398–2407.
14. Weekes E, Elia M. Resting energy expenditure and body composition following cerebro-vascular accident. *Clin Nutr*. 1992;11(1): 18–22.
15. Finestone HM, Greene-Finestone LS, Foley NC, et al. Measuring longitudinally the metabolic demands of stroke patients: Resting energy expenditure is not elevated. *Stroke*. 2003;34(2):502–507.
16. Bardutzky J, Georgiadis D, Kollmar R, et al. Energy demand in patients with stroke who are sedated and receiving mechanical ventilation. *J Neurosurg*. 2004;100(2):266–271.
17. The SAFE Study Investigators. A comparison of albumin and saline for fluid resuscitation in the intensive care unit. *N Engl J Med*. 2004;350:2247–2256.
18. The SAFE Study Investigators. Saline or albumin for fluid resuscitation in patients with traumatic brain injury. *N Engl J Med*. 2007;357:874–884.
19. Bivins BA, Twyman DL, Young AB. Failure of nonprotein calories to mediate protein conservation in brain-injured patients. *J Trauma*. 1986;26(11):980–986.
20. Rhoney DH, Parker D Jr. Considerations in fluids and electrolytes after traumatic brain injury. *Nutr Clin Pract*. 2006;21(5):462–478.
21. Prough DS, Zornow MH. Hypertonic maintenance fluids for patients with cerebral edema: Does the evidence support a "phase ii" trial? *Crit Care Med*. 1998;26(3):421–422.
22. Tommasino C. Fluids and the neurosurgical patient. *Anesthesiol Clin N Am*. 2002;20(2):329–346.
23. D'Alecy LG, Lundy EF, Barton KJ, et al. Dextrose containing intravenous fluid impairs outcome and increases death after eight minutes of cardiac arrest and resuscitation in dogs. *Surgery*. 1986;100 (3):505–511.
24. de Courten-Myers G, Myers RE, Schoolfield L. Hyperglycemia enlarges infarct size in cerebrovascular occlusion in cats. *Stroke*. 1988;19(5):623–630.
25. Pulsinelli WA, Waldman S, Rawlinson D, et al. Moderate hyperglycemia augments ischemic brain damage: a neuropathologic study in the rat. *Neurology*. 1982;32(11):1239–1246.
26. Lam AM, Winn HR, Cullen BF, et al. Hyperglycemia and neurological outcome in patients with head injury. *J Neurosurg*. 1991;75(4):545–551.
27. Young B, Ott L, Dempsey R, et al. Relationship between admission hyperglycemia and neurologic outcome of severely brain-injured patients. *Ann Surg*. 1989;210(4):466–473.
28. Pentelenyi T, Kammerer L, Stutzel M, et al. Alterations of the basal serum insulin and blood glucose in brain-injured patients. *Injury*. 1979;10(3):201–208.
29. Merguerian PA, Perel A, Wald U, et al. Persistent nonketotic hyperglycemia as a grave prognostic sign in head-injured patients. *Crit Care Med*. 1981;9(12):838–840.
30. Cook AM, Peppard A, Magnuson B. Nutrition considerations in traumatic brain injury. *Nutr Clin Pract*. 2008;23:608–620.
31. Marsh WR, Anderson RE, Sundt TM Jr. Effect of hyperglycemia on brain ph levels in areas of focal incomplete cerebral ischemia in monkeys. *J Neurosurg*. 1986;65(5):693–696.
32. Kushner M, Fieschi C, Alavi A, et al. Local cerebral metabolic changes in acute ischemic strokes. *Gerontol*. 1987;33(3–4):265–267.
33. Zygun DA, Steiner LA, Johnston AJ, et al. Hyperglycemia and brain tissue ph after traumatic brain injury. *Neurol*. 2004;55(4):877–882.
34. Kinoshita K, Kraydieh S, Alonso O, et al. Effect of posttraumatic hyperglycemia on contusion volume and neutrophil accumulation after moderate fluid-percussion brain injury in rats. *J Neurotrauma*. 2002;19(6):681–692.
35. Li P-A, Liu G-J, He QP, et al. Production of hydroxyl free radical by brain tissues in hyperglycemic rats subjected to transient forebrain ischemia. *Free Radic Biol Med*. 1999;27(9/10):1033–1040.
36. Suchner U. Enteral versus parenteral nutrition: effects of gastrointestinal function and metabolism. *Nutrition*. 1998;14(1):76–81.
37. Mackay LE, Morgan AS, Bernstein BA. Swallowing disorders in severe brain injury: risk factors affecting return to oral intake. *Arch Phys Med Rehabil*. 1999;80:365–371.
38. Runions S, Rodrigue N, White C. Practice on an acute stroke unit after implementation of a decision-making algorithm for dietary management of dysphagia. *J Neurosci Nurs*. 2004;36(4):200–207.
39. Logemann JA. Swallowing disorders. *Best Pract Res Clin Gastroenterol*. 2007;21(4):563–573.
40. Lind CD. Dysphagia: evaluation and treatment. *Gastroenterol Clin N Am*. 2003;32(2):553–575.
41. Gordon C, Hewer RL, Wade DT. Dysphagia in acute stroke. *Br Med J*. 1987;295:411–414.
42. National Dysphagia Diet Task Force. *National Dysphagia Diet: Standardization for Optimal Care*. Chicago, IL: American Dietetic Association; 2002.
43. Long CL, Schaffel N, Geiger JW, et al. Metabolic response to injury and illness: Estimation of energy and protein needs from indirect calorimetry and nitrogen balance. *J Parenter Enter Nutr*. 1979;3(6): 452–456.
44. Kolpek JH, Ott LG, Record KE, et al. Comparison of urinary urea nitrogen excretion and measured energy expenditure in spinal

cord injury and nonsteroid-treated severe head trauma patients. *J Parenter Enteral Nutr*. 1989;13(3):277–280.
45. McClave SA, Martindale RG, Vanek VW, et al. Guidelines for the provision and assessment of nutrition support therapy in the adult critically ill patient. *J Parenter Enteral Nutr*. 2009;33(3):277–316.
46. McCall M, Jeejeebhoy K, Pencharz P, et al. Effect of neuromuscular blockade on energy expenditure in patients with severe head injury. *J Parenter Enteral Nutr*. 2003;27(1):27–35.
47. Dempsey DT, Guenter P, Mullen JL, et al. Energy expenditure in acute trauma to the head with and without barbiturate therapy. *Surg Gynecol Obstet*. 1985;160(2):128–134.
48. Fried RC, Dickerson RN, Guenter PA, et al. Barbiturate therapy reduces nitrogen excretion in acute head injury. *J Trauma*. 1989; 29(11):1558–1564.
49. Cox SA, Weiss SM, Posuniak EA, et al. Energy expenditure after spinal cord injury: An evaluation of stable rehabilitating patients. *J Trauma*. 1985;25(5):419–423.
50. Rodriguez DJ, Clevenger FW, Osler TM, et al. Obligatory negative nitrogen balance following spinal cord injury. *J Parenter Enteral Nutr*. 1991;15(3):319–322.
51. Bauman WA, Spungen AM, Wang J, et al. The relationship between energy expenditure and lean tissue in monozygotic twins discordant for spinal cord injury. *J Rehabil Res Dev*. 2004; 41(1):1–8.
52. Monroe MB, Tataranni PA, Pratley R, et al. Lower daily energy expenditure as measured by a respiratory chamber in subjects with spinal cord injury compared with control subjects. *Am J Clin Nutr*. 1998;68(6):1223–1227.
53. Gater DR Jr. Obesity after spinal cord injury. *Phys Med Rehabil Clin N Am*. 2007;18(2):333–351, vii.
54. Groah SL, Nash MS, Ljungberg IH, et al. Nutrient intake and body habitus after spinal cord injury: an analysis by sex and level of injury. *J Spinal Cord Med*. 2009;32(1):25–33.
55. Weaver FM, Collins EG, Kurichi J, et al. Prevalence of obesity and high blood pressure in veterans with spinal cord injuries and disorders: a retrospective review. *Am J Physic Med Rehab*. 2007;86(1): 22–29.
56. Kolpek JH, Ott LG, Record KE, et al. Comparison of urinary urea nitrogen excretion and measured energy expenditure in spinal cord injury and nonsteroid-treated severe head trauma patients. *J Parenter Enteral Nutr*. 1989;13(3):277–280.
57. Yoo SH, Kim JS, Kwon SU, et al. Undernutrition as a predictor of poor clinical outcomes in acute ischemic stroke patients. *Arch Neurol*. 2008;65(1):39–43.
58. Dennis M, Lewis S, Cranswick G, et al. Food: a multicentre randomised trial evaluating feeding policies in patients admitted to hospital with a recent stroke. *Health Technol Assess*. 2006;10(2): iii–iv, ix–x, 1–120.
59. Foley N, Finestone H, Woodbury MG, et al. Energy and protein intakes of acute stroke patients. *J Nutr Health Aging*. 2006;10(3): 171–175.
60. Azcue MP, Zello GA, Levy LD, et al. Energy expenditure and body composition in children with spastic quadriplegic cerebral palsy. *J Pediatr*. 1996;129(6):870–876.
61. Stallings VA, Zemel BS, Davies JC, et al. Energy expenditure of children and adolescents with severe disabilities: a cerebral palsy model. *Am J Clin Nutr*. 1996;64(4):627–634.
62. Bandini LG, Puelzl-Quinn H, Morelli JA, et al. Estimation of energy requirements in persons with severe central nervous system impairment. *J Pediatr*. 1995;126(5 Pt 1):828–832.
63. Bell KL, Davies PS. Energy expenditure and physical activity of ambulatory children with cerebral palsy and of typically developing children. *Am J Clin Nutr*. 2010;92(2):313–319.
64. Dickerson RN, Brown RO, Gervasio JG, et al. Measured energy expenditure of tube-fed patients with severe neurodevelopmental disabilities. *J Am Coll Nutr*. 1999;18(1):61–68.
65. Dickerson RN, Brown RO, Hanna DL, et al. Effect of upper extremity posturing on measured resting energy expenditure of nonambulatory tube-fed adult patients with severe neurodevelopmental disabilities. *J Parenter Enteral Nutr*. 2002;26(5):278–284.
66. Dickerson RN, Brown RO, Hanna DL, et al. Validation of a new method for estimating resting energy expenditure of non-ambulatory tube-fed patients with severe neurodevelopmental disabilities. *Nutr*. 2002;18(7–8):578–582.
67. Dickerson RN, Brown RO, Hanna DL, et al. Energy requirements of non-ambulatory, tube-fed adult patients with cerebral palsy and chronic hypothermia. *Nutr*. 2003;19(9):741–746.
68. Slaughter MH, Lohman TG, Boileau RA, et al. Skinfold equations for estimation of body fatness in children and youth. *Human Biol*. 1988;60(5):709–723.
69. Johnson RK, Goran MI, Ferrara MS, et al. Athetosis increases resting metabolic rate in adults with cerebral palsy. *J Am Dietet Assoc*. 1996;96(2):145–148.
70. Foley NC, Martin RE, Salter KL, et al. A review of the relationship between dysphagia and malnutrition following stroke. *J Rehabil Med*. 2009;41(9):707–713.
71. Daniels SK, Brailey K, Priestly DH, et al. Aspiration in patients with acute stroke. *Arch Phys Med Rehab*. 1998;79(1):14–19.
72. Mann G, Hankey GJ, Cameron D. Swallowing function after stroke: prognosis and prognostic factors at 6 months. *Stroke*. 1999;30(4):744–748.
73. Kidd D, Lawson J, Nesbitt R, et al. The natural history and clinical consequences of aspiration in acute stroke. *QJM*. 1995;88(6): 409–413.
74. Aviv JE, Martin JH, Sacco RL, et al. Supraglottic and pharyngeal sensory abnormalities in stroke patients with dysphagia. *Ann Otol Rhinol Laryngol*. 1996;105(2):92–97.
75. DePippo KL, Holas MA, Reding MJ, et al. Dysphagia therapy following stroke: a controlled trial. *Neurol*. 1994;44(9):1655–1660.
76. McClave SA, Heyland DK. The physiologic response and associated clinical benefits from provision of early enteral nutrition. *Nutr Clin Pract*. 2009;24(3):305–315.
77. Hartl R, Gerber LM, Ni Q, et al. Effect of early nutrition on deaths due to severe traumatic brain injury. *J Neurosurg*. 2008;109(1):50–56.
78. Marik PE, Pinsky M. Death by parenteral nutrition. *Intensive Care Med*. 2003;29:867–869.
79. Magnuson B, Hatton J, Williams S, et al. Tolerance and efficacy of enteral nutrition for neurosurgical patients in pentobarbital coma. *Nutr Clin Pract*. 1999;14:131–134.
80. Adrogue HJ, Madias NE. Hyponatremia. *N Engl J Med*. 2000; 342(21):1581–1589.
81. Singh S, Bohn D, Carlotti AP, et al. Cerebral salt wasting: truths, fallacies, theories, and challenges. *Crit Care Med*. 2002;30(11): 2575–2579.
82. Zanchi NE, Nicastro H, Lancha AH Jr. Potential antiproteolytic effects of l-leucine: Observations of in vitro and in vivo studies. *Nutr Metab (Lond)*. 2008;5:20.
83. Aquilani R, Viglio S, Iadarola P, et al. Peripheral plasma amino acid abnormalities in rehabilitation patients with severe brain injury. *Arch Phys Med Rehabil*. 2000;81(2):176–181.
84. Potenza MA, Nacci C, Mitolo-Chieppa D. Immunoregulatory effects of l-arginine and therapeutical implications. *Curr Drug Targets Immune Endocr Metabol Disord*. 2001;1(1):67–77.
85. Shang HF, Wang YY, Lai YN, et al. Effects of arginine supplementation on mucosal immunity in rats with septic peritonitis. *Clin Nutr*. 2004;23(4):561–569.

86. Muhling J, Fuchs M, Fleck C, et al. Effects of arginine, l-alanyl-l-glutamine or taurine on neutrophil (pmn) free amino acid profiles and immune functions in vitro. *Amino Acids*. 2002;22(1):39–53.
87. Lorente JA, Landin L, De Pablo R, et al. L-arginine pathway in the sepsis syndrome. *Crit Care Med*. 1993;21(9):1287–1295.
88. Argaman Z, Young VR, Noviski N, et al. Arginine and nitric oxide metabolism in critically ill septic pediatric patients. *Crit Care Med*. 2003;31(2):591–597.
89. Kalil AC, Danner RL. L-arginine supplementation in sepsis: beneficial or harmful? *Curr Opin Crit Care*. 2006;12(4):303–308.
90. Cherian L, Hlatky R, Robertson CS. Nitric oxide in traumatic brain injury. *Brain Pathol*. 2004;14(2):195–201.
91. Bak LK, Schousboe A, Waagepetersen HS. The glutamate/gaba-glutamine cycle: Aspects of transport, neurotransmitter homeostasis and ammonia transfer. *J Neurochem*. 2006;98(3):641–653.
92. Schulman AS, Willcutts KF, Claridge JA, et al. Does the addition of glutamine to enteral feeds affect patient mortality? *Crit Care Med*. 2005;33(11):2501–2506.
93. Boelens PG, Houdijk AP, Fonk JC, et al. Glutamine-enriched enteral nutrition increases in vitro interferon-gamma production but does not influence the in vivo specific antibody response to klh after severe trauma. A prospective, double blind, randomized clinical study. *Clin Nutr*. 2004;23(3):391–400.
94. Holecek M. Relation between glutamine, branched-chain amino acids, and protein metabolism. *Nutr*. 2002;18(2):130–133.
95. Conejero R, Bonet A, Grau T, et al. Effect of a glutamine-enriched enteral diet on intestinal permeability and infectious morbidity at 28 days in critically ill patients with systemic inflammatory response syndrome: a randomized, single-blind, prospective, multicenter study. *Nutr*. 2002;18(9):716–721.
96. Garrel D, Patenaude J, Nedelec B, et al. Decreased mortality and infectious morbidity in adult burn patients given enteral glutamine supplements: a prospective, controlled, randomized clinical trial. *Crit Care Med*. 2003;31(10):2444–2449.
97. Vermeulen MA, van de Poll MC, Ligthart-Melis GC, et al. Specific amino acids in the critically ill patient—exogenous glutamine/arginine: a common denominator? *Crit Care Med*. 2007;35(9 Suppl):S568–S576.
98. Benarroch EE. Glutamate transporters: diversity, function, and involvement in neurologic disease. *Neurol*. 2010;74(3):259–264.
99. Yang DL, Xu JF. Effect of dipeptide of glutamine and alanine on severe traumatic brain injury. *Chin J Traumatol*. 2007;10(3):145–149.
100. Berg A, Bellander BM, Wanecek M, et al. Intravenous glutamine supplementation to head trauma patients leaves cerebral glutamate concentration unaffected. *Intensive Care Med*. 2006;32(11):1741–1746.
101. Berg A, Bellander BM, Wanecek M, et al. The pattern of amino acid exchange across the brain is unaffected by intravenous glutamine supplementation in head trauma patients. *Clin Nutr*. 2008;27(6):816–821.
102. Fontani G, Corradeschi F, Felici A, et al. Cognitive and physiological effects of omega-3 polyunsaturated fatty acid supplementation in healthy subjects. *Eur J Clin Invest*. 2005;35(11):691–699.
103. Yuen AW, Sander JW, Fluegel D, et al. Omega-3 fatty acid supplementation in patients with chronic epilepsy: a randomized trial. *Epilepsy Behav*. 2005;7(2):253–258.
104. Mazza M, Pomponi M, Janiri L, et al. Omega-3 fatty acids and antioxidants in neurological and psychiatric diseases: an overview. *Prog Neuropsychopharmacol Biol Psychiatry*. 2007;31(1):12–26.
105. Mills JD, Bailes JE, Sedney CL, et al. Omega-3 fatty acid supplementation and reduction of traumatic axonal injury in a rodent head injury model. *J Neurosurg*. 2011;114(1):77–84.
106. Mills JD, Hadley K, Bailes JE. Dietary supplementation with the omega-3 fatty acid docosahexaenoic acid in traumatic brain injury. *Neurosurgery*. 2011;68(2):474–481; discussion 481.
107. Heller AR, Stehr SN, Litz RJ. Omega-3 alpha linolenic acid does not reflect the entire omega-3 fatty acid family. *Anesth Analg*. 2006;102(4):1289; author reply 1290.
108. Pontes-Arruda A, Martins LF, de Lima SM, et al. Enteral nutrition with eicosapentaenoic acid, gamma-linolenic acid and antioxidants in the early treatment of sepsis: results from a multicenter, prospective, randomized, double blinded and controlled study - intersept study. *Crit Care*. 2011;15(3):R144.
109. Gadek JE, DeMichele SJ, Karlstad MD, et al. Effect of enteral feeding with eicosapentaenoic acid, gamma-linolenic acid, and antioxidants in patients with acute respiratory distress syndrome. *Crit Care Med*. 1999;27(9):1409–1420.
110. Rice TW, Wheeler AP, Thompson BT, et al. Enteral omega-3 fatty acid, gamma-linolenic acid, and antioxidant supplementation in acute lung injury. *JAMA*. 2011;306(14):1574–1581.
111. Minard G, Kudsk KA, Melton S, et al. Early versus delayed feeding with an immune-enhancing diet in patients with severe head injuries. *J Parenter Enter Nutr*. 2000;24(3):145–149.
112. Heyland D, Dhaliwal R. Immunonutrition in the critically ill: From old approaches to new paradigms. *Intensive Care Med*. 2005;31(4):501–503.
113. Young B, Ott L, Kasarskis E, et al. Zinc supplementation is associated with improved neurologic recovery rate and visceral protein levels of patients with severe closed head injury. *J Neurotrauma*. 1996;13(1):25–34.
114. Sano M, Ernesto C, Thomas RG, et al. A controlled trial of selegiline, alpha-tocopherol, or both as treatment for Alzheimer's disease. *N Engl J Med*. 1997;336(17):1216–1222.
115. Young AB, Ott LG, Beard D, et al. The acute-phase response of the brain-injured patient. *J Neurosurg*. 1988;69:375–380.
116. Loan T. Metabolic/nutritional alterations of traumatic brain injury. *Nutr*. 1999;15:809–812.
117. Hatton J, Rapp RP, Kudsk KA, et al. Intravenous insulin-like growth factor-i (igf-1) in moderate-to-severe head injury: a phase ii safety and efficacy trial. *J Neurosurg*. 1997;86:779–786.
118. Schneider M, Schneider HJ, Stalla GK. Anterior pituitary hormone abnormalities following traumatic brain injury. *J Neurotrauma*. 2005;22(9):937–946.
119. McCullough G, Pelletier C, Steele C. National dysphagia diet: what to swallow? The ASHA Leader [serial on the Internet]; 2003. www.asha.org/Publications/leader/2003/031104/f031104c/. Accessed March 23, 2012.
120. American Dietetics Association. Level 2 nutrition therapy for dysphagia: mechanically altered foods [online]. http://nutritioncaremanual.org/vault/editor/Docs/Level%202%20NT%20for%20Dysphagia_MechAltered.pdf. Accessed March 23, 2012.
121. American Dietetics Association. Level 3 nutrition therapy for dysphagia: advanced foods [online]. http://nutritioncaremanual.org/vault/editor/Docs/Level%203%20NT%20for%20Dysphagia_Advanced.pdf. Accessed March 23, 2012.
122. American Dietetics Association. National dysphagia level 1: pureed nutrition therapy [online]. http://nutritioncaremanual.org/vault/ editor/Docs/National%20Dysphagia%20Level% 201%20Pureed%20Nutrition%20Therapy.pdf. Accessed March 23, 2012.

123. Hatton J. Pharmacotherapy and nutrition. In: Carter BL, ed. *Pharmacotherapy Self-Assessment Program*. 3 ed. Kansas City, MO: American College of Clinical Pharmacy; 1999: c157–178.
124. Doak KK, Haas CE, Dunnigan KJ, et al. Bioavailability of phenytoin acid and phenytoin sodium with enteral feedings. *Pharmacotherapy*. 1998;18(3):637–645.
125. Thomson FC, Naysmith MR, Lindsay SA. Managing drug therapy in patients receiving enteral and parenteral nutrition. *Hospital Pharmacist*. 2000;7(6):155–164.
126. Schelosky L, Raffauf C, Jendroska K, et al. Kava and dopamine antagonism. *J Neurol Neurosurg Psychiatry*. 1995;58(5):639–640.
127. Package insert. Carbamazepine suspension 100mg/5ml. Novartis; 2003.

23 Critical Care Sepsis

Keith Miller, MD, Laszlo Kiraly, MD, and Robert G. Martindale, MD, PhD

CONTENTS

Background 378
Definitions 378
Pathophysiology 379
Metabolic Responses During Sepsis 379
Carbohydrate Metabolism 379
Protein Metabolism 380
Lipid Metabolism 380
Nutrition Assessment in Sepsis and Critical Care 380
Energy Expenditure 381
Route of Feeding 381
Timing of Nutrition Support 383
Complications of Enteral Feeding in the Intensive Care Unit 384
Complications of Parenteral Feeding in the Intensive Care Unit 384
Nutritional Requirements 385
Energy 385
Carbohydrate 385
Lipid 385
Protein 386
Arginine and Glutamine 386
Antioxidants 387
Host Immunity 387
References 388

Objectives

1. Define infection and sepsis.
2. Describe the pathophysiology of inflammatory metabolism.
3. Review the route of feeding for enteral versus parenteral, and the pros and cons of each.
4. Describe the quantity and quality of appropriate macronutrients in the septic patient.
5. Delineate options for feeding the septic patient.
6. Describe nutritional adjuncts that may improve outcomes in septic patients.
7. Recognize the impact of nutrition support in host immunity.

Test Your Knowledge Questions

1. Which of the following characterizes the current understanding of systemic inflammation?
   A. Overstimulated immune system
   B. Mixture of immune stimulation and suppression
   C. Initial immune suppression followed by stimulation
   D. Immune suppression

2. Why is hemodynamic stability an important consideration before initiating enteral nutrition (EN)?
   A. To avoid overfeeding.
   B. Hemodynamic instability is an indication for parenteral nutrition (PN).
   C. Gastrointestinal perfusion may be compromised.
   D. To avoid underfeeding.
3. What is the best reason to prescribe energy in nutrition support regimens conservatively?
   A. Glycemic control
   B. To facilitate permissive underfeeding
   C. Cost containment
   D. To achieve goal infusions more efficiently

Test Your Knowledge Answers

1. The correct answer is **B**. Current understanding of inflammation has evolved from interpreting the condition as one of an overstimulated immune system and altered metabolic reaction to infection and trauma to a combination, depending on clinical and individual attributes, of both overstimulation of metabolic and immune responses and also a compensatory reaction causing immune metabolic suppression. In fact, decreased immunity may predominate depending on the source of inflammation, the timing, and the clinical status of the patient.
2. The correct answer is **C**. Gastrointestinal perfusion is compromised during septic states, particularly in conditions of hemodynamic instability. Feeding into the gastrointestinal tract may initiate an ischemic event. Once adequately resuscitated, enteral feeding may in fact help preserve gastrointestinal perfusion. In any case, EN should be started as early as possible under conditions of hemodynamic stability.
3. The correct answer is **A**. Hyperglycemia is associated with adverse outcomes in critical care populations including increased incidence of infections. Conservative energy prescription including gradual increase of infusion rates to goal energy requirements assists in controlling serum glucose levels.

Background

Sepsis continues to be a major health care problem in the United States. From 2000 to 2008, the rate of hospitalization has doubled.[1] Sepsis is the eleventh leading cause of death in the United States, and this figure does not include the common diagnosis of pneumonia and influenza.[2] A study of eight academic tertiary care centers indicated that the hospital-wide incidence of sepsis syndrome is 2.0 ± 0.2 cases per 100 admissions, or 2.8 ± 0.2 per 1000 patient-days, and patients in the intensive care unit (ICU) account for 59% of cases.[3] A retrospective analysis in the surgical ICU indicated that in 78% of the patients who died of sepsis and multiple system organ failure, the main source of infection was either the respiratory or gastrointestinal tract.[4] Anti-infective agents have had little impact on mortality in sepsis in the last century.[5] The majority of the decrease in mortality from sepsis resulted from public health measures such as immunization, establishment of public health departments, and the pasteurization of milk.[5] The major influence of antibiotics has, in fact, been to change the source of bacteria causing sepsis from exogenous environmental sources to endogenous sources. Specialized nutrition therapy including appropriate substrate prescription delivered at the most suitable time and via the optimal route may have significant influence on the endogenous microbial population virulence and quantity. This chapter discusses our current understanding of nutrition therapy in sepsis and infection, and the multiple benefits appropriate nutrition intervention can offer in sepsis management.

Definitions

The term "sepsis" encompasses a spectrum of diseases ranging from systemic inflammatory response syndrome (SIRS) to severe sepsis and multiple organ failure. It is no longer considered a disease with a specific definition but a group of diseases based on the predisposition of the patient, the severity of insult, the physiological or pathophysiological response of the host, and the number and extent of organ involvement. The terms "sepsis" and "infection or inflammation" are commonly misused in the critically ill population. Standardized definitions have been published by the American College of Chest Physicians and Society of Critical Care Medicine Consensus Conference of 1992.[6] These definitions help to clarify the differences between "sepsis" and "infection," and can be readily applied to patients in different stages of infection or inflammation.

Sepsis is the systemic response to infection. Historically, sepsis described a life-threatening condition characterized by fever, tachycardia, tachypnea, and organ dysfunction, and was frequently associated with shock and death. It was also often associated with a bacterial, fungal, or viral infection, which could be either localized or systemic in nature. However, other conditions, such as severe trauma, pancreatitis, hemorrhage, ischemia, and burn injury, can produce the same clinical findings in the absence of an identified infectious source. This constellation of fever, tachycardia, tachypnea, and organ dysfunction has come to be known as SIRS. That is, SIRS is a clinical syndrome that can be caused by a variety of insults, including sepsis.

The exact definition of sepsis is variable but generally is defined as the presence or presumed presence of an infectious source accompanied by SIRS, as described previously. Severe sepsis is defined as the presence of sepsis with one or more organ dysfunction. Septic shock is defined as the presence of sepsis and hemodynamic instability. This is primarily refractory hypotension with systolic peak pressures less than 90 mm Hg, mean arterial pressures less than 65 mm Hg, or a drop of greater than 40 mm Hg from baseline. These blood pressures noted are unresponsive to crystalloid volume resuscitation of at least 20 to 40 mL/kg.[3,7,8]

Additionally, the concept of sepsis has evolved since the 1992 definition to recognize that it is the interaction of several factors that determines the severity of the septic response and also influences the response to treatment. The multifactor model of sepsis is known as predisposition, insult, response, and organ dysfunction (PIRO).[8] "Predisposition" encompasses a range of genetic, biological, and cultural factors that influence the risk of development of SIRS as well as the potential to benefit from various interventions. "Insult" refers to the nature of the inciting event, specifically the microbiology and location of an infection, or a noninfectious source. "Response" is the physiological, biochemical, and biological changes that occur as a result of the insult. "Organ dysfunction" measures the degree of failure of the major organ systems: neurological, respiratory, cardiac, renal, and, of course, gastrointestinal. This model has been likened to the tumor, node, and metastasis staging system for malignancies, which stratifies the severity and guides therapy for many different kinds of cancers. Further studies are needed to develop a scoring system based on the PIRO model to predict outcomes (such as overall survival) in SIRS. The PIRO model allows us to begin to model a therapy plan, including a nutritional plan, more focused to the individual rather than the "one-size-fits-all" model commonly practiced today.

Pathophysiology

The metabolic response to sepsis is in many ways similar to the response that follows major surgery or trauma (see Chapter 24). Increases in energy expenditure, protein catabolism, and oxidation of stored lipids along with significant alterations in the body's ability to metabolize carbohydrate make the responses very similar.[9]

A series of events requiring multiple organ systems are required for the progression from localized infection to sepsis, severe sepsis, and septic shock. The initial reaction of the host is localized to the site of infection or injury. The process begins with cellular activation at the endothelial level of macrophages, monocytes, and neutrophils. Various microbial components such as cell wall structures, proteins, or deoxyribonucleic acid bind to specific receptors on the surface of white cells called pattern recognition receptors including toll-like receptors and others.[10] These cells then start a cascade of events, including activation of the complement system leading to vasodilatation and increased capillary permeability, which leads to increased interstitial fluid, and chemoattractrants in the local area. Additional macrophages are attracted to the area; these, in turn, then orchestrate the intensity of the inflammatory response. In the presence of infection, the macrophages undergo accelerated phagocytic activity with elaboration of tumor necrosis factor (TNF), interleukin (IL)-1, IL-2, IL-6, and multiple other proinflammatory cytokines, which can, if in high enough concentration, "spill over" into the systemic circulation to influence the entire systemic response. Once systemic activation has begun, microvascular coagulation is noted; platelets, mast cells, and local vasodilators result in generalized edema, accelerated oxygen free radical production, and eventual organ injury. This initial septic response is proinflammatory. This proinflammatory phase is followed by a compensatory anti-inflammatory response.[2,5] Virtually all major organs are involved but disruption in cardiac, pulmonary, renal, and hepatic function is most commonly observed clinically. Although at first glance it would appear that the systemic response is destructive to the host, these systemic manifestations of the "septic response" are in effect related to attempts to contain the infection.[2,5] It is only when the cascade of events becomes overwhelming to the host that it is destructive and not protective. It is important to remember that immune suppression is a major part of the later phases of sepsis, making this period a perfect target for nutritional intervention.[5]

The hallmark of the management of sepsis includes the timely use of appropriate antimicrobial agents and early drainage or removal of purulent foci to achieve rapid bacterial or fungal eradication. Support of the septic patient also includes administration of early goal-directed therapy with crystalloid and colloid solutions, blood products (including red blood cells and fresh frozen plasma), inotropic and vasoactive agents, and mechanical ventilation to ensure hemodynamic stability and oxygenation of vital tissues.[5,11,12] Data would also support intense management of hyperglycemia and corticosteroids for the appropriate patient.[5]

Recently, the understanding of sepsis has become somewhat more complicated than described previously as an initial proinflammatory phase followed by compensatory anti-inflammatory stage. In fact, anti-inflammatory cytokines (IL-4 and IL-10) may predominate rather than proinflammatory cytokines (TNF-α, IL-2, interferon-γ) depending on the initial stimulus of inflammation, polymorphisms in genes for cytokines, and clinical status, including age. Thus, susceptible patients may be immune suppressed, causing host inability to eradicate the pathogen adequately.[5] Outcome in sepsis is extremely difficult to predict or affect because the timing of intervention is so variable in relation to the host inflammatory response.[9] To date, attempting blockade of targeted mediators of the inflammatory response has been uniformly unsuccessful.[2,13] Over 30 years of dedicated efforts to reverse sepsis with various broad-spectrum antibiotics (alone or in combination) and monoclonal antibodies has, at best, only shown modest benefit and in fact been harmful in some cases.[2] Appropriate nutritional therapy during sepsis and severe infections is essential because it plays a key role in modulating the inflammatory response, maintaining immune function, abrogating skeletal muscle catabolism, improving wound healing, and maintaining gastrointestinal and pulmonary mucosal barrier function.

Metabolic Responses During Sepsis

Carbohydrate Metabolism

Under normal conditions, glucose homeostasis (see Chapter 3) is regulated by several control mechanisms to match the uptake and production of glucose. These mechanisms maintain "normal" blood glucose concentrations under a wide range of conditions. However, hyperglycemia and significant insulin resistance is a clinical characteristic uniformly found in sepsis. Proinflammatory cytokines potentiate the release of catabolic hormones (glucagon, catecholamines, and cortisol). These catabolic hormones stimulate glycogenolysis and gluconeogenesis to mobilize glucose. Glucagon-stimulated glycogenolysis, for example, is one of the most sensitive and reproducible metabolic effects of hormones on any tissue.[14,15] Following the onset of sepsis, glycogen stores are depleted within hours, and endogenous lipid and protein become the major source of oxidative energy substrate.[16]

Sepsis results in hyperglycemia secondary to alterations in endogenous glucose production, decreased glucose uptake, and insulin resistance.[16,17] Moderate or severe infection is associated with a 150% to 200% increase in the glucose production rate, and circulating glucose levels tend to be correspondingly high. Dahn and colleagues reported hepatic glucose production in trauma and sepsis is sixfold greater than in trauma alone.[18] Gluconeogenesis increases with progressive organ failure, as does the level and production of gluconeogenic precursors (lactate, pyruvate, alanine, and glycerol). As sepsis progresses, reduced splanchnic blood flow and severe end-stage hepatic dysfunction eventually leads to decreased glucose production and hypoglycemia at the final stages of life.

Protein Metabolism

Although protein breakdown and synthesis both continue to occur at accelerated rates during sepsis, patients remain in generalized net-negative nitrogen balance for variable periods even after the inciting insult has been resolved.[16] The accelerated peripheral muscle protein breakdown noted in sepsis is accompanied with diminished amino acid uptake by muscle, leading to the net flux of amino acids away from the periphery to the liver.[19] The ureagenesis rate is increased, as well as the synthesis rates of creatinine, uric acid, and ammonia. All are excreted in increased amounts in the urine during sepsis. The nitrogen loss of severe sepsis complicating recovery from trauma may exceed 30 g/d.[19,20] The primary sites of this amino acid efflux are from the "labile" amino acid pools in skeletal muscle, connective tissue, and unstimulated gut. It is important to keep in mind the mammalian species has no "storage" of protein and that any protein utilized during catabolic stress of any kind comes at the expense of other tissues that are more labile. During sepsis, hepatic uptake of amino acids and hepatic protein synthesis are increased, which allows a substrate for gluconeogenesis and production of acute-phase proteins. However, the increase in hepatic protein synthesis is not uniform. Although positive acute-phase protein, such as haptoglobin and C-reactive protein concentrations in serum increase in response to stress, synthesis of negative acute-phase proteins such as albumin and prealbumin falls.[21] This concept is often referred to as hepatic reprioritization.

Under these catabolic circumstances, patients who receive adequate exogenous amino acids to maintain production of acute-phase proteins are more likely to survive.[22] Nonetheless, adequate nutrition support can only attenuate the response and will not completely ablate the catabolic effects and response.[22] In an elaborate series of metabolic studies by Plank et al., it was reported that in septic patients, 13.5% of total body protein was lost in the first 21 days following a single septic or traumatic insult. This was despite receiving adequate nutritional support. The metabolic rate was still elevated above baseline at 21 days.[21]

As the systemic response to sepsis progresses, protein catabolism increases, and the failure of synthetic processes to keep up with the breakdown rate results in severe losses of skeletal protein. In an unfed, stressed patient, up to 250 g of lean body mass will be broken down each day.[15] Some of the amino acids thus mobilized provide oxidative substrate for gluconeogenesis, but even in the face of seemingly adequate exogenous glucose supplies, there is obligate mobilization of amino acids.[15] In addition to supplying amino acid for acute-phase protein synthesis, a driving force for the mobilization of amino acids during sepsis and other significant stress is thought to be the host attempting to provide glutamine to enterocytes and leukocytes.[23] Unfortunately, prolonged catabolism of skeletal muscle protein compromises respiratory function, impairs wound healing, exacerbates immunosuppression, accelerates the loss of strength and endurance necessary for recovery, and increases ventilator dependency time and ICU stay, the risk of thromboembolic disease, recovery time, and mortality incidence.

Lipid Metabolism

The catabolic hormones epinephrine, norepinephrine, and glucagon are the predominant stimulators of the hydrolysis of stored triglycerides (lipolysis) via direct stimulation hormone-sensitive lipase. In early sepsis, catabolic hormones outweigh the effects of anabolic hormones such as insulin and growth hormone, and result in the breakdown of stored triglycerides to glycerol and free fatty acids (FFAs).[24] In addition to the increased rate of lipolysis of peripheral adipose stores observed in sepsis, intracellular transport metabolism is also affected.[24] The ability of the cell to transport long-chain FFAs from the cytosol into mitochondria via the acylcarnitine carrier is impaired. Consequently, long-chain FFA esters accumulate within the cell and can inhibit the function of pyruvate dehydrogenase complex directly. This will result in intracellular acidosis and the accumulation of lactate and pyruvate.[25,26] This is a major reason for the decrease in aerobic respiration and the cells' ability to use the Krebs cycle for efficient energy production. Furthermore, in addition to impaired FFA utilization, sepsis impairs ketogenesis. The keto acids are an important source of oxidative fuel for several organs during starvation. Finally, the activity of lipoprotein lipase, which is responsible for the conversion of triglycerides to FFAs in peripheral cells, is suppressed in sepsis. Consequently, hyperlipidemia, hyperglycemia, hyperlactatemia, and high levels of circulating β-hydroxybutyrate often are observed in severe sepsis.[24,25]

Nutrition Assessment in Sepsis and Critical Care

Traditional methods of nutrition assessment are not as useful in the septic or critically ill patient as in the general hospitalized patient. Critically ill patients suffer from significant fluid shifts and metabolic abnormalities related to the inflammatory response that deem anthropometric and biochemical measures unreliable. Hepatically synthesized proteins such as albumin and prealbumin are commonly misused in severely ill patients as markers of nutrition status when in fact their levels are indicative of reprioritization of hepatic protein synthesis and increased vascular permeability during the inflammatory response. [21] In addition, an inability to obtain nutrition history from the patient directly also makes it difficult to perform and interpret nutrition assessment criteria. A thorough weight and diet history must often be pieced together from the available medical record history and family members. In absence of validated tools for assessment, the Society of Critical Care Medicine and American Society for Parenteral and Enteral Nutrition recommends evaluating weight loss and nutrition history prior to admission, level of disease severity, and gastrointestinal function.[27] Thereafter, an ongoing meticulous review of the patient's current physical and metabolic status including weight changes, abdominal exam, gastrointestinal function, evidence of wounds, line, drain and tube placements, ventilation parameters, vital signs, hemodynamics, and laboratory values provides the information necessary to apply the appropriate nutrition intervention. Chapter 9 discusses in detail the use of nutrition assessment tools as well as the drawbacks of their use in the critically ill patient.

Energy Expenditure

Literature evaluating energy expenditure in sepsis has been limited by heterogeneity of the population studied and the rather loose definitions of sepsis used in most studies. Elaborate metabolic studies following the onset of sepsis in patients with peritonitis indicated that resting energy expenditure progressively increases over the first 7 days and remains elevated for up to 21 days even when the sepsis has been adequately addressed and treated.[21] These data are partially clouded by the thermogenic influence of the nutrition delivery itself, which is noted when nutrition support is started. The very early stages of sepsis are also characterized by decreased mitochondrial energy utilization.[28] The clinical importance of this early phase, however, is largely unknown.

In summary, metabolism during sepsis is associated with a significant increase in energy expenditure estimated to be from 20% to 60% above basal energy expenditure.[21] The increase in energy expenditure is associated with amplified protein muscle catabolism, as well as an increased reliance on lipid stores for oxidative fuel. Initially, these metabolic alterations may be beneficial to mobilize adequate endogenous substrate to support the immune and wound healing processes, but when prolonged, become detrimental to host survival. This supply may be even more important after the early phase of sepsis as the cellular "machinery" recovers. Although PN support cannot alter the rate of catabolism, EN and use of anti-inflammatory lipids (eicosapentaenoic acid [EPA] and docosahexaenoic acid [DHA]) can attenuate the catabolic response to stress.[27] Supplying substrates for enhanced acute-phase protein synthesis has the potential to improve conditions for enhanced survival.

Route of Feeding

Early administration of enteral nutrients has been shown to offer outcome benefits in critical care populations when compared to PN.[29,30] Numerous mechanisms have been proposed to explain the benefits observed including maintaining mucosal integrity, improving visceral blood flow, supporting the gut-associated lymphoid tissue (GALT), among others.

The gastrointestinal tract and the liver are susceptible to ischemia during sepsis secondary to the shunting of blood flow away from the splanchnic bed. Gut ischemia, in turn, leads to mitochondrial dysfunction, mucosal acidosis, progressive cell injury, and death.[31–33] Practitioners are often concerned that EN may increase the ischemic injury during states of decreased perfusion of the splanchnic organs in septic patients, especially if the patient is receiving vasoactive medications.[31] Laboratory evidence provides support for the opposing view: namely, that EN provides protection and even enhances perfusion during septic states.[34] For example, Gosche and colleagues used in vivo microvascular techniques to examine the effect of mucosally applied glucose on intestinal microvascular blood flow during *Escherichia coli* sepsis in the rat.[35] Blood flow was rapidly restored to above-baseline values after glucose was added, showing that the hyperemia induced by direct application of glucose to the mucosal surface of the small intestine is able to overcome the flow-restrictive effect of gram-negative bacteremia. The authors suggest that this direct hyperemic effect of transmucosal absorption of nutrients on the intestinal microvasculature is a factor that accounts for the improved maintenance of mucosal integrity associated with EN.[35] Khalid et al. recently reported the results of early enteral feeding in over 1000 patients requiring ventilation for over 48 hours and on vasopressors to maintain blood pressure. They showed a decrease in mortality in those patients fed early despite the use of pressors.[36]

Generally, vasopressors shunt flow away from the splanchnic bed, although not all the vasopressors have the same influence on the visceral blood flow, and each agent must be considered in relation to the clinical situation in which it is being used.[31] Revelly et al. evaluated EN in a group of hemodynamically unstable critically ill patients requiring vasoactive medications and concluded that vasopressors increased visceral blood flow and that nutrient absorption was not adversely influenced.[37] Nonetheless, because splanchnic circulation is one of the major vascular beds affected by vasoactive agents, even at low doses, care must be taken when providing EN to patients in septic shock.[33] The vasoconstrictive effects of vasopressors may prevent a normal increase in splanchnic blood flow during enteral feeding, even though the gastrointestinal tract may seem to be functional and without evidence of paralytic ileus. This can lead to an ischemic state and result in jejunal feeding associated small bowel necrosis.[38–41]

Several approaches can be taken to maximize gut function in sepsis and inflammatory states such as critical illness. These include maintaining visceral perfusion, which can usually be done by providing adequate resuscitation; glycemic control; correction of acidosis and electrolyte abnormalities; minimizing the use of anticholinergic medications, narcotics, and other medications that decrease intestinal motility; and instituting EN, even at low rates, within the first 24 to 48 hours of the onset of SIRS or sepsis. Currently available data support enteral feeding in the septic patient, but only after the patient has been adequately volume resuscitated and has shown to be at goal perfusion pressures[12,41] (Practice Scenario 23-1). Most clinicians rightfully approach feeding the resuscitated septic patient still requiring vasoactive agents with trepidation. These patients need close monitoring and frequent exams to ensure they do not suffer the devastating complications of bowel ischemia.

One of the foremost benefits of EN may not be in the treatment, but rather the prevention of serious infections.[42] Once sepsis has been well established, EN has unproven efficacy compared to PN, or even no nutritional support, in improving outcome. For example, if EN is delayed until 4 to 6 days after the onset of injury, sepsis, or ICU admission, as in the study of ICU patients by Eyer and colleagues, it does not prevent progression to multiple organ system dysfunction or alter the risk of mortality.[43] Evaluations of EN in patients with sepsis are rare. Most papers addressing the benefits of enteral feeding are in mixed critical care populations with a portion of the studied patients having sepsis. As discussed in the previous section, the enteral route is the preferred route of administration of nutritional therapy in critically ill patients whenever feasible.[42,44] However, during sepsis, EN may be complicated by lack of access or by gastrointestinal dysfunction. Lack of access (see Chapter 12) should not be used as an excuse for not utilizing the gastrointestinal tract. Numerous protocols have recently been described reporting 75% to 80% success in obtaining enteral access in severely ill patients.[45,46] Furthermore, centers with protocols including tube placement and promotility agents have demonstrated significantly higher nutrition adequacy and lower utilization of PN in critically ill patients.[47] When true gastrointestinal intolerance or dysfunction prevents adequate nutrient delivery via the enteral route, PN should be considered (Practice Scenario 23-2). The institution of PN when EN is not tolerated is controversial, but starting PN earlier than 5 to 7 days has not proven to be of benefit.[27] If low infusion rates of EN can be safely administered, it can be combined with PN in attempts to maintain gut mucosal integrity and GALT.[47–49] Despite these theoretical benefits of PN, a large recent randomized trial comparing ICU patients treated with early (48 hours) versus late (8 days) PN noted higher mortality, organ failure, and infections in the early group.[50]

Practice Scenario 23-1

Question: What is he best approach to EN initiation and feeding in an acutely septic trauma patient?

Scenario: A 58-year-old male is involved in a motorcycle collision. He is brought to the emergency department for evaluation. Workup reveals a brain injury and bilateral rib fractures, pulmonary contusions, and a moderate spleen injury. The spleen injury is managed nonoperatively. No nutrition therapy is started. He requires intubation for worsening mental status and hypoxia. After 48 hours of ventilator support, the patient develops fever of 38.7°C and hypotension. His minute ventilation is 15 L. A chest x-ray reveals a left lower lobe infiltrate. He is started on vasopressors and antibiotics. That morning, he has a blood pressure of 80/60 despite moderate doses of norepinephrine and vasopressin. A nutrition consult is obtained given his lack of nutrition delivery in the past 48 hours. His height is 175 cm, and his weight is 80 kg.

Intervention: Feeding was not initiated immediately as the patient was unstable. The patient was further resuscitated, and his vasopressor requirement decreased. Tube feeding was started at a low rate (20 mL/hr). Frequent exams were performed to ensure the patient was tolerating the regimen. By the next day, the patient's hemodynamics were much improved. The tube feeds were advanced at a rate of 20 mL each 4 hours to the goal rate of 100 mL/hr.

Answer: The energy requirement is approximately 2300 estimated by the recently validated Penn State equation.[157] The estimated protein requirement was ~140 g (1.8 g/kg). An immune-enhancing (isotonic, lactose-free, low-residue) tube feeding formulation was selected given his history of trauma and sepsis. The specialized formula provided ~60 g of protein/L, thus in order to meet the patient's estimated nutrition needs, a final goal rate of 100 mL/h would be necessary. Enteral feeding should not be started in the setting of acutely worsening hemodynamics. Once his status improved, feeding was started carefully and advanced.

Rationale: Enteral tube feeds could have been started shortly after admission. The patient likely had an orogastric tube placed shortly after endotracheal intubation. Given the evidence for early tube feeding (< 48 hours), admission would have been an ideal time to start. Starting tube feeds earlier also gives the opportunity to "troubleshoot" patients who may not tolerate initial regimens (prokinetic agents, postpyloric tubes, etc.). The patient required further stabilization with resuscitation. Good communication with the ICU team allowed nutrition therapy to be started quickly.

Practice Scenario 23-2

Question: What is the best approach to PN initiation and feeding in an acutely septic patient?

Scenario: A 74-year-old woman is admitted with a 3-day history of diarrhea, abdominal pain, and lethargy. She has an extremely tender abdomen. She has a history of type 2 diabetes mellitus and atrial fibrillation. Laboratory examination indicated her blood glucose level was 542 mg/dL and white blood cell count was 22,100 cells/mm^3. Given her status and very concerning exam, she is taken to the operating room. The surgery team finds 100 cm of nonviable infracted jejunum. A small bowel anastomosis is performed. She initially improves but again worsens with high fevers and high white blood cell count. A computed tomography scan is performed 7 days postoperatively revealing a fluid collection around the anastomosis. She was taken to the operating room, her anastomosis was repaired, and drains were placed. Her blood cultures grew *E. coli* and *Pseudomonas aeruginosa*. She was begun on broad-spectrum antibiotics. She improved but soon after develops evidence of a proximal small bowel fistula from her surgically placed drains.

Intervention: PN was selected over EN because she had a proximal intestinal fistula, diarrhea, and sepsis. A predictive equation was used to calculate her requirement. After several days, indirect calorimetry was used to reevaluate.

Answer: This patient had not received nutrition for over 7 days and was malnourished. EN would not be absorbed reliably. PN would offer the best chance of her fistula closing spontaneously. Her estimated energy expenditure using the Mifflin-St. Joer predictive equation is ~1650 calories. Protein requirements are approximately 1.5 g/kg/d. A mixed fuel system was preferred because she was hyperglycemic and dextrose alone was inadequate to provide enough energy. In addition to hyperglycemia, she was likely insulin resistant, as is the case in most septic patients. Furthermore, infusion of more than 5 mg/kg/min will likely exceed maximal glucose oxidation and lead to no additional protein synthesis. Exogenous lipids can be effectively used as a fuel source during sepsis. The patient received 1700 with 1.5 g/kg of amino acid from PN and tolerated it well. During the next 3 days post surgery, her body temperature and white blood cell count gradually decreased. Blood sugar level was maintained below 180 mg/dL. Indirect calorimetry was performed 5 days post surgery and observed to be 1150 kcal. To improve hyperglycemia and avoid other deleterious effects of overfeeding, the decision was made to lower the caloric level of PN. The patient's nutritional status was monitored using daily weights, in and out fluid records, and serum glucose and electrolyte levels. Indirect calorimetry was repeated once or twice weekly as part of monitoring.

Rationale: The patient was at significant risk for complications secondary to her comorbidities and malnutrition. Her gut could not be reliably used, and PN was selected. She was given an increased protein allowance given her wound and sepsis. Her energy requirements were estimated, reassessed, and then adjusted throughout her course.

Timing of Nutrition Support

The optimal time to start nutrition support is influenced by a host of factors including age, premorbid conditions, route of nutrient delivery, metabolic state, and organ function.[51,52] As previously noted, literature evaluating nutritional support for critically ill patients has analyzed heterogeneous populations, which contain patients with sepsis. Nevertheless, these studies yield important concepts for feeding the patient with sepsis.[15] The reported benefits of early EN are, among others, prevention of adverse structural and functional alterations in the mucosal barrier, augmentation of visceral blood flow, and enhancement of local and systemic immune response.[29,30] The clinical benefits of early EN have recently been the focus of three meta-analyses, which report a benefit of reducing infections and length of hospital stay with minimal risk and virtually no increase in major morbidity.[29,30,53] Despite these acknowledged benefits, nutrition support remains suboptimal in a significant percentage of critically ill patients.

Acknowledging that the early initiation of nutrition support is the superior and accepted practice, a multidisciplinary approach to determining appropriate timing in the individual patient cannot be overemphasized. This entails the combined efforts of all involved health care providers acknowledging the unique skills and expertise that each brings to the care of the patient. Enteral feeding should not proceed until appropriate resuscitation has been undertaken. Resuscitation remains a cornerstone of the three-armed approach to the management of sepsis comprised of source control, early antibiotic administration, and resuscitation. Early and aggressive resuscitation, or "early goal-directed therapy," involves the placement of invasive lines including central venous catheters with continuous venous oxygen saturation monitoring, arterial lines, etc., in order to evaluate the overall volume status of the patient. Fluid resuscitation is continued with set central venous pressure goals, at which point vasopressor medications are added in the hypotensive (mean arterial pressures < 65 mm Hg), vasodilated patient.[12] A single laboratory or hemodynamic parameter signaling the successful resuscitation of the critically ill patient in shock remains elusive. Generally, trends in hemodynamic parameters, including mean arterial pressures, central venous pressures, and vasopressor requirements in conjunction with urine output, arterial base deficit, serum lactate, and venous oxygen saturations, are utilized in order to determine the relative success of resuscitation. Splanchnic circulation increases by as much as 40% to 60% in the setting of enteral feeding and increases the metabolic demand required of the gastrointestinal tract.[54] If supply falls short of demand, rare but devastating complications can ensue. Fortunately, nonocclusive mesenteric ischemia (NMI) remains an uncommon complication following the early initiation of enteral feeding in the underresuscitated patient. NMI is a low flow state that most commonly affects the distribution of the superior mesenteric artery, which can result in irreversible ischemia and necrosis of the associated small and large bowel. Hypovolemia and underresuscitation can exaggerate the already hypoperfused and dysregulated splanchnic circulation in the setting of sepsis. Enteral feeding in the hemodynamically unstable patient should be undertaken with extreme caution. Treatment of NMI is usually supportive. Hemodynamic status is optimized, and intraarterial vasodilators can be used as an adjunct. Patients that go on to require laparotomy and resection of nonviable bowel have very poor outcomes with mortality rates reported as high as 80%.[55] Following resuscitation and assuming no other absolute contraindication to enteral feeding exist (ie, bowel obstruction), enteral support should be initiated as soon as possible.

Recent reports support the concept that bowel sounds and evidence of bowel function, that is, passing flatus or stool, is not required for EN.[56] The approach of waiting for these signs can contribute to further delays in feeding. In a randomized trial, Suehiro et al. initiated oral feeding within 48 hours of gastrectomy, thereby demonstrating a proof of concept with regards to early feeding without awaiting traditional predictors of tolerance.[57] They reported no increase in morbidity and successfully reduced hospital stays. A recent meta-analysis examining 15 studies and 1240 patients with gastrointestinal anastomoses demonstrated reduced postoperative complications when fed within 24 hours of operation.[53] Other meta-analyses specifically in ICU and trauma patients now report significant decrease in mortality as well as infectious complications.[58,59]

Although the benefits of early EN have been reported in many populations, feeding immediately after the initial diagnosis of sepsis is made yields an entirely different set of problems. Gastrointestinal dysfunction in ICU ranges from 30% to 70%, depending on the diagnosis, premorbid condition, ventilation mode, medications, and metabolic state.[52,60] Proposed mechanisms of ICU and postoperative gastrointestinal dysfunction can be separated into three general categories: mucosal barrier disruption, altered motility, and atrophy of the mucosa and GALT. Barrier disruption seems to most commonly be associated with splanchnic hypoperfusion, which is precipitated by numerous factors in the critical care setting and immediate postoperative period, including hypovolemia, increased catecholamines, increased proinflammatory cytokines, and decreased cardiac output. All ultimately lead to reduced mucosal blood flow, barrier disruption, altered gastrointestinal motility, and changes in the bacterial flora and virulence of the organisms.[61–64] In sepsis, specific protein interactions continue to be more fully elucidated. Membrane toll-like receptors have been implicated in altered motility with resultant changes in intestinal bacterial flora and the potential for translocation. Lipopolysaccharide, or endotoxin, has been demonstrated to stimulate toll-like receptor-4, resulting in impaired smooth muscle function in the gastrointestinal tract, which may contribute to dysmotility.[65]

Kalff et al. recently described the mechanism inducing postoperative ileus.[61] Although this is not a septic model, similar mechanisms are extrapolated. In an elaborate series of human and animal studies, these investigators described the sequence of events following bowel manipulation. Following visceral manipulation, activation of transcription factors is noted, with up-regulation of intracellular adhesion molecule-1 on the endothelium of the muscularis vessels. Leukocyte extravasation into the muscularis occurs, with resultant up-regulation of inducible nitric oxide synthase, cyclooxygenase-2, IL-6, and signal transducer and activator of transcription-3 protein phosphorylation. This inflammatory focus then decreases contractile response and alters electrical activity, resulting in ileus.

As previously stated, recent approaches to maximize gut function in the postoperative and critical care settings include maintenance of visceral perfusion; glycemic control; electrolyte correction; early EN; and minimization of medications that alter gastrointestinal function, such as anticholinergic agents, narcotics, and high-dose vasopressors.[56] Gastrointestinal intolerance should be continually reassessed and can manifest clinically in a variety of forms including abdominal distension, increased gastric residual volumes or nasogastric output, abdominal pain, or diarrhea. The segmental contractility of the gastrointestinal tract should be assessed as dysmotility can be focal (affecting predominately either the proximal or distal bowel) or diffuse. Impaired gastric and proximal GI motility can be addressed efficiently through the placement of postpyloric feeding tubes, and this can be done successfully at the bedside in more than 80% of patients.[66]

Prokinetic agents can be utilized early and are helpful in some patients. Erythromycin acts on motilin receptors resulting in increased motility and can be utilized on a short-term basis but is limited due to tachyphylaxis. Metoclopramide, a $5HT_4$ receptor agonist, works via cholinergic stimulation and is most efficacious in the proximal gut. Alvimopan, a peripherally acting mu-antagonist, has demonstrated some success in the setting of dysmotility associated with narcotic administration in the postoperative setting.[67] No single prokinetic agent will have uniform success in the ICU, and the factors contributing to gastrointestinal dysmotility in each individual patient must be considered. Caution should be used when using prokinetic agents on patients at high risk for bowel necrosis or obstruction.

Early EN can be accomplished in the ICU and postoperative settings using standardized protocols with little morbidity and a gastrointestinal tolerance rate in the 70% to 85% range.[47] A recent study by Barr et al., in which they implemented a standardized, evidence-based enteral feeding protocol, reported shortened duration of mechanical ventilation and a reduced mortality.[46]

Complications of Enteral Feeding in the Intensive Care Unit

In addition to the previously discussed NMI and gastrointestinal intolerance, other complications of nutrition support include aspiration and feeding tube malplacement. These complications are not specific to patients with sepsis but are commonly encountered in the ICU and warrant mention.

Aspiration can cause significant respiratory compromise and is likely related to an increased incidence of pneumonia. In addition to serial reassessment of the need for analgesics and sedatives, simple maneuvers such as electrolyte correction, elevation of the head of the bed, and routine oropharyngeal care can dramatically reduce the incidence of aspiration and pneumonia. Once again, the level of infusion in patients receiving enteral support can also be important. A recent restrospective review by Metheny et al. demonstrated a 12%, 13%, and 18% lower incidence of aspiration events as the position of the feeding tube was advanced to the first, second/third, and fourth portions of the duodenum, respectively, when compared to feeding in the stomach.[68] This suggests that postpyloric feeding should be the goal in patients that are at high risk for aspiration. Despite these findings, most literature does not suggest a clear benefit to routine postpyloric feeding for pneumonia prevention in all patients in the ICU.[69]

Complications associated with nasoenteric feeding tube placement include malpositioning of the tube into the respiratory tract, epistaxis, tube clogging, sinusitis, and displacement of an appropriately placed tube. Positioning of the tube should be confirmed by radiographic assessment prior to the initiation of feeding. Patients requiring prolonged enteral access (> 4 weeks) should be evaluated for potential percutaneous gastric or jejunal access, and complications of these procedures are discussed elsewhere.[70]

Complications of Parenteral Feeding in the Intensive Care Unit

In patients with clear contraindications to enteral support or who present with preexisting malnutrition, parenteral support may be appropriate. Several studies have demonstrated an increased risk of infectious complications in patients receiving parenteral support, but it has proven difficult to ascertain the exact etiology. The most common nosocomial infection associated with PN remains the catheter-related bloodstream infection (CRBSI) due to the required central venous access for administration. In a recent prospective trial, patients receiving PN were still four times as likely to develop CRBSI as their counterparts despite superior glycemic control.[71] Preventive measures taken to avoid this complication are often "bundled" in the ICU, resulting in a reduced incidence of CRBSI and include appropriate education with regards to sterile technique, hand hygiene, prudent choices of insertion sites, and meticulous line care.[72]

Nutritional Requirements

Energy

Estimating energy requirements in patients with sepsis is difficult. As previously noted, energy expenditure studies report increases in expenditure over basal of 20% to 60%.[21] The ability to utilize the calories delivered in the early phases of sepsis is a second issue.[20] The caloric requirement estimates for the septic and critically ill patient is evolving, as illustrated by the concept of hypocaloric or "permissive underfeeding" in the first few days of care in critically ill populations.[73–75] Several studies in critically ill obese patients have used a hypocaloric high-protein regimen with beneficial outcome[75,76] (see Chapter 35). This morbidly obese population is often treated separately in terms of energy prescriptions in the ICU. Generally, extreme caloric restriction (less than 20% of estimated caloric goals) has been cited as detrimental to the critically ill patient.[77] A teleological argument for permissive underfeeding during times of severe illness and stress states that a relative "anorexia of illness" develops with significant infection and that supply of nutrients during this period induces a more proinflammatory state, which then exacerbates the condition. This concept has led several investigators to hypothesize that hypocaloric feeding in the early phases of critical illness and sepsis may be beneficial to patients. Retrospective and prospective studies have evaluated caloric delivery and outcome, suggesting a possible benefit for relative hypocaloric feeding regimens.[78,79] These earlier trials may have had numerous confounding factors. Specifically, retrospective studies tended to include healthier patients without prescribed nutrition therapy in the hypocaloric groups, thus improving their mortality. Currently, caloric delivery is considered safe is in the range of 20 to 30 kcal/kg/d (excluding the morbidly obese). However, more recent trials have examined the association of outcomes and caloric deficit in critically ill patients. Villet et al. observed that patients with a negative total caloric energy balance had worse outcomes at one week.[80] In a larger multi-institutional ICU study, Heyland et al. grouped patients by proportion of prescribed nutrition support received.[81] This study demonstrated decreased mortality in patients receiving a larger proportion of their prescribed nutrition support. This newer data suggests a benefit to full delivery of nutrition support throughout the hospital course. Interestingly, however, even with aggressive delivery protocols, the prescribed calories delivered are often reported at around 80% in the ICU.[82] In actual practice, this results in hypocaloric nutrition delivery despite best efforts to feed to goal calories.

Carbohydrate

Glucose oxidation is increased in sepsis and, to a certain extent, can provide the appropriate route of disposal for exogenously administered glucose.[83] The infusion of glucose is associated with no significant activation of the sympathetic nervous system and therefore carries a negligible thermogenic response.[84] Wolfe et al., in an elaborate series of studies, concluded that nonprotein calorie provision in patients with sepsis should be largely in the form of carbohydrate, with exogenous insulin added to stimulate cellular protein anabolism.[85] However, glucose administration rates in excess of 4 to 6 mg/kg/min result in excess lipogenesis and lead to hyperglycemia. Carbohydrate administration should supply 50% to 60% of the total energy prescription to avoid exceeding the maximum contribution of glucose oxidation and contributing to excess lipogenesis.[83] Excess carbohydrate administration is also more likely to result in poor control of blood glucose levels. Studies have investigated strict control of blood glucose levels between 80 and 110 mg/dL in the ICU population. Initial large prospective, randomized trials demonstrated decreased ICU stay and in-hospital mortality rates, and had 46% fewer episodes of septicemia compared to patients who had blood glucose levels maintained in the 180 to 200 mg/dL range.[17] In a subsequent study by the same group, significant hepatic mitochondrial abnormalities were noted in the control group not receiving meticulous glucose control. The mitochondrial abnormalities noted in these critically ill populations no doubt have significance in the patients' ability to oxidize nutrient substrates.[86]

However, a more recent larger ICU trial with longer follow-up demonstrated a higher mortality in the group receiving very strict blood glucose control.[87] In the wake of these findings, there has been a shift to moderation in glucose control in the ICU. Thus carbohydrate administration and glucose control continues to be a moving target in the care of the critically ill.

Lipid

Exogenous lipids can be effectively used as a fuel source during sepsis, although the optimal composition of the various lipid sources continues to be controversial.[25,88] There are two characteristics of lipids that make them a valuable energy source for patients with sepsis. First, lipids are energy-dense, containing 9 kcal/g; this allows for delivery of more calories in less volume. This is advantageous for patients in whom volume restriction is important (eg, in the setting of renal failure or pulmonary edema). Second, the respiratory quotient is lower for lipids than carbohydrates (0.7 vs. 1.0, respectively). This implies that lipid oxidation produces less carbon dioxide than metabolism of carbohydrates, which may reduce blood concentrations of carbon dioxide. Although theoretically this seems appealing, no prospective, randomized studies have shown significant benefit of high-fat diets in the patient with sepsis.

Intravenous fat emulsions in critical care and sepsis should not exceed 1.0 g/kg/d where soybean oil (18-carbon, omega-6 fatty acid) is the source of lipid such as is the only option in the United States.[25,89] The majority of the rest of the world has several much more physiologic and less inflammatory intravenous lipid emulsions available including olive oil, fish oil, and medium-chain fatty acid sources.

Enteral lipid delivery should follow guidelines similar to those of parenteral lipid provision. This level (1.0 g/kg/d) can be liberalized when enteral lipids include lipid substrates containing omega-3 fatty acids, medium-chain fatty acids, and short-chain fatty acids. As discussed previously, the route and makeup of the lipid substrate is critical, and a mixture of lipid fuels should be delivered whenever possible. Sepsis results in a decrease in cellular ability to transport long-chain fatty acids across the mitochondrial membrane secondary to a sepsis-induced alteration in the acylcarnitine carrier.[25] Medium-chain fatty acids do not require carnitine for transport into the mitochondria.[90] Data supporting benefits of short-chain fatty acids (butyrate and propionate) produced from the bacterial oxidation of soluble fibers in the gastrointestinal lumen have been reported.[91,92] Benefits range from maintaining optimal gastrointestinal mucosal membrane integrity to systemically enhancing immune function via receptors on multiple cell types including white blood cell lines.[93]

Omega-3 fatty acids when delivered as fish oils (DHA and EPA) have beneficial effects in patients with sepsis, including modulation of leukocyte function and regulation of cytokine release through nuclear signaling and gene expression.[94,95] Leukotrienes, thromboxane, and prostaglandins derived from omega-6 fatty acids are proinflammatory compared to metabolites associated with the omega-3 fatty acids.[96] EPA and DHA lipids have recently been reported to enhance the production of a group of prostaglandin derivatives called resolvins and neuroprotectins,[89] which play a role in accelerating the resolution of the proinflammatory state. Abundant data report the influence of EPA and DHA on nuclear signaling and gene expression.[97] For example, polyunsaturated fatty acids interact with various nuclear receptor proteins such as peroxisome proliferator-activated receptor, which then alters nuclear factor-kB and gene expression. By decreasing nuclear factor-kB migration into the nucleus, omega-3 fatty acids downregulate the proinflammatory response to stressful stimuli.[96] The route of delivery of omega-3 fatty acids may also be of importance. Utilizing the enteral route, approximately 2 to 3 days are required to achieve adequate omega-3 fat levels in the cellular membrane to elicit the beneficial effects on the prostaglandin cascade. However, when given parenterally, a clinically relevant response can be achieved in 1 to 3 hours depending on the dose and tissue being evaluated.[98,99] Heller et al. recently published a large randomized trail in 661 patients receiving intravenous omega-3 PN admixtures showing a decrease in antibiotic, length of hospital stay, and a trend toward lowering mortality.[100] Intravenous omega-3 fatty acids are currently unavailable in parenteral emulsions in the United States.

Respiratory failure is common in patients with sepsis. EPA has been recently reported to have beneficial influence on preventing the loss of diaphragm function in sepsis.[101] In addition, one report suggests that EPA can enhance resistance to gram negative pathogens such as pseudomonas.[102] Multiple prospective trials have demonstrated improved mortality and lung-related outcomes in the setting of acute lung injury/acute respiratory distress syndrome with the use of formula containing EPA, DHA, and antioxidants.[103–106] Recently, however, a larger prospective trial found no benefit when patients with lung injury were treated with supplemental fatty acids and antioxidants.[107] This discrepancy highlights the need for further research in regards to method of delivery of these adjuncts. These reports are consistent with the concept that EPA and DHA can be thought of as not just passively modulating the inflammatory process but as actively involved in the resolution of inflammation. The use of enteral formulations containing anti-inflammatory lipids, primarily EPA and DHA, can be used as pharmacologic agents to modulate the hyperdynamic response and outcomes in septic and critically ill patients.

Other general functions of lipids important to nutrition support include carrying fat-soluble vitamins, forming structural units in cell membranes, providing precursors to eicosanoids, cytokine production, and interaction with gene expression.[25,98,100] The optimal lipid for the septic patient remains to be determined, but certainly a blend of n-3 and n-6 lipid sources would seem to be more appropriate for critically ill and septic patients than the predominant n-6 source provided by soy oil used in parenteral emulsions in the United States.[89,100]

Protein

Optimal protein delivery during sepsis is estimated to be between 1.5 to 2 g/kg/d.[15,19] However, requirements may be higher in patients with excessive nitrogen losses, such as in burns and large open wounds.[108] Recent data would also support increasing protein requirements in patients with sepsis during tight glucose control. Conversely, the amount and quality of protein may be altered for patients with hepatic and acute renal failure. Recent data would support the use of whey and casein protein sources in critically ill populations.[109–111] The biological value, protein efficiency ratio, and net protein utilization all are superior for whey and casein rather than soy.

Arginine and Glutamine

Amino acids supplements used to improve outcome or limit morbidity and mortality in the critically ill and septic populations remain controversial.[112] Arginine and glutamine have been the most extensively studied. Regarding arginine, one school of thought indicates that arginine is potentially toxic,[113] while another argument is that arginine is deficient in sepsis and should be supplemented.[114] Arginine is critical in the nitric oxide production pathway. Arginine levels are also dramatically reduced in the septic state.[115] Nitric oxide has been reported to have numerous beneficial effects including decrease in hepatic and splanchnic injury following ischemic insult, increasing myocardial perfusion and preventing endothelial damage via platelet and leukocyte adherence changes noted in sepsis.[113–118] On the other hand, investigators have feared that increasing arginine levels with supplementation would lead to worsening hypotension and outcomes secondary to uncontrolled nitric oxide production. However, in a small study of patients with severe sepsis, large-dose L-arginine infusion did not have hemodynamic consequences.[119] In the clinical setting, one published study demonstrated a dramatically increased mortality with arginine-containing enteral feeding versus PN in a subgroup analysis of a small number of patients with sepsis.[120] However, several trials studying arginine formulas demonstrated improved outcomes for general ICU patients, including those with sepsis.[121,122] The largest trial published on septic patients specifically demonstrated a mortality benefit with the use of arginine formula.[123] As noted previously, enterally feeding the patient with severe sepsis or septic shock must be done cautiously. However, recent prospective trials delivering arginine to septic patients has shown absolutely no harm. It appears that additional arginine at least partially overcomes the elevated asymmetric dimethyl arginine, which causes vasoconstriction, consequently improving perfusion to underperfused tissues.[124–127] Several investigators in the area believe arginine may be deficient in sepsis. In summary, the overwhelming bulk of the current literature suggests arginine-containing formulas are safe and reduce complications in sepsis.

Glutamine, like arginine, is considered conditionally essential in the stressed individual. Sepsis results in a rapid and precipitous drop in both plasma and muscle glutamine concentrations.[128] Over the past 20 years, glutamine has been reported to offer a number of biochemical and clinical benefits, including maintenance of acid-base balance, provision of primary fuel for rapidly proliferating cells (ie, enterocytes and lymphocytes), integrity of gastrointestinal mucosa, decreased clinical infections and gram-negative bacteremia, synthesis of glutathione and arginine, lowering of insulin resistance, and inflammatory response, and function as a key substrate for gluconeogenesis.[118,129,130] Recent evidence that glutamine can induce heat shock protein is yet another beneficial molecular effect of this amino acid.[131] Heat shock protein is a class of cellular chaperone proteins that support appropriate protein folding as they come off the ribosome. These proteins prevent poorly folded intracellular proteins from irreversible degradation by endogenous cellular proteolytic enzyme systems.[132] Supplemental glutamine increases production of heat shock protein, enhancing cellular ability to protect itself from subsequent stress. Singleton et al. reported in a septic animal model that glutamine could decrease lung injury and mortality.[133] In a randomized, controlled clinical trial in ICU patients, of which 71% were septic, glutamine supplementation resulted in a 24% decrease in mortality.[134] These results are supported by the meta-analysis of glutamine use in the ICU showing reduced length of hospital stay, lower infectious complications in surgical patients, and improved mortality in critically ill patients.[135]

Antioxidants

Evidence indicates that sepsis significantly increases production of reactive oxygen species (ROS) by multiple cell lines.[136] Oxidant injury occurs with loss of balance between endogenous antioxidant defenses and cellular production of ROS. ROS generated by activated phagocytic cells results in a host of signal transduction and gene activation events, resulting in a proinflammatory state. Free radicals may injure cell membranes directly by forming lipid peroxides or may damage intracellular proteins, nucleic acids, and organelles, leading to cell death.[136]

During normal physiological conditions and inspiration of 21% oxygen, humans have adequate defenses against ROS produced in routine metabolic processes. Cellular injury occurs when overproduction of ROS overwhelms the host's ability to detoxify the generated ROS. Once the endogenous antioxidant defenses, such as glutathione, superoxide dismutase, and antioxidant vitamins, are overwhelmed, injury occurs.[137] Nathens et al. reported in a large prospective, randomized trial of 595 ICU patients (91% trauma) that addition of 3 g/d of intravenous vitamin C and 3000 IU enterally delivered vitamin E could decrease ICU stay and ventilator time.[138] Collier et al. studied high-risk trauma patients before and after initiation of an antioxidant protocol. The study demonstrated a modest mortality benefit after implementation of the protocol.[139] The exact ratio of antioxidant cocktail has yet to be determined for the septic population. To date, at least 22 randomized, prospective trials of various antioxidants in severely stressed and septic patients have been reported with variable results, the majority showing benefit.[128] Several trials have investigated selenium supplementation specifically in patients with sepsis.[140–144] A majority of these studies demonstrated some benefit. A notable exception is the Forceville et al. study which used doses of up to 4000 mcg. Based on the current literature, moderate doses around 500 mcg daily may have a mortality benefit for the septic population. Larger prospective trials are needed to confirm the benefit and address dosing specifics. A second unknown variable is the duration of therapy. Published protocols have demonstrated a range from 7 to 28 days. Though there is no clear data comparing different intervals, a logical approach would be to continue therapy as long as the patient is at high risk for infectious complications (ie, continued ICU admission).

Host Immunity

The progression from sepsis to septic shock and ultimate death results from the imbalance of a vast array of interrelated hormones, cytokines, altered substrate utilization, and the subsequent host response to the infection. A frequently quoted reference from Lewis Thomas describes inflammation as follows: "Our arsenals for fighting off bacteria are so powerful . . . that we are more in danger from them than the invaders."[145]

The development of malnutrition is rapid in the critically ill and septic patient because of the complex metabolic changes induced by cytokine mediators and a wide array of hormones. Malnutrition is clearly linked to derangements in both humoral and cellular immunity, resulting in increased susceptibility to infection.[64,146] Many studies indicate that adequate nutrition is necessary to support a functional immune system and reduce septic morbidity and mortality.[5,146,147]

If appropriate nutrition support is not maintained during the management of sepsis, the gut can also fail, contributing to multiple organ failure.[148,149] Gut failure is manifested as feeding intolerance as well as loss of the gut barrier to intestinal flora. The results of a prospective study investigating associations between bacterial translocation, gastric microflora, and septic morbidity in critically ill patients indicate that proximal gut colonization is associated with both increased bacterial translocation and septic morbidity.[150,151]

Bacterial translocation from the intestinal lumen to gut lymphatics or the portal venous system most likely occurs in all individuals, but is not clinically significant in the immune-competent host.[152] Destruction of translocated bacteria in mesenteric lymph nodes is dependent on the immunological function of the host and individual bacterial virulence factors. Studies have suggested that early enteral feeding may protect the mucosal barrier from dysfunction.[153,154] In addition to the nutrients previously discussed as having potentially beneficial effects in septic patients, probiotics have recently shown promise in sepsis in immunocompromised hosts.[155,156]

At the present time, no specific biological immunomodulators (eg, antibodies to E5 and HA-1A moieties of gram-negative cell walls, to IL-2 receptors, or to soluble TNF-α receptor) or pharmacological therapies (eg, naloxone, pentoxifylline, bradykinin antagonists, and N-acetylcysteine) with the exception of drotrecogin alfa (activated) have improved survival of septic patients.[1,9] Maintenance of host immunity is still the most valuable defense to reduce septic complications and mortality. The recent data utilizing immune-modulating nutrients via both the enteral and parental formulations show promise. Nutrition support is one of the most effective ways to reach this goal.

References

1. Hall MJ, Williams SN, DeFrances CJ, et al. Inpatient care for septicemia or sepsis: A challenge for patients and hospitals. *NCHS Data Brief.* 2011;62.
2. Kochanek KD, Xu, J, Murphy SL, et al. Deaths: preliminary data for 2009. *National Vital Statistics Reports.* 2011:59(4).
3. Sands KE, Bates DW, Lanken PN, et al. Epidemiology of sepsis syndrome in eight academic medical centers. *JAMA.* 1997;278: 234–240.
4. Manship L, McMillin RD, Brown JJ. The influence of sepsis and multisystem organ failure on mortality in the surgical intensive care unit. *Am Surg.* 1984;50:94–101.
5. Hotchkiss RS, Karl IE. The pathophysiology and treatment of sepsis. *N Engl J Med.* 2003;348:138–150.
6. Bone RC, Balk RA, Cerra FB, et al. "Definitions for sepsis and organ failure and guidelines for the use of innovative therapies in sepsis. The ACCP/SCCM Consensus Conference Committee. American College of Chest Physicians/Society of Critical Care Medicine. 1992." *Chest.* 2009 Nov; 136 (5 Suppl):1644–1655.
7. Calandra T, Cohen J. The international sepsis forum consensus conference on definitions of infection in the intensive care unit. *Crit Care Med.* 2005;33:1538–1548.
8. Levy MM, Fink MP, Marshall JC, et al. 2001 SCCM/ ESICM/ACCP/ ATS/SIS international sepsis definitions conference. *Crit Care Med.* 2003;31:1250–1256.
9. Rice TW, Bernard GR. Therapeutic intervention and targets for sepsis. *Ann Rev Med.* 2005;56:225–248.
10. Cinel I, Opal SM. Molecular biology of inflammation and sepsis: a primer. *Crit Care Med.* 2009;37(1):291–304.
11. Dellinger RP, Carlet JM, Masur H, et al. Surviving sepsis campaign guidelines for management of severe sepsis and septic shock. *Crit Care Med.* 2004;32:858–873.
12. Rivers E, Nguyen B, Havstad S, et al. Early goaldirected therapy in the treatment of severe sepsis and septic shock. *N Engl J Med.* 2001;345:1368–1377.
13. Meisner M. Biomarkers of sepsis: clinically useful? *Curr Opin Crit Care.* 2005;11:473–480.
14. Rusavy Z, Sramek V, Lacigova S, et al. Influence of insulin on glucose metabolism and energy expenditure in septic patients. *Crit Care.* 2004;8:R213–R220.
15. Martindale R, Shikora S, Nishikawa R, et al. The metabolic response to stress and alterations in nutrient metabolism. In: Shikora S., Martindale R, eds. *Nutritional Considerations in the Intensive Care Unit.* Dubuque, IA: Kendall Hunt Publishing, pp. 11–20.
16. Plank LD, Hill GL. Sequential metabolic changes following induction of systemic inflammatory response in patients with severe sepsis or major blunt trauma. *World J Surg.* 2000;24:630–638.
17. Van Den Berghe G, Wouters P, Weekers F, et al. Intensive insulin therapy in the critically ill patients. *N Engl J Med.* 2001;345: 1359–1367.
18. Dahn MS, Mitchell RA, Lange MP, et al. Hepatic metabolic response to injury and sepsis. *Surgery.* 1995;117:520–530.
19. Shaw JH, Wildbore M, Wolfe RR. Whole body protein kinetics in severely septic patients: the response to glucose infusion and total parenteral nutrition. *Ann Surg.* 1987;205:288–294.
20. Streat SJ, Beddoe AH, Hill GL. Aggressive nutritional support does not prevent protein loss despite fat gain in septic intensive care patient. *J Trauma.* 1987;27:262–266.
21. Plank LD, Connolly AB, Hill GL. Sequential changes in the metabolic response in severely septic patients during the first 23 days after onset of peritonitis. *Ann Surg.* 1998;228(2):146–158.
22. Cerra FB. Hypermetabolism, organ failure, and metabolic support. *Surgery.* 1987;101:1–14.
23. Ziegler T, Bazargan N, Leader L, Martindale R. Glutamine and the gastrointestinal tract. *Curr Opin Clin Nutr Metab Care.* 2000;3: 355–362.
24. Martinez A, Chiolero R, Bollman M, et al. Assessment of adipose tissue metabolism by means of subcutaneous microdialysis in patients with sepsis or circulatory failure. *Clin Physiol Funct Imaging.* 2003;23:286–292.
25. Hasselmann M, Reimund JM. Lipids in the nutritional support of critically ill patients. *Curr Opin Crit Care.* 2004;10:449–455.
26. Bansal V, Syres KM, Makarenkova V, et al. Interactions between fatty acids and arginine metabolism: implications for the design of immune-enhancing diets. *J Parenter Enteral Nutr.* 2005;29: S75–80.
27. Martindale RG, McClave SA, Vanek VW, McCarthy M, Roberts P, Taylor B, Ochoa JB, Napolitano L, Cresci G; American College of Critical Care Medicine; A.S.P.E.N. Board of Directors. Guidelines for the provision and assessment of nutrition support therapy in the adult critically ill patient: Society of Critical Care Medicine and American Society for Parenteral and Enteral Nutrition: executive summary. *Crit Care Med.* 2009;37(5):1757–1761.
28. Ruggieri AJ, Levy RJ, Deutschman CS, et al. Mitochondrial dysfunction and resuscitation in sepsis. *Crit Care Clin.* 2010;26(3): 567–575.
29. Marik PE, Zaloga GP. Early enteral nutrition in acutely ill patients: a systemic review. *Crit Care Med.* 2001;29:2264–2270.
30. Heyland DK, Dhaliwal R. Early enteral nutrition vs. early parenteral nutrition: an irrelevant question for the critically ill? *Crit Care Med.* 2005;33:260–261.
31. Zaloga GP, Roberts PR, Marik P. Feeding the hemodynamically unstable patient: a critical evaluation of the evidence. *Nutr Clin Pract.* 2003;18:285–293.
32. Clemmesen O, Ott P, Larsen FS. Splanchnic metabolism in acute liver failure and sepsis. *Curr Opin Crit Care.* 2004;10:152–155.
33. McClave SA, Chang WK. Feeding the hypotensive patient: does enteral feeding precipitate or protect against ischemic bowel? *Nutr Clin Pract.* 2003;18:279–284.
34. Moore-Olufemi SD, Kozar RA, Moore FA, et al. Ischemic preconditioning protects against gut dysfunction and mucosal injury after ischemia/reperfusion injury. *Shock.* 2005;23:258–263.
35. Gosche JR, Garrison RN, Harris PD, Cryer HG. Absorptive hyperemia restores intestinal blood flow during Escherichia coli sepsis in the rat. *Arch Surg.* 1990;125:1573–1576.
36. Khalid I, Doshi P, DiGiovine B. Early enteral nutrition and outcomes of critically ill patients treated with vasopresors and mechanical ventilation. *Am J Crit Care.* 2010;19(3):261–268.
37. Revelly JP, Tappy L, Berger MM, et al. Early metabolic and splanchnic responses to enteral nutrition in postoperative cardiac surgery patients with circulatory compromise. *Intensive Care Med.* 2001; 21:540–547.
38. Myers JG, Page CP, Stewart RM, et al. Complications of needle catheter jejunostomy in 2022 consecutive applications. *Am J Surg.* 1995;170:547–551.

39. Schunn CD, Daly JM. Small bowel necrosis associated with postoperative jejunal tube feeding. *J Am Coll Surg*. 1995;180:410–416.
40. Smith-Choban P, Max MH. Feeding jejunostomy: a small bowel stress test? *Am J Surg*. 1988;155:112–117.
41. Marvin RG, McKinley BA, McQuiggan M, et al. Nonocclusive bowel necrosis occurring in critically ill trauma patients receiving enteral nutrition manifests no reliable clinical signs for early detection. *Am J Surg*. 2000;179:7–12.
42. Zaloga GP. Parenteral nutrition in adult inpatients with functioning gastrointestinal tracts: assessment of outcomes. *Lancet*. 2006;367:1101–1111.
43. Eyer SD, Micon LT, Konstantinides FN, et al. Early enteral feeding does not attenuate metabolic response after blunt trauma. *J Trauma*. 1993;34:639–644.
44. Jacobs DG, Jacobs DO, Kudsk KA, et al. Practice management guidelines for the nutritional support of the trauma patient. *J Trauma*. 2004;57:660–679.
45. Barr J, Hecht M, Flavin KE, et al. Outcomes in critically ill patients before and after the implementation of an evidence-based nutritional management protocol. *Chest*. 2004;125:1446–1457.
46. Kozar RA, McQuiggan MM, Moore EE, et al. Postinjury enteral tolerance is reliably achieved by a standardized protocol. *J Surg Res*. 2002;104:70–75.
47. Heyland DK, Cahill NE, Dhaliwal R, et al. Impact of enteral feeding protocols on enteral nutrition delivery: results of a multicenter observational study. *J Parenter Enteral Nutr*. 2010;34(6):675–684.
48. Alpers DH. Why, how, and to which part of the gastrointestinal tract should forced enteral feeding be delivered in patients? *Curr Opin Gastroenterol*. 2004;20:104–109.
49. Hammarqvist F. Can it all be done by enteral nutrition? *Curr Opin Clin Nutr Metab Care*. 2004;7:183–187.
50. Caesaer MP, Mesotten D, Hermans G, et al. Early versus late parenteral nutrition in critically ill adults. *New Engl J Med*. 2011; 365(6):506–517.
51. Lewis SF, Egger M, Sylvester PA, et al. Early enteral feeding versus "nil by mouth" after gastrointestinal surgery: systematic review and meta-analysis of controlled trials. *Br Med J*. 2001;323:1–5.
52. Mutlu GM, Mutlu EA, Factor P. Prevention and treatment of gastrointestinal complications in patients on mechanical ventilation. *Am J Respir Med*. 2003;2:395–411.
53. Osland E, Yunus RM, Khan S, Memon MA. Early versus traditional postoperative feeding in patients undergoing resectional gastrointestinal surgery: a meta-analysis. *J Parenter Enteral Nutr*. 2011; 35(4):473–487.
54. Revelly JP, Tappy L, Berger MM, et al. Early metabolic and splanchnic responses to enteral nutrition in postoperative cardiac surgery patients with circulatory compromise. *Intensive Care Med*. 2001;27:540–547.
55. Park WM, Gloviczki P, Cherry KJ Jr, et al. Contemporary management of acute mesenteric ischemia: Factors associated with survival. *J Vasc Surg*. 2002;35:445–452.
56. Caddell, KA, Martindale R, McClave SA, et al. Can the intestinal dysmotility of critical illness be differentiated from postoperative ileus? *Curr Gatroenterol Rep*. 2011;13(4):358–367.
57. Suehiro T, Matsumata T, Shikada Y, Sugimachi K. Accelerated rehabilitation with early postoperative oral feeding following gastrectomy. *Hepatogastroenterology*. 2004;51:1852–1855.
58. Doig GS, Heighes PT, Simpson F, et al. Early enteral nutrition, provided within 24 h of injury or intensive care unit admission, significantly reduces mortality in critically ill patients: a meta-analysis of randomized controlled trials. *Intensive Care Med*. 2009;35(12):2018–2027.
59. Doig GS, Heighes PT, Simpson F, et al. Early enteral nutrition reduces mortality in trauma patients requiring intensive care: a meta-analysis of randomized controlled trials. *Injury*. 2011; 42(1):50–56.
60. Schmidt H, Martindale RG. The gastrointestinal tract in critical illness: nutritional implications. *Curr Opin Nutr Metab Care*. 2003; 6:587–591.
61. Kalff JC, Turler A, Schwartz NT, et al. Intraabdominal activation of a local inflammatory response with the human muscularis externa during laparotomy. *Ann Surg*. 2003;237:301–315.
62. Ritz MA, Fraser R, Tam W, et al. Impacts and patterns of disturbed gastrointestinal function in critically ill patients. *Am J Gastroenterol*. 2000;95:3044–3052.
63. Alverdy J, Zaborina O, Wu L. The impact of stress and nutrition on bacterial–host interactions at the intestinal epithelial surface. *Curr Opin Clin Nutr Metab Care*. 2005;8:205–209.
64. Ayala A, Chung CS, Grutkoski PS, et al. Mechanisms of immune resolution. *Crit Care Med*. 2003;31:S558–S571.
65. Scirocco A, Matarrese P, Petitta C, et al. Exposure of toll-like receptors 4 to bacterial lipopolysaccharide (LPS) impairs human colonic smooth muscle cell function. *J Cell Phys*. 2010;223(2):442–450.
66. Gatt M, MacFie J. Bedside postpyloric feeding tube placement: a pilot series to validate this novel technique. *Crit Care Med*. 2009;37(2):523–527.
67. Wolff BG, Michelassi F, Gerkin TM, et al.; Alvimopan Postoperative Ileus Study Group. Alvimopan, a novel, peripherally acting mu opioid antagonist: results of a multicenter, randomized, double-blind, placebo-controlled, phase III trial of major abdominal surgery and postoperative ileus. *Ann Surg*. 2004;240(4):728–734.
68. Metheny NA, Stewart BJ, McClave SA. Relationship between feeding tube site and respiratory outcomes. *J Parenter Enteral Nutr*. 2011;35(3):346–355.
69. Marik PE, Zaloga GP. Gastric versus post-pyloric feeding: a systematic review. *Crit Care*. 2003;7(3):R46–51.
70. Itkin M, DeLegge MH, Fang JC, et al. Multidisciplinary practical guidelines for gastrointestinal access for enteral nutrition and decompression from the Society of Interventional Radiology and American Gastroenterological Association Institute, with endorsement by Canadian Interventional Radiological Association and Cardiovascular and Interventional Radiological Society of Europe. *Gastroenterology*. 2011;141:742–765.
71. Matsushima K, Cook A, Tyner T, et al. Parenteral nutrition: a clear and present danger unabated by tight glucose control. *Am J Surg*. 2010;200(3):386–390.
72. Kim JS, Holtom P, Vigen C. Reduction of catheter-related bloodstream infections through the use of a central venous line bundle: epidemiologic and economic consequences. *Am J Infect Control*. 2011;39(8):640–646.
73. Heyland DK, Dhaliwal R, Drover JW, et al. Canadian clinical practice guidelines for nutrition support in the mechanically ventilated, critically ill adult patients. *J Parenter Enteral Nutr*. 2003;27:355–373.
74. Zaloga GP, Robert P. Permissive underfeeding. *New Horiz*. 1994;2: 257–263.
75. Grimble RF. Dietary manipulation of the inflammatory response. *Proc Nutr Soc*. 1992;51:285–294.
76. McGinnis C, Fischer J, Larson G. Nutrition support in the morbidly obese critically ill patient. *Nutr Clin Pract*. 2004;19:290–296.
77. Rubinson L, Diette GB, Song X, et al. Low caloric intake is associated with nosocomial bloodstream infections in patients in the medical intensive care unit. *Crit Care Med*. 2004;32:350–357
78. Krishnan JA, Parce PB, Martinez A, et al. Caloric intake in medical ICU patients. *Chest*. 2003;124:297–305.

79. McCowen KC, Friel C, Sternberg J, et al. Hypocaloric total parenteral nutrition: effectiveness in prevention of hyperglycemia and infectious complications—a randomized clinical trial. *Crit Care Med.* 2000;28:3606–3611.
80. Villet S, Chiolero RL, Bollmann MD, et al. Negative impact of hypocaloric feeding and energy balance on clinical outcome in ICU patients. *Clin Nutr.* 2005;24(4):502–509.
81. Heyland DK, Cahill N, Day AG. Optimal amount of calories for critically ill patients: depends on how you slice the cake! *Crit Care Med.* 2011;39(12):2619–2626.
82. Heyland DK, Cahill NE, Dhaliwal R, et al. Enhanced protein-energy provision via the enteral route in critically ill patients: a single center feasibility trial of the PEP uP protocol. *Crit Care.* 2010;14(2):R78.
83. Long CL. Fuel preferences in the septic patient: glucose of lipid. *J Parenter Enteral Nutr.* 1987;11:333–335.
84. Carlson GL, Gray P, Arnold J, et al. Thermogenic, hormonal and metabolic effects of intravenous infusion in human sepsis. *Br J Surg.* 1997;84:1454–1459.
85. Wolfe RR. Substrate utilization/insulin resistance in sepsis/trauma. *Baillieres Clin Endocrinol Metab.* 1997;11:645–657.
86. Vanhorebeek I, De Vos R, Mesotten U, et al. Protection of hepatocyte mitochondrial ultrastructure and function by strict blood glucose control with insulin in critically ill patients. *Lancet.* 2005;365:53–59.
87. Finfer S, Chittock DR, Su SY, et al. Intensive versus conventional glucose control in critically ill patients. *N Engl J Med.* 2009; 360(13):1283–1297.
88. Garnacho-Montero J, Ortiz-Leyba C, Jimeniz-Jimeniz FJ, et al. Clinical and metabolic effects of two lipid emulsions on the parenteral nutrition of septic patients. *Nutrition.* 2002;18:134–138.
89. Serhan CN. Novel eicosanoid and docosanoid mediators: resolvins, docosatrienes, and neuroprotectins. *Curr Opin Nutr Metab Care.* 2005;8:115–121.
90. Calabrese C, Myer S, Munson S, et al. A cross-over study of the effect of a single oral feeding of medium chain triglyceride oil vs. canola oil on post-ingestion plasma triglyceride levels in healthy men. *Altern Med Rev.* 1999;4:23–28.
91. Sanderson IR. Nutritional factors and immune functions of the gut epithelium. *Proc Nutr Soc.* 2001;60:443–447.
92. Bengmark S, Martindale R. Prebiotics and synbiotics in clinical medicine. *Nutr Clin Pract.* 2005;20:244–261.
93. Bengmark S. Synbiotics and the mucosal barrier in critically ill patients. *Curr Opin Gastroenterol.* 2005;21:712–716.
94. Calder PC, Grimble RF. Polyunsaturated fatty acids, inflammation and immunity. *Eur J Clin Nutr.* 2002;56:S14–19.
95. Sweeney B, Puri P, Reen DJ. Modulation of immune cell function by polyunsaturated fatty acids. *Pediatr Surg Int.* 2005;21:335–340.
96. Mayer K, Grimm H, Grimminger F, Seeger W. Parenteral nutrition with n-3 lipids in sepsis. *Br J Nutr.* 2002;87:S69–S75.
97. Calder PC. N-3 polyunsaturated fatty acids and inflammation: from molecular biology to the clinic. *Lipids.* 2003;38:343–352.
98. Roy CC, Bouthillier L, Seidman E, Levy E. New lipids in enteral feeding. *Curr Opin Clin Nutr Metab Care.* 2004;7:117–122.
99. Mayer K, Gokorsch S, Fegbeutel C, et al. Parenteral nutrition with fish oil modulates cytokine response in patients with sepsis. *Am J Respir Crit Care Med.* 2003;167:1321–1328.
100. Heller AR, Rossler S, Litz RJ, et al. Omega-3 fatty acids improve the diagnosis-related clinical outcome. *Crit Care Med.* 2006;34: 972–979.
101. Supinski GS, Vanags J, Callahan LA, et al. Eicosapentaenoic acid preserves diaphragm force generation following endotoxin administration. *Crit Care.* 2010;14(2):R35.
102. Tiesset H, Pierre M, Desseyn JL, et al. Dietary polyunsaturated fatty acids affect the kinetics of pro- and anti-inflammatory responses in mice with Pseudomonas aeruginosa lung infection. *J Nutr.* 2009;139(1):82–89.
103. Pontes-Arruda A, Aragão AM, Albuquerque JD. Effects of enteral feeding with eicosapentaenoic acid, gamma-linolenic acid, and antioxidants in mechanically ventilated patients with severe sepsis and septic shock. *Crit Care Med.* 2006;34(9):2325–2333.
104. Gadek JE, DeMichele SJ, Karlstad MD, et al. Effect of enteral feeding with eicosapentaenoic acid, gamma-linolenic acid, and antioxidants in patients with acute respiratory distress syndrome. *Crit Care Med.* 1999;27:1409–1420.
105. Singer P, Theilla M, Fisher H, et al. Benefit of an enteral diet enriched with eicosapentaenoic acid and gamma-linolenic acid in ventilated patients with acute lung injury. *Crit Care Med.* 2006;34(4):1033–1038.
106. Moran V, Grau T, de Lorenzo AC, et al. Effect of an enteral feeding with eicosapentaenoic and gamma-linoleic acids on the outcome of mechanically ventilated critically ill septic patients. *Clin Nutr.* 2011 Oct; 30(5):578–584.
107. Rice TW, Wheeler AP, Thompson BT, et al. Enteral omega-3 fatty acid, gamma-linolenic acid, and antioxidant supplementation in acute lung injury. *JAMA.* 2011;306(14):1574–1581.
108. Verbruggen SC, Coss-Bu J, Wu M, Schierbeek H, Joosten KF, Dhar A, van Goudoever JB, Castillo L. Current recommended parenteral protein intakes do not support protein synthesis in critically ill septic, insulin-resistant adolescents with tight glucose control. *Crit Care Med.* 2011;39(11):2518–2525.
109. Lefton J, Lopez PP. Macronutrient requirements: carbohydrate, protein, and lipid. In: Cresci G, ed. *Nutritional Support for the Critically Ill Patient.* Boca Raton, FL: Taylor and Francis; 2005:99–108.
110. Katsanos CS, Kobayashi H, Sheffield-Moore M, et al. A high proportion of leucine is required for optimal stimulation of the rate of muscle protein synthesis by essential amino acids in the elderly. *Am J Physiol Endocrinol Metab.* 2006;291:E111–E117.
111. Tipton KD, Elliott TA, Cree MG, et al. Ingestion of casein and whey proteins result in muscle anabolism after resistance exercise. *Med Sci Sports Exerc.* 2004;36:2073–2081.
112. Furst P, Stehle P. What are the essential elements needed for the determination of amino acid requirements in humans? *J Nutr.* 2004;134:1558S–1565S.
113. Heyland DK, Samis A. Does immunonutrition in patients with sepsis do more harm than good? *Intensive Care Med.* 2003;29: 669–671.
114. Luiking YC, Poeze M, Dejong CH, et al. Sepsis: an arginine deficiency state? *Crit Care Med.* 2004;32:2135–2145.
115. Davis JS, Anstey NM. Is plasma arginine concentration decreased in patients with sepsis? A systematic review and meta-analysis. *Crit Care Med.* 2011;39:380–385.
116. Suchner U, Heyland DK, Peter K. Immune-modulatory actions of arginine in the critically ill. *Br J Nutr.* 2002;87:S121–S132.
117. Chiarla C, Giovannini I, Siegel JH. Plasma arginine correlations in trauma and sepsis. *Amino Acids.* 2005;30:81–86.
118. Grimble RF. Immunonutrition. *Curr Opin Gastroenterol.* 2005; 21:216–222.
119. Luiking YC, Poeze M, Hendrikx M, et al. "Continuous L-arginine infusion does not deteriorate the haemodynamic condition in patients with severe sepsis." *Europ J Gastrol Hepatol.* January 2006; 18(1):A8.
120. Bertolini G, Iapichino G, Radrizzani D, et al. Early enteral immunonutrition in patients with severe sepsis: results of an interim analysis of a randomized multicentre clinical trial. *Intensive Care Med.* 2003;29(5):834–840.

121. Caparros T, Lopez J, Grau T. Early enteral nutrition in critically ill patients with a high protein diet enriched with arginine, fiber, and antioxidants compared with a standard high-protein diet. The effect on nosocomial infections and outcome. *J Parenter Enteral Nutr*. 2001;25(6):299–308.
122. Atkinson S, Sieffert E, Bihari D. A prospective, randomized, double-blind, controlled clinical trial of enteral immunonutrition in the crtically ill. Guy's Hospital Intensive Care Group. *Crit Care Med*. 1998;26(7):1164–1172.
123. Galban C, Montejo JC, Mesejo A, et al. An immune-enhancing enteral diet reduces mortality rate and episodes of bacteremia in septic intensive care unit patients. *Crit Care Med*. 2000;28(3):643–648.
124. Luiking YC, Poeze M, Ramsay G, Deutz NE. Reduced citrulline production in sepsis is related to diminished de novo arginine and nitric oxide production. *Am J Clin Nutr*. 2009;89(1):142–152.
125. Kao CC, Bandi V, Guntupalli KK, Wu M, Castillo L, Jahoor F. Arginine, citrulline and nitric oxide metabolism in sepsis. *Clin Sci (Lond)*. 2009;2;117:23–30.
126. Boger RH. The pharmacodynamics of L-arginine. 6th Amino Acid Assessment Workshop. *J Nutr*. 2007;137:1650S–1655S.
127. Zhou M, Martindale RG. Immune-modulating enteral formulations: optimum components, appropriate patients, and controversial use of arginine in sepsis. *Curr Gastroenterol Rep*. 2007;9:329–337.
128. Coeffier M, Dechelotte P. The role of glutamine in intensive care unit patients: mechanisms of action and clinical outcome. *Nutr Rev*. 2005;63:65–69.
129. Wischmeyer PE, Lynch J, Leidel J, et al. Glutamine administration reduces Gram-negative bacteremia in severely burned patients: prospective, randomized, double-blind trial versus isonitrogenous control. *Crit Care Med*. 2001;29:2075–2080.
130. Newsholme P, Procopio J, Lima MM, et al. Glutamine and glutamate—their central role in cell metabolism and function. *Cell Biochem Funct*. 2003;21:1–9.
131. Ziegler TR, Ogden LG, Singleton KD, et al. Parenteral glutamine increases serum heat shock protein 70 in critically ill patients. *Intensive Care Med*. 2005;31(8):1079–1086.
132. Macario AJ, Conway de Macario E, et al. Sick chaperones, cellular stress, and disease. *N Engl J Med*. 2005;353:1489–1501.
133. Singleton KD, Serkova N, Beckey VE, Wischmeyer PE. Glutamine attenuates lung injury and improves survival after sepsis: role of enhanced heat shock protein expression. *Crit Care Med*. 2005;33:1206–1213.
134. Griffiths RD, Jones C, Palmer TE. Six-month outcome of critically ill patients given glutamine-supplemented parenteral nutrition. *Nutr*. 1997;13:295–302.
135. Novak F, Heyland DK, Avenell A, et al. Glutamine supplementation in serious illness: a systematic review of the evidence. *Crit Care Med*. 2002;30:2022–2029.
136. Macdonald J, Galley HF, Webster NR. Oxidative stress and gene expression in sepsis. *Br J Anaesth*. 2003;90:221–232.
137. Heyland DK, Dhaliwal R, Suchner U, Berger MM. Antioxidant nutrients: a systemic review of trace elements and vitamins in the critically ill patient. *Intensive Care Med*. 2005;31:327–337.
138. Nathens AB, Neff MJ, Jurkovich GJ, et al. Randomized, prospective trial of antioxidant supplementation in critically ill surgical patients. *Ann Surg*. 2002;236:814–822.
139. Collier BR, Giladi A, Dossett LA, et al. Impact of high-dose antioxidants on outcomes in acutely injured patients. *J Parenter Enteral Nutr*. 2008;32(4):384–388.
140. Zimmermann T, Albrecht S, Kuhne H, et al. Selenium administration in patients with sepsis. A prospective randomized study. *Med Klin (Munich)*. 1997;15:92.
141. Angstwurm MW, Schottdorf J, Schopohl J, et al. Selenium replacement in patients with severe systemic inflammatory response syndrome improves clinical outcome. *Crit Care Med*. 1999;27(9):1807–1813.
142. Angstwurm MW, Engelmann L, Zimmermann T, et al. Selenium in Intensive Care (SIC): results of a prospective randomized, placebo-controlled, multiple-center study in patients with severe systemic inflammatory response syndrome, sepsis, and septic shock. *Crit Care Med*. 2007;35(1):118–126.
143. Mishra V, Baines M, Perry SE, et al. Effect of selenium supplementation on biochemical markers and outcome in critically ill patients. *Clin Nutr*. 2007;26(1):41–50.
144. Forceville X, Laviolle B, Annane D, et al. Effects of high doses of selenium, as sodium selenite, in septic shock: a placebo-controlled, randomized, double-blind, phase II study. *Crit Care*. 2007;11(4):R73.
145. Thomas L. *The Lives of a Cell: Notes of a Biology Watcher*. New York, NY: Viking Press; 1974.
146. Riedemann NC, Guo RF, Ward PA. The enigma of sepsis. *J Clin Invest*. 2003;112:460–467.
147. Martindale RG, Cresci G. Preventing infectious complications with nutrition intervention. *J Parenter Enteral Nutr*. 2005;29:S53–S56.
148. Moore EE, Moore FA, Harken AH, et al. The two-event contruct of postinjury multiple organ failure. *Shock*. 2005;24:S71–S74.
149. Wheeler AP, Bernard GR. Treating patients with severe sepsis. *N Engl J Med*. 1999;340:207–214.
150. Shimizu K, Orgura H, Goto M, et al. Altered gut flora and environment in patients with severe sepsis. *J Trauma*. 2006;60:126–133.
151. MacFie J, O'Boyle C, Mitchell C, et al. Gut origin of sepsis: a prospective study investigating associations between bacterial translocation, gastric microflora, and septic morbidity. *Gut*. 1999;45:223–228.
152. De-Souza DA, Greene LJ. Intestinal permeability and systemic infections in critically ill patients: effect of glutamine. *Crit Care Med*. 2005;33:1125–1135.
153. Magnotti LJ. Deitch EA. Burns, bacterial translocation, gut barrier function, and failure. *J Burn Care Rehab*. 2005;26:383–391.
154. MacFie J. Enteral vs. parenteral nutrition: the significance of bacterial translocation and gut-barrier function. *Nutr*. 2000;16: 606–611.
155. Besselink MG, Timmerman HM, van Minnen LP, et al. Prevention of infectious complications in surgical patients: potential role of probiotics. *Dig Surg*. 2005;22:234–244.
156. Madden JAJ, Plummer SF, Tang J, et al. Effect of probiotics on preventing disruption of the intestinal microflora following antibiotic therapy: a double-blind, placebo-controlled pilot study. *Int Immunopharmacol*.2005;5:1091–1097.
157. Frankenfield DC, Coleman A, Alam S, et al. "Analysis of estimation methods for resting metabolic rate in critically ill adults." *JPEN* 2009 33:27–36.

24 Trauma, Surgery, and Burns

Bryan R. Collier, DO, FACS, CNSC, Jill R. Cherry-Bukowiec, MD, MS, FACS, and Mary E. (Beth) Mills, MS, RD, CNSC, LDN

CONTENTS

Background 393
Incidence 393
Severity of Injury 394
Physiological Response to Stress 394
Neuroendocrine Response and Systemic Inflammation 394
Reperfusion Injury/Low-Flow States 394
Malnutrition in the Intensive Care Unit 395
Nutrition Assessment 396
Screening and Anthropometrics 396
Biochemical Measures 397
Nutrition Requirements 399
Determination of Nutrient Requirements 399
Energy 399
Protein 400
Carbohydrate 400
Fat 401
Fluid and Electrolytes 401
Vitamins, Trace Elements, and Minerals 402
Route of Nutrition Support 402
Feeding Access 403
Enteral Access 403
Gastric Access 403
Small Bowel Access 403
Transitioning to Oral Nutrition 403
Adjunctive Therapies 404
Glutamine 404
Arginine 404
Omega-3 Fatty Acids 404
Antioxidants and Trace Minerals 404
Prebiotics, Probiotics, and Synbiotics 405
Formula Selection/Immunonutrition 405
Perioperative Nutrition Provision 406
Burns 406
Acknowledgments 406
References 406

Objectives

1. Recognize how injury and inflammation alter metabolism.
2. Understand how injury-related malnutrition differs from starvation-related malnutrition.
3. Assess nutritional risk and determine nutrient requirements for trauma, surgery, and burn patients.
4. Discuss the role of parenteral, enteral, and oral nutrition therapy in trauma, burn, and surgical patients.
5. Select the best adjunct nutritional therapies for the trauma, surgical, and burned patient.
6. Describe a perioperative process improvement, including nutrition, to optimize the elective surgical patient.

Test Your Knowledge Questions

1. Which of the following is the most important consideration to starting early enteral nutrition (EN) after trauma?
   A. Addressing protein-calorie malnutrition before it is severe
   B. Preventing negative nitrogen balance
   C. Modulating the immune process and supporting the gastrointestinal (GI) tract
   D. Preventing severe hyperglycemia
2. For routine colon surgery, which of the following components of enhanced recovery after surgery (ERAS) contributes to the improved outcomes?
   A. Keep the patient nothing by mouth after midnight to avoid aspiration on induction of general anesthesia.
   B. Provide a glucose-rich supplementation 6 and 2 hours prior to surgery.
   C. Utilize a bowel prep to prevent wound infections.
   D. Limit mobility of the patient to prevent wound dehiscence.
3. Which of the following antioxidants have not been shown to benefit trauma patients?
   A. Vitamin C
   B. Vitamin E
   C. Selenium
   D. Zinc

Test Your Knowledge Answers

1. The correct answer is **C**. Negative nitrogen balance frequently occurs despite adequate energy provision as a result of the counterregulatory hormone and cytokine changes that occur from traumatic insult. Epinephrine, glucagon, and growth hormones are elevated, resulting in increased lipolysis and increased glycerol and free fatty release. Circulating levels of insulin are elevated in most metabolically stressed patients, but the responsiveness of tissues to insulin, especially skeletal muscle, is severely blunted. Insulin resistance is believed to be caused by the effects of the counterregulatory hormones and causes hyperglycemia regardless of nutrition provision. The hormonal milieu normalizes only after the injury or metabolic stress has resolved. By providing early EN, the cytokine storm and counterregulatory hormone secretion is attenuated. As a result, critically ill patients experience fewer infections despite not obtaining protein and calorie goals within the first few days of nutrition provision.
2. The correct answer is **B**. The principles of a perioperative plan to improve outcomes in elective colon surgery have included avoiding starvation, limiting intravenous fluids, and increasing mobility. Providing a carbohydrate-enhanced drink preoperatively as part of a complex perioperative plan has improved outcomes. Patients consuming 800 mL of a carbohydrate-rich liquid (100 g of carbohydrate) at midnight and 400 mL 2 hours prior to surgical intervention demonstrate a faster recovery, fewer infectious complications, and no increased aspirations. By providing this fluid and nutritional supplementation without a preoperative bowel prep, patients received less intravenous fluids, which improved recovery. In addition, a decrease in insulin resistance has been observed that has been shown to be associated with decreased complications and mortality.
3. The correct answer is **D**. Numerous studies have evaluated antioxidants in the critically ill; however, few have focused on trauma patients. Vitamins C and E combined have demonstrated some improvement in a prospective trial with trauma patients. In a large but retrospective study of strictly trauma patients, lower mortality was associated with the use of vitamins C and E, and selenium in combination. Zinc administration has not demonstrated improved outcomes in trauma patients.

Background

Incidence

Injury represents the most common cause of death between the ages of 1 and 35, accounting for over 150,000 deaths per year, or 7% of all deaths. In addition, over 1.9 million hospitalizations will occur with approximately 16% of those injured missing at least 6 days of work; approximately 33% will suffer time lost from school.[1] Projections for 2020 reveal traffic injuries will rise to the 3rd most common cause of death worldwide, while interpersonal violence is projected to rise to the 12th most common.[2]

Overall, trauma patients have experienced improved mortality; however, those who survive often suffer the morbidity related to protein-calorie malnutrition. There are two major nutrition tenets that must be addressed when treating patients who are not only admitted to various surgical wards and critical care units, but also undergo one or more surgical interventions. The first tenet is that these patients will be in negative nitrogen balance and suffer weight loss, weakness, and a long duration of rehabilitation prior to return to baseline.[3] The second tenet is that early administration of nutrition and nutrition supplements is needed as the patient is being admitted and going to the operating room within minutes of evaluation in the emergency department. These early decisions could not only affect surgical infections and hospital length of stays, but also the time the patient spends returning to baseline.[4–8]

Severity of Injury

Trauma can be differentiated as blunt versus penetrating injury, with burns considered separately. The severity of trauma/burns has been described with multiple scoring systems (Injury Severity Score, Glasgow Coma Scale, Penetrating Abdominal Trauma Index, and total body surface area [TBSA] burn affected) that attempt to not only predict mortality but also predict who will benefit from aggressive nutrition therapy.

In general, all of these patients undergo a systemic inflammatory response syndrome (SIRS), which entails the presence of two out of four abnormal systems (heart rate, respiratory rate, temperature, white blood cell count). When at least two SIRS criteria are met, the local injury of trauma or burn is producing a systemic reaction.[9] During this "flow" phase originally described by Cuthbertson, amino acid mobilization occurs for gluconeogenesis, immunologic properties, and the initiation of healing. The magnitude of the flow phase or SIRS suggests the degree of inflammation.[10] Not only is there a greater risk of death (infectious and noninfectious), but for those who do survive, a greater negative nitrogen balance, longer hospital stay, more weight loss, and a more difficult time returning to the life prior to the injury is seen.[11]

Physiological Response to Stress

Neuroendocrine Response and Systemic Inflammation

The immediate goal following major trauma is to maintain oxygen delivery and to diminish the *systemic* inflammation that is a result of the insult. Though nutrition support is often considered on post trauma days 1 to 3, consideration of access and initiation of various modes of nutrition support (enteral tube feeds, immunomodulating formulas, antioxidants, etc.) must be addressed as soon as resuscitation is complete. Otherwise, the goal of early (within 24 hours of insult) EN and antioxidant provision will not be achieved, thereby producing worse outcomes.[2,12–14] However, aggressive nutrition provision has associated risks (ie, small bowel necrosis), albeit low, that must be taken into consideration after complete resuscitation.

After injury, the neuroendocrine and cytokine response activates a cascade of events resulting in what has been termed the systemic inflammatory response (see Chapter 23), which was described previously. The response includes an increase in heart rate and minute ventilation to meet tissue demands for increased oxygen requirements. In addition, a rapid shift occurs from a state of storing protein, lipid, and glycogen to a catabolic state with mobilization of these nutrients for energy utilization. There is a direct correlation between the severity of the injury and the degree of substrate mobilization. Tissue catabolism is mediated through the release of cytokines such as tumor necrosis factor; interleukins-1, -2, and -6; and the counterregulatory hormones such as epinephrine, norepinephrine, glucagon, and cortisol.[15] These hormones are labeled counterregulatory because they oppose the anabolic effects of insulin and other anabolic hormones. Circulating levels of insulin are elevated in most metabolically stressed patients, but the responsiveness of tissues to insulin, especially skeletal muscle, is severely blunted. This relative insulin resistance is believed to be caused by the effects of counterregulatory hormones (Figure 24-1).[16] The hormonal milieu normalizes only after the injury or metabolic stress has resolved (see Chapter 23).

With appropriate resuscitation maneuvers, the SIRS abates. These maneuvers include source control (stopping the bleeding, controlling bowel content spillage, debriding necrotic tissues) and oxygen delivery (ventilator management, fluid and vasopressor resuscitation). In the last decade, nutrition support literature has focused its benefit(s) toward reducing systemic inflammation (Figure 24-2). Primarily, this support comes in the form of early (< 36 hours) initiation of EN.[4,13,14,17] Current evidence suggests that caloric and protein goals need not be met initially. These early nutrition therapies are less likely to address protein-calorie malnutrition and more likely to address the modulation of the immune function.[18]

Reperfusion Injury/Low-Flow States

Significant insults, such as sepsis and hemorrhage, decrease splanchnic blood flow and increase oxygen consumption. In human studies, removing as much as 3% to 5% of the blood volume can result in a 50% to 70% shunt of visceral blood flow.[19] Other events, such as routine general anesthesia and midline abdominal incisions can lower visceral blood flow by approximately 40% to 50%.[20] Gut ischemia can lead to mitochondrial disruption, mucosal acidosis, progressive cell injury, and cell destruction (see Chapter 23). Mucosal acidosis, a measure of reduced intraoperative splanchnic perfusion, is associated with exaggerated local and systemic immune responses, increased intestinal permeability, an increase in septic complications, and a trend toward increased multiorgan dysfunction syndrome.[21] The presence of luminal nutrients increases GI blood flow, a phenomenon termed postprandial hyperemia.[22]

Inadequate splanchnic blood flow is thought to play a pivotal role in the development of multiorgan dysfunction syndrome. When splanchnic perfusion is compromised, feeding that increases intestinal metabolic demand poses a theoretical risk of intestinal ischemia.[23,24] In these conditions, some suggest that EN may cause nonocclusive bowel necrosis.[25,26] Nonocclusive bowel necrosis has an estimated incidence varying from 0.3% to 8.5% in the intensive care unit (ICU) and remains a concern.[25,27]

The literature does not clarify whether EN increases the potential for complications or whether increased blood flow associated with EN protects the mucosa. Over the past decade, several investigators using large and small animal models of shock states have reported that nutrient delivery enhances visceral blood perfusion in these low-flow states.[28–33] In addition, clinical and laboratory evidence suggests that EN is not necessarily contraindicated with the use of vasoactive agents.[27] However, care must be taken in providing EN to patients in shock (see Chapter 23). In a review of the literature of jejunal feeding associated with small bowel necrosis, virtually all patients experienced distention, and half had pneumatosis, abdominal pain, hypotension, and increased nasogastric output.[34] Use of EN in hemodynamically unstable or low-flow state critically ill

FIGURE 24-1 Mechanisms of Hyperglycemia during States of Stress and Inflammation[16]

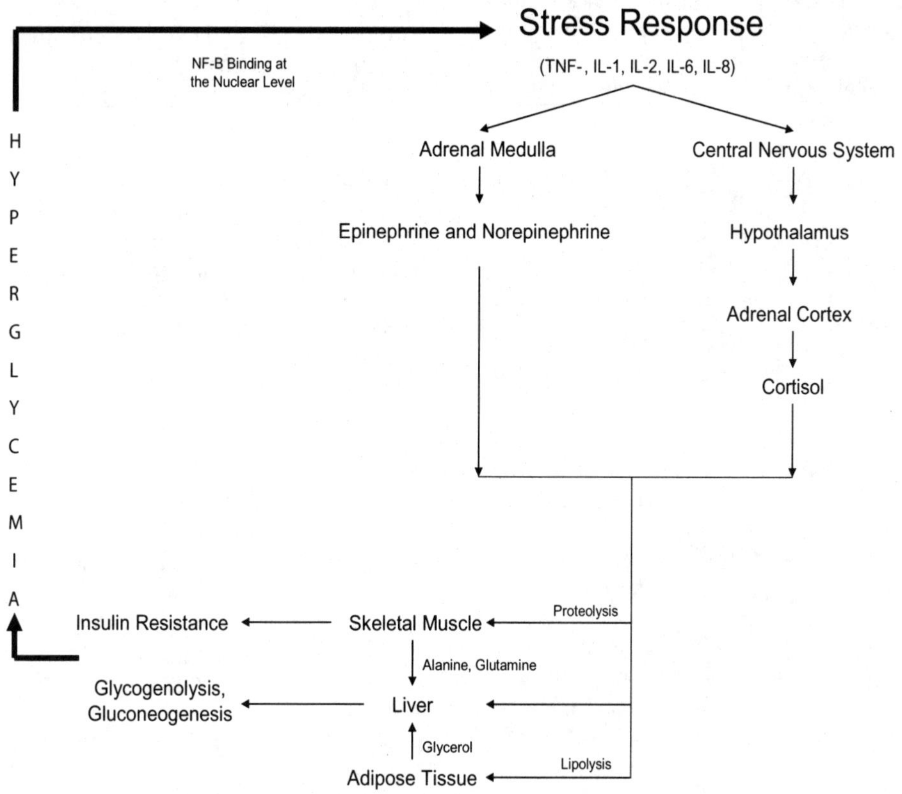

IL, interleukin); NF-κB, nuclear factor-kappa B; TNF-α, tumor necrosis factor-alpha.

FIGURE 24-2 Key Components in the Treatment of the Systemic Inflammatory Response Syndrome

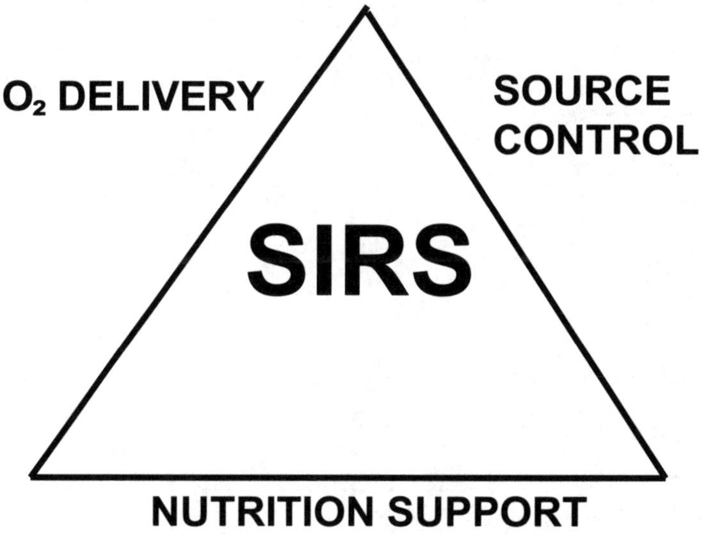

Effective treatment of the systemic inflammatory response syndrome (SIRS) requires a focus on three strategies: the delivery of oxygen (O_2) to vital tissues, source control (control of bleeding, necrotic, and infected tissues), and provision of nutritional support. Control of the patient's global inflammatory response is crucial for achieving euglycemia.

patients requires consideration of the feeding location, delivery rate, and bowel motility. Use of EN in such patients should be conservative (low infusion rate) until they are adequately resuscitated, with the EN advanced only when the patient demonstrates tolerance. Following adequate resuscitation, EN may protect the GI tract, especially the mucosa, from relatively low levels of ischemia.

Malnutrition in the Intensive Care Unit

Traditionally, malnutrition was defined on the basis of inadequate intake or starvation. Patients with malnutrition have a lower resting energy expenditure, a preferred fat utilization as the body's fuel, and minimal mobilization of protein. Whereas the malnutrition related to a surgical or traumatic stress stems from an increased resting energy expenditure and tremendous mobilization of the body's various protein deposits. Such a process is driven by systemic inflammation.

Inflammation has gained recognition as the prime factor in the pathophysiology of chronic disease states. Whether the inflammation is acute or chronic, it promotes cytokine-driven protein catabolism of the skeletal muscle.[35,36] This systemic inflammation can drive catabolism to the severity of affecting cardiac mass and function.[37] Once muscle is catabolized to the degree that it alters functional level, most experts would agree malnutrition is present. However, when this level of skeletal muscle depletion is observed in the outpatient setting or with patients with chronic inflammatory states, severe protein calorie malnutrition is noted and aggressive measures to address the disease state and the malnutrition are warranted. Unfortunately, inflammation and its metabolic consequences start immediately, rapidly depleting even the well-nourished critically injured or ill patient. This inflammatory response and subsequent protein catabolism provides the environment for adverse outcomes.

International experts have proposed changes to the nomenclature of malnutrition due to our current understanding of the links between inflammatory metabolism and catabolic depletion of body habitus. Recently, Jensen and colleagues developed a consensus statement delineating the different states of malnutrition: (1) chronic starvation without inflammation, (2) chronic diseases with mild to moderate inflammation, and (3) acute disease states (trauma, burns, major infections) with a tremendous burden of inflammation and subsequent malnutrition.[38] This "acute disease– or injury-related malnutrition" gives nomenclature to the phenomenon of elevated resting energy expenditure, increased nitrogen excretion, and subsequent increased caloric and protein requirements. This occurs over the first hours to days after the patient is admitted. However, this inflammation and subsequent nitrogen excretion continues for weeks to months after the patient is discharged from the ICU (Figure 24-3).[39] In addition, this inflammation, which continues to drive the protein catabolism, drives the anorexia that prevents appropriate intake.

Nutrition Assessment

Screening and Anthropometrics

Up to 40% of hospitalized patients are malnourished, and malnutrition has been linked to immunosuppression, impaired wound healing, increased hospital costs, greater length of hospital stay, and even increased mortality.[40]

Screening for malnutrition risk within 24 to 48 hours of hospital admission followed by nutritional assessment (when required) and timely intervention has been mandated by multiple national advisory organizations. Such practice has been identified as a national standard by The Joint Commission (see Chapter 9).[40] Multiple nutrition screening tools have been developed for hospitalized populations; however, most patients requiring admission to a hospital for trauma, surgery, or burn have increased caloric and protein requirements, putting them at risk for malnutrition, as previously described. This is especially true for critically ill patients in a surgical ICU.

Surgical ICU patients typically fall into three main categories: postoperative major elective surgery, major injury (eg, burns and trauma), and serious sepsis. The patients who undergo major elective surgery are often moderately depleted of body protein preoperatively because of their disease process. In addition, these patients can lose approximately 5% or 43 g/d of body protein during the first two weeks postoperatively.[41,42] Up to 20% of total body protein is metabolized in critically ill patients in the first three weeks following trauma or illness.[43] The severity of illness can be compounded by preexisting medical conditions, such as liver disease and associated alcohol abuse, renal dysfunction, cardiac failure, obesity, pulmonary

FIGURE 24-3 Metabolic Response to Injury and Illness: Estimation of Energy and Protein Needs from Indirect Calorimetry and Nitrogen Balance

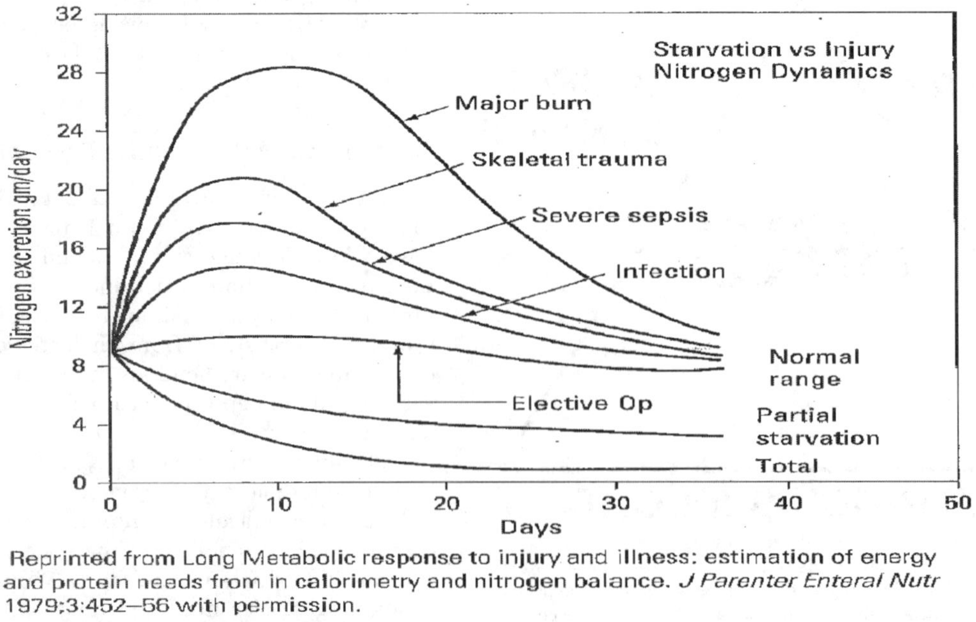

Reprinted from Long with permission (JPEN 1979;3:452–456).

dysfunction and failure requiring mechanical ventilation, and diabetes. All of these factors contribute to nutritional risk. Additionally, extensive wounds, infections, and burns significantly increase the body's energy requirements.

These conditions not only place patients at increased risk of malnutrition, but also make assessment of body composition and caloric and protein requirements challenging. In such patients, nutrition assessment data (eg, medical/surgical history, medication, nutrition intake; see Chapter 9) is often obtained from family members or caregivers.[44] Generally, anthropometric data such as height and weight are not as valuable as an index of functional capacity or metabolic health in critically/acutely ill patients.[45] Resuscitative fluids and capillary permeability cause generalized body edema, anasarca, and elevated body weights. Hill demonstrated that over a four-week period, critically ill patients had a net accumulation of 4.7 to 12.5 L of fluid.[42] Therefore, body weight measured in the ICU is not a valid indicator of body cell mass. Often, weight must be estimated using historical information provided by family members, with consideration of clinical events affecting body compartment fluid shifts. Ideally, weight changes should be monitored weekly. Acute weight changes are most likely due to fluid shifts, as 1 L of fluid is equal to 1 kg body weight.[46] Loss of limb(s), bulky dressings, and other attached supportive materials required for critical care must be factored into interpretation of body weight (see Chapter 9).

Biochemical Measures

Protein biochemical markers traditionally used in nutrition assessment, such as albumin, prealbumin, transferrin, and retinol-binding protein, do not accurately reflect the nutrition status of critically ill patients.[47] During liver dysfunction, inflammation, and physical stress, the liver decreases the synthesis of transport proteins and increases the synthesis of positive acute phase response proteins such as C-reactive protein.[15,48] Additionally, fluid shifts and increased vascular permeability change the proportion of fluid to protein, effectively changing the measured concentration of serum proteins. Therefore, in patients with acute illness, inflammation, or injury (such as in the early postoperative period and in trauma and burn patients), transport proteins cannot reliably be regarded as a marker of nutrition status, but can only be interpreted as a marker of severity of illness and inflammation.[47] This concept is illustrated in the burn scenario (Practice Scenario 24-1).

Nitrogen balance (see Chapter 9) has historically been used as an additional indicator of adequacy of whole body protein delivery, calculated by measuring the amount of nitrogen provided as nutrition support (protein intake) and subtracting the total body nitrogen loss. A positive nitrogen balance would indicate that the patient is receiving enough nitrogen to meet or exceed the body's demand. In acute illness, injury, and burn, it can be difficult to quantify all sources of protein loss (stool, wounds, abdominal drains, urine, dialysate, etc.).[53] Additionally, in the early stages of a severe burn, injury, postoperative setting, or sepsis, patients are severely catabolic. Until their catabolic drive has passed, a positive nitrogen balance may not be achievable due to intrinsic protein synthesis and breakdown cycles. Therefore, measuring nitrogen balance to determine adequacy of nutrient delivery is infrequently performed in the clinical setting.

Practice Scenario 24-1

Question: How does the practitioner prescribe nutrition therapy for a complex burn patient?

Scenario: A 39-year-old male involved in a house fire was transferred from the emergency room to the burn unit within 2 hours (a total of 4 hours out from the scene). Physical assessment revealed an injury involving 75% TBSA burn, 60% full thickness. Although the patient's lungs were clear, bronchoscopy via the endotracheal tube showed significant erythema in the airways. In addition, the partial pressure of oxygen in arterial blood:fraction of inspired oxygen ratio of 280 was diagnostic for inhalation injury. The patient was measured at 178 cm in height and weighed 78 kg (dry weight) per bed scale. A nasogastric tube was connected to intermittent low wall suction. Bowel sounds were absent in all four quadrants. Intravenous resuscitative fluids were provided to maintain urine output at 30 to 50 mL/h.

Intervention: Within 8 hours of admission, an enteric feeding tube was placed fluoroscopically into the proximal duodenum. Once adequate urine output was accomplished and cardiopulmonary resuscitation was complete, a high protein enteral formula was started and increased to goal over the next 72 hours. As the patient required multiple surgeries, EN was provided through the immediate perioperative period. Once the patient was able to tolerate oral intake, EN was cycled to a 12-hour nighttime regimen. The enteral feeds were discontinued when the patient consistently consumed greater than 60% of nutrition requirements.

Answer: Energy requirement (measured energy expenditure) was determined by indirect calorimetry to be 2886 kcal/d. Protein needs are estimated at 20% to 25% of this caloric goal, which correlates to 144 to 180 g of protein/d. As calorie needs change over the course of treatment, protein needs are adjusted accordingly. The patient required a product that is of high biological, intact protein. The total nonprotein calorie-to-nitrogen ratio of the product choice should have been low (100:1 or less). The formula should also have been moderately low in fat. The presence of arginine, glutamine, and omega-3 fatty acids could be considered (see Chapter 11). Because burn patients need a large volume of fluid, a 1.5 to 2.0 kcal/mL formula was not considered. Osmolality was not a significant factor in the decision of formula type.

For the first week off the ventilator, the patient consumed mostly liquids with a few bites of solids. Over the next week, he gradually improved, consuming approximately 25% of calorie needs orally. As a result, tube feedings were withheld 2 hours (1 hour before and 1 hour during) at mealtime. As a result of supplementation, his oral calorie intake improved to 75% of goal, and the feeding tube was discontinued. The patient's intake continued to improve; however, approximately 25% of his intake was supported by high-calorie oral supplements.

Rationale: Energy need is influenced by numerous variables (see Chapter 2). Indirect calorimetry incorporates the stage of recovery

TABLE 24-1 Predictive Equations for Energy Expenditure

Author	Patient Characteristics	Predictive Equations	Modifiers	
HBE[162]	Male Female	66.47 + (13.75 × wt) + (5 × ht) − (6.75 × age) 655.09 + (9.56 × wt) + (1.84 × ht) − (4.67 × age)	Weight in kg Height in cm	Age in years
American College of Chest Physicians[163]		25 kcal/usual body wt/day 20–25 kcal/actual body wt/day	Weight in kg Weight in kg	
European Society for Clinical Nutrition and Metabolism guidelines[160]				
Brandi et al.[164]		HBE (0.96) + HR (7) + Ve (48) − 702	HR beats/minute Ve = minute ventilation in L/min	
Curreri et al.[166]		25 × actual weight + 40 × (% TBSA burn)	Weight in kg	
Davies and Lilijedahl[167]		(20 × actual weight) + (70 × %TBSA burn)	Weight in kg	
Fusco et al.[168]		(−983) − 4 × (age) + 32 × (ht) + 11 × (wt)	Age in years Height in inches	Weight in kg
Ireton-Jones et al. (1992)[169]		1925 − 10(age) + 5(actual wt) + 281(s) + 292(t) + 851(b)	Age in yrs s = sex male = 1 female = 0 t = trauma present = 1 absent = 0 b = burn present = 1 absent = 0	
Ireton-Jones et al. (1997)[170]		Wt(5) − age(11) + male (244) + trauma(239) + burn(851) + 1784	Age in yrs s = sex male = 1 female = 0 t = trauma present = 1 absent = 0 b = burn present = 1 absent = 0	
Kleiber[171]	Male Female	71.2 × (wt) × (0.75) × [1 + 0.004 × (30 − age) + 0.01 × (ht/wt) × (1/3) − 43.4] 65.8 × (wt) × (0.75) × [1 + 0.004 × (30 − age) + 0.018 × (cm/Kg) × (1/3) − 42.1]	Age in years Height in cm Weight in kg	
Liu et al.[172]		13.88 × wt + 4.16 × ht − 3.43 × age − 112.4 × s + 54.34	Height in cm Weight in kg Age in years	s = sex Male = 0 Female = 1
Long[173]		(66.47 + 13.7 actual weight + 5.0 height − 6.76 age) × 1.2 × 2.0	Weight in kg Height in cm	Age in years
Mifflin-St. Jeor[174]	Male Female	9.99 × (wt) + 6.25 × (ht) − 4.92 × (age) + 5 9.99 × (wt) + 6.25 × (ht) − 4.92 × (age) − 161	Weight in kg Height in cm	Age in years
Penn State (1998)[175]		HBE × (1.1) + (Ve32) + (Tmax × 140) − 5340	Ve = minute ventilation in L/min	
Penn State (2003)[176]		HBE × (0.85) + (Ve × 33) + (Tmax × 175) − 6433	Tmax = maximum temperature in C°	
Penn State (2003)[177]		Mifflin × (0.96) + Tmax(167) + Ve (31) − 6212		

(continued)

as well as changes in clinical status and, therefore, is the best tool for determining energy requirements. However, many facilities lack access to indirect calorimetry measurement. Alternatively, there are equations used in critical care populations (Table 24-1). Once wounds are completely covered, and the patient enters convalescence, identifying and reaching the feeding is imperative.

In general, protein amounting to 20% to 25% of overall calories is recommended. This translates to about 2.5 g/kg/d of protein in the early postburn course, and up to 4 g/kg/d during the extended flow period.

A growing number of institutions are safely providing continuous enteral feedings to burn patients in the perioperative period.[27] The tube-feeding regimen is minimally interrupted and nutrient provision is maximized.

The assessment of protein status based upon prealbumin must factor inflammatory processes (see Chapters 9 and 23) into the review. Serum prealbumin is a negative acute-phase reactant; therefore, levels are affected by the burn process and additional inflammatory factors such as surgical intervention and infection throughout the recovery course.[45,46] Protein is also lost through the plasma of the open wound, further depleting stores. Prealbumin levels are generally inversely related to C-reactive protein during inflammatory metabolism.

Nutrition Requirements

Determination of Nutrient Requirements

Assessment of nutrition requirements can be quite difficult in critically ill patients.[54] Critical illness and its treatment can profoundly alter metabolism and significantly increase or decrease energy expenditure. Determination of energy expenditure is necessary to ensure that energy needs are provided without over- or underfeeding (see Chapter 2). Overfeeding is associated with many complications including hepatic steatosis, hyperglycemia, and pulmonary compromise.[55] Prolonged periods of undernutrition can lead to poor wound healing, impaired organ function, altered immunological status, and increased risk of mortality.[56] To adequately assess a patient's nutrition requirements, one must first determine the amount of calories needed to meet the patient's daily energy expenditure.

Energy

The clinical "gold standard" of determining energy (caloric) requirements is by measurement with an indirect calorimeter (also sometimes referred to as a "metabolic cart") (see

TABLE 24-1 Predictive Equations for Energy Expenditure *(continued)*

Author	Patient Characteristics	Predictive Equations	Modifiers
Roza and Shizgal[178]	Male	88.362 + 4.799 × (ht) + 13.397 × (wt) 5.677 × (age)	Height in cm; Age in years; Weight in kg
	Female	447.593 + 3.098 × (ht) + 9.247 × (kg) − 4.330 × age	
Faisy et al.[179]		8 × (wt) +14 × (ht) + 32 × (Ve) + 94 × (Temp) − 4834	Weight in kg; Height in cm; Tmax = maximum temperature in C°; Ve = minute ventilation in L/min
Schofield[180]	Male		Weight in kg
	18–30 yrs	15 × (wt) + 690	
	30–60 yrs	11.4 × (wt) + 870	
	> 60 yrs	11.7 × (wt) + 585	
	Female		
	18–30 yrs	14.8 × (wt) + 485	
	30–60 yrs	8.1 × (wt) + 842	
	> 60 yrs	9.0 × (wt) + 656	
Swinamer[181]		945 (BSA) − 6.4 (age) + 108 (Temp) + 24.2 (RR) + 81.7 (VT) − 4349	BSA in m^2; Age in years; Temp in C°; RR in breaths/min; VT = tidal volume in L/min
Food and Agriculture Organization/World Health Organization/ United Nations University[182]	18–30 yrs	13.3 × (wt) + 334 × (ht/100) + 35	Weight in kg
	30–60 yrs	8.7 × (wt) − 25 × (ht/100) + 865	Height in cm
	> 60 yrs	9.2 × (wt) + 637 × (ht/100) − 302	

BMI, body mass index; BSA, body surface area; HBE, Harris-Benedict equation; HR, heart rate; RR, respiratory rate; TBSA, total body surface area.

Chapter 2). Indirect calorimetry measures energy expenditure through analysis of respiratory gases (oxygen consumption, carbon dioxide production) and uses a modified Weir equation to determine energy expenditure.[57] Although indirect calorimetry is considered the gold standard, with the best accuracy for measuring energy requirements in the clinical setting, it is expensive to perform routinely, and many facilities do not have the technology or trained personnel to conduct the studies. Also, indirect calorimetry can be inaccurate under a variety of circumstances that commonly affect critically ill patients, such as those receiving > 60% fraction of inspired oxygen in a gas mixture or those with leaking chest tubes or endotracheal tubes in which the ventilated gas is not completely captured.[58]

Most institutions do not have access to a metabolic cart and rely instead on predictive equations to determine energy requirements. Early in the last century, Harris and Benedict developed one of the first widely accepted predictive equations derived from metabolic research performed on healthy men and women with no extremes of weight or age. Over 200 similar equations have been reported in the literature since, with many of these equations still in use. As medicine has evolved over the last century, we have created a need for ICUs to manage a patient population that is older, more critically ill, and has sustained more invasive surgery. Patients are surviving tremendous trauma and burn injuries. Through research, we now have a better understanding of how these processes alter metabolic demands. We have responded to these changes by adding modifiers to the Harris-Benedict equations and by creating new equations in attempt to better estimate energy requirements of specific populations. Some of the more common equations are listed in Table 24-1. A more detailed description of these equations is provided in Chapter 2.

Despite slightly more accurate equations, estimating caloric requirements in surgical, critically ill, injured, and burn patients is challenging. The estimates are often inaccurate, particularly in very obese patients, very underweight patients, and in patients with acute or chronic liver disease. These findings are reflected in recent guidelines published by the Society of Critical Care Medicine (SCCM) and the American Society for Parenteral and Enteral Nutrition (A.S.P.E.N.), which recommend measuring resting energy expenditure via indirect calorimetry when available in these patient populations (see Chapter 2). Even when caloric requirements are accurately determined, most ICU patients do not receive their estimated energy needs.[56,65,66]

One of the most important aspects of monitoring a patient receiving EN or parenteral nutrition (PN) is to assess delivery of estimated nutritional needs. An astute clinician should evaluate whether or not the patient has attained prescribed enteral feeding goals. If not, one should determine impediments, then troubleshoot and develop new recommendations for attainment of goals. Many methods have been utilized to improve the daily amount of calories and protein provided to patients. Examples include compensatory goal feeding rate increases, avoidance of unnecessary cessation of tube feedings for repositioning patients, reduction in the time patients with protected airways are made nothing by mouth prior to procedures or surgeries, and the bridling of feeding tubes.[59–62] Heyland et al. have completed a pilot study assessing a new feeding protocol known as "the PEP uP protocol." This protocol is driven by the bedside nurse and utilizes daily volume-based goals, liberalization of the gastric residual volume threshold, and initiating protein supplementation with motility agents on Day 1 of a patient's ICU stay.[63] In addition, another method to promote adequate enteral provision is early initiation of EN infusion after percutaneous endoscopic gastrostomy tube placement. In adults, current practice recommendations indicate that after a percutaneous endoscopic gastrostomy tube is placed, it may be utilized for feeding within two hours instead of the routine 24-hour delay.[64]

Protein

Despite optimal nutrition support, patients sustaining major injury lose a large amount of protein via wound exudate and urine during the first ten days following injury (~110 g/d).[41] Surgical ICU patients often have preexisting nutritional depletion as a result of other medical conditions (eg, diabetes, renal failure, cancer, hepatic failure), multiple operations, or prolonged admissions. Large losses of lean body mass (~150 g/d) typically occur in septic patients despite aggressive nutrition support sufficient to result in a gain in total body fat.[41] Because of the increased protein loss that is associated with critical illness and injury, protein needs are elevated.[67] Although catabolism is not reversed by provision of energy and protein, the protein synthetic rate is partially responsive to amino acid infusion.[68,69] The current recommendation for stressed patients, including burns, is that 20% to 25% of total nutrient intake be provided as protein. This equates to roughly 1.5 to 2.0 g/kg/d, with the higher range to promote nitrogen equilibrium, or at least to minimize nitrogen deficit. Administration of 2 g/kg of ideal body weight per day has been suggested for obese patients with a body mass index of > 30. In patients with large surface area burns, higher protein loads (3 to 4 g/kg/d) may be required.[67,70,71] Protein administration in excess of these amounts has not been shown to be beneficial and, in fact, may cause azotemia.[72] It has also been suggested that ICU patients receiving continuous renal replacement therapy should receive 2.0 to 2.5 g/kg/d to overcome protein losses in the dialysate.[73] See Chapter 6 for further detailed discussion of protein requirements.

Carbohydrate

Glucose is the primary fuel for the central nervous system and blood cells, with a minimum of about 120 g/d necessary to maintain central nervous system function. In the metabolically stressed adult, the maximum rate of glucose oxidation is 4 to 7 mg/kg/min, roughly equivalent to 400 to 700 g/d in a 70-kg person.[74] In the hypermetabolic patient, a large portion of oxidized glucose is derived from amino acid substrates via gluconeogenesis yielding up to 2 to 3 mg/kg/min of glucose. This endogenous production is poorly suppressed by exogenous glucose administration. Therefore, providing large amounts of exogenous carbohydrate can cause hyperglycemia and hyperinsulinemia. Complications of excess glucose administration include hyperosmolar states, excess carbon dioxide production, hepatic steatosis, and hyperglycemia.[72]

Studies have revealed admission hyperglycemia to be a prognostic indicator in trauma patients with elevations correlating with increased morbidity and mortality.[75–77] Insulin therapy, where patients are kept normoglycemic with continuous insulin infusion, has been shown to prevent excessive inflammation in critically ill patients.[78] The single institution prospective randomized trial performed on parenterally fed surgical patients in Leuven, Belgium by Van den Berghe and colleagues initially showed significant benefit from maintaining tight glucose control (blood glucose concentration of 80 to 110 mg/dL [4.4 to 6.1 mmol/L]) in cardiac surgery patients.[79] However, subsequent studies failed to show benefit in general surgery or vascular surgery patients. More recent studies, such as the international multicenter Normoglycemia in Intensive Care Evaluation-Survival Using Glucose Algorithm Regulation trial, differed from the Van den Berghe trial, demonstrating increased morbidity and mortality when glucose levels were tightly controlled in mixed ICU patients (who were mostly fed enterally).[80,81] In addition, the Efficacy of Volume Substitution and Insulin Therapy in Severe Sepsis multicenter German trial was stopped early for concerns of an unacceptably high incidence of hypoglycemia.[82] Because of these findings and similar findings in smaller trials, a more moderate blood glucose control regimen, such as 144 to 180 mg/dL (8 to 10 mmol/L) is recommended.[83] Others have adopted a simpler goal of < 150 mg/dL.[84]

Fat

Lipid metabolism is altered in the critically ill patient as a result of alterations in hormonal and cytokine mediators.[85–87] Enhanced mobilization of adipose tissue triglyceride stores, despite increased plasma levels of glucose and insulin, is characteristic of the metabolic response to severe stress.[88] Linoleic acid and a-linolenic acid are essential fatty acids required for proper body metabolism and are provided to all patients. However, research to determine how much and which lipid preparation should be provided to critically ill patients is ongoing.

Polyunsaturated fatty acids are major structural components of cell membranes. The two main types of polyunsaturated fatty acids are omega-6s (linoleic acid [18:2 n-6]), and omega-3s (a-linolenic acid [18:3 n-3]). Both omega-6s and omega-3s are converted to biologically active long-chain triglycerides (eicosanoids). The omega-6 eiconsanoids (such as arachidonic acid [20:4 n-6] and docosapentaenoic acid [22:5 n-6]) tend to have proinflammatory and prothrombotic effects. Omega-3 polyunsaturated fatty acids (such as eicosapentaenoic acid [20:5 n-3] and docosahexaenoic acid [22:6 n-3]) tend to produce anti-inflammatory and antithrombotic effects. The recent meta-analysis by Marik and Zaloga[89] concluded that critically ill patients receiving EN formulas with high concentrations of omega-3 polyunsaturated fatty acids from fish oil had decreased infection rates, hospital length of stay, and mortality. Medium-chain triglycerides are attractive in that they are small and water-soluble and can thereby be absorbed without requiring bile salts. Most available commercial EN formulations contain mixtures of both long-chain triglycerides and medium-chain triglycerides. In contrast, commercially available intravenous lipid emulsions in the United States are soy-based and have a high percentage of omega-6 long-chain triglycerides.

Fluid and Electrolytes

Surgery, trauma, and burns disrupt normal fluid and electrolyte homeostasis as a result of resuscitative fluid delivery and fluid compartmental shifts. Calculations for the resuscitation and maintenance fluid requirements for early burn patients have been well described. The most commonly used method to determine adult fluid resuscitation requirements is the Parkland formula, traditionally used for patients with > 15% TBSA second- and third-degree burns. The formula calls for 4 mL of lactated Ringer's for each kilogram of body weight times the TBSA. One half of this total amount is administered in the first eight hours after the burn. The remaining amount is administered over the subsequent 16 hours, followed by maintenance fluids. Monitoring urine output is an essential part of providing fluid to thermal injury patients, as the patient should make a minimum of 0.3 to 0.5 mL/kg per hour.[90] Rates of fluid administration should be adjusted to assure adequate fluid volume resuscitation. Clinicians should be cognizant of the fact that overresuscitation of fluids can also increase morbidity and mortality in these patients by increasing the chances of respi-

TABLE 24-2 Electrolyte Recommendations for Critically Ill Patients

Electrolyte	Daily Needs (mEq/d)	Reasons for Increased Needs	Reasons for Decreased Needs
Sodium	70–100	Loop diuretics, cerebral salt wasting, wound losses	Hypertension, fluid overload
Potassium	70–100	Refeeding syndrome, diuretic therapy, amphotericin wasting, wound losses	Renal failure
Chloride	80–120	Wound or prolonged gastric losses	Acid-base balance
Phosphorus	10–30 mmol/d	Refeeding syndrome	Renal failure
Magnesium	8–24	Refeeding syndrome, diuretic therapy, gastrointestinal or wound losses	——
Calcium	5–20	↑ Blood products, wound losses	——

Adapted with permission from Cresci GA, Martindale RG. Nutrition support in trauma. In: Gottschlich MM, ed. *The Science and Practice of Nutrition Support: A Case-based Core Curriculum*. Dubuque, IA: Kendall/Hunt Publishing Co; 2001:445–464.

ratory failure, total body edema, and abdominal and/or extremity compartment syndromes. Respiratory failure is of greatest concern in inhalation injuries and in the patient who suffers both burn and traumatic injuries (such as pulmonary contusions). Many institutions have begun to incorporate colloid administration into their burn resuscitation protocols in efforts to reduce "fluid creep" (a phenomenon where burn patients require progressively increasing crystalloid fluid requirements in an attempt to avoid adverse outcomes associated with excessive fluid administration). The large volume fluid resuscitations required in burn victims can lead to electrolyte imbalances. Electrolyte levels should be monitored closely and replaced when necessary. Electrolytes can be safely provided in doses specified in Table 24-2. See Chapter 7 for further discussion of fluid and electrolytes. Pediatric burn centers also often use the Parkland formula; however, they use a goal urine output of 1 to 2 mL/kg of patients weighing < 30 to 50 kg.[90] Colloid administration has also been described in the pediatric population.

Vitamins, Trace Elements, and Minerals

Currently, there are no specific guidelines regarding vitamin and mineral requirements in the critically ill patient. Presumably, needs are increased post injury because of increased metabolic demands. However, objective data to support specific recommendations for supplementation are lacking. The antioxidant vitamins and minerals have received the most recent attention. Oxidative metabolites or reactive oxygen species are theoretically overproduced during critical illness (eg, trauma, surgery, reperfusion injury, acute respiratory distress syndrome, infection, burns). Release of cytokines and initiation of an acute-phase response most likely mediate this response.[91] Reactive oxygen species induce tissue injury through peroxidation of plasma membranes, oxidation of critical enzymatic or structural proteins, induction of apoptosis, and activation of nuclear factor-kappa B, leading to the induction of genes critical to the initiation and perpetuation of the systemic inflammatory response. Along with increased levels of reactive oxygen species, decreased levels of circulating vitamins C and E have been found after surgery, trauma, burns, sepsis, and long-term PN.[92–96] Both retrospective and prospective studies, specifically in trauma patients, have demonstrated improved outcomes utilizing antioxidant supplementation with vitamin C, vitamin E, and selenium.[12,97]

Current recommendations are to provide at minimum the dietary reference intake for vitamins and minerals in the critically ill patient.[98] EN formulations contain recommended allowances when provided at specified volumes. If those volumes are not tolerated, patients may require additional supplementation enterally or intravenously—keeping in mind that supratherapeutic doses present the risk of side effects and toxicity. See Table 24-3 for suggested guidelines for vitamin/mineral supplementation in burns.[98,99] In addition, hypovitaminosis D is common in critically ill patients and has been associated with increased mortality. Therefore, clinical monitoring with appropriate supplementation may be warranted. Further studies are needed before the true efficacy of vitamin D replacement in the critically ill can be determined.[100–104] See Chapter 8 for further discussion of micronutrients.

TABLE 24-3 Recommended Vitamin and Mineral Supplementation for Burns

> 20% TBSAB
- One multivitamin daily
- 500 mg of ascorbic acid twice daily[a]
- 10,000 IU of vitamin A daily
- 45–50 mg of zinc daily[a]

< 20% TBSAB or reconstructive patient
- One multivitamin daily

TBSAB, total body surface area burned.
[a]Recommended delivery in suspension for tube feeding because oral vitamin C and zinc in large doses may precipitate nausea or vomiting.
Adapted with permission from Gottschlich and Warden.[99]

Route of Nutrition Support

For those individuals unable to consume adequate nutrients (at least 60% of nutritional needs) orally, EN or PN should be considered. EN is the preferred route of feeding the critically ill patient and should be initiated in the hemodynamically stable patient within 24 to 48 hours of admission.[52] In the past several years, the emphasis in critical care nutrition has moved away from PN toward EN. Although PN has been lifesaving in short bowel syndrome and intestinal failure, and has been successful in reversing malnutrition in many disease states (see Chapter 14), the narrow risk/benefit ratio for PN limits its use in critically ill patients in an ICU setting. Current PN formulations (see Chapter 15) available in the United States may, in fact, be immunosuppressive. PN has also been associated with an increased incidence of hyperglycemia, adding to patient immunocompromise with decreased neutrophil chemotaxis, phagocytosis, oxidative burst, and superoxide production. Comparisons of PN to EN have revealed that PN is associated with increasing the metabolic stress response, alterations in gut flora, gut atrophy, and contributing to systemic immunocompromise (see Chapter 16).[52]

Assessment of the patient's disease state, the extent of functional GI anatomy, the expected duration of EN support, and the ability to safely access the GI tract (via radiological, surgical, or endoscopic techniques) should be considered when selecting an enteral access device.[105] The SCCM/A.S.P.E.N. practice guidelines for the ICU patient population indicate that either gastric or small bowel feeding is acceptable. Neither the presence or absence of bowel sounds nor evidence of passage of flatus or stool is required prior to the initiation of EN feeding.[52]

Meta-analyses comparing PN with EN after trauma have revealed PN to be associated with a higher relative risk of infection, even accounting for catheter sepsis, complication rates, and mortality.[106,107] Studies by Moore et al. in 1986 and 1989 compared early EN to early PN in trauma patients with an abdominal trauma index between 15 to 40.[7,13] These two prospective, randomized clinical trials showed that patients randomized to receive EN had reduced major septic complications (abdominal abscesses and pneumonia) compared to those randomized to no supplemental feeding or PN. A study by the same group in trauma patients showed a blunting of the hepatic stress response, with higher constitutive proteins and lower acute-phase proteins in the EN group than the PN group.[17] These findings were later confirmed by different investigators in patients with a penetrating abdominal trauma index > 15 who were randomized to either early EN (< 24 hours) or early PN.[4] Those receiving early EN experienced significantly fewer major septic complications (eg, pneumonias, intra-abdominal abscesses, line sepsis) than those receiving PN (14% versus 38%). The benefits were seen most in the severely injured patients and those with penetrating injuries. A subsequent meta-analysis of eight prospective, randomized trials comparing EN to PN in a total of 230 high-risk surgical patients found that enterally fed trauma patients had significantly fewer septic complications.[14] Given the overwhelming data, EN should be given primary consideration for all trauma, surgery, and burn patients with an intact GI system.[47]

In the previously well-nourished patient, PN support should be reserved and initiated only after efforts to provide nutrition via the enteral route have failed to advance EN to meet 100% of target goal calories for 7 to 10 days.[52] A recent prospective, randomized, controlled multicenter trial of early versus late PN in critically ill adults conducted in Europe resulted in the recommendation to delay the addition of supplemental PN until day 8 of hospitalization.[108] This study also supports findings from the Glue Grant that showed critically ill trauma patients who received PN to supplement EN calories during the first week had worse outcomes regarding infections and mortality.[109] This would indicate that an increasing caloric deficit does not justify the use of early PN, even when the enteral route does not meet goal requirements.

Exceptions to the delay of PN initiation are patients expected to undergo elective major upper GI surgery who have preexisting severe malnutrition. For these patients who are unable to receive EN, it is recommended that 5 to 7 days of preoperative PN be provided with continued PN postoperatively. However, in the malnourished GI surgery patient who did not receive preoperative PN, it is recommended to delay initiation of PN postoperatively for 5 to 7 days if EN continues to be contraindicated. PN provided for < 5 days has not shown benefit.[47]

Feeding Access

Enteral Access

The intention to start EN early can be challenging because not all GI access methods (see Chapter 12) are suitable for the critically ill patient. The optimal access site for EN in the critically ill is not yet clear. As described previously, decisions have to be made based on the clinical condition and individualized for each patient. Patients may be unstable and too high risk to transport to radiology or endoscopy suites, or to tolerate procedures at the bedside.[110] Many studies report successful early EN in trauma patients with the use of a feeding jejunostomy tube placed at the time of laparotomy.[4,7,17] However, not every critically ill or trauma patient requires laparotomy, so this method may not be employed in the majority of ICU patients.

Gastric Access

While it is easy to obtain gastric access, critically ill patients fed gastrically may be predisposed to aspiration, regurgitation, and reflux. Many critically ill, injured, and postoperative patients have delayed gastric emptying, potentially limiting their ability to tolerate gastric feedings.[111,112] Approximately 40% to 79% of gastrically fed medical/surgical ICU patients exhibit some degree of upper digestive intolerance caused by impaired gastric emptying.[113,114] Many diagnoses commonly seen in the ICU (eg, pneumonia, pancreatitis, sepsis, peritonitis, elevated intracranial pressures, and altered hemodynamics) are associated with gut dysmotility.[115]

However, delayed gastric emptying and gastric feeding in critically ill patients do not automatically lead to pulmonary aspiration. Studies have shown that while the risk of aspiration decreases as the level of formula infusion descends the GI tract, similar rates of pneumonia are seen whether patients are fed in the stomach or small bowel.[89,116] These results are limited by small sample sizes and lack of determination as to whether patients aspirated tube feeding formula or their own oral secretions. Regurgitation and pulmonary aspiration may occur despite extremely low gastric residuals (30 to 35 mL).[117] Others advocate small bowel feeding in critically ill patients because it is associated with decreased gastroesophageal reflux, reduced aspiration, an increase in nutrient delivery, and a shorter time to achieve desired nutrient delivery.[118]

Small Bowel Access

A clinically rational approach to EN in the critically ill patient is to feed into the small bowel in patients at high risk for aspiration and gut dysmotility. High-risk patients include those who have sustained severe blunt and penetrating torso and abdominal injuries, severe head injuries, major burns, those who have undergone major intra-abdominal surgery, had a previous episode of aspiration or emesis, persistent high gastric residuals (> 500 mL), are unable to protect the airway, require prolonged supine or prone positioning, or are anticipated to have multiple surgical procedures. Blind-bedside small-bore feeding tube placement has frequent complications of 1% to 2% airway placement, with a 30% mortality, which has been reported. Recently, blind-bedside small bowel feeding tube placement methods and protocols have been reported to decrease these noted complications.[119] The advantages of these methods are that they are less traumatic to the patient, do not require patient transport, are minimally invasive, and are less costly if performed by trained personnel. Success rates when trained personnel follow a protocol for bedside placement of a feeding tube range from 80% to 95%.[120,121]

Transitioning to Oral Nutrition

Clinicians should strive to transition patients to partial or full oral nutrition whenever the patient's clinical course will permit. Nighttime cycling of EN has been considered when patients are meeting > 60% of target calories by the oral route prior to discontinuing EN. Oral dietary restrictions are discouraged to maximize intake.[52]

Adjunctive Therapies

A variety of individual nutrients provided in supraphysiologic quantities have been studied over the past several decades. Recent publications provide details on the mechanisms of actions of omega-3 fatty acids,[122] glutamine,[123] arginine[124] and antioxidants (vitamins C and E, and selenium) in trauma,[12] burn, and critically ill surgical patients. Wischmeyer's excellent review of nutritional pharmacology in surgery and critical care divides several nutrients into major categories of immune-modulating, anti-inflammatory, and cell protective pharmaconutrients. The following provides background information on the clinical effects of pharmaconutrients in specific states of critical illness, trauma, and surgery.[125]

Glutamine

Glutamine, the most abundant amino acid in blood and preferred fuel source for rapidly dividing cells such as the enterocyte, seems to prevent intestinal mucosal damage and enhance neutrophil function in critical illness and trauma.[126,127] Increased mortality in critically ill patients has been associated with a severe reduction in plasma glutamine levels[128,129] due to the body's inability to keep up with the accelerated rate of glutamine utilization during critical illness or injury.[123,129,130] Some explanations postulated for the increased demand for glutamine during stress and critical illness are that glutamine serves as a fuel source for rapidly dividing cells,[123] as a precursor for synthesis of nucleic acids,[123] and has a role in renal acid buffering.[123] Proposed mechanisms through which glutamine exerts its protective effects in critical illness are improved tissue protection, immune regulation, preservation of glutathione and antioxidant capacity, and preservation of cellular metabolism post injury.[123,131] Glutamine decreases intestinal permeability and maintains the physiologic barrier (thereby reducing the frequency of infections).[132] Glutamine's beneficial effect of tissue protection involves induction of heat shock proteins, which may have an antiapoptotic effect on gut epithelial cells.[123,131,133] Enhanced heat shock protein expression provides stress tolerance and protection from continued injury that could cause cell death or impaired recovery.[123,131] SCCM/A.S.P.E.N. guidelines recommend enteral glutamine supplementation of 0.3 to 0.5 g/kg/d given in two or three divided doses in trauma and critically ill surgery patients if they are not already receiving an immune-modulating enteral formula.[52] Parenteral glutamine should be considered in the critical care setting. Doses of > 0.35 to 0.5 g/kg/d of glutamine have been suggested.[123]

Arginine

Zhu describes arginine starvation as a mechanism of immune control. Plasma arginine levels are reported to drop by 50% or more and remain depressed for days to weeks within hours of trauma or surgery.[124] T-lymphocyte function and nitric oxide production are two arginine-dependent processes.[124] Decreased T-cell proliferation, anergic responses to antigen recall, decreased interleukin-2 and interferon-γ production, and loss of ζ chain are characteristics of T-lymphocyte dysfunction after injury.[124] The inducible enzyme arginase 1 in myeloid cells is expressed after injury.[124] Arginase 1 increases destruction of arginine by metabolizing arginine to ornithine and urea, leading to a decrease in circulating arginine within a few hours after injury.[124] The myeloid cells induced by injury become immunosuppressor cells (termed myeloid-derived suppressor cells) and are thought to be a cause of arginine depletion, resulting in T-cell suppression.[124] This arginine deficiency caused by myeloid-derived suppressor cells can be treated with dietary arginine supplementation. Also, an increase in circulating nitric oxide metabolites and evidence of improved microcirculation with arginine supplementation after injury have been demonstrated.[124] SCCM/A.S.P.E.N. guidelines recommend arginine supplementation in major surgery, trauma, and burn patients.[47] Amounts of arginine supplementation that have been studied are in the range of 8 to 30 g/d, which is much higher than the normally ingested amounts of natural arginine of approximately 3 to 5 g/d.[124]

Omega-3 Fatty Acids

Stapleton et al. recently reviewed the mechanisms and clinical applications of omega-3 fatty acids (fish oil) in critical illness. Specifically, they examined the mechanisms of action by which omega-3 fatty acids may affect inflammation by enteral or parenteral administration. Omega-3 fatty acids incorporated into the phospholipids present in the membranes of immune cells (macrophages, monocytes, and neutrophils) can influence membrane fluidity-affecting the activity of membrane-bound enzymes, receptors, transporters, and lipid-based second messenger systems.[122] Also fish oils, due to their eicosapentaenoic acid and docosahexanoic acid content, have been shown to decrease production of arachidonic acid–derived eicosanoid inflammatory mediators. Lipid mediators derived from eicosapentaenoic acid and docosahexanoic acid with potent proresolving, anti-inflammatory, and neuroprotective properties called resolvins, protectins, and maresins have been found to play a role in the repair and resolution of inflammation. However, further research is needed to determine clinical benefit before recommendations for supplementation of omega-3 fatty acids (administered as bolus or by continuous infusion) are made.[122] Of late, bolus omega-3 fatty acid supplementation was not shown to provide benefit to critically ill medical patients.[134] For the patient with acute lung injury/acute respiratory distress syndrome, current guidelines from all the professional nutrition societies (SCCM/A.S.P.E.N., Canadian Critical Care Practice Guidelines, European Society for Clinical Nutrition and Metabolism) recommend the use of continuously administered enteral omega-3 fatty acids.[125]

Antioxidants and Trace Minerals

Ascorbic acid, ascorbate, or vitamin C, a water-soluble organic compound, acts as a cofactor in many enzymatic and chemical pathways and as a powerful aqueous-phase antioxidant.[135] Vitamin C functions as a cofactor in many enzymes including those involved with the metabolism of cholesterol to bile acids, carnitine, and norepinephrine biosynthesis, and the hydroxylation of collagen and cortisol.[135] As an antioxidant, vitamin C scavenges both reactive oxygen and nitrogen species and is considered a therapeutic supplement in various clinical conditions. Fukushima et al.[135] reported that vitamin C levels decreased after surgery, possibly due to increased demand. Supplementation with > 500 mg/day is suggested for uncomplicated surgical patients. In severely stressed patients, even higher doses may be needed. In burn patients, supplementation levels as high as 66 mg/kg/hour every 24 hours have been advocated to diminish fluid resuscitation.[136,137] Further investigation is required to define clinical benefit and optimal doses for supplementation.[135]

Collier et al. investigated high-dose antioxidants (intravenous vitamin C 1000 mg every 8 hours, 1000 IU vitamin E via naso- or orogastric tube every 8 hours, and intravenous selenium 200 μg per day) in acutely injured patients and found a significant reduction in both hospital and ICU length of stay, as well as a 28% relative risk reduction in mortality.[12]

SCCM/A.S.P.E.N. guidelines recommend that a combination of antioxidant vitamins and trace minerals (specifically including selenium) should be provided to all critically ill patients receiving specialized nutrition therapy.[52] The Canadian Critical Care Practice Guidelines state that the use of supplemental combined vitamins and trace elements should be considered in critically ill patients based on three Level 1 and thirteen Level 2 studies.[138]

Prebiotics, Probiotics, and Synbiotics

The SCCM/A.S.P.E.N. guidelines support the administration of probiotic agents in specific critically ill patient populations involving transplantation, major abdominal surgery, and severe trauma. A grade C recommendation was given for evidence of the studies reviewed, due to the differences in bacterial strains, variability of dosing, and the heterogeneity of the ICU population studied. However, the Canadian Critical Care Practice Guidelines report that there are insufficient data to make a recommendation on the use of prebiotic, probiotics, or synbiotics in critically ill patients.[138] See Chapter 4 for further discussion.

Formula Selection/Immunonutrition

The appropriate selection of an EN formula following injury requires individualized consideration of patient age, GI function, clinical condition, nutrient requirements, patient tolerance, product efficacy, and cost. Relevant to patients with trauma, surgery, and burns is the emergence of EN products formulated to modulate the immune system, wound healing, inflammation, and/or organ function.[139–142] Despite considerable research, such formulas continue to be the subject of controversy. In addition to the previous discussions of adjunctive (nutrient) therapies, refer to Chapter 11, which provides a current review of EN formulas and their applications. Practice Scenario 24-2 describes clinical exercises involved in the selection of appropriate enteral products in trauma.

Practice Scenario 24-2

Question: How does the practitioner prescribe nutrition therapy for a complex trauma patient?

Scenario: A 42-year-old male sustained a sternal fracture, right rib fractures, pulmonary contusion, lumbar spine fracture (L1–L3), open pelvic fracture, left femur fracture, right open tibia/fibula fractures, right open ankle fracture, right sinus fracture, and a closed head injury from a motor vehicle accident. After stabilization in the emergency department, he arrived in the shock/trauma ICU chemically sedated and intubated. The patient was wearing a cervical collar and because of his spinal injury was in a supine position and was under log roll only orders. Chest radiograph showed fluffy infiltrates in the right lung. A neurological exam revealed a Glasgow Coma Scale score of 10. He had an orogastric tube to low intermittent wall suction and was receiving intravenous fluids of normal saline at 120 mL/h.

Intervention: A member of the surgical nutrition support team placed a feeding tube at bedside. The tube was passed through the mouth instead of the naris because of the patient's sinus fracture. The tube position was confirmed by abdominal radiograph to be in the fourth portion of the duodenum. An immune-enhancing formula was initiated at 30 mL/h within 24 hours of admission, after resuscitation was complete. A goal regimen was achieved on post trauma day 4, approximately 72 hours after EN initiation.

Answer: After resuscitation, it is imperative to provide an initial tube feed prescription (~50% goal) within 24 to 48 hours. To avoid ongoing protein calorie deficit, nutrition goals should subsequently be met within the first week of admission.

Rationale: While most patients are suited for a standard, isotonic enteral feeding formula, there are a number of patients in which a disease-specific formula may be indicated. There are commercially available immune-modulating formulas that contain combinations of added arginine, glutamine, omega-3 fatty acids, and nucleotides. Numerous prospective, randomized, controlled trials have studied the efficacy and safety of immune formulations in a variety of clinical settings, including trauma.[8,49–51] These studies have documented that trauma patients receiving the immune formula had fewer nosocomial infections, reduced intra-abdominal abscesses and multiple organ failure, decreased days receiving antibiotics, and decreased hospital length of stay.

The patient is at risk for gastric feeding intolerance, reflux, and pulmonary aspiration because of supine positioning, high fraction of inspired oxygen in a gas mixture, and absence of bowel sounds. Additionally, the patient will require multiple operative interventions in the forthcoming days. Studies indicate that patients fed postpylorically do not necessarily have a decrease in gastroesophageal regurgitation, time to achieve nutritional goals, or increased nutrient delivery. But patients who may require multiple interruptions in feeds for procedures, such as operative interventions, may benefit from postpyloric feeds to reduce the preoperative nothing by mouth time required by anesthesia. Most critically ill patients may be enterally fed via the stomach safely.[52]

Indirect calorimetry provides the most accurate determination of energy requirements. However, logistics and resources often do not allow for the use of indirect calorimetry. Therefore, recommendations for moderately to severely injured patients are to provide 25 to 30 kcal/kg/d or 120% to 140% of the energy expenditure derived from predictive equations, and to meet high protein requirements (1.5 to 2 g/kg/d) (Table 24-1).

Perioperative Nutrition Provision

Perioperative nutrition support can be divided into four principal categories in the literature: preoperative PN, preoperative EN, postoperative PN, and postoperative EN. Postoperative PN and EN are the more important groups because surgery often cannot (and should not) be delayed.[143] However, surgeons have recognized the association between nutritional status and morbidity and mortality for many years. In 1936, Studley reported that chronic peptic ulcer patients undergoing gastrectomy had a 3.5% mortality rate if they had 20% preoperative weight loss and a 33% mortality rate with > 20% weight loss.[144] In fact, recognition of this problem drove Dr. Rhoads' efforts[78] that led to the development of PN.

In 1991, a prospective trial randomized 395 preoperative malnourished patients to receive PN or not.[145] Results of the study demonstrated that only severely malnourished patients benefited from preoperative PN, with significant reductions in noninfectious complications. In fact, those patients who were only borderline or mildly malnourished had higher infection rates if PN was utilized.

Trials have also compared early postoperative PN to EN in surgical populations, most notably trauma and acute pancreatitis populations. In general, the trauma studies have reported fewer postoperative infections, improved protein or nitrogen balance studies, and shorter hospital stays in subjects who received EN.[4,8,13] Patients with pancreatitis who received EN suffered fewer infections, decreased hospitalization, and faster disease resolution.[146–149]

There are relatively few (compared to PN) preoperative EN reports. In 1984, an Indian group reported reduced postoperative mortality and wound infections in malnourished subjects receiving EN ten days before surgery versus controls (routine hospital diet).[150] Gastric and colorectal cancer patients randomized to PN or EN for ten days before surgery had a significant decrease in postoperative intra-abdominal abscesses, with either form of preoperative nutrition compared to "controls" who went directly to surgery.[151]

Two meta-analyses of nine studies both concluded that while PN had no effect on mortality, increased morbidity was seen (mostly septic complications).[106,107,138,143,152] The latest nutrition guidelines stated that PN should be reserved and initiated only after the first seven days of hospitalization in patients without preadmission malnutrition.[52]

Most recently, collaborators of ERAS have introduced an elaborate pre- and postoperative care program involving elective colon resection patients. The principles of the program are to avoid starvation, to decrease the physiological stress of surgery (which induces insulin resistance), and to limit postoperative intravenous fluids, while optimizing pain control, GI function, and mobilization.[153] All of these principles are in an effort to decrease insulin resistance, which has been shown in multiple studies to be associated with increased complications (such as infections, increased hospitalization, and mortality).[154]

The nutritional components to the ERAS program are progressive. The first component is to avoid preoperative fasting. Solid meals are provided up until six hours before surgery. In addition, 800 mL (~100 grams; 400 calories) of a carbohydrate-rich clear liquid is given at midnight and 400 mL of the same formula is given again two hours prior to surgical intervention. The ERAS pathway meta-analysis (452 patients) demonstrated a decrease in complications (infectious and noninfectious) by approximately 50%, and a > 2-day reduction in length of hospitalization, with no change in readmissions (in view of earlier discharges) or mortality (from aspiration) when the program is used.[155,156]

By providing the preoperative carbohydrate nutrition/fluid administration in combination to withholding a routine bowel prep, patients receive less intravenous fluids and experience less postoperative complications (such as wound dehiscence).[157–159] As adherence to the program increased to over 70%, symptoms, morbidity, hospital length of stay, and readmissions all improved.[159] It remains unclear if ERAS, which was designed for elective colon resection patients, is applicable to other operative interventions or whether further improvements can be made with administration of antioxidants or other macronutrients.

Burns

For the burn patient, European Society for Clinical Nutrition and Metabolism guidelines report insufficient data to recommend routine supplementation of omega-3 fatty acids, arginine, glutamine, or nucleotides.[160] The same guidelines did recommend that the trace elements copper, selenium, and zinc be supplemented at higher than standard doses.[160] Daily doses of 40.4 μmol copper, 2.9 μmol selenium, and 406 μmol zinc for 30 days after burn injury have been associated with a reduction in the length of hospital stay and the number of bronchopneumonic infections.[160] A summary article on immunonutrition in burn injury care[161] reports that there is insufficient data to support routine use of immunonutrients (such as arginine and fish oil) in combination therapies or for individual supplementation. Kurmis et al. recommend use of enteral glutamine supplementation for patients with severe burn injury, but state that questions remain on the ideal dosage, timing, and duration of therapy.[161] The SCCM/A.S.P.E.N. guidelines recommend enteral glutamine supplementation of 0.3 to 0.5g/kg/d given in two or three divided doses in burn patients.

Acknowledgments

Material from the first and second editions was also contributed by Robert G. Martindale, PhD, MD, Gail Cresci, MS, RD, LD, CNSD, Michele Gottschlich, PhD, RD, LD, CNSD, Theresa Mayes, RD, LD, and Charles Mueller, PhD, RD, CD, CNSD.

References

1. U.S. Centers for Disease Control and Prevention. *Injury in the US: 2007 Chartbook*. CDC website. Accessed May 31, 2011. http://www.odo.gov/injury/
2. Murray CJ, Lopez AD. Alternative projections of mortality and disability by cause 1990-2020: Global Burden of Disease Study. *Lancet*. 1997;349(9064):1498–1504.
3. Wilmore DW. Alterations in protein, carbohydrate, and fat metabolism in injured and septic patients. *J Am Coll Nutr*. 1983;2(1):3–13.
4. Kudsk KA, Croce MA, Fabian TC, et al. Enteral versus parenteral feeding. Effects on septic morbidity after blunt and penetrating abdominal trauma. *Ann Surg*. 1992;215(5):503–511.

5. Kudsk KA. Clinical applications of enteral nutrition. *Nutr Clin Pract.* 1994;9(5):165–171.
6. Kudsk KA, Minard G, Croce MA, et al. A randomized trial of isonitrogenous enteral diets after severe trauma. An immune-enhancing diet reduces septic complications. *Ann Surg.* 1996 ;224(4):531–540.
7. Moore FA, Moore EE, Jones TN, McCroskey BL, Peterson VM. TEN versus TPN following major abdominal trauma—reduced septic morbidity. *J Trauma.* 1989;29(7):916–922.
8. Moore FA, Moore EE, Kudsk KA, et al. Clinical benefits of an immune-enhancing diet for early postinjury enteral feeding. *J Trauma.* 1994;37(4):607–615.
9. American College of Chest Physicians/Society of Critical Care Medicine. Consensus Conference: definitions for sepsis and organ failure and guidelines for the use of innovative therapies in sepsis. *Crit Care Med.* 1992;20(6):864–874.
10. Cuthbertson DP. Second annual Jonathan E. Rhoads Lecture. The metabolic response to injury and its nutritional implications: retrospect and prospect. *J Parenter Enteral Nutr.* 1979;3(3):108–129.
11. Malone DL, Kuhls D, Napolitano LM, McCarter R, Scalea T. Back to basics: validation of the admission systemic inflammatory response syndrome score in predicting outcome in trauma. *J Trauma.* 2001;51(3):458–463.
12. Collier BR, Giladi A, Dossett LA, Dyer L, Fleming SB, Cotton BA. Impact of high-dose antioxidants on outcomes in acutely injured patients. *J Parenter Enteral Nutr.* 2008;32(4):384–388.
13. Moore EE, Jones TN. Benefits of immediate jejunostomy feeding after major abdominal trauma—a prospective, randomized study. *J Trauma.* 1986;26(10):874–881.
14. Moore FA, Feliciano DV, Andrassy RJ, et al. Early enteral feeding, compared with parenteral, reduces postoperative septic complications. The results of a meta-analysis. *Ann Surg.* 1992;216(2): 172–183.
15. Gabay C, Kushner I. Acute-phase proteins and other systemic responses to inflammation. *N Engl J Med.* 1999;340(6):448–454.
16. Collier B, Dossett LA, May AK, Diaz JJ. Glucose control and the inflammatory response. *Nutr Clin Pract.* 2008;23(1):3–15.
17. Moore EE, Moore FA. Immediate enteral nutrition following multisystem trauma: a decade perspective. *J Am Coll Nutr.* 1991;10(6): 633–648.
18. Todd SR, Kozar RA, Moore FA. Nutrition support in adult trauma patients. *Nutr Clin Pract.* 2006;21(5):421–429.
19. Ohri SK, Somasundaram S, Koak Y, et al. The effect of intestinal hypoperfusion on intestinal absorption and permeability during cardiopulmonary bypass. *Gastroenterology.* 1994;106(2):318–323.
20. Fink MP. Adequacy of gut oxygenation in endotoxemia and sepsis. *Crit Care Med.* 1993;21(2 Suppl):S4–S8.
21. Holland J, Carey M, Hughes N, et al. Intraoperative splanchnic hypoperfusion, increased intestinal permeability, down-regulation of monocyte class II major histocompatibility complex expression, exaggerated acute phase response, and sepsis. *Am J Surg.* 2005; 190(3):393–400.
22. Matheson PJ, Wilson MA, Garrison RN. Regulation of intestinal blood flow. *J Surg Res.* 2000;93(1):182–196.
23. Ceppa EP, Fuh KC, Bulkley GB. Mesenteric hemodynamic response to circulatory shock. *Curr Opin Crit Care.* 2003;9(2):127–132.
24. Sigalet DL, Mackenzie SL, Hameed SM. Enteral nutrition and mucosal immunity: implications for feeding strategies in surgery and trauma. *Can J Surg.* 2004;47(2):109–116.
25. Marvin RG, McKinley BA, McQuiggan M, Cocanour CS, Moore FA. Nonocclusive bowel necrosis occurring in critically ill trauma patients receiving enteral nutrition manifests no reliable clinical signs for early detection. *Am J Surg.* 2000;179(1):7–12.
26. Munshi IA, Steingrub JS, Wolpert L. Small bowel necrosis associated with early postoperative jejunal tube feeding in a trauma patient. *J Trauma.* 2000;49(1):163–165.
27. Gottschlich MM, Jenkins ME, Mayes T, Khoury J, Kagan RJ, Warden GD. The 2002 Clinical Research Award. An evaluation of the safety of early vs delayed enteral support and effects on clinical, nutritional, and endocrine outcomes after severe burns. *J Burn Care Rehabil.* 2002;23(6):401–415.
28. Bortenschlager L, Roberts PR, Black KW, Zaloga GP. Enteral feeding minimizes liver injury during hemorrhagic shock. *Shock.* 1994; 2(5):351–354.
29. Gielkens HA, van Oostayen JA, Onkenhout W, Lamers CB, Masclee AA. Effect of amino acids on mesenteric blood flow in humans. *Scand J Gastroenterol.* 1997;32(12):1230–1234.
30. Gosche JR, Garrison RN, Harris PD, Cryer HG. Absorptive hyperemia restores intestinal blood flow during Escherichia coli sepsis in the rat. *Arch Surg.* 1990;125(12):1573–1576.
31. Inoue S, Lukes S, Alexander JW, Trocki O, Silberstein EB. Increased gut blood flow with early enteral feeding in burned guinea pigs. *J Burn Care Rehabil.* 1989;10(4):300–308.
32. Kazamias P, Kotzampassi K, Koufogiannis D, Eleftheriadis E. Influence of enteral nutrition-induced splanchnic hyperemia on the septic origin of splanchnic ischemia. *World J Surg.* 1998; 22(1):6–11.
33. Purcell PN, Davis K Jr, Branson RD, Johnson DJ. Continuous duodenal feeding restores gut blood flow and increases gut oxygen utilization during PEEP ventilation for lung injury. *Am J Surg.* 1993; 165(1):188–193.
34. Schunn CD, Daly JM. Small bowel necrosis associated with postoperative jejunal tube feeding. *J Am Coll Surg.* 1995;180(4):410–416.
35. Jensen GL. Inflammation as the key interface of the medical and nutrition universes: a provocative examination of the future of clinical nutrition and medicine. *J Parenter Enteral Nutr.* 2006; 30(5):453–463.
36. Jensen GL, Bistrian B, Roubenoff R, Heimburger DC. Malnutrition syndromes: a conundrum vs continuum. *J Parenter Enteral Nutr.* 2009;33(6):710–716.
37. Hill AA, Plank LD, Finn PJ, et al. Massive nitrogen loss in critical surgical illness: effect on cardiac mass and function. *Ann Surg.* 1997;226(2):191–197.
38. Jensen GL, Mirtallo J, Compher C, et al. Adult starvation and disease-related malnutrition: a proposal for etiology-based diagnosis in the clinical practice setting from the International Consensus Guideline Committee. *J Parenter Enteral Nutr.* 2010;34(2): 156–159.
39. Long CL, Schaffel N, Geiger JW, Schiller WR, Blakemore WS. Metabolic response to injury and illness: estimation of energy and protein needs from indirect calorimetry and nitrogen balance. *J Parenter Enteral Nutr.* 1979;3(6):452–456.
40. Barker LA, Gout BS, Crowe TC. Hospital malnutrition: prevalence, identification and impact on patients and the healthcare system. *Int J Environ Res Public Health.* 2011;8(2):514–527.
41. Hill GL. Jonathan E. Rhoads Lecture. Body composition research: implications for the practice of clinical nutrition. *J Parenter Enteral Nutr.* 1992;16(3):197–218.
42. Hill GL. Implications of critical illness, injury, and sepsis on lean body mass and nutritional needs. *Nutrition.* 1998;14(6):557–558.
43. Plank LD, Hill GL. Sequential metabolic changes following induction of systemic inflammatory response in patients with severe sepsis or major blunt trauma. *World J Surg.* 2000;24(6):630–638.
44. Cresci G. Patient history. In: Charney P, Malone A, eds. *ADA Pocket Guide to Nutrition Assessment.* Chicago, IL: American Dietetic Association; 2004:23–40.

45. Winkler M. Nutrition assessment and monitoring. In: Cresci G, ed. *Nutrition Support for the Critically Ill Patient: A Guide to Practice.* Boca Raton, FL: CRC Press; 2005:71–81.
46. Cresci G. Nutrition assessment and monitoring. In: Shikora S, Martindale R, Schwaitzberg S, eds. *Nutritional Considerations in the Intensive Care Unit.* Dubuque, IA: Kendall/Hunt Publishing; 2002:21–30.
47. Martindale RG, McClave SA, Vanek VW, et al. Guidelines for the provision and assessment of nutrition support therapy in the adult critically ill patient: Society of Critical Care Medicine and American Society for Parenteral and Enteral Nutrition: Executive Summary. *Crit Care Med.* 2009;37(5):1757–1761.
48. Ritchie RF, Palomaki GE, Neveux LM, Navolotskaia O, Ledue TB, Craig WY. Reference distributions for the negative acute-phase serum proteins, albumin, transferrin and transthyretin: a practical, simple and clinically relevant approach in a large cohort. *J Clin Lab Anal.* 1999;13(6):273–279.
49. Brown RO, Hunt H, Mowatt-Larssen CA, Wojtysiak SL, Henningfield MF, Kudsk KA. Comparison of specialized and standard enteral formulas in trauma patients. *Pharmacotherapy.* 1994;14(3):314–320.
50. Kudsk KA, Minard G, Croce MA, et al. A randomized trial of isonitrogenous enteral diets after severe trauma. An immune-enhancing diet reduces septic complications. *Ann Surg.* 1996;224(4):531–540.
51. Weimann A, Bastian L, Bischoff WE, et al. Influence of arginine, omega-3 fatty acids and nucleotide-supplemented enteral support on systemic inflammatory response syndrome and multiple organ failure in patients after severe trauma. *Nutrition.* 1998;14(2):165–172.
52. McClave SA, Martindale RG, Vanek VW, et al. Guidelines for the Provision and Assessment of Nutrition Support Therapy in the Adult Critically Ill Patient: Society of Critical Care Medicine (SCCM) and American Society for Parenteral and Enteral Nutrition (A.S.P.E.N.). *J Parenter Enteral Nutr.* 2009;33(3):277–316.
53. Cheatham ML, Safcsak K, Brzezinski SJ, Lube MW. Nitrogen balance, protein loss, and the open abdomen. *Crit Care Med.* 2007;35(1):127–131.
54. Flancbaum L, Choban PS, Sambucco S, Verducci J, Burge JC. Comparison of indirect calorimetry, the Fick method, and prediction equations in estimating the energy requirements of critically ill patients. *Am J Clin Nutr.* 1999;69(3):461–466.
55. Fontaine E, Muller MJ. Adaptive alterations in metabolism: practical consequences on energy requirements in the severely ill patient. *Curr Opin Clin Nutr Metab Care.* 2011;14(2):171–175.
56. Drover JW, Cahill NE, Kutsogiannis J, et al. Nutrition therapy for the critically ill surgical patient: we need to do better! *J Parenter Enteral Nutr.* 2010;34(6):644–652.
57. Weir JB. New methods for calculating metabolic rate with special reference to protein metabolism. *J Physiol.* 1949;109(1-2):1–9.
58. Witte MK. Metabolic measurements during mechanical ventilation in the pediatric intensive care unit. *Respir Care Clin N Am.* 1996;2(4):573–586.
59. Lichtenberg K, Guay-Berry P, Pipitone A, Bondy A, Rotello L. Compensatory increased enteral feeding goal rates: a way to achieve optimal nutrition. *Nutr Clin Pract.* 2010;25(6):653–657.
60. Metheny N. Turning tube feeding off while repositioning patients in bed. *Crit Care Nurse.* 2011;31(2):96–97.
61. Pousman RM, Pepper C, Pandharipande P, et al. Feasibility of implementing a reduced fasting protocol for critically ill trauma patients undergoing operative and nonoperative procedures. *J Parenter Enteral Nutr.* 2009;33(2):176–180.
62. Seder CW, Stockdale W, Hale L, Janczyk RJ. Nasal bridling decreases feeding tube dislodgment and may increase caloric intake in the surgical intensive care unit: a randomized, controlled trial. *Crit Care Med.* 2010;38(3):797–801.
63. Heyland DK, Cahill NE, Dhaliwal R, et al. Enhanced protein-energy provision via the enteral route in critically ill patients: a single center feasibility trial of the PEP uP protocol. *Crit Care.* 2010;14(2):R78.
64. Bankhead R, Boullata J, Brantley S, et al. Enteral nutrition practice recommendations. *J Parenter Enteral Nutr.* 2009;33(2):122–167.
65. Kan MN, Chang HH, Sheu WF, Cheng CH, Lee BJ, Huang YC. Estimation of energy requirements for mechanically ventilated, critically ill patients using nutritional status. *Crit Care.* 2003;7(5):R108–R115.
66. McClave SA, Lowen CC, Kleber MJ, et al. Are patients fed appropriately according to their caloric requirements? *J Parenter Enteral Nutr.* 1998;22(6):375–381.
67. ASPEN Board of Directors and Clinical Guidelines Task Force. Guidelines for the use of parenteral and enteral nutrition in adult and pediatric patients. *J Parenter Enteral Nutr.* 2002;26(1 Suppl):1SA–138SA.
68. Cerra FB, Siegel JH, Coleman B, Border JR, McMenamy RR. Septic autocannibalism. A failure of exogenous nutritional support. *Ann Surg.* 1980;192(4):570–580.
69. Shaw JH, Wildbore M, Wolfe RR. Whole body protein kinetics in severely septic patients. The response to glucose infusion and total parenteral nutrition. *Ann Surg.* 1987;205(3):288–294.
70. Alexander JW, MacMillan BG, Stinnett JD, et al. Beneficial effects of aggressive protein feeding in severely burned children. *Ann Surg.* 1980;192(4):505–517.
71. Jacobs DG, Jacobs DO, Kudsk KA, et al. Practice management guidelines for nutritional support of the trauma patient. *J Trauma.* 2004;57(3):660–678.
72. Cerra FB. Hypermetabolism, organ failure, and metabolic support. *Surgery.* 1987;101(1):1–14.
73. Scheinkestel CD, Kar L, Marshall K, et al. Prospective randomized trial to assess caloric and protein needs of critically Ill, anuric, ventilated patients requiring continuous renal replacement therapy. *Nutrition.* 2003;19(11-12):909–916.
74. Wolfe RR, Allsop JR, Burke JF. Glucose metabolism in man: responses to intravenous glucose infusion. *Metabolism.* 1979;28(3):210–220.
75. Collier B, Diaz J Jr, Forbes R, et al. The impact of a normoglycemic management protocol on clinical outcomes in the trauma intensive care unit. *J Parenter Enteral Nutr.* 2005;29(5):353–358.
76. Laird AM, Miller PR, Kilgo PD, Meredith JW, Chang MC. Relationship of early hyperglycemia to mortality in trauma patients. *J Trauma.* 2004;56(5):1058–1062.
77. Yendamuri S, Fulda GJ, Tinkoff GH. Admission hyperglycemia as a prognostic indicator in trauma. *J Trauma.* 2003;55(1):33–38.
78. Hansen TK, Thiel S, Wouters PJ, Christiansen JS, Van den Berghe G. Intensive insulin therapy exerts antiinflammatory effects in critically ill patients and counteracts the adverse effect of low mannose-binding lectin levels. *J Clin Endocrinol Metab.* 2003;88(3):1082–1088.
79. Van den Berghe G, Wouters P, Weekers F, et al. Intensive insulin therapy in the critically ill patient. *N Engl J Med.* 2001;345(19):1359–1367.
80. Finfer S, Chittock DR, Su SY, et al. Intensive versus conventional glucose control in critically ill patients. *N Engl J Med.* 2009;360(13):1283–1297.

81. Griesdale DE, de Souza RJ, van Dam RM, et al. Intensive insulin therapy and mortality among critically ill patients: a meta-analysis including NICE-SUGAR study data. *CMAJ*. 2009;180(8): 821–827.
82. Brunkhorst FM, Engel C, Bloos F, et al. Intensive insulin therapy and pentastarch resuscitation in severe sepsis. *N Engl J Med*. 2008;358(2):125–139.
83. Egi M, Finfer S, Bellomo R. Glycemic control in the ICU. *Chest*. 2011;140(1):212–220.
84. Dellinger RP, Levy MM, Carlet JM, et al. Surviving Sepsis Campaign: international guidelines for management of severe sepsis and septic shock: 2008. *Crit Care Med*. 2008;36(1):296–327.
85. Carpentier YA, Scruel O. Changes in the concentration and composition of plasma lipoproteins during the acute phase response. *Curr Opin Clin Nutr Metab Care*. 2002;5(2):153–158.
86. Gottschlich MM, Alexander JW. Fat kinetics and recommended dietary intake in burns. *J Parenter Enteral Nutr*. 1987;11(1): 80–85.
87. Nordenstrom J, Carpentier YA, Askanazi J, et al. Free fatty acid mobilization and oxidation during total parenteral nutrition in trauma and infection. *Ann Surg*. 1983;198(6):725–735.
88. Shaw JH, Wolfe RR. An integrated analysis of glucose, fat, and protein metabolism in severely traumatized patients. Studies in the basal state and the response to total parenteral nutrition. *Ann Surg*. 1989;209(1):63–72.
89. Marik PE, Zaloga GP. Gastric versus post-pyloric feeding: a systematic review. *Crit Care*. 2003;7(3):R46–R51.
90. Warden GD. Burn shock resuscitation. *World J Surg*. 1992;16(1): 16–23.
91. Goode HF, Webster NR. Free radicals and antioxidants in sepsis. *Crit Care Med*. 1993;21(11):1770–1776.
92. Crimi E, Liguori A, Condorelli M, et al. The beneficial effects of antioxidant supplementation in enteral feeding in critically ill patients: a prospective, randomized, double-blind, placebo-controlled trial. *Anesth Analg*. 2004;99(3):857–863, table.
93. Goode HF, Cowley HC, Walker BE, Howdle PD, Webster NR. Decreased antioxidant status and increased lipid peroxidation in patients with septic shock and secondary organ dysfunction. *Crit Care Med*. 1995;23(4):646–651.
94. Lemoyne M, Van GA, Kurian R, Jeejeebhoy KN. Plasma vitamin E and selenium and breath pentane in home parenteral nutrition patients. *Am J Clin Nutr*. 1988;48(5):1310–1315.
95. Louw JA, Werbeck A, Louw ME, Kotze TJ, Cooper R, Labadarios D. Blood vitamin concentrations during the acute-phase response. *Crit Care Med*. 1992;20(7):934–941.
96. Schorah CJ, Downing C, Piripitsi A, et al. Total vitamin C, ascorbic acid, and dehydroascorbic acid concentrations in plasma of critically ill patients. *Am J Clin Nutr*. 1996;63(5):760–765.
97. Nathens AB, Neff MJ, Jurkovich GJ, et al. Randomized, prospective trial of antioxidant supplementation in critically ill surgical patients. *Ann Surg*. 2002;236(6):814–822.
98. Prelack K, Sheridan RL. Micronutrient supplementation in the critically ill patient: strategies for clinical practice. *J Trauma*. 2001;51(3):601–620.
99. Gottschlich MM, Warden GD. Vitamin supplementation in the patient with burns. *J Burn Care Rehabil*. 1990;11(3):275–279.
100. Gottschlich MM, Mayes T, Khoury J, Warden GD. Hypovitaminosis D in acutely injured pediatric burn patients. *J Am Diet Assoc*. 2004;104(6):931–941, quiz.
101. Klein GL, Langman CB, Herndon DN. Vitamin D depletion following burn injury in children: a possible factor in post-burn osteopenia. *J Trauma*. 2002;52(2):346–350.
102. Lee P, Nair P, Eisman JA, Center JR. Vitamin D deficiency in the intensive care unit: an invisible accomplice to morbidity and mortality? *Intensive Care Med*. 2009;35(12):2028–2032.
103. Lucidarme O, Messai E, Mazzoni T, Arcade M, du CD. Incidence and risk factors of vitamin D deficiency in critically ill patients: results from a prospective observational study. *Intensive Care Med*. 2010;36(9):1609–1611.
104. Melamed ML, Michos ED, Post W, Astor B. 25-hydroxyvitamin D levels and the risk of mortality in the general population. *Arch Intern Med*. 2008;168(15):1629–1637.
105. Ukleja A, Freeman KL, Gilbert K, et al. Standards for nutrition support: adult hospitalized patients. *Nutr Clin Pract*. 2010;25(4): 403–414.
106. Heyland DK, MacDonald S, Keefe L, Drover JW. Total parenteral nutrition in the critically ill patient: a meta-analysis. *JAMA*. 1998;280(23):2013–2019.
107. Koretz RL, Lipman TO, Klein S. AGA technical review on parenteral nutrition. *Gastroenterology*. 2001;121(4):970–1001.
108. Casaer MP, Mesotten D, Hermans G, et al. Early versus late parenteral nutrition in critically ill adults. *N Engl J Med*. 2011; 365(6):506–517.
109. Sena MJ, Utter GH, Cuschieri J, et al. Early supplemental parenteral nutrition is associated with increased infectious complications in critically ill trauma patients. *J Am Coll Surg*. 2008;207(4): 459–467.
110. Shirley PJ, Bion JF. Intra-hospital transport of critically ill patients: minimising risk. *Intensive Care Med*. 2004;30(8): 1508–1510.
111. Heyland DK, Tougas G, Cook DJ, Guyatt GH. Cisapride improves gastric emptying in mechanically ventilated, critically ill patients. A randomized, double-blind trial. *Am J Respir Crit Care Med*. 1996;154(6 Pt 1):1678–1683.
112. Jooste CA, Mustoe J, Collee G. Metoclopramide improves gastric motility in critically ill patients. *Intensive Care Med*. 1999;25(5): 464–468.
113. Mentec H, Dupont H, Bocchetti M, Cani P, Ponche F, Bleichner G. Upper digestive intolerance during enteral nutrition in critically ill patients: frequency, risk factors, and complications. *Crit Care Med*. 2001;29(10):1955–1961.
114. Montejo JC. Enteral nutrition-related gastrointestinal complications in critically ill patients: a multicenter study. The Nutritional and Metabolic Working Group of the Spanish Society of Intensive Care Medicine and Coronary Units. *Crit Care Med*. 1999; 27(8):1447–1453.
115. Mutlu GM, Mutlu EA, Factor P. GI complications in patients receiving mechanical ventilation. *Chest*. 2001;119(4):1222–1241.
116. Neumann DA, DeLegge MH. Gastric versus small-bowel tube feeding in the intensive care unit: a prospective comparison of efficacy. *Crit Care Med*. 2002;30(7):1436–1438.
117. McClave SA, Lukan JK, Stefater JA, et al. Poor validity of residual volumes as a marker for risk of aspiration in critically ill patients. *Crit Care Med*. 2005;33(2):324–330.
118. Heyland DK, Drover JW, Dhaliwal R, Greenwood J. Optimizing the benefits and minimizing the risks of enteral nutrition in the critically ill: role of small bowel feeding. *J Parenter Enteral Nutr*. 2002;26(6 Suppl):S51–S55.
119. Koopmann MC, Kudsk KA, Szotkowski MJ, Rees SM. A team-based protocol and electromagnetic technology eliminate feeding tube placement complications. *Ann Surg*. 2011;253(2):287–302.
120. Cresci G, Martindale R. Bedside placement of small bowel feeding tubes in hospitalized patients: a new role for the dietitian. *Nutrition*. 2003;19(10):843–846.

121. Zaloga GP. Bedside method for placing small bowel feeding tubes in critically ill patients. A prospective study. *Chest*. 1991; 100(6):1643–1646.
122. Stapleton RD, Martin JM, Mayer K. Fish oil in critical illness: mechanisms and clinical applications. *Crit Care Clin*. 2010;26(3): 501–514, ix.
123. Weitzel LR, Wischmeyer PE. Glutamine in critical illness: the time has come, the time is now. *Crit Care Clin*. 2010;26(3):515–551, x.
124. Zhu X, Herrera G, Ochoa JB. Immunosupression and infection after major surgery: a nutritional deficiency. *Crit Care Clin*. 2010;26(3):491–500, ix.
125. Wischmeyer P. Nutritional pharmacology in surgery and critical care: "you must unlearn what you have learned." *Curr Opin Anaesthesiol*. 2011;24(4):381–388.
126. de Aguilar-Nascimento JE. The role of macronutrients in gastrointestinal blood flow. *Curr Opin Clin Nutr Metab Care*. 2005; 8(5):552–556.
127. Saito H, Furukawa S, Matsuda T. Glutamine as an immunoenhancing nutrient. *J Parenter Enteral Nutr*. 1999;23(5 Suppl): S59–S61.
128. Kelly D, Wischmeyer PE. Role of L-glutamine in critical illness: new insights. *Curr Opin Clin Nutr Metab Care*. 2003;6(2):217–222.
129. Bongers T, Griffiths RD, McArdle A. Exogenous glutamine: the clinical evidence. *Crit Care Med*. 2007;35(9 Suppl):S545–S552.
130. Melis GC, ter Wengel N, Boelens PG, van Leeuwen PA. Glutamine: recent developments in research on the clinical significance of glutamine. *Curr Opin Clin Nutr Metab Care*. 2004;7(1):59–70.
131. Wischmeyer PE. Glutamine: mode of action in critical illness. *Crit Care Med*. 2007;35(9 Suppl):S541–S544.
132. De-Souza DA, Greene LJ. Intestinal permeability and systemic infections in critically ill patients: effect of glutamine. *Crit Care Med*. 2005;33(5):1125–1135.
133. Alpers DH. Glutamine: do the data support the cause for glutamine supplementation in humans? *Gastroenterology*. 2006;130(2 Suppl 1):S106–S116.
134. Rice TW, Wheeler AP, Thompson BT, deBoisblanc BP, Steingrub J, Rock P. Enteral omega-3 fatty acid, gamma-linolenic acid, and antioxidant supplementation in acute lung injury. *JAMA*. 2011; 306(14):1574–1581.
135. Fukushima R, Yamazaki E. Vitamin C requirement in surgical patients. *Curr Opin Clin Nutr Metab Care*. 2010;13(6):669–676.
136. Kahn SA, Beers RJ, Lentz CW. Resuscitation after severe burn injury using high-dose ascorbic acid: a retrospective review. *J Burn Care Res*. 2011;32(1):110–117.
137. Kremer T, Harenberg P, Hernekamp F, et al. High-dose vitamin C treatment reduces capillary leakage after burn plasma transfer in rats. *J Burn Care Res*. 2010;31(3):470–479.
138. Heyland DK, Dhaliwal R, Drover JW, Gramlich L, Dodek P. Canadian clinical practice guidelines for nutrition support in mechanically ventilated, critically ill adult patients. *J Parenter Enteral Nutr*. 2003;27(5):355–373.
139. Gadek JE, DeMichele SJ, Karlstad MD, et al. Effect of enteral feeding with eicosapentaenoic acid, gamma-linolenic acid, and antioxidants in patients with acute respiratory distress syndrome. Enteral Nutrition in ARDS Study Group. *Crit Care Med*. 1999; 27(8):1409–1420.
140. Gottschlich MM, Jenkins M, Warden GD, et al. Differential effects of three enteral dietary regimens on selected outcome variables in burn patients. *J Parenter Enteral Nutr*. 1990;14(3): 225–236.
141. Nelson JL, DeMichele SJ, Pacht ER, Wennberg AK. Effect of enteral feeding with eicosapentaenoic acid, gamma-linolenic acid, and antioxidants on antioxidant status in patients with acute respiratory distress syndrome. *J Parenter Enteral Nutr*. 2003;27(2):98–104.
142. Pacht ER, DeMichele SJ, Nelson JL, Hart J, Wennberg AK, Gadek JE. Enteral nutrition with eicosapentaenoic acid, gamma-linolenic acid, and antioxidants reduces alveolar inflammatory mediators and protein influx in patients with acute respiratory distress syndrome. *Crit Care Med*. 2003;31(2):491–500.
143. Howard L, Ashley C. Nutrition in the perioperative patient. *Annu Rev Nutr*. 2003;23:263–282.
144. Studley HO. Percentage of weight loss: a basic indicator of surgical risk in patients with chronic peptic ulcer. *Nutr Hosp*. 2001; 16(4):141–143.
145. Perioperative total parenteral nutrition in surgical patients. The Veterans Affairs Total Parenteral Nutrition Cooperative Study Group. *N Engl J Med*. 1991;325(8):525–532.
146. Abou-Assi S, Craig K, O'Keefe SJ. Hypocaloric jejunal feeding is better than total parenteral nutrition in acute pancreatitis: results of a randomized comparative study. *Am J Gastroenterol*. 2002; 97(9):2255–2262.
147. McClave SA. Nutrition support in acute pancreatitis. *Gastroenterol Clin North Am*. 2007;36(1):65–74, vi.
148. O'Keefe SJ, Broderick T, Turner M, Stevens S, O'Keefe JS. Nutrition in the management of necrotizing pancreatitis. *Clin Gastroenterol Hepatol*. 2003;1(4):315–321.
149. Olah A, Pardavi G, Belagyi T, Nagy A, Issekutz A, Mohamed GE. Early nasojejunal feeding in acute pancreatitis is associated with a lower complication rate. *Nutrition*. 2002;18(3):259–262.
150. Shukla HS, Rao RR, Banu N, Gupta RM, Yadav RC. Enteral hyperalimentation in malnourished surgical patients. *Indian J Med Res*. 1984;80:339–346.
151. von Meyenfeldt MF, Meijerink WJ, Rouflart MM, Builmaassen MT, Soeters PB. Perioperative nutritional support: a randomised clinical trial. *Clin Nutr*. 1992;11(4):180–186.
152. Heyland DK, Montalvo M, MacDonald S, Keefe L, Su XY, Drover JW. Total parenteral nutrition in the surgical patient: a meta-analysis. *Can J Surg*. 2001;44(2):102–111.
153. Fearon KC, Ljungqvist O, Von MM, et al. Enhanced recovery after surgery: a consensus review of clinical care for patients undergoing colonic resection. *Clin Nutr*. 2005;24(3):466–477.
154. Sato H, Carvalho G, Sato T, Lattermann R, Matsukawa T, Schricker T. The association of preoperative glycemic control, intraoperative insulin sensitivity, and outcomes after cardiac surgery. *J Clin Endocrinol Metab*. 2010;95(9):4338–4344.
155. Varadhan KK, Lobo DN, Ljungqvist O. Enhanced recovery after surgery: the future of improving surgical care. *Crit Care Clin*. 2010;26(3):527–547, x.
156. Varadhan KK, Neal KR, Dejong CH, Fearon KC, Ljungqvist O, Lobo DN. The enhanced recovery after surgery (ERAS) pathway for patients undergoing major elective open colorectal surgery: a meta-analysis of randomized controlled trials. *Clin Nutr*. 2010; 29(4):434–440.
157. Brandstrup B, Tonnesen H, Beier-Holgersen R, et al. Effects of intravenous fluid restriction on postoperative complications: comparison of two perioperative fluid regimens: a randomized assessor-blinded multicenter trial. *Ann Surg*. 2003;238(5):641–648.
158. Gustafsson UO, Hausel J, Thorell A, Ljungqvist O, Soop M, Nygren J. Adherence to the enhanced recovery after surgery protocol and outcomes after colorectal cancer surgery. *Arch Surg*. 2011;146(5):571–577.
159. Lobo DN, Bostock KA, Neal KR, Perkins AC, Rowlands BJ, Allison SP. Effect of salt and water balance on recovery of gastrointestinal function after elective colonic resection: a randomised controlled trial. *Lancet*. 2002;359(9320):1812–1818.

160. Kreymann KG, Berger MM, Deutz NE, et al. ESPEN Guidelines on Enteral Nutrition: Intensive care. *Clin Nutr*. 2006;25(2):210–223.
161. Kurmis R, Parker A, Greenwood J. The use of immunonutrition in burn injury care: where are we? *J Burn Care Res*. 2010;31(5): 677–691.
162. Harris JA, Benedict FG. A biometric study of human basal metabolism. *Proc Natl Acad Sci U S A*. 1918;4(12):370–373.
163. Cerra FB, Benitez MR, Blackburn GL, et al. Applied nutrition in ICU patients. A consensus statement of the American College of Chest Physicians. *Chest*. 1997;111(3):769–778.
164. Brandi LS, Bertolini R, Calafà M. Indirect calorimetry in critically ill patients: clinical applications and practical advice. *Nutrition*. 1997;13(4):349–358.
165. Cole TJ, Henry CJ. The Oxford Brookes basal metabolic *rate database—a reanalysis. *Public Health Nutr*. 2005;8:1202–1212.
166. Curreri PW, Richmond D, Marvin J, Baxter CR. Dietary requirements of patients with major burns. *J Am Diet Assoc*. 1974;65(4): 415–417.
167. Davies JWL, Liljedahl SL. Metabolic consequences of an extensive burn. In: Polk, Stone, eds. *Contemporary Burn Management*. Boston: Little, Brown & Company; 1971:151–169.
168. Fusco MA, Mills ME, Nelson LD. Predicting caloric requirements with emphasis on avoiding overfeeding. *J Parenter Enteral Nutr*. 1995;19(suppl):18S (abstr).
169. Ireton-Jones CS, Turner WW Jr, Liepa GU, Baxter CR. Equations for the estimation of energy expenditures in patients with burns with special reference to ventilatory status. *J Burn Care Rehabil*. 1992;13(3):330–333.
170. Ireton-Jones C, Jones JD. Improved equations for predicting energy expenditure in patients: the Ireton-Jones equations. *Nutr Clin Pract*. 2002;17(1):29–31.
171. Kleiber M. *The Fire of Life: A Introduction to Animal Energetics*. Huntington, NY: Robert E. Krieger Publishing Co.; 1975.
172. Liu HY, Lu YF, Chen WJ. Predictive equations for basal metabolic rate in Chinese adults: a cross-validation study. *J Am Diet Assoc*. 1995;95:1403–1408.
173. Long CL, Schaffel N, Geiger JW, Schiller WR, Blakemore WS. Metabolic response to injury and illness: estimation of energy and protein needs from indirect calorimetry and nitrogen balance. *J Parenter Enteral Nutr*. 1979;3(6):452–456.
174. Mifflin MD, St Jeor ST, Hill LA, Scott BJ, Daugherty SA, Koh YO. A new predictive equation for resting energy expenditure in healthy individuals. *Am J Clin Nutr*. 1990;51(2):241–247.
175. Frankenfield DC, Muth ER, Rowe WA. The Harris-Benedict studies of human basal metabolism: history and limitations. *J Am Diet Assoc*.1998;98(4):439–445.
176. Frankenfield DC, Rowe WA, Smith JS, Cooney RN. Validation of several established equations for resting metabolic rate in obese and nonobese people. *J Am Diet Assoc*. 2003;103(9): 1152–1159.
177. Frankenfield DC, Rowe WA, Smith JS, Cooney RN. Validation of several established equations for resting metabolic rate in obese and nonobese people. *J Am Diet Assoc*. 2003;103(9): 1152–1159.
178. Roza AM, Shizgal HM. The Harris Benedict equation re-evaluated: resting energy requirements and the body cell mass. *Am J Clin Nutr*. 1984;40(1):168–182.
179. Faisy C, Guerot E, Diehl JL, Labrousse J, Fagon JY. Assessment of resting energy expenditure in mechanically ventilated patients. *Am J Clin Nutr*. 2003;78(2):241–249.
180. Schofield WN. Predicting basal metabolic rate, new standards and review of previous work. *Hum Nutr Clin Nutr*. 1985; 39(Suppl 1):5–41.
181. Swinamer DL, Grace MG, Hamilton SM, Jones RL, Roberts P, King EG. Predictive equation for assessing energy expenditure in mechanically ventilated critically ill patients. *Crit Care Med*. 1990;18(6):657–661.
182. Food and Agriculture Organization/Whole Health Organization/United Nations University. Energy and protein requirements: report of a joint FAO/WHO/UNU expert consultation. *World Health Organization Technical Report Series*. 1985;724: 1–206.

25 Pulmonary Failure

Krista L. Turner, MD, FACS

CONTENTS

Introduction 413
Pulmonary Function 413
Structure and Physiology 413
Ventilator Modes 413
Types of Pulmonary Failure 414
Acute Pulmonary Failure 414
Acute Lung Injury/Acute Respiratory Distress Syndrome 414
Prolonged Mechanical Ventilation 414
Chronic Critical Illness 415
Nutrition Consideration per Type of Failure 415
Medication Consideration 417
Nutrition Assessment 417
History and Physical Exam 417
Predictive Equations and Indirect Calorimetry 417
Underfeeding 418
Overfeeding 418
Obesity 419
Nutrition Support 419
Macronutrients 419
Micronutrients 419
Enteral Nutrition 419
Aspiration and Ventilator-Associated Pneumonia 420
Ventilator-Associated Pneumonia Prevention Strategies 420
Parenteral Nutrition 422
Immunonutrition 422
Omega-3 Fatty Acids 422
Summary 424
References 424

Objectives

1. Compare and contrast nutrition strategies for acute versus chronic pulmonary failure with regard to estimation of caloric needs, selection of mode of nutrition support therapy, and utilization of immunonutrition.
2. Understand how overfeeding hinders ventilator weaning for patients with pulmonary failure.
3. Apply enteral nutrition (EN) strategies which limit potential for aspiration.
4. Appraise emerging data regarding lipid provision and immunonutrition for acute lung injury (ALI) or acute respiratory distress syndrome (ARDS).

Test Your Knowledge Questions

1. The strategy of permissive hypercapnia is applicable to which disease process?
   A. Brain injury
   B. ARDS
   C. Pulmonary embolism
   D. Acute renal failure
2. Which of the following in excess contributes the most to carbon dioxide (CO_2) production?
   A. Carbohydrate
   B. Fat
   C. Protein
   D. Calories
3. All of the following are components of the ventilator-associated pneumonia (VAP) bundle except:
   A. Early parenteral nutrition (PN)
   B. Elevating the head of the bed to 45 degrees
   C. Decreasing oral flora
   D. Gastric ulcer prophylaxis

Test Your Knowledge Answers

1. The correct answer is **B**. Permissive hypercapnia refers to the strategy of limiting further lung barotrauma by decreasing tidal volumes and allowing the serum CO_2 levels to rise. This practice is most important to patients with ARDS, in which barotrauma exacerbates inflammation at the level of the alveoli. In this setting, excessive production of CO_2 by overfeeding may limit this strategy, making liberation from the ventilator more difficult. Permissive hypercapnia is not utilized in patients with brain injury as high CO_2 levels can increase brain swelling. For patients with renal failure, permissive hypercapnia worsens their existing acidosis. The primary problem in pulmonary embolism is oxygenation, so this strategy is not indicated.
2. The correct answer is **D**. Total excess calories, not particular substrates, are responsible for increased production of CO_2. Overfeeding calories can be detrimental to patients with pulmonary failure as the work of breathing is increased in an effort to remove excess CO_2 from the body. Indirect calorimetry may be helpful to estimate caloric needs.
3. The correct answer is **A**. VAP is a morbid but preventable complication of EN. Strategies to minimize the risk of VAP are designed to limit aspiration of stomach and oral contents into the airway. Components of VAP "bundles" include elevating the head of the bed 45 degrees, reducing oral flora with chlorhexidine wash, subglottic drainage of secretions, and reducing the risk of upper gastrointestinal ulceration and bleeding with acid-reducing agents. Despite concerns for aspiration, EN is essential to patients with pulmonary failure, and PN should not be used in an effort to prevent VAP.

Introduction

The implementation of nutrition support therapy in the critically ill population has received much attention as a therapeutic modality. As one of the defining parameters of critical illness, pulmonary failure requires special attention for multiple reasons. The profound catabolism that accompanies pulmonary failure and critical illness must be considered, the provision of calories should be tailored with attention to prevent overfeeding, and the safe delivery of nutrition support must be carefully monitored. Malnutrition is a risk factor for the onset of pulmonary failure, and once established, pulmonary failure can further worsen nutrition status. Administration of nutrition can affect pulmonary function in several ways: via muscle function, CO_2 production, and immune modulation. Fluid balance, micronutrient needs, electrolyte homeostasis, and acid-base balance affect pulmonary function and must also be considered in the nutrition plan. While pulmonary-specific formulas and adjuncts are increasingly available, successful support and recovery from pulmonary failure relies on accurately estimating changing caloric requirements, determining micronutrient deficiencies, early EN, and reassessing for tolerance.

Pulmonary Function

Structure and Physiology

The pulmonary system is responsible for the oxygenation of blood and removal of the metabolic byproduct CO_2. Essential components of this system include respiratory drive, airway patency, lung expansion, gas exchange at the alveoli, and pulmonary blood flow.

Primary muscles of respiration are the diaphragm and intercostal muscles. Accessory muscles include the sternocleidomastoid and scalene muscles, the use of which may indicate increased work of breathing. Movement of air into the lungs depends on adequate strength of these muscles, in addition to the unobstructed flow of air into the pharynx, trachea, bronchi, and smaller airways. Gas exchange then takes place functionally at the level of the alveoli in the lungs, as illustrated in Figure 25-1. Provided the unobstructed flow of blood through the pulmonary circulation, oxygenated blood may then circulate systemically in the body to provide fuel for aerobic metabolism. Carbon dioxide will likewise diffuse from the blood into the airways for elimination. Exhalation depends on the elastic recoil of the lungs and the ribcage, as well as patency of the upper airway.

Ventilator Modes

The failure of any of these components of the pulmonary function may require supplemental support. Patients with low oxygen levels due to pneumonia, edema, inflammation, or mild chronic pulmonary disease may only require supplemental oxygen in the form of a nasal cannula or mask. Patients with impairment of CO_2 exhalation (ventilation) may require positive pressure ventilation in the form of an airtight mask. Transient forms of CO_2 retention can occur at night in patients with obstructive sleep apnea or in patients with mild muscular weakness during acute illness. These patients can often be treated with noninvasive ventilation in which a machine provides a constant positive pressure and supplemental oxygen, while the patient initiates the breath.

FIGURE 25-1 Lung Alveoli and Gas Exchange

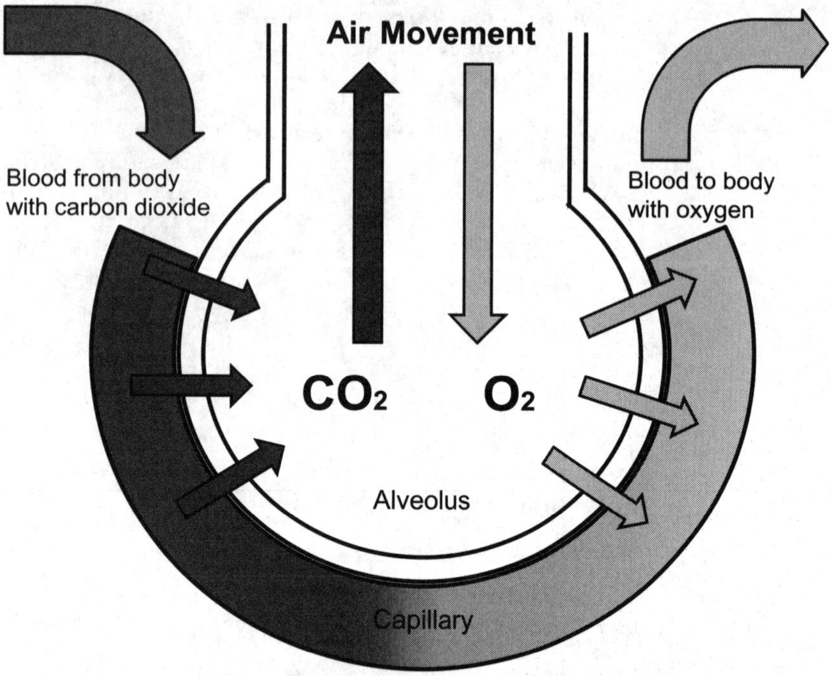

Lungs are comprised of numerous air sacs called alveoli. These sacs are surrounded by pulmonary capillaries. Blood flows into the pulmonary circulation that is high in CO_2 and low in oxygen. Inspired oxygen diffuses across the alveolar and capillary membranes to bind with red blood cells in the capillary (eg, oxygenation). CO_2 diffuses from the capillary into the alveolus where it is expired via the airway (eg, ventilation).

For patients with more severe forms of hypoxemia or hypercapnia, more invasive modes of ventilator support are required. This constitutes the placement of an endotracheal tube into the airway and complete pulmonary support via mechanical ventilation. Various modes of ventilation may be employed by setting desired combinations of respiratory rate, tidal volume, positive inspiratory pressure, positive end expiratory pressure, inspiratory time, expiratory time, and fraction of inspired oxygen (Table 25-1 for definitions of commonly used terms). These variables are manipulated based on the primary problem (hypoxemia vs. hypercapnia), lung compliance, and patient-ventilator synchrony. Various modes of ventilation are listed in Table 25-2. Further discussion of mechanical ventilation is beyond the scope of this chapter, and the reader is directed to further references as desired.

Types of Pulmonary Failure

Pulmonary failure requiring supplemental oxygen or mechanical ventilator support occurs when any of the previously mentioned components falters, as outlined in Table 25-3. Failure may occur for a variety of reasons and with varying severity and anticipated duration. The underlying cause and expected duration of pulmonary failure will often determine the details of the nutrition regimen. As it applies to nutrition support therapy, pulmonary failure will be described here in the categories of acute (short-term) versus chronic failure.

Acute Pulmonary Failure

Acute pulmonary failure is often a manifestation of a systemic disease process. Neurologic injury, altered mental status, or airway obstruction are conditions that often necessitate airway protection provided by endotracheal intubation. While the lungs themselves are not the source of pathology in these patients, consideration should be given to the mechanics of providing EN in this situation. These patients will still require provision of EN via tube feeds with attendant aspiration precautions taken. Likewise, the presence of a tube in the airway provides another opportunity for iatrogenic infection, so anergy and infection prevention via adequate nutrition support therapy are paramount.

Acute Lung Injury/Acute Respiratory Distress Syndrome

Acute pulmonary failure may also manifest from inflammatory conditions, the most important of which is ALI or ARDS. This is defined as the acute onset of diffuse bilateral pulmonary infiltrates by chest radiograph, as seen in Figure 25-2; a partial pressure of oxygen in blood/fraction of inspired oxygen < 300 for ALI and < 200 for ARDS; and a pulmonary artery wedge pressure < 18 mm Hg or no clinical evidence of fluid overload.[1] The partial pressure of oxygen in blood/fraction of inspired oxygen value is a measure of the amount of oxygen in the blood per amount of oxygen delivered to the patient, with a smaller ratio indicating more severe hypoxemia. The normal pulmonary artery wedge pressure value establishes that the infiltrates seen are inflammatory in nature and not the result of pulmonary edema.

The clinical disorders that give rise to ALI/ARDS can be divided into those associated with direct injury to the lung (eg, aspiration, pneumonia, pulmonary contusion, fat emboli, and smoke or toxic gas inhalation) and those that cause indirect lung injury by inciting a systemic inflammatory response (eg, sepsis, traumatic shock, pancreatitis, cardiopulmonary bypass, and blood transfusions). In the acute phase, leakage of edema into the lung and inflammatory cellular infiltrates causes ventilation-perfusion mismatch, which is clinically manifested as hypoxemia. After the acute phase, some patients progress into a fibroproliferative phase, during which chronic inflammation and fibrosis take place, requiring prolonged ventilator support.

Prolonged Mechanical Ventilation

Prolonged mechanical ventilation (PMV) is defined as ventilator dependence for greater than 21 days for at least 6 hours per day.[2] Unlike acute pulmonary failure, chronic pulmonary failure is often secondary to primary pulmonary pathology.

TABLE 25-1 Pulmonary Failure Terminology

Pulmonary Mechanics
Respiratory rate (frequency): The number of breaths delivered per minute. **Tidal volume:** The volume of gas, either inhaled or exhaled, during a breath. **Minute ventilation:** The tidal volume multiplied by the respiratory rate. **Vital capacity:** The volume change of the lung between a full inspiration and a maximal expiration. **Functional residual capacity:** The volume of air present in the lungs at the end of passive expiration. At functional residual capacity, the elastic recoil forces of the lungs and chest wall are equal but opposite, and there is no exertion by the diaphragm or other respiratory muscles.
Mechanical Ventilator
Mechanical ventilator: A machine designed to provide all or part of the work required to move gas into and out of the lungs to satisfy the body's respiratory needs. **End expiratory pressure:** The pressure at the end of the expiratory phase, measured relative to atmospheric pressure. For mechanical ventilation, this is a positive pressure referred to as positive end-expiratory pressure. **Pressure control:** The delivery of a predetermined inspiratory pressure throughout inspiration. Also termed pressure support. **Volume control:** The delivery of a predetermined inspiratory volume despite changing respiratory system mechanics or ventilatory muscle activity. **Assisted breath:** A breath for which all or part of the inspiratory or expiratory flow is generated by the ventilator doing work for the patient. A mandatory breath is assisted. A spontaneous breath may be assisted or unassisted. **Spontaneous breath:** A breath that is patient triggered. **Mandatory breath:** A breath that is ventilator triggered. **Breath sequence:** A particular pattern of mandatory and/or spontaneous breaths (CMV, IMV, or CSV). **CMV:** A breath sequence in which all ventilator-delivered breaths are mandatory and delivered at a set minimum frequency, but in which any inspiratory effort by the patient during the expiratory phase may trigger the next breath. Also termed assist control. **IMV:** A ventilatory pattern in which spontaneous breaths are permitted between mandatory breaths. When the mandatory breath is patient triggered, it is commonly referred to as synchronized intermittent mandatory ventilation. **CSV:** A breath sequence in which all breaths are spontaneous (assisted or unassisted). **Ventilator mode:** A specific combination of control variables and breath sequence. There are five possible ventilatory patterns: VC-CMV, VC-IMV, PC-CMV, PC-IMV, PC-CSV.

CMV, continuous mandatory ventilation; CSV, continuous spontaneous ventilation; IMV, intermittent mandatory ventilation; PC, patient-controlled; VC, ventilator-controlled.

Chronic neuromuscular disease is also a common underlying cause. Neuromuscular diseases compromise the ability to ventilate via progressive respiratory muscle weakness and/or diminished respiratory drive due to central neurologic sequelae. Patients with anticipated PMV often have a tracheostomy performed to increase the level of comfort, provide for better oral care, reduce rates of pneumonia, and decrease dead space ventilation.[3]

Of the primary pulmonary disorders requiring PMV, those of an obstructive nature can be the most difficult to treat. Chronic obstructive pulmonary disease (COPD) is the most common of these disorders. Obstructive or restrictive diseases manifest as a primarily ventilator defect, with hypercapnia the end result. Oxygenation may also be affected due to perfusion defect. Decline in respiratory muscle function cannot compensate for the progressive increase in inspiratory volumes and overdistention that is classic with COPD, leading to worsening ventilator dependence.[2] Prevalence of malnutrition in the COPD population can be as high as 35% in those with the worst form of disease.[4] This correlates directly with increased ventilator requirement and mortality.[5] Severe malnutrition can result in decreased respiratory muscle strength and reduced endurance.

Chronic Critical Illness

Inclusive of PMV, a condition resulting from the sequelae of surviving acute critical illness has recently been described. Labeled as chronic critical illness, this syndrome manifests as constellation of metabolic and immunologic derangements, of which ventilator dependence and malnutrition are central components. Characteristics of the syndrome include profound muscle weakness, neuropathy, anasarca, endocrine dysfunction, hyperglycemia, depression, skin abnormalities, and depressed endocrine axis function.[6] This parallels the concept of compensatory anti-inflammatory response syndrome, in which anergy and increased risk of infection occurs during the nadir after an acute proinflammatory response. While this syndrome may only occur in 5% to 10% of all critically ill patients,[7] the associated morbidity is profound, with only 50% of patients achieving ventilator liberation and only 4% of patients with eventual discharge home.[6]

Nutrition Consideration per Type of Failure

Patients with acute pulmonary failure typically will exhibit catabolism requiring aggressive early nutrition support therapy.

TABLE 25-2 Hierarchy of Mechanical Ventilation

Least Advanced → Most Advanced	Mode	Variables
Non-invasive	**Nasal Cannula, Face Mask**	Oxygen
	CPAP/BiPAP	Oxygen Continuous Pressure
Invasive (ETT or trach)	**PSV**	Oxygen Inspiratory Pressure PEEP
	SIMV	Oxygen Inspiratory Pressure Tidal Volume PEEP Respiratory rate
	CMV/AC	Oxygen Tidal Volume PEEP Respiratory rate
	BiLevel/APRV	Oxygen High and Low Pressure ± Inspiratory and Expiratory Time
	HFOV	Oxygen Mean Airway Pressure Frequency Amplitude

Least Advanced → **Most Advanced**

The various modes of pulmonary support are listed with the basic variables available for manipulation. As the modes of support become more advanced, they require a greater degree of invasiveness (endotracheal intubation), as well as sedation to overcome discomfort and ventilator dyssynchrony. Typically, the more advanced modes of ventilation are reserved for severe lung injury and acute respiratory distress syndrome. Escalation and weaning from the ventilator typically occur in the sequence shown, although this may vary. HFOV is reserved for patients with refractory hypoxemia and is not utilized for hypercapnia. AC, assist control; APRV, airway pressure release ventilation; BiPAP, bilevel positive airway pressure; CMV, controlled mechanical ventilation; CPAP, continuous positive airway pressure; HFOV, high frequency oscillatory ventilation; PEEP, positive end-expiratory pressure; PSV, pressure support ventilation; SIMV, synchronized intermittent mandatory ventilation.

TABLE 25-3 Sources of Pulmonary Failure by Components of Function

Component	Pathologic Process
Respiratory drive	Brain or spinal cord injury, stroke, respiratory depressant medications (narcotics, benzodiazepines)
Airway patency	Craniofacial or neck injury, neck or lung mass, tracheal collapse, upper airway soft tissue (obstructive sleep apnea), reactive airway disease (asthma)
Lung expansion	Neuromuscular diseases, muscle weakness, obesity, chest wall burns or dressings, rib cage injury, restrictive lung disease
Alveolar diffusion	Infection (pneumonia), inflammation (acute lung injury or acute respiratory distress syndrome), pulmonary edema, pulmonary contusion (trauma)
Capillary flow	Pulmonary embolism, vasculitis

FIGURE 25-2 Chest Radiograph of Patient with Acute Respiratory Distress Syndrome

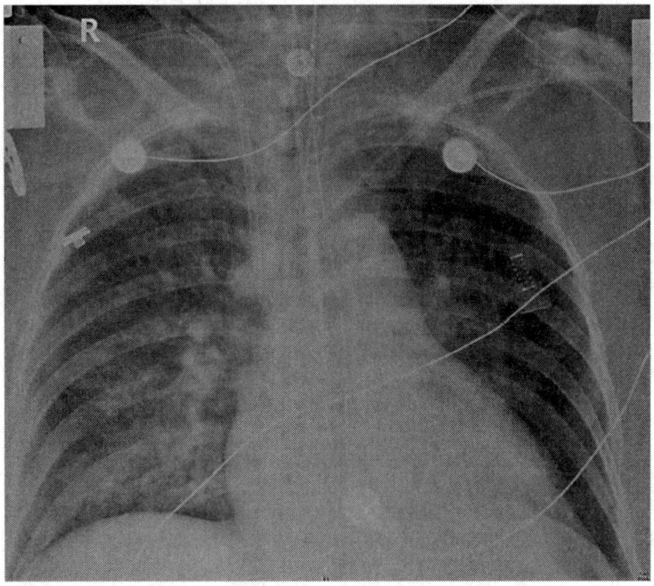

This chest radiograph demonstrates diffuse bilateral infiltrates characteristic of acute lung injury/acute respiratory distress syndrome.

This is often performed in the setting of ongoing resuscitation, whether from surgery, trauma, or sepsis, and should therefore be carefully monitored for signs of intolerance, hyperglycemia, and changing caloric needs. Adjuvant therapy for patients with acute failure should be tailored to the underlying disorder with consideration for associated organ failure. For example, trauma or postsurgical patients may benefit from arginine-based immunonutrition, and patients with renal failure need a reduced amount of volume and electrolyte solutions. Specific recommendations for these populations can be found elsewhere in the text.

Patients with chronic critical illness suffer from metabolic disorders such as insulin resistance with hyperglycemia, hypothyroidism, diminished growth hormone release, vitamin D deficiency, hypophosphatemia, and adrenal insufficiency. The net effect of these disorders results in preferential utilization of protein from muscle, with profound weakness particularly of the respiratory muscles.[7] Careful attention must be paid monitoring for these derangements, as well as frequent reassessment of nutrition status and metabolic demands.

Medication Consideration

Medications used during either acute or chronic pulmonary failure may alter the nutrition plan. Patients with severe ALI/ARDS are often heavily sedated and even paralyzed to assist with ventilator synchrony. While paralytics do not limit gut peristalsis, the ability to assess the patient for abdominal pain is severely limited when they are used. If EN is provided while the patient is paralyzed or heavily sedated, close attention should be paid to other signs of intolerance such as changes in stool, abdominal distention, changes in appearance of the bowel pattern on x-ray, or unexplained acidemia. Use of the sedative propofol should be recognized when calculating total calories provided as it is delivered in a lipid emulsion.

Patients with acute pulmonary failure may also have ongoing shock with necessary catecholamine vasopressor administration. High doses of vasopressors can cause splanchnic vasoconstriction, which could lead to bowel ischemia when EN is delivered. This practice has been challenged, with inconsistent agreement on what dose of vasopressor is prohibitive.[8]

Acute and chronic pulmonary failure patients often receive either inhaled or oral steroids to help control inflammatory components of the disease. This should be considered when providing vitamin supplementation and preventing hyperglycemia.

Nutrition Assessment

History and Physical Exam

Establishing preexisting malnutrition in patients with pulmonary failure is the first step in assessment. A thorough history should be performed, assessing for recent weight loss, poor appetite, decreased ability to take in food, and recurrent infections. Particular attention should be given to comorbidities that are often present with a pulmonary disease process. These include renal failure, diabetes, and other endocrine disorders. Associated cardiac disease is also common in the form of hypertension, congestive heart failure, and coronary artery disease. Physical exam should focus on ratio of lean muscle mass, condition of the skin and nails, unhealed wounds, as well as signs of abdominal pathology such as ascites, scars, or organomegaly.

Malnutrition as defined by body mass index (BMI) has been associated with impairment in respiratory function, particularly hyperinflation of the lungs.[9] Fat-free mass index (FFMI) is considered as an alternative and perhaps better indicator of nutrition in this population. Low FFMI is positively correlated with airway obstruction, lung hyperinflation, and inspiratory load.[10] Low FFMI, but not BMI, has also been shown to be an independent predictor of long-term survival in patients requiring long-term supplemental oxygen or PMV.[11]

Predictive Equations and Indirect Calorimetry

Predictive equations are often used to determine initial calorie requirements for pulmonary failure patients. Although the resting energy expenditure is based on lean body mass, several factors influence the metabolic demand. Ventilated patients typically have many if not most of these factors, including infection, recent surgery, trauma, systemic inflammation, anasarca, and obesity.

When available, indirect calorimetry is a valuable tool for assistance with determining resting energy expenditure, as well as calculating the respiratory quotient. In the ventilated patient, indirect calorimetry may have technical limitations and should not be used with elevated fraction of inspired oxygen or positive end-expiratory pressure (PEEP) levels or when an air leak in the circuit is present. For further reading on predictive equations and indirect calorimetry, refer to Chapter 2.

Underfeeding

Inadequate provision of nutrients can have devastating effects for the patient with pulmonary failure. This occurs either from underestimation of needs, inadequate delivery, or poor tolerance in the case of EN. Underfeeding results in poor wound healing, diminished muscle strength, and inadequate protein for recovery from acute illness. For the patient on the ventilator, this translates to decreased ability to respond to hypoxemia and hypercapnia, with resultant diminished weaning capacity.[12,13]

Conceptually, permissive underfeeding during acute illness gained attention due to studies showing improved clinical outcomes.[14,15] More recent work examining cumulative caloric deficits in the critically ill calls this practice into question. Accumulating a caloric debt from time of intensive care unit (ICU) admission has been associated with immunosuppression, increased infection rates, length of stay, days of mechanical ventilation, and mortality.[16] The size of the deficit dramatically affects outcome: for those on the ventilator, a debt of greater than 10,000 calories leads to longer ICU stay and prolonged ventilator weaning. For ventilated patients, establishing early enteral feeding of any amount should be the goal. Every effort should be made to achieve target caloric intake via EN.

Overfeeding

Similar to underfeeding, overfeeding patients with pulmonary failure has substantial consequences. One of the key therapeutic strategies for ventilated patients is the concept of limiting tidal volumes to prevent further inflammation and barotrauma. In doing so, the arterial CO_2 is allowed to rise above the normal level as long as the pH is maintained above 7.2. This is known as permissive hypercapnia. For this reason, the minute ventilation for some patients with pulmonary failure, from ALI/ARDS and COPD in particular, cannot be increased as readily by adjusting the tidal volume. With this CO_2 release mechanism limited, it is even more imperative to tightly regulate the amount of CO_2 produced by substrate metabolism.

The amount of substrate delivered via nutrition support therapy can impact CO_2 production. Overfeeding can lead to increased lipogenesis, increased glucose levels, hepatic dysfunction, and inability to wean from the ventilator. Those patients most affected by overfeeding are typical of the critical care population: hypermetabolic, nutritionally depleted, stressed, and those unable to eliminate CO_2. Patients with prolonged mechanical ventilator support also suffer from overfeeding, with as many as 58% overfed based on indirect calorimetry studies.[17]

Studies suggest the administration of PN is more likely to lead to overfeeding than provision of EN, likely due to absorption, initiation, and tolerance limitations of EN.[18] PN may prohibit ventilator weaning when administration is not carefully adjusted, with some experts advocating underfeeding to only 80% of resting energy expenditure when utilizing PN alone.[19,20]

Carbohydrates were initially implicated with hypercapnia and overfeeding. Previous studies demonstrated that limiting carbohydrate administration resulted in reduced CO_2 elaboration, reduced the respiratory quotient, and improved respiratory outcomes.[21,22] A more recent trial by Talpers et al. helped clarify this issue.[23] When isocaloric diets were administered with varying concentrations of carbohydrate, CO_2 production was unchanged. With increasing caloric loads at a steady state carbohydrate concentration (60%), the CO_2 increased significantly. This study demonstrated that caloric overfeeding, not excess carbohydrate, causes excess CO_2 production (Practice Scenario 25-1).

If overfeeding is suspected, indirect calorimetry may help establish an accurate energy requirement. Indirect calorimetry is particularly helpful for the patient in this example because she is underweight at baseline and has acute organ failure. Her daily intake of calories is further complicated by the administration of propofol, which is delivered in a 10% lipid emulsion. Reduction in total macronutrient provision should be performed when overfeeding is suspected.

Practice Scenario 25-1

Question: How is overfeeding determined in the pulmonary failure patient?

Scenario: A 56-year-old thin woman (5′3″ tall and 52 kg in weight) with a history of Crohn's disease is admitted to the surgical ICU after undergoing abdominal exploration and small bowel resection for infarcted and perforated jejunum. She remains on mechanical ventilation and requires renal replacement therapy. On day 3, she is started on PN at a goal of 2200 kcal/day. She does not require vasopressors, but is sedated with continuous propofol. On day 6, she still requires mechanical ventilation despite adequate oxygenation and has worsening tachypnea (rapid breathing) with elevated CO_2 levels on her arterial blood gas.

Intervention: A nutrition support team is consulted. Indirect calorimetry is obtained which reveals a measured energy expenditure of 1500 kcal/day. The patient is taken off of the propofol, and the PN is decreased to provide 1500 kcal/day. The patient's tachypnea resolves, and she is weaned off of the ventilator over the next few days.

Answer: Overfeeding may be suspected in patients who are difficult to wean off of the ventilator. The patients may exhibit tachypnea, failed spontaneous breathing trials, and increased levels of plasma CO_2.

Rationale: Overfeeding is often not suspected when patients have difficulty weaning off of the ventilator. Patients who are being fed excessive calories will typically exhibit elevated plasma CO_2 levels without a preceding history of COPD (in which CO_2 is chronically retained). This elevation in CO_2 triggers an increased respiratory rate so that a normal pH is maintained. Tachypnea hinders the weaning process and further weakens the patient. Other causes of tachypnea must be ruled out, including hypoxia, pain, and anxiety.

Obesity

Numerous studies have examined outcomes of obese mechanically ventilated patients in the ICU. A meta-analysis found that BMI was a risk factor for increased length of stay and longer duration of ventilator dependence, although no change in mortality was noted.[24] Several factors associated with obesity affect ventilator and nutrition management. Obese patients have reduced functional reserve capacity and smaller lung volumes due to the extra weight extrinsically compressing the chest. Preexisting alveolar-arterial gradients are exacerbated with inflammatory respiratory failure, often necessitating higher PEEP and plateau pressures. Careful attention must be paid to maintaining appropriate positioning of the endotracheal tube, as reestablishing an airway can be difficult.

The obese similarly have difficulty with glycemic control. Caloric restriction can improve glycemic control, while also reducing the hypercapnia and fluid retention. Protein adequacy and hypocaloric energy provision should therefore be a priority, as this promotes endogenous fat oxidation.[25] Consensus documents endorse hypocaloric feeding for the obese patient with goals of 60% to 70% of target or 11 to 14 kcal/g calculated for ideal body weight.[26–28] Critically ill obese patients with a BMI of 30 to 40 kg/m^2 should likewise receive 2.0 g/kg/day protein for ideal body weight, with an increase to 2.5 g/kg/day for those with a BMI > 40 kg/m^2 (see Chapter 35 for further information).

Nutrition Support

Nutrition support therapy for mechanically ventilated patients has been set forth in the American Society for Parenteral and Enteral Nutrition (A.S.P.E.N.)/Society of Critical Care Medicine (SCCM) guidelines. These guidelines are intended to guide practitioners in caring for the average patient with pulmonary failure.[28] A summary of these guidelines is outlined in Tables 25-4 and 25-5.

Macronutrients

Provision of carbohydrates, protein, and lipids should be given to the pulmonary failure patient in a manner similar to that of most critically ill patients. As previously noted, overfeeding and hypercapnia are more a function of excessive total calories as opposed to carbohydrate load. High fat nutrition strategies should therefore be avoided. Protein should be given as 1.5 to 2.0 g//kg/day to accommodate the elevated catabolism for these patients. Further information regarding substrate provision can be found in Chapters 3, 5, and 6.

Micronutrients

Micronutrient deficiencies can adversely affect patients with acute or chronic pulmonary failure. Electrolytes such as phosphorus, calcium, and magnesium should be replenished aggressively as depleted levels have been associated with reduced diaphragm and respiratory muscle strength.[19] Antioxidant properties of vitamins A, C, and E are recognized, but their use in critically ill patients is not well established.

TABLE 25-4 Summarized American Society for Parenteral and Enteral Nutrition (A.S.P.E.N.)/Society of Critical Care Medicine (SCCM) Guidelines for Pulmonary Failure Patients: Assessment and Enteral Nutrition

Assessment and Plan
Evaluate weight loss, previous intake, disease severity, comorbidities, GI function
Indirect calorimetry should be used when available for estimation of energy goal
Provide supplemental protein to achieve 1.2–2.0 g/kg/day; 2.0–2.5 g/kg/day for obese
Hypocaloric feeding recommended for obese (11–14 kcal/kg(actual weight)/day)
EN
EN preferred when the gut is functional
Start EN early (24–48 hours) after the patient is resuscitated
Target 65% of goal EN within the first week
Polymeric formula preferred, peptide-based formula reserved for intolerance
Tolerance of EN
Evaluate for signs of intolerance such as abdominal pain, distention, or diarrhea
Presence of bowel sounds, flatus, or stool not required to initiate EN
Soluble fiber administration encouraged for management of diarrhea in normal gut

EN, enteral nutrition; GI, gastrointestinal.
Highlighted recommendations from the *Guidelines for the Provision and Assessment of Nutrition Support Therapy in the Adult Critically Ill Patient.*[28]
Aspiration precautions included in Table 25-6.

Deleterious effects of trace mineral deficits are also recognized, particularly with zinc and selenium. In a systematic review of antioxidants in critical illness, Heyland et al. found that selenium supplementation may be associated with a reduction in mortality.[29] Results of the Scottish Intensive Care Glutamine or Selenium Evaluative Trial likewise demonstrated reduction in infection in critically ill patients who received more than 5 days of continuous parenteral selenium.[30] A combination of micronutrients is often provided with commercial EN formulas and in parenteral formulations, making the effect of an individual component uncertain. The reader is referred to Chapter 8 for further discussion.

Enteral Nutrition

The benefits of EN for pulmonary failure are well established (ie, preservation of gut mucosa and immune function). EN is considered the route of choice for patients on the ventilator due to significantly reduced rates of infection (compared to PN).[31] Stimulation of gut-associated lymphoid tissue by EN has been reported to increase immunoglobulin A, which is protective against airway infections.[32] EN may also provide gut

TABLE 25-5 Summarized American Society for Parenteral and Enteral Nutrition (A.S.P.E.N.)/Society of Critical Care Medicine (SCCM) Guidelines for Pulmonary Failure Patients: Parenteral Nutrition and Adjuvants

PN
Malnourished patients who cannot tolerate EN should start PN after resuscitation
If goal EN cannot be met by day 7–10, consider supplemental PN
In patients receiving PN, mild permissive underfeeding (80% goal) initially
Withhold soy-based lipids during the first week
When PN provided, supplementation with IV glutamine recommended
Adjuvants
Provide enteral glutamine for burn, trauma, and mixed critical care populations
Immune-modulating diets may be used in mechanically ventilated patients
Arginine should be used with caution in patients with severe sepsis
High-lipid/low-carbohydrate formulas not encouraged for patients with pulmonary failure
Provide fish oil/borage oil/antioxidant supplement to patients with ARDS
Provide antioxidants and trace minerals
Provide at least 50% of goal for immune modulating diet efficacy
Other Recommendations
Fluid restricted formulas considered for pulmonary failure patients
Aggressive replacement of phosphorus in patients with normal renal function
Moderately strict insulin therapy should be provided

ARDS, acute respiratory distress syndrome; EN, enteral nutrition; IV, intravenous; PN, parenteral nutrition.
Highlighted recommendations from the *Guidelines for the Provision and Assessment of Nutrition Support Therapy in the Adult Critically Ill Patient.*[28] Aspiration precautions included in Table 25-6.

prophylaxis against gastrointestinal bleeding, a complication that is frequently associated with mechanical ventilation.[33]

EN should be used in the setting of a functional gut and should commence as soon as resuscitation is complete. Administration of 100% of calculated amount of calories should be the goal. The amount received, however, often depends on the ability to achieve access, interruptions of feeding, and tolerance.[34–36] Provision of "trophic" tube feeds (ie, the amount of substrate necessary to provide gut stimulation and prevent permeability and infection) is typically carried out when tolerance may be an issue. As noted previously, however, every effort should be made to achieve goal rates as early as possible for best outcomes.

Aspiration and Ventilator-Associated Pneumonia

Despite the numerous protective benefits of EN, one of the greatest concerns in patients with pulmonary failure is its potential causality with aspiration and pneumonia or pneumonitis.[37,38] VAP complicates the care in up to 30% of patients on mechanical ventilation.[39] The pathogenesis of VAP is complex, but it is thought to involve the colonization of the aerodigestive tract with bacteria and microaspiration of secretions containing pathogenic bacteria. As illustrated in Figure 25-3, the presence of an endotracheal tube stent opens the vocal cords and allows for the passage of these secretions into the respiratory tract, providing a surface for biofilm formation. Similarly, patients may suffer from aspiration pneumonitis, a condition in which gastric contents are aspirated into the respiratory tract, causing a chemical inflammatory reaction without secondary infection. Both conditions are devastating to mechanically ventilated patients.

Patients with pulmonary failure have an increased risk of aspiration secondary to sedation and analgesia, positioning, gastric dysmotility, and altered oral and gastrointestinal flora from shock and aggressive antibiotic use. Likewise, increased levels of PEEP with ventilator therapy may increase this risk. Patients with long-term pulmonary failure who have tracheotomies suffer from frequent aspiration up to 80% of the time.[40] Once extubated, the aspiration risk in this patient population is high, with persistence of dysphagia in 40% of patients.[41]

Ventilator-Associated Pneumonia Prevention Strategies

Effective VAP prevention strategies target modifiable risk factors for colonization and aspiration, including elevation of the head of the bed, subglottic secretion draining, oral care with chlorhexidine, limiting time of mechanical ventilation, in addition to other aspiration precautions as listed in Table 25-6.[42] Reduction of gastroesophageal reflux should be achieved with more distally placed tubes for administration of nutrition, with a nasogastric or orogastric tube used for stomach decompression.[34] The North American Summit on Aspiration in the Critically Ill Patient recommends small bowel feedings for patients at high risk of aspiration,[35] as delivery of EN to the jejunum is associated with reduced rates of VAP compared to gastric or duodenal placement.[36] Prokinetic agents such as metoclopramide or erythromycin are often used to assist with gastric emptying and bowel motility. Further discussion of feeding tube placement and complications are discussed in Chapter 13.

Positioning strategies to prevent aspiration are simple and effective. Generally interpreted as having the head of bed at 30 degrees, true semirecumbent positioning requires 45-degree elevation as recommended by the Centers for Disease Control and Prevention and other societies.[43,44] Patients with advanced pulmonary failure and severe hypoxia may occasionally be placed in the prone position.[45] While gastric feeds are poorly tolerated in this position, there is no difference in clinical pneumonia when comparing prone to supine positioning.[46,47] Compared to a semirecumbent position, however, prone feeding did demonstrate higher rates of pneumonia and longer duration of ventilation.[48] Safe enteral feeding can be achieved in the prone position, as long as the practitioner is vigilant to signs of intolerance or aspiration (Practice Scenario 25-2).

FIGURE 25-3 Upper Aerodigestive Tract

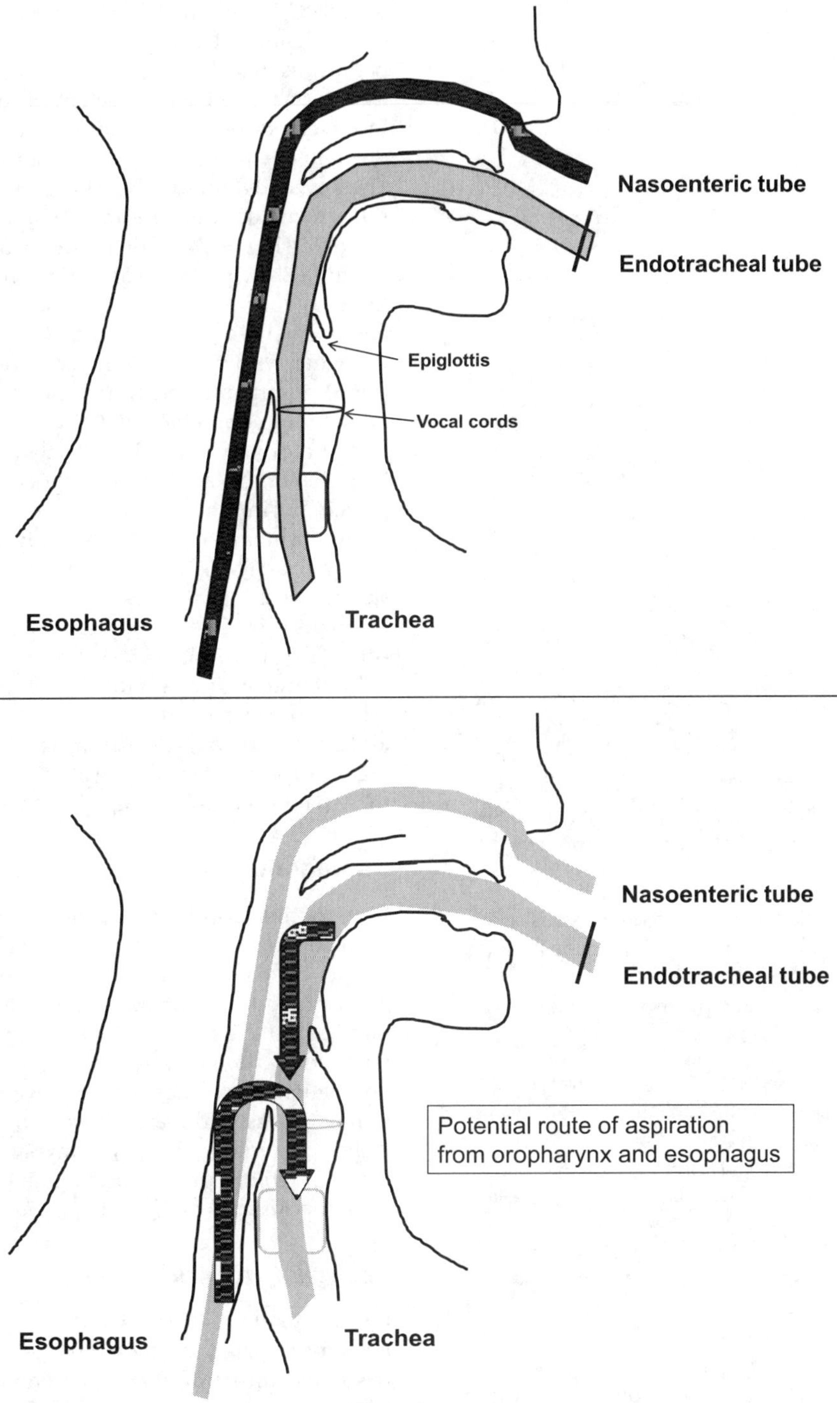

The natural anatomic defenses to regurgitation and aspiration are stented open by nasoenteric tubes (upper esophageal sphincter) and endotracheal tubes (epiglottis and vocal cords), providing a potential route of passage for secretions.

TABLE 25-6 Ventilator-Associated Pneumonia Prevention

Maintain head of bed > 45 degrees
Chlorhexidine oral wash
Peptic ulcer prophylaxis
Continuous small bowel tube feeds
Subglottic suctioning of secretions
Prokinetic agents
Daily spontaneous breathing trial
Daily sedation holiday
Limit ventilator days
Limit transfusions
Limit antibiotics

Practice Scenario 25-2

Question: How are VAP precautions applied in a clinical setting?

Scenario: A 78-year-old well-nourished man with a history of stroke and gastric reflux is admitted to the surgical ICU after suffering pulmonary contusions in a motor vehicle accident. He also has severe head injury and requires mechanical ventilation for his lung injury. A nasoenteric tube is inserted blindly at the bedside and appears to terminate in the pylorus on x-ray. Tube feeds are initially started within the first 24 hours in the ICU. The bedside nurse notices a large amount of tube feeding coming out of the nasogastric tube on the second day, with questionable amounts noticed in the endotracheal tube. Metoclopramide is ordered at a scheduled dose; however, the patient develops seizure activity and the drug is stopped. The bedside nurse wants to know if PN should be started.

Intervention: Erythromycin is started with no change in gastric tube feed output. An endoscopically placed nasojejunal tube is placed with distal tip in the jejunum. The head of bed is also elevated to 45 degrees. Tube feeds are restarted with advancement to goal per protocol.

Answer: VAP prevention involves the expertise of multiple disciplines within the ICU setting. While interventions such as chlorhexidine mouth decontamination and subglottic suctioning are left to the bedside nurse and respiratory therapist, the administration of enteral nutrition in a safe manner is essential to prevent aspiration.

Rationale: Patients at high risk for aspiration should never be excluded from the provision of EN for that reason alone. This patient is at high risk for VAP due to age, pulmonary contusions, history of stroke, and immunosuppressed state after trauma. While it may be tempting to not risk aspiration of tube feeds and simply order PN, the benefits of maintaining gut integrity and avoiding complications of PN highly outweigh the risks. Patients who do not tolerate gastric or duodenal tube feeds may benefit from placement of enteric access more distal in the gastrointestinal tract. Prokinetics such as erythromycin and metoclopramide may also be used, but may lose efficacy and, in the case of metoclopramide, cause neurologic sequelae. The simple measure of elevating the head of the bed can reduce gravitational pooling of gastric contents in the oropharynx.

Parenteral Nutrition

Although the benefits of EN on immune function are well described,[49] patients with acute pulmonary failure may have other significant morbidities such a nonfunctional gut and peritonitis that can preclude provision of EN. Likewise, inability to keep up with energy deficits accrued early in illness results in increased morbidity and mortality for these patients.[50] As noted in the Algorithms for Critical-Care Enteral and Parenteral Therapy study, survival benefits ensue when larger amounts of nutrient are delivered more consistently.[51]

A growing body of literature in Europe advocates supplementing EN with PN.[52] The European Society of Parenteral and Enteral Nutrition guidelines for nutrition support therapy endorse initiating supplemental PN at day 4 if 60% of goal EN is not met within 3 days.[53] This is a controversial practice, however. A recent multicenter trial comparing provision of EN with or without supplemental PN demonstrated a trend toward greater mortality with added PN whether administered early or late despite the significantly higher provision of calories and protein.[54] Timing of administration may be part of the issue. A multicenter trial comparing early (within 48 hours) versus late (after day 8) PN supplementation to early EN demonstrated fewer infections and decreased duration of mechanical ventilation when PN supplementation occurred later in the course of critical illness.[55] Although supplemental PN may be helpful in reducing the cumulative caloric deficit, this concept requires further clarification regarding composition, timing, and amount before advocating its use in pulmonary failure. As previously stated, EN should always be promoted primarily for these patients in the setting of a functional gut.

Immunonutrition

Immunonutrition is the concept of providing nutrition substrate for the purpose of modulating immune function. Various substances have been investigated for this purpose, with the effect of reducing inflammation, enhancing healing, reducing rates of infection, and decreasing pulmonary morbidity as reflected by time required for mechanical ventilation. Patient populations recommended to receive immunonutrition include trauma, burns, perioperative, oncology, and septic with varying degree of certainty.[56] Agents investigated for these purposes include prebiotics, probiotics, arginine, glutamine, antioxidants, nucleic acids, and omega-3 fatty acids.

Omega-3 Fatty Acids

Omega-3 fatty acids (n-3) and omega-6 fatty acids (n-6) have been investigated for their anti- and proinflammatory properties. n-3s consist of docosahexaenoic acid (DHA) and eicosapentaenoic acid (EPA), which are found predominantly in fish oils, as well as α-linolenic acid found in walnut and flax seed oils. These polyunsaturated fatty acids are metabolized to 3-series prostaglandins and 5-series leukotrienes, substances that reduce inflammation and eicosanoid production.[57] n-6s and omega-9 fatty acids (n-9) are found predominantly in animal fat and consist of linolenic acid, dihomo-γ-linolenic acid, and arachidonic acid. Via a common enzyme pathway (Figure 25-4), n-6s are metabolized to 2-series prostaglandins,

FIGURE 25-4 Omega-3 and Omega-6 Fatty Acid Metabolism

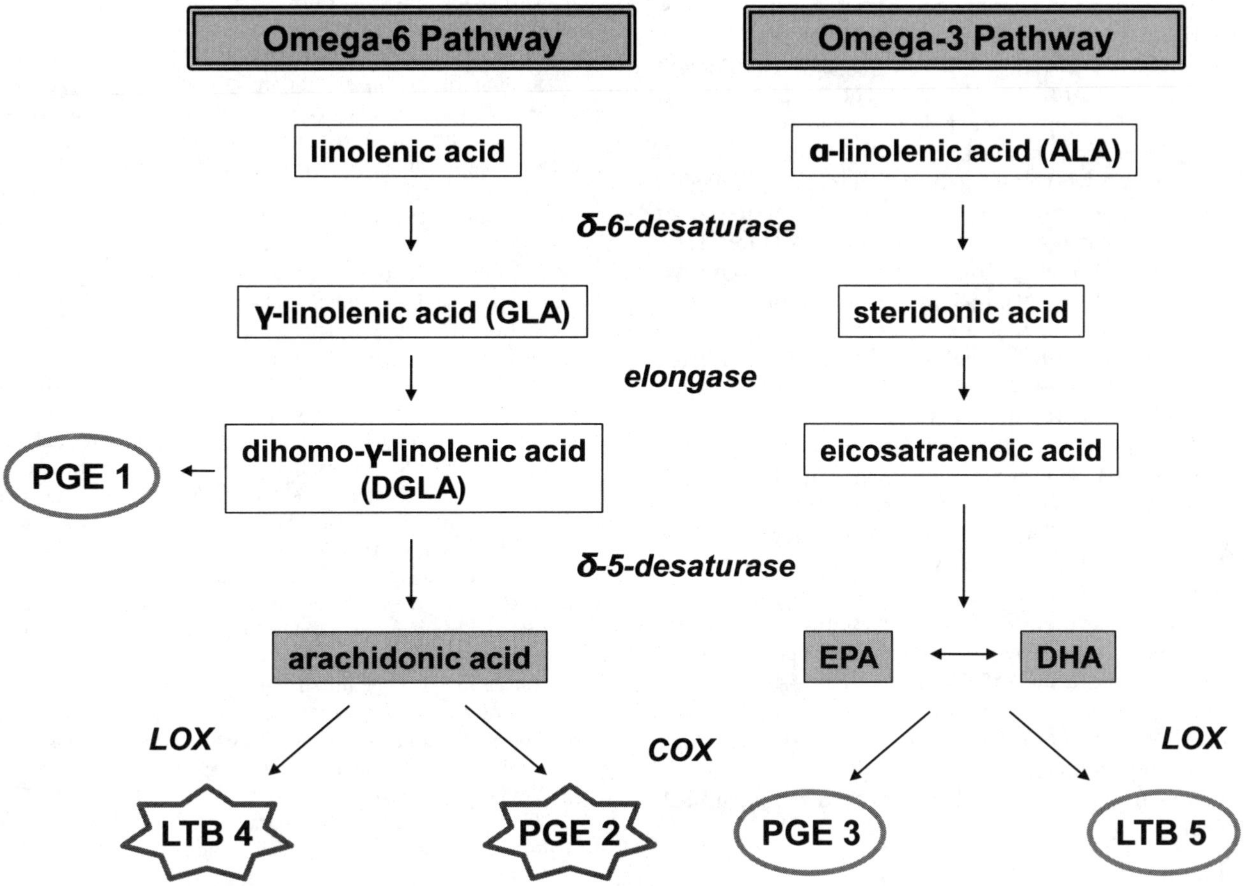

The two pathways for omega-6 (n-6) and omega-3 (n-3) polyunsaturated fatty acid metabolism are shown. Enzymes listed in italics are common for each substrate as noted. The final end-products of the n-3 pathway are the 3-series of prostaglandins (PGE 3) and the 5-series of leukotrienes (LTB 5), which are anti-inflammatory in nature. The final end-products of the n-6 pathway are the 2-series of prostaglandins (PGE 2) and the 4-series of leukotrienes (LTB 4). These are proinflammatory in nature, signaling leukocyte adhesion, cytokine production, vasodilation, and platelet aggregation. Prostaglandin E-1 (PGE 1) is a direct derivative of dihomo-gamma-linolenic acid (DGLA) and is responsible for pulmonary vascular vasodilation. COX, cyclo-oxygenase; DHA, docosahexaenoic acid; EPA, eicosapentaenoic acid; LOX, lipoxygenase.

thromboxanes, and 4-series leukotrienes. These substances are proinflammatory in nature, influencing cytokine production, platelet aggregation, vasodilation, and vascular permeability.[58] As an intermediate in the n-6 pathway, γ-linolenic acid (GLA) causes in increase in arachidonic acid levels. When GLA is administered with EPA, however, the terminal enzyme is blocked, reducing the resultant arachidonic acid production. This combination also leads to an increased production of prostaglandin E_1, a potent pulmonary vasodilator.[59]

As a primary inflammatory disorder, ALI/ARDS lends themselves well to potential modulation by immunonutrition. Early animal studies utilizing enteral administration of EPA and GLA plus antioxidants demonstrated decreased production of eicosanoids, improved gas exchange, and decreased pulmonary microvascular permeability in sepsis-mediated lung injury.[60,61] Based on these findings, a landmark paper published by Gadek et al. in 1999 utilized this same commercial formulation of EPA, DHA, borage oil (containing GLA), and antioxidants for patients with ARDS.[62] This study reported improved oxygenation and decreased ICU length of stay for patients receiving continuous infusion of the n-3–based formula versus a standard commercial pulmonary formula. Subsequent randomized controlled trials utilizing the same high n-3 ratio formula were published that likewise demonstrated improved pulmonary physiology, decreased ICU length of stay, decreased new organ failures, and decreased mortality.[63,64] These findings lead to a grade A (highest) recommendation for use of n-3 fatty acids in patients with ARDS by the A.S.P.E.N./SCCM guidelines.[28]

Despite the initial enthusiasm for this n-3 formula for treatment of ARDS, numerous questions were raised. Of primary concern, the control group in these studies received a formula with a higher n-6 to n-3 ratio, exaggerating the potential anti-inflammatory effect of the n-3 supplementation. Likewise, it is unknown which component of the formula was responsible for the improved outcomes: EPA, DHA, GLA, antioxidants, or a particular combination of each. Additionally, lung protective ventilation strategies, which decrease systemic inflammation,[65] were not universally applied to all patients in these initial studies and could influence the effects of further anti-inflammatory agents.

Subsequent trials were designed to address these questions. The investigators in a multicenter study randomized ALI/ARDS patients to receive either an n-3/GLA/antioxidant supplement or an isocaloric control supplement.[66] The supplement was given enterally as a bolus twice daily independently of provision of EN by protocol. Despite an eightfold increase in plasma EPA levels, patients who received the n-3 supplements failed to demonstrate any improvement in pulmonary physiology or clinical outcomes such as ventilator-free days, ICU-free days, organ failures, or mortality. This study was halted for futility after accrual of 272 patients, making determination of potential harmful effects of the n-3 supplement uncertain.

An additional randomized controlled trial was completed during this same time period utilizing DHA and EPA supplements alone for patients with ALI/ARDS.[67] This trial compared the n-3 supplements with saline placebo in a bolus fashion. No sources of GLA or antioxidants were administered. Additional EN or PN provided was at the discretion of the clinician. This study likewise achieved significant serum levels of EPA; however, similar to the Omega-3 Fatty Acid Therapy in Patients With Ventricular Tachyarrhythmias trial, no differences in clinical outcomes were achieved. Additionally, serum and lung biomarkers of inflammation were unchanged in the study group.

Discordance among the initial and later trials requires further elucidation by larger trials. Questions about n-3 supplementation remain regarding timing and route of administration, duration of use, and optimal dose. Likewise, the specific effects of each component of the n-3-based formula need to be identified.

Summary

Pulmonary failure in the critically ill patient is a significant source of disability and mortality. Nutrition support therapy for these patients may attenuate the catabolic state and optimize respiratory muscle strength for ventilator weaning. Estimating caloric requirements can be difficult due to comorbidities and secondary diagnoses common to this population, and should be reassessed frequently to avoid overfeeding. EN is preferred, with appropriate aspiration precautions vigilantly followed. PN may be appropriate for patients with baseline malnutrition or for whom EN is not feasible. Inflammatory pulmonary conditions such as ALI/ARDS may be appropriate for immunonutrition with n-3 fatty acids and antioxidants, although further clarification of dose, selection of components, and timing is needed.

References

1. Wheeler AP, Bernard GR. Acute lung injury and the acute respiratory distress syndrome: a clinical review. *Lancet*. 2007;369(9572):1553–1564.
2. Jubran A, Tobin MJ. Pathophysiologic basis of acute respiratory distress in patients who fail a trial of weaning from mechanical ventilation. *Am J Respir Crit Care Med*. 1997;155(3):906–915.
3. Engels PT, Bagshaw SM, Meier M, et al. Tracheostomy: from insertion to decannulation. *Can J Surg*. 2009;52(5):427–433.
4. Wilson DO, Rogers RM, Wright EC, et al. Body weight in chronic obstructive pulmonary disease. The National Institutes of Health Intermittent Positive-Pressure Breathing Trial. *Am Rev Respir Dis*. 1989;139(6):1435–1438.
5. Vitacca M, Clini E, Porta R, et al. Acute exacerbations in patients with COPD: predictors of need for mechanical ventilation. *Eur Respir J*. 1996;9(7):1487–1493.
6. Nelson JE, Meier DE, Litke A, et al. The symptom burden of chronic critical illness. *Crit Care Med*. 2004;32(7):1527–1534.
7. Mechanick JI, Brett EM. Nutrition and the chronically critically ill patient. *Curr Opin Clin Nutr Metab Care*. 2005;8(1):33–39.
8. Khalid I, Doshi P, DiGiovine B. Early enteral nutrition and outcomes of critically ill patients treated with vasopressors and mechanical ventilation. *Am J Crit Care*. 2010;19(3):261–268.
9. Budweiser S, Heinemann F, Meyer K, et al. Weight gain in cachectic COPD patients receiving noninvasive positive-pressure ventilation. *Respir Care*. 2006;51(2):126–132.
10. Budweiser S, Meyer K, Jörres RA, et al. Nutritional depletion and its relationship to respiratory impairment in patients with chronic respiratory failure due to COPD or restrictive thoracic diseases. *Eur J Clin Nutr*. 2008;62(3):436–443.
11. Hitzl AP, Jörres RA, Heinemann F, et al. Nutritional status in patients with chronic respiratory failure receiving home mechanical ventilation: impact on survival. *Clin Nutr*. 2010;29(1):65–71.
12. Larca L, Greenbaum DM. Effectiveness of intensive nutritional regimes in patients who fail to wean from mechanical ventilation. *Crit Care Med*. 1982;10(5):297–300.
13. Doekel RC Jr, Zwillich CW, Scoggin CH, et al. Clinical semi-starvation: depression of hypoxic ventilatory response. *N Engl J Med*. 1976;295(7):358–361.
14. Jeejeebhoy KN. Permissive underfeeding of the critically ill patient. *Nutr Clin Pract*. 2004;19(5):477–480.
15. Owais AE, Bumby RF, MacFie J. Review article: permissive underfeeding in short-term nutritional support. *Aliment Pharmacol Ther*. 2010;32(5):628–636.
16. Villet S, Chiolero RL, Bollmann MD, et al. Negative impact of hypocaloric feeding and energy balance on clinical outcome in ICU patients. *Clin Nutr*. 2005;24(4):502–509.
17. McClave SA, Lowen CC, Kleber MJ, et al. Are patients fed appropriately according to their caloric requirements? *J Parenter Enteral Nutr*. 1998;22(6):375–381.
18. Liposky JM, Nelson LD. Ventilatory response to high caloric loads in critically ill patients. *Crit Care Med*. 1994;22(5):796–802.
19. Benotti PN, Bistrian B. Metabolic and nutritional aspects of weaning from mechanical ventilation. *Crit Care Med*. 1989;17(2):181–185.
20. McClave SA. Indirect calorimetry: relevance to patient outcome. *Respir Care Clin N Am*. 2006;12(4):635–650, vii.
21. 9th Clinical Congress Proceedings: American Society for Parenteral and Enteral Nutrition, Inc. January 21-24, 1984, Aspen. Abstracts. *J Parenter Enteral Nutr*. 1985;9(1):106–131.
22. Baker JP, Detsky AS, Stewart S, et al. Randomized trial of total parenteral nutrition in critically ill patients: metabolic effects of varying glucose-lipid ratios as the energy source. *Gastroenterology*. 1984;87(1):53–59.
23. Talpers SS, Romberger DJ, Bunce SB, et al. Nutritionally associated increased carbon dioxide production. Excess total calories vs high proportion of carbohydrate calories. *Chest*. 1992;102(2):551–555.
24. Akinnusi ME, Pineda LA, El Solh AA. Effect of obesity on intensive care morbidity and mortality: A meta-analysis. *Crit Care Med*. 2008;36(1):151–158.
25. Dickerson RN. Hypocaloric feeding of obese patients in the intensive care unit. *Curr Opin Clin Nutr Metab Care*. 2005;8(2):189–196.
26. Frankenfield DC, Rowe WA, Smith JS, et al. Validation of several established equations for resting metabolic rate in obese and nonobese people. *J Am Diet Assoc*. 2003;103(9):1152–1159.

27. Port AM, Apovian C. Metabolic support of the obese intensive care unit patient: a current perspective. *Curr Op Clin Nutr Metab Care.* 2010;13(2):184–191.
28. McClave SA, Martindale RG, Vanek VW, et al. Guidelines for the provision and assessment of nutrition support therapy in the adult critically ill patient: Society of Critical Care Medicine (SCCM) and American Society for Parenteral and Enteral Nutrition (A.S.P.E.N.). *J Parenter Enteral Nutr.* 2009;33(3):277–316.
29. Heyland DK, Dhaliwal R, Suchner U, et al. Antioxidant nutrients: a systematic review of trace elements and vitamins in the critically ill patient. *Intensive Care Med.* 2005;31(3):327–337.
30. Andrews PJD, Avenell A, Noble DW, et al. Randomised trial of glutamine, selenium, or both, to supplement parenteral nutrition for critically ill patients. *BMJ.* 2011;342:d1542.
31. Griffiths RD. Is parenteral nutrition really that risky in the intensive care unit? *Curr Opin Clin Nutr Metab Care.* 2004;7(2): 175–181.
32. King BK, Kudsk KA, Li J, et al. Route and type of nutrition influence mucosal immunity to bacterial pneumonia. *Ann Surg.* 1999; 229(2):272–278.
33. McClave SA, Chang W-K. When to feed the patient with gastrointestinal bleeding. *Nutr Clin Pract.* 2005;20(5):544–550.
34. Lien HC, Chang CS, Chen GH. Can percutaneous endoscopic jejunostomy prevent gastroesophageal reflux in patients with preexisting esophagitis? *Am J Gastroenterol.* 2000;95(12):3439–3443.
35. McClave SA, DeMeo MT, DeLegge MH, et al. North American Summit on Aspiration in the Critically Ill Patient: consensus statement. *J Parenter Enteral Nutr.* 2002;26(6 Suppl):S80–S85.
36. Heyland DK, Drover JW, Dhaliwal R, et al. Optimizing the benefits and minimizing the risks of enteral nutrition in the critically ill: role of small bowel feeding. *J Parenter Enteral Nutr.* 2002; 26(6 Suppl):S51–S55; discussion S56–S57.
37. Metheny NA. Preventing respiratory complications of tube feedings: evidence-based practice. *Am J Crit Care.* 2006;15(4):360–369.
38. Artinian V, Krayem H, DiGiovine B. Effects of early enteral feeding on the outcome of critically ill mechanically ventilated medical patients. *Chest.* 2006;129(4):960–967.
39. Rello J, Ollendorf DA, Oster G, et al. Epidemiology and outcomes of ventilator-associated pneumonia in a large US database. *Chest.* 2002;122(6):2115–2121.
40. Elpern EH, Borkgren Okonek M, Bacon M, et al. Effect of the Passy-Muir tracheostomy speaking valve on pulmonary aspiration in adults. *Heart Lung.* 2000;29(4):287–293.
41. Leder SB, Ross DA. Confirmation of no causal relationship between tracheotomy and aspiration status: a direct replication study. *Dysphagia.* 2010;25(1):35–39.
42. Blot S, Rello J, Vogelaers D. What is new in the prevention of ventilator-associated pneumonia? *Curr Opin Pulm Med.* 2011;17(3): 155–159.
43. Guidelines for prevention of nosocomial pneumonia. Centers for Disease Control and Prevention. *MMWR Recomm Rep.* 1997; 46(RR-1):1–79.
44. Dodek P, Keenan S, Cook D, et al. Evidence-based clinical practice guideline for the prevention of ventilator-associated pneumonia. *Ann Intern Med.* 2004;141(4):305–313.
45. Gattinoni L, Tognoni G, Pesenti A, et al. Effect of prone positioning on the survival of patients with acute respiratory failure. *N Engl J Med.* 2001;345(8):568–573.
46. Reignier J, Thenoz-Jost N, Fiancette M, et al. Early enteral nutrition in mechanically ventilated patients in the prone position. *Crit Care Med.* 2004:94–99.
47. Mancebo J, Fernández R, Blanch L, et al. A multicenter trial of prolonged prone ventilation in severe acute respiratory distress syndrome. *Am J Respir Crit Care Med.* 2006;173(11):1233–1239.
48. Alexiou VG, Ierodiakonou V, Dimopoulos G, et al. Impact of patient position on the incidence of ventilator-associated pneumonia: a meta-analysis of randomized controlled trials. *J Crit Care.* 2009;24(4):515–522.
49. Peter JV, Moran JL, Phillips-Hughes J. A metaanalysis of treatment outcomes of early enteral versus early parenteral nutrition in hospitalized patients. *Crit. Care Med.* 2005;33(1):213–220; discussion 260–261.
50. Villet S, Chiolero RL, Bollmann MD, et al. Negative impact of hypocaloric feeding and energy balance on clinical outcome in ICU patients. *Clin Nutr.* 2005;24(4):502–509.
51. Martin CM, Doig GS, Heyland DK, et al. Multicentre, cluster-randomized clinical trial of algorithms for critical-care enteral and parenteral therapy (ACCEPT). *CMAJ.* 2004;170(2):197–204.
52. Preiser JC, Berré J, Carpentier Y, et al. Management of nutrition in European intensive care units: results of a questionnaire. Working Group on Metabolism and Nutrition of the European Society of Intensive Care Medicine. *Intensive Care Med.* 1999;25(1):95–101.
53. Kreymann KG, Berger MM, Deutz NEP, et al. ESPEN Guidelines on Enteral Nutrition: Intensive care. *Clin Nutr.* 2006;25(2):210–223.
54. Kutsogiannis J, Alberda C, Gramlich L, et al. Early use of supplemental parenteral nutrition in critically ill patients: Results of an international multicenter observational study. *Crit Care Med.* 2011;39:2691–2699.
55. Casaer MP, Mesotten D, Hermans G, et al. Early versus late parenteral nutrition in critically ill adults. *N Engl J Med.* 2011;365(6): 506–517.
56. Marik PE, Zaloga GP. Immunonutrition in critically ill patients: a systematic review and analysis of the literature. *Intensive Care Med.* 2008;34(11):1980–1990.
57. Calder PC. Polyunsaturated fatty acids, inflammation, and immunity. *Lipids.* 2001;36(9):1007–1024.
58. Bulger EM, Maier RV. Lipid mediators in the pathophysiology of critical illness. *Crit Care Med.* 2000;28(4 Suppl):N27–N36.
59. Barham JB, Edens MB, Fonteh AN, et al. Addition of eicosapentaenoic acid to gamma-linolenic acid-supplemented diets prevents serum arachidonic acid accumulation in humans. *J Nutr.* 2000; 130(8):1925–1931.
60. Murray MJ, Kumar M, Gregory TJ, et al. Select dietary fatty acids attenuate cardiopulmonary dysfunction during acute lung injury in pigs. *Am J Physiol.* 1995;269(6 Pt 2):H2090–H2099.
61. Mancuso P, Whelan J, DeMichele SJ, et al. Dietary fish oil and fish and borage oil suppress intrapulmonary proinflammatory eicosanoid biosynthesis and attenuate pulmonary neutrophil accumulation in endotoxic rats. *Crit Care Med.* 1997;25(7):1198–1206.
62. Gadek JE, DeMichele SJ, Karlstad MD, et al. Effect of enteral feeding with eicosapentaenoic acid, gamma-linolenic acid, and antioxidants in patients with acute respiratory distress syndrome. Enteral Nutrition in ARDS Study Group. *Crit Care Med.* 1999;27(8):1409–1420.
63. Singer P, Theilla M, Fisher H, et al. Benefit of an enteral diet enriched with eicosapentaenoic acid and gamma-linolenic acid in ventilated patients with acute lung injury. *Crit Care Med.* 2006; 34(4):1033–1038.
64. Pontes-Arruda A, Aragão AMA, Albuquerque JD. Effects of enteral feeding with eicosapentaenoic acid, gamma-linolenic acid, and antioxidants in mechanically ventilated patients with severe sepsis and septic shock. *Crit Care Med.* 2006;34(9):2325–2333.
65. Parsons PE, Eisner MD, Thompson BT, et al. Lower tidal volume ventilation and plasma cytokine markers of inflammation in patients with acute lung injury. *Crit Care Med.* 2005;33(1):1–6; discussion 230–232.
66. Rice TW, Wheeler AP, Thompson BT, et al. Enteral omega-3 fatty acid, gamma-linolenic acid, and antioxidant supplementation in acute lung injury. *JAMA.* 2011;306(14):1574–1581.
67. Stapleton RD, Martin TR, Weiss NS, et al. A phase II randomized placebo-controlled trial of omega-3 fatty acids for the treatment of acute lung injury. *Crit Care Med.* 2011;39(7):1655–1662.

26 Gastrointestinal Disease

David Frantz, MD, MS, Craig Munroe, MD, Carol Rees Parrish, MS, RD, Joseph Krenitsky, MS, RD, Kate Willcutts, MS, RD, CNSC, and Amy Fortune, RD, PA-C

CONTENTS

Background 428

Stomach Disorders 428
- Gastric Resections 428
  - Partial Gastric Resection 428
  - Vagotomy 428
  - Roux-en-Y Total Gastric Resection 429
  - Nutritional Assessment 429
  - Postgastrectomy Syndrome 429
  - Dumping Syndrome 429
  - Fat Maldigestion 429
  - Gastric Stasis 429
  - Lactose Intolerance 430
  - Afferent Limb Syndrome, Alkaline Reflux Gastritis, and Postvagotomy Diarrhea 430
  - General Treatment Principles after Gastrectomy 430
  - Nutrient Deficiencies 430
    - Anemia 430
    - Pernicious Anemia 430
    - Folate Deficiency 430
    - Iron Deficiency 431
    - Metabolic Bone Disease 431
  - Pancreaticoduodenectomy (Whipple Procedure) 431
- Gastroparesis 432
  - Nutritional Assessment 432

Laboratory Data 433
- Serum Glucose and Hemoglobin A1C 433
- Ferritin 433
- Vitamin B12 434
- Vitamin D 434

Factors That Influence Gastric Emptying 434

Factors That Can Affect Oral Intake 434
- Nausea and Vomiting 434
- Small Bowel Bacterial Overgrowth 434
- Bezoar Formation 434

Nutritional Management 434
- Oral Nutrition Guidelines 434
- Enteral Nutrition 435
- Formula Selection/Delivery 436
- Parenteral Nutrition 436
- Additional Resources 436

Small Bowel and Colon 436
- Small Bowel Bacterial Overgrowth 436
  - Diagnosing Small Bowel Bacterial Overgrowth 437
  - Treatment 437
- Celiac Disease 437

Dermatitis Herpetiformis ... 438
Nutritional Implications ... 438
Diagnosis ... 438
Serological Testing ... 438
Small Bowel Biopsy ... 438
Refractory Celiac Disease ... 439
Nutritional Management ... 439
Inflammatory Bowel Disease ... 440
Crohn's Disease ... 440
Nutritional Assessment ... 440
Calorie and Protein Requirements ... 440
Nutrition Intervention ... 440
Fiber ... 440
Lactose ... 440
Enteral Nutrition ... 441
Parenteral Nutrition ... 441
Specific Nutrient Issues ... 441
Vitamin and Mineral Deficiencies ... 441
Fish Oil ... 442
Ulcerative Colitis ... 442
Specific Nutrients ... 442
Protein-Losing Enteropathy ... 442
Short Bowel Syndrome ... 443
Physiological Changes in Short Bowel Syndrome ... 444
Assessment/Monitoring ... 445
Nutrition Intervention ... 446
Oral Diet ... 446
Enteral Nutrition ... 447
Parenteral Nutrition/Intravenous Fluids ... 447
Long-Term Monitoring ... 447
Future Directions ... 447
Enterocutaneous Fistulas ... 447
Etiology ... 447
Diagnosis ... 448
Nutrition Intervention ... 448
Specific Nutrient Issues ... 449
Hydration and Electrolytes ... 449
Vitamin and Mineral Supplementation ... 449
Intestinal Urinary Diversions ... 449
Acknowledgments ... 449
References ... 450

Objectives

1. Outline main digestive maladies and nutritional complications associated with abnormalities of the stomach, small intestine, and colon
2. Outline common metabolic, immunologic, and idiopathic conditions related to maldigestion
3. Help the reader to recognize the common nutrient deficiencies and intolerances that are associated with postsurgical anatomy
4. Outline appropriate indications of enteral nutrition (EN) and parenteral nutrition (PN) support in many of these conditions

Test Your Knowledge Questions

1. A 66-year-old male with history of heavy alcohol use (2 pints of hard liquor per day for the last 30 years) presents to your clinic with weight loss and abdominal pain. The patient has abstained from alcohol for the last 6 months, but has had a 20-lb weight loss over that time. The patient also complains of foul smelling stools that "stick to the toilet bowl" and that are yellow and oily in color and consistency. Liver function tests, including bilirubin, are normal. A 72-hour fecal fat analysis reveals a fat content of 60 g. The patient is vitamin D deficient and was incidentally found to have an international

normalized ratio of 1.9. The most likely cause of this patient's symptoms is:
A. Acute pancreatitis
B. Chronic pancreatitis
C. Pancreatic cancer
D. *Clostridium difficile* infection
E. Acute alcoholic hepatitis

2. A 35-year-old Caucasian female presents to the clinic with diarrhea, weight loss, and abnormal liver function tests. Her primary care physician also noted that the patient was vitamin D and iron deficient with anemia. On physical exam, the patient has a very pruritic maculopapular rash with vesicular eruptions on her lower legs. An upper endoscopy is performed, and a mosaic pattern with nodularity is noted in the second portion of the duodenum. The most likely cause of the patient's symptoms is:
   A. Crohn's disease
   B. Celiac disease (CD)
   C. Whipple disease
   D. Peptic ulcer disease
   E. Irritable bowel syndrome
3. The patient is a 33-year-old female who underwent Roux-en-Y gastric bypass procedure for morbid obesity. Her body mass index prior to surgery was 52. She was prediabetic and hypertensive prior to the operation. She comes in today 2 years after her surgery. She is exercising regularly and currently has a body mass index of 29. The patient states she was found to have low iron levels as well as a low calcium on her routine physical blood work with her primary care physician. The patient reports normal menses and states she drinks two glasses of milk a day and eats a balanced diet high in "nutrients" from the health food store. The most likely explanation for the patient's laboratory findings is:
   A. Duodenal exclusion after Roux-en-Y procedure
   B. Heavy menstruation
   C. Malnutrition from only eating certain foods ("selective eating")
   D. Gastric hypersecretion after Roux-en-Y procedure
   E. Laboratory error

Test Your Knowledge Answers

1. The correct answer is **B**. This patient has chronic pancreatitis. Signs of chronic pancreatitis in this patient include abdominal pain and weight loss. Weight loss in this case is likely related to fat malabsorption, which in this context is most likely related to steatorrhea from pancreatic insufficiency as witnessed by the patient's elevated fecal fat. The patient does not likely have a pancreatic cancer at this time as the liver function tests remain normal, but chronic pancreatitis is a risk factor for pancreatic adenocarcinoma.
2. The correct answer is **B**. The patient has classic CD. In addition to the mosaic pattern seen on endoscopy, the patient has both vitamin D and iron deficiency, findings consistent with CD. The rash on the legs likely represents dermatitis herpetiformis, again a classic finding of celiac syndrome. Abnormal liver function tests and abdominal pain are also commonly seen in CD.
3. The correct answer is **A**. This patient suffers from calcium and iron deficiency as a result of duodenal exclusion. Calcium and iron are primarily absorbed in the duodenum. After Roux-en-Y surgery, the duodenum is effectively excluded, putting the patient at risk for these findings.

Background

Nutrition status and the digestive tract are inescapably linked. Some of the most persistent nutrition myths relate to diseases of the digestive tract. Research into digestive diseases has also produced some of the earliest evidence-based nutrition recommendations. A thorough understanding of the digestive process, and the interaction between gastrointestinal (GI) pathology and nutrition is essential to a proper understanding of nutrition support (see Chapter 1). The most common GI disorders and their nutritional ramifications are presented here.

Stomach Disorders

Gastric Resections

Improved medical therapy for ulcer disease and declining cancer rates has reduced the need for gastric resection. Gastric resection is reserved for patients with peptic ulcer disease that has failed to respond to medical therapy or those with malignant disease. Nevertheless, it is not uncommon for clinicians to treat patients with a history of gastric resection. Gastric resections fall into one of two categories: partial, or subtotal, gastrectomy (PG) and total gastrectomy (TG). The nutritional complications that result are similar for both categories.

Partial Gastric Resection

A PG may be performed for recurrent ulcers or malignancy limited to the antrum. PG involves removal of the gastrin-secreting antrum, which includes up to 75% of the distal stomach. Reconstruction is performed with anastomosis of the remaining gastric segment to the duodenum (Billroth I [BI]) or jejunum (Billroth II [BI]). During a BI anastomosis, the surgeon creates an end-to-end anastomosis of the duodenum to the remaining gastric body. This procedure is not as common as it once was. A BII reconstruction consists of a side-to-side anastomosis of the gastric body to the jejunum approximately 15 cm distal to the ligament of Treitz. The duodenal stump is preserved in the BII to allow continued flow of bile salts and pancreatic enzymes.

Vagotomy

BI and BII operations may or may not involve a vagotomy. Furthermore, the type of vagotomy may differ. A truncal vagotomy severs the vagus nerve on the distal esophagus and significantly reduces acid secretion; this creates gastric stasis and poor gastric emptying and is, therefore, combined with a gastric drainage procedure (pyloroplasty or gastrojejunostomy). A selective vagotomy divides and severs the vagus nerve branches that supply the parietal cells while preserving those that innervate the antrum and pylorus. Because of this, a gastric drainage procedure is unnecessary.[1] A PG as treatment for cancer is similar to a BII but only denervates the part of the vagus nerve associated with the resected area of the stomach.

Roux-en-Y Total Gastric Resection

TG is performed for gastric malignancies that affect the middle or upper part of the stomach. The entire stomach is resected, and standard reconstruction is usually via the Roux-en-Y method. Doubling the end of the Roux limb is sometimes used to create a "stomach pouch." The Roux limb is of sufficient length so that the esophageal anastomosis will be at least 40 cm above the subsequent jejunojejunostomy.[2] Diagrams of the various procedures are available elsewhere.[3] TG, by nature, involves a functional vagotomy, removing cholinergic drive and eliminating acid production.

Nutritional Assessment

Weight loss of 10% to 30% of preoperative weight is not uncommon following PG and TG.[4] Reasons for this loss are multifactorial and are often attributed to insufficient oral intake, malabsorption, rapid intestinal transit time, and bacterial overgrowth.[5] Nevertheless, weight gain after surgery is possible.[6] Nutritional assessment should focus on actual dietary intake and weight history. Specifically, the clinician should ask about postprandial complaints, including early satiety, epigastric fullness, nausea, vomiting, symptoms of dumping syndrome (DS), diarrhea (steatorrhea), or lactose intolerance.

Postgastrectomy Syndrome

Postgastrectomy syndrome encompasses nutritional intolerances and deficiencies. The most common intolerances include early satiety, DS, fat maldigestion, gastric stasis, and lactose intolerance. Specific nutrient deficiencies develop months to years after gastric resections, often resulting in serious consequences. Anemia and bone disease are the most common manifestations of nutrient deficiencies seen in patients who have undergone gastric resections. Rarer postgastrectomy symptoms include afferent and efferent limb syndrome, alkaline reflux gastritis, and postvagotomy diarrhea.

Dumping Syndrome

Loss of the gastric reservoir, altered secretion of GI hormones, and accelerated gastric emptying of hyperosmolar contents into the proximal small bowel resulting in release of vasoactive hormones contribute to DS.[7] DS can be divided into early and late symptoms. Early dumping occurs within approximately 30 minutes of eating when hyperosmotic fluids enter the small bowel and cause rapid fluid shifts.[8] Symptoms associated with early dumping include abdominal cramping, nausea, diarrhea, and palpitations. In contrast, late dumping occurs up to 3 hours after eating and is characterized by symptoms typically associated with hypoglycemia. Late dumping syndrome results from rapid absorption of simple sugars in the small bowel, which triggers an exaggerated release of insulin resulting in a reactive hypoglycemia. Patients complain of sweating, dizziness, tachycardia, irritability, hunger, and syncopal symptoms. The percentage of patients who develop DS after gastrectomy has been reported to range from 1% to 75%.[4] DS symptoms are more prevalent in the immediate postoperative period and frequently resolve over time.[9] Approximately 1% of patients will develop persistent, debilitating symptoms.[10] DS unresponsive to diet manipulation may require use of gut-slowing medication.[9] Guidelines for an antidumping diet can be found in Table 26-1.

Fat Maldigestion

Exocrine pancreatic insufficiency and increased fecal fat excretion (steatorrhea) have been demonstrated following both PG and TG.[5] The etiology of fat malabsorption is multifactorial. First, an accelerated transit time prevents sufficient mixing of food with digestive enzymes and bile salts. Second, decreased enzyme production reduces the ratio of enzymes to food.[11] Finally, before loss of the distal stomach, and hence its sieving function, larger-than-normal food particles empty into the jejunum, making their degradation by enzymes more difficult.[12] The addition of exogenous pancreatic enzymes has been shown to reduce fecal fat excretion in some patients.[13] Prolonged steatorrhea may necessitate monitoring and replacement of fat-soluble vitamins.[9]

Gastric Stasis

Three to five percent of patients with truncal vagotomy are reported to experience problems with gastric stasis. Poor

TABLE 26-1 Antidumping Diet Guidelines[3]

- Eat six or more small meals a day.
- Eat slowly, and chew all foods thoroughly.
- Sit upright while eating.
- Avoid or limit high sugar foods and beverages including the following:
  - Kool-aid, juice, soda, Ensure (Ross Products, Abbott Park, IL), Boost (Novartis, Basel, Switzerland), cakes, pies, candy, doughnuts, cookies, etc.
- Limit fluid consumption at meals. Drink liquids 30 to 60 minutes either before or after meals.
- Eat a protein-containing food with each meal. High-protein foods include the following: eggs, meat, poultry, fish, lunch meat, nuts, milk, yogurt, cottage cheese, cheese, peanut butter, dried beans, lentils, and tofu.
- If you have difficulty maintaining your weight, you may need to drink a nutritional supplement for extra calories. You can try low-sugar over-the-counter supplements. These include no-sugar-added Carnation Instant Breakfast, sugar-free Nutrishakes, or Glucerna weight loss shakes; lactose-free products are also available.
- Choose high-fiber foods when possible. These include whole wheat bread, fruits, vegetables, and beans (pinto, black, brown, kidney).

emptying may manifest as postprandial bloating, discomfort, or fullness lasting many hours. Emesis of undigested food consumed hours to days before may also be present. These patients are at a higher risk for bezoar formation, bacterial overgrowth, and intolerance to solid food. Liquids may be processed normally or rapidly.[12] Diet manipulation and/or prokinetic drugs may be effective to varying degrees (see section on gastroparesis).

Lactose Intolerance

Lactase, the enzyme required for lactose absorption, is found primarily on villi in the jejunum.[14] Most gastrectomized patients have an intact jejunum. Patients complaining of abdominal cramping or pain, bloating, diarrhea, flatulence, and distention after consumption of lactose may benefit from decreasing or avoiding it in the diet. Tolerance to lactose is typically dose dependent and may improve over time.[14]

Afferent Limb Syndrome, Alkaline Reflux Gastritis, and Postvagotomy Diarrhea

Gastrojejunostomy reconstruction with a BII reconstruction results in the formation of an afferent and efferent limb of the small bowel attached to the gastric remnant. In rare cases, the afferent limb, which drains the biliary system, can become obstructed due to malpositioning, stricture, radiation enteritis, or adhesions.[15] Afferent limb syndrome is a late-term complication of partial gastrectomy where the afferent limb is positioned in a dependent position, allowing it to fill with food during a meal. A dilated afferent limb on imaging is diagnostic, and symptoms of pain and cramping are attributed to limb distension. Patients describe relief with vomiting which temporarily clears or decompresses the afferent limb. Treatment usually consists of surgical revision.

Alkaline reflux gastritis can occur after BII reconstruction because the bile stream must pass through the anastomosis of gastrojejunostomy to reach the efferent limb. Bile salts are irritating to the gastric and esophageal mucosa. Patients often complain of dyspepsia and bile reflux. Evidence of gastritis and esophagitis are seen on endoscopic exam. Treatment is generally conservative as with other cases of gastritis and should include an empiric trial of cholestyramine, which binds bile salts. Surgical reconstruction could be considered in refractory cases.[16]

Postvagotomy diarrhea results from unclear mechanisms in patients who have undergone a truncal vagotomy. A study looking at patients who had undergone vagotomy found an increased incidence of diarrhea after fluid meals and a significant decrease in intestinal motility in response to dry meals.[11] Treatment is conservative.

General Treatment Principles after Gastrectomy

Although diet therapy may be beneficial in treating nutritional intolerances, it is important to minimize diet restrictions and encourage frequent tolerable meals. Undue restrictions can further aggravate weight loss. If weight loss persists, despite dietary management, nonelemental enteral feedings for supplemental nutrition should be initiated. In cases where a small gastric remnant precludes gastrostomy tube placement, a surgically or endoscopically placed jejunostomy tube may be considered. PN should be used only as a last resort.

Nutrient Deficiencies

Anemia

Nutritional anemias, resulting from vitamin B_{12}, folate, or iron deficiency, are common in patients with gastric resections. Because consequences of anemia can be severe, baseline and periodic monitoring are important. Patients with a distant history of gastric resection may be at greater risk because anemia often presents as a late complication.

Pernicious Anemia

Megaloblastic anemia results from either vitamin B_{12} or folate deficiency. B_{12} deficiency in patients with a history of gastric resection can occur for several reasons. In the patient with unaltered anatomy, intrinsic factor is complexed to B_{12} and facilitates its absorption by the terminal ileum. A lack of intrinsic factor from the stomach and overall reduced gastric acidity in gastrectomized patients impairs cleavage of protein bound B_{12} and its attachment to intrinsic factor.[1] Bacterial overgrowth and reduced intake of B_{12}-rich foods may also contribute to a deficiency. The incidence of B_{12} deficiency has been reported in patients with PG (10% to 43%) and TG (theoretically 100%). Although deficiencies have been found as early as 1 year postoperatively, they are more common in the late postoperative state.[4] Clinical features, while useful in the diagnosis of megaloblastic anemia, can often be nonspecific or absent in some patients[17]; therefore, periodic serum monitoring and supplementation of B_{12} is prudent. Measuring metabolic intermediaries such as methylmalonic acid and homocysteine concurrently with B_{12} monitoring may lead to higher sensitivity in detecting early deficiency.[18] A study investigating the effects of either oral or intramuscular B_{12} supplementation in patients with TG found that enteral B_{12} treatment increased serum concentration rapidly.[19] Symptom resolution was comparable in patients who received enteral or parenteral supplementation. It is possible that the body adapts after TG and may produce intrinsic factor in the duodenum and jejunum.[19] The decision to supplement B_{12} orally or via intramuscular injection should be based on expected patient compliance. It may be prudent to start with intramuscular injections initially when neurologic function is impaired or until compliance has been established.

Folate Deficiency

Folate deficiency may develop after gastric surgery but is not well studied. Causes of folate deficiency likely include malabsorption and impaired digestion.[12] Folate is absorbed in the proximal small bowel. Tests for serum folate represent short-term balance and fluctuate according to meals. Red blood cell folate (*not* serum folate) represents long-term balance and more accurately reflects body stores. A daily dose of 5 mg folate is recommended in deficiency states. The 100 mcg dose supplied in a daily multivitamin should be sufficient for maintenance.[19]

Iron Deficiency

Iron deficiency is the most common anemia following gastric resection.[12] The reported incidence varies tremendously. Alterations in digestion and absorption are thought to be responsible for iron deficiency in patients with TG and PG. The duodenum, the primary site for iron absorption, is bypassed (except in BI), and reduced gastric acidity impairs the conversion of ferric iron to the more absorbable ferrous form.[12] Poor iron intake may also play a role. In a multistudy review by Fischer, 5% to 62% of patients with BII were found to be iron deficient.[20] Indeed, at 10 years post gastrectomy, iron deficiency was noted to be the most frequent nutrient deficiency.[4] Iron deficiency may manifest more quickly in BII procedures, as compared with BI operations, presumably because of lack of duodenal continuity with the BII procedure.[21] Ferritin levels in the nonacute-phase setting are an accurate indicator of iron stores.[17] Guidelines for iron repletion are available elsewhere.[3]

Metabolic Bone Disease

Bone disease, as osteoporosis, osteopenia, or osteomalacia, is commonly reported in patients with PG or TG. The prevalence of metabolic bone disease, defined as having a low bone mineral density (BMD), is approximately 27% to 44%.[22,23] The etiology of metabolic disease in gastrectomy patients is poorly understood. Bone remodeling occurs throughout a patient's lifetime, and appropriate bone mass and strength is maintained through a closely regulated homeostatic relationship between bone reabsorption and formation.[24] Bone disease is usually attributed to decreased formation of new bone, often as a result of vitamin and mineral deficiency. However, an increased rate of bone reabsorption can also result in net bone loss. For example, one study found that osteomalacia was present in up to 18% of patients with PG despite the finding that the majority of these patients had normal serum calcium, alkaline phosphatase, and 25-hydroxyvitamin D (25-OHD) levels.[25] Homeostatic dysregulation, in addition to impaired mineral and vitamin absorption, may play an important role in the development of metabolic bone disease after gastric resection.[24] Because of these findings, it has been postulated that older studies relying solely on laboratory values have underestimated the prevalence of osteomalacia in gastric resection patients.[22] Klein et al. found that vertebral body fractures were three times as common in men who had undergone a BII procedure when compared to controls.[25] It is important to note that age and bone status at the time of surgery play a role in overall bone disease independent of gastric resection, and most patients who undergo gastric resection are older.

However, patients who have undergone gastric resection are at higher risk of malabsorption despite their age. The loss of the duodenal surface area, an increased transit time, and alterations in diet all play a role in the development of malnutrition after gastrectomy.[26] Some patients may require dietary supplementation to overcome the effects of malnutrition. One study demonstrated an increase in 25-OHD when patients with TG and PG were supplemented with 400 IU of vitamin D daily.[26] Another study found statistically significant increases in 25-OHD in patients with PG supplemented with 400 to 600 IU of vitamin D_2.[22] Currently, there are no accepted supplementation guidelines for calcium and vitamin D in postgastrectomy states. For patients with bone disease, 1500 mg of calcium and 800 IU of vitamin D daily is recommended. Patients should be encouraged to include calcium-rich foods in their diet as tolerated.

Dual energy x-ray absorptiometry provides an inexpensive, reproducible method to determine BMD.[27] It is reasonable to monitor BMD, even in the setting of normal laboratory values, at baseline and then every 1 to 2 years. Prompt initiation of antiresorptive agents (calcium, vitamin D, calcitonin, and bisphosphonates) and bone-formation agents (recombinant parathyroid hormone) may need to be considered in severe cases. Continuous nutrition assessment and intervention is an effective tool to prevent or minimize dietary intolerances and manifestations of nutrient deficiencies. Table 26-2 provides a summary of nutrition management guidelines following gastric resection. A more comprehensive review on managing the nutrition consequences following gastrectomy is available elsewhere.[3]

Pancreaticoduodenectomy (Whipple Procedure)

Limited literature exists for the nutrition care of patients with pancreatic cancer. Survival statistics for patients with pancreatic cancer are grim. The 5-year survival for patients with stage IA cancer is 31.4%; for stage IV, it is 4.5%.[28] Tumor resection offers the best chance of survival and varies depending on tumor location. However, the most common procedure is the pancreaticoduodenectomy (Whipple procedure). The conventional Whipple involves removal of the distal stomach, gallbladder, common bile duct, portion of the duodenum, and usually the head of the pancreas. Today, the preferred variation on the procedure is the pylorus-preserving pancreaticoduodenectomy. This procedure preserves the entire stomach, pylorus, and a 2-cm piece of the duodenum, thus maintaining a more normal GI tract.

Delayed gastric emptying is the most common complication after a Whipple procedure, but weight loss, dumping syndrome, diabetes mellitus, and malabsorption due to pancreatic exocrine insufficiency may also occur.[29] The pathophysiological mechanisms that are involved in gastric stagnation are multifactorial and not fully understood. Patients experiencing delayed gastric emptying often require a nasogastric tube because of intractable nausea and vomiting. Treating acid hypersecretion with a proton pump inhibitor (PPI; versus an H_2 receptor antagonist) postoperatively can significantly improve gastric stagnation.[30] Pharmacological treatment with prokinetic agents is also common. Pancreatic exocrine deficiency usually presents with steatorrhea, but DS and bile salt diarrhea can complicate the diagnosis. Measurements of fecal fat as well as fecal elastase can aid in the diagnosis. In patients who develop pancreatic enzyme deficiency, pancreatic enzyme replacement therapy with periodic testing of fat-soluble vitamin levels may be warranted. Nutrient deficiencies and

TABLE 26-2 Summary of Nutrition Management Guidelines Following Gastric Resection[3]

Maintain Optimal Nutritional Status
• Determine cause(s) of weight loss through careful diet history • Provide diet education to minimize symptoms of dumping syndrome and lactose intolerance, if present • Daily multivitamin with minerals • Additional calcium and vitamin D supplementation as warranted • Continued nutrition intervention for at-risk patients
Treat Fat Malabsorption
• Determine if steatorrhea present (ensure patient consuming ≥ 100 g fat/day when checking qualitative or quantitative fecal fat) • Consider use of pancreatic enzymes • Use gut-slowing agents if needed • Treat bacterial overgrowth if present • Monitor and supplement fat soluble vitamins as needed • Daily multivitamin with minerals
Prevent Nutritional Anemias
• Monitor – Vitamin B_{12} – Red blood cell folate – Ferritin • Supplement as needed
Prevent and Treat Metabolic Bone Disease
• Monitor 25-hydroxyvitamin D – 1,25-dihydroxyvitamin D *is not* a good indicator of vitamin D status (it can be normal, high, or low in vitamin D deficiency—the most commonly used and most sensitive index is 25-hydroxyvitamin D). • Supplement with 1500 mg of calcium – 500 mg doses three times a day – 800 IU vitamin D daily • Monitor bone mineral density (dual-energy x-ray absorptiometry scan) • Evaluate need for antiresorptive and bone formation agents
Gastric Stasis
• Treat bezoars[25] • Treat bacterial overgrowth[24] • Treat gastroparesis[27]

nutrient guidelines post-Whipple procedure are similar to those found in patients who have undergone gastrectomy.[3]

Gastroparesis

Gastroparesis (GP), or delayed gastric emptying, is also known as gastric stasis or diabetic gastropathy or enteropathy (in patients with diabetes mellitus). GP has many origins (Table 26-3), although the most common are diabetes mellitus, postvagotomy syndrome, postviral GP, and narcotics or other agents that slow motility. Clinically, GP will wax and wane, depending on the underlying etiology.

Symptoms of GP (Table 26-4) range from mild to severely debilitating, and even life-threatening. In severe cases, patients can develop severe dehydration and electrolyte imbalances such as hypokalemia and hypochloremia. Glucose control can worsen. Patients with protracted nausea and vomiting often require an alternate means of nutrition and hydration to combat weight loss and dehydration. During this period, early nutritional support can reverse significant malnutrition. In fact, many patients with refractory GP related to postviral or posttraumatic syndrome that initially requires enteral feeding eventually resume adequate oral intake.[28] Patients presenting with clinical symptoms of GP (especially when coupled with one of the conditions listed in Table 26-3) should be evaluated for altered gastric motility. Motility agents such as metoclopramide, erythromycin, and domperidone (not approved by the U.S. Food and Drug Administration for use in the United States) are used with limited success. It is important to review a patient's medication list whenever GP is suspected. Numerous drugs, including the now widespread use of narcotics, can result in GP. Colonic inertia and pelvic floor dyssynergia can result in severe constipation that can also lead to GP which can be easily reversed with initiation of a bowel regimen.

In patients undergoing a gastric emptying study, a 4-hour solid-phase gastric scintigraphic study is recommended. Liquid-phase emptying can actually be accelerated in patients with diabetes or neuropathy, leading to a false negative test. Patients must be off motility-slowing agents and undergo a sufficient washout period for the test to be valid. International control values using a low-fat meal have been established.[31] Gastric retention of > 10% of the test meal at 4 hours is indicative of delayed gastric emptying. In some situations, symptoms may be present with or without delayed gastric emptying. Regardless, many clinicians treat based on a patient's symptoms, especially when the patient is faced with nutritional compromise. General conservative measures include counseling on maintaining a food log; small frequent meals per day (usually six); intake of low residue foods that are easily cleared from the stomach such as ground meats, starches, and liquids; and avoidance of foods that are more difficult to clear such as fatty foods, raw vegetables, and fruits that are high in insoluble fibers.

Nutritional Assessment

Nutritional screening and evaluation of the patient with GP will help to distinguish the adequately nourished patient who can tolerate further GI evaluation from a malnourished patient who requires immediate nutritional support. Unintentional weight loss over time is probably the most important noninvasive parameter by which to determine overall nutritional status. A thorough diet history can help identify those patients for whom diet manipulation may be advantageous. For example, a patient who develops nausea while eating three large meals per day may benefit by simply instituting smaller,

TABLE 26-3 Clinical Conditions Associated With Gastroparesis[31,32]

Mechanical Obstruction	Metabolic/Endocrine Disorders
Duodenal ulcer Pancreatic carcinoma or pseudocyst Gastric carcinoma Superior mesenteric artery syndrome	Diabetes mellitus Hypothyroidism Hyperthyroidism Hyperparathyroidism Adrenal insufficiency (Addison disease)
Acid-Peptic Disease	**Gastritis**
Gastric ulcer Gastroesophageal reflux disease	Atrophic gastritis Viral gastroenteritis
Postgastric Surgery	**Disorders of Gastric Smooth Muscle**
Vagotomy Antrectomy Subtotal gastrectomy Roux-en-Y gastrojejunostomy Fundoplication	Scleroderma Polymyositis Muscular dystrophy Amyloidosis Chronic idiopathic pseudo-obstruction Dermatomyositis Systemic lupus erythematosus
Psychogenic Disorders	**Neuropathic Disorders**
Anorexia Bulimia Depression	Parkinson disease Paraneoplastic syndrome Central nervous system disorders High cervical cord lesions (C4 and above)

more frequent meals. In contrast, the patient with severe GP who has significant vomiting after ingestion of water may require gastric decompression and enteral jejunal feeding to provide symptom relief, nutrients, fluids, and medications. When obtaining a diet history, be sure to evaluate for:

- Changes in appetite and nausea/vomiting/diarrhea
- Problems chewing and/or swallowing, which can affect one's ability to ingest certain foods
- The patient's typical daily dietary intake
- The use of supplemental nutrition (oral, enteral, or parenteral)
- Food intolerances or allergies
- Use of supplements, such as vitamins, minerals, herbs, or protein powders
- Use of stool-bulking agents or laxatives
- History of severe constipation
- Medications known to slow gastric emptying (Table 26-5)

TABLE 26-4 Clinical Symptoms of Gastroparesis

- Decreased appetite/anorexia
- Nausea and vomiting
- Bloating
- Fullness (especially in the morning after an overnight fast)
- Early satiety
- Halitosis
- Postprandial hypoglycemia or fluctuating glucose levels in an otherwise well-controlled patient with diabetes mellitus

Used with permission. University of Virginia Health System, Nutrition Support Traineeship Syllabus; Charlottesville, VA; Updated July 2010 @ www.ginutrition.virginia.edu.

Laboratory Data

Intolerance to various foods, as well as malabsorption, can lead to nutrient deficiencies. While intolerances can often be managed with dietary manipulation, nutrient deficiencies—particularly those resulting in anemia and metabolic bone disease—require ongoing monitoring and supplementation.

Serum Glucose and Hemoglobin A1C

Hyperglycemia—especially if widely fluctuating—can cause transient GP in some patients; however, this delayed emptying responds to normalization of serum glucose levels.[32,33] In addition, hyperglycemia has been shown to attenuate the prokinetic effect of erythromycin.[34] Glycemic control must be evaluated at the initial nutritional assessment and monitored continually. Periodic monitoring of glycosylated hemoglobin ensures that optimal glucose control is maintained.

Ferritin

Iron-deficiency anemia is common in this patient population, and the etiology is likely multifactorial. First, many patients with GP limit iron-rich food (ie, red meat) because of intolerance. Second, acid reflux, often associated with GP, is commonly treated with acid-suppressive medications such as PPIs. This reduced gastric acidity impairs the conversion of dietary ferric iron to the more absorbable ferrous form.[12] Third, elevated gastric pH and poor motility can increase the risk of developing small bowel bacterial overgrowth, which can significantly decrease duodenal iron absorption.

Iron deficiency must be carefully monitored in patients receiving jejunal EN because the duodenum (the primary site for iron absorption) is bypassed.[12] While ferritin is an accurate indicator of iron stores over time, it is an acute-phase reactant and should therefore be checked in the nonacute setting.[17] Oral iron supplementation is the preferred method of replacement and is available as ferrous sulfate, gluconate, or fumarate.[9] Iron is constipating, and attention to symptoms and prompt treatment is important to prevent worsening symptoms. Taking iron with a beverage containing vitamin C, which is acidic, will enhance iron absorption.[35]

TABLE 26-5 Medications Known to Delay Gastric Emptying[32,35]

Aluminum-containing antacids	Diphenhydramine	Narcotics
Anticholinergics	Ethanol	Nicotine
Atropine	Glucagon	Potassium salts
Beta-agonists	Interleukin-1	Progesterone
Calcitonin	L-Dopa	Sucralfate
Calcium channel blockers	Lithium	Tricyclic antidepressants
Dexfenfluramine	Octreotide	Selective serotonin reuptake inhibitors
	Ondansetron	

Vitamin B12

Some patients with GP have a history of gastric resection and therefore are at risk for vitamin B_{12} deficiency (see gastric resections). Clinical features of B_{12} deficiency are nonspecific and often absent in deficient patients. Baseline and periodic monitoring, in addition to supplementation when necessary, are therefore important.

Vitamin D

Osteoporosis affects patients with GP and with a history of subtotal gastrectomy. Evaluation of 25-OHD levels (*not* 1,25-OHD vitamin D) and BMD is important. After vitamin D is absorbed by the intestine, it is rapidly converted to 25-OHD in the liver. In vitamin D-deficient states, calcium levels drop resulting in hyperparathyroidism and the release of parathyroid hormone, which increases the rate at which the limited 25-OHD is converted to 1,25-OHD. As a result, calcium bone loss increases despite the finding of a normal level of 1,25-OHD. Patients with bone disease are recommended to take 1500 mg of elemental calcium and 800 IU of vitamin D daily. To maximize absorption, calcium should be administered in single doses no greater than 500 mg.

Factors That Influence Gastric Emptying

Volume of food consumed, liquids versus solids, medications, hyperglycemia, fiber, fat, and osmolality are all factors that may affect gastric emptying. However, their *clinical significance* has yet to be proved in prospective, randomized, controlled trials. A patient's diet history can help determine which factors may respond the most to dietary manipulation. Modifying one or two parameters at a given time will prevent an overzealous intervention that often results in unnecessary dietary limitations.

Factors That Can Affect Oral Intake

Nausea and Vomiting

Empiric trials of antiemetics and prokinetic agents can be used to attempt to reduce symptoms in patients with significant nausea and vomiting.[36,37] Scheduled dosing (versus as-needed dosages) and liquid preparations or alternate dosing methods such as suppositories provide the most consistent symptom control. Special attention is warranted when using prokinetic agents. Metoclopramide (Reglan) now carries a black-box warning because of its association with tardive dyskinesia that may not resolve on discontinuation of the drug. Intravenous erythromycin has been used off-label as a prokinetic; however, the drug quickly loses effectiveness and can only be used for short periods of time. High doses are associated with macrolide toxicity including hearing loss, a prolonged QT-interval, and antibiotic resistance. Cisapride (Propulsid) has been associated with ventricular arrhythmias and as a result is now only available in the United States through an investigational limited access program through Janssen Pharmaceuticals. Domperidone (Motillium) is not approved for use in the United States. The U.S. Food and Drug Administration recommends that physicians who wish to prescribe domperidone for patients with refractory GP establish an investigational new drug application. Information is available by contacting the U.S. Food and Drug Administration directly.

Small Bowel Bacterial Overgrowth

Patients with GP are at a high risk of developing small bowel bacterial overgrowth (SBBO)[38] (see section on SBBO).

Bezoar Formation

Bezoars, which are retained concretions of indigestible foreign material, accumulate in the stomach and may be caused by nondigestible food material (phytobezoars) or medications (pharmacobezoars). Patients with altered GI motility are at an increased risk for bezoar formation. The symptoms associated with bezoars often mimic those of GP: patients may present with early satiety, nausea, and vomiting. Fiber intake and some medications have been implicated in the formation of bezoars.[28] Treatment of gastric phytobezoars includes enzymatic therapies such as cellulase and lavage with or without endoscopic intervention.[39] Infusions of Coca Cola™ or acetylcysteine have also appeared effective in case studies.[40–43] Use of meat tenderizer that contains papain—a protease with broad activity—has been reported in the literature, but because it breaks down normal tissue, its use is associated with peptic ulcer disease, esophagitis, and gastritis, and it should be avoided. Long-term prokinetic therapy to treat and prevent bezoar formation may also be beneficial. In refractory cases, surgery to remove the bezoar provides definitive treatment.

Nutritional Management

Oral Nutrition Guidelines

Patients and clinicians alike prefer nutrition via the oral route. If the patient is not malnourished, a trial of dietary manipulation in the patient with GP is worthwhile (Table 26-6). Patients should keep a food diary to provide a more objective

TABLE 26-6 Summary of Oral Nutrition Intervention in the Patient With Gastroparesis

1. Advise patients to eat smaller, more frequent meals.
2. Use more liquid calories.
   - If solid foods cause increased symptoms, begin with a liquid/puréed diet to promote gastric emptying.
   - If symptoms increase over the course of the day, try solid food meals in the morning, switching to more liquid meals later in the day.
   - Chew foods well.
   - Suggest that the patient sit up during meals and for 1 to 2 hours afterward.
3. Glucose control:
   - If gastroparesis is a result of diabetes mellitus, maximize glucose control.
   - Monitor the need to change the timing of, or the overall requirements for, insulin in order to have consistent delivery of nutrients with optimal total calories ingested.
   - Expect an increase in insulin requirements because improved symptom control will likely result in an increase in total calories ingested.
   - In general, dietary restrictions (eg, diabetic or heart healthy diets) should be lifted during the trial.
4. Medications:
   - Prokinetics and antiemetics should be given in regular scheduled doses (rather than "as-needed" doses) and may be best tolerated in liquid form.
   - Avoid use of medications that alter gastric motility (Table 26-5).
   - Review and delete any "unnecessary" meds (they can always be added back later).
5. Fat:
   - Fat in liquids should be tolerated; so before restricting them, implement steps 1 to 4.
6. Fiber
   - Fiber, fermented by short bowel bacterial obstruction if present, may cause gas, cramping, and bloating, aggravating symptoms of gastroparesis.
   - If bezoar formation is a concern, avoid the following high-fiber foods and medications:
     - Oranges, persimmons, coconuts, berries, green beans, figs, apples, sauerkraut, brussels sprouts, potato peels, and legumes.
   - Fiber supplements such as Metamucil, Perdiem, Benefiber, Fibercon, Citrucel, etc.
7. Treat bacterial overgrowth if suspected/symptomatic.
8. Monitor and replace as needed: iron, vitamin B_{12}, vitamin D, and calcium.
   - If the patient is significantly malnourished, a daily standard vitamin/mineral elixir can be used for 1 month or longer or until stores are replete.
   - If patient has gastric intolerance to iron, try smaller doses; some is better than none. Liquid iron may be a better choice in some patients. Consider giving iron with vitamin C.

Used with permission. University of Virginia Health System, Nutrition Support Traineeship Syllabus; Charlottesville, VA; Updated July 2010 @ www.ginutrition.virginia.edu.

determination of actual oral intake. It is prudent to define a target weight goal and the timeframe over which this must be achieved. If weight gain is achieved through diet manipulation, continue oral nutrition. If weight gain is not achieved, proceed to EN support. Comprehensive oral dietary suggestions for GP patients are also available at www.medicine.virginia.edu/clinical/departments/medicine/divisions/digestive-health/nutrition-support-team/patient-education.

Enteral Nutrition

When significant malnutrition prevails in spite of maximal diet manipulation, a trial of EN should be pursued. Most clinicians prefer a trial of nasojejunal feeding before endoscopically or surgically placed enteral access in order to rule out chronic idiopathic intestinal pseudo-obstruction. Unfortunately, it is not uncommon for refractory patients to dislodge the nasojejunal tube with a bout of emesis. Nasogastric-jejunal tubes, which allow gastric venting concomitantly with jejunal feedings, are also used; however, patient acceptance of these tubes is poor because of discomfort caused by the tube's large diameter. Patients should remain on nothing by mouth orders during initiation of EN until tolerance is established. This will prevent intolerance to oral intake from being mistaken as EN intolerance. Finally, in patients with significant weight loss, clinicians should anticipate refeeding syndrome and initiate EN judiciously.[44]

Long-term jejunal access can be achieved by various methods including percutaneous endoscopic gastrostomy-jejunostomy, separate venting percutaneous endoscopic gastrostomy (PEG) with a percutaneous endoscopic jejunostomy, or a surgical jejunostomy. Motility specialists do not agree on the best approach to feed these patients—clinical trials are greatly needed in this area to determine if one technique is better than others with regard to patient preference, symptom improvement, and complications. A more in-depth discussion is available elsewhere.[28]

Formula Selection/Delivery

The majority of patients—including those with diabetes mellitus—tolerate standard, polymeric formulas based on available research to date (see Chapter 11).[45] Because the stomach is bypassed, a formula that contains fiber may be tolerated; however, indigestible fiber may aggravate symptoms if SBBO is a chronic problem. Powdered pancreatic enzymes can be added to enteral feedings or dosed periodically during infusion in those patients with a PG and poor mixing of tube feeding with pancreatic enzymes.

The small bowel is volume sensitive and generally does not tolerate bolus feeding. Jejunal feeding may be administered via a cycled pump or gravity infusion, typically over 8 to 14 hours. Enteral feedings need not be diluted; the flow rate can be increased from 125 mL to 160 mL per hour as tolerated; some patients may tolerate rates even > 160 mL per hour.

Intolerance of jejunal EN is variable in patients with GP. Often, the side effects associated with EN can be explained physiologically and are relatively simple to resolve.[46] See Table 26-7 for summary and problem-solving guidelines for enteral intervention.

Parenteral Nutrition

PN is rarely necessary for the patient with GP and should be considered a last resort for patients with a functional GI tract distal to the stomach. Exceptions include patients with chronic intestinal pseudo-obstruction, end-stage scleroderma, or other dysmotility disorders that include both the small bowel and the stomach.

Additional Resources

For an excellent patient and professional resource for GP see the GP and Dysmotilities Association at http://digestivedistress.com. In addition, a consensus document on the diagnosis and treatment of GP is available.[37]

Small Bowel and Colon

Small Bowel Bacterial Overgrowth

A wide variety of bacteria colonize the small intestine. Ordinarily, the concentration of bacteria in the small bowel is significantly lower than that found in the colon. A number of factors prevent the overgrowth of bacteria within the small intestine including gastric acid, intestinal peristalsis, the ileocecal valve, bile acids, the enteric immune system, and pancreatic enzyme secretion.[38] Clinical conditions that impair one or more of these defenses may allow bacteria to proliferate within the small bowel (Table 26-8). SBBO was traditionally thought to occur primarily in the setting of surgical blind loops, small bowel diverticula, or in small bowel motility disorders. However, research has demonstrated that SBBO is common in the setting of diarrhea-predominant irritable bowel syndrome, end-stage liver disease, pancreatic insufficiency, and even in end-stage kidney failure.[47–51]

Bacterial colonization of the small bowel results in deconjugation of bile salts and impaired micelle formation, resulting in fat malabsorption. Intestinal bacteria also compete with the host for available nutrients. SBBO can produce an inflammatory

TABLE 26-7 Enteral Nutrition Summary and Problem-Solving Suggestions for the Patient With Gastroparesis

- Use standard, polymeric formulas.
- If there is a high suspicion of oral intake, we ask our patients to tell us what, rather than if, they are eating and drinking on a daily basis.
- Reiterate periods of strict nothing by mouth status (except for a few ice chips) during initiation of EN to avoid confusing oral intolerance with EN intolerance, until tube feeding tolerance is established.
- If the patient experiences increased nausea/vomiting after initiating EN, try decreasing the rate of infusion for a few days (this could be from the ileal brake).
- Maximize the use of liquid prokinetic agents and antiemetics with delivery via the jejunostomy tube (scheduled versus as-needed dosing and liquid preparations may be beneficial). Gastric delivery of medications in a patient requiring gastric decompression will be ineffective.
- Consider enteral treatment of bacterial overgrowth utilizing antibiotics given via the jejunostomy tube.
- If bacterial overgrowth is a chronic problem, try a nonfiber-containing formula.
- Check tube placement—specifically for backward migration of a jejunostomy tube into the stomach.
- Seek to reposition the tube.
- If nausea and vomiting increase after the placement of a surgical jejunostomy tube (assuming it has an internal bumper) and ileus is ruled out, a fluoroscopic study with oral contrast (swallowed, not administered via the jejunostomy tube) can determine if the internal balloon is obstructing the lumen.
- Decreasing the volume of saline in the balloon will alleviate the mechanical obstruction.
- Use a more calorically dense formula to decrease total volume of EN required to meet calorie needs. *Note:* Be sure to increase hydration with more calorically dense tube-feeding formulas.
- Maximize glucose control (glucose levels > 200 mg/dL may aggravate gastroparesis).

EN, enteral nutrition.
Used with permission. University of Virginia Health System, Nutrition Support Traineeship Syllabus; Charlottesville, VA; Updated July 2010 @ www.ginutrition.virginia.edu.

TABLE 26-8 Patients at Risk for Bacterial Overgrowth

Anatomic defects
Duodenal or jejunal diverticula
Strictures/obstructions/adhesions/cancer
Gastrocolic/jejunal-colic fistulas
Vagotomy
Resection of ileocecal valve
Surgical blind loops (Billroth II, Roux-en-Y, total gastrectomy, Whipple, etc.)
Segmented dilation of the ileum
Leiomyosarcoma
Motility disorders
Diabetic autonomic neuropathy
Gastroparesis
Diabetes mellitus
Intestinal pseudo-obstruction
Intestinal stasis
Fibrosis of the intestinal wall
Scleroderma
Radiation enteritis
Irritable bowel syndrome
Amyloidosis
Reduced mucosal defense mechanism
Hypochlorhydria/achlorhydria
Atrophic gastritis
Loss of ileocecal valve
Immune deficiency syndrome
Mucosal disease (Crohn's, etc.)
Pancreatic insufficiency
Other
Drug-induced (proton pump inhibitors, narcotics, etc.)
Cirrhosis
Pancreatitis
Cystic fibrosis
Hypothyroidism

Used with permission. University of Virginia Health System, Nutrition Support Traineeship Syllabus; Charlottesville, VA; Updated July 2010 @ www.ginutrition.virginia.edu.

process that impairs nutrient absorption or can cause a protein-losing enteropathy (PLE).[52] Bacterial metabolism produces short-chain fatty acids (SCFAs). SCFAs may decrease luminal pH, denature intestinal enzymes, and increase the overall osmotic load. The result is rapid gut transit, maldigestion, and malabsorption.

The symptoms of SBBO include gas, bloating, abdominal distension/discomfort, nausea, diarrhea, weight loss, and an overall decline in nutritional status. The possibility of SBBO is often underappreciated in patients with other GI pathology. Testing for and treatment of SBBO should be considered in those patients who have persistent GI symptomatology despite adequate therapy of their primary GI disorder.

Diagnosing Small Bowel Bacterial Overgrowth

A noninvasive hydrogen breath test is one way to assay for SBBO. The patient is administered an oral sugar load (either lactulose or glucose); a characteristic delayed release of hydrogen from the bacterial fermentation of the sugar is diagnostic of bacterial overgrowth of the small bowel. Unfortunately, not all hospitals have the capability to perform this test.[53] Also, up to 15% of the population do not harbor the bacteria required to produce hydrogen. In contrast, radiolabeled carbon incorporated into xylose can be used, and the release of labeled carbon dioxide in the patient's breath is diagnostic of SBBO. However, this is a more involved technique and fewer facilities have this testing capability. The traditional gold standard test for bacterial overgrowth is an ileal aspirate and culture. However, this is invasive and requires special culture methods. In practice, it is not uncommon for clinicians to empirically treat for SBBO based on symptoms, and an underlying diagnosis that would predispose the patient to SBBO.

Treatment

Enteral antibiotics are the treatment of choice for SBBO.[38,54] The most frequently used antibiotics are metronidazole, ciprofloxacin, amoxicillin/clavulanate, or doxycycline. However, rifaximin is being used with increasing frequency.[55] Patients with persistent SBBO may require monthly rotating antibiotics to prevent reoccurrence of symptoms.

Celiac Disease

CD, also known as celiac sprue, nontropical sprue, and gluten-sensitive enteropathy, is an immune-mediated enteropathy caused by gluten. CD differs from immunoglobulin (Ig)E-mediated food allergies. It is characterized by a chronic, T-lymphocyte–mediated inflammatory response affecting the proximal small intestinal mucosa in response to ingested gluten.[56,57] It results from a genetic predisposition, exposure to gluten, and an inappropriate T-cell response against ingested gluten. CD is significantly underappreciated in the United States; it is more prevalent than Crohn's disease, ulcerative colitis (UC), and cystic fibrosis combined. Its reported prevalence is 1:100–300 people,[56] and there are numerous areas in the United States where it is still considered a rare disease and as such, it is *not considered* in the differential diagnosis. Currently, the estimated time to diagnosis in the United States is 11 years.[57] See Table 26-9 for clinical features that may be indicative of CD.

One of the reasons CD is difficult to diagnose is the diverse way in which it can present to the clinician. The classic presentation is diarrhea (steatorrhea), weight loss, iron-deficiency anemia, and fat-soluble vitamin deficiencies. However, it is now recognized that CD may present differently and in some patients remains asymptomatic except for conditions such as unexplained iron deficiency, dermatitis herpetiformis, rising serum transaminases (aspartate aminotransferase/alanine aminotransferase), and problems with infertility.[58–61] It is important to

TABLE 26-9 Clinical Features Encountered in Celiac Disease

- Diarrhea/weight loss/failure to thrive
- Iron deficiency anemia
- Macrocytic anemia (folate or B_{12})
- Short stature
- Osteopenia/bone pain/pathological fractures
- Recurrent abdominal pain/bloating
- Infertility/recurrent miscarriages
- Recurrent aphthous stomatitis
- Rising serum transaminases
- Fatigue/lassitude
- Depression

maintain a high index of suspicion. See Table 26-10 for disorders associated with CD.

Dermatitis Herpetiformis

Dermatitis herpetiformis (DH), a skin manifestation of CD, affects 10% to 20% of patients. Only 20% of patients with DH exhibit clinical symptoms,[57] while nearly 100% will have varying degrees of enteropathy.[56] Frequently, many patients are treated with medication and are never advised to also follow a gluten-free (GF) diet. The frontline treatment for the skin lesions of DH is dapsone, a sulfone antibiotic medication, which relieves the pruritic rash within 48 to 72 hours. However, only a GF diet will clear both the intestinal and skin lesions.[57] After following 133 patients with DH who consumed a GF diet, Garioch et al. reported the following advantages to following a GF diet in those with DH including: (1) need for medication is reduced or abolished; (2) resolution of enteropathy; (3) a general feeling of well-being; and (4) a potentially protective effect against development of lymphoma.[62]

Nutritional Implications

Patients with newly diagnosed CD should be evaluated for nutritional deficiencies. They are at risk for significant nutritional compromise not only as a result of their CD, but also because of the length of time it often takes to make the diagnosis. The classic presentation of CD has been described as a patient with significant weight loss, diarrhea (steatorrhea), and iron deficiency. In addition, there is an increased risk of fat-soluble vitamin and folate deficiency.[57] B_{12} deficiency, which at one time was thought to be uncommon in CD, was found in up to 41% of patients in one prospective study.[63]

Iron-deficiency may be the sole manifestation of CD in the absence of diarrhea; in fact, iron-deficiency anemia is the most common clinical presentation of CD, resolving after initiation of a GF diet.[58,64,65] Up to 8% of cases of iron-deficiency anemia resistant to oral iron supplementation can be attributed to CD.[66] Osteoporosis is another consequence of untreated CD, affecting up to 75% of patients.[67] The reasons are multifactorial and include decreased calcium absorption, precipitating secondary hyperparathyroidism, increased bone resorption turnover and loss, malabsorption of vitamin D and calcium secondary to a decreased absorptive surface area, inadequate intake from avoidance of milk products because of lactose intolerance, and finally, the patient may never have achieved peak bone mass at baseline.

Bone density should be measured in all adults after initial diagnosis of CD.[68] In patients with demonstrable bone loss, aggressive intervention is warranted. Improved BMD was seen after 1 year on a GF diet with standard amounts of oral calcium and 25-hydroxycholecalciferol.[67] In those patients who present with diarrhea/steatorrhea, a lactose restriction might be beneficial for a short period. It is not uncommon for patients with symptoms attributed to lactose intolerance to be ultimately diagnosed with untreated CD.[61]

TABLE 26-10 Disorders Associated With Celiac Disease

• Type I diabetes mellitus (3% to 8%) • Autoimmune thyroid disease Hyper- and hypo-thyroidism • Dermatitis herpetiformis • Addison disease • Autoimmune hepatitis • Systemic lupus erythematosus • Connective tissue disease • Sjögren syndrome • Atrophic gastritis	• Alopecia • Rheumatoid arthritis • Primary biliary cirrhosis • Down syndrome • Turner syndrome • William syndrome • Congenital heart defects • Immunoglobulin A deficiency • Psoriasis

Diagnosis

Serological Testing

Serology testing for CD is used to help identify patients who should undergo small bowel biopsy. As in all laboratory testing, false positives and false negatives are not uncommon. In particular, children under 2 years of age, those on a strict GF diet for > 4 to 6 weeks, and IgA-deficient individuals (as most of the serological tests are IgA based) may require a more sensitive screening test. The endomysial antibody and tissue transglutaminase (TTG-IgA) are both highly sensitive and specific, and have been recommended as the best serological screening tests at this time.[59] Selective IgA deficiency is the most common immunodeficiency in humans and may have a higher prevalence in patients with CD for unknown reasons. It is common to order IgA levels when ordering celiac serologies. In patients in whom an IgA deficiency is suspected, IgG anti-tissue transglutaminase and IgG antideaminated gliadin peptide testing should be ordered and patients should undergo small bowel biopsy.

Small Bowel Biopsy

To confirm the serological findings of CD, a small bowel biopsy, the "gold standard" for diagnosis, may be performed. Small bowel biopsy is not without limitations: multiple biopsies (six to eight) from the proximal duodenum including the bulb are required, as is correct orientation of the sample on the slide that is read by a pathologist trained in identifying CD. The patient needs to have consumed gluten within the past 6 weeks. If not, a gluten challenge (ie, three to four slices of bread/d) until symptoms develop (serology becomes positive or 3 to 6 months have passed) may be necessary before the biopsy is performed.

Refractory Celiac Disease

True refractory CD is a rare complication of CD.[69] The most common cause of seemingly refractory CD is noncompliance or inadvertent gluten ingestion. In fact, the single most important threat to disease remission is dietary noncompliance, with rates reported at 50% to 80%.[70,71] Hence, in nonresponders, intentional or inadvertent gluten ingestion must be excluded, and a TTG-IgA level checked in non–IgA-deficient individuals. Consider reevaluating the diagnosis after 6 to 9 months if symptoms persist with adherence to a GF diet. Collagenous sprue, ulcerative jejunitis, and small bowel T-cell lymphoma may have symptoms similar to that of CD. Table 26-11 lists conditions and symptoms that can mimic CD.

Nutritional Management

The only treatment for CD is lifelong elimination of gluten. Even small amounts of gluten can lead to mucosal changes on intestinal biopsy.[61] This translates into the restriction of wheat, rye, barley, and all derivatives of these grains from foods, beverages, and medications.[71,72] The inclusion of oats in the GF diet remains controversial. In patients with stable CD, the decision to include oats should be determined on an individual basis between the clinician and patient.[59] Lactose may need to be restricted initially, but often can be resumed after approximately 1 month on a strict GF diet after the mucosa has begun to heal.

A good mnemonic to help clinicians remember important mainstays of treatment is CELIAC[60]: *c*onsultation with a skilled dietician, *e*ducation about CD, *l*ifelong adherence to a GF diet, *i*dentification and treatment of nutrition deficiencies, *a*ccess to a support group, *c*ontinuous long-term follow-up. The mnemonic is important because it reminds providers that adherence to a GF diet is difficult, and continued support and education is necessary for success. Foods that patients would not normally think of containing gluten often contain fillers and additives that may contain gluten. Two common examples are ketchup and ice cream. Another common source of gluten exposure is from contamination of GF foods as they are processed in manufacturing plants that also process gluten-containing products. A complete list of dietary recommendations is beyond the scope of this chapter.

It is imperative that patients are referred early to a dietitian with expertise in CD; the longer the interval between diagnosis and nutritional counseling, the greater the chance the patient will receive misinformation from family, friends, and the Internet.[73] There are many surveys describing the dissatisfaction of patients with CD when they have spent time with physicians or dietitians not well trained in the nutritional management of CD, only to find that their support group provides the most accurate and helpful information.[74,75] The clinician should be sensitive to the emotional, lifestyle, and relationship infringements that a GF diet imposes, such as food situations at work, school, or social events, grocery shopping, when traveling, or just going out to eat, and the unwanted attention this diet sometimes brings.[76]

Although CD is not a wheat allergy, wheat comprises the majority of gluten in the diet. Recently, the U.S. Food and Drug Administration proposed new rules on voluntary use of GF labeling. This new labeling mandate will help the celiac community tremendously in the identification of safe versus toxic foods.

In patients with newly diagnosed CD, baseline red blood cell folate, ferritin, 25-OH D, vitamin A, and vitamin B_{12} should be checked, especially in those who present with diarrhea or significant weight loss. Initial supplementation with a therapeutic vitamin/mineral while initiating a GF diet may be important. The levels should be rechecked in 2 to 3 months to ensure efficacy of supplementation.

Symptomatic improvement is expected within 2 weeks in 70% to 95% of patients after the initiation of a GF diet.[58,77] However, histology may not recover completely for months to years, despite clinical normalization. Endomysial antibody or TTG-IgA antibody titers should be negative after 4 to 6 months of following a strict GF diet, although elevated TTG-IgA levels may persist because of various causes. The 2004 National Institutes of Health consensus conference developed six key elements for management of individuals with CD (Table 26-12).

Nutrition support is rarely necessary in a patient with CD. For patients who fail to respond to a GF diet and are at

TABLE 26-11 Conditions with Similar Symptoms to Celiac Disease

• Agammaglobulinemia	• Intestinal allergy to nongluten proteins such as milk, egg, soy
• Acquired immunodeficiency syndrome enteropathy	• Intestinal lymphoma
• Amyloidosis	• Irritable bowel syndrome
• Autoimmune enteropathy	• Microscopic colitis
• Bacterial overgrowth	• Pancreatic insufficiency
• Eosinophilic gastroenteritis	• Lactose intolerance
• Giardiasis	• Tropical sprue
• Inflammatory bowel disease	• Whipple disease
• Intestinal lymphangiectasia	

TABLE 26-12 Key Elements for Managing Patients with Celiac Disease[156]

1. **C**onsultation with a dietitian skilled in celiac disease
2. **E**ducation about the disease
3. **L**ifelong adherence to a gluten-free diet
4. **I**dentification and treatment of nutritional deficiencies
5. **A**ccess to an advocacy group
6. **C**ontinuous long-term follow-up by a multidisciplinary team

significant nutritional risk, a trial of a GF oral or enteral feeding as the sole source of intake may be beneficial (and diagnostic). This intervention will help to determine a true refractory patient versus one who is getting inadvertent gluten in his or her diet. In severe cases, an elemental diet may even be worthwhile, at least initially.[78]

Periodic reassessment of the GF diet by the physician and dietitian are also important to update patients on any new information and to review diet compliance. Support groups are one of the mainstays of treatment for patients with CD. To locate a support group, go to www.celiac.com. See Table 26-13 for professional resources.

Inflammatory Bowel Disease

Crohn's Disease

Crohn's disease is characterized by transmural inflammation of the digestive tract, with disease activity appearing anywhere from the mouth to the anus. The precise etiology of Crohn's disease remains unknown. There is evidence that inflammation results from excessive T-helper cell type 1 response to bacteria within normal GI flora. There is no single test that is absolute for the diagnosis for Crohn's disease or UC. Diagnosis of inflammatory bowel disease is based on a combination of clinical presentation, findings on endoscopy, and biopsy evaluation. Serological markers for inflammatory bowel disease, including antineutrophil cytoplasmic antibody and antisaccharomyces cerevisiae antibody, remain controversial, in part because of their low sensitivity.[79]

TABLE 26-13 Professional Resources

National Support Groups

- Gluten Intolerance Group www.gluten.net/
- Celiac Disease Foundation www.celiac.org
- Canadian Celiac Association www.celiac.ca
- American Celiac Alliance www.americanceliac.org

More Resources

- NIH Proceedings of the Consensus Conference http://digestive.niddk.nih.gov/ddiseases/pubs/celiac/
- North American Society for Pediatric Gastroenterology, Hepatology and Nutrition www.naspghan.org/assets/diseaseInfo/pdf/Celiac-E.pdf
- Entire Supplement 2 of *Gastroenterology* April 2005 is dedicated to celiac disease
- Best Practice & Research Clinical Gastroenterology www.elsevier.com/locate/issn/15216918 Volume 19, Issue 3, Pages 311–487 (June 2005) Coeliac Disease
- World Gastroenterology Organisation www.worldgastroenterology.org/guidelines/guide13 (February 2005)

Nutritional Assessment

Malnutrition occurs frequently in patients with inflammatory bowel disease. It is estimated that 65% to 75% of inpatients and over 50% of outpatients with Crohn's disease experience significant weight loss.[80] Weight loss is seen as a result of decreased oral intake caused by abdominal pain, diarrhea, nausea, or small bowel strictures. Sitophobia (fear of eating) can develop because of previous experience with diarrhea, abdominal pain, and/or oral pain with food intake.[80] Finally, malabsorption may contribute to malnutrition in patients with extensive intestinal resection(s).

Calorie and Protein Requirements

Energy expenditure is not significantly elevated in patients with inactive Crohn's disease.[81] Resting energy expenditure is increased during active inflammation although total energy expenditure is not significantly elevated—this may be related to decreased physical activity during periods of disease exacerbation.[82] Standard prediction equations used to predict calorie requirements may be employed, with appropriate adjustments for activity level and comorbidities. Initial feedings should be provided at a decreased calorie level to those patients with malnutrition to reduce the incidence of refeeding syndrome.[46]

Protein requirements may be elevated in Crohn's disease because of increased losses related to intestinal inflammation or fistulas. Patients in the postoperative setting or those with short bowel syndrome (SBS) may benefit from an increase in protein intake. Protein recommendations for those with Crohn's disease are 1 to 1.5 g/kg,[83] although there are no randomized trials that have investigated optimum protein intake in this population.

Nutrition Intervention

Fiber

There is no specific dietary regimen with proven efficacy in Crohn's disease. It is common for patients with stricturing Crohn's disease to follow a low-fiber diet. A reduced fiber intake is without known adverse effects. However, there are no controlled trials that demonstrate a low-fiber diet leads to symptom improvement, decreased admissions, or decreased incidence of small bowel obstruction.

Lactose

There is inadequate evidence to support withholding lactose-containing foods in patients with Crohn's disease who are not symptomatic after ingestion of normal amounts of lactose. A study by Park and coworkers has suggested that there is not an increased incidence of lactose intolerance in patients with Crohn's disease compared to the general public, based on jejunal lactase levels.[84] In contrast, two studies of breath hydrogen in response to lactose ingestion documents a significantly increased incidence of lactose intolerance in patients with Crohn's disease as compared to healthy controls.[85,86] However, the clinical significance of this increased breath hydrogen response is unclear. Many patients with lactose intolerance and Crohn's disease tolerate normal amounts of dairy products.[87]

Enteral Nutrition

EN effectively reverses malnutrition and supports growth (in pediatric patients) in those with Crohn's disease and adequate bowel length. EN is also significantly more efficacious than placebo in inducing remission in those patients who remain compliant with therapy.[88] However, EN is not as effective as corticosteroid therapy in inducing remission. There are no significant differences between elemental, semielemental, or polymeric formulas in terms of effectiveness.[89,90] Reduced-fat formulas may offer improved efficacy compared to formulas with increased amounts of long-chain triglycerides, but formulas with increased amounts of medium-chain triglycerides provided remission rates that were the same as low-fat formulas.[91,92] Controlled trials have demonstrated that there is no clinical benefit of supplemental glutamine or glutamine-rich enteral formulas to patients with inflammatory bowel disease.[93–95] Please see Practice Scenario 26-1 for a discussion on the use of PEG tube placement in patients with Crohn's disease.

Practice Scenario 26-1

Question: Is it appropriate to place a PEG tube in a patient with Crohn's disease and SBS?

Scenario: A 31-year-old male with a history of inflammatory bowel disease presents to the outpatient clinic for a nutrition consultation. Ten years ago, he underwent a total abdominal colectomy with end-ileostomy after presenting with "abdominal sepsis." At first, he was thought to have ulcerative colitis based on pancolonic involvement of the inflammatory process. Three years later, however, he presented to the emergency room with abdominal pain. Conservative measures with pain medications and fluids were unsuccessful. Evidence of small bowel disease was seen on computed tomography scan. The diagnosis for the patient was changed to Crohn's enteritis. He was started on corticosteroids and an aminosalicylic acid compound with partial resolution of symptoms. Over the next 12 months, the patient seemed to improve overall after switching to stronger immunosuppressive therapy with infliximab and azathioprine therapy. The patient presented again 2 years ago with severe pain, fever, decreased ostomy output, nausea, vomiting, and confusion. An abdominal film revealed Crohn's disease with a spontaneous bowel perforation. The patient became critically ill, requiring aggressive management with antibiotics and fluid volume resuscitation, and ended up proceeding to the operating room for exploratory laparotomy. The patient had to be transfused 10 units of blood intraoperatively, and an extensive small bowel resection was performed. Postoperatively, the patient was estimated to have approximately 200 cm of remaining small intestine. He had a central venous catheter placed and was started on PN. While his weight fluctuated on PN, his main problem has been recurrent central line infections and the need to frequently replace his central line catheter. He presents now to the clinic for a nutrition consultation and further management.

Intervention: A PEG tube was placed and the patient was started on EN with a small peptide/medium-chain triglyceride formula. Use of a small portable pump carried in a fanny pack allowed the patient to feed 24 hours a day. Gradually over 4 months, the patient was weaned off PN. Oral intake was allowed ad lib, as tolerated by volume of ostomy output. The patient was encouraged to use oral rehydration solutions and small frequent meals with no fat restriction, separating fluid intake from the solid meals. Six months later, his weight is stable at 10 pounds over his ideal body weight.

Answer: In the past, Crohn's disease was thought to be a relative contraindication to placement of a PEG tube in a disease process characterized by fistula formation and intraperitoneal adhesion formation. The chance of perforating an intervening loop of small bowel caught in an adhesion or creating an intentional enterocutaneous fistula with the PEG tube placement in a disease process prone to fistula formation was thought to be a high risk poor management strategy. In tough cases, though, placement of a PEG tube may be the key strategy that allows the patient to finally achieve gut autonomy and live off PN.

Rationale: In difficult cases with severe Crohn's disease requiring continued immunosuppressive therapy to keep the disease process in remission, the patient is at high risk for recurrent central line infection. With each infection, the central line has to be changed. The patient may lose weight in the interim, and the risk of running out of intravenous access sites in the future increases. In general, gut autonomy may be achieved with as little as 70 to 90 cm of small bowel in patients with SBS who still have their colon intact. In the absence of a colon, greater length of small bowel is required (at least 120 to 150 cm) to achieve autonomy. In this patient who should have enough bowel length to achieve autonomy, however, the remaining 200 cm of small bowel may be compromised by continued Crohn's disease activity and suboptimal absorption. While the patient is instructed to follow diet recommendations for severe SBS, these measures may not be sufficient to achieve gut autonomy. Provision of a semielemental formula at a slow rate through the entire 24 hours each day optimizes efficiency of absorption.

Parenteral Nutrition

PN does not have a role as primary therapy in patients with Crohn's disease.[96,97] The indications for PN in Crohn's disease are similar to those in other disease states. These include SBS, persistent small bowel obstruction, inability to tolerate EN for extended periods, or enteric fistula originating in a location that does not allow EN distal to the fistula site. In rare circumstances, patients have been put on PN for short periods to try to help induce remission through bowel rest, but this is not standard therapy.

Specific Nutrient Issues

Vitamin and Mineral Deficiencies

Several micronutrient deficiencies occur frequently in Crohn's disease. Iron deficiency anemia is frequently related to blood loss. However, iron supplements should not be provided unless a patient has a documented iron deficiency. Enteral iron supplements may result in increased GI symptoms.[98] Parenteral iron carries the (infrequent) risk of anaphylactic reactions.

Patients with Crohn's disease are at increased risk of osteopenia and osteoporosis. Recent reports have estimated the incidence of osteopenia in populations with Crohn's disease between 35% to 40%.[99,100] Periodic exposure to corticosteroids is believed to be a primary etiologic factor, although inflammatory cytokines and malabsorption are potential contributors. Supplemental calcium to reach a total intake of 1500 mg elemental calcium and 800 to 1000 IU of vitamin D is recommended to those with frequent use of corticosteroids. Supplemental calcium of 500 mg and vitamin D of 400 IU per day for 2 years in patients with Crohn's disease resulted in significant increase in BMD.[101] One nutrient that is frequently underappreciated in terms of osteoporosis risk is vitamin K. Vitamin K is essential to form osteocalcin. Populations with Crohn's disease have a decreased dietary intake of vitamin K,[102] and malabsorption may increase vitamin K losses.

Patients with Crohn's disease have a high incidence of hyperhomocysteinemia (associated with increased risk of cardiovascular disease) that is related to decreased serum levels of vitamin B_{12} and folate.[98,103] Ileal resections increase the risk of vitamin B_{12} deficiency, while use of methotrexate and/or decreased intake of leafy green vegetables increase the risk of folate deficiency. Patients with high-output enterocutaneous (EC) fistulas and those with frequent diarrhea are at increased risk of zinc deficiency.[104] Inflammatory conditions can result in temporary decreases in serum zinc that may not represent a true deficiency. Patients with excessive GI fluid losses or those with documented zinc deficiency should receive supplemental zinc (see short bowel section for micronutrient dosing).

Fish Oil

Fish oils are rich in omega-3 fatty acids that have anti-inflammatory effects through their ability to modify production of prostaglandins, leukotrienes, and thromboxanes. The results of studies with fish oil supplements in Crohn's disease have been conflicting. A recent systematic review and meta-analysis concluded that there is insufficient data to recommend the use of omega-3 fatty acids for maintenance of remission in inflammatory bowel disease.[105]

Ulcerative Colitis

UC is a chronic inflammatory disease of the colon. The incidence of protein–calorie malnutrition in UC is less than that seen in Crohn's disease because the primary nutrient absorptive area (small bowel) is not affected.

There is no evidence to support the use of EN (elemental, semielemental, or polymeric) as primary therapy in the treatment of UC.[99,106] Two studies have demonstrated that EN is tolerated during acute flares of UC.[105,107] Gonzalez-Huix[107] reported that polymeric EN maintained nutrition status with fewer infectious complications compared to PN during severe acute flares of UC. The use of EN in severe UC in this study was associated with similar rates of remission and need for surgery compared to PN. Patients who required surgery had significantly fewer postoperative infections after EN compared to those who received PN. In clinical practice, however, it is rare for patients with severe exacerbations of UC with large-volume stool output to be placed on EN support.

Specific Nutrients

The incidence of iron deficiency anemia related to GI blood loss is higher in UC than in Crohn's disease. It is estimated that up to 80% of patients with UC may develop iron-deficiency anemia.[108]

Folic acid adequacy has special relevance in UC because of its link to cancer prevention because patients with long-standing disease are known to be at increased risk of colon cancer. Two case control studies and a retrospective review have suggested that folate supplementation may have a protective role in cancer prevention in this patient population.[109]

The incidence of osteopenia reported in UC is 25% to 32%, which is somewhat less than that seen in Crohn's disease.[101] Recommendations for increased calcium and vitamin D intake are similar: 1500 mg of elemental calcium and 800 to 1000 IU of vitamin D.

SCFAs (butyrate, acetate, propionate) are fermented in the colon from dietary fiber by colonic microorganisms. SCFAs serve as fuel for the colonocytes and promote water and sodium absorption in the colon.[98,110] Butyrate enemas reduced inflammation in UC, and when combined with 5-aminosalicylic acid resulted in more patients with remission than with 5-aminosalicylic acid alone.[110] Increased dietary fiber increases colonic butyrate production, and several studies with increased fiber diets or supplements have suggested improved symptoms in UC.[111-113]

Protein-Losing Enteropathy

PLE is a disorder that is associated with a number of different disease states that results in a loss of serum proteins into the GI tract (Table 26-14). The pathologies that may cause PLE are often grouped into two major categories: (1) disorders of the GI mucosa, and (2) disorders of lymphatic flow. Patients with PLE frequently present with edema caused by decreased serum proteins resulting in a decrease in plasma oncotic pressure.

In the past, PLE was a diagnosis of exclusion, requiring that other possible sources of hypoalbuminemia be ruled out. Currently, the most common methods of diagnosing PLE is a fecal measurement of alpha-1 antitrypsin or technetium 99m–labeled human serum albumin.[114,115] Alpha 1-antitrypsin is an endogenous protein that is not present in food that has a molecular weight similar to albumin. It is not actively secreted, absorbed, or digested in a healthy GI tract.

In PLE, the GI loss of albumin and other plasma proteins occur faster than the body can synthesize new proteins.[116] Consequently, it is not possible to reverse the hypoalbuminemia simply by providing additional protein to the patient.

Intestinal lymphangiectasia is associated with compromised flow of lymph with increased pressure in the lymphatic system. The absorption of long-chain fat increases intestinal lymph flow, increasing pressure in the intestinal lymphatics, resulting in protein leakage into the intestinal lumen. A very

TABLE 26-14 Disorders Associated With Protein-Losing Gastroenteropathies[114,115]

Disorders of the Mucosa	
Without Erosions or Ulceration	*With Erosions or Ulceration*
• Acquired immunodeficiency syndrome–associated gastroenteropathy	• Alpha-chain disease
• Acute viral gastroenteritis	• Amyloidosis, Behçet disease
• Allergic enteritis	• Carcinoid syndrome
• Celiac disease	• Crohn's disease
• Collagenous colitis	• Duodenitis
• Eosinophilic gastroenteritis	• Erosive gastritis
• Hypertrophic hypersecretory gastropathy	• Gastrointestinal carcinomas
• Small intestinal bacterial overgrowth	• Graft-versus-host disease
• Parasitic diseases:	• Helicobacter pyloric gastritis
– Malaria, giardiasis, schistosomiasis, nematodiasis	• Idiopathic ulcerative jejunoileitis
• Lymphocytic colitis	• Infectious diarrhea:
• Tropical sprue	– *Clostridium difficile, Shigella*
• Vascular ectasia (gastric, colonic)	• Kaposi sarcoma
• Whipple disease	• Lymphoma
	• Neurofibromatosis
	• Ulcerative colitis
	• Waldenström macroglobulinemia
Disorders of Lymphatic Flow	
Intestinal endometriosis	
Intestinal lymphangiectasia (congenital, acquired)	
Lymphenteric fistula	
Lymphoma	
Mesenteric venous thrombosis	
Mesenteric tuberculosis and sarcoidosis	
Portal hypertensive gastroenteropathy	
Posttransplant lymphoproliferative disease	
Sclerosing mesenteritis	
Systemic lupus erythematosus	
Whipple disease	
Retroperitoneal fibrosis	
Increased central venous pressure	
Constrictive pericarditis	
Congestive heart failure	

low-fat diet (< 20 g to start) may relieve pressure in the lymphatic system with a reduction in protein losses.[117] Alternatively, enteral formulations high in medium-chain fatty acids may be empirically tried. These fats are not absorbed through the lymphatics and are transported across the mucosa directly into the portal system. Patients are at increased risk of essential fatty acid deficiency and fat-soluble vitamin deficiencies, and plasma triene/tetraene ratio along with vitamin A, D, E, and K status should be monitored.

PN may be indicated in those patients with failure to thrive or with no symptom improvement on very low-fat EN. There are no randomized trials aimed at determining the optimum nutrition regimen for those with PLE because of the varied nature and infrequent occurrence of this disorder. The goal is to help restore protein balance when possible. The available data are in the form of retrospective reviews, which suggests that enteral therapy is an effective way to provide nutrition for some patients with PLE.[118]

Short Bowel Syndrome

SBS is broadly defined as inadequate absorptive capacity resulting from loss of bowel length and/or bowel function. In practice, remaining SBS occurs when there is < 200 cm of small bowel length. Managing SBS is complex and best managed by a multispeciality team consisting of surgeons, dieticians, and doctors trained in nutrition. There are three phases of accommodation each presenting with a unique set of challenges. The first phase occurs right after surgery. This period is characterized by hypersecretion of gastric fluids and significant fluid losses. PN and fluid resuscitation is life-saving during this period. Over the next 2 years, the remaining gut goes through a period of accommodation when the absorptive ability and surface area of mucosa of the small bowel increases. Patients are transitioned from total PN to enteral feeding. This is the time that patients learn dietary and lifestyle changes that will help determine if they are able to achieve gut autonomy. After approximately 2 years, a maintenance period begins when further accommodation is not possible and hopefully patients can maintain relatively normal oral intake. Nutritional support is tailored to the patient's needs.

In general, patients with ≥ 70 to 90 cm of small bowel and an intact colon are able to gain autonomy from total PN. Patients need approximately 130 to 150 cm of small bowel when the colon is also removed. Nevertheless, inadequate bowel function to support nutrient and fluid requirements, regardless of the length of the GI tract, can be termed SBS. The etiology of SBS is multifactorial and can occur at any age[119–121]; however, surgical resection is the most common. Table 26-15 lists common causes in both children and adults.

The primary goal in managing SBS is to regain as much gut function as possible. During this process, PN and/or EN will be necessary to maintain adequate nutrients, water, and electrolytes to maintain health and growth.[122,123] Factors affecting adaptation include length of the remaining bowel, section of bowel resected, overall health of the remaining bowel, and the length of time that has elapsed since the initial surgery or insult. The age of the patient and any other GI organ involvement may also play a role. Additional factors affecting bowel adaptation include:

- Stimulation by intraluminal nutrients
- Stimulation by bile and pancreatic secretions
- Trophic effects of gut hormones
- Altered intestinal blood flow
- Altered bowel innervations

To improve the chance for successful weaning from PN or intravenous fluids, it is essential to increase nutrient and fluid absorption by slowing intestinal transit time, controlling gastric acid hypersecretion, and enhancing the mixing of pancreatic enzymes and bile salts. It is equally important to use as much of the remaining surface area as possible to avoid osmotic agents and to treat bacterial overgrowth when necessary. Dehydration is common in these patients, and it is important that they be trained in the use of oral rehydration solutions to minimize recurrent hospitalizations.

TABLE 26-15 Etiology of Short Bowel Syndrome in Children and Adults[121–123]

Children	Adults
• Necrotizing enterocolitis • Intestinal atresia Volvulus Hernia Intussusception • Congenital short bowel syndrome • Trauma • Gastroschisis • Apple peel anomaly • Crohn's disease • Abdominal tumors • Radiation enteritis • Hirschsprung's disease	• Massive surgical resection • Crohn's disease • Malignancy • Radiation enteritis • Trauma • Vascular catastrophes Embolism/thrombus • Volvulus • Strangulated hernias • Small bowel fistulas • Surgical bypass • Surgical error or obesity treatment • Chronic intestinal pseudo-obstruction

Physiological Changes in Short Bowel Syndrome

After significant resection of the small bowel, gastric hypersecretion (particularly problematic when jejunal surface area is lost) must be addressed.[123] Worse in the first few weeks after surgery and lasting up to 6 months or longer postoperatively, gastric hypersecretion increases the sheer volume of secretions entering the small bowel, lowers the pH of the proximal gut, damages the duodenal mucosa, and stimulates peristalsis. The added volume of secretions contributes to an already significant stool output. Furthermore, the acidic environment denatures pancreatic enzymes and precipitates bile salts, both of which function optimally at a pH of 7 to 8, impairing pancreatic enzyme activity and disrupting micelle formation.

Both histamine$_2$-receptor antagonists (H_2-blockers) and PPIs have been used to treat gastric hypersecretion; however, PPIs suppress significantly more acid than H_2-blockers.[122] Fifty centimeters of jejunum are necessary to absorb PPIs.[124] Intravenous H_2-blockers or PPIs may be indicated if the oral route proves unsuccessful. In patients whose GI fluid output is driven by secretory processes, octreotide may be useful during this time. Unfortunately, octreotide must be given subcutaneously, it is expensive, and tachyphylaxis develops rather quickly. Suggested dosing of antisecretory medications can be found elsewhere.[125]

Transit of food from the stomach into the proximal gut is regulated by feedback mechanisms along the GI tract; one of the most important is the terminal ileum, which is often lost in SBS. The ileal brake is recruited in response to undigested nutrients that have escaped absorption in the upper gut and reached the ileum, primarily carbohydrate and fat.[126] The response is a slowing of gastric motility and peristalsis in the upper gut, thereby giving greater nutrient exposure to the mucosa for absorption. Loss of the ileum, and hence the ileal brake mechanism, contributes to gastric hypersecretion and accelerated small bowel transit.

In addition, when the ileocecal valve is removed, the bowel becomes one continuous conduit and all patients develop SBBO to some degree. Bacterial overgrowth can contribute to malabsorption and diarrhea. Antibiotics can be given when patients experience symptoms of bloating and flatulence for symptom relief. Unfortunately, diarrhea associated with SBS does not respond as well to antibiotics as do the symptoms of bloating.

Antimotility agents are the primary treatment to slow intestinal transit in the clinical setting. Patients should receive a trial of less potent (eg, loperamide [Imodium]) gut-slowing medications with a plan to titrate up or change to more potent, prescription agents (eg, diphenoxylate [Lomotil], opiates such as codeine or tincture of opium) if needed. It is important to dose these medications at a time when there is no competition for mucosal receptors (eg, 30 minutes or so before meals and/or bedtime snack) in order to maximize their efficacy in a shortened GI tract. It is not uncommon to use a combination of agents in these patients.[127]

Following bowel resection, patients are often at higher risk for SBBO. Factors that increase this risk include loss of the ileocecal valve, the presence of blind loops, decreased motility, acid suppression, and other underlying disease processes (see section on SBBO).

Bile salts are required for the absorption of fat, fat-soluble vitamins, and some medications. Bile salts are primarily reabsorbed in the terminal ileum and transported back to the liver for reuse. Enterohepatic circulation of bile salts is such an efficient system that approximately 90% of the bile salt pool is maintained this way. When the terminal ileum is lost, bile salt reabsorption is impaired and bile salts enter the colon, which can contribute to a choleric diarrhea.

Cholestyramine can be administered in an effort to try to help control the diarrhea, but there are some caveats for its use. If < 100 cm of functional distal ileum is resected, bile salt reabsorption will be impacted, but the remaining bowel can accommodate and maintain adequate enterohepatic circulation. Cholestyramine can be helpful in these patients because it reduces the colon's exposure to free bile salts while enterohepatic circulation is maintained. In contrast, patients who lose > 100 cm of terminal ileum have difficulty reabsorbing and maintaining adequate bile salt stores through enterohepatic circulation. The liver must increase bile salt production in an effort to maintain adequate fat absorption. A trial of cholestyramine in these patients results in initial improvement of diarrhea, but its use rapidly depletes the bile salt pool. Loss of the bile salt pool leads to impaired micelle formation, thereby decreasing solubilization of fat in the lumen, resulting in steatorrhea, which worsens the diarrhea. In patients without a colon, cholestyramine has little benefit.[127]

Osteoporosis is a significant problem in patients with SBS. Malabsorption of vitamin D and calcium, a persistent inflammatory state, and chronic metabolic acidosis from stool bicarbonate loss are all contributing factors. A dual energy x-ray absorptiometry scan should be obtained on all patients with SBS and followed regularly. Monitoring vitamin D levels is essential even in patients routinely receiving vitamin D in PN. Assessment of 25-OHD (not 1,25-OHD) should be performed at baseline with a serum goal of 25 to 30 ng/mL. Checking serum parathyroid hormone will help with early identification of those patients who need more intensive intervention. Treatment should be aimed at the provision of adequate vitamin D, eliminating metabolic acidosis if present, and replacement of magnesium if necessary (see section on hypomagnesemia). Additional bicarbonate, in the form of acetate, may be needed in the PN solution to correct metabolic acidosis.

Nephrolithiasis from calcium oxalate stones are especially problematic for patients with an intact colonic segment.[128] Stone formation is multifactorial but is primarily due to accelerated absorption of oxalate in the remaining colon. Normally, calcium preferentially binds to oxalate, forming an unabsorbable complex that is excreted in the stool. In the presence of steatorrhea, free fatty acids have a higher affinity for calcium, thereby allowing the readily absorbable free dietary oxalate to be taken up by the colonic mucosa. Ultimately, the oxalate binds to calcium in the kidney and the calcium oxalate is excreted via the kidney. The risk of nephrolithiasis is compounded by volume depletion, metabolic acidosis, and hypomagnesemia. Maintaining a urine output of > 1200 mL/d is the most important intervention to avoid this complication.[129–132] A diet low in oxalate may be also be helpful.[129] Oral calcium supplements of 800 to 1200 mg/d, in divided doses not exceeding more than 500 mg, are used in an effort to compete with fatty acids in the lumen to bind oxalate.

Fat restriction in SBS is controversial. Some feel that with an intact colon fat restriction may be of some benefit to control diarrhea. If the colon is removed, there is no need for fat restriction. Other providers feel that fat restriction is only good for short segment resections and that in major resection, fat restriction does not change diarrhea substantially. Rather, patients with SBS need the calories that fat provides. SBS patients must often eat 200% or more of the normally required calories in order to obtain sufficient nutrients to meet their needs.

Assessment/Monitoring

It is essential to determine not only the length of bowel resected but also the length of bowel remaining, the presence or absence of the terminal ileum, and the amount of remaining colon. Operative reports and a small bowel follow-through should be reviewed.

For some patients going home on PN, a 72-hour quantitative fecal fat collection may be necessary to document malabsorption.[133] For results to be accurate, patients must consume enough fat, either by mouth or feeding tube. Specific guidelines for a quantitative fat collection and 100 g of fat diet are available elsewhere.[125]

It is important to know the exact medications prescribed, including the dosage, timing, and frequency. All these factors are important in patients with SBS. For example, PPIs and gut-slowing medications should always be given 30 minutes to 1 hour *before* meals and bedtime. Check for, and avoid using, sustained release medications in this patient population.

Ideally, have the patient record 3 to 5 days of typical oral intake, including all fluids ingested. The consumption of any highly osmotic beverage such as high-calorie shakes, sodas, or juice or the use of other nutritional products, such as protein powders, herbals, or vitamins, needs to be determined.

Vitamin and mineral levels need to be monitored at least annually in patients with SBS. Baseline levels should be checked at the first clinic visit or 3 months out from the initial surgery or insult. Patients with SBS are most at risk for deficiency of fat-soluble vitamins (A, D, E, K), as well as vitamin B_{12}.[129] Loss of the ileum, gastric hypersecretion, and its effects on R protein, and/or bacterial overgrowth can all contribute to vitamin B_{12} deficiency.

Severe zinc losses are of concern to the clinician in patients with SBS. The presumption is that zinc losses will be high in this patient population secondary to the high stool volume typically associated with SBS. It is also based on the theory that replacing losses is necessary to prevent symptoms of zinc deficiency. These recommendations were based on a 3-week study of 24 patients with SBS on total PN in whom zinc balance was measured.[106] They determined that, as a whole, 12 mg of zinc per day would be sufficient to achieve positive zinc balance.

Excessive loss of sodium through GI secretions leads to hypotension and prerenal azotemia. Hyperaldosteronism is not uncommon in this patient population in an effort to decrease sodium losses in the urine. Sodium losses are greater in ileostomy effluent compared to jejunostomy effluent (120 versus 90 mEq/L, respectively); however, net jejunostomy sodium losses are often greater given the higher volume of stool lost each day.[132] To detect sodium depletion, check a random urine sodium (make sure the patient is not receiving diuretics). A urine sodium of < 5 to 10 mmol/L is indicative of maximal sodium conservation and hence, sodium depletion. The urine sodium should be maintained > 20 mmol/L. Salt should be added to meals and snacks.

To assess dehydration in this population, patients should be taught to self-monitor for rapid weight loss (> 0.5 to 1.0 kg/d) and symptoms of orthostatic hypotension such as tachycardia and decreased urine output. The blood urea nitrogen and creatinine may remain low until the late stages of dehydration. Maintaining a patient's hydration status is often difficult. Some patients will benefit from the use of oral rehydration therapy (ORT).[134] Water is absorbed in the small bowel through simple diffusion and passive transport. Transport can by improved with the addition of sodium and glucose. The addition of these molecules in oral rehydration solutions increases the active absorption of water through their respective sodium and glucose transporters. In other patients (with very little jejunum remaining), ORT will increase the stool or ostomy output. Ideally, patients will sip ORT over the course of the day instead of other fluids. Another option is to try giving ORT as a nocturnal infusion, first via a nasogastric tube, and if successful, through a PEG. This may allow some patients to avoid intravenous fluids.[135] See Table 26-16 for tips on assessing and maximizing hydration. Commercial ORT solutions as well as recipes are available elsewhere.[131]

Hypomagnesemia is common in patients with SBS. Hyperaldosteronism caused by sodium and water depletion increases urinary magnesium losses. Magnesium deficiency can precipitate a serum calcium deficiency due to impaired release of parathyroid hormone; this results in greater urinary loss of calcium, along with insufficient 1,25-OHD production, ultimately reducing calcium and magnesium absorption in the gut.[136] See Table 26-17 for guidelines to treat hypomagnesemia.

TABLE 26-16 Assessing and Maximizing Hydration

- Maintain urine output > 1200 mL (have patients measure their urine output periodically).
- Serial weights: if patient loses > 0.5 lb/d or 1 kg/wk, add or increase intravenous fluids.
- A rise in blood urea nitrogen/creatinine ratio is a late indicator in ostomates; use other indicators such as blood pressure, signs of tachycardia, or drop in urine output.
- Patients with end jejunostomies: Drink/sip higher sodium, carbohydrate-containing, relatively isotonic beverages (no sweet drinks); also avoid hypotonic fluids such as water, tea, coffee, and alcohol.
- Patients with colon intact can handle a wider range of fluids, but avoidance of very hypertonic fluids is still beneficial.
- Try oral rehydration therapy. (*Note:* Gatorade and other sports drinks are not oral rehydration therapy.)
- Avoid nephrolithiasis.
- Avoid foods high in oxalate.
- Consider avoiding large doses of vitamin C supplementation (> 500 mg)—theoretical; there is no data to support (converts to oxalate endogenously).
- Try calcium citrate supplements to bind oxalate and alkalinize urine.

Used with permission from Shugar Publishing, Parrish CR. The clinician's guide to short bowel syndrome. *Pract Gastroenterol.* 2005;XXIX(9):67.

Nutrition Intervention

Oral Diet

Stimulation of the residual bowel with macronutrient exposure is an important part of the adaptive process. It is accepted that patients with SBS should consume whole food diets and/or use a polymeric formula for maximum intestinal stimulation and adaptation.[132] A high-fat diet can contribute to nutrient loss by aggravating steatorrhea. To potentially gain freedom from PN, patients with SBS may need to eat 200% to 400% over their dietary needs to surmount the malabsorption that occurs.[137] It is also suggested that diets should differ somewhat in patients with a colonic segment versus those without. A diet rich in carbohydrate and lower in fat is preferable in patients with a colon as compared to a higher-fat, lower-carbohydrate diet in patients with a jejunostomy to reduce total fluid losses.[133,138] A diet high in simple carbohydrate will pull water into the lumen of the GI tract, precipitating net fluid/nutrient loss. Avoiding simple sugars such as sweets, fruit juices, and sodas are one of the few beneficial dietary restrictions in this patient population. In addition, liquid and solid components of meals should be

TABLE 26-17 Treatment of Hypomagnesemia

- Correct water and sodium depletion (and thus secondary hyperaldosteronism).
- Use an oral magnesium preparation (eg, 12 mmol magnesium oxide) at night when transit may be slowest, and the patient is on nothing by mouth to avoid competition with other medications/foods.[133]
- Reduce lipid in diet because a high-fat diet binds magnesium increasing stool losses.
- Trial calcitriol or rocaltrol (active vitamin D analog)
- Give intravenous magnesium over as many hours as possible →> 8 hours minimum; continuous is best, to decrease renal wasting.
- Try adding injectable magnesium to oral rehydration therapy for sipping: magnesium sulfate—5 mEq/mL (Abbott Pharmaceuticals, Inc., Abbott Park, Illinois, USA).
- Replete magnesium until normal urinary magnesium is achieved.

Nightingale JM, ed. *Intestinal Failure.* London, UK: Greenwich Medical Media Limited; 2001:188. Reprinted with the permission of Cambridge University Press.

TABLE 26-18 Diet Guidelines for Short Bowel Syndrome

General Guidelines

- Patients with jejunostomies/ileostomies (higher fat): approximately 20% to 30% carbohydrate, 20% to 30% protein, 50% to 60% fat.
- Patients with intact colon (higher carbohydrate): approximately 50% to 60% carbohydrate, 20% to 30% protein, 20% to 30% fat.
- Avoid concentrated sweets and fluids.
- Chew foods well.
- Add salty meals and snacks if no colon.
  - Eat smaller meals, more often.
- Decrease total nutrient load over the day and space out over time.
- Trial of oral rehydration solutions.
- Limit fluids with meals; drink isotonic beverages.
- Separate solids and liquids at meals as much as possible (solids before liquids).
  - Solids slow emptying.
  - Too much liquid creates a column effect (imagine the swelling of a stream when it rains and the increased flow generated).
- Use medium-chain triglyceride–containing beverages if necessary versus medium-chain triglyceride oil.
- Lactose restriction if necessary (may try Lactaid).
- Avoid high oxalate foods in patients with kidney stones.
- Liquid or chewable vitamin/mineral supplements if necessary.
- Limit or avoid enteral stimulants such as alcohol and caffeine.

Used with permission. University of Virginia Health System, Nutrition Support Traineeship Syllabus; Charlottesville, VA; Updated July 2010 @ www.ginutrition.virginia.edu.

ingested separately to maximize absorption. Oral dietary guidelines can be found in Table 26-18.

Enteral Nutrition

If EN support is necessary, it should be infused into the most proximal location to maximize the absorption surface area. Isotonic, or near isotonic (300 mOsm), polymeric formulas with some medium-chain triglycerides are appropriate. EN should be infused at low rates over time in order to saturate transporters to decrease nutrient load delivered per centimeter of bowel. If unsuccessful, a semielemental formula may be tried. Elemental formulas should be avoided because they are hypertonic and have not demonstrated a physiological advantage.[139–141] Fiber-containing formulas are advantageous in patients with remaining colon because of colon "salvage." Bacteria in the remaining colon can ferment otherwise nondigestible fiber into SCFAs that do not require bile salts for absorption. These fats diffuse across the mucosa and enter the enterohepatic circulation where they can contribute up to 500 cal/d.[133,142] Colonic salvage is an important way for dieticians to get extra calories into patients with SBS, and these extra calories can make up the difference in patients who are close to regaining gut autonomy.

Parenteral Nutrition/Intravenous Fluids

The need for PN may be permanent in some patients. In preparation for home, imitate the anticipated regimen for a few days before discharge. Should the patient require fluid above and beyond the maximum volume possible in home PN bags (3 to 4 L), additional intravenous fluids can be sent. Most home patients infuse their PN over 10 to 12 hours overnight, allowing them time off during the day to participate in desired activities; infusion rates of 250 to 350 mL/h are not uncommon in the home setting. If frequent urination at night interferes with sleep, review the PN prescription for potential excess fluid volume. Backpacks to transport the PN solution and the intravenous pump are also available to allow daytime infusion with increased mobility.

Long-Term Monitoring

Patients with SBS require ongoing monitoring. Periodic measurements of 24-hour urine and stool output should be conducted to ensure continued success of the nutrition regimen. Urine outputs < 1 L/d and serial weight loss should prompt the clinician to intervene in order to prevent renal stone development with the potential for detrimental effects to the kidney over time.[135] A sudden increase in stool or ostomy output requires evaluation.[131] Periodic assessment of vitamin and mineral indices, as discussed previously, are also necessary. Routinely review the patient's medication list to check for the addition of new medications (especially over-the-counter, herbals, vitamins, etc.). It is important to consistently assess the patient's overall functional status and quality of life. Comprehensive clinical guidelines for short bowel syndrome are available.[131]

Future Directions

Hormonal therapy, specifically the use of growth hormone, is still considered experimental; nevertheless, its use is increasing primarily in major teaching hospitals to enhance bowel adaptation.[143] Another agent, glucagon-like peptide 2, is actively being investigated because of its intestinotrophic effects, including mucosal cell growth and proliferation.[144]

Enterocutaneous Fistulas

Etiology

EC fistulas are defined as abnormal communication between the intestine and the skin. They are classified by output volume, etiology, site of origin, and number of fistula tracts. Most of them (75% to 85%) occur after surgery, within the first 7 to 10 days postoperatively.[145,146] Unfortunately, good data regarding incidence are unavailable. The surgical procedures most commonly associated with EC fistula development are lysis of adhesions and bowel resection for inflammatory bowel disease, cancer, or pancreatitis. Emergent surgery or surgery on previously radiated

TABLE 26-19 Conditions Associated with Fistula Formation

Causes of Surgical Fistulas	Causes of Spontaneous Fistulas
• Lysis of adhesions • Bowel resection for inflammatory bowel disease • Bowel resection for cancer • Surgery for pancreatitis • Surgery on radiated bowel • Gastrointestinal surgery in malnourished patient	• Radiation • Inflammatory bowel disease • Diverticular disease • Appendicitis • Ischemic bowel • Perforation of duodenal ulcers • Pancreatic and gynecologic malignancies • Intra-abdominal abscesses • Abdominal penetrating trauma

TABLE 26-20 Potential Complications of Fistulas

- Sepsis
- Fluid/electrolyte imbalance
- Hemorrhage
- Pain
- Anxiety/poor body image
- Expense
- Death

bowel can increase the risk of fistula formation. Anecdotally, some surgeons consider malnourished patients at higher risk of fistula formation. Tables 26-19 and 26-20 list conditions associated with, and potential complications of, fistula development.[147]

Diagnosis

Patients may present with abdominal pain, fever, and/or leukocytosis. Enteric drainage begins within 24 to 48 hours after the appearance of cellulitic skin. Initially, the odor, color, consistency, and volume of the fluid draining can help identify the part of the bowel where the fistula originates. Blue dye or methylene blue can be given in the bowel proximal to the fistula in order to confirm that the source of the fistula is indeed the GI tract. Definitive assessment of the fistula source, fistula route, and presence of obstructions or abscesses is essential in determining the appropriate medical intervention, including the method of feeding. Computed tomography imaging and magnetic resonance imaging are diagnostic tests to determine the presence of obstructions or abscess formation; however, a fistulogram is considered the gold standard for identifying the location and route of the fistulous tract.

Nutrition Intervention

Before the use of specialized nutrition support, malnutrition was a major determinant of adverse outcomes in patients with EC fistulas; high-output fistulas in malnourished patients were 100% fatal. With specialized nutrition support, mortality in high-output fistulas decreased to 20% by 1989.[147] The presence of a fistula increases morbidity and likelihood of malnutrition by reducing the patient's desire to eat, increasing the loss of nutrients via fistula drainage (if located in the proximal gut), and/or by increasing energy and protein needs because of sepsis. Scientific literature regarding EC fistulas and nutrition include only retrospective case reports or studies that include a small number of subjects. Robust evidence is difficult to obtain because of the significant variation in patient comorbidities, the many different types of fistulas, and the relatively low numbers of fistulas treated at any single institution.

Traditionally, PN has been used in the treatment of EC fistulas. Spontaneous closure of fistulas may take only 4 to 6 weeks (Table 26-21). Enteral feeding may be possible in low output fistulas ($<$ 500 mL/d), esophageal, gastric, duodenal, or proximal jejunal fistulas with distal enteral access, or distal ileal or colonic fistulas. To minimize fistula output in patients with distal fistulas, a fiber-free formula or a low-fiber diet should be used, and the patient should be fed as proximally as possible to the fistula to maximize absorptive surface area. If the fistula is proximal to the site where feedings enter the bowel, a fiber-containing formula can be used. There are published reports of using elemental formulas in hopes of reducing GI secretions and pancreatic enzyme concentration in fistula output.[147,148] Gastric or duodenally delivered elemental formulas may not stimulate pancreatic secretions as much as standard enteral formulas; however, no outcome trials exist to support more rapid fistula closure.[149] If significant amounts of the pancreatobiliary secretions are lost from the fistula site and cannot or are not reinfused, elemental or semielemental feedings may be beneficial. Powdered pancreatic enzymes can be mixed with intact protein formulas to enhance absorption.[150] There are no controlled clinical trials comparing elemental or semielemental feedings to standard tube feedings, or comparing standard formulas with added enzymes to standard formulas in fistula patients. Depending on the overall patient care goals, creative methods of feeding may be necessary; for example, the fistula can be used as the access site for a feeding tube if spontaneous closure is not the goal.[151]

The ability to contain fistula drainage adequately to prevent skin breakdown around the fistula is essential. To accomplish this, the expertise of a certified continence ostomy wound nurse is very valuable. If, despite the efforts of a certified continence ostomy wound nurse, the surrounding skin continues to be exposed to fistula drainage, EN (tube feeding and/or oral diet) may need to be held and PN administered until output can be adequately contained. Once the drainage is controlled, another trial of EN may be warranted.

Many patients with fistulas require PN.[152] Interestingly, the first reported use of PN in humans was in 1968 in a 52-year-old male with multiple fistulas secondary to Crohn's disease who had lost 80 lb before receiving PN.[153] PN is more likely to be utilized in patients with fistulas that originate in the pancreas, high-output fistulas located in the jejunum or ileum, proximal fistulas where distal enteral access is not feasible, or any type of fistula where the output cannot be collected in a manner that protects the skin.[147]

TABLE 26-21 Factors Affecting Likelihood of Fistula Closure

Factor	Likely to Close	Unlikely to Close
Anatomic location	Oropharyngeal	Gastric
	Esophageal	
	Duodenal stump	Ligament of Treitz
	Pancreatobiliary	Ileal
	Jejunal	
Nutritional status	Well nourished	Malnourished
Sepsis	Absent	Present
Etiology	Appendicitis	Crohn's disease
	Diverticulitis	Cancer
	Postoperative	Radiation
		Foreign body (such as a stent, mesh, or staple)
Condition of bowel	Health of adjacent tissue	Total disruption
	Small leak	Distal obstruction
	No abscess	Abscess
	Quiescent disease	Active disease, such as Crohn's or tumor
Other	Tract > 2 cm long	Tract < 2 cm, epithelialization

With data from Maykel JA, Fischer JE. Current management of intestinal fistulas. In: Tompkins RK, ed. *Advances in Surgery*. Orlando, FL: Mosby; 2003: 283–299.[148]

Specific Nutrient Issues

Hydration and Electrolytes

Fluid balance must be monitored very carefully to prevent dehydration. If possible, fistula output and urine and stool/ostomy output should be measured. A drop in urine volume can be a sign of dehydration; immediate measures should be taken to rehydrate the patient. To accomplish this, intravenous fluids may be needed. Electrolyte content of the fistula output varies depending on the origin of the fistula in the bowel (see Chapter 7).

Vitamin and Mineral Supplementation

Patients with high-output fistulas who are not on PN may require extra vitamin and mineral supplementation. Loss of zinc and copper, in particular, can be excessive from proximal EC fistula drainage.[148,152] However, there is no evidence regarding replacement doses of these micronutrients. Patients with ostomies or fistulas that drain above the ileum and who are not receiving intravenous multivitamins will require intravenous or nasal vitamin B_{12} supplementation.

Intestinal Urinary Diversions

Urinary diversions and bladder reconstruction/replacement (ileal conduits, ureterosigmoidostomies, ileocecal pouches, ileal bladder augmentation, neobladder) using intestinal (usually ileum and/or colon) segments are performed for intractable incontinence or following cystectomy, most commonly for bladder cancer. Nutrition-related problems associated with these surgeries may include metabolic acidosis and vitamin B_{12} deficiency. The mechanism for the metabolic acidosis is not known. However, because it is a hyperchloremic metabolic acidosis, the theory is that it is caused by increased absorption of chloride and ammonium in the bowel segment, as well as increased losses of bicarbonate. Acidosis increases calcium excretion in the urine and also has a direct effect on bone causing an increase in osteoclastic activity. These changes raise concern over the bone health of patients with intestinal urinary diversions.

Metabolic acidosis is believed to be less common with newer surgical techniques because of reduced time the urine is in contact with the bowel mucosa. Patients who have had the older procedure, the ureterosigmoidostomy, may be more likely to have significant acidosis. However, data establishing clinical relevancy for the concern over metabolic acidosis causing bone problems is currently lacking. After a thorough review of the research to date, Roosen et al.[147] stated that there is limited evidence for any clinically significant change in acid-base balance: only a few published cases of bone demineralization were found, and each case was asymptomatic. In addition, despite up to 30 years of follow-up, bone changes were not seen, even in those cases with metabolic acidosis.

Standard practice includes early correction of base deficit (> -2.5) with sodium citrate or sodium bicarbonate. Patients at risk for long-term bone problems include children, adolescents, and patients with renal dysfunction. They may require follow-up (dual energy x-ray absorptiometry scans) to ensure that metabolic acidosis is not contributing to bone demineralization.[148]

If terminal ileum is used for the urinary diversion, there is the potential for the patient to develop vitamin B_{12} deficiency. Annual screening is recommended.[148]

Acknowledgments

Gastrointestinal material from the previous The A.S.P.E.N. Nutrition Support Core Curriculum: A Case-Base Approach—The Adult Patient was contributed by Carol Parrish, MS, RD, Joe Krenitsky, MS, RD, Kate Willcutts, MS, RD, CNSD, and Amy E. Radigan, RD, CNSD.

References

1. Rege RV, Jones DB. Current role of surgery in peptic ulcer disease. In: Feldman M, Friedman LS, Sleisenger MH, eds. *Gastrointestinal and Liver Disease*. 7th ed. New York, NY: Elsevier Science; 2002:CD ROM, Chapter 42.
2. Bodai BI, Kuehner CR. The small intestine. In: Bodai BI, ed. *Synopsis of Common Surgical Procedures*. Malvern, PA: Lea & Febiger; 1993:177–178.
3. Radigan A. Post-gastrectomy: managing the nutrition fall-out. *Pract Gastroenterol.* 2004;XXVIII(6):63.
4. Tovey F, Godfrey J, Lwein M. A gastrectomy population: 25–30 years on. *Postgrad Med J.* 1990;66:450–456.
5. Grant J, Chapman G, Russell M. Malabsorption associated with surgical procedures and its treatment. *Nutr Clin Pract.* 1996;11:43–52.
6. Braga M, Zuliani W, Foppa L, et al. Food intake and nutritional status after total gastrectomy: results of a nutritional follow-up. *Br J Surg.* 1988;75:477–480.
7. Ukleja A. Dumping syndrome: pathophysiology and treatment. *Nutr Clin Pract.* 2005;20(5):517–525.
8. Abell TL, Minocha A. Gastrointestinal complications of bariatric surgery: diagnosis and therapy. *Am J Med Sci.* 2006;331(4):214–218.
9. Harju E. Metabolic problems after gastric surgery. *Int Surg.* 1990; 75:27–35.
10. Gray JL, Debas HT, Mulvhill SJ. Control of dumping symptoms by somatostatin analogue in patients after gastric surgery. *Arch Surg.* 1991;126:1231–1236.
11. McKelvey ST. Gastric incontinence and post-vagotomy diarrhoea. *Br J Surg.* 1970;57:741–747.
12. Meyer J. Chronic morbidity after ulcer surgery. In: Sleisenger MH, Fordtran JS, eds. *Gastrointestinal Diseases*. 5th ed. Philadelphia, PA: Saunders; 1994:731–744.
13. Bae J, Park J, Yang H, Kim J. Nutritional status of gastric cancer patients after total gastrectomy. *World J Surg.* 1998;22:254–261.
14. McCray S. Lactose intolerance: considerations for the clinician. *Pract Gastroenterol.* 2003;XXVII(2):21.
15. Pannala R, Brandabur JJ, Gan SI, et al. Afferent limb syndrome and delayed GI problems after pancreaticoduodenectomy for pancreatic cancer: single-center, 14-year experience. *Gastrointestinal Endoscopy.* 2011;74(2):295–302.
16. Yamada T, Alpers DH. *Textbook of Gastroenterology*. 5th ed. Hoboken, NJ: Blackwell Publishing; 2009.
17. Pawson R, Mehta A. Review article: the diagnosis and treatment of haematinic deficiency in gastrointestinal disease. *Aliment Pharmacol Ther.* 1998;12:687–698.
18. Lindenbaum J, Savage DG, Stabler SP, Allen RH. Diagnosis of cobalamin deficiency: II. Relative sensitivities of serum cobalamin, methylmalonic acid, and total homocysteine concentrations. *Am J Hematol.* 1990;34(2):99–107.
19. Adachi S, Kawamoto T, Otsuka M, et al. Enteral vitamin B_{12} supplements reverse postgastrectomy B_{12} deficiency. *Ann Surg.* 2000;232: 199–201.
20. Fischer AB. Twenty-five years after Billroth II gastrectomy for duodenal ulcer. *World J Surg.* 1984;8:293–302.
21. Friess H, Bohm J, Muller M, et al. Maldigestion after total gastrectomy is associated with pancreatic insufficiency. *Am J Gastroenterol.* 1990;91:341–347.
22. Bisballe S, Eriksen EF, Melsen F, et al. Osteopenia and osteomalacia after gastrectomy: interrelations between biochemical markers of bone remodeling, vitamin D metabolites, and bone histomorphometry. *Gut.* 1991;32:1303–1307.
23. Vestegaard P. Bone loss associated with gastrointestinal disease: prevalence and pathogenesis. *Euro J Gastroenterol Hepat.* 2003;15: 851–856.
24. Bisballe S, Buus S, Lund B, et al. Food intake and nutritional status after gastrectomy. *Hum Nutr: Clin Nutr.* 1986;40C:301–308.
25. Klein KB, Orwoll ES, Liberman DA, et al. Metabolic bone disease in asymptomatic men after partial gastrectomy with Billroth II anastomosis. *Gastroenterology.* 1987;92:608–616.
26. Bernstein C, Leslie W. The pathophysiology of bone disease in gastrointestinal disease. *Euro J Gastroenterol Hepat.* 2003;15: 857–864.
27. Arden NK, Cooper C. Assessment of the risk of fracture in patients with gastrointestinal disease. *Euro J Gastroenterol Hepat.* 2003;15: 865–868.
28. Bilimoria KY, Bentrem DJ, Ko CY, et al. Validation of the 6th edition AJCC Pancreatic Cancer Staging System: report from the National Cancer Database. *Cancer.* 2007;110(4):738–744.
29. Redlich PN, Steven AA, Pitt HA. Tumors of the pancreas, gallbladder, and bile ducts. In: Lenhard RE, Osteen RT, Gansler T, eds. *The American Cancer Society's Clinical Oncology*. Atlanta, GA: The American Cancer Society; 2001:373–394.
30. Toyota N, Takada T, Yasuda H, et al. The effects of omeprazole, a proton pump inhibitor, on early gastric stagnation after a pylorus-preserving pancreaticoduodenectomy: results of a randomized study. *Hepato-Gastroenterology.* 1998;45:1005–1010.
31. Tougas G, Eaker EY, Abell TL, et al. Assessment of gastric emptying using a low fat meal: establishment of international control values. *Am J Gastroenterol.* 2000;95(6):1456–1462.
32. Horowitz M, Harding PE, Maddox AF, et al. Gastric and esophageal emptying in patients with type II (non-insulin dependent) DM. *Diabetologia.* 1989;32(3):151–159.
33. MacGregor IL, Gueller R, Watts HD, et al. The effect of acute hyperglycemia on gastric emptying in man. *Gastroenterology.* 1976;70: 190–197.
34. Rayner CK, Su YC, Doran SM, et al. The stimulation of antral motility by erythromycin is attenuated by hyperglycemia. *Am J Gastroenterol.* 2000;95(9):2233–2341.
35. Hallberg L, Brune M, Rossander-Hulthen L. Is there a physiologic role of vitamin C in iron absorption? *Ann NY Acad Sci.* 1987;498: 324–332.
36. American Gastroenterological Association. American Gastroenterological Association medical position statement: nausea and vomiting. *Gastroenterology.* 2001;120(1):261–262.
37. Abell TL, Bernstein VK, Cutts T, Farrugia G, et al., Treatment of gastroparesis: a multidisciplinary clinical review. *Neurogastroenterol Motility.* 2006;18:263–283.
38. Zaidel O, Lin HC. Uninvited guests: the impact of small intestinal bacterial overgrowth on nutritional status. *Pract Gastroenterol.* 2003;XXVII(7):27. 27. Parrish CR, Yoshida C. Nutrition intervention for the patient with gastroparesis: an update. *Pract Gastroenterol.* 2005;XXIX(8):29.
39. Sanders MK. Bezoars. from mystical charms to medical and nutritional management. *Pract Gastroenterol.* 2004;XXVIII(1):37.
40. Hayashi K, Ohara H, Naitoh I, et al. Persimmon bezoar successfully treated by oral intake of Coca-Cola: a case report. *Cases J.* 2008;1(1):385.
41. Lin CS, Tung CF, Peng YC, Chow WK, Chang CS, Hu WH. Successful treatment with a combination of endoscopic injection and irrigation with coca cola for gastric bezoar-induced gastric outlet obstruction. *JCMA.* 2008;71(1):49–52.
42. Silva FG, Goncalves C, Vasconcelos H, Cotrim I. Endoscopic and enzymatic treatment of gastric bezoar with acetylcysteine. *Endoscopy.* 2002;34(10):845.
43. Schlang HA. Acetylcysteine in removal of bezoar. *JAMA.* 1970; 214(7):1329.
44. McCray S, Walker S, Parrish CR. Much ado about refeeding. *Pract Gastroenterol.* 2004;XXVIII(12):26.

45. Malone AM. Enteral formula selection: a review of selected product categories. *Pract Gastroenterol.* 2005;XXIX(6):44.
46. Parrish CR. Enteral feeding: the art and the science. *Nutr Clin Pract.* 2003;18:76–85.
47. Lin HC. Small intestinal bacterial overgrowth: a framework for understanding irritable bowel syndrome. *JAMA.* 2004;18;292(7): 852–858.
48. Teo M, Chung S, Chitti L, et al. Small bowel bacterial overgrowth is a common cause of chronic diarrhea. *J Gastroenterol Hepatol.* 2004;19(8):904–909.
49. Strid H, Simren M, Stotzer PO, et al. Patients with chronic renal failure have abnormal small intestinal motility and a high prevalence of small intestinal bacterial overgrowth. *Digestion.* 2003; 67(3):129–137.
50. Gunnarsdottir SA, Sadik R, Shev S, et al. Small intestinal motility disturbances and bacterial overgrowth in patients with liver cirrhosis and portal hypertension. *Am J Gastroenterol.* 2003;98(6): 1362–1370.
51. Trespi E, Ferrieri A. Intestinal bacterial overgrowth during chronic pancreatitis. *Curr Med Res Opin.* 1999;15(1):47–52.
52. Su J, Smith MB, Rerknimitr R, et al. Small intestine bacterial overgrowth presenting as protein-losing enteropathy. *Dig Dis Sci.* 1998; 43(3):679–681.
53. Van Citters GW, Lin HC. Management of small intestinal bacterial overgrowth. *Curr Gastroenterol Rep.* 2005;7(4):317–320.
54. Di Stefano M, Miceli E, Missanelli A, et al. Treatment of small intestine bacterial overgrowth. *Eur Rev Med Pharmacol Sci.* 2005;9: 217–222.
55. Di Stefano M, Malservisl S, Veneto G, et al. Rifaximin versus chlortetracycline in the short-term treatment of small bowel intestinal bacterial overgrowth. *Aliment Pharmacol Ther.* 2000;14(5): 551–556.
56. Fasano A, Catassi C. Current approaches to diagnosis and treatment of celiac disease: an evolving spectrum. *Gastroenterology.* 2001; 120(3):636–651.
57. Murray JA. The widening spectrum of celiac disease. *Am J Clin Nutr.* 1999;69:354–363.
58. Hill ID, Dirks MH, Liptak GS, et al. Guideline for the diagnosis and treatment of celiac disease in children: recommendations of the North American Society for Pediatric Gastroenterology, Hepatology and Nutrition. *J Pediatr Gastroenterol Nutr.* 2005, Jan;40(1):1–19.
59. Alaedini A, Green PHR. Narrative review: celiac disease: understanding a complex autoimmune disorder. *Ann Intern Med.* 2005; 142:289–298.
60. See J, Murray JA. Gluten-free diet: the medical and nutrition management of celiac disease. *Nutr Clin Pract.* 2006;21(1):1–15.
61. Duggan JM, Duggan AE. Systematic review: the liver in celiac disease. *Aliment Pharmacol Ther.* 2005;21:515–518.
62. Garioch JJ, Lewis HM, Sargent SA, et al. 25 years' experience of a gluten-free diet in the treatment of dermatitis herpetiformis. *Br J Dermatol.* 1994;131(4):541–545.
63. Dahele A, Ghosh S. Vitamin B_{12} deficiency in untreated celiac disease. *Am J Gastroenterol.* 2001;96(3):745–750.
64. Fasano A, Berti I, Gerarduzzi T. Prevalence of celiac disease in at-risk and not-at-risk groups in the United States. *Arch Intern Med.* 2003;163:286–292.
65. Murray JA. Celiac disease in patients with an affected member, Type I diabetes, iron-deficiency, or osteoporosis? *Gastroenterology.* 2005;128:S52–S56.
66. Hoffman RJ, Dhaliwal G, Gilden DJ, et al. Special cure. *N Engl J Med.* 2004;351:1997–2002.
67. Corazza RG, Di Stefano M, Mauriño E, et al. Bones in coeliac disease: diagnosis and treatment. *Best Pract Res Clin Gastroenterol.* 2005;19(3):311–487.
68. NIH Consensus Development Conference on Celiac Disease. National Institutes of Health. Consensus Development Conference Statement. June 28–30, 2004. http://digestive.niddk.nih.gov/ddiseases/pubs/celiac/. Accessed November 1, 2005.
69. Abdulkarim AS, Murray JA. Celiac disease. *Curr Treatment Options Gastroenterol.* 2002;5:27–38.
70. Ciclitira PJ, Ellis HJ, Lundin KEA. Gluten-free diet—what is toxic? *Best Pract Res Clin Gastroenterol.* 2005;19(3):359–371.
71. Ciacci C, Cirillo M, Cavallaro R, et al. Long-term follow-up of celiac adults on gluten-free diet: prevalence and correlates of intestinal damage. *Digestion.* 2002;66:178–185.
72. Case S. *Gluten-Free Diet: A Comprehensive Resource Guide.* 2006 ed. www.glutenfreediet.ca. Accessed July 21, 2006.
73. Case S. The gluten-free diet: how to provide effective education and resources. *Gastroenterology.* 2005;128(4 Suppl 1):S128–S134.
74. Zarkadas M, Cranney A, Case S, et al. The impact of a gluten-free diet on adults with celiac disease: results of a national survey. *J Hum Nutr Dietet.* 2006;19:41–49.
75. Green PHR, Stavropoulos SN, Panagi SG, et al. Characteristics of adult celiac disease in the USA: results of a national survey. *Am J Gastroenterol.* 2001;96:126–131.
76. Sverker A, Hensing G, Hallert C. "Controlled by food"—lived experiences of celiac disease. *J Hum Nutr Diet.* 2005;18:171–180.
77. Murray JA, Watson T, Clearman B, et al. Effect of a gluten-free diet on gastrointestinal symptoms in celiac disease. *Am J Clin Nutr.* 2004;79:669–673.
78. Mandal A, Mayberry J. Elemental diet in the treatment of refractory coeliac disease. *Eur J Gastroenterol Hepatol.* 2001;13(1): 79–80.
79. Sandborn WJ, Loftus EV Jr, Colombel JF, et al. Evaluation of serologic disease markers in a population-based cohort of patients with ulcerative colitis and Crohn's disease. *Inflamm Bowel Dis.* 2001;7:192–201.
80. Krok KL, Lichtenstein GR. Nutrition in Crohn's disease. *Curr Opin Gastroenterol.* 2003;19:148–153.
81. Chan AT, Fleming CR, O'Fallon WM, et al. Estimated versus measured basal energy requirements in patients with Crohn's disease. *Gastroenterology.* 1986;91(1):75–78.
82. Stokes MA, Hill GL. Total energy expenditure in patients with Crohn's disease: measurement by the combined body scan technique. *J Parenter Enteral Nutr.* 1993;17:3–7.
83. Eiden K. Nutritional considerations in inflammatory bowel disease. *Pract Gastroenterol.* 2003;XXVII(5):33.
84. Park RH, Duncan A, Russell RI. Hypolactasia and Crohn's disease: a myth. *Am J Gastroenterol.* 1990;85:708–710.
85. von Tirpitz C, Kohn C, Steinkamp M, et al. Lactose intolerance in active Crohn's disease: clinical value of duodenal lactase analysis. *J Clin Gastroenterol.* 2002;34:49–53.
86. Mishkin B, Yalovsky M, Mishkin S. Increased prevalence of lactose malabsorption in Crohn's disease patients at low risk for lactose malabsorption based on ethnic origin. *Am J Gastroenterol.* 1997;92: 1148–1153.
87. Pironi L, Callegari C, Cornia GL, et al. Lactose malabsorption in adult patients with Crohn's disease. *Am J Gastroenterol.* 1988; 83:1267–1271.
88. Zachos M, Tondeur M, Griffiths AM. Enteral nutritional therapy for inducing remission of Crohn's disease. *Cochrane Database Syst Rev.* 2001;(3):CD000542.
89. Griffiths AM, Ohlsson A, Sherman PM, et al. Meta-analysis of enteral nutrition as a primary treatment of active Crohn's disease. *Gastroenterology.* 1995;108:1056–1067.
90. Makola, D. Elemental and semi-elemental formulas: are they superior to polymeric formulas? *Pract Gastroenterol.* 2005;XXIX(12): 59-72.

91. Gassull MA, Fernandanares F, Cabre E, et al. European Group on Enteral Nutrition in Crohn's Disease. Fat composition may be a clue to explain the primary therapeutic effect of enteral nutrition in Crohn's disease: results of a double blind randomised multicentre European trial. *Gut.* 2002;51:164–168.
92. Sakurai T, Matsui T, Yao T, et al. Short-term efficacy of enteral nutrition in the treatment of active Crohn's disease: a randomized, controlled trial comparing nutrient formulas. *J Parenter Enteral Nutr.* 2002;26:98–103.
93. Akobeng AK, Miller V, Stanton J, et al. Double-blind randomized controlled trial of glutamine-enriched polymeric diet in the treatment of active Crohn's disease. *J Pediatr Gastroenterol Nutr.* 2000; 30(1):78–84.
94. Den Hond E, Hiele M, Peeters M, et al. Effect of long-term oral glutamine supplements on small intestinal permeability in patients with Crohn's disease. *J Parenter Enteral Nutr.* 1999;23:7–11.
95. Ockenga J, Borchert K, Stuber E, et al. Glutamine-enriched PN in patients with inflammatory bowel disease. *Eur J Clin Nutr.* 2005; 59:1302–1309.
96. Goh J, O'Morain CA. Review article: nutrition and adult inflammatory bowel disease. *Aliment Pharmacol Ther.* 2003;17: 307–320.
97. A.S.P.E.N. Board of Directors and the Clinical Guidelines Task Force. Guidelines for the use of parenteral and enteral nutrition in adult and pediatric patients. *J Parenter Enteral Nutr.* 2002;26: 73SA–74SA.
98. Erichsen K, Ulvik RJ, Nysaeter G, et al. Oral ferrous fumarate or intravenous iron sucrose for patients with inflammatory bowel disease. *Scand J Gastroenterol.* 2005;40:1058–1065.
99. Vestergaard P. Prevalence and pathogenesis of osteoporosis in patients with inflammatory bowel disease. *Minerva Med.* 2004; 95:469–480.
100. Schulte CM. Review article: bone disease in inflammatory bowel disease. *Aliment Pharmacol Ther.* 2004;20(suppl 4):43–49.
101. Siffledeen JS, Fedorak RN, Siminoski K, et al. Randomized trial of etidronate plus calcium and vitamin D for treatment of low bone mineral density in Crohn's disease. *Clin Gastroenterol Hepatol.* 2005;3:122–132.
102. Duggan P, O'Brien M, Kiely M, et al. Vitamin K status in patients with Crohn's disease and relationship to bone turnover. *Am J Gastroenterol.* 2004;99:2178–2185.
103. Chowers Y, Sela BA, Holland R, et al. Increased levels of homocysteine in patients with Crohn's disease are related to folate levels. *Am J Gastroenterol.* 2000;95:3498–3502.
104. Wolman SL, Anderson H, Marliss EB, et al. Zinc in total parenteral nutrition: requirements and metabolic effects. *Gastroenterology.* 1979;76:458–467.
105. Klaassen J, Zapata R, Mella JG, et al. Enteral nutrition in severe ulcerative colitis: digestive tolerance and nutritional efficiency. *Rev Med Chil.* 1998;126:899–904.
106. Gassull MA. Nutrition and inflammatory bowel disease: its relation to pathophysiology, outcome and therapy. *Dig Dis.* 2003;21: 220–227.
107. Gonzalez-Huix F, Fernandez-Banares F, Esteve-Comas M, et al. Enteral versus parenteral nutrition as adjunct therapy in acute ulcerative colitis. *Am J Gastroenterol.* 1993;88:227–232.
108. Wilson A, Reyes E, Ofman J. Prevalence and outcomes of anemia in inflammatory bowel disease: a systematic review of the literature. *Am J Med.* 2004;116(suppl 7A):44S–49S.
109. Diculescu M, Ciocirlan M, Ciocirlan M, et al. Folic acid and sulfasalazine for colorectal carcinoma chemoprevention in patients with ulcerative colitis: the old and new evidence. *Rom J Gastroenterol.* 2003;12:283–286.
110. Vernia P, Annese V, Bresci G, et al. Topical butyrate improves efficacy of 5-ASA in refractory distal ulcerative colitis: results of a multicentre trial. *Eur J Clin Invest.* 2003;33:244–248.
111. Seidner DL, Lashner BA, Brzezinski A, et al. An oral supplement enriched with fish oil, soluble fiber, and antioxidants for corticosteroid sparing in ulcerative colitis: a randomized, controlled trial. *Clin Gastroenterol Hepatol.* 2005;3:358–369.
112. Hallert C, Bjorck I, Nyman M, et al. Increasing fecal butyrate in ulcerative colitis patients by diet: controlled pilot study. *Inflamm Bowel Dis.* 2003;9:116–121.
113. Fernandez-Banares F, Hinojosa J, Sanchez-Lombrana JL, et al. Spanish Group for the Study of Crohn's Disease and Ulcerative Colitis. Randomized clinical trial of Plantago ovata seeds (dietary fiber) as compared with mesalamine in maintaining remission in ulcerative colitis. *Am J Gastroenterol.* 1999;94:427–433.
114. Karbach U, Singe CC, Ewe K. Simplified determination of intestinal protein excretion based on alpha 1-antitrypsin clearance. *Z Gastroenterol.* 1988;26:169–173.
115. Chiu NT, Lee BF, Hwang SJ, et al. Protein-losing enteropathy: diagnosis with (99m)Tc-labeled human serum albumin scintigraphy. *Radiology.* 2001;219:86–90.
116. Takeda H, Ishihama K, Fukui T, et al. Significance of rapid turnover proteins in protein-losing gastroenteropathy. *Hepatogastroenterology.* 2003;50:1963–1965.
117. McCray S, Parrish CR. When chyle leaks: nutrition intervention. *Pract Gastroenterol.* 2004;XXVIII(5):60.
118. Aoyagi K, Iida M, Matsumoto T, et al. Enteral nutrition as a primary therapy for intestinal lymphangiectasia: value of elemental diet and polymeric diet compared with PN. *Dig Dis Sci.* 2005; 50:1467–1470.
119. Purdum PP, Kirby DF. Short-bowel syndrome: a review of the role of nutrition support. *J Parenter Enteral Nutr.* 1991;15:93–101.
120. Vanderhoof JA, Langnas AN. Short-bowel syndrome in children and adults. *Gastroenterology.* 1997;113:1767–1778.
121. Abad-Sinden A, Sutphen J. Nutritional management of pediatric short bowel syndrome. *Pract Gastroenterol.* 2003;XXVII(12):28.
122. Jeppesen PB, Staun M, Tjellesen L, et al. Effect of intravenous ranitidine and omeprazole on intestinal absorption of water, sodium, macronutrients in patients with intestinal resection. *Gut.* 1998;43:763–769.
123. A.S.P.E.N. Board of Directors. Guidelines for the use of parenteral and enteral nutrition in adult and pediatric patients. *J Parenter Enteral Nutr.* 2002;26:70SA–73SA.
124. Buchman AL, Scolapio J, Fryer J. AGA technical review on short bowel syndrome and intestinal transplantation. *Gastroenterology.* 2003;124(4):1111–1134.
125. Parrish CR. The clinician's guide to short bowel syndrome. *Pract Gastroenterol.* 2005;XXIX (9):67.
126. Van Citters GW, Lin HC. The ileal brake: a fifteen-year progress report. *Curr Gastroenterol Rep.* 1999;1(5):404-409.
127. Thompson CRV. Nephrocalcinosis and nephrolithiasis. In: Nightingale JM, ed. *Intestinal Failure.* London, UK: Greenwich Medical Media Limited; 2001:237.
128. Nightingale JMD, Lennard-Jones JE, Gertner DJ, et al. Colonic preservation reduces need for parenteral therapy, increases the incidence of renal stones, but does not change high prevalence of gallstones in patients with short bowel. *Gut.* 1992;33:1493–1497.
129. Sundaram A, Koutkia P, Apovian CM. Nutritional management of short bowel syndrome in adults. *J Clin Gastroenterol.* 2002; 34(3):207–220.
130. Hoppe B, Leumann E, von Unruh G, et al. Diagnostic and therapeutic approaches in patients with secondary hyperoxaluria. *Frontiers Biosci.* 2003;8:437–443.

131. Bambach CP, Robertson WG, Peacock M, et al. Effect of intestinal surgery on the risk of urinary stone formation. *Gut.* 1981;22: 257–263.
132. Wilmore DW. Indications for specific therapy in the rehabilitation of patients with the short-bowel syndrome. *Best Pract Res Clin Gastroenterol.* 2003;17(6):895–906.
133. Nordgaard I, Hensen BS, Mortensen PB. Colon as a digestive organ in patients with short bowel. *Lancet.* 1994;343:373–376.
134. Kelly D, Nadeau J. Oral rehydration solution: a "low-tech" oft neglected therapy. *Pract Gastroenterol.* 2004;XXVIII(10):51.
135. Nauth J, Chang CW, Mobarhan S, et al. A therapeutic approach to wean total parenteral nutrition in the management of short bowel syndrome: three cases using nocturnal enteral rehydration. *Nutr Rev.* 2004;62(5):221–231.
136. Fleming CR, George L, Stoner G, et al. The importance of urinary magnesium values in gut failure patients [abstract]. *21st Clinical Congress Syllabus.* San Antonio, TX: American Society for Parenteral and Enteral Nutrition; 1994:A21S–A30.
137. Jeppesen PB, Mortensen PB. Intestinal failure defined by measurements of intestinal energy and wet weight absorption. *Gut.* 2000;46:701–706.
138. Byrne TA, Veglia L, Camelio M, et al. Beyond the prescription: optimizing the diet of patients with short bowel syndrome. *Nutr Clin Pract.* 2000;15:306–311.
139. Levy E, Frileux P, Sandrucci S, et al. Continuous enteral nutrition during the early adaptive stage of the short bowel syndrome. *Br J Surg.* 1988;75:549–553.
140. McIntyre PB, Fitchew M, Lennard-Jones JE. Patients with a high jejunostomy do not need a special diet. *Gastroenterology.* 1986;91: 25–33.
141. Bosaeus I, Carlsson NG, Andersson H. Low-fat versus medium-fat enteral diets: effects on bile salt excretion in jejunostomy patients. *Scand J Gastroenterol.* 1986;21:891–896.
142. Nordgaard I, Hansen BS, Mortensen PB. Importance of colonic support for energy absorption as small-bowel failure proceeds. *Am J Clin Nutr.* 1996;64:222–231.
143. Matarese LE, O'Keefe SJ, Kandil HM, et al. Short bowel syndrome: clinical guidelines for nutrition management. *Nutr Clin Pract.* 2005;20(5):493–502.
144. Jeppesen PB. Clinical significance of GLP-2 in short-bowel syndrome. *J Nutr.* 2003;133(11):3721–3724.
145. Berry SM, Fischer JE. Classification and pathophysiology of enterocutaneous fistulas. *Surg Clin North Am.* 1996;76:1009–1018.
146. Gonzalez-Pinto I, Gonzalez EM. Optimizing the treatment of upper gastrointestinal fistulas. *Gut.* 2001;49(suppl 4):22–31.
147. Willcutts K, Scarano K, Eddins C. Ostomies & fistulas: a collaborative approach. *Pract Gastroenterol.* 2005;XXIX(11):63.
148. Maykel JA, Fischer JE. Current management of intestinal fistulas. In: Tompkins RK, ed. *Advances in Surgery.* Orlando, FL: Mosby; 2003:283–299.
149. Keith RG. Effect of a low fat elemental diet on pancreatic secretion during pancreatitis. *Surgery.* 1980;151:227–343.
150. Yoder A. Nutrition support in pancreatitis: beyond parenteral nutrition. *Pract Gastroenterol.* 2003;XXVII(1):19.
151. Voitk AJ, Echave V, Brown RA, et al. Elemental diet in the treatment of fistulas of the alimentary tract. *Surg Gynecol Obstet.* 1973;137:68–72.
152. A.S.P.E.N. Board of Directors. Guidelines for the use of parenteral and enteral nutrition in adult and pediatric patients. *J Parenter Enteral Nutr.* 2002;26:76SA–77SA.
153. Dudrick SJ. A 45-year obsession and passionate pursuit of optimal nutrition support: puppies, pediatrics, surgery, geriatrics, home tpn, ASPEN, et cetera. *J Parenter Enteral Nutr.* 2005;29: 272–297.
154. Roosen A, Gerharz EW, Roth S, et al. Bladder, bowel and bones-skeletal changes after intestinal urinary diversion. *World J Urol.* 2004;22:200–209.
155. Levy E, Frileux P, Cugnenc PH, et al. High-output external fistula of the small bowel: management with continuous enteral nutrition. *Br J Surg.* 1989;76:676–679.
156. Farrell RJ, Kelly CP. Celiac sprue. *N Engl J Med.* 2002;346: 180–188.

27 Liver Disease

Thomas H. Frazier, MD, Benjamin E. Wheeler, MD, Craig J. McClain, MD, and Matthew Cave, MD

CONTENTS

Background 455
Pathogenesis, Malnutrition, and Nutritional Aspects of Liver Disease 456
Alcoholic Liver Disease 457
Nonalcoholic Fatty Liver Disease and Nonalcoholic Steatohepatitis 458
Viral Hepatitis 459
Hereditary Hemochromatosis 459
Wilson Disease 459
Cholestatic Liver Diseases 460
Malnutrition in Chronic Liver Disease 460
Energy Expenditure in Chronic Liver Disease 461
Metabolism in Chronic Liver Disease 461
Nutritional Assessment 462
Anthropometrics 462
Laboratory Measurements 462
Other Nutritional Assessment Tools 462
Provision of Nutrients 462
Patients with Compensated Liver Disease 462
Patients with Decompensated Liver Disease 464
Complementary and Alternative Medicine Agents and Selected Micronutrients 465
Vitamin E 465
Glutathione Prodrugs and Combined Antioxidants 465
S-Adenosylmethionine/Betaine 466
Zinc 466
Silymarin 466
Branched-Chain Amino Acids 467
Miscellaneous Vitamin and Mineral Deficiencies Complicating Cirrhosis 467
Monitoring and Treating Complications 467
Summary 468
Acknowledgment 468
References 468

Objectives

1. Understand the pathogenesis of various liver diseases with an emphasis on how pathogenesis relates to nutrition and malnutrition.
2. Review the difficulty in assessing nutritional status in patients with liver disease and identify possible solutions to these problems.
3. Identify important micronutrient deficiencies and toxicities in patients with liver disease.
4. Determine the energy and protein requirements for patients with both acute and chronic liver diseases.
5. Identify and learn how to address barriers to the delivery of nutrition in patients with liver disease.

Test Your Knowledge Questions

1. Which of the following is an accurate marker of nutritional status in all patients with chronic liver disease with portal hypertension?
   A. Serum albumin
   B. Serum prealbumin
   C. Retinol-binding protein
   D. Anthropometry
   E. None of the above
2. Which of the following statement(s) is false regarding alcoholic hepatitis?
   A. Virtually all patients with alcoholic hepatitis have some degree of malnutrition.
   B. The severity of liver disease generally correlates with the degree of malnutrition.
   C. Caloric intake correlates with mortality.
   D. Protein delivery should be reduced to prevent portal systemic encephalopathy (PSE).
3. Which of the following statements is true regarding total parenteral nutrition (TPN) in the care of the inpatient with liver disease?
   A. There is no role for TPN in nutrition in liver disease.
   B. TPN should be initiated in all hospitalized patients with liver disease.
   C. In a patient unable to tolerate enteral feeding TPN can provide necessary nutrition, but should be discontinued in favor of enteral nutrition as soon as possible.
   D. Once a patient is unable to tolerate enteral nutrition they should continue on TPN for the duration of their hospitalization.

Test Your Knowledge Answers

1. The correct answer is **E**. There are no consistently accurate measures of malnutrition in patients with significant liver disease. Visceral proteins such as albumin, prealbumin, and retinol-binding protein are made in the liver and better correlate with the severity of liver disease rather than the degree of malnutrition. Anthropometry can be inaccurate in the setting of edema and/or ascites.
2. The correct answer is **D**. The Veterans Health Administration Cooperative Studies Program demonstrated that virtually all patients with alcoholic hepatitis have some degree of malnutrition. In addition, the severity of liver disease generally correlated with the degree of malnutrition. Study subjects consuming > 3000 kcal per day had near zero mortality, whereas those consuming less than 1000 kcal per day had > 80% mortality. Thus, food intake correlated with 6-month mortality. Protein requirements in patients with alcoholic hepatitis are increased and the delivery of protein is not a significant precipitant of PSE. Restriction of protein is not recommended in alcoholic hepatitis (or any other liver disease, for that matter) and should only be implemented in the setting of PSE refractory to medical treatment.
3. The correct answer is **C**. The goal should always be to provide enteral nutrition to patients with liver disease. In certain patients, such as those without a functional gut, it is necessary to provide nutrition in the form of TPN. This should be continued for the minimal period possible. Enteral feeding is always preferred to TPN when enteral feeding is possible.

Background

Nutritional support for patients with liver diseases is a complex topic. The liver is pivotal in many metabolic processes. It normally has considerable metabolic reserve. Despite this, patients with decompensated liver disease can develop significant nutritional deficiencies. A complicating factor for providing nutritional support is the tremendous variability in the causes and severity of liver disease among patients. In addition, traditional methods of assessing nutritional status are often unreliable. These issues make it difficult to provide a "blanket" recommendation for nutritional therapy in liver disease patients.

Perfused by both the portal vein and hepatic artery, the liver has a unique dual blood supply and consists of multiple cell types having differing functions. Hepatocytes make up over 80% of the total liver mass and play a critical role in the metabolism of amino acids and ammonia; in the detoxification of a variety of drugs, vitamins, and hormones; and in the biochemical oxidation reactions. Hepatic Kupffer cells, the largest reservoir of fixed macrophages in the body, play a protective role against gut-derived toxins that have escaped into the portal circulation. These cells are major producers of cytokines, which can markedly influence nutritional status. The liver also contains hepatic stellate cells, which play an important role in collagen formation following liver injury and are the major storehouse for vitamin A in the body. There are a host of additional cell types located in the liver, each with distinctive functions (eg, bile duct epithelium in bile flow, sinusoidal endothelial cells in adhesion molecule expression and endocytosis).

The liver plays an essential role in the metabolism of proteins, carbohydrates, and fats. Plasma proteins, nonessential amino acids, urea (for ammonia excretion), glycogen, and critical hormones such insulinlike growth factor-1 are synthesized in the liver. The liver is also a chief site for the metabolism of fatty acids. In addition, bile from the liver is needed for fat absorption from the intestine. Thus, a properly functioning liver is imperative for achieving and maintaining appropriate nutritional status.

Acute hepatitis is usually a self-limited liver disease characterized by the elevation of serum transaminases (alanine aminotransferase (ALT) and aspartate aminotransferase (AST)). Acute hepatitis is most frequently caused by a viral infection, medication/toxicant, Wilson disease, or shock. Malnutrition and the presence of chronic liver diseases, such as nonalcoholic fatty liver disease (NAFLD), may predispose patients to acute liver injury. The functional reserve of the liver is so great that 80% to 90% of liver cells must be injured before physiologic functions are impaired. Destruction of a large proportion of the hepatocytes results in acute liver failure, which is characterized by deterioration in hepatic synthetic function (eg, jaundice, coagulopathy, hypoalbuminemia) and manifestations of portal hypertension (eg, ascites, hyponatremia, esophageal varices). Hepatic encephalopathy (HE) can range from subtle behavioral changes to disorientation and deep coma.

Two epidemics are fueling the most recent increase in the prevalence of chronic liver disease, namely, hepatitis C virus (HCV) and NAFLD/nonalcoholic steatohepatitis (NASH). Approximately 2% of Americans are infected with HCV. NAFLD, the hepatic manifestation of metabolic syndrome/insulin resistance, has become the most common liver disease in the United States. Both of these diseases can progress to cirrhosis in a significant percentage of patients. Cirrhosis, characterized by dense collagen accumulation, or fibrosis, may lead to end-stage (or decompensated) liver disease, which may also be accompanied by synthetic dysfunction and portal hypertension as well as hepatocellular carcinoma. However, in its early stages, chronic liver disease may be asymptomatic. Serologic tests may reveal abnormal liver enzymes in either a hepatocellular (AST/ALT) or a cholestatic pattern (alkaline phosphatase). Progressive fibrosis develops in some but not all patients with chronic liver disease resulting in cirrhosis.

Pathogenesis, Malnutrition, and Nutritional Aspects of Liver Disease

There are multiple etiologies of liver disease (Table 27-1). Although often difficult to diagnose, patients with advanced liver disease are often at risk for malnutrition.[1] Although the pathophysiology of how liver dysfunction causes malnutrition is unclear, local and systemic neurohormonal mechanisms are likely involved in causing delayed gastric emptying, small bowel dysmotility and bacterial overgrowth, and constipation.[2-6] Further complicating this picture are increased renal losses of micronutrients, such as zinc, in conditions such as alcoholic liver disease.[7]

TABLE 27-1 Causes of Liver Disease

Toxins
• Ethanol
• Medications
• Industrial chemicals (vinyl chloride)
• Aflatoxins
• Other (eg, *Amanita* sp. mushroom)
Metabolic causes
• Obesity (NAFLD)
• Wilson disease
• Hemochromatosis
• Alpha-1-antitrypsin deficiency
Infectious
• Viral (eg, hepatitis A, B, C, E)
• Bacterial
Immune mediated
• Autoimmune hepatitis
• Primary biliary cirrhosis
• Primary sclerosing cholangitis
• Sarcoidosis
Other
• Budd-Chiari syndrome

NAFLD, nonalcoholic fatty liver disease.

Maldigestion and malabsorption may occur in liver disease and may play an important role in causing malnutrition. Typical gastrointestinal disturbances in liver disease include dysgeusia, anorexia, nausea, and early satiety. Concomitant complications typical of liver disease such as upper gastrointestinal bleeding, portal systemic encephalopathy, and sepsis also cause prolonged periods of poor oral intake. Dietary management of fluid retention with salt and water restriction; and carbohydrate and lipid restrictions used in patients with diabetes mellitus, chronic pancreatic insufficiency, and cholestatic liver disease can all affect diet palatability and can severely restrict patients' food choices.

Impaired lipid metabolism is multifactorial in liver disease. Decreased intraluminal bile salts, small bowel bacterial overgrowth, coexistent pancreatic insufficiency or intestinal disease (inflammatory bowel disease, sprue), and mucosal vascular hypertension and edema can worsen maldigestion and malabsorption. Cholestatic liver disorders are associated with decreased intraluminal concentration of bile salts, resulting in lipid and lipid-soluble vitamin malabsorption.[8]

The loss of glycogen stores that occurs in patients with advanced liver disease predisposes them to enter a starvation state within a few hours of fasting.[9,10] This can lead to peripheral muscle proteolysis to provide amino acids for gluconeogenesis, thus contributing to protein malnutrition. Liver disease patients with portal hypertension and ascites and those with acute alcoholic hepatitis are at increased risk of developing a hypermetabolic state (resting energy expenditure > 110% of its expected value), which also contributes to overall malnutrition.[11-13]

Dysregulated cytokine metabolism (eg, elevated tumor necrosis factor [TNF]) is well documented in many forms of liver disease.[14] Low-grade endotoxemia, facilitated by portal hypertension and gut bacterial translocation, leads to increases in proinflammatory cytokines and further affects nutrient management and overall metabolism.[15] Increased levels of cytokines have been postulated to cause many of the metabolic and nutritional abnormalities observed in liver disease, especially in acute alcoholic hepatitis and in chronic decompensated liver disease.[14] Thus, abnormalities such as fever, anorexia, muscle breakdown, and wasting and altered mineral metabolism are likely to be at least partially cytokine mediated.

Despite the increased frequency of malnutrition in patients with alcoholic or viral liver disease, one cannot assume that all of these patients are at nutritional risk. Moreover, obesity and the metabolic syndrome are increasingly recognized as a major cause of abnormal liver enzymes and can also coexist with and worsen liver diseases of other etiologies. Consequently, both undernutrition and obesity play important roles in liver disease. For this reason, an accurate assessment of nutritional status in patients with liver disease is essential. Patients with alcoholic liver disease are also at risk for complications of alcohol use such as pancreatitis and myopathy. It is not clear, however, what contribution a diminished nutritional status plays in the incidence of these complications. Although the role of nutrition in the pathogenesis, progression, and treatment of specific forms of liver disease (Table 27-1) is clearly beyond the scope of this chapter, some etiologies clearly deserve special focus because they are prevalent or closely linked to nutrition. These include alcoholic liver disease, nonalcoholic fatty liver disease, viral hepatitis, hemochromatosis, Wilson disease, and cholestatic diseases including primary sclerosing cholangitis and primary biliary cirrhosis.

Alcoholic Liver Disease

The liver is the main organ responsible for ethanol metabolism; other organs, such as the stomach, contribute to a much lesser degree. The pathogenesis is complex and involves numerous mechanisms that are variably well understood. Acetaldehyde (one of the metabolites of ethanol) is postulated to play an etiologic role in alcoholic liver disease (ALD). Other mechanisms such as oxidative stress (through both direct injury and cell signaling); mitochondrial dysfunction; hypoxia; impaired proteasome function; abnormal metabolism of methionine, *S*-adenosylmethionine (SAM), and folate; Kupffer cell activation; dysregulated cytokine production; immune responses to altered hepatocellular proteins; and genetic/epigenetic mechanisms are all thought to be involved in the development and progression of ALD.[16] Importantly, many are directly modifiable through nutritional interventions (eg, oxidative stress).

The most extensive studies involving interactions between nutritional status and liver disease have been in patients with ALD. The most detailed of these studies derive from the U.S. Department of Veterans Affairs (VA) Cooperative Studies Program in patients with alcoholic hepatitis.[17-20] In these and other studies it is clear that malnutrition is a major complication of ALD. Importantly, malnutrition worsens clinical outcomes in ALD, and nutritional support improves nutritional status and may improve clinical outcome (Practice Scenario 27-1).

The first of the VA Cooperative Studies (Study #119) established that nearly every patient with alcoholic hepatitis had some degree of malnutrition.[19] This study categorized 284 patients with complete nutritional assessments into groups with mild, moderate, or severe alcoholic hepatitis (based on clinical and biochemical parameters). Mean alcohol consumption among all patients was 228 g per day, with almost 50% of energy intake coming from alcohol. As a result, although caloric intake for many patients was adequate, there was often a deficient intake of protein and critical micronutrients. The severity of liver disease generally correlated with the severity of malnutrition. Similar data were generated in a follow-up VA study on alcoholic hepatitis (Study #275).[21]

In both of these studies, patients were carefully monitored by a dietitian and encouraged to eat a balanced 2500-kcal hospital diet. In the second study, patients in the therapy arm of the protocol also received oxandrolone 80 mg per day and an enteral nutritional support product high in branched-chain amino acids (BCAAs). Caloric intake correlated in a stepwise fashion with 6-month mortality data. Those patients who consumed $<$ 1000 kcal per day had $>$ 80% 6-month mortality, whereas those who voluntarily consumed $>$ 3000 kcal per day had virtually no mortality.[17] Furthermore, the degree of malnutrition correlated with the development of serious complications such as encephalopathy, ascites, and hepatorenal syndrome.[17] Although it is possible that nutrition prevented mortality, it is also possible that the inability to eat was simply a marker of disease severity. Nonetheless, many centers, including our own, provide enteral nutritional support to patients with severe acute alcoholic hepatitis who are unable to voluntarily consume sufficient calories.

In the VA Cooperative Studies, the chronic alcohol-consuming control population without liver disease also frequently had some degree of protein-energy malnutrition. This contradicts other data indicating that only alcoholics with underlying liver disease demonstrated significant protein-energy malnutrition. Although the VA studies evaluated patients with acute alcoholic hepatitis, patients with stable alcoholic cirrhosis without alcoholic hepatitis have been studied as well. One such investigation of patients with compensated alcoholic cirrhosis (not actively drinking) revealed indicators of malnutrition almost as severe as those in patients with alcoholic hepatitis (eg, a creatinine-height index of 71% of normal).[22] Supplemental micronutrients such as SAM and zinc have a potential therapeutic role in alcoholic liver disease and are subsequently discussed as CAM agents later in this chapter.

Practice Scenario 27-1

Question: How important is enteral nutrition in the management of acute alcoholic hepatitis?

Scenario: A 55–year-old male with a past medical history of alcoholism presents with a 2-week history of nausea, vomiting, increasing abdominal girth, and jaundice. Until 2 weeks ago the patient was drinking one-fifth of vodka per day, but since has been unable to tolerate anything by mouth. A physical examination reveals scleral icterus, jaundice, and a tense abdomen with a positive fluid wave consistent with ascites. The patient's memory is normal and there is no asterixis. His weight is 70 kg and his height is 68 in. Diagnostic studies, including laboratory and radiologic investigations, reveal severe alcoholic hepatitis, normal renal function, and new onset ascites. The original diet order is a 2 g sodium diet. Despite aggressive supportive care and corticosteroids, over the next 48 hours the patient develops worsening renal function consistent with hepatorenal syndrome, and an assessment of diet intake reveals the patient is consuming 10% of goal calories and protein.

Intervention: Given the inadequacy of the patient's caloric and protein intake, nasogastric access is obtained and the patient is started on a standard polymeric enteral formula. Enteral nutrition is increased slowly with close attention to his risk of refeeding syndrome. By day 5 of the hospitalization, the patient is receiving 40 kcal per kilogram per day and tolerating 1.5 g of protein per kilogram per day. Over the next several days, the patient begins tolerating oral feeding and is discharged in stable condition 1 week later.

Answer: Early and aggressive enteral nutrition improves outcomes in patients with alcoholic hepatitis. Nasoenteral access is generally required given the many obstacles to enteral feeding in patients with severe liver disease (eg, anorexia, nausea, vomiting). These patients are at risk of refeeding syndrome.

Rationale: The Veterans Health Administration Cooperative Studies Program demonstrated that virtually all patients with alcoholic hepatitis have some degree of malnutrition.[17-20] In addition, the severity of liver disease generally correlated with the degree of malnutrition. Study subjects consuming > 3000 kcal per day had near zero mortality, whereas those consuming less than 1000 kcal per day had > 80% mortality. Thus, food intake correlated with 6-month mortality. A major multicenter study demonstrated that enteral nutrition, when compared to corticosteroids, has similar short-term mortality rates, improved 1-year mortality rates, and reduced infectious complications. Restricting protein is not recommended in alcoholic hepatitis (or any other liver disease, for that matter) and should only be implemented in the setting of PSE refractory to medical treatment.

Nonalcoholic Fatty Liver Disease and Nonalcoholic Steatohepatitis

An estimated 65% of Americans are either overweight or obese. Some estimates predict that close to 100% of Americans will be overweight by the year 2030, placing them at increased risk for development of the metabolic syndrome (see Chapter 35).

NAFLD, the hepatic manifestation of the metabolic syndrome, is a consequence of inappropriate hepatic management of lipids resulting in the abnormal accumulation of fat in the hepatocytes. This phenomenon, although not completely understood, seems to be a consequence of increased free fatty acid delivery to the liver from visceral sources coupled with hyperinsulinemia-related inadequate formation and the export of very low-density lipoproteins (VLDL) out of the hepatocyte.

Although steatosis alone does not usually result in progressive fibrosis, approximately 10% to 20% of patients with NAFLD experience a "second hit," of unknown nature, that induces an inflammatory response to the fat-laden hepatocytes. This inflammation, in turn, can lead to liver cell injury, death, and replacement by scarring (fibrosis). As this necroinflammatory response progresses, it can and frequently does lead to cirrhosis. NASH-related cirrhosis can lead to liver failure and has been associated with the development of hepatocellular carcinoma.

Most NAFLD/NASH patients are obese. As with other obese patients, nutritional assessment is often difficult and complicated, and standard estimates of nutritional needs based on weight and anthropometric measurements are often misleading.[23-26] Additionally, patients with NAFLD/NASH are often diabetic (see Chapter 34) and have varying degrees of diabetic nephropathy and associated proteinuria, which can lead to low serum albumin levels.

When patients' fatty liver disease advances to cirrhosis with serologic hepatic dysfunction, hepatic production of proteins is often impaired. Furthermore, because cirrhosis often results in a catabolic state, a patient's nutritional needs, especially with respect to protein requirements, can be underestimated. Cirrhotic NASH patients are often malnourished and protein deprived despite being obese.

Evidence indicating that specific dietary components play a role in the development/progression of NAFLD is continually emerging. Mechanisms such as lipotoxicity, oxidative stress, endotoxemia, dysregulated cytokines/adipokines, and alterations in gut microflora appear to be involved in triggering both steatosis and steatohepatitis. These mechanisms are also linked with specific dietary habits (eg, obesity, high fat diets [HFDs], excess fructose, diets low in omega-3 fatty acids). HFDs have often been implicated in NAFLD. In fact, many animal models use a HFD (71% of energy from fat) to induce NAFLD.[27] Importantly, HFDs result in a number of metabolic derangements, including oxidative stress, alterations in postprandial triglyceride metabolism, increased TNF-α, circulating free fatty acids (FFAs), and insulin resistance that likely play an etiologic role in NAFLD.

Although the amount of dietary fat certainly appears to be important in the development of NAFLD, there is emerging evidence that the type and ratios of dietary fats can also contribute. An increased fat intake with an excessive amount of omega-6 fatty acids has been implicated in promoting necroinflammation.[28] On the other hand, a diet containing medium-chain triglycerides (MCTs) in the absence of long-chain triglycerides (LCTs) has been reported to be hepatoprotective.[29] There are also studies demonstrating the role of fructose in the pathogenesis of NAFLD.[30,31] Indeed, specific sources of fructose, such as soft drinks, have also been implicated. Recent animal studies have confirmed that high fructose diets induce the metabolic syndrome with intrahepatic accumulation of triglycerides. In these models, fructose-induced NAFLD was associated with intestinal bacterial overgrowth and increased intestinal permeability, subsequently leading to an endotoxin-dependent activation of hepatic Kupffer cells and increased monocyte chemotactic protein-1 (MCP-1) and tumor necrosis factor alpha (TNF-α).[32,33]

Diet and physical activity for weight reduction and weight loss surgery for extreme obesity are the current standard recommendations for the treatment of NAFLD. There is recent evidence that intensive lifestyle intervention in patients with type 2 diabetes can reduce steatosis and the incidence of NAFLD.[34] Caloric restriction can result in significant changes in both liver fat and volume within a few days. Another area of increasing interest is the use of low carbohydrate diets in NAFLD. A low carbohydrate, ketogenic diet in patients with NASH led to significant weight loss and histologic improvement of fatty liver disease at 6 months.[35] Dietary avoidance of lipogenic, simple sugars (ie, fructose) seems to be universally recommended. A reduction in the consumption of sweetened beverages can also lead to significant weight loss owing to a reduction in total calories consumed.[36] Regarding exercise, vigorous exercise may be most beneficial, because it appears that exercise intensity may be more important than duration.[37] Weight loss by bariatric surgery attenuates both steatosis and steatohepatitis, but data supporting improvements in fibrosis are limited.[38] Despite intensive research, there remains no U.S. Food and Drug Administration (FDA)-approved therapy for NAFLD. However, the PIVENS study demonstrated a benefit with vitamin E therapy (800 IU daily), which has become standard practice in many areas of the country. The PIVENS study is further discussed in the CAM section of this chapter.

Patients with NASH-related decompensated cirrhosis pose other challenges. Despite their often marked obesity and because of the catabolic nature of cirrhosis, these patients are often significantly malnourished with protein deficits.[39,40] Although weight reduction is still beneficial, all efforts should be made to ensure adequate protein needs are supplied. As is the case with cirrhotics in general, there is rarely, if ever, an indication to limit protein intake to subnormal levels in patients with NAFLD. In fact, there are emerging data that high protein intake may lead to better outcomes in patients with cirrhosis with liver failure.[41]

Viral Hepatitis

Viral hepatitis consists of five distinct entities (A to E). Hepatitis A is an RNA virus that is transmitted via the fecal–oral route. It is an uncommon infection in the United States, but has higher prevalence in areas of low socioeconomic status, such as Africa, Asia (excluding Japan), the Mediterranean basin, Eastern Europe, the Middle East, Mexico, Central and South America, and parts of the Caribbean. In the United States, this disease is most often encountered in individuals that have emigrated from or traveled to these locations without receiving appropriate vaccinations.[42] This virus does not cause chronic infection. Management of acute hepatitis A consists of supportive care; there are no specific recommendations for dietary restrictions or support, aside from abstinence from alcohol intake.[43]

Hepatitis B is a DNA virus that is transmitted most commonly via perinatal, percutaneous, and sexual routes. The disease is endemic in sub-Saharan Africa and Asia where as much as 25% of the population have an active hepatitis B infection. Rates of infection in the United States are substantially lower. It is estimated that 0.1% to 0.2% of the population has chronic hepatitis B infection, whereas 200,000 to 300,000 new cases of hepatitis B infection occur annually.[44] In the United States, the majority of cases can be attributed to intravenous (IV) drug use and high risk sexual practices. Low rates in developed countries are largely due to preventative measures, specifically, vaccination against the virus. In young, otherwise healthy individuals, the virus will be cleared with complete recovery 95% to 99% of the time. The infection is more likely to become chronic in newborns who contract the virus during birth and in young children who contract the virus. The disease will only become chronic in 1% to 5% of adults that contract the virus.[44] Chronic infection can lead to inflammation and fibrosis leading to cirrhosis. Chronic hepatitis B virus is associated with the highest risk for the subsequent development of hepatocellular carcinoma among viral hepatitis. Concomitant exposure to dietary aflatoxins, particularly in Asia, has been associated with a greater risk for the development of cirrhosis and hepatocellular carcinoma in patients with hepatitis B.[45] Preliminary liver cancer chemoprevention trials have been performed in these patients using broccoli extracts, which are shown to activate the antioxidant response element.[46]

Hepatitis C is the most common blood-borne infection in the United States with an estimated 3.2 million people suffering from chronic hepatitis C infection.[47] The peak incidence of the disease occurs in individuals between the ages of 40 and 49. Approximately 30,000 new cases are diagnosed each year with the vast majority of infections having been contracted decades prior to presentation.[47] Infection with hepatitis C is most commonly acquired via IV drug use, but also occurs in transfusion recipients (most often those who received transfusions prior to 1992), hemodialysis patients, Vietnam veterans, and in health care workers due to accidental sticks with infected needles. Sexual and perinatal transmission of the disease is far less common.[47] Hepatitis C usually results in chronic infection and cirrhosis develops over 20 to 25 years in an estimated 20% of patients. Acute hepatitis C is typically asymptomatic, although signs such as fever, nausea, and jaundice can occur 1 to 3 months after exposure.[48]

Supplement use is common with chronic hepatitis C infection. In the most rigorously designed study to date, highly purified silymarin (milk thistle) was recently found to have no effect on liver enzymes in patients with chronic hepatitis C, but the use of this over-the-counter supplement remains widespread.[49] In contrast, multiple studies demonstrate that vitamin D supplementation increases sustained virologic response (cure) rates in patients on HCV therapy with pegylated interferon (IFN) and ribavirin.[50] Likewise, preliminary studies indicate that SAM may lead to increased sustained viral response (SRV) rates, but its clinical use is uncertain given the recent introduction of HCV protease inhibitors.[51] St. John's wort, a CAM agent commonly used for depression, is absolutely contraindicated in patients taking HCV protease inhibitors because it may lead to increased metabolism and subsequent loss of efficacy of these medications.

Hereditary Hemochromatosis

Hereditary hemochromatosis is a genetic disorder of iron overload classically occurring as an autosomal recessive disorder in individuals heterozygous for the C282Y mutation in the human hemochromatosis (HFE) gene. The disease is common, with an incidence of 1 in 250 people. Penetrance is incomplete, with clinical disease presenting more commonly in Caucasian males.[52] The resulting iron accumulation affects the liver, as well as the heart, endocrine system, and musculoskeletal systems. The disease results in cirrhosis in its late stages. However, if the disease is caught before the onset of cirrhosis, it can essentially be cured. The most effective treatment for hemochromatosis is therapeutic phlebotomy, initially scheduled weekly, with maintenance phlebotomy performed as need based on serum ferritin levels.[53] It is essential to limit dietary iron intake in patients with a diagnosis of hereditary hemochromatosis. In addition, alcohol consumption should be limited in patients with hemochromatosis, because intake greater than 60 g per day is associated with increased rates of cirrhosis.[52] Excess vitamin C supplementation should also be avoided because this vitamin may lead to increased dietary iron absorption.

Wilson Disease

Wilson disease is an important, but rare, heterogeneous inborn disorder of copper metabolism occurring due to mutations in the *ATP7B* gene. Copper accumulation leads to hepatic and neurologic disease resulting from improper hepatocellular use and biliary excretion of copper. Wilson disease occurs in 1:30,000 people and usually becomes clinically apparent before the age of 40.[54] Wilson disease can also affect the eyes (Kayser-Fleischer rings) and kidneys and has been associated with hemolysis. The disease may present with either neuropsychiatric symptoms or liver disease (chronic liver disease and cirrhosis or acute liver failure). A variety of tests (serum ceruloplasmin, 24-hour urine copper, slit-lamp eye examination, and liver biopsy with hepatic copper quantification) are used to diagnose suspected Wilson disease.[55] Treatment involves the use of chelating agents to remove tissue copper and to allow excretion in the urine. The most commonly used chelating agents are penicillamine and trientine. Patients receiving penicillamine therapy require the replacement of vitamin B6. Zinc acetate has also been approved by the FDA for the treatment of Wilson disease. Zinc induces metallothionein and reduces dietary copper absorption. A recent report demonstrated that there may be more "nonresponders" to zinc than chelation therapy.[56] The authors proposed that combination therapy with zinc plus a chelator could be considered, particularly if monotherapy fails to normalize liver enzymes. Wilson disease patients should also be instructed to avoid foods high in copper, including liver, chocolate, shellfish, and nuts.[55]

Cholestatic Liver Diseases

In contrast to the aforementioned hepatocellular liver diseases, primary biliary cirrhosis (PBC) and primary sclerosing cholangitis (PSC) are the most prevalent etiologies of chronic cholestatic liver disease. Cholestatic liver diseases pose unique challenges in nutrition. In PBC, the initial damage occurs in the biliary tree due to T-cell–mediated destruction of the intrahepatic bile ducts. Over time, the damage becomes severe enough to cause cholestasis, which results in a universal end point of cirrhosis and end-stage liver disease.[57] The disease most commonly presents with pruritus and alkaline phosphatase elevation in middle-aged women. Striking hypercholesterolemia may accompany PBC, but curiously, hypercholesterolemia in PBC has not been definitively linked to increased atherosclerosis. The only approved treatment in the United States for PBC is ursodeoxycholic acid (UDCA), which alters bile cholesterol composition.[58]

PSC is characterized by inflammation and sclerosis of the intrahepatic and/or extrahepatic bile ducts. PSC has a more rapid and severe course than PBC, however, with median time from diagnosis to time of death ranging between 9 and 12 years. As the disease progresses, complete obstruction of the biliary tree occurs, leading to cirrhosis and the development of end-stage liver disease.[59] PSC has been associated with both inflammatory bowel disease and autoimmune hepatitis (especially in children). PSC carries an increased risk of cholangiocarcinoma with estimates of risk between 8% and 15% over a patient's lifetime.[60] UCDA does not appear to be effective for PSC.[61] Endoscopic treatment (endoscopic retrograde cholangiography) of dominant biliary strictures may be performed to exclude cholangiocarcinoma and to relieve obstruction.

Regardless of its etiology, chronic cholestasis may cause calcium- and lipid-soluble vitamin malabsorption. Fat malabsorption is usually associated with a decrease in dietary calcium absorption and an increase in oxalate absorption. This is because FFAs bind to calcium in the digestive tract, making it unavailable for absorption. Calcium malabsorption may be worsened by vitamin D deficiency. The liver usually activates vitamin D into its active compound 1,25-dihydroxyvitamin D. Most patients with chronic cholestasis have osteoporosis, but osteomalacia is rare. These bone problems are known as metabolic bone disease and are responsible for significant morbidity. Calcium usually binds oxalates in the intestine, therefore fatty acid malabsorption results in an increase in free oxalates that are easily absorbed and predispose the patient to kidney stones. In PBC, 23% of patients have a decrease in their vitamin K plasma levels, which does not correlate with the prothrombin time (PT).[62] Vitamin A, D, and E deficiencies are usually present together with vitamin K deficiency. The prevalence of lipid-soluble vitamin deficiencies correlates with bilirubin levels.

In chronic cholestatic diseases, such as PBC and PSC, parenteral supplementation of lipid soluble vitamins (A, D, E, and K) may be necessary if steatorrhea greater than 10 g per day is present. Oral calcium supplements are also recommended. The progression of PBC-related osteodystrophy can be slowed by supplementing with calcium, 1,25-dihydroxyvitamin D, and calcitonin.[63] In patients with weight loss, supplements containing MCTs (MCT oil) can be given to provide extra calories because they do not need bile acids to be absorbed.

Malnutrition in Chronic Liver Disease

There is a high prevalence of protein-calorie malnutrition (PCM) in cirrhosis, which appears to correlate better with the severity rather than the etiology of the chronic liver disease.[64–68] The literature reports malnutrition in 34% to 82% patients with alcoholic cirrhosis.[20] In nonalcoholic cirrhosis, the prevalence of PCM ranges from 27% to 87%.[20] Because of the difficulties with nutrition assessment in cirrhosis, these prevalence figures are based on anthropometric data only.

In general, malnutrition in cirrhosis has many causes; these can be classified into three groups: (1) causes that limit oral intake; (2) causes that decrease the digestion and absorption of nutrients; and (3) causes that interfere with the metabolism of nutrients (Table 27-2). A majority of cirrhotic patients suffer

TABLE 27-2 Causes of Malnutrition in Cirrhosis

Decrease in oral intake
- Anorexia
- Nausea
- Vomiting
- Early satiety
- Taste abnormalities
- Alcohol abuse
- Iatrogenic due to restrictive diets or NPO status
- Medications

Maldigestion and malabsorption
- Fat malabsorption due to cholestasis or chronic pancreatitis
- Water-soluble vitamin malabsorption due to alcohol abuse
- Calcium and lipid-soluble vitamin malabsorption due to cholestasis

Metabolic abnormalities
- Glucose intolerance
- Increased protein and lipid catabolism similar to sepsis
- Trauma or other catabolic states

Associated renal diseases
- Urinary micronutrient losses
- Hepatorenal syndrome
- Viral hepatitis associated glomerulonephritis (MPGN in HCV, membranous glomerulonephritis in HBV)

NPO, nothing by mouth; MPGN, membranoproliferative glomerulonephritis; HCV, hepatitis C virus; HBV, hepatitis B virus.

from gastrointestinal symptoms such as anorexia, early satiety secondary to ascites, taste dysfunction, nausea, and vomiting, which limit their nutrient intake. The prevalence of weight loss, nausea, and anorexia among cirrhotic patients were reported to be 60%, 55%, and 87%, respectively.[69] Taste abnormalities have been associated with zinc and magnesium deficiencies.[70] Steatorrhea (fat malabsorption) has been reported in 40% of cirrhotics, and 10% have severe steatorrhea (more than 30 g per day), usually caused by concomitant pancreatic insufficiency. Side effects of medications and diets with excessive protein and salt restriction seem to be a common cause of malnutrition in cirrhosis, but studies evaluating the magnitude of this problem are not available.

Regardless of the etiology of cirrhosis, poor nutritional status is associated with a poor prognosis for survival. This has been shown in decompensated cirrhotic patients as well as those awaiting liver transplantation and undergoing abdominal surgery.[71,72] Whether PCM is an independent predictor of survival or just a reflection of the severity of liver insufficiency is still a subject of controversy.

Energy Expenditure in Chronic Liver Disease

Patients with chronic liver disease can develop serious metabolic abnormalities that mimic a state of catabolism similar to sepsis or trauma.[69] Measurements of the basal energy expenditure in cirrhotics have not shown a statistically significant difference from healthy controls when energy expenditure is expressed in calories per kilogram of body weight.[73–75] The prediction of the Resting Energy Expenditure (REE) by the Harris–Benedict equation (see Chapter 2) is not accurate in more than 50% of patients with cirrhosis.[74] The presence of ascites has been noted to increase the REE by 10%.[76] Given that body cell mass is decreased even in early stages of cirrhosis, the energy expenditure per unit of metabolically active tissue is thought to be increased.

Regardless of the absolute rates of energy expenditure, the type of fuel preferred by cirrhotic patients is altered. Cirrhotic patients have Respiratory Quotient (RQs) that are significantly lower than controls after an overnight fast. This indicates that cirrhotic patients are using more fat as a fuel, which is similar to what occurs to a normal subject after 72 hours of starvation.[75] In other words, the metabolism of cirrhotic patients, after an overnight fast, mimics that of starving controls. However, as opposed to a starving patient in whom the energy expenditure decreases over time, cirrhotic patients continue to have normal or increased energy expenditures, leading to progressive loss of muscle and fat mass, and resulting in PCM.

Metabolism in Chronic Liver Disease

Studies on carbohydrate metabolism in cirrhosis have shown that the prevalence of glucose intolerance in cirrhosis is high.[77] The pathogenesis of this abnormality is not well defined, but it seems to be caused by a postreceptor intracellular abnormality in both the liver and muscle. Associated with this insulin resistance are the decreased storage of glycogen in the liver and muscle and the early use of lipids and protein as fuel sources, manifested as a low RQ. Abnormalities in lipid metabolism have also been described in cirrhosis. The levels of fatty acids and ketone bodies are increased, and there is an increase in ketone body production.[69] There is evidence of impairment of fatty acid storage in the form of triglycerides, which is likely caused by lipoprotein lipase inhibition and a decrease in the availability of glycerol phosphate in the adipocyte. This imbalance between fat synthesis and catabolism results in depletion of the reserves in adipose tissue. In addition, leptin levels in cirrhotics are inappropriately elevated for their fat mass.[78] This excessive leptin production by the adipose tissue is postulated to decrease appetite and increase energy expenditure in these patients. Both insulin resistance and hepatic steatosis have been associated with HCV infection and with viral replication and resistance to antiviral therapy.

Perhaps the most remarkable metabolic abnormality of patients with end-stage liver disease is in amino acid metabolism. Urine nitrogen losses are increased in cirrhotic patients with a normal renal function, suggesting a catabolic state. The catabolism of protein is increased and fails to decrease normally in response to feeding.[79] In cirrhosis, the plasma levels of BCAAs (leucine, valine, and isoleucine) are low, and the levels of aromatic amino acids (phenylalanine, tyrosine, and tryptophan) are high. This serum amino acid imbalance is also seen in sepsis and trauma, and is probably mediated by an alteration in the balance between insulin and other regulatory hormones.

The role of skeletal muscle in amino acid metabolism has gained prominence. Skeletal muscle constitutes the largest metabolic organ of the body and actively takes up BCAAs that are used to synthesize glutamine and alanine. These amino acids are, in turn, released into the bloodstream and taken up by the liver to become the substrates for hepatic gluconeogenesis. Glutamine is a carrier for ammonia that is converted to urea by the liver and excreted by the kidneys. In cirrhosis, excessive glutamine is synthesized in the skeletal muscle, while hepatic urea synthesis is impaired. This leads to an increase in renal glutamine uptake and constitutes a back up mechanism for ammonia elimination through the kidneys. Studies have shown that cirrhotic patients with decreased skeletal muscle mass are more prone to develop hepatic encephalopathy.[80] This underscores the importance of preserving the skeletal muscle mass in cirrhotic patients as a means of preventing chronic hepatic encephalopathy.

In summary, cirrhotic patients have decreased carbohydrate use and storage capacity plus an increase in fat and protein catabolism, which lead to a chronic catabolic state resulting in the depletion of protein and lipid reserves. These abnormalities, combined with a decrease in food intake and nutrient absorption, constitute the basis of the pathogenesis of PCM in end-stage liver disease. Without question, dysregulated cytokine levels are intimately involved in many of the metabolic and nutritional abnormalities observed in liver disease, especially in acute alcoholic hepatitis and in more decompensated liver disease.[14] More specifically, cirrhotic patients have increased levels of TNF and interleukin(IL)-1 and -6, which have catabolic effects in muscle, adipose tissue, and the liver.[81] Endotoxin produced by intestinal gram-negative bacteria is often present in the blood of cirrhotic patients.[82] Cirrhotic patients have an increase in intestinal permeability that allows the leakage of endotoxin from the intestine to the lymphatics and the bloodstream.[83]

Endotoxin triggers the release of cytokines and nitric oxide, which may be mediators of the catabolic state as well as the hyperdynamic circulation of cirrhotics.[84]

Nutritional Assessment

All of the previous data suggest that a proper assessment of nutritional status in patients with liver disease is important. This helps to determine the goals for nutritional support. Although there is a common recognition of the importance of accurate nutrition assessments in patients with liver disease, there are several issues that make a nutritional assessment in these patients difficult (Table 27-3).

Anthropometrics

Height and weight are normally a good starting point for a nutritional assessment, but because of fluid abnormalities such as ascites, patients with liver disease may have a normal or greater than normal body weight in relation to their height and still have decreased protein and muscle mass. This is the result of excess fluid such as ascites, which increases weight without increasing protein stores. Because the excess fluid weight provides no structural protein for strength and activities of daily living, it makes a physical examination in a patient with liver disease essential. In this examination, the clinician must determine if the patient has muscle wasting in the extremities, the upper body, and the temporal areas despite a weight greater than the ideal weight.

Laboratory Measurements

Laboratory values can also be misleading in these patients. Because of ongoing liver disease, albumin and prealbumin may be moderately or very low, even in the presence of good nutritional status.[85] This is due to the decreased production by the diseased liver. One method of determining muscle mass is to collect a 24-hour urine sample for creatinine. A normal value of 18 mg per kilogram of ideal weight in females and 23 mg per kilogram of ideal weight in males would suggest normal muscle mass, and decreased values would suggest decreased muscle mass. This technique is limited to patients with normal renal function, and requires an accurate 24-hour urine collection, which can be challenging in an ambulatory setting.

TABLE 27-3 Nutrition Assessment in Advanced Liver Diseases

Method	Reliable	Unreliable
Weight for height		X
Plasma proteins: albumin, prealbumin		X
Delayed skin reactions and total lymphocyte count		X
24-h creatinine: height ratio	X (only with normal renal function)	
Bioelectric impedance		X
Anthropometry: triceps skinfold and mid-arm muscle area or Subjective Global Assessment	X	

Other Nutritional Assessment Tools

Other methods of nutrition assessment (see Chapter 9) may be more accurate in these patients, such as a subjective global assessment (Table 27-4). This method evaluates patient performance during daily activities and includes a physical exam and may provide a more accurate assessment of the nutrition status of a patient with liver disease.[85] A physical and functional examination is essential in assessing the nutritional status of patients with liver disease.

Provision of Nutrients

Patients with Compensated Liver Disease

Interest in nutritional therapy in cirrhosis began when Patek et al.[86] showed that a nutritious diet improved the 5-year outcomes compared to control subjects consuming an inadequate diet. Although these patients had alcoholic liver disease, several recent studies further support the concept of improved outcomes with nutritional support in patients with cirrhosis due to any cause. Hirsch et al.[87] demonstrated that outpatients supplementing their diet with an enteral nutritional support product (1000 kcal [4.2 MJ], 34 g protein) had significantly improved protein intake and significantly fewer hospitalizations. This group then provided an enteral supplement to outpatients with alcoholic cirrhosis and observed an improvement in nutritional status and immune function.[87] In the VA Cooperative Study on nutritional support in alcoholic liver disease using the anabolic steroid oxandrolone and an enteral nutritional supplement, an improvement in mortality was seen with the combination of oxandrolone plus nutritional supplementation in patients who had moderate protein-energy malnutrition.[17] Those with severe malnutrition did not significantly benefit from therapy. This was possibly due to their disease being so severe that no intervention could improve their outcome. Studies by Kearns et al.[88] showed that patients with alcoholic liver disease who were hospitalized for treatment and given an enteral nutritional supplement via a feeding tube had significantly improved serum bilirubin levels and liver function as assessed by antipyrine clearance. A multicenter randomized study of enteral nutrition versus steroids in patients with alcoholic hepatitis showed similar overall short-term results.[89] Moreover, those receiving enteral nutrition (rich in BCAAs) had a better long-term outcome with fewer infection-related deaths. Thus, nutritional supplementation clearly improved nutritional status and, in some instances, hepatic function and other indicators of outcome in cirrhosis.

An important component of the dietary management of the patient with advanced liver disease is to minimize periods without food intake because patients rapidly enter into starvation mode with decreased glucose oxidation and increased protein and fat catabolism.[90] To prevent this, the diet should, optimally,

TABLE 27-4 Subjective Global Assessment

(Select the appropriate category with a check mark, or enter numerical value where indicated by "#".)

A. History

1. Weight change
   Overall loss in past 6 mos: amount = # __________ kg; % loss = # __________
   Change in past 2 wks: _____ increase, _____ no change, _____ decrease
2. Dietary intake change (relative to normal)
   __________ No change
   __________ Change __________ duration = # __________ weeks
   __________ Type: _____ suboptimal solid diet _____ full liquid diet
   _____ hypocaloric liquids _____ starvation
3. Gastrointestinal symptoms (that persisted for >2 wks)
   _____ none _____ nausea _____ vomiting _____ diarrhea _____ anorexia
4. Functional capacity
   __________ No dysfunction (eg, full capacity)
   __________ Dysfunction __________ duration = # __________ wks
   __________ Type: _____ working suboptimally
   _____ ambulatory
   _____ bedridden
5. Disease and its relation to nutritional requirements
   Primary diagnosis (specify) ____________________
   Metabolic demand (stress): ______ no stress ______ low stress
   ______ moderate stress ______ high stress

B. Physical
(for each trait specify 0 = normal, 1+ = mild, 2+ = moderate, 3+ = severe)
__________ loss of subcutaneous fat (triceps, chest)
__________ muscle wasting (quadriceps, deltoids)
__________ ankle edema
__________ sacral edema
__________ ascites

C. SGA rating (select one)
____________ A = Well nourished
____________ B = Moderately malnourished (or suspected of being malnourished)
____________ C = Severely malnourished

SGA, Subjective Global Assessment. Reprinted from Detsky AJ, McLaughlin JR, Baker JP, et al. What is subjective global assessment of nutritional status? *J Parenter Enteral Nutr.* 1987;11:8–14.

be divided into three meals (the first of which should be early in the morning), three snacks, plus one bedtime supplement. The early breakfast improves cognitive function in patients with subclinical (minimal) hepatic encephalopathy and the bedtime supplement improves body protein stores.[91] Importantly, an improvement in muscle mass with nighttime supplements was demonstrated by Plank et al.,[9] who randomized 103 cirrhotic patients to receive two cans of Ensure Plus (710 kcal with 26 g of protein) or two cans of Diabetic Resource (500 kcal with 30 g of protein) either during the day or at bedtime, for a total of 12 months. Only the patients who received the supplements at bedtime gained lean muscle mass (2 kg) over 12 months (Practice Scenario 27-2). Unfortunately, there is a long tradition of protein restriction for patients with advanced liver disease who also have hepatic encephalopathy. This tradition has no solid scientific basis, and recent studies do not support this approach. Cordoba et al.,[92] in a prospective randomized study, treated 30 cirrhotic patients who suffered episodic overt hepatic encephalopathy with either a low-protein enteral formula (with increased protein every 3 days [0 g, then 12 g, 24 g, and 48 g]) or a normal protein formula (1.2 g per kilogram per day) from the first day. Both formulas provided 30 kcal per kilogram per day. The outcome of hepatic encephalopathy was similar with both formulas. In a second study, Gheorghe et al.[93] treated 153 consecutive cirrhotic patients with overt HE with a diet providing 30 kcal per kilogram per day with 1.2 g of protein per kilogram per day, divided into five meals from 8:00 AM to 10:00 PM. Most patients improved their HE, with the best results seen in the more severe HE patients.[93] The HE should be treated with FDA-approved medications such as lactulose or rifaximin, if needed. If the HE persists despite maximal medical therapy and an evaluation for other causes of changes in mentation, then protein intake can be decreased to the maximal tolerated, and a BCAA-enriched formula supplement can be administered to complete the nitrogen needs. These studies highlight the need to maintain caloric intake in patients with liver disease at 25 to 30 kcal per kilogram via enteral feeds and, more specifically, the importance of maintaining protein intake at 1.0 to 1.5 g per kilogram per day (Table 27-5).[94]

Practice Scenario 27-2

Question: What is the appropriate meal schedule to provide optimal nutrition to the outpatient with chronic liver disease?

Scenario: A 57-year-old female with a history of cirrhosis secondary to PBC presents to the clinic for consultation regarding her nutrition. The patient states that she has had trouble maintaining her weight despite her best efforts to eat an appropriate amount. The patient states that she feels progressively weaker and feels that she has been losing muscle mass. In addition, the patient reports that her husband notices that she tends to function more slowly in the mornings. The patient has never received any education regarding proper nutrition in the setting of her liver disease. She requests that some intervention be made to help her maintain or increase her weight and to improve her mentation.

Intervention: The patient is started on a diet consisting of three meals per day with one early morning meal. In addition, the patient begins to eat three snacks per day, as well as a late night snack before bed. Over the course of the next 6 months the patient gains 5 pounds and notes improvement in her strength and mentation.

Answer: Nutrition is essential to improve both lean muscle mass and overall function in patients with liver disease. This patient should be educated regarding the importance of consuming an appropriate number of calories. The emphasis should be on consumption of three meals per day beginning with an early morning breakfast. The patient should also be instructed to consume three small snacks in between meals. Additionally, the patient should be encouraged to consume a late night snack before bed. This will improve her overall functioning, but more importantly, will increase lean muscle mass.

Rationale: An important component of the dietary management of the patient with advanced liver disease is to minimize periods without food intake because patients rapidly enter into starvation mode, with decreased glucose oxidation and increased protein and fat catabolism.[90] To prevent this, the diet should, optimally, be divided into three meals (the first of which should be early in the morning), three snacks, plus one bedtime supplement. The early breakfast improves cognitive function in patients with subclinical (minimal) hepatic encephalopathy and the bedtime supplement improves body protein stores.[91] Importantly, an improvement in muscle mass with nighttime supplements was demonstrated by Plank et al.,[62] who randomized 103 cirrhotic patients to receive two cans of Ensure Plus (710 kcal with 26 g of protein) or two cans of Diabetic Resource (500 kcal with 30 g of protein) either during the day or at bedtime, for a total of 12 months. Patients who received supplements at bedtime gained lean muscle mass (2 kg) over 12 months,[9] demonstrating the importance of late night snacking in maintaining muscle mass in patients with cirrhosis.

Patients with Decompensated Liver Disease

Patients with decompensated liver disease can be very challenging to manage because of the presence of ascites, encephalopathy, and the increased frequency of diminished renal function. Decompensated cirrhosis is defined as cirrhosis with ascites and/or encephalopathy. Liver chemistries usually show albumin < 3 g per deciliter and total bilirubin > 2.5 mg per deciliter. Patients with PSE may present with behavioral changes, reversal of sleep pattern, slurred speech, disorientation, or coma. The nutritional requirements mentioned earlier in this chapter do still apply to the decompensated patient, and it is more difficult to provide proper nutrition to patients with decompensated liver disease. It is recommended that if patients fail to achieve the recommended 35 to 40 kcal per kilogram and 1.0 to 1.5 g per kilogram of protein on their own, supplemental enteral nutrition in the form of nasogastric or orogastric tube feeds should be considered.[94,95] Enteral nutrition is preferred over parenteral nutrition because of cost, the risk of sepsis of the parenteral nutrition line, the preservation of the integrity of the gut mucosa, and the prevention of bacterial translocation and multiple organ failure. Moreover, total parenteral nutrition can, in some instances, cause liver disease as one of its complications. If enteral nutrition is not possible, parenteral nutrition can be used with the knowledge that it is important to return to the enteral route as soon as the small bowel shows evidence of recovered function. Parenteral nutrition can be started with a standard amino acid formula in amounts that are increased until nitrogen needs are met. If the patient develops PSE, then standard therapy with FDA-approved medications should be given. If the patient is still unable to tolerate the amount of amino acids needed to satisfy nitrogen requirements, then the standard amino acids can be replaced by a BCAA-enriched solution specifically designed for liver disease.[96,97] It is unusual to require either parenteral nutrition or BCAA formulas, and the primary goal is always aggressive enteral support (Practice Scenario 27-3).

TABLE 27-5 Nutritional Therapy in Cirrhosis

- Early assessment of nutritional status along with regular follow-up.
- Total energy can be estimated by the following formula: 1.2–1.4 × resting energy expenditure.
- Protein requirement: 1.0–1.5 g/kg/day.
- Fat requirement: 30%–40% of nonprotein calories.
- Replace vitamins and minerals as needed (eg, zinc, vitamin D, avoid excess iron and copper intake).
- Use enteral supplementation (ie, tube feeds) to complement other enteral intake (may use parenteral nutrition for shortest time possible if necessary).

Practice Scenario 27-3

Question: What are the appropriate nutritional interventions to institute in a malnourished inpatient with liver disease?

Scenario: A 60-year-old male with hepatitis C cirrhosis is admitted with portal systemic encephalopathy. In addition to his encephalopathy, a physical exam reveals ascites as well as bitemporal wasting and muscle atrophy. The patient is admitted and a nasoenteric tube is placed for enteral access and the administration of lactulose and rifaximin. An interview of the patient's wife reveals that the patient has had poor appetite for several years, but particularly in the last 3 to 4 weeks. He is currently on lactulose and rifaximin at home, but does not take any additional nutritional supplements, including no vitamin or mineral supplements.

Intervention: This patient shows characteristic signs of malnutrition (bitemporal wasting and muscle atrophy). In addition, his ascites and encephalopathy reveal that he has decompensated disease. As such, the patient is started on enteral tube feeding with additional protein modules to provide 1.2 g per kilogram of protein per day. The patient is also given nutritional supplements, including zinc.

Answer: Patients with malnutrition as a result of their liver disease require the early institution of nutritional supplementation. Patients with liver disease are likely to have protein calorie malnutrition. Adequate calories, specifically protein calories, must be given as soon as possible. In addition, patients with liver disease are known to be deficient in a variety of vitamins and minerals. Supplementation of these vitamins and minerals should also be a priority.

Rationale: It is recommended that, in patients unable to achieve the recommended 35 to 40 kcal per kilogram and 1.0 to 1.2 g per kilogram of protein on their own, supplemental enteral nutrition in the form of nasogastric or orogastric tube feeds should be considered.[95] Zinc is an essential trace element that participates in cellular function through hundreds of zinc proteins, including zinc metalloenzymes and critical zinc transcription factors. Zinc may be a helpful adjunctive therapy in hepatic encephalopathy.[121]

Complementary and Alternative Medicine Agents and Selected Micronutrients

A recent major change in therapy for liver disease has been supplementation with individual nutrients, or the use of CAM. A detailed discussion of CAM is necessary because estimates indicate that > 40% of the U.S. population uses CAM, and patients with chronic disease processes such as cirrhosis are frequent users of CAM. Moreover, CAM use is frequently not reported to physicians. A variety of forms of CAM have been used effectively to treat or prevent liver injury in animal models, and preliminary data with some agents suggest efficacy in human liver disease. It is the responsibility of health care workers to be aware of the potential benefits and toxicities of these agents and to demand well-designed randomized human trials on such products. The specific CAM agents that will be reviewed in relation to liver disease include vitamin E, glutathione (GSH) prodrugs and antioxidant cocktails, SAM and betaine, silymarin (milk thistle), and herbals. Selected other miscellaneous vitamin and mineral deficiencies frequently complicating chronic liver disease are also discussed.

Vitamin E

Vitamin E is a potent antioxidant that is widely used as a nutritional supplement. In patients with alcoholic liver disease and in experimental models of liver disease, depressed serum and hepatic levels of vitamin E have been documented. Vitamin E has been used extensively to protect against experimental models of liver injury, such as that induced by carbon tetrachloride via the inhibition of nuclear factor kappa B (NF-κB) activation.[98] Hill et al.[99] treated human peripheral blood monocytes and rat Kupffer cells in vitro with vitamin E, inhibiting both NF-κB activation and TNF production.[99] Vitamin E also inhibits the activation of hepatic stellate cells and collagen production in vitro.

Vitamin E was initially reported to have beneficial effects in some but not all studies of patients with fatty liver (NASH).[100–102] A pilot study in children showed improvement in liver enzymes, and a study from Japan showed that vitamin E not only improved liver enzymes but also decreased serum levels of the profibrotic cytokine, transforming growth factor beta (TGF-β).[100,101] Notably, a study in patients with alcoholic hepatitis showed improvement in hyaluronic acid, a marker of fibrosis. That same study did not demonstrate improvement in mortality, however.[103] The most important and compelling vitamin E data are from a large multicenter National Institutes of Health (NIH)-funded trial, which assigned 247 adults with NASH (without diabetes) to receive pioglitazone at a dose of 30 mg daily (80 subjects), vitamin E at a dose of 800 IU daily (84 subjects), or placebo (83 subjects) for 96 weeks.[102] Vitamin E therapy, as compared with placebo, was associated with a significantly higher rate of improvement in NASH (43% versus 19%, $p = .001$). Serum alanine and aspartate aminotransferase levels were reduced with vitamin E and with pioglitazone, as compared to placebo ($p < .001$ for both comparisons). No treatment demonstrated an improvement in fibrosis. Subjects who received pioglitazone gained more weight than did those who received vitamin E or placebo. In conclusion, vitamin E improved liver histology and liver enzymes, was not associated with the weight gain seen with pioglitazone, and at this time, 800 IU of vitamin E is the preferred "drug" therapy for NASH at some centers.

Glutathione Prodrugs and Combined Antioxidants

GSH is a tripeptide synthesized from glutamate, cysteine, and glycine. GSH, in its reduced form, is the main nonprotein thiol in cells and has an important role in the detoxification of electrophiles and in protection against reactive oxygen toxicity. This includes protection against intracellular free radicals, reactive oxygen intermediates, and several endogenous and exogenous toxins.[104] GSH also protects against toxicity from certain drugs (eg, acetaminophen). GSH cannot be taken up by hepatocytes, but a number of pharmacologic agents have been devised to enhance intracellular pools (eg, N-acetylcysteine, 2-oxothiazolidine-4-carboxylic acid). There are two distinct intercellular GSH pools: cytosolic (approximately 80%) and mitochondrial (approximately 20%). Mitochondrial GSH detoxifies hydrogen peroxide and other organic peroxides produced in mitochondria. Chronic alcohol consumption has been reported to deplete GSH levels.[104] Moreover, alcohol causes a marked depletion of GSH in the mitochondrial pool, with at least part of that depletion attributed to its impaired transport from the cytosolic pool. This depletion renders hepatocytes more vulnerable to oxidative stress. The molecular basis for the impaired GSH transport into mitochondria is unclear, but it has been reported that exogenous SAM, but not N-acetylcysteine (NAC) or other pro-GSH molecules, restores mitochondrial function, enhances mitochondrial transport, and corrects mitochondrial GSH deficiency.

GSH precursors also can regulate the production of proinflammatory cytokines, such as TNF and IL-8, by Kupffer cells and monocytes, with increased GSH levels decreasing cytokine production.[105] This occurs, at least in part, through the inhibition of the oxidative-stress–sensitive transcription factor NF-κB, which plays a central role in lipopolysaccharide-stimulated TNF production.

The glutathione precursor NAC has been used clinically for decades to treat acute acetaminophen overdose with good results if administered early (optimally within 12 hours of acetaminophen ingestion). A recent study evaluated the effects of an IV NAC on transplant-free survival in patients with non-acetaminophen-related acute liver failure.[106] The 173 patients received either NAC or a placebo. In patients with early stage nonacetaminophen-related acute liver failure, NAC improved transplant-free survival. This important study supports the use of IV NAC in patients with acute liver failure. Unfortunately, combined trials of antioxidants that not only increase GSH but also provide other antioxidant effects have not shown efficacy in patients with chronic alcoholic liver disease. In contrast to administering exogenous antioxidants, an alternative approach uses CAM agents to stimulate the endogenous production of antioxidants. This approach (broccoli extracts) has been evaluated in preliminary hepatocellular carcinoma chemoprevention studies in Asian patients exposed to aflatoxins.[46] Thus, there is a scientific rationale for an antioxidant approach, but defining appropriate clinical populations and doses appear to be major challenges.

S-Adenosylmethionine/Betaine

Elevated methionine and decreased methionine clearance represent possible therapeutic targets for liver disease, especially ALD. In animal models of liver injury, decreased levels of SAM and elevated levels of S-adenosylhomocysteine are regularly observed. In human studies of alcoholic hepatitis and cirrhosis, abnormal hepatic gene expression occurs and contributes to decreased hepatic SAM, cysteine, and glutathione levels. Rodent and primate studies demonstrate that SAM depletion occurred in early stages of fatty liver infiltration in alcoholic liver disease, and decreased SAM concentration, liver injury, and mitochondrial damage could be reversed with SAM supplementation.[107] SAM attenuated oxidative stress and hepatic stellate cell activation in an ethanol-LPS–induced fibrotic rat model.[108] Most importantly, a randomized double-blind trial was performed in 123 patients with alcoholic cirrhosis treated with SAM (1200 mg per day, orally) or placebo for 2 years.[109] When Child class C cirrhotics were excluded from the analysis, the overall mortality/liver transplantation rate was significantly greater in the placebo group than in the SAM group (20% versus 12%), and differences between the 2-year survival curves of the two groups (defined as the time to death or liver transplantation) were also statistically significant. A subsequent Cochrane review of SAM and ALD could not find evidence supporting or refuting the use of SAM for patients with alcoholic liver diseases.[110] Further studies and long-term, high-quality randomized trials are clearly needed.

Betaine (trimethylglycine) is a key nutrient in humans and is obtained from a variety of foods and nutritional supplements. In the liver, betaine can transfer one methyl group to homocysteine to form methionine. This process removes toxic metabolites (homocysteine and S-adenosylhomocysteine), restores SAM levels, reverses steatosis, prevents apoptosis, and reduces both damaged protein accumulation and oxidative stress. Betaine also appears to attenuate alcoholic steatosis by restoring phosphatidylcholine generation via the phosphatidylethanolamine methyltransferase pathway.[111] Unfortunately, the most definitive human trial thus far (in NASH patients) showed no benefit.[112]

Zinc

Zinc is an essential trace element that participates in cellular function through hundreds of zinc proteins, including zinc metalloenzymes and critical zinc transcription factors. Zinc deficiency has also been well examined in liver disease.[113–115] Zinc deficiency can present as angular (perioral) cheilosis, muscle cramps, and neurosensory defects.[116] An altered zinc metabolism with zinc deficiency and decreased serum zinc is noted in most forms of clinical liver disease, especially ALD. Stress/inflammation caused by a variety of factors, including lipopolysaccharide/tumor necrosis factor (LPS/TNF), also causes an internal redistribution of zinc, with loss of zinc from some tissues (deficiency) and redirection to other tissues or organs such as the liver (redistribution). Importantly, zinc deficiency was recently shown to be induced by oxidative stress, in which thiol oxidation of zinc-finger transcription factors resulted in zinc loss, leading to a loss of DNA-binding activity.[117–119]

Recent studies from Kang and Zhou[114] provide major new insights into the molecular mechanisms of altered zinc metabolism in the development and progression of experimental ALD, with important potential therapeutic implications for ALD and other forms of chronic liver disease. In both acute and chronic alcohol-induced hepatotoxicity, alcohol intake and oxidative stress disrupt tight junctions in the intestine, leading to the translocation of bacterial products such as endotoxin.[113,117] Endotoxin activates Toll-like receptor 4 (TLR-4) and TNF production, with subsequent oxidative stress and liver injury. Endotoxin and TNF also play critical roles in liver fibrosis. The disruption of tight-junction proteins occurs not only in the intestine but also in the lung and likely at the blood–brain barrier, thus potentially predisposing the patient to lung injury and hepatic encephalopathy.[113] Zinc treatment in experimental animals with ALD attenuated the increased gut permeability, endotoxemia, TNF production, oxidative stress, and liver injury, while improving the activity of key zinc transcription factors. [113,114,117,118] Thus, zinc supplementation targets most postulated mechanisms for the development of ALD and certain other forms of chronic liver disease such as NAFLD.

A recent human pilot trial also suggests that zinc may stabilize or cause the regression of hepatic fibrosis.[120] Polaprezinc, a synthetic zinc-containing compound with 34 mg of elemental zinc, was administered daily for 24 weeks to patients with chronic hepatitis or cirrhosis, and zinc-supplemented patients significantly improved their serum zinc levels and markers of fibrosis. Zinc may also be effective in the treatment of hepatic encephalopathy.[121] There are no strict parameters for zinc replacement. Zinc can be replaced in patients with liver disease as 50 mg elemental zinc by mouth.[116] If higher doses are used, copper deficiency with cytopenias may ensue.

Silymarin

Silymarin, the active ingredient extracted from *Silybum marianum* (also known as milk thistle), was shown in experimental animals to protect against multiple types of liver injury, including that induced by carbon tetrachloride, acetaminophen, and iron overload, and, very importantly, mushroom poisoning.[122] Silymarin is probably the most widely used form of CAM in the treatment of liver disease. Clinically, it has been suggested to have hepatoprotective effects in various forms of toxic hepatitis, fatty liver, cirrhosis, ischemic injury, and viral-induced liver disease.[122] It has antioxidant activities, protects against lipid peroxidation, has anti-inflammatory effects, and has antifibrotic effects. Large controlled trials performed in Europe of silymarin have had variable results.[123,124] Silymarin has become one of the most popular forms of CAM therapy for liver disease because it has a good safety profile, has been extensively investigated in multiple forms of experimental liver injury in animals, and some positive results have been reported in humans. However, the results of a Cochrane analysis questioned the beneficial effects of milk thistle for patients with alcoholic and/or hepatitis B or C virus liver diseases and highlighted the lack of high quality evidence to support this intervention.[125] A recently reported, high quality, randomized clinical trial of highly purified milk thistle found no beneficial effects on chronic HCV.[49]

Branched-Chain Amino Acids

An additional consideration in the management of individuals with cirrhosis is the addition of oral BCAAs. In addition to hepatic encephalopathy, the effects of BCAA supplementation have been studied on survival and hepatocellular carcinoma (HCC). In one study,[126] high doses of oral BCAA (12 g per day) were given to individuals with cirrhosis, but without a history of HCC. After 6 months of therapy, the patients receiving BCAAs had a lower incidence of HCC, as well as fewer medical complications related to their cirrhosis.[126] Additional support for BCAA supplementation was demonstrated in a study involving the administration of an identical dose of BCAA for 2 years. Patients given high-dose BCAAs were found to have an improved quality of life, increased event-free survivals, and improved serum albumin concentrations.[127] Benefits were also seen in patients undergoing a partial hepatectomy for HCC. In one study,[128] patients were given 14 days of IV nutritional therapy that consisted of 35% BCAAs. When compared to a control group undergoing the same procedure, the group receiving BCAAs had decreased postoperative morbidity, including less weight loss, less ascites, and fewer infectious complications.[128] Based on this evidence, BCAAs should be a consideration in the management of patients with cirrhosis.

Miscellaneous Vitamin and Mineral Deficiencies Complicating Cirrhosis

A substantial number of patients with liver disease, regardless of etiology, are known to be deficient in vitamin D.[129,130] This should prompt an assessment of vitamin D status in the form of a serum 25-OH vitamin D level. Although guidelines for the replacement of vitamin D in liver disease have not been completely delineated, replacement to achieve a 25-OH vitamin D level > 32 ng per milliliter has been suggested.[131] Importantly, vitamin D supplementation increases sustained virologic response (cure) rates in patients on HCV therapy with pegylated IFN and ribavirin.[50] Patients with cholestatic liver diseases may be at particularly high risk for vitamin D deficiency.

Thiamine deficiency may complicate chronic alcoholism and bariatric surgery.[132] This increases the risk of serious neurologic consequences, specifically Wernicke encephalopathy (WE), and should be treated aggressively. Likewise, alcoholics and bariatric surgery patients may also be at risk for refeeding syndrome.[133] Iron deficiency anemia may occur in some patients with chronic gastrointestinal blood loss due to portal hypertensive gastropathy or gastric antral vascular ectasia; iron should be replaced in these patients.[134]

Monitoring and Treating Complications

Many of the complications of liver disease can be effectively managed as long as there is an appropriate monitoring of signs and symptoms. This can begin with simple physical exam findings. Patients with decompensated liver disease often have ascites that are easily assessed by increased abdominal girth. There are simple nutritional interventions that can decrease the occurrence of ascites. Institution of a 2 g per day sodium diet is an important step in preventing the recurrence of ascites.[135] Hypervolemic hyponatremia is common in cirrhotic patients, but fluid restriction is not necessary in treating most patients because severe hypernatremia (< 125 mmol per liter) is relatively rare.[135] Practice guidelines indicate that fluid restriction for serum sodium < 125 mmol per liter is reasonable.[135] However, our practice is to institute a 1.5 to 2 L fluid restriction in patients with serum sodium concentrations < 130 mmol per liter, particularly if they are candidates for liver transplantation to avoid potential complications from intraoperative fluid shifts. Two calorie per microliter formulas may be used in cirrhotic patients with hyponatremia who are receiving enteral nutrition.

Furthermore, patients with decompensated cirrhosis present several unique challenges to the delivery of enteral nutrition. Patients in a hepatic coma will likely require nasoenteric tube placement for the delivery of medications as well as nutrition. Thrombocytopenia and coagulopathy typically accompany decompensated liver disease, and in this setting, epistaxis may complicate nasoenteric tube placement. Epistaxis in a patient with compromised airway protection due to hepatic encephalopathy can result in aspiration. Likewise, inadvertent tube displacement is not uncommon in patients with hepatic encephalopathy. Although we could find no published guidelines on these issues, our practice is to carefully place soft-tipped, fine-bore nasogastric tubes often accompanied by commercially available magnetic string-type bridles in these patients. Unless patients have a history of epistaxis and/or significant thrombocytopenia or coagulopathy, we do not routinely transfuse platelets or fresh frozen plasma prior to a nasoenteric tube placement. Anecdotally, we have administered topical vasoconstrictor sprays intranasally (such as oxymetazoline) prior to tube placement in an effort to reduce the likelihood of epistaxis. Although we could find no published data to support this practice, oxymetazoline did prevent epistaxis prior to nasotracheal intubation.[136]

A second potential problem confounding nasoenteric tube placement is esophageal varices. The risk that the placement of a soft-tipped, fine-bore nasally or orally placed feeding tube will precipitate varicocele hemorrhage (in nonbleeding varices) is low and should typically not preclude tube placement.[137] One important exception occurs during (or immediately following the treatment of) bleeding gastroesophageal varices. Bleeding esophageal varies are typically managed by an endoscopic band ligation. A tube could, theoretically, prematurely dislodge the band from the varices and precipitate rebleeding. There is also a theoretical risk that enteral nutrition could increase intestinal blood flow and portal pressures. Although one small study found an increased risk of rebleeding when enteral nutrition was initiated within 72 hours of varicocele hemorrhage,[138] other authors advise holding enteral nutrition for the first 48 hours.[137] There is high mortality with percutaneous gastrostomy tube placement (PEG) in patients with cirrhosis, and especially those with ascites.[139] Therefore, PEG is contraindicated in patients with ascites. Patients with liver disease may also be intolerant of intragastric feeding due to nausea, vomiting, or increased gastric residuals. Although this may necessitate alteration in the delivery of nutritional supplementation, it should not lead to cessation. This issue can be addressed with use of postpyloric tube feeds.

Summary

Liver disease encompasses a heterogeneous group of disorders with diverse clinical outcomes ranging from acute hepatitis, acute liver failure, asymptomatic chronic elevation of liver enzymes, compensated cirrhosis, and end-stage liver disease. In many cases, poor nutrition has been linked to the pathogenesis and progression of liver disease. Likewise, data indicate that nutrition therapy my favorably impact the course of many liver disease cases. Therefore, nutrition support providers have a unique opportunity to positively affect the lives of these patients.

Acknowledgment

Liver disease material from the previous *Core Curriculum* was contributed by Philip C. Delich, MD; John K Siepler, PharmD; and Patricia Parker, PharmD.

References

1. Santolaria F, Perez-Manzano JL, Milena A, et al. Nutritional assessment in alcoholic patients. Its relationship with alcoholic intake, feeding habits, organic complications and social problems. *Drug Alcohol Depend.* 2000;59(3):295–304.
2. Galati JS, Holdeman KP, Bottjen PL, Quigley EM. Gastric emptying and orocecal transit in portal hypertension and end-stage chronic liver disease. *Liver Transpl Surg.* 1997;3(1):34–38.
3. Galati JS, Holdeman KP, Dalrymple GV, Harrison KA, Quigley EM. Delayed gastric emptying of both the liquid and solid components of a meal in chronic liver disease. *Am J Gastroenterol.* 1994; 89(5):708–711.
4. Isobe H, Sakai H, Satoh M, Sakamoto S, Nawata H. Delayed gastric emptying in patients with liver cirrhosis. *Dig Dis Sci.* 1994; 39(5):983–987.
5. Thuluvath PJ, Triger DR. Autonomic neuropathy and chronic liver disease. *Q J Med.* 1989;72(268):737–747.
6. Quigley EM. Gastrointestinal dysfunction in liver disease and portal hypertension. Gut-liver interactions revisited. *Dig Dis Sci.* 1996;41(3):557–561.
7. Yoshida Y, Higashi T, Nouso K, et al. Effects of zinc deficiency/zinc supplementation on ammonia metabolism in patients with decompensated liver cirrhosis. *Acta Med Okayama.* 2001;55(6): 349–355.
8. Vlahcevic ZR, Buhac I, Farrar JT, Bell CC Jr, Swell L. Bile acid metabolism in patients with cirrhosis. I. Kinetic aspects of cholic acid metabolism. *Gastroenterology.* 1971;60(4):491–498.
9. Plank LD, Gane EJ, Peng S, et al. Nocturnal nutritional supplementation improves total body protein status of patients with liver cirrhosis: a randomized 12-month trial. *Hepatology.* 2008;48(2): 557–566.
10. Swart GR, Zillikens MC, van Vuure JK, van den Berg JW. Effect of a late evening meal on nitrogen balance in patients with cirrhosis of the liver. *BMJ.* 1989;299(6709):1202–1203.
11. Dolz C, Raurich JM, Ibanez J, et al. Ascites increases the resting energy expenditure in liver cirrhosis. *Gastroenterology.* 1991; 100(3):738–744.
12. Muller MJ, Lautz HU, Plogmann B, et al. Energy expenditure and substrate oxidation in patients with cirrhosis: the impact of cause, clinical staging and nutritional state. *Hepatology.* 1992;15(5): 782–794.
13. John WJ, Phillips R, Ott L, Adams LJ, McClain CJ. Resting energy expenditure in patients with alcoholic hepatitis. *JPEN J Parenter Enteral Nutr.* 1989;13(2):124–127.
14. McClain CJ, Song Z, Barve SS, Hill DB, Deaciuc I. Recent advances in alcoholic liver disease. IV. Dysregulated cytokine metabolism in alcoholic liver disease. *Am J Physiol Gastrointest Liver Physiol.* 2004;287(3):G497–502.
15. McClain CJ, Barve S, Deaciuc I, Kugelmas M, Hill D. Cytokines in alcoholic liver disease. *Semin Liver Dis.* 1999;19(2):205–219.
16. Sleisenger MH, Feldman M, Friedman LS, Brandt LJ. *Sleisenger and Fordtran's Gastrointestinal and Liver Disease: Pathophysiology, Diagnosis, Management.* 9th ed. Philadelphia, PA: Saunders/Elsevier; 2010.
17. Mendenhall C, Roselle GA, Gartside P, Moritz T. Relationship of protein calorie malnutrition to alcoholic liver disease: a reexamination of data from two Veterans Administration Cooperative Studies. *Alcohol Clin Exp Res.* 1995;19(3):635–641.
18. Mendenhall CL, Tosch T, Weesner RE, et al. VA cooperative study on alcoholic hepatitis. II: Prognostic significance of protein-calorie malnutrition. *Am J Clin Nutr.* 1986;43(2):213–218.
19. Mendenhall CL, Anderson S, Weesner RE, Goldberg SJ, Crolic KA. Protein-calorie malnutrition associated with alcoholic hepatitis. Veterans Administration Cooperative Study Group on Alcoholic Hepatitis. *Am J Med.* 1984;76(2):211–222.
20. Mendenhall CL, Moritz TE, Roselle GA, et al. Protein energy malnutrition in severe alcoholic hepatitis: diagnosis and response to treatment. The VA Cooperative Study Group #275. *JPEN J Parenter Enteral Nutr.* 1995;19(4):258–265.
21. Mendenhall CL, Moritz TE, Roselle GA, et al. A study of oral nutritional support with oxandrolone in malnourished patients with alcoholic hepatitis: results of a Department of Veterans Affairs cooperative study. *Hepatology.* 1993;17(4):564–576.
22. Antonow DR MC. Nutrition in alcoholism. In: Tarter RE, Van Thiel DH, eds. *Alcohol and the Brain: Chronic Effects.* New York, NY: Plenum; 1985:81–120.
23. Gloria L, Cravo M, Camilo ME, et al. Nutritional deficiencies in chronic alcoholics: relation to dietary intake and alcohol consumption. *Am J Gastroenterol.* 1997;92(3):485–489.
24. Corrao G, Ferrari PA, Galatola G. Exploring the role of diet in modifying the effect of known disease determinants: application to risk factors of liver cirrhosis. *Am J Epidemiol.* 1995;142(11):1136–1146.
25. Srivastava S, Younossi ZM. Morbid obesity, nonalcoholic fatty liver disease, and weight loss surgery. *Hepatology.* 2005;42(2):490–492.
26. Blackburn GL, Mun EC. Effects of weight loss surgeries on liver disease. *Semin Liver Dis.* 2004;24(4):371–379.
27. Lieber CS, Leo MA, Mak KM, et al. Model of nonalcoholic steatohepatitis. *Am J Clin Nutr.* 2004;79(3):502–509.

28. Cortez-Pinto H, Jesus L, Barros H, et al. How different is the dietary pattern in non-alcoholic steatohepatitis patients? *Clin Nutr.* 2006; 25(5):816–823.
29. Lieber CS, DeCarli LM, Leo MA, et al. Beneficial effects versus toxicity of medium-chain triacylglycerols in rats with NASH. *J Hepatol.* 2008;48(2):318–326.
30. Lim JS, Mietus-Snyder M, Valente A, Schwarz JM, Lustig RH. The role of fructose in the pathogenesis of NAFLD and the metabolic syndrome. *Nat Rev Gastroenterol Hepatol.* 2010;7(5):251–264.
31. Ouyang X, Cirillo P, Sautin Y, et al. Fructose consumption as a risk factor for non-alcoholic fatty liver disease. *J Hepatol.* 2008;48(6): 993–999.
32. Spruss A, Kanuri G, Wagnerberger S, et al. Toll-like receptor 4 is involved in the development of fructose-induced hepatic steatosis in mice. *Hepatology.* 2009;50(4):1094–1104.
33. Sanchez-Lozada LG, Mu W, Roncal C, et al. Comparison of free fructose and glucose to sucrose in the ability to cause fatty liver. *Eur J Nutr.* 2010;49(1):1–9.
34. Lazo M, Solga SF, Horska A, et al. Effect of a 12-month intensive lifestyle intervention on hepatic steatosis in adults with type 2 diabetes. *Diabetes Care.* 2010;33(10):2156–2163.
35. Tendler D, Lin S, Yancy WS Jr, et al. The effect of a low-carbohydrate, ketogenic diet on nonalcoholic fatty liver disease: a pilot study. *Dig Dis Sci.* 2007;52(2):589–593.
36. Zivkovic AM, German JB, Sanyal AJ. Comparative review of diets for the metabolic syndrome: implications for nonalcoholic fatty liver disease. *Am J Clin Nutr.* 2007;86(2):285–300.
37. Kistler KD, Brunt EM, Clark JM, et al. Physical activity recommendations, exercise intensity, and histological severity of nonalcoholic fatty liver disease. *Am J Gastroenterol.* 2011;106(3):460–468.
38. Rafiq N, Younossi ZM. Effects of weight loss on nonalcoholic fatty liver disease. *Semin Liver Dis.* 2008;28(4):427–433.
39. Dickerson RN. Hypocaloric feeding of obese patients in the intensive care unit. *Curr Opin Clin Nutr Metab Care.* 2005;8(2):189–196.
40. Choban PS, Flancbaum L. Nourishing the obese patient. *Clin Nutr.* 2000;19(5):305–311.
41. Guglielmi FW, Panella C, Buda A, et al. Nutritional state and energy balance in cirrhotic patients with or without hypermetabolism. Multicentre prospective study by the 'Nutritional Problems in Gastroenterology' Section of the Italian Society of Gastroenterology (SIGE). *Dig Liver Dis.* S2005;37(9):681–688.
42. Martin A, Lemon SM. Hepatitis A virus: from discovery to vaccines. *Hepatology.* 2006;43(2 Suppl 1):S164–172.
43. Taylor RM, Davern T, Munoz S, et al. Fulminant hepatitis A virus infection in the United States: Incidence, prognosis, and outcomes. *Hepatology.* 2006;44(6):1589–1597.
44. Lok AS, McMahon BJ. Chronic hepatitis B. *Hepatology.* 2007; 45(2):507–539.
45. Wild CP, Montesano R. A model of interaction: aflatoxins and hepatitis viruses in liver cancer aetiology and prevention. *Cancer Lett.* 2009;286(1):22–28.
46. Yates MS, Kensler TW. Keap1 eye on the target: chemoprevention of liver cancer. *Acta Pharmacol Sin.* 2007;28(9):1331–1342.
47. Armstrong GL, Wasley A, Simard EP, et al. The prevalence of hepatitis C virus infection in the United States, 1999 through 2002. *Ann Intern Med.* 2006;144(10):705–714.
48. Conry-Cantilena C, VanRaden M, Gibble J, et al. Routes of infection, viremia, and liver disease in blood donors found to have hepatitis C virus infection. *N Engl J Med.* 1996;334(26):1691–1696.
49. Fried M, Navarro V, Afdhal N, et al. A randomized, placebo-controlled trial of oral silymarin (milk thistle) for chronic hepatitis C: final results of the SYNCH multicenter study. *Hepatology (Baltimore, Md.)* 2011;54(S1):119A.
50. Gutierrez JA, Parikh N, Branch AD. Classical and emerging roles of vitamin D in hepatitis C virus infection. *Semin Liver Dis.* 2011; 31(4):387–398.
51. Feld JJ, Modi AA, El-Diwany R, et al. S-adenosyl methionine improves early viral responses and interferon-stimulated gene induction in hepatitis C nonresponders. *Gastroenterology.* 2011; 140(3):830–839.
52. Pietrangelo A. Hereditary hemochromatosis—a new look at an old disease. *N Engl J Med.* 2004;350(23):2383–2397.
53. Adams PC. Review article: the modern diagnosis and management of haemochromatosis. *Aliment Pharmacol Ther.* 2006;23(12): 1681–1691.
54. Ala A, Walker AP, Ashkan K, Dooley JS, Schilsky ML. Wilson's disease. *Lancet.* 2007;369(9559):397–408.
55. Roberts EA, Schilsky ML. A practice guideline on Wilson disease. *Hepatology.* 2003;37(6):1475–1492.
56. Weiss KH, Gotthardt DN, Klemm D, et al. Zinc monotherapy is not as effective as chelating agents in treatment of Wilson disease. *Gastroenterology.* 2011;140(4):1189–1198, e1181.
57. Kaplan MM, Gershwin ME. Primary biliary cirrhosis. *N Engl J Med.* 2005;353(12):1261–1273.
58. Corpechot C, Carrat F, Bahr A, et al. The effect of ursodeoxycholic acid therapy on the natural course of primary biliary cirrhosis. *Gastroenterology.* 2005;128(2):297–303.
59. Maggs JR, Chapman RW. Sclerosing cholangitis. *Curr Opin Gastroenterol.* 2007;23(3):310–316.
60. Kim WR, Therneau TM, Wiesner RH, et al. A revised natural history model for primary sclerosing cholangitis. *Mayo Clin Proc.* 2000;75(7):688–694.
61. Lindor KD, Kowdley KV, Luketic VA, et al. High-dose ursodeoxycholic acid for the treatment of primary sclerosing cholangitis. *Hepatology (Baltimore, Md).* 2009;50(3):808–814.
62. Kowdley KV, Emond MJ, Sadowski JA, Kaplan MM. Plasma vitamin K1 level is decreased in primary biliary cirrhosis. *Am J Gastroenterol.* 1997;92(11):2059–2061.
63. Floreani A, Zappala F, Fries W, et al. A 3-year pilot study with 1,25-dihydroxyvitamin D, calcium, and calcitonin for severe osteodystrophy in primary biliary cirrhosis. *J Clin Gastroenterol.* 1997; 24(4):239–244.
64. Sarin SK, Dhingra N, Bansal A, Malhotra S, Guptan RC. Dietary and nutritional abnormalities in alcoholic liver disease: a comparison with chronic alcoholics without liver disease. *Am J Gastroenterol.* 1997;92(5):777–783.
65. Caregaro L, Alberino F, Amodio P, et al. Malnutrition in alcoholic and virus-related cirrhosis. *Am J Clin Nutr.* 1996;63(4):602–609.
66. Lolli R, Marchesini G, Bianchi G, et al. Anthropometric assessment of the nutritional status of patients with liver cirrhosis in an Italian population. *Ital J Gastroenterol.* 1992;24(8):429–435.
67. Thuluvath PJ, Triger DR. Evaluation of nutritional status by using anthropometry in adults with alcoholic and nonalcoholic liver disease. *Am J Clin Nutr.* 1994;60(2):269–273.
68. DiCecco SR, Wieners EJ, Wiesner RH, et al. Assessment of nutritional status of patients with end-stage liver disease undergoing liver transplantation. *Mayo Clin Proc.* 1989;64(1):95–102.
69. McCullough AJ, Tavill AS. Disordered energy and protein metabolism in liver disease. *Semin Liver Dis.* 1991;11(4):265–277.
70. Madden AM, Bradbury W, Morgan MY. Taste perception in cirrhosis: its relationship to circulating micronutrients and food preferences. *Hepatology.* 1997;26(1):40–48.
71. Kalman DR, Saltzman JR. Nutrition status predicts survival in cirrhosis. *Nutr Rev.* 1996;54(7):217–219.
72. Selberg O, Bottcher J, Tusch G, et al. Identification of high- and low-risk patients before liver transplantation: a prospective cohort

study of nutritional and metabolic parameters in 150 patients. *Hepatology.* 1997;25(3):652–657.
73. Heymsfield SB, Waki M, Reinus J. Are patients with chronic liver disease hypermetabolic? *Hepatology.* 1990;11(3):502–505.
74. Shanbhogue RL, Bistrian BR, Jenkins RL, et al. Resting energy expenditure in patients with end-stage liver disease and in normal population. *JPEN J Parenter Enteral Nutr.* 1987;11(3):305–308.
75. Merli M, Riggio O, Romiti A, et al. Basal energy production rate and substrate use in stable cirrhotic patients. *Hepatology.* 1990; 12(1):106–112.
76. Campillo B, Bories PN, Pornin B, Devanlay M. Influence of liver failure, ascites, and energy expenditure on the response to oral nutrition in alcoholic liver cirrhosis. *Nutrition.* 1997;13(7–8):613–621.
77. Petrides AS, Vogt C, Schulze-Berge D, Matthews D, Strohmeyer G. Pathogenesis of glucose intolerance and diabetes mellitus in cirrhosis. *Hepatology.* 1994;19(3):616–627.
78. McCullough AJ, Bugianesi E, Marchesini G, Kalhan SC. Gender-dependent alterations in serum leptin in alcoholic cirrhosis. *Gastroenterology.* 1998;115(4):947–953.
79. Mullen KD, Denne SC, McCullough AJ, et al. Leucine metabolism in stable cirrhosis. *Hepatology.* 1986;6(4):622–630.
80. Mullen KD, Weber FL Jr. Role of nutrition in hepatic encephalopathy. *Semin Liver Dis.* 1991;11(4):292–304.
81. Khoruts A, Stahnke L, McClain CJ, Logan G, Allen JI. Circulating tumor necrosis factor, interleukin-1 and interleukin-6 concentrations in chronic alcoholic patients. *Hepatology (Baltimore, Md.).* 1991;13(2):267–276.
82. Bigatello LM, Broitman SA, Fattori L, et al. Endotoxemia, encephalopathy, and mortality in cirrhotic patients. *Am J Gastroenterol.* 1987;82(1):11–15.
83. Teran JC, Mullen KD, McCullough AJ. Glutamine—a conditionally essential amino acid in cirrhosis? *Am J Clin Nutr.* 1995;62(5): 897–900.
84. Guarner C, Soriano G, Tomas A, et al. Increased serum nitrite and nitrate levels in patients with cirrhosis: relationship to endotoxemia. *Hepatology.* 1993;18(5):1139–1143.
85. Lieber CS. Relationships between nutrition, alcohol use, and liver disease. *Alcohol Res Health.* 2003;27(3):220–231.
86. Patek AJ Jr, Post J, et al. Dietary treatment of cirrhosis of the liver; results in 124 patients observed during a 10 year period. *J Am Med Assoc.* 1948;138(8):543–549.
87. Hirsch S, de la Maza MP, Gattas V, et al. Nutritional support in alcoholic cirrhotic patients improves host defenses. *J Am Coll Nutr.* 1999;18(5):434–441.
88. Kearns PJ, Young H, Garcia G, et al. Accelerated improvement of alcoholic liver disease with enteral nutrition. *Gastroenterology.* 1992;102(1):200–205.
89. Cabre E, Rodriguez-Iglesias P, Caballeria J, et al. Short- and long-term outcome of severe alcohol-induced hepatitis treated with steroids or enteral nutrition: a multicenter randomized trial. *Hepatology (Baltimore, Md.)* 2000;32(1):36–42.
90. Owen OE, Trapp VE, Reichard GA Jr, et al. Nature and quantity of fuels consumed in patients with alcoholic cirrhosis. *J Clin Invest.* 1983;72(5):1821–1832.
91. Vaisman N, Katzman H, Carmiel-Haggai M, Lusthaus M, Niv E. Breakfast improves cognitive function in cirrhotic patients with cognitive impairment. *Am J Clin Nutr.* 2010;92(1):137–140.
92. Cordoba J, Lopez-Hellin J, Planas M, et al. Normal protein diet for episodic hepatic encephalopathy: results of a randomized study. *J Hepatol.* J2004;41(1):38–43.
93. Gheorghe L, Iacob R, Vadan R, Iacob S, Gheorghe C. Improvement of hepatic encephalopathy using a modified high-calorie high-protein diet. *Rom J Gastroenterol.* 2005;14(3):231–238.
94. Brown Bowman BA, Russell R, International Life Sciences Institute. *Present Knowledge in Nutrition.* 9th ed. Washington, DC: International Life Sciences Institute; 2006.
95. Plauth M, Cabre E, Riggio O, et al. ESPEN Guidelines on Enteral Nutrition: Liver disease. *Clinical nutrition.* 2006;25(2):285–294.
96. Marchesini G, Bianchi G, Merli M, et al. Nutritional supplementation with branched-chain amino acids in advanced cirrhosis: a double-blind, randomized trial. *Gastroenterology.* 2003;124(7): 1792–1801.
97. Charlton M. Branched-chain amino acid-enriched supplements as therapy for liver disease: Rasputin lives. *Gastroenterology.* 2003; 124(7):1980–1982.
98. Liu SL, Degli Esposti S, Yao T, Diehl AM, Zern MA. Vitamin E therapy of acute CCl4-induced hepatic injury in mice is associated with inhibition of nuclear factor kappa B binding. *Hepatology.* 1995;22(5):1474–1481.
99. Hill DB, Devalaraja R, Joshi-Barve S, Barve S, McClain CJ. Antioxidants attenuate nuclear factor-kappa B activation and tumor necrosis factor-alpha production in alcoholic hepatitis patient monocytes and rat Kupffer cells, in vitro. *Clin Biochem.* 1999; 32(7):563–570.
100. Lavine JE. Vitamin E treatment of nonalcoholic steatohepatitis in children: a pilot study. *J Pediatr.* 2000;136(6):734–738.
101. Hasegawa T, Yoneda M, Nakamura K, Makino I, Terano A. Plasma transforming growth factor-beta1 level and efficacy of alpha-tocopherol in patients with non-alcoholic steatohepatitis: a pilot study. *Aliment Pharmacol Ther.* 2001;15(10):1667–1672.
102. Sanyal AJ, Chalasani N, Kowdley KV, et al. Pioglitazone, vitamin E, or placebo for nonalcoholic steatohepatitis. *New Engl J Med.* 2010;362(18):1675–1685.
103. Mezey E, Potter JJ, Rennie-Tankersley L, Caballeria J, Pares A. A randomized placebo controlled trial of vitamin E for alcoholic hepatitis. *J Hepatol.* 2004;40(1):40–46.
104. Lauterburg BH, Velez ME. Glutathione deficiency in alcoholics: risk factor for paracetamol hepatotoxicity. *Gut.* 1988;29(9): 1153–1157.
105. Pena LR, Hill DB, McClain CJ. Treatment with glutathione precursor decreases cytokine activity. *JPEN J Parenter Enteral Nutr.* 1999;23(1):1–6.
106. Lee WM, Hynan LS, Rossaro L, et al. Intravenous N-acetylcysteine improves transplant-free survival in early stage non-acetaminophen acute liver failure. *Gastroenterology.* 2009;137(3):856–864, e851.
107. Lieber CS. S-Adenosyl-L-methionine and alcoholic liver disease in animal models: implications for early intervention in human beings. *Alcohol.* 2002;27(3):173–177.
108. Karaa A, Thompson KJ, McKillop IH, Clemens MG, Schrum LW. S-adenosyl-L-methionine attenuates oxidative stress and hepatic stellate cell activation in an ethanol-LPS-induced fibrotic rat model. *Shock.* 2008;30(2):197–205.
109. Mato JM, Camara J, Fernandez de Paz J, et al. S-adenosylmethionine in alcoholic liver cirrhosis: a randomized, placebo-controlled, double-blind, multicenter clinical trial. *J Hepatol.* 1999; 30(6):1081–1089.
110. Rambaldi A, Gluud C. S-adenosyl-L-methionine for alcoholic liver diseases. *Cochrane Database Syst Rev.* 2006(2):CD002235.
111. Kharbanda KK, Mailliard ME, Baldwin CR, et al. Betaine attenuates alcoholic steatosis by restoring phosphatidylcholine generation via the phosphatidylethanolamine methyltransferase pathway. *J Hepatol.* 2007;46(2):314–321.
112. Abdelmalek MF, Sanderson SO, Angulo P, et al. Betaine for nonalcoholic fatty liver disease: results of a randomized placebo-controlled trial. *Hepatology.* 2009;50(6):1818–1826.

113. Joshi PC, Mehta A, Jabber WS, Fan X, Guidot DM. Zinc deficiency mediates alcohol-induced alveolar epithelial and macrophage dysfunction in rats. *Am J Respir Cell Mol Biol.* 2009;41(2):207–216.
114. Kang YJ, Zhou Z. Zinc prevention and treatment of alcoholic liver disease. *Mol Aspects Med.* 2005;26(4–5):391–404.
115. McClain CJ, Antonow DR, Cohen DA, Shedlofsky SI. Zinc metabolism in alcoholic liver disease. *Alcohol Clin Exp Res.* 1986; 10(6):582–589.
116. Kugelmas M. Preliminary observation: oral zinc sulfate replacement is effective in treating muscle cramps in cirrhotic patients. *J Am Coll Nutr.* 2000;19(1):13–15.
117. Zhong W, McClain CJ, Cave M, Kang YJ, Zhou Z. The role of zinc deficiency in alcohol-induced intestinal barrier dysfunction. *Am J Physiol Gastrointest Liver Physiol.* 2010;298(5):G625–633.
118. Kang X, Zhong W, Liu J, et al. Zinc supplementation reverses alcohol-induced steatosis in mice through reactivating hepatocyte nuclear factor-4alpha and peroxisome proliferator-activated receptor-alpha. *Hepatology.* Oct 2009;50(4):1241–1250.
119. Zhou Z, Kang X, Jiang Y, et al. Preservation of hepatocyte nuclear factor-4alpha is associated with zinc protection against TNF-alpha hepatotoxicity in mice. *Exp Biol Med (Maywood).* 2007; 232(5):622–628.
120. Takahashi M, Saito H, Higashimoto M, Hibi T. Possible inhibitory effect of oral zinc supplementation on hepatic fibrosis through downregulation of TIMP-1: A pilot study. *Hepatol Res.* 2007;37(6):405–409.
121. Takuma Y, Nouso K, Makino Y, Hayashi M, Takahashi H. Clinical trial: oral zinc in hepatic encephalopathy. *Aliment Pharmacol Ther.* Nov 2010;32(9):1080–1090.
122. Luper S. A review of plants used in the treatment of liver disease: part 1. *Altern Med Rev.* 1998;3(6):410–421.
123. Ferenci P, Dragosics B, Dittrich H, et al. Randomized controlled trial of silymarin treatment in patients with cirrhosis of the liver. *J Hepatol.* 1989;9(1):105–113.
124. Pares A, Planas R, Torres M, et al. Effects of silymarin in alcoholic patients with cirrhosis of the liver: results of a controlled, double-blind, randomized and multicenter trial. *J Hepatol.* 1998;28(4): 615–621.
125. Rambaldi A, Jacobs BP, Iaquinto G, Gluud C. Milk thistle for alcoholic and/or hepatitis B or C virus liver diseases. *Cochrane Database Syst Rev.* 2005(2):CD003620.
126. Hayaishi S, Chung H, Kudo M, et al. Oral branched-chain amino acid granules reduce the incidence of hepatocellular carcinoma and improve event-free survival in patients with liver cirrhosis. *Dig Dis.* 2011;29(3):326–332.
127. Muto Y, Sato S, Watanabe A, et al. Effects of oral branched-chain amino acid granules on event-free survival in patients with liver cirrhosis. *Clin Gastroenterol Hepatol.* 2005;3(7):705–713.
128. Fan ST, Lo CM, Lai EC, et al. Perioperative nutritional support in patients undergoing hepatectomy for hepatocellular carcinoma. *N Engl J Med.* 1994;331(23):1547–1552.
129. Barchetta I, Angelico F, Del Ben M, et al. Strong association between non alcoholic fatty liver disease (NAFLD) and low 25(OH) vitamin D levels in an adult population with normal serum liver enzymes. *BMC Med.* 2011;9(1):85.
130. Malham M, Jorgensen SP, Ott P, et al. Vitamin D deficiency in cirrhosis relates to liver dysfunction rather than aetiology. *World J Gastroenterol.* 2011;17(7):922–925.
131. Pappa HM, Bern E, Kamin D, Grand RJ. Vitamin D status in gastrointestinal and liver disease. *Curr Opin Gastroenterol.* 2008; 24(2):176–183.
132. Zahr NM, Kaufman KL, Harper CG. Clinical and pathological features of alcohol-related brain damage. *Nat Rev Neurol.* May 2011;7(5):284–294.
133. Khan LU, Ahmed J, Khan S, Macfie J. Refeeding syndrome: a literature review. *Gastroenterol Res Pract.* 2011;2011.
134. Ripoll C, Garcia-Tsao G. Management of gastropathy and gastric vascular ectasia in portal hypertension. *Clin Liver Dis.* May 2010;14(2):281–295.
135. Runyon BA. Management of adult patients with ascites due to cirrhosis: an update. *Hepatology (Baltimore, Md.)* 2009;49(6): 2087–2107.
136. Katz RI, Hovagim AR, Finkelstein HS, et al. A comparison of cocaine, lidocaine with epinephrine, and oxymetazoline for prevention of epistaxis on nasotracheal intubation. *J Clin Anesth.* 1990;2(1):16–20.
137. Hebuterne X, Vanbiervliet G. Feeding the patients with upper gastrointestinal bleeding. *Curr Opin Clin Nutr Metab Care.* Mar 2011;14(2):197–201.
138. de Ledinghen V, Beau P, Mannant PR, et al. Early feeding or enteral nutrition in patients with cirrhosis after bleeding from esophageal varices? A randomized controlled study. *Dig Dis Sci.* Mar 1997;42(3):536–541.
139. Baltz JG, Argo CK, Al-Osaimi AM, Northup PG. Mortality after percutaneous endoscopic gastrostomy in patients with cirrhosis: a case series. *Gastrointest Endosc.* Nov 2010;72(5):1072–1075.

28 Pancreatitis

Carol Rees Parrish, MS, RD, Joseph Krenitsky, MS, RD, and Stephen A. McClave, MD

CONTENTS

Background ... 473
Acute Pancreatitis ... 474
Definition and Pathophysiology ... 474
Incidence ... 474
Etiology ... 474
Nutritional Implications of Acute Pancreatitis ... 475
Role of the Gut in Systemic Inflammatory Response Syndrome and Benefits of Enteral Nutrition ... 476
The Importance of Pancreatic Rest ... 476
Providing Nutritional Support ... 476
Provision of Enteral Nutrition Support ... 478
Nasogastric Versus Nasojejunal ... 479
Formula Choices for Enteral Nutrition ... 479
Troubleshooting Enteral Nutrition ... 479
Parenteral Nutrition ... 479
Intravenous Lipid Emulsions ... 480
The Resumption of Oral Intake ... 480
Chronic Pancreatitis ... 480
Introduction ... 480
Epidemiology ... 481
Etiology ... 481
Hypertriglyceridemia ... 482
Pathophysiology and Clinical Presentation ... 482
Factors Promoting Protein/Calorie Malnutrition ... 482
Treatment ... 483
Nutritional Management ... 483
Oral Diet ... 483
Nutrition Support ... 484
Pancreatic Insufficiency ... 484
References ... 487

Objectives

1. Differentiate the etiology and the clinical presentation between acute and chronic pancreatitis.
2. Identify nutritional issues associated with both acute and chronic pancreatitis.
3. Determine the best route for nutrition support based on the evidence.
4. Surmount barriers to nutrition repletion in patients with pancreatitis.
5. Identify long-term nutritional issues in those with chronic pancreatitis.

Test Your Knowledge Questions

1. A consult was called on the 2nd day of hospitalization with regard to initiating nutrition support in a patient who presented with severe acute pancreatitis. The patient continued to require mechanical ventilation and a recent dynamic contrast-enhanced computed tomography (CT) scan revealed necrosis involving 30% of the pancreatic gland and a small 4-cm pseudocyst in the tail of the gland. Which of the following would you recommend?
   A. Continue nothing by mouth (NPO) status with no tube feeds, noting that the necrosis may require surgical intervention.
   B. Start the patient on parenteral nutrition (PN) because the patient is mechanically ventilated and has a pseudocyst.
   C. Place a nasojejunal tube and begin enteral tube feeds, providing no more than 10 to 20 mL/h.
   D. Place a nasojejunal tube, begin tube feeds, and advance to goal over the first 24 to 48 hours.
2. Which of the following nutrition regimens is appropriate for a patient with <2 Ranson Criteria and an APACHE II score of <9 (nonsevere), who has no pancreatic necrosis on a CT scan?
   A. Begin volume resuscitation, provide narcotic analgesia, and advance to an oral diet as soon as tolerated.
   B. Begin PN in the first 24 hours of admission because the patient has acute pain.
   C. Keep the patient NPO for at least 7 days.
   D. Use PN in the first 24 hours, then switch to an oral diet.
3. Which of the following is true?
   A. The immune response of the gut remains intact if the patient can be maintained on PN.
   B. Failure to use the gastrointestinal tract causes loss of gut integrity and exacerbates the stress response associated with pancreatitis.
   C. Loss of gut integrity may allow bacteria of gut origin to infect distant organ sites, but this is improved with bowel rest.
   D. Enteral feedings should be stopped if the ileus is noted radiographically.

Test Your Knowledge Answers

1. The correct answer is **D**. Complications such as pancreatic ascites, fistulas, or pseudocysts are part of the natural disease course of acute pancreatitis. Information from mostly retrospective case series indicates that the use of the enteral route is safe and allows for the resolution of these complications in most circumstances. The patient has severe pancreatitis, confirmed by 30% necrosis on a CT scan, and thus will benefit from placement on EN.
2. The correct answer is **A**. This patient has mild-to-moderate pancreatitis. Such patients have a mortality rate of 0% to 1.5%, a 6% rate of complications, and an 81% chance of advancing to an oral diet within 7 days. These patients may also be supported with intravenous fluid resuscitation and analgesia without added specialized nutrition support.
3. The correct answer is **B**. Loss of gut integrity has been demonstrated in patients hospitalized for pancreatitis who are maintained on PN and gut disuse while awaiting surgery. Over time, the villi in these patients become shortened, then lost. In contrast to pancreatitis patients kept on enteral tube feeding, pancreatitis patients placed on PN with gut disuse have been shown to have greater exposure to endotoxins and greater oxidant stress.

Background

The pancreas is a major organ involved in the digestion and absorption of food. It is a soft globular gland with no external capsule, located in the retroperitoneum between the duodenal c-loop and the hilum of the spleen. The pancreas is really two glands in one. Structurally, the endocrine portion involves the islets of Langerhans, and is responsible for producing insulin, glucagon, and somatostatin. The exocrine portion of the gland is structurally comprised of the acini and the ductal system, and is responsible for the secretion of multiple digestive enzymes including amylase, lipase, carboxypeptidase, phospholipase-α, chymotrypsin, aminopeptidase, trypsinogen, and cholesterase. The gland produces 1.0 to 2.5 L of exocrine secretions per day, which include bicarbonate, fluid volume, electrolytes, and enzymes.[1] The pancreatic exocrine secretions drain through the ductal system and join with biliary secretions in the common bile duct just prior to emptying into the duodenum through the major ampulla (ampulla of Vater). The shared tract for pancreatic and biliary secretions can be a source of pancreatitis if biliary stones or sludge occludes the common duct and prevents the drainage of pancreatic exocrine secretions. In approximately 10% of the population, the dorsal and ventral ducts do not fuse during embryonic development (pancreas divisum), and the majority of pancreatic secretions drain into the duodenum via the minor ampulla.[2] The digestive enzymes are stored in inactive precursor forms inside zymogen granules contained within the acinar cells. The activation of enzymes is prevented by protease inhibitors. The brush border enzyme enterokinase activates trypsinogen to trypsin. Once activated, trypsin is capable of activating all the other enzymes. The pancreatic exocrine secretion is influenced by a variety of stimulatory factors involving neural (vagus nerve), chemical (acid, fat, protein), mechanical (gastric distention), and hormonal agents (gastrin, secretin, vasoactive intestinal peptide, and cholecystokinin).[1] Three phases of stimulation exist. In the cephalic phase, the sight, smell, taste, and even the anticipation of food leads to the vagal stimulation of pancreatic enzyme secretion. In the gastric phase, food entering the stomach leads to the release of gastrin and the stimulation of acid output (both of which are stimulants of pancreatic secretion). Distention of the gastric wall with food leads to stimulation of the pancreas through vagal nerve input. In the intestinal phase, protein and fat entering the duodenum, along with acid, cause the release of cholecystokinin and secretin, which stimulate the release of pancreatic enzyme, fluid volume, and bicarbonate. Also in the intestinal phase, inhibitory factors are released (such as peptide YY, somatostatin, glucagon, pancreatic polypeptide, bile salts, luminal proteases, and increasing pH), all of which decrease pancreatic exocrine secretion. In the fasted state, the volume of pancreatic exocrine output is decreased, but the pancreas continues to secrete a basal flow of exocrine secretions.[1]

Acute Pancreatitis

Definition and Pathophysiology

Acute pancreatitis is an inflammatory process initiated in the pancreas with immune activation caused by active pancreatic enzymes damaging pancreatic tissue with variable involvement of other regional tissues and remote organ systems.[3–5] A poorly defined trigger event initiates the process, leading to premature activation of proteolytic digestive enzymes.[6] The initial insult results in the activation and release of trypsin into the cytoplasm of the acinar cell. This results in an amplification process, which in turn leads to a release of cytokines, inflammatory mediators, and inflammatory cell recruitment.[6] The onset of pain usually occurs 24 to 36 hours after the peak of cytokine production, with the onset of systemic manifestations and distant organ failure occurring 1 to 3 days later.[7]

Incidence

The incidence of acute pancreatitis is estimated at 40 cases per 100,000 adults in the United States, with a conservative estimate of $2.2 billion annual direct medical costs.[8] In the United States and a number of other countries, the incidence of acute pancreatitis has substantially increased in the last decade.[8–10] The increasing incidence of pancreatitis may be in part due to the increased incidence of obesity and the increased incidence of gallstone pancreatitis in older women.[9]

Etiology

Worldwide, the most common etiologies of acute pancreatitis involve alcohol (ETOH) abuse, biliary tract disease (passage of common bile duct stone), or idiopathic pancreatitis, accounting for 90% of all cases.[8–12] The distribution among these main etiologies varies with country and region, as well as the sex and age of the patients, with gallstone pancreatitis more common in women, and alcohol-related pancreatitis more common in men.[9–11] The remaining 10% of pancreatitis cases is accounted for by a variety of disorders such as pancreas divisum, trauma, hypoparathyroidism, hypercalcemia, hyperlipidemia, postendoscopic retrograde cholangiopancreatography (post-ERCP), medications, and biliary dyskinesia.[9–11] The majority of all admissions for acute pancreatitis (80% to 85%) are of mild-to-moderate severity, which is a self-limiting process with a low risk of complications (<6%) and negligible mortality. Over 80% of patients with uncomplicated, mild-to-moderate pancreatitis successfully advance to an oral diet within 1 week of hospitalization.[13–17]

Severe acute pancreatitis represents 15% to 20% of admissions, and the burden of disease in these patients is considerable.[13–17] The mean hospital length of stay is approximately 1 month, organ failure occurs in at least 16% to 33% of cases, and infection complicates the disease course in 30% to 50%. Mortality alone is 19% to 30%, but may range up to as high as 80% if organ failure or sepsis complicates the disease process.[13–17] The likelihood for advancement to an oral diet within 1 week of hospitalization for acute severe pancreatitis is close to 0%.[17] The overall disease severity is determined by the adequacy of fluid resuscitation, the presence and extent of necrosis within the gland, the presence of obesity, infection within the gland, failure of at least one organ system, and the route of nutrition support.[7,13,18,19] Pathophysiological processes outside the pancreas, primarily related to the integrity of the gastrointestinal (GI) tract, may also contribute to the level of the systemic inflammatory response syndrome (SIRS) and the rate of complications.[20–22] Severe acute pancreatitis may be identified by objective scoring systems (Acute Physiology and Chronic Health Evaluation [APACHE] II score and Ranson Criteria), and the presence of necrosis on a CT scan (Tables 28-1 to 28-3). Serum amylase or lipase greater than three times the upper limit of normal in the setting of severe abdominal pain is consistent with a diagnosis of pancreatitis. However, the severity of pancreatitis does not correlate with the degree of enzyme elevation and increased serum amylase and lipase can occur due to other intra-abdominal processes.[11,23] Additionally, the normalization (or lack of normalization) of serum amylase and lipase is not a sensitive or specific marker for the resolution of pancreatitis. A study of patients with acute pancreatitis reported that a serum lipase greater than 3 times normal the day before restarting an oral diet was significantly associated with an increased likelihood of pain relapse upon

TABLE 28-1 Differentiating Severe From Mild to Moderate Acute Pancreatitis[13,16,17]

	APACHE II ≤9 Rans Crit ≤2	APACHE II ≥10 Rans Crit ≥3
Degree of pancreatitis	Mild/moderate	Severe
CT scan	No necrosis	Necrosis
Mortality	0%	19%
PO diet in 7 days	81%	0%
Management	Supportive	EN/PN

Not exclusions: Necrosis, pseudocyst, ascites, surgery.
Exclusions: Intolerance.
CT, computed tomography; PO, by mouth; EN, enteral nutrition; PN, parenteral nutrition; Rans Crit, Ranson Criteria; APACHE, acute physiology and chronic health evaluation.

TABLE 28-2 Computed Tomography Grading System of Balthazar

Grade A	Normal-appearing pancreas
Grade B	Focal or diffuse enlargement of the pancreas
Grade C	Pancreatic gland abnormalities accompanied by mild parapancreatic inflammatory changes
Grade D	Fluid collection in a single location, usually within the anterior pararenal space
Grade E	Two or more fluid collections near the pancreas or gas either within the pancreas or within parapancreatic inflammation

Adapted with permission from Balthazar EJ, Freeny PC, van Sonneberg E. Imaging and interventions in acute pancreatitis. *Radiology.* 1994;193:297–306.

TABLE 28-3 Computed Tomography Severity Index of Balthazar and Ranson Criteria

Computed Tomography (CT) Grade	Quantity of Necrotic Pancreas
Grade A = 0	<33% necrosis = 2
Grade B = 1	
Grade C = 2	33%–50% necrosis = 4
Grade D = 3	
Grade E = 4	>50% necrosis = 6

Total Score = CT Grade (0–4) + Necrosis (0–6)
Mortality increased with score ≥7.
Reprinted by permission from Macmillan Publishers Ltd: *Am J Gastroenterol.* Banks PA. Practice guidelines in acute pancreatitis. 1997;92:377–386.

TABLE 28-4 Factors Causing Deterioration of Nutritional Status in Acute and Chronic Pancreatitis

	Acute	Chronic
Hypermetabolism	++	+
Skeletal muscle catabolism	++	+
Increased oxidative stress	++	+
Reduced oral intake	++	+
Nausea, vomiting	++	+
Errors in carbohydrate, fat metabolism	++	+
Abdominal pain	++	++
Food aversion	++	++
Protein loss (diarrhea, fistulas, inflammation)	++	++
Delayed gastric emptying	+	++
Continued ETOH abuse	+	++
Maldigestion, malabsorption	+	++
Gastric outlet obstruction	+	++

+ moderate; ++ significant; ETOH, alcohol

oral refeeding.[24] However, serum amylase and lipase after food introduction were not consistently different between the groups that tolerated oral refeeding compared to those that experienced pain. There is no data to support holding enteral feeding due to elevated serum amylase or lipase without other signs of clinical exacerbation of pancreatitis.[11,23]

The course and ultimate resolution of severe acute pancreatitis can be complicated by the effects of damage to pancreatic and surrounding tissue and the secondary response to this injury. One or more areas of the pancreatic parenchyma can become devitalized, resulting in necrotic pancreatitis. If the necrotic areas of the pancreas become infected, the risk of mortality is substantially increased, and surgical intervention is often indicated.[11] Early in the course of severe acute pancreatitis, extravasation of pancreatic fluid into the extrapancreatic space and fluid from the inflammatory and immune response to enzyme-rich pancreatic secretions can form acute peripancreatic fluid collections.[25] After several weeks, these fluid collections can be enclosed by a nonepithelialized wall of fibrinous or granulation tissue, creating a pancreatic pseudocyst.[25] Acute peripancreatic fluid collections and pseudocysts are at risk of becoming infected, and medical management frequently involves draining the fluid collections via endoscopic or percutaneous means. A circumscribed collection of obviously infected peripancreatic fluid (pus) that does not contain necrotic pancreatic tissue is termed a pancreatic abscess.[25]

Nutritional Implications of Acute Pancreatitis

Severe acute pancreatitis represents a hypermetabolic, hyperdynamic disease process very similar to sepsis (see Chapter 23).[26,27] The process generates increased oxidative stress, exaggerated catabolism, a systemic inflammatory response, and the rapid deterioration of nutritional status (Table 28-4).[3,4] Energy expenditure (see Chapter 2) may be increased by as much as 139% of that predicted by the Harris–Benedict equation.[28] More patients with acute pancreatitis are hypermetabolic than those patients with chronic pancreatitis (61% vs. 33%, respectively).[28] Sepsis complicating pancreatitis can further raise energy expenditure by a mean of 15%.[28] The catabolic stress state generates increased muscle catabolism and proteolysis, causing the loss of lean muscle mass. Accelerated ureagenesis occurs, and glutamine levels are decreased both in muscle and in serum.[29] A number of consequences in addition to exaggerated catabolism promote the deterioration of nutritional status. Reduced oral intake can occur from abdominal pain, food aversion, nausea, vomiting, gastric atony with paralytic ileus, continued ethanol abuse, or partial obstruction of the duodenum from enlargement of the pancreatic gland. Nutrient losses may be increased because of maldigestion from reduced enzyme output, malabsorption of luminal nutrients, or excessive protein loss caused by diarrhea, pancreatic fistulas, or inflammation of peritoneal and retroperitoneal surfaces. No studies have compared the effect of different calorie or protein provisions on patient outcomes in acute pancreatitis. Nutrition goals in the early stage of severe pancreatitis are to avoid overfeeding and provide adequate protein to support acute-phase protein synthesis (Table 28-6). Calorie provision may need to be increased if recurrent infections maintain elevated energy expenditure, or to support increased physical activity and positive nitrogen balance when the acute phase of illness has passed.

Stress hyperglycemia and insulin resistance occur in 40% to 90% of patients with severe acute pancreatitis.[30,31] Insulin resistance and persistent gluconeogenesis are a result of critical illness (see Chapter 23) and can be compounded in pancreatitis when there is sufficient necrosis of parenchymal tissue with decreased insulin production.[31] Errors in fat metabolism (see Chapter 4) with hypertriglyceridemia occur in 12% to 15% of cases.[29,31,32] Hypertriglyceridemia is frequently seen in association with inadequate glucose control due to the downregulation of lipoprotein lipase in hyperglycemia.[33] Achieving adequate glucose control is essential to decrease serum triglyceride levels when hypertriglyceridemia is secondary to poor glucose control.[33,34] Electrolyte and micronutrient alterations (see Chapters 7 and 8) are common, especially hypocalcemia, which can occur in up to 25% of cases.[32] A reduction in calcium levels are related to decreased parathyroid hormone release, increased calcitonin, decreased magnesium levels, hypoalbuminemia, and saponification of calcium with unabsorbed free fatty acids. Long-term ethanol abuse can lead to decreases in zinc, magnesium, thiamin, and folate levels.[29,31,32]

Role of the Gut in Systemic Inflammatory Response Syndrome and Benefits of Enteral Nutrition

The provision of enteral nutrition (EN) to patients with severe acute pancreatitis helps maintain gut integrity by preventing increases in permeability and keeping the functional tight junctions between the intestinal epithelial cells closed (Table 28-5).[35–37] EN stimulates blood flow to the gut, which prevents ischemia/reperfusion injury. EN stimulates the release of secretory immunoglobulin A (IgA) and bile salts, which coat bacteria and prevent their adherence to the intestinal epithelium.[35–37] EN maintains the mass of gut-associated lymphoid tissue (GALT), which in turn supports the mass of mucosal-associated lymphoid tissue (MALT) at distant organ sites.[35-39] EN supports the role of commensal bacteria, which prevent colonization of the gut by pathogenic organisms.[35,40] Colonization of the gut with commensal organisms may reduce the likelihood for contact-dependent activation of intestinal epithelial cells by pathogenic organisms. Such a process can lead to increases in gut permeability from cell apoptosis and opening of the tight junctions, activation of neutrophils, and the release of inflammatory cytokines.[35,40] A small scale study suggested that a probiotic preparation may potentiate the action of commensal bacteria.[41] However, a large multicenter randomized study demonstrated no decrease in infectious complications and significantly increased mortality from ischemic bowel from a high-dose multispecies probiotic preparation in severe pancreatitis.[42]

A provision of EN attenuates the stress response compared to patients who receive parenteral nutrition (PN).[20] Patients placed on EN with severe acute pancreatitis demonstrate increases in antioxidant capacity, faster decreases in C-reactive protein levels, and faster resolution of SIRS compared to patients who are placed on PN. [20] Time to resolution of the disease process, as evidenced by the resolution of abdominal pain, the near normalization of amylase, and the successful advancement to a clear liquid diet is reduced by half with the use of EN compared to PN.[43] As a result of the differential effect of the gut in response to starvation versus feeding, it should not be surprising that the provision of EN has a dramatic impact on patient outcome compared to a provision of PN.[22,44] Two meta-analyses, involving seven prospective randomized trials in patients admitted for acute pancreatitis, showed that the use of EN reduces infection by as much as 52% ($p<.05$), hospital length of stay by as much as 4 days ($p<.05$), the need for surgical intervention by as much as 52% ($p<.05$), and a trend toward reduced organ failure by as much as 41% ($p=.06$), when compared to the use of PN.[22,44] No difference in mortality was seen between the two routes of nutrition support.[22,44]

TABLE 28-5 Benefits of Early Enteral Feeding in Acute Severe Pancreatitis

Maintains gut integrity (reduce bacterial challenge)
Sets the tone for systemic immunity (downregulate immune response)
Attenuates oxidative stress
Lessens disease severity
Promotes a faster resolution of the disease process
Reduces complications (less infections and need for surgical interventions, shorter hospital length of stays, and possibly less multiple organ failures)

The Importance of Pancreatic Rest

The clinician's perspective on the need for pancreatic rest and its overall clinical significance has changed dramatically over the last 15 years. In the past, early use of the gut and the advancement to an oral diet was thought to increase the risk for late complications, primarily pancreatic abscess. Prospective randomized trials have failed to confirm this fear.[22,44] Instead, the clinical consequences of early use of the enteral route seem to involve one of three possible scenarios: a clinically silent increase in pancreatic enzyme output,[45] an uncomplicated exacerbation of symptoms (which occurs in approximately 21% of patients),[45,46] or an exacerbation of the disease process itself with an increase in SIRS (in 4% of cases).[45,46] Usually subtle changes in the manner by which EN is provided are sufficient to reduce the exacerbation, promote tolerance, and continue feeding without an overall deleterious impact on the patient. Experience from the literature suggests that efforts to promote pancreatic rest as the sole management strategy to treat pancreatitis (through the use of nasogastric suction, somastatin, acid-reducing agents, etc.) is ineffective and does not have an impact on patient outcomes.[29] It seems now that reducing pancreatic enzyme output to basal unstimulated levels is not required to allow for the resolution of inflammation within the gland, but that reducing output to subclinical levels may be sufficient. The concept of putting the pancreas to rest and using the gut are not incompatible; both may be accomplished simultaneously in the same patient.

Providing Nutritional Support

The options for nutritional support in patients with acute pancreatitis are threefold: the provision of EN, the placement on PN, or the use of standard therapy (STD) in which no specialized nutritional support is provided (and patients are on their own to advance to an oral diet with the delivery of food on a tray). The choice among these options is determined by disease severity, timing, and tolerance (Figure 28-1 and Tables 28-6 and 28-7).

The patients with the greatest need for specialized nutritional support, who are most likely to experience a benefit in a clinical outcome from the provision of EN, are those patients with greater severity of pancreatitis. Intestinal permeability is increased in patients with severe pancreatitis, compared to those patients with mild pancreatitis (and controls with no pancreatic disease).[47] Patients with severe pancreatitis complicated by organ failure have greater increases in permeability above that seen in patients with severe but uncomplicated

FIGURE 28-1 Algorithm for the Nutritional Management of Acute Pancreatitis

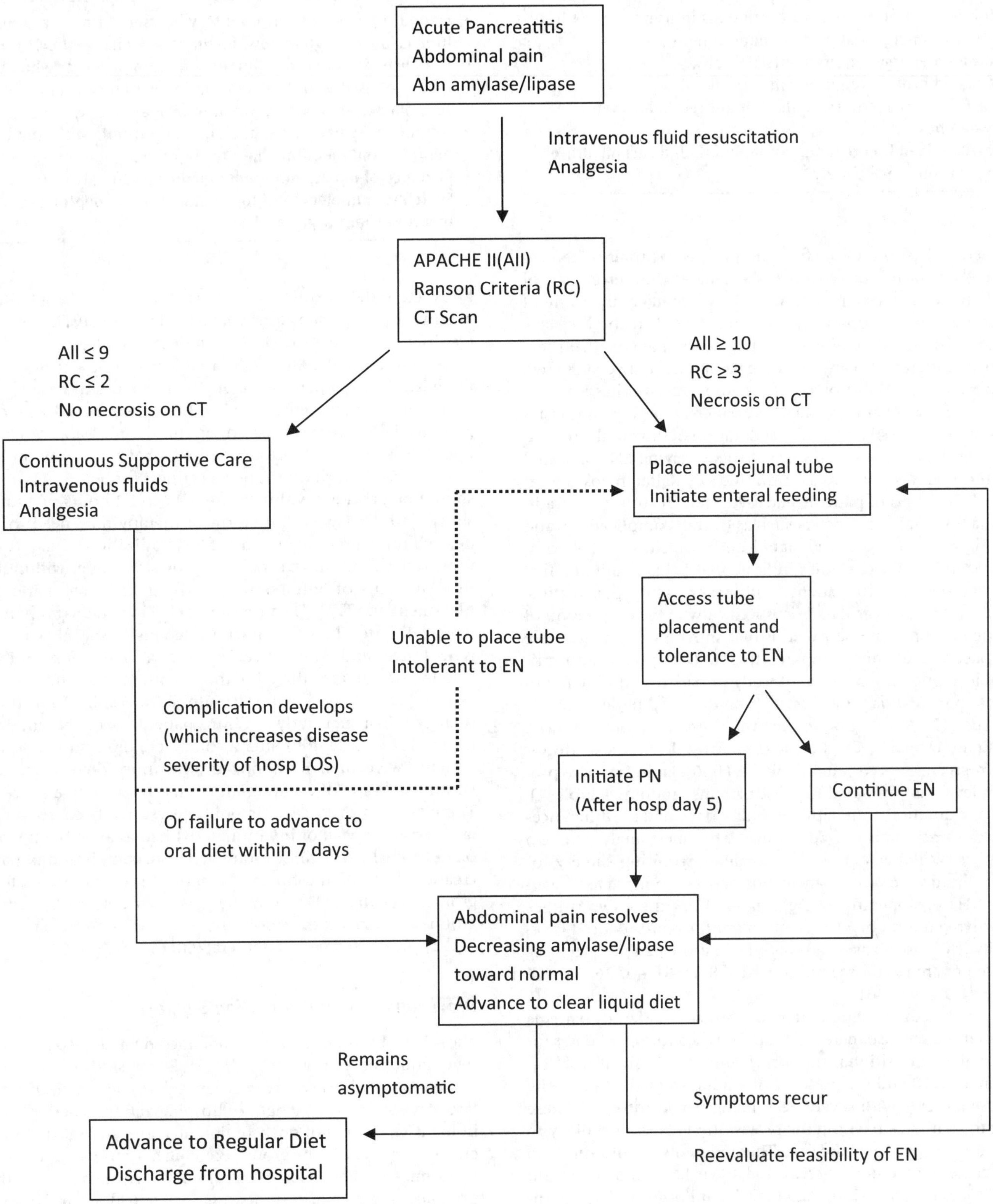

APACHE, acute physiology and chronic health evaluation; CT, computerized tomography; EN, enteral nutrition; PN, parenteral nutrition; hosp, hospital; LOS, length of stay;

TABLE 28-6 The Initiation of Enteral Nutrition in Severe Acute Pancreatitis

Initiate nutrition support by continuous infusion over 24 h/d to meet energy and protein requirements
Estimated energy requirements 25 kcal/kg/d
Estimated protein requirements 1.5 g/kg/d
Measure energy requirements with indirect calorimetry when possible
Provide mixed fuel regimen (protein, fat, and carbohydrate)
Monitor tolerance closely

TABLE 28-7 The Selection of Enteral Formula in Severe Acute Pancreatitis

• Standard polymeric formula: May be used if tip of feeding tube is low enough (below ligament of Treitz) in the GI tract.
• Evidence of intolerance (increase in pain, fever, or white blood cell [WBC] count in association with increases in serum amylase, lipase): Switch to elemental very low fat formula or switch to a semielemental formula with small peptides and medium-chain triglycerides.
• Evidence of malassimilation (diarrhea and/or steatorrhea): Switch to semielemental formula with small peptides and medium-chain triglycerides.

pancreatitis.[48] Out of the first four prospective trials of EN versus PN in acute pancreatitis, the greater the percentage of patients with severe pancreatitis, the more likely the route of feeding had an impact on outcome.[20,43,46,49] In the McClave study,[46] where 19% of patients had severe pancreatitis, there was no difference in any outcome parameters between the two groups. In the Windsor[20] and the Abou-Assi studies,[43] where 35% to 38% of patients had severe pancreatitis, there was faster resolution of SIRS and a shorter duration of time to the resolution of the disease process in patients receiving EN compared to those on PN. Only in a fourth study by Kalfarentzos et al.,[48] in which 100% of patients had severe pancreatitis, were traditional outcome parameters such as overall complications and septic morbidity reduced significantly with use of EN compared to PN. These studies indicate that EN is clearly the first choice over PN in patients with severe acute pancreatitis. Unfortunately, little data exist specifically in the population of patients with acute pancreatitis that show EN has a favorable impact on outcome compared to STD (no specialized nutritional support). In one small study in patients admitted with acute pancreatitis, Powell et al.[49] randomized patients to EN versus STD. A reduction in the overall stress response in those patients receiving EN was suggested by decreases in tumor necrosis factor (TNF), interleukin-6 (IL-6), and C-reactive protein levels as compared to those patients randomized to STD, but the duration of therapy was only 4 days, and the differences did not reach statistical significance.[49] In a meta-analyses of two studies by Pupelis et al.,[22,50,51] patients requiring surgery for complications of acute pancreatitis were randomized to EN versus STD postoperatively. Aggregating from these two studies involving a total of 71 patients, a trend toward reduced mortality (by as much as 74%) was seen in those patients receiving EN compared to those randomized to STD (RR = 0.26; 95% CI 0.06; 1.09; p – .06).[22]

An objective scoring system may be used to identify patients with more severe pancreatitis, who are therefore candidates for specialized nutritional support (Figure 28-1). An APACHE II score of ≥10 and the presence of ≥3 Ranson Criteria identify those patients with severe necrotizing pancreatitis.[14–16] These are the patients in whom the provision of EN is most likely to have an impact on outcome. These patients should undergo placement of enteral access and have EN initiated within 48 hours of admission. Patients with mild-to-moderate pancreatitis may be identified by APACHE II scores of ≤9 and the presence of ≤2 Ranson Criteria.[13–16] These patients would not be expected to have outcomes affected by the provision of EN, and may be supported alone with STD, intravenous fluid resuscitation, and the provision of narcotic analgesia. Not all patients tolerate EN. Although variable from one institution to the next, a certain percentage of patients may still require the provision of PN. Placement on PN should be reserved for those patients with severe disease in whom the provision of EN is poorly tolerated or not feasible (see Chapter 14). The timing of specialized nutrition support is critical for both EN (which should be provided within the first 48 to 72 hours of admission), and PN (where initiation of therapy may need to be delayed until after the 5th day of hospitalization). In an early prospective randomized trial, the provision of PN within the first 24 hours of admission caused net harm compared to placement on STD.[17] The provision of PN in patients with mild pancreatitis resulted in a hospital length of stay that was 1 week longer and a rate of central line catheter infection that was tenfold greater than for those patients receiving intravenous fluid volume support without specialized nutrition therapy.[17] In a later study in China, patients were not randomized to PN or STD until after a complete fluid resuscitation.[52] Patients were then randomized, and nutrition was started within 48 hours of completion of that resuscitative process. The provision of PN at this point (presumably several days later, past the peak of inflammation) had a favorable impact on outcome by reducing mortality, overall complications, pancreatic infection, and hospital length of stay, compared to a group receiving STD (outcome was even better for a third group of patients in the study who were randomized to receive PN supplemented with parenteral glutamine).[52]

Provision of Enteral Nutrition Support

The safety of jejunal EN is now well documented in 10 prospective randomized trials.[20,43,46,48,53–58] Every study end point related to the clinical outcome (days to normalization of amylase, days to oral diet, length of hospitalization, length of stay in the ICU, percent of nosocomial infection, and mortality) is equal to or better in the group receiving EN compared to those randomized to PN.[22] Complications of pancreatitis (such as the presence of a pseudocyst, abscess, or ascites) are not a contraindication to EN. EN may continue to be provided as long as tolerance is demonstrated.

Nasogastric Versus Nasojejunal

Several studies have suggested that nasogastric feeding may be an effective means to provide nutrition support to patients with severe acute pancreatitis.[59,60] However, there continues to be some controversy about the appropriateness of gastric enteral feeding for severe pancreatitis. There is concern that several studies compared gastric feeding with distal duodenal, not jejunal feeding.[61] Duodenal feeding may actually result in greater pancreatic stimulation than gastric feeding.[62,63] Additionally, in one study,[59] the median pain score and use of narcotic pain medications was near zero by the 3rd day of feeding (study day 5) in both groups, which appears inconsistent with severe pancreatitis and the relatively high mortality rate in the study. In the sole study that has randomized patients to receive either gastric EN or PN, there were significantly more complications in the EN group, despite the greater incidence of hyperglycemia in the PN group.[64] Despite the ongoing questions, there does appear to be a number of patients that apparently tolerated early semielemental gastric EN. Gastric feeding access is easier to achieve than jejunal placed tubes and has the potential advantage of allowing earlier EN in severe pancreatitis. Currently, the preponderance of data supporting EN over PN in severe pancreatitis have provided EN beyond the ligament of Treitz (LOT), but there is a clear need for additional studies of gastric EN.

Fluoroscopy and endoscopy are frequently used to assist and ensure the placement of feeding tubes due to the difficulty in achieving blind placement of tubes beyond the LOT. Magnetic guidance, the use of modified feeding tubes that generate an electromagnetic signal recognized by an external receiver, and self-advancing feeding tubes have all been reported to assist with small bowel feeding tube placement.[65–67] However, there is limited data about their effectiveness for placement of feeding tubes beyond the LOT, especially in patients prone to duodenal compression from an inflamed pancreas. It is advisable for clinicians to recognize the location of feeding ports in relation to the tip of the feeding tube used at their facility. Feeding tubes that have feeding ports proximal to the tip (frequently seen with weighted tubes) may appear to be positioned beyond the LOT, whereas in reality, the feeding ports remain in the duodenum.

Formula Choices for Enteral Nutrition

Standard polymeric enteral feeding formulas may be used when feeding distal to the LOT. Several of the studies that have demonstrated the superiority of jejunal EN over PN used polymeric formulas,[20,51,68] and when polymeric formulas were infused 40 to 60 cm distal to LOT there was actually an inhibition of pancreatic secretions compared to PN.[63] However, patients with extensive pancreatic necrosis or those demonstrating signs of maldigestion/malabsorption may benefit from a semielemental or elemental feeding after the most common causes of diarrhea (sorbitol-containing medications and *Clostridium difficile*) are excluded. A review of 127 patients with complicated pancreatitis receiving jejunal feeding documented that 30% of the patients tested had a positive fecal fat result indicating steatorrhea.[69]

Troubleshooting Enteral Nutrition

Patients that experience intolerance to EN infusion (increased abdominal pain, exacerbation of SIRS) should have the position of the feeding tube rechecked or advanced further beyond the LOT. In the study by McClave,[46] a patient tolerant of a jejunal infusion of formula flared with an exacerbation of SIRS when the same formula was infused into the stomach (after the tip of the tube was displaced proximally in the GI tract). Patients with severe pancreatitis frequently experience abdominal pain, and it is important to distinguish persistent pain from pancreatitis from acute increase in pain associated with starting EN initiation when evaluating tolerance.

However, increased nausea due to pain medications, functional gastric outlet obstructions, or an ileal brake from jejunal feeding should not be a contraindication to continued jejunal EN.[72] Double lumen tubes, which allow feeding through a distal opening and simultaneous gastric decompression through the proximal opening, may be useful to decrease nausea without the need for a second nasal tube for nasogastric decompression. One potential disadvantage of double lumen tubes is that in order to maintain an external diameter that is relatively comfortable for the patient (14 to 16 Fr), the jejunal portion of the tube is usually 6 to 9 Fr and may be prone to frequent clogging.

The institutional variation in the tolerance of EN in pancreatitis may be related to local expertise in achieving enteral access, the existence of a multidisciplinary nutrition support team, and the aggressiveness with which the institution initiates EN. At one institution, only 5 patients out of 16 randomized to EN demonstrated problems with ileus (requiring decreases in the rate of infusion but not of the cessation of feeding).[20] In a separate institution in the same city, attempts to initiate EN were successful in only 53% of patients admitted for pancreatitis; 47% were unsuccessful and had to be placed on PN or STD.[72] The duration of ileus before the initiation of EN may be a factor in tolerance. In a study from Portugal, patients in whom the duration of ileus was ≥6 days did not tolerate EN and had to be placed on PN.[48] If the duration of ileus was limited to ≤5 days, 50% of patients tolerated EN, whereas ileus limited to ≤2 days resulted in a 92% tolerance of EN.[72,73]

Parenteral Nutrition

Although the majority of patients appear to tolerate EN in severe acute pancreatitis, there are patients in whom EN is not feasible and PN is required to prevent severe malnutrition. Persistent ileus or small bowel obstruction, especially in patients admitted with compromised nutrition status, are indications for PN. Additionally, there are occasional patients that experience exacerbations of pancreatitis symptoms even with a proper jejunal placement of feeding tubes and elemental EN infusion. In two different studies, some patients failed to tolerate EN in a situation where the tube was placed well below the LOT.[43,46] The physiologic reasons why some individual patients are unable to tolerate EN in pancreatitis remains unclear, but EN is considered contraindicated if it is clearly exacerbating disease morbidity.

Intravenous Lipid Emulsions

Intravenous lipid emulsions do not exacerbate the symptoms of pancreatitis that has not been caused by hypertriglyceridemia, and a mixed fuel source (carbohydrate CHO, protein, lipid) PN is recommended.[74,75] Hypertriglyceride-induced pancreatitis generally occurs only in susceptible individuals with triglyceride >1000 mg/dL, and a lipid emulsion can be safely restarted when triglycerides decrease below 400 mg/dL. When the quantity of lipids in PN is limited to less than 1 g of fat per kilogram, and glucose control is maintained, the occurrence of hypertriglyceridemia during PN is limited.[76] When hypertriglyceridemia occurs in the setting of pancreatitis, it is frequently related to familial dyslipidemia and/or hyperglycemia.[77]

The Resumption of Oral Intake

There is limited data to guide the resumption of oral intake following an episode of acute pancreatitis. Most clinicians take into consideration the presence or absence of pain, the severity of pancreatitis, biochemical markers, and radiologic improvement based on a CT scan. Pancreatitis that has been complicated by a pseudocyst or sterile necrosis is increasingly managed with conservative therapy. It is unclear if extending the period of nil per oris (nothing by mouth) with longer term jejunal feeding offers benefits over standard care in the conservative management of complicated pancreatitis. Some facilities have reported favorable outcomes in retrospective reviews with long-term access for jejunal feeding in patients with more chronic or complicated pancreatitis.[69,78]

In mild acute pancreatitis, there does not appear to be any advantage to starting diets with liquids or a low-fat oral intake.[79–81] In fact, it appears that allowing patients free-choice regarding when to begin oral intake and the self-selection of foods may offer the advantage of decreasing the length of hospitalization without increasing the rate of relapse or abdominal pain.[79–81] (Practice Scenario 28-1)

Practice Scenario 28-1

Question: How should the patient with severe acute pancreatitis receive nutrition support?

Scenario: A 57-year-old female is admitted with a sudden acute onset of bilateral upper quadrant abdominal pain, nausea, and vomiting accompanied by fever. Initial laboratory results reveal an elevated amylase and lipase, suggesting acute pancreatitis. Over the first 12 hours of hospitalization, the patient developed respiratory distress and hypoxemia, requiring placement on mechanical ventilation. Height, 5′2″; weight, 165 lb (calculated body mass index [BMI], 30.2). Temperature was elevated at 103°F, with a blood pressure of 180/70 mm Hg, and a heart rate of 135. The patient's abdomen is obese, distended, and bowel sounds are hypoactive. She has voluntary guarding. Examination of her extremities reveal mild edema. Current medications include acetaminophen, a proton pump inhibitor, meperidine, and promethazine hydrochloride. Initial laboratories reveal an elevated WBC of 21,000, hemoglobin of 10.5, hematocrit of 32.8, blood urea nitrogen (BUN) of 55 mg/dL, creatinine of 2.5 mg/dL, serum potassium of 3.4 mmol/L, and sodium of 155 mmol/L. Her glucose is 186 mg/dL, albumin is 3.0 g/dL, and calcium is 7.8 mg/dL. The patient's serum lactate dehydrogenase was elevated at 400 IU/L. The patient underwent a CT scan, which revealed an enlarged edematous pancreas, necrosis involving 35% of the gland, surrounding inflammatory changes, and free fluid in the lesser sac. An abdominal ultrasound revealed a prominent common bile duct with possible choledocholithiasis. The patient's urinalysis was remarkable for increased specific gravity, but no evidence of infection. Blood cultures and urine cultures were obtained and were negative. The patient was admitted to the intensive care unit (ICU), and a central line was placed and started on intravenous volume resuscitation with normal saline.

Intervention: On day 2 of admission, the patient had a small bore orojejunal tube placed via fluoroscopy with the feeding ports distal to the LOT.

Answer: With a feeding tube placed well below the LOT, a standard polymeric feeding formula may be initiated. Hypocaloric protein-sparing feedings would be appropriate in a patient with a BMI of 30, and the use of a high-nitrogen 1 calorie per milligram formula would help to meet calorie-protein goals without excessive protein supplement administration. A reduced-electrolyte "renal" formulation should not be necessary unless clinically relevant hyperkalemia occurs on a standard formula due to the patient's renal compromise; protein should not be restricted. Considering the severity of the pancreatitis and extensive pancreatic necrosis, it is possible that the patient may require a semielemental or very low fat elemental formula to prevent steatorrhea. If the patient experiences distention or nausea, the decompression of endogenous gastric and/or biliary secretions with a nasogastric or orogastric tube may be necessary.

Rationale: This patient presents with classic, acute pancreatitis as evidenced by abdominal pain, elevated amylase and lipase, and an early SIRS response. The patient had three Ranson Criteria (WBC >16,000, lactate dehydrogenase >350, and serum calcium level <8.0 mg/dL) and the admission APACHE II score was 16, indicating severe pancreatitis. There was also >30% necrosis of the gland per the CT scan and evidence of multiple organ failure. The severe and complicated pancreatitis indicates that the patient has a 40% chance of having a complication, a 6% chance of mortality, and her chance of advancing successfully to an oral diet within 7 days was close to zero. This patient's clinical outcome could have a favorable impact by the placement of a jejunal tube and the initiation of EN. If endoscopic intervention is delayed due to critical illness, then the fluoroscopic placement of a feeding tube would be appropriate to initiate timely enteral nutrition.

Chronic Pancreatitis

Introduction

Chronic pancreatitis (CP) is an insidious and very debilitating disorder that comes at a very high cost—socially, financially, and to the individual experiencing it. The health care cost is difficult to quantify given the myriad of comorbidities (diabetes, alcoholic liver disease, smoking related diseases, etc.) associated with CP. The total estimated cost for all pancreatitis for nonfederal institutions and physicians was reported as $3.7 billion in 2004. The number of hospital admissions and ambulatory visits where pancreatitis was listed as the first diagnosis were 277,000 and 475,000, respectively. Pancreatitis ranked eighth in overall health care costs to society and seventh in hospital admissions and charges among all digestive disorders.[82] CP has a high mortality rate of approximately 50% within 20 to 25 years of onset[83]; pancreatic cancer looms at 3 to 5 times the expected incidence.[84] There is no consensus on the best treatment for CP; therefore, primary treatment is aimed at symptom control. Abdominal pain is one of the outstanding features of CP; hence, analgesia is frontline treatment. Pain management and problems arising from use of pain medications are often a component of the care of patients with CP. Newer therapies, however, such as the use of micronutrients and antioxidants, are emerging.[85]

Epidemiology

The reported yearly incidence of CP varies considerably and ranges from 3 to 8 new cases per 100,000. [85] There is a significant gender difference in those with CP, which is by far predominated by men and reported to be between 73% to 91%.[83] This is no surprise given the high proportion of men with alcoholism. In fact, 90% to 95% of alcohol-induced CP may be male, presenting in the 4th or 5th decade of life. The only country where this sex difference does not hold true is in the United States, where there is almost an even split between the sexes in hospital admissions for CP.[83] Overall, the data suggest that the incidence of CP is rising worldwide; it is surmised that rising alcohol use in addition to an improvement in diagnostic techniques are responsible. Smoking is associated with a fourfold increase in the risk of acute pancreatitis progressing to CP.[86]

Etiology

Although CP has many origins (Table 28-8), the clinical presentation of CP reveals a geographical variation, with alcohol being the most common etiology in the industrialized world, and tropical or idiopathic forms dominating the developing world. Although alcohol has long been touted as the leading cause of CP worldwide, less than 10% of those who drink in excess develop the disease process.[83] In the United States, chronic alcohol consumption was thought to be the leading cause of CP; however, a new hypothesis is emerging, the sentinel acute pancreatitis event (SAPE) hypothesis, which suggests acute pancreatitis, and especially recurrent bouts, are prerequisites for developing CP—an "end-stage" if you will, of recurrent AP.[87] A large, multicenter questionnaire was completed by physicians and patients to evaluate the combinations of risk factors, which together, defined an immune-medicated pathologic process or pathway.[87] Those who present with CP, presumably as a result of alcohol consumption, report an intake of ≥50 to 150 g/day over 6 to 12 years.[83,88] See Table 28-9 for grams of alcohol in commonly consumed libations.

TABLE 28-8 Causative Factors[88]

Toxic Xenobiotics
- Alcohol
- Cigarette smoke
- Occupational volatile hydrocarbons
- Drugs: valproate, phenacetin, thiazide, estrogen, azathioprine

Endogenous
- Hypercalcemia, hyperparathyroidism
- Hyperlipidemia, lipoprotein lipase deficiency
- Chronic renal failure

Infection or Infestation
- HIV, mumps virus, Coxsackie virus
- *Echinococcus, Cryptosporidium*

Genetic[a]
- *CFTR* mutation
- *PRSS1* mutation
- *SPINK1* mutation

Obstruction of Main Pancreatic Duct
- Cancer
- Posttraumatic scarring
- Postduct destruction in a severe attack
- Pancreatic divisum

Recurrent Acute Pancreatitis
- Postnecrotic
- Vascular diseases/ischemic
- Postirradiation

Autoimmune
- Isolated autoimmune chronic pancreatitis
- Syndromic autoimmune chronic pancreatitis (Sjögren syndrome, inflammatory bowel disease, and primary biliary cirrhosis-associated chronic pancreatitis)

Miscellaneous
- Gallstones
- Posttransplant
- Postirradiation
- Vascular disease
- ERCP-induced

Idiopathic
- Early or late onset
- Tropical

CFTR, cystic fibrosis transmembrane conductance regulator; PRSS1, protease serine cationic trypsinogen; SPINK1, serine protease inhibitor Kazal-type 1; ERCP, endoscopic retrograde cholangiopancreatography.
[a]Other, less common mutations have been described.
Adapted from *The Lancet*, 377, Braganza JM, Lee SH, McCloy RF, McMahon MJ, Chronic Pancreatitis, 1184–1197. Copyright 2011, with permission from Elsevier.

TABLE 28-9 Alcohol Content of Common Libations

Beverage	Alcohol (%)	g/100 mL (3.3 oz)
Beers (lager)	3.2–4	3.2–4
Ales	4.5	4.5
Porter	6	6
Stout	6–8	6–8
Malt Liquor	3.2–7	3.2–7
Sake	14–16	14–16
Table wines	7.1–14	7.1–14
Sparkling wines	8–14	8–14
Brandies	40–43	40–43
Whiskies	40–75	40–75
Vodkas	40–50	40–50
Gin	40–48.5	40–48.5
Rum	40–95	40–95
Tequila	45–50.5	–50.5

Hypertriglyceridemia

Hypertriglyceridemia, specifically a triglyceride (TG) level >1000 mg/dL, is associated with pancreatitis; recurrent bouts are reported if TG are not adequately controlled.[89,90] Patients at particular risk for hypertriglyceride-induced pancreatitis include those with type I, IV, or V hyperlipoproteinemia, diabetes mellitus (DM), ETOH abuse, obesity, and pregnancy. The age of onset also provides clues as to the etiology of CP. The median age of onset for alcoholic, idiopathic, familial, and tropical CP is reported as 40.8, 27.0, 18.8, and 9.8 years, respectively.[83]

Pathophysiology and Clinical Presentation

CP is a progressive, inflammatory process in which pancreatic tissue is slowly destroyed and replaced by fibrotic, calcified tissue. Traditionally, CP was considered distinctly different from acute pancreatitis, an event after which the pancreas fully recovers. CP, however, was thought to be a condition characterized by permanent and irreversible damage. Now it is thought that CP may be on a continuum where recurrent acute pancreatic injury is occurring (either overtly or subclinically), but may be subclinical with genetics and the environment playing a significant role.[87] As structural changes occur over time, functional alterations follow, primarily endocrine and exocrine.

The hallmark features of CP include abdominal pain (85% to 90% of cases); in some, episodes of acute pain and inflammation occur in a previously injured pancreas ("acute on chronic"). Pain can be intermittent, constant, or superimposed with acute flares. Some will have weight loss from an inability to eat, malabsorption, and poorly controlled diabetes, if present, and there are some who may be asymptomatic for years. Diagnosis relies on symptoms, radiographic evidence, CT scans, and elevated amylase and lipase (in those who have enough functioning pancreatic tissue left to synthesize and secrete it).[88] Complications of CP include bile duct stricture, duodenal stricture, portal hypertension, pseudocysts, pancreatic fistulas and ascites; mortality is nearly 50% within 20 to 25 years of the disease onset.[91]

Factors Promoting Protein/Calorie Malnutrition

Recurrent flares of CP invoke similar mechanisms for promoting the deterioration of nutritional status as seen in acute pancreatitis, with increased caloric and protein requirements, decreased oral intake, and greater nutrient losses.[92] However, multiple problems develop, specifically as a complication of CP and set the stage for progressive malnutrition (Table 28-10). Between bouts or flares of CP, persistent abdominal pain may generate anorexia, decreased intake due to fear of exacerbating symptoms, fat-restricted diets (either self-imposed or by health care professionals),[93,94] and weight loss.[95] Continued alcohol consumption is an independent risk factor itself in promoting malnutrition. Gastric dysmotility is common with up to 44% of patients having gastroparesis.[96] A large pseudocyst, diffuse inflammation, or scarring in the head of the gland can contribute to gastric outlet obstruction. Exocrine insufficiency occurs in about 50% of patients, developing 10 to 12 years after the onset of CP, and 90% or more of the exocrine pancreatic tissue is destroyed. It manifests clinically as diarrhea, steatorrhea, and malassimilation.[97] Steatorrhea is defined as the quantitative appearance of >7 g of fat per day after consuming or having infused 100 g of fat. Patients need to consume enough dietary fat before and during a fecal fat test to avoid false negative results (one must receive enteral fat in order to malabsorb it). It is important to note, however, that these patients may be on enough narcotic analgesia to prevent diarrhea,

TABLE 28-10 Factors Promoting Protein/Calorie Malnutrition in Patients with Chronic Pancreatitis[110]

- Recurrent flares/hospital admissions and NPO status
- Abdominal pain
- Increased caloric requirements, especially in those with low BMI, have higher lean body mass/fat ratio
- Anorexia
- Pancreatic insufficiency
- Alterations in bile salt efficacy due to decreased bicarbonate secretion in those not acid suppressed
- Motility changes from inflammation, duodenal compression, scarring
- Gastroparesis from hyperglycemia
- Continued alcohol misuse
- Small bowel bacterial overgrowth
- Self-imposed dietary restrictions caused by the fear of inducing pain
- Fat restricted diets

NPO, nothing by mouth; BMI, body mass index. Used with permission from the University of Virginia Health System Nutrition Support Traineeship Manual, July 2010.

and constipation may occur. Carbohydrate absorption is usually fairly well preserved. Due to decreased bicarbonate output from the pancreas with a resultant loss of gastric acid neutralization, the bile salts and what few pancreatic enzymes that are secreted become inactivated by gastric acid, which serves to worsen the maldigestion.[98] Small bowel bacterial overgrowth has been reported in 34% to 40% of patients with chronic pancreatitis.[99,100,101]

Maldigestion in itself increases the risk for vitamin and trace element deficiencies. Vitamin B12 deficiency is fairly common, because of the lack of production of the proteolytic enzyme secreted from the pancreas that is required to cleave the R-protein from intrinsic factor.[102] Patients with CP are at risk for the malabsorption of fat-soluble vitamins (A, D, E, and K), but isolated deficiencies are somewhat rare. The bone mineral density of patients with CP has been shown to be markedly decreased compared to controls.[103,104] In another study, low trauma fracture was found to be comparable with high-risk GI disease states that have osteoporosis screening guidelines in place.[105] Consider a dual-emission X-ray absorptiometry (DXA, previously DEXA) at the diagnosis of CP to identify those who might require more aggressive intervention to maximize bone health.

Persistent or intermittent hypermetabolism occurs in one-third of patients and may be a factor in continued weight loss. In one study, 65% of patients with CP who had weight loss showed an energy expenditure $>110\%$ of what was predicted by the Harris–Benedict equation, whereas only 20% of the CP patients with normal weight demonstrated such findings.[106] The increased energy expenditure may be related to continued ethanol ingestion or the persistent secretion of cytokines and catabolic hormones.

Diabetes mellitus is the major late sequelae of CP and is an independent risk factor for mortality in patients with CP. In a prospective study of 500 patients with CP, the cumulative rates of the appearance of diabetes mellitus since the onset of CP were 50% and 83% at 10 and 25 years, respectively; insulin requirement was 26% and 53% at 10 and 25 years, respectively.[107] These patients with CP behave as if they have "brittle" diabetes, with wildly fluctuating glucose levels and a propensity for hypoglycemia.[97,108] Diabetes alone may contribute further to underlying gastroparesis.

Several mechanisms may be involved in the persistent pain experienced by patients with CP.[109] Because of distorted ductal anatomy resulting from scar tissue, pancreatic stimulation may lead to elevated pancreatic ductal pressure. Increases in ductal pressure may, in turn, compromise blood flow to pancreatic parenchyma, producing ischemia and worsening abdominal pain. The obstruction of normal flow through the pancreatic duct may force enzymes into the parenchyma, resulting in autodigestion of the pancreatic tissue.[109]

Treatment

The causes of CP are diverse (Table 28-8), and as such, it is important that the underlying cause be identified to target interventions accordingly in an effort to reduce recurrent injury and delay or to stop further damage to the pancreas from occurring. In order to successfully maintain or replete the patient with CP, absolute abstinence from alcohol in those misusers, and sufficient pain control is necessary. In patients who are able to abstain from alcohol, symptoms tend to progress less rapidly, 75% of whom may expect to achieve symptomatic relief with the cessation of alcohol.[111] Pancreatic enzyme supplementation in high doses has been evaluated in an effort to provide pain relief in patients with CP. However, evidence to date has failed to show consistent benefit.[112]

Oxidative stress has been implicated in the pathophysiology of CP and is theorized to initiate cell damage in the following manner: either directly by cell membrane destruction, depleting the cells of antioxidants or by toxicity from free radical peroxidation products; or through altering signaling pathways, including redox regulation of genes. Morris-Stiff et al.[113] evaluated antioxidant profiles of patients with recurrent acute or chronic pancreatitis and found evidence of multiple antioxidant deficiencies. Zinc status in its relationship to chronic pancreatitis and oxidative stress has also received attention.[114,115] As a result of these and other findings, an emerging therapy in the treatment of pain (that might also arrest the development of chronic pancreatitis in high-risk groups) is the use of micronutrients/antioxidants.[85] The mechanism of pain relief by antioxidants is thought to be mediated through a reduction in oxidative stress and pancreatic inflammation. A recent study from India evaluating daily doses of 600 mcg organic selenium, 0.54 g ascorbic acid, 9000 IU beta-carotene, 270 IU alpha-tocopherol, and 2 g methionine concluded that antioxidant supplementation was effective in relieving abdominal pain in patients with CP.[116] This study has been criticized due to postrandomization dropouts, the high prevalence of tropical pancreatitis in the patient population studied, and hence the generalizability to other patient populations with CP.[117,118] Although some clinicians prescribe antioxidants in practice, larger studies to determine which antioxidants, dose, and length of therapy might be most efficacious, and if there are differences between the treatment effect and the underlying etiology of chronic pancreatitis.

Other interventions include counseling the individual in alcohol and smoking cessation, controlling hypertriglyceridemia by way of glycemic control, or lipid lowering agents as necessary; if hyperparathyroidism is present creating hypercalcemic-induced pancreatitis needs to be brought under control, and eradicating and preventing the further development of gallstones.[119] Control of pain should increase appetite and nutrient intake.

Nutritional Management

Oral Diet

In some patients, modifications of oral intake may reduce abdominal pain and reverse early changes of malnutrition. Although high fat diets are more likely to induce pancreatic enzyme secretion than high carbohydrate diets, there are no randomized trials that have investigated a low fat versus high fat diet in this patient population; in some, a low fat diet may further accelerate the calorie deficit that often plagues these patients. Still, some clinicians feel this is a worthwhile intervention to control pain, as long as overall nutritional status is monitored. Substituting medium-chain triglyceride (MCT) oil for long-chain fat has been shown to decrease cholecystokinin (CCK) levels and pancreatic stimulation in normal volunteers; it also improved persistent pain in patients with CP.[120] However, the study group was not tried on a standard enteral formulation for comparison. In a small study of patients with severe pancreatic insufficiency, Caliari et al.[121] found that MCT was absorbed better than long-chain triglycerides, but required pancreatic enzymes for optimal absorption. The authors concluded that no advantage is to be expected from replacing usual dietary fats with MCTs if pancreatic supplements are used.[121] In a recent study by Singh et al.,[94] dietary counseling was demonstrated to be as effective as the use of an oral liquid supplement.

Nutrition Support

For the 5% to 15% of patients with a more difficult, refractory disease course, more invasive nutritional therapy may be required. Unlike those with acute pancreatitis based on evidence to date, patients with CP may be tried on gastric feeding first; in those who do not tolerate gastric feedings, the provision of EN through jejunal access should be pursued. The jejunal placement of the feeding tube may be achieved by nasojejunal placement, the nasogastric–jejunal extension tube (NG-J),[122] the conversion of a percutaneous endoscopic gastrostomy (PEG) tube to a percutaneous endoscopic gastrojejunostomy (PEG/J) tube, or by the placement of a direct percutaneous jejunostomy tube (DPEJ). Endoscopic, radiological, and surgical techniques are described for such procedures in Chapter 12. In retrospective studies, the use of prolonged nasojejunal feedings resulted in fewer complications, a lesser need for surgical intervention, and fewer readmissions to the hospital than placement on an oral diet.[123,124] In one case series, long-term enteric feeding through a PEG/J or DPEJ tube over 6 months resulted in a significant reduction in the incidence of abdominal pain (96% to 24%), and in the number of patients requiring narcotic analgesia (91% to 28%).[78] In those with pancreatic insufficiency, pancreatic enzymes may be used with standard products; however, the microspheres make it difficult to administer, and the cost of doing so can increase the financial burden over the use of a semielemental or elemental product (Table 28-11). See Practice Scenario 28-2 for an example of a patient with chronic pancreatitis and malnutrition.

Practice Scenario 28-2

Question: Is this patient a candidate for nutrition support (EN or PN)?

Scenario: A 42-year-old male presented for his sixth admission this year to the hospital with an exacerbation of chronic abdominal pain. The pain was described as a penetrating, deep epigastric pain, radiating to the back, and made worse by eating. The patient had a history of chronic ethanol abuse, and admitted to an episode of binge drinking 1 week before admission. On a review of the systems, the patient complained of soft, runny, "greasy" stools with increased bloating. He reported extreme thirst, frequent urination, nausea, and anorexia since his abdominal pain had worsened. Physical examination revealed a thin Caucasian male appearing older than his stated age. Height was 5′8″ and weight was 128 lb (BMI 19.8), down from his original weight of 153 lb 1 year prior. Current laboratory tests for the patient revealed a normal leukocyte count, with a mild elevation in alkaline phosphatase, and a mildly elevated bilirubin. The patient had normal amylase and lipase, most likely due to his calcified pancreas and insufficient functional pancreatic tissue for synthesizing and secreting these enzymes. Repeat glucose levels were >250 mg/dL with a glycated hemoglobin (HbA1c) of 10; diabetes mellitus had not been clinically apparent in this patient until this admission.

Intervention: Jejunal feedings were initiated at a refeeding level early in the hospital admission.

Answer/Rationale: Because of frequent hospitalizations over the past year, his persistent weight loss in the setting of continued oral (gastric) intake, the low likelihood that a male alcoholic will get symptom relief from enzyme supplementation, and the severity of damage to the gland (as evidenced by endoscopic ultrasound (EUS) and endoscopic retrograde cholangiopancreatography (ERCP) findings and endocrine and exocrine insufficiency), the patient is a good candidate for jejunal EN.[127] If the patient is cooperative, a trial of nasojejunal feeding at home may provide the opportunity to determine a response to this management strategy. More permanent enteral access would be achieved by DPEJ or PEG/J placement. This procedure may be performed in the outpatient setting and should not be difficult in a thin patient with no previous abdominal scars, surgeries, or ascites. The successful placement of a DPEJ or PEG/J and the initiation of jejunal feeds would be expected to improve nutritional status, increase the likelihood for symptomatic relief, and reduce the frequency for subsequent hospitalizations in the future. This patient is at a significant risk for refeeding syndrome, accelerated in fact, as his hyperglycemia is brought under control.[128] He will need to be started at a refeeding level of calories between 15 to 20 kcal/kg while his glucose is carefully controlled. Electrolytes will need to be carefully monitored and replaced. Ultimately, this patient may need >35 kcal/kg/d to achieve weight gain with good glycemic control and adequate hydration. As current pancreatic enzyme preparations are not able to be used with jejunal feeding tubes without significant clogging potential, the patient will need a semielemental formula, and if unsuccessful due to persistent steatorrhea and failed clinical response, an elemental product.

Pancreatic Insufficiency

Pancreatic enzyme supplementation is a key factor in maximizing absorption in the patient with CP; however, it does not completely abolish steatorrhea.[126] Enzymes typically contain various concentrations of lipase, protease, and amylase. The dose of enzymes usually required to treat steatorrhea should contain the concentration of enzymes that approximates 10%

TABLE 28-11 MCT Containing and Very Low Fat Commercial Enteral Formulas[125]

Enteral Product	Kcal/mL	$ Cost /1500 kcal	Total g fat/ 1500 kcal	MCT/LCT %		MCT:LCT/ 1500 kcal (g)	
Optimental[a]	1.0	36.70	42	28	72	11.9	30.7
Peptamen[b]	1.0	42.48	59	70	30	41	17.5
Peptamen AF[b]	1.2	40.85	68.5	50	50	62.5	62.5
Peptamen 1.5[b]	1.5	36.67	55	70	30	39	16.8
Perative[a]	1.3	13.23	56	40	60	22.4	33.6
Portagen[c](powder)[e]	1.0	19.28	75	87	13	62.2	9.3
Vital HN[a] (powder)	1.0	36.50	16.5	48	52	7.2	7.8
Vital HN 1.5[a]	1.5	30.01	57.1	47	53	26.8	30.3
Vivonex TEN[b] (powder)	1.0	41.65	4.2	n/a	n/a	–	–

[a]Abbott Nutrition: 800-227-5767 or www.abbottnutrition.com
[b]Nestle Nutrition:800-422-2752 or www.nestle-nutrition.com/Public/Default.aspx
[c]Mead Johnson Nutrition: 800-222-9123 or www.meadjohnson.com
[e]Per Mead Johnson: "Portagen powder is not nutritionally complete. If used long term, supplementation of essential fatty acids and ultra-trace minerals should be considered."
Reproduced with permission. McCray, S, Parrish CR. Nutritional Management of Chyle Leaks: An Update. *Practical Gastroenterology.* 2011;XXXV(4):12.

of what the pancreas would normally produce and achieve maximum efficacy at a pH of 7 to 8. Such a dosage is usually accomplished by orally taking (30,000 IU of lipase) per meal.[93] Enteric-coated enzyme preparations resist degradation by gastric acid and are absorbed after passage into the small bowel.

TABLE 28-12 Factors That May Affect the Efficacy of Pancreatic Enzyme Replacement

- Compliance
- Dosing of enzymes (Table 28-13)
- Timing of enzymes
  - Enzymes should be taken with meals, and no more than 30 minutes prior to eating in order to have maximum effectiveness and ideally in smaller amounts throughout meal for best mixing.
  - Needs to be given with snacks also
- Acidic gastric environment
  - Decreased bicarbonate secretion and increased gastric acidity may reduce enzyme activity by delaying the release of enzyme in the proximal duodenum.
  - The enteric coating that protects the digestive enzyme is not dissolved until pH approaches 6.
  - If this does not occur early in the duodenum, it may be helpful to add adjunct therapies such as proton pump inhibitors, H2 blockers, or bicarbonate tablets, all of which help to raise the pH of gastric secretions higher in the duodenum, increasing the efficacy of enzymes.
- Slow gastric emptying
  - Consider prokinetic, if appropriate
- Exposure of enzymes to heat during storage
  - Enzymes stored in an exceptionally hot environment (such as in an automobile during the summer), may lose efficacy.

Used with permission from the University of Virginia Health System Nutrition Support Traineeship Manual, July 2010.

If uncoated enzymes were to be used, gastric acid suppression is typically necessary to prevent the inactivation of lipase. Currently, there are no uncoated preparations on the market in the United States. Enteric-coated enzymes were designed to avoid this problem; however, fat malabsorption often persists in CP due to an insufficient bicarbonate secretion needed to neutralize the gastric acidic entering the proximal small bowel unless acid suppression is used.[97] The lipase contained in these enteric-coated products requires a luminal pH of at least >5.0; bile acids will also become deactivated at an acidic pH adding to malabsorption.

TABLE 28-13 Methods Used to Dose Pancreatic Enzymes

- 500–2500 U lipase/kg/meal
- <10,000 U lipase/kg/day
- 1000–4000 U lipase/1 g dietary fat per day at meals and snacks
  - Assessing lipase units per gram of fat in the diet is useful in those situations where the per kilogram enzyme dose appears higher than recommendations, but the diet and symptoms suggest a need for increased lipase.
- Swallow beads without crushing or chewing to maintain the enteric coating
  - Fat malabsorption may persist in CP due to insufficient bicarbonate secretion needed to neutralize acidic stomach contents that enter the proximal small bowel. The lipase contained in enteric-coated products requires a luminal pH of at least >5.0; bile acids will also become deactivated at an acidic pH adding to malabsorption.
- Consider adding to enteral feeding or bolusing in set doses every few hours; also see www.ginutrition.virginia.edu under Resources for the Nutrition Support Clinician.

CP, chronic pancreatitis. Used with permission from the University of Virginia Health System Nutrition Support Traineeship Manual, July 2010.

Nonenteric preparations, if available, should be given with an acid-reducing agent, such as a proton pump inhibitor or an H2 blocker to avoid degradation by gastric acid.[97,129] Enzymes should be taken with meals and snacks, so that the enzymes are timed to be present when the food passes into the small bowel.[97] Poor tolerance of enzyme supplements may occur in some patients, as evidenced by nausea, bloating, cramping, constipation, and diarrhea. Failure to respond to initial enzyme therapy usually is related to noncompliance, inadequate dosing, insufficient acid suppression, or poor timing (Table 28-12). Changing to a different enzyme preparation, increasing the dose, or decreasing the fat in the diet may improve response. Restricting fat in the diet is required only if symptoms (especially weight maintenance, diarrhea, and steatorrhea) are poorly controlled on enzyme therapy or if pain persists on both enzyme supplementation and narcotic analgesia.

The U.S. Food and Drug Administration (FDA) recently determined that pancreatic enzyme supplements currently on the market varied in composition, enzyme activity, formulation, stability, and bioavailability differences leading to variable therapeutic performance. As a result, all preparations were required to undergo new drug applications to demonstrate efficacy by April 28, 2010, or be removed from the marketplace. Table 28-14 provides those pancreatic enzymes that obtained, or have pending FDA approval as of April 21, 2011. For more information see http://www.fda.gov/OHRMS/DOCKETS/98fr/04-9652.htm.

TABLE 28-14 FDA-Approved Pancreatic Enzyme Replacement Therapy[130]

Name	Amylase Units	Lipase Units	Protease Units	Contact
Creon 6000	30,000	6000	19,000	Abbott (Solvay) www.abbottgrowth-us.com (800) 241-1643
Creon 12,000	60,000	12,000	38,000	Abbott (Solvay) www.abbottgrowth-us.com (800) 241-1643
Creon 24,000	120,000	24,000	76,000	Abbott (Solvay) www.abbottgrowth-us.com (800) 241-1643
Pancreaze	n/a	1000	n/a	Ortho-McNeil www.mcneilpediatrics.net (800) 526-7736
Zenpep 5000	27,000	5000	17,000	Eurand www.zenpep.com (800) 716-6507
Zenpep 10,000	55,000	10,000	34,000	Eurand www.zenpep.com (800) 716-6507
Zenpep 15,000	82,000	15,000	51,000	Eurand www.zenpep.com (800) 716-6507
ZenPep 20,000	109,000	20,000	68,000	Eurand www.zenpep.com (800) 716-6507

Pancreatic Enzyme Products **PENDING** FDA approval[a]

- Ultrase Capsules
- Ultrase MT 12 Capsules
- Ultrase MT 18 Capsules
- Ultrase MT 20 Capsules
- Viokase 8 Tablet
- Viokase 16 Tablet

*Contact: Axcan www.axcan.com (800) 950-8085

[a]All are oral, delayed release capsules. Capsules cannot be chewed or crushed. Capsules can be opened and contents sprinkled: (www.epocrates.com) (www.rx-list.com)

Resource: www.fda.gov/Drugs/DrugSafety/PostmarketDrugSafetyInformationforPatientsandProviders/ucm204745.htm

Reproduced with permission. Quatrara B. FDA-approved pancreatic enzyme replacement therapy. *Practical Gastroenterology.* 2011;XXXV(5):19.

Acknowledgments

The authors of this chapter would like to thank Amy Tiu, MD, for her prior contributions.

References

1. Corcoy R, Ma Sanchez J, Domingo P, Net A. Nutrition in the patient with severe acute pancreatitis. *Nutrition.* 1998;4:269–275.
2. Varshney S, Johnson CD. Pancreas divisum. *Int J Pancreatol.* 1999; 25(2):135–141.
3. Bradley EL III. A clinically based classification system for acute pancreatitis. *Arch Surg.* 1993;128:586–590.
4. Bradley EL III. Acute pancreatitis: clinical classification and terminology. *Pract Gastroenterol.* 1996;20:8–24.
5. Soergel KH. Acute pancreatitis. In: Sleisenger MH, Fordtran JS, eds. *Gastrointestinal Disease - Pathophysiology, Diagnosis, Management.* Philadelphia, PA: Saunders; 1989:1814–1842.
6. Saluja AK, Steer MLP. Pathophysiology of pancreatitis. Role of cytokines and other mediators of inflammation. *Digestion.* 1999;60(suppl 1):27–33.
7. Norman JG. New approaches to acute pancreatitis: role of inflammatory mediators. *Digestion.* 1999;60(suppl 1):57–60.
8. Khan AS, Latif SU, Eloubeidi MA. Controversies in the etiologies of acute pancreatitis. *JOP.* 2010;11(6):545–552.
9. Tonsi AF, Bacchion M, Crippa S, Malleo G, Bassi C. Acute pancreatitis at the beginning of the 21st century: the state of the art. *World J Gastroenterol.* 2009;15(24):2945–2959.
10. Satoh K, Shimosegawa T, Masamune A, et al. Nationwide epidemiological survey of acute pancreatitis in Japan. *Pancreas.* 2011; 40(4):503–507.
11. Whitcomb DC. Clinical practice. Acute pancreatitis. *N Engl J Med.* 2006;354(20):2142–2150.
12. Holt S. Chronic pancreatitis. *South Med J.* 1993;86:201–207.
13. Banks PA. Pancreatitis for the endoscopist. ASGE Postgraduate Course; Digestive Disease Week; May 23–24, 1996; San Francisco, CA.
14. Larvin M, McMahon MJ. APACHE-II score for assessment and monitoring of acute pancreatitis. *Lancet.* 1989;2:201–205.
15. Corfield AP, Cooper MJ, Williamson RC, et al. Prediction of severity in acute pancreatitis: prospective comparison of three prognostic indices. *Lancet.* 1985;2:403–407.
16. Wilson C, Heath DI, Imrie CW. Prediction of outcome in acute pancreatitis: a comparative study of APACHE II, clinical assessment and multiple factor scoring systems. *Br J Surg.* 1990;77: 1260–1264.
17. Sax HC, Warner BW, Talamini MA, et al. Early total parenteral nutrition in acute pancreatitis: lack of beneficial effects. *Am J Surg.* 1987;153:117–124.
18. Bradley EL III. Operative vs. nonoperative therapy in necrotizing pancreatitis. *Digestion.* 1999;60(suppl 1):19–21.
19. Gardner TB, Vege SS, Chari ST, et al. Faster rate of initial fluid resuscitation in severe acute pancreatitis diminishes in-hospital mortality. *Pancreatology.* 2009;9(6):770–776.
20. Windsor AC, Kanwar S, Li AG, et al. Compared with parenteral nutrition, enteral feeding attenuates the acute phase response and improves disease severity in acute pancreatitis. *Gut.* 1998;42: 431–435.
21. Doig CJ, Sutherland LR, Sandham JD, et al. Increased intestinal permeability is associated with the development of multiple organ dysfunction syndrome in critically ill ICU patients. *Am J Respir Crit Care Med.* 1998;158:444–451.
22. McClave SA, Chang WK, Dhaliwal R, Heyland DK. Nutrition support in acute pancreatitis: a systematic review of the literature. *J Parenter Enteral Nutr.* 2006;30:143–156.
23. Swaroop VS, Chari ST, Clain JE. Severe acute pancreatitis. *JAMA.* 2004;291(23):2865–2868.
24. Levy P, Heresbach D, Pariente EA, et al. Frequency and risk factors of recurrent pain during refeeding in patients with acute pancreatitis: a multivariate multicentre prospective study of 116 patients. *Gut.* 1997;40: 262–266.
25. Andrén-Sandberg A, Dervenis C. Pancreatic pseudocysts in the 21st century. Part I: classification, pathophysiology, anatomic considerations and treatment. *JOP.* 2004 Jan;5(1):8–24.
26. Di Carlo V, Nespoli A, Chiesa R, et al. Hemodynamic and metabolic impairment in acute pancreatitis. *World J Surg.* 1981;5:329–339.
27. Shaw JH, Wolfe RR. Glucose, fatty acid, and urea kinetics in patients with severe pancreatitis. *Ann Surg.* 1986;204:665–672.
28. Dickerson RN, Vehe KL, Mullen JL, Feurer ID. Resting energy expenditure in patients with pancreatitis. *Crit Care Med.* 1991;19: 484–490.
29. Helton WS. Intravenous nutrition in patients with acute pancreatitis. In: Rombeau JL, ed. *Clinical Nutrition: Parenteral Nutrition.* Philadelphia, PA: Saunders; 1990:442–461.
30. Marulendra S, Kirby D. Nutrition support in pancreatitis. *Nutr Clin Pract.* 1995;10:45–53.
31. Havala T, Shronts E, Cerra F. Nutritional support in acute pancreatitis. *Gastroenterol Clin North Am.* 1989;18:525–542.
32. Kohn CL, Brozenec S, Foster PF. Nutritional support for the patient with pancreatobiliary disease. *Crit Care Nurs Clin North Am.* 1993;5:37–45.
33. Kovár J, Fejfarová V, Pelikánová T, Poledne R. Hyperglycemia downregulates total lipoprotein lipase activity in humans. *Physiol Res.* 2004;53:61–68.
34. Mesotten D, Swinnen JV, Vanderhoydonc F, Wouters PJ, Van den Berghe G. Contribution of circulating lipids to the improved outcome of critical illness by glycemic control with intensive insulin therapy. *J Clin Endocrinol Metab.* 2004;89:219–226.
35. DeWitt RC, Kudsk KA. The gut's role in metabolism, mucosal barrier function, and gut immunology. *Infect Dis Clin North Am.* 1999;13:465–481.
36. Kagnoff MF. Immunology of the intestinal tract. *Gastroenterology.* 1993;105:1275–1280.
37. Jabbar A, Chang WK, Dryden GW, McClave SA. Gut immunology and the differential response to feeding and starvation. *Nutr Clin Pract.* 2003;18:461–482.
38. Targan SR, Kagnoff MF, Brogan MD, Shanahan F. Immunologic mechanisms in intestinal diseases. *Ann Intern Med.* 1987;106: 853–870.
39. Dobbins WO. Gut immunophysiology: a gastroenterologist's view with emphasis on pathophysiology. *Am J Physiol.* 1982;242:G1–8.
40. Alverdy JC, Laughlin RS, Wu L. Influence of the critically ill state on host-pathogen interactions within the intestine: gut-derived sepsis redefined. *Crit Care Med.* 2003;31:598–607.
41. Oláh A, Belágyi T, Issekutz A, Gamal ME, Bengmark S. Randomized clinical trial of specific lactobacillus and fibre supplement to early enteral nutrition in patients with acute pancreatitis. *Br J Surg.* 2002;89(9):1103–1107.
42. Besselink MG, van Santvoort HC, Buskens E, et al. Probiotic prophylaxis in predicted severe acute pancreatitis: a randomised, double-blind, placebo-controlled trial. *Lancet.* 2008;371(9613):651–659.
43. Abou-Assi S, Craig K, O'Keefe SJ. Hypocaloric jejunal feeding is better than total parenteral nutrition in acute pancreatitis: results of a randomized comparative study. *Am J Gastroenterol.* 2002;97: 2255–2262.

44. Marik PE, Zaloga GPL. Meta-analysis of parenteral nutrition versus enteral nutrition in patients with acute pancreatitis. *BMJ.* 2004;328:1407–1412.
45. O'Keefe SJ, Broderick T, Turner M, et al. Nutrition in the management of necrotizing pancreatitis. *Clin Gastroenterol Hepatol.* 2003;1:315–321.
46. McClave SA, Greene LM, Snider HL, et al. Comparison of the safety of early enteral vs parenteral nutrition in mild acute pancreatitis. *J Parenter Enteral Nutr.* 1997;21:14–20.
47. Ammori BJ, Leeder PC, King RF, et al. Early increase in intestinal permeability in patients with severe acute pancreatitis: correlation with endotoxemia, organ failure, and mortality. *J Gastrointest Surg.* 1999;3:252–262.
48. Kalfarentzos F, Kehagias J, Mead N, et al. Enteral nutrition is superior to parenteral nutrition in severe acute pancreatitis: results of a randomized prospective trial. *Br J Surg.* 1997;84: 1665–1669.
49. Powell JJ, Murchison JT, Fearon KC, et al. Randomized controlled trial of the effect of early enteral nutrition on markers of the inflammatory response in predicted severe acute pancreatitis. *Br J Surg.* 2000;87:1375–1381.
50. Pupelis G, Austrums E, Jansone A, et al. Randomised trial of safety and efficacy of postoperative enteral feeding in patients with severe pancreatitis: preliminary report. *Eur J Surg.* 2000;166: 383–387.
51. Pupelis G, Selga G, Austrums E, Kaminski A. Jejunal feeding, even when instituted late, improves outcomes in patients with severe pancreatitis and peritonitis. *Nutrition.* 2001;17:91–94.
52. Xian-LI H, Qing-Jiu M, Jian-Guo L, et al. Effect of total parenteral nutrition (TPN) with and without glutamine dipeptide supplementation on outcome in severe acute pancreatitis (SAP). *Clin Nutri Suppl.* 2004;1:43–47.
53. Louie B, Noseworthy T, Hailey D, et al. Enteral or parenteral nutrition for severe pancreatitis: a health technology assessment. *J Parenter Enteral Nutr.* 2002;26:S32.
54. Gupta R, Patel K, Calder PC, et al. A randomised clinical trial to assess the effect of total enteral and total parenteral nutritional support on metabolic, inflammatory and oxidative markers in patients with predicted severe acute pancreatitis (APACHE II > or = 6). *Pancreatology.* 2003;3:406–413.
55. Petrov MS, Kukosh MV, Emelyanov NV. A randomized controlled trial of enteral versus parenteral feeding in patients with predicted severe acute pancreatitis shows a significant reduction in mortality and in infected pancreatic complications with total enteral nutrition. *Dig Surg.* 2006;23(5–6):336–345.
56. Doley RP, Yadav TD, Wig JD, et al.Enteral nutrition in severe acute pancreatitis. *JOP.* 2009 Mar 9;10(2):157–162.
57. Wu XM, Ji KQ, Wang HY, et al. Total enteral nutrition in prevention of pancreatic necrotic infection in severe acute pancreatitis. *Pancreas.* 2010 Mar;39(2):248–251.
58. Casas M, Mora J, Fort E, et al. Total enteral nutrition vs. total parenteral nutrition in patients with severe acute pancreatitis. *Rev Esp Enferm Dig.* 2007;99(5):264–269.
59. Eatock FC, Chong P, Menezes N, et al. A randomized study of early nasogastric versus nasojejunal feeding in severe acute pancreatitis. *Am J Gastroenterol.* 2005;100:432–439.
60. Kumar A, Singh N, Prakash S, Saraya A, Joshi YK. Early enteral nutrition in severe acute pancreatitis: a prospective randomized controlled trial comparing nasojejunal and nasogastric routes. *J Clin Gastroenterol.* 2006 May-Jun;40(5):431–434.
61. O'Keefe SJ. Jejunal feeding is the best approach to early enteral feeding in patients with acute pancreatitis. *AGA Perspectives.* 2006;2:5–19.
62. Ledeboer M, Masclee AA, Biemond I, Lamers CB. Effect of intragastric or intraduodenal administration of a polymeric diet on gallbladder motility, small-bowel transit time, and hormone release. *Am J Gastroenterol,* 1998;93:2089–2096.
63. Kaushik N, Pietraszewski M, Holst JJ, O'Keefe SJ. Enteral feeding without pancreatic stimulation. *Pancreas.* 2005;31:353–359.
64. Eckerwall GE, Axelsson JB, Andersson RG. Early nasogastric feeding in predicted severe acute pancreatitis: A clinical, randomized study. *Ann Surg.* 2006 Dec;244(6):959–965.
65. Gabriel SA, Ackermann RJ. Placement of nasoenteral feeding tubes using external magnetic guidance. *JPEN J Parenter Enteral Nutr.* 2004;28(2):119–122.
66. Holzinger U, Kitzberger R, Bojic A, et al. Comparison of a new unguided self-advancing jejunal tube with the endoscopic guided technique: a prospective, randomized study. *Intensive Care Med.* 2009;35(9):1614–1618.
67. Gray R, Tynan C, Reed L, et al. Bedside electromagnetic-guided feeding tube placement: an improvement over traditional placement technique? *Nutr Clin Pract.* 2007;22(4):436–444.
68. Modena JT, Cevasco LB, Basto CA, Vicuna AO, Ramirez MP. Total enteral nutrition as prophylactic therapy for pancreatic necrosis infection in severe acute pancreatitis. *Pancreatology.* 2006;6: 58–64.
69. Makola D, Krenitsky J, Parrish C, et al. Efficacy of enteral nutrition for the treatment of pancreatitis using standard enteral formula. *Am J Gastroenterol.* 2006;101(10):2347–2355.
70. Lin HC, Zhao XT, Wang L. Jejunal brake: inhibition of intestinal transit by fat in the proximal small intestine. *Dig Dis Sci.* 1996;41(2):326–329.
71. Van Citters GW, Lin HC. The ileal brake: a fifteen-year progress report. *Curr Gastroenterol Rep.* 1999;1(5):404–409.
72. Cravo M, Camilo ME, Marques A, Pinto Coneia J. Early tube feeding in acute pancreatitis: a prospective study. *Clin Nutr.* 1989; 8(suppl):14.
73. Schneider H, Boyle N, McCluckie A, Beal R, Atkinson S. Acute severe pancreatitis and multiple organ failure: total parenteral nutrition is still required in a proportion of patients. *Br J Surg.* 2000;87:362–373.
74. Stabile BE, Borzatta M, Stubbs RS, et al. Intravenous mixed amino acids and fats do not stimulate exocrine pancreatic secretion. *Am J Physiol.* 1984;246:G274–G280.
75. Burns GP, Stein TA. Pancreatic enzyme secretion during intravenous fat infusion. *J Parenter Enteral Nutr.* 1987;11:60–62.
76. Willcutts K, Krenitsky J, Banh L, et al. Is monitoring of serum triglycerides indicated in all parenterally fed patients? [abstract] *Nutr Clin Pract.* 2005;20:142–N055.
77. Ewald N, Hardt PD, Kloer HU. Severe hypertriglyceridemia and pancreatitis: presentation and management. *Curr Opin Lipidol.* 2009 Dec;20(6):497–504.
78. Giger U, Stanga Z, DeLegge MH. Management of chronic pancreatitis. *Nutr Clin Pract.* 2004;191:37–49.
79. Moraes JM, Felga GE, Chebli LA, et al. A full solid diet as the initial meal in mild acute pancreatitis is safe and results in a shorter length of hospitalization: results from a prospective, randomized, controlled, double-blind clinical trial. *J Clin Gastroenterol.* 2010;44(7):517–522.
80. Teich N, Aghdassi A, Fischer J, et al. Optimal timing of oral refeeding in mild acute pancreatitis: results of an open randomized multicenter trial. *Pancreas.* 2010;39(7):1088–1092.
81. Eckerwall GE, Tingstedt BB, Bergenzaun PE, Andersson RG. Immediate oral feeding in patients with mild acute pancreatitis is safe and may accelerate recovery—a randomized clinical study. *Clin Nutr.* 2007 Dec;26(6):758–763.

82. Everhart JE, Ruhl CE. Burden of digestive diseases in the United States Part III: Liver, biliary tract, and pancreas. *Gastroenterology.* 2009;136:1134–1144.
83. Jupp J, Fine D, Johnson CD. The epidemiology and socioeconomic impact of chronic pancreatitis. *Best Pract Res Clin Gastroenterol.* 2010;24(3):219–231.
84. Andersson R, Tingstedt B, Xia J. Pathogenesis of chronic pancreatitis: a comprehensive update and a look into the future. *Scand J Gastroenterol.* 2009;44(6):661–663.
85. Braganza JM, Dormandy TL. Micronutrient therapy for chronic pancreatitis: rationale and impact. *JOP.* 2010;11(2):99–112.
86. Lankisch PG, Breuer N, Bruns A, et al. Natural history of acute pancreatitis: a long-term population-based study. *Am J Gastroenterol.* 2009;104(11):2797–2805.
87. Whitcomb DC, Yadav D, Adam S, et al. Multicenter approach to recurrent acute and chronic pancreatitis in the United States: the North American Pancreatitis Study 2 (NAPS2). *Pancreatology.* 2008;8(4–5):520–531.
88. Braganza JM, Lee SH, McCloy RF, et al. Chronic pancreatitis. *Lancet.* 2011;377(9772):1184–1197.
89. Lloret Linares C, Pelletier AL, Czernichow S, et al. Acute pancreatitis in a cohort of 129 patients referred for severe hypertriglyceridemia. *Pancreas.* 2008;37(1):13–20.
90. Tsuang W, Navaneethan U, Ruiz L, et al. Hypertriglyceridemic pancreatitis: presentation and management. *Am J Gastroenterol.* 2009;104(4):984–991.
91. Barrett KE, Boitano S, Barman SM, Brooks HL. Overview of gastrointestinal function and regulation and digestion and absorption. In: Barrett KE, Barman SM, Boitano S, Brooks H, eds. *Review of Medical Physiology,* 23rd ed. New York: Lange Medical Books/ McGraw-Hill; 2010:467–478.
92. Duggan S, O'Sullivan MO, Feehan S, et al. Nutrition treatment of deficiency and malnutrition in chronic pancreatitis: a review. *Nutr Clin Pract.* 2010;25:362–370.
93. Domínguez-Muñoz JE. Pancreatic enzyme replacement therapy for pancreatic exocrine insufficiency: when is it indicated, what is the goal and how to do it? *Adv Med Sci.* 2011 Mar 30:1–5.
94. Singh S, Midha S, Singh N, Joshi YK, Garg PK. Dietary counseling versus dietary supplements for malnutrition in chronic pancreatitis: a randomized controlled trial. *Clin Gastroenterol Hepatol.* 2008;6(3):353–359.
95. Ammann RW, Muellhaupt B. The natural history of pain in alcoholic chronic pancreatitis. *Gastroenterology.* 1999;116: 1132–1140.
96. Chowdhury RS, Forsmark CE, Davis RH, et al. Prevalence of gastroparesis in patients with small duct chronic pancreatitis. *Pancreas.* 2003;26:235–238.
97. Krishnamurty DM, Rabiee A, Jagannath SB, Andersen DK. Delayed release pancrelipase for treatment of pancreatic exocrine insufficiency associated with chronic pancreatitis. *Ther Clin Risk Manag.* 2009;5(3):507–520.
98. Petersen JM, Forsmark CE. Chronic pancreatitis and maldigestion. *Semin Gastrointest Dis.* 2002;13:191–199.
99. Trespi E, Ferrieri A. Intestinal bacterial overgrowth during chronic pancreatitis. *Curr Med Res Opin.* 1999;15:47–52.
100. Lembcke B, Kraus B, Lankisch PG. Small intestinal function in chronic relapsing pancreatitis. *Hepatogastroenterology* 1985;32: 149–151.
101. Pezzilli R. Chronic pancreatitis: maldigestion, intestinal ecology and intestinal inflammation. *World J Gastroenterol.* 2009;15(14): 1673–1676.
102. Taubin HL, Spiro HM. Nutritional aspects of chronic pancreatitis. *Am J Clin Nutr.* 1973;26:367–373.
103. Mann ST, Stracke H, Lange U, et al. Alterations of bone mineral density and bone metabolism in patients with various grades of chronic pancreatitis. *Metabolism.* 2003;52:579–585.
104. Dujsikova H, Dite P, Tomandl J, Sevcikova A, Precechtelova M. Occurrence of metabolic osteopathy in patients with chronic pancreatitis. *Pancreatology.* 2008;8:583–586.
105. Tignor AS, Wu BU, Whitlock TL, et al. High prevalence of low-trauma fracture in chronic pancreatitis. *Am J Gastroenterol.* 2010;105:2680–2686.
106. Hebuterne X, Hastier P, Peroux JL, et al. Resting energy expenditure in patients with alcoholic chronic pancreatitis. *Dig Dis Sci.* 1996;41:533–539.
107. Malka D, Hammel P, Sauvanet A, et al. Risk factors for diabetes mellitus in chronic pancreatitis. *Gastroenterology.* 2000;119: 1324–1332.
108. Latifi R, McIntosh JK, Dudrick SJ. Nutritional management of acute and chronic pancreatitis. *Surg Clin North Am.* 1991;71:579–595.
109. Owyang C. Negative feedback control of exocrine pancreatic secretion: role of cholecystokinin and cholinergic pathway. *J Nutr.* 1994;124(8 suppl):1321S–1326S.
110. Parrish CR, Krenitsky J, McCray S. University of Virginia Health System Nutrition Support Traineeship Syllabus; University of Virginia Health System, Charlottesville, VA. Revised July 2010.
111. Trapnell JE. Chronic relapsing pancreatitis: a review of 64 cases. *Br J Surg.* 1979;66:471–475.
112. Brown A, Hughes M, Tenner S, et al. Does pancreatic enzyme supplementation reduce pain in patients with chronic pancreatitis: a meta-analysis. *Am J Gastroenterol* 1997;92: 2032–2035.
113. Morris-Stiff GJ, Bowrey DJ, Oleesky D, et al. The antioxidant profiles of patients with recurrent acute and chronic pancreatitis. *Am J Gastroenterol.* 1999;94(8):2135–2140.
114. Girish BN, Rajesh G, Vaidyanathan K, Balakrishnan V. Zinc status in chronic pancreatitis and its relationship with exocrine and endocrine insufficiency. *JOP.* 2009;10(6):651–656.
115. Girish BN, Rajesh G, Vaidyanathan K, Balakrishnan V. Assessment of oxidative status in chronic pancreatitis and its relation with zinc status. *Indian J Gastroenterol.*2011;30(2): 84–88.
116. Bhardwaj P, Garg PK, Maulik SK, et al. A randomized controlled trial of antioxidant supplementation for pain relief in patients with chronic pancreatitis. *Gastroenterology.* 2009;136(1): 149–159.
117. Romagnuolo J. Postrandomization dropouts and other issues threaten validity of trial results of antioxidants in chronic pancreatitis. *Gastroenterology.* 2009;137(1):391–392.
118. Forsmark CE. Antioxidants for chronic pancreatitis. *Curr Gastroenterol* Rep. 2009;11(2):91–92.
119. Lieb JG 2nd, Forsmark CE. Review article: pain and chronic pancreatitis. *Aliment Pharmacol Ther.* 2009;29(7):706–719.
120. Shea JC, Bishop MD, Parker EM, et al. An enteral therapy containing medium-chain triglycerides and hydrolyzed peptides reduces postprandial pain associated with chronic pancreatitis. *Pancreatology.* 2003;3:36–40.
121. Caliari S, Benini L, Sembenini C, Gregori B, Carnielli V, Vantini I. Medium-chain triglyceride absorption in patients with pancreatic insufficiency. *Scand J Gastroenterol.* 1996;31(1): 90–94.
122. O'Keefe SJ. A guide to enteral access procedures and enteral nutrition. *Nat Rev Gastroenterol Hepatol.* 2009 Apr;6(4):207–215.
123. Hamvas J, Schwab R, Pap A. Jejunal feeding in chronic pancreatitis with severe necrosis. *JOP.* 2001;2:112–116.

124. Gonzalez C, Silverman W. The impact of prolonged nasojejunal tube feeding in patients with refractory pancreatitis and abdominal pain: a five year retrospective review. *Gastroenterology*. 2003;124:A401.
125. McCray, S, Parrish CR. Nutritional management of chyle leaks: an update. *Practical Gastroenterol.* 2011;XXXV(4):12. Available at: www.ginutrition.virginia.edu.
126. Waljee AK, Dimagno MJ, Wu BU, et al. Systematic review: pancreatic enzyme treatment of malabsorption associated with chronic pancreatitis. *Aliment Pharmacol Ther.* 2009;29(3): 235–246.
127. Al-Omran M, Albalawi ZH, Tashkandi MF, et al. Enteral versus parenteral nutrition for acute pancreatitis. *Cochrane Database Syst Rev.* 2010 Jan 20;(1):CD002837.
128. McCray S, Walker S, Parrish CR. Much ado about refeeding. *Practical Gastroenterol.* 2004;XXVIII(12):26. Available at: www.GInutrition.virginia.edu
129. Graham DY. Pancreatic enzyme replacement: the effect of antacids or cimetidine. *Dig Dis Sci.* 1982;27(6):485–490.
130. Quatrara B. FDA-approved pancreatic enzyme replacement therapy. *Practical Gastroenterol.* 2011;XXXV(5):19. Available at: www.ginutrition.virginia.edu

29 Renal Disease

Robert Wolk, PharmD, and Charles J. Foulks, MD, FACP, FACN

CONTENTS

Background 492
Normal Renal Function 492
Acute Kidney Injury 493
Definition, Incidence, and Impact of Acute Kidney Injury 493
Metabolic Abnormalities Associated with Acute Kidney Injury 494
Chronic Kidney Disease 494
Definition, Incidence, and Impact of Chronic Kidney Disease 494
Metabolic Abnormalities Associated with Chronic Kidney Disease 495
Renal Replacement Therapy 495
Hemodialysis 496
Peritoneal Dialysis 496
Continuous Renal Replacement Therapies 496
Nutrition Assessment 497
Nutrition Requirements 499
Energy 499
Protein 501
Fluid and Sodium Requirements 502
Electrolytes and Minerals 502
Guidelines for Phosphorus Evaluation and Management 502
Guidelines for Calcium Evaluation and Management 503
Acid–Base Balance 503
Vitamins 503
Water-Soluble Vitamins 503
Fat-Soluble Vitamins 504
Trace Elements 504
Zinc 504
Trace Elements in Renal Replacement Therapy 504
Aluminum 504
Iron 504
Carnitine 505
Nutrition Therapy 505
Oral Diets 505
Enteral Nutrition 505
Parenteral Nutrition 506
Intradialytic Parenteral Nutrition 508
References 508

Objectives

1. Describe the anatomical features and physiological function of the kidney.
2. List the major causes of acute kidney injury (AKI) and chronic kidney disease (CKD).
3. Review the nutritional requirements of patients with CKD and discuss how these needs change once dialysis is initiated.
4. Construct a parenteral nutrition (PN) formula that considers the metabolic changes that occur in AKI.
5. Compare the calorie needs in AKI to those seen in CKD.

Test Your Knowledge Questions

1. Which of the following metabolic alterations is most commonly observed in AKI?
   A. Decreased energy expenditure
   B. Metabolic acidosis
   C. Decreased serum magnesium concentration
   D. Metabolic alkalosis
2. Which of the following parenteral amino acid preparations is most appropriate for a dialysis-dependent patient with renal failure (RF)?
   A. Essential amino acids only
   B. Nonessential amino acids only
   C. Mixtures of essential and nonessential amino acids
   D. High branched-chain amino acids (BCAAs)
3. Which of the following is a measurement of body iron stores?
   A. Total iron-binding capacity (TIBC)
   B. Ferritin
   C. Transferrin
   D. Ceruloplasmin
4. What percentage of instilled dextrose is typically absorbed from peritoneal dialysate with a 6-hour dwell time?
   A. 25%
   B. 50%
   C. 75%
   D. 100%

Test Your Knowledge Answers

1. The correct answer is **B**. In AKI, a metabolic acidosis develops from organic and inorganic acid accumulation. Serum potassium concentrations increase as obligate renal clearance is reduced.
2. The correct answer is **C**. Essential and nonessential amino acids are lost via dialysis solutions used for hemodialysis (HD) and peritoneal dialysis (PD). The ability to synthesize nonessential amino acids is reduced in patients with acute renal insufficiency. Therefore, a solution containing both essential and nonessential amino acids is preferred in this clinical setting. Enriched BCAA solutions have been studied in AKI and have not been shown to improve clinical outcome.
3. The correct answer is **B**. Ferritin is a serum protein that binds iron and serves as a reliable indicator of total iron stores. Low levels of this protein are typically seen with iron deficiency anemia, while high values occur with iron overload from an excessive intake of iron or the presence of hemochromatosis. Ferritin is an acute-phase protein and is also increased with acute inflammatory diseases of the liver. In CKD, ferritin should be > 100 ng/dL and the transferrin saturation should be $> 20\%$. The TIBC is a measure of serum iron and various proteins that transport iron within the circulation. A saturation index for these proteins is a measure of the available iron within the bloodstream. Transferrin is a circulating transport protein that carries iron that can be used in hematopoiesis. Ceruloplasmin is a serum transport protein that binds zinc and copper. It is not involved in the transport of iron.
4. The correct answer is **C**. In 6 hours, approximately 75% to 80% of the instilled dextrose of the dialysate solution is absorbed. This can provide a significant source of calories to the patient.

Background

The kidney is responsible for clearing nitrogenous waste and other metabolic byproducts and also regulates fluid, electrolyte, and acid–base balance; eliminates certain drugs; and synthesizes and metabolizes certain hormones. Because of these functions, the development of AKI or CKD can have a profound effect on the nutritional and metabolic status of patients. In AKI, an increase in protein and energy requirements parallels those seen in patients who experience trauma, serious infection, and other acute inflammatory illnesses. Patients with CKD may experience a series of metabolic changes that result in the development of protein–calorie malnutrition (PCM). The advent of renal replacement therapy (RRT) has vastly improved the management of AKI and CKD by improving survival in patients with AKI, enhancing the quality of life in patients with CKD, and by making it possible to provide adequate protein and energy to these patients. When provided in sufficient amounts, nutrition support can reverse PCM (in the absence of injury, inflammation, or the presence of cancer), reduce nutrition-related complications, and perhaps improve overall survival in patients with kidney disease. This chapter reviews the physiological changes that occur in patients with a decreased glomerular filtration rate (GFR), examines the impact of renal replacement therapies on these changes, and discusses the nutritional requirements of patients with RF and how to apply these principles to the provision of nutrition support.

Normal Renal Function

The major function of the kidney is to excrete most end products of metabolism, to regulate the body concentrations of electrolytes and minerals, and to regulate fluid and acid–base balance.[1,2] Other functions include gluconeogenesis, regulation of calcium–phosphorus balance, vitamin activation and metabolism, hormone synthesis and elimination, and drug metabolism and clearance.

The kidneys are two fist-sized organs located in the retroperitoneal space and are attached to the lower portion of the aorta and vena cava by the renal arteries and veins, respectively.[1] Each kidney is composed of approximately 1 million nephrons, the term used for the filtering, secreting, and reabsorbing part of the kidneys. The nephron can be divided into several functional segments that include the glomerulus through which blood is filtered; the proximal tubule through which various substances are actively or passively reabsorbed, secreted, or metabolized; the distal tubule and loop of Henle that are involved in the secretion of potassium and hydrogen ion, and the regulation of volume and water; and the medulla, where urine is concentrated (Figure 29-1).[3] The majority of fluid and solute reabsorption occurs by active transport in the proximal and distal tubule and by passive transport, which relies on the development of an osmotic gradient that varies along the length of the loop of Henle and collecting tubule. This entire process results in the formation of urine, an ultrafiltrate of plasma.

The nephron functions in conjunction with the liver to clear the plasma of metabolic end products including urea, creatinine, uric acid, and organic and inorganic acids. Electrolytes (sodium, potassium, chloride), minerals (calcium, phosphorus, magnesium), and micronutrients (zinc, selenium) are filtered through the glomeruli and may be reabsorbed or excreted, depending on the metabolic needs of the body.[1,2] Small nutrients that are filtered through the glomerulus, such as glucose, small proteins, amino acids, and vitamins, are reabsorbed by active transport in the proximal tubule.[1]

FIGURE 29-1 Functional Nephron

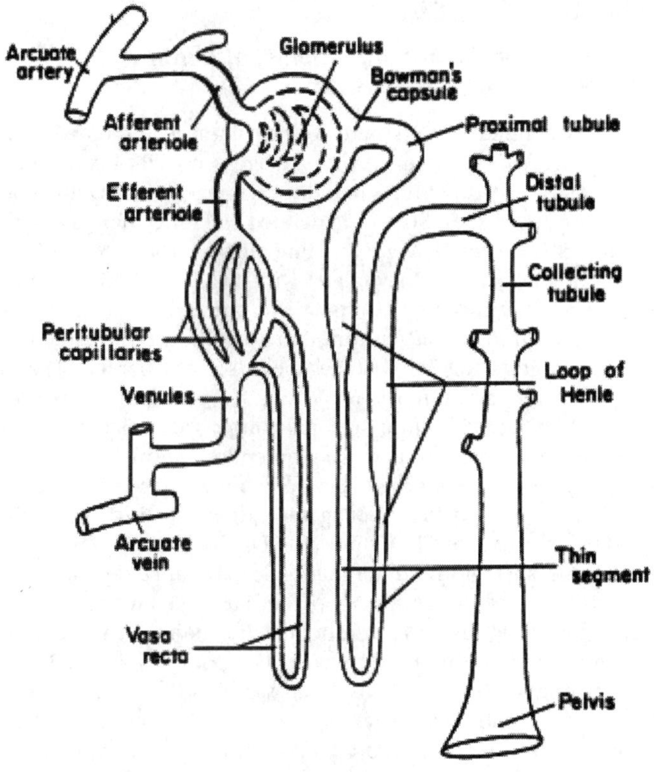

Reprinted with permission Guyton A, ed. *Basic Human Physiology*. Philadelphia, PA: Saunders; 1971:271–287.

Acute Kidney Injury

Definition, Incidence, and Impact of Acute Kidney Injury

AKI is defined as an abrupt decline in kidney function over at least 24 to 48 hours that leads to a reduction of both glomerular filtration and tubular function.[4,5] Clinically, the diagnosis is made by observing a rise in the serum creatinine (Cr) often in association with a decrease in urine output.[6] When severe enough to reduce renal function below 30% of normal, a number of complications may occur including hyperkalemia, hyperphosphatemia, glucose intolerance, fluid overload, acidosis, and azotemia.[4,6] The causes of AKI may be divided into three broad categories depending on the injury. Intrinsic RF occurs with a direct injury to the kidney such as with glomerulonephritis. Prerenal RF results when there is reduced renal blood flow that can be caused by any renal hemoperfusion such as volume depletion, congestive heart failure, shock, acute myocardial injury, nephrotic syndrome, or cirrhosis. Post-RF is caused by a blockage of the urinary drainage such as ureteral obstruction or prostatic hypertrophy.[7,8] A list of the most common etiologies of AKI is presented in Table 29-1.

TABLE 29-1 Causes of Acute Kidney Injury

Category and Disorder	Example
Prerenal	
Hypovolemia	Skin, gastrointestinal, or renal volume loss
	Hemorrhage
	Sequestration
Cardiovascular failure	Congestive heart failure
	Cardiac tamponade
	Capillary leak during sepsis or anaphylaxis
Renal/intrinsic	
Glomerulonephritis	Poststreptococcal, bacterial endocarditis
Acute tubular necrosis	Hemolysis
	Rhabdomyolysis
	Medications
Interstitial nephritis	Drug allergy
Arterial disorder	Hemolytic uremic syndrome
	Malignant hypertension
	Hypotension/shock
	Thrombotic thrombocytopenic purpura
Postrenal	
Ureteral obstruction	Nephrolithiasis
	Neoplasm
Venous occlusion	Renal vein thrombosis
	Neoplasm
Urethral obstruction	Prostatitis
	Foreign object
	Neoplasm

AKI occurs in approximately 0.37% to 5% of all hospitalized patients and is most often caused by a combination of events including sepsis, hypotension, and exposure to nephrotoxic drugs and therapeutic agents.[4,9,10] AKI is associated with a 30% to 80% mortality rate, and the cause of death is usually the result of multisystem organ failure or uncontrolled sepsis, and is generally not directly related to the RF per se.[1,2,4] AKI that occurs in patients in the intensive care unit (ICU) carries a higher mortality than AKI that occurs in patients who are not receiving care in an ICU.[11]

Metabolic Abnormalities Associated with Acute Kidney Injury

Patients with AKI occasionally are both hypermetabolic and hypercatabolic as a result of the neurohumoral responses associated with acute injury.[9] The metabolic complications that occur in AKI are listed in Table 29-2 and include the loss of glucose homeostasis, muscle wasting, protein catabolism, electrolyte imbalance, and the development of metabolic acidosis.[10,12]

TABLE 29-2 Metabolic Complications of Renal Failure

Glucose intolerance
Insulin resistance
Hyperglycemia
Lipid abnormalities
Hypercholesterolemia
Hypertriglyceridemia
Protein and amino acid abnormalities
Decreased protein and amino acid synthesis
Increased protein catabolism
Azotemia
Fluid and electrolyte
Volume expansion and contraction
Hypo- or hypernatremia
Hyper- or hypokalemia
Hyper- or hypophosphatemia
Hypocalcemia
Metabolic acidosis
Gastrointestinal
Anorexia
Nausea and vomiting
Altered taste acuity
Gastroenteritis
Peptic ulceration
Ascites
Endocrine
Renal osteodystrophy
Secondary hyperparathyroidism
Amenorrhea
Infertility
Other
Anemia
Vitamin deficiencies
Hypertension
Atherosclerosis

Muscle wasting may be more obvious in elderly patients due to their inherent scarcopenia.[13] Protein catabolism can result in an accumulation of several byproducts of protein metabolism including an elevated blood urea nitrogen (BUN), and is referred to as azotemia. Besides urea, Cr, aromatic and aliphatic amines, guanidines, and indoles are elevated in the blood of these patients compared to those with normal kidney function.[14] Tissue catabolism also releases intracellular electrolytes such as potassium, phosphorus, magnesium, and protein-bound acids such as sulfuric acid (from sulfur-containing methionine and cysteine) and hydrochloric acid (from the chloride salt amino acids).[14] This accumulation can lead to metabolic acidosis and electrolyte imbalance. Metabolic acidosis increases skeletal muscle release of BCAA that are preferentially used for gluconeogenesis, worsening protein catabolism.

Nutrition support plays an important role in the setting of AKI and may influence the patient's course and ultimately clinical outcome.[4,15–17] Some authors have suggested that nutrition support may promote renal functional recovery.[14,15,18] Sufficient nutrition may decrease the degree of protein catabolism and decrease the severity of negative nitrogen balance.[10,15,16] Although it might seem necessary to achieve a positive nitrogen balance to enhance survival in patients with AKI, achieving positive energy balance and neutral nitrogen balance seems to be more important. As with all forms of nutrition support, the success of this therapy depends on the ability to reverse or control the patient's underlying illness, and positive protein balance cannot be attained in patients with AKI or CKD until all acute inflammatory processes are controlled.

Chronic Kidney Disease

Definition, Incidence, and Impact of Chronic Kidney Disease

CKD is defined as persistent kidney damage for more than 3 months that is associated with a decreased GFR or confirmed by renal biopsy or markers of kidney damage.[19,20] CKD is classified into five stages. Stage 1 is defined as kidney damage with GFR > 90 mL/min/1.73 m^2 and that ranges through Stages 2, 3, and 4 to Stage 5 as kidney failure with a GFR of < 15 mL/min/1.73 m^2. CKD currently affects one in nine Americans or more than 20 million people with another 20 million at increased risk of developing CKD.[19,20] Diabetes mellitus (see Chapter 34) and hypertension account for 65% to 80% of all new cases of CKD.[2,10,20] The remaining 20% are comprised of patients with primary renal diseases such as a glomerulonephritis, adult polycystic kidney disease, progressive CKD from a preceding episode of AKI, and some patients with genitourinary obstruction. A limited list of causes of CKD is presented in Table 29-3.

Diminished glomerular function leads to altered renal fluid, electrolyte, and mineral metabolism. Metabolism or clearance of certain drugs and the production of certain hormones and vitamins may be reduced as well. If a patient has CKD, the remaining nephrons increase their workload in an attempt to maintain the highest level of renal function possible. This increase in single-nephron GFR results in intraglomerular hypertension, stretching of the mesangial supporting cells, and an increase in oxygen-free radicals and other inflammatory

TABLE 29-3 Causes of Chronic Kidney Disease

Diabetes mellitus
Hypertension
Intrinsic renal disease
  Glomerulonephritis
  Vasculitis
Urinary tract obstruction
  Malformation
  Tumors
Vascular disease
Hemolytic uremic syndrome

metabolic products. This causes progressive scarring of the remaining glomeruli.[21] Protein restriction is a mainstay in the therapeutic armamentarium in the management of CKD.[15,20,21] This is largely based on the concept that a low protein intake may preserve renal function by reducing intraglomerular pressure, solute load, mesangial stretch, toxic products of metabolism, and overall nephron activity. However, the only firm result of protein restriction in patients with CKD is to prevent or postpone the development of uremic symptoms.

Metabolic Abnormalities Associated with Chronic Kidney Disease

There are multiple contributors to the development of protein energy wasting (PEW) in CKD.[22–26] Cytokines such as tumor necrosis factor, interleukin-1, and other neuroendocrine factors are effectors (see Chapter 23). Abnormalities reported to occur with CKD include reduced protein synthesis and increased protein breakdown, glucose intolerance with a diabetic-like state, and abnormal lipid metabolism with hypertriglyceridemia.[23]

Many of the metabolic complications of CKD are similar to those seen with AKI (Table 29-2). These complications include impaired electrolyte clearance, abnormal acid–base status, and altered fluid status.[1] Calcium and phosphorus metabolism is altered as a result of decreased conversion of 25-hydroxy- to 1,25-dihydroxyvitamin D, a fall in proximal tubular phosphate clearance, and changes in parathyroid responses to serum calcium concentrations. Anemia is common and is in part due to decreased erythropoietin synthesis and a decrease in the erythrocyte life span. Patients treated with HD and PD are prone to the development of water-soluble vitamin deficiency, and those treated with HD are subject to iron deficiency as a result of chronic blood loss. Patients treated with PD also can develop iron deficiency secondary to the required blood loss associated with repetitive blood sampling (30 to 60 mL/month depending on the patient's underlying disease processes). Uremia can secondarily worsen PEW through the development of anorexia, food intolerance, nausea, and vomiting.[25,26] Inflammatory factors associated with chronic RF (CRF) and other comorbid conditions can worsen PEW.[25,26] These factors should be considered when developing a nutrition program for individuals with CKD.

Renal Replacement Therapy

There are three main types of RRT: HD, PD, and continuous RRT (CRRT).[1,2] The decision to perform RRT and the type of RRT depends on a number of factors including the patient's condition, the availability of RRT, vascular and peritoneal access, the serum levels of various electrolyte and metabolic waste products, and the characteristics of the RRT methodology. Nutritionally, 8% of patients with RF have cachexia, adding to the practitioner's challenge.[13] Dietary protein restriction and RRT have been used together to reduce azotemia and signs and symptoms of uremia in CKD.[21,24] Dietary protein restriction decreases the severity of uremic symptoms, can delay the onset of dialysis need, and preserves GFR.[20,23] The type of RRT selected can also have an impact on the nutritional status of the patient. The characteristics of the various forms of RRT are outlined in Table 29-4.

TABLE 29-4 Features of Various Renal Replacement Therapy Methods

	Typical Regimen		Typical Use		Clearance of Fluid and Solutes						
	Time (h)	Frequency	ARF	CRF	Fluid	Urea (ml/min)	E'lytes[a]	Pro	AA	Quantitative Pro + AA	Effect on Calorie Needs
HD	3–6	2–4/wk	Y	Y	> 1 L/h	100–250	++	+	++	10–13 g/d	Increase
Peritoneal Dialysis											
CAPD	24	daily	Y	Y	≤ 1 L/d	20	++	+	+++	5–24 g/d	Decrease
Continuous RRT											
CAVHF/CVVHF	24	daily	Y	N	≥ 20 L/d	5–15	+	++	+		V[b]
CAVHD/CVVHD	24	daily	Y	N	≥ 20 L/d	20	+	++	+		V[c]
SCUF	24	daily	Y	N	≥ 20 L/d	20	+	++	+		V[d]

AA, amino acids; ARF, acute renal failure; CAPD, continuous ambulatory peritoneal dialysis; CAVHD, continous arteriovenous hemodialysis; CAVHF, continuous arteriovenous hemofiltration; CRF, chronic renal failure; CCCHD; CVVHF; E'lytes, electrolytes; HD,hemodialysis; N, no; Pro, protein; RRT, renal replacement therapy; SCUF, slow continuous ultrafiltration; V, variable; Y, yes.
[a]Specifically potassium, magnesium, and phosphorus.
[b]Depends on dextrose use in replacement intravenous fluids.

Hemodialysis

HD is highly effective in treating uremia and other metabolic complications associated with AKI and CKD.[1,2] While this therapy can be provided in-center or at home (home hemodialysis), in-center HD accounts for 80% of all RRT used to manage patients with end-stage renal disease (ESRD). Dialysis is used in RF to maintain fluid and electrolyte balance, and to prevent the accumulation of nitrogen waste products. This form of dialysis can also remove a variety of medications that would otherwise be excreted by the kidney and thus prevents the accumulation and potentially toxic effects of these drugs. In HD, blood is removed from a venous catheter or arteriovenous fistula, and is pumped through a filter that contains a semipermeable membrane.[27] A dialysate solution is pumped through the filter on the other side of the membrane in the opposite direction. The dialysate is an isotonic sodium chloride solution with calcium, magnesium, potassium, bicarbonate, and dextrose. Modern dialysis machines allow hypertonic concentrations of sodium to be attained that can stabilize the blood pressure in some patients on HD who are prone to the development of hypotension across the HD procedure. The counter-current flow of dialysate to blood increases dialysis efficiency. Solutes such as urea, creatinine, and potassium are cleared by diffusion or convective transport and in general, molecular substances with a size < 5000 daltons can be efficiently removed with HD. Excess volume (the equivalent of isotonic saline) is removed by the application of a pressure gradient across the dialysis membrane. HD clears amino acids and small peptides from the blood with losses as high as 10 to 13 g per session.[28] HD also removes some water-soluble vitamins (such as vitamin C and pyridoxine), minerals, and electrolytes.

Magnesium is dialyzable and phosphorus can be removed as well. Calcium, potassium, sodium, and bicarbonate concentrations in the dialysate can be adjusted as needed based on the patient's condition. In ESRD, HD is typically administered 3 to 4 hours per day, 3 days per week to provide effective RRT.

Peritoneal Dialysis

PD is useful for the management of CKD.[29,30] Although this form of RRT is quite effective, only 15% of dialysis patients use PD because of access problems, difficulty complying with the prescription and thus achieving adequate clearance of solute, the potential for peritonitis, and hyperglycemia.[1] PD has the advantage of being relatively "low-tech," portable, and useful for home therapy.[1] The peritoneum acts as a semipermeable membrane where solute and water cross between the blood and peritoneal fluid. Elevated concentrations of urea and other solutes pass from the blood into the dialysate, which is initially free of urea. Potassium, urea, glucose, and other electrolytes pass between the peritoneal capillaries and the dialysate by diffusion based on the concentration gradient.[2] Hypokalemia (see Chapter 7) can occur on occasion because most commercially available solutions do not contain potassium. Potassium can be added to the dialysate, usually in amounts ranging from 3 to 5 mEq/L of solution to prevent or treat hypokalemia.

Water crosses from the blood to the dialysate as of the result of a glucose-mediated osmotic pressure gradient that is provided by using a dextrose-based dialysis solution. Commercially prepared dialysis solutions contain dextrose in concentrations of 1.5 to 4.25 g/dL or 1500 to 4250 mg/dL, which is considerably higher than the normal serum glucose of 60 to 110 mg/dL. As water moves from the blood into the peritoneal dialysate, solutes transfer to the peritoneal fluid based on their size and electrical charge. This transfer is termed convection or solvent drag, and is responsible for a large part of the clearance of small molecules from the uremic patient on PD. Although PD is not as efficient as HD per unit of time in removing solutes and water from the body, its application on a continuous basis allows it to be as effective as HD as a chronic therapy. Continuous ambulatory PD (CAPD) is the most commonly used form of PD.[29] Adult patients will typically instill (and drain) 2 to 3 L of dialysate four to five times each day with dwell times of 4 to 6 hours. Another form of PD is continuous cycling PD (CCPD) that uses a cycling machine that automatically fills and drains the patient's abdomen of dialysate usually over the nighttime while the patient sleeps. The machine is set up with the appropriate amount of peritoneal dialysate, and the patient connects to the dialysate circuit. The cycler warms the peritoneal fluid, measures and delivers the prescribed amount of dialysis fluid, controls the time that the dialysate dwells in the abdomen, and drains the abdomen of dialysate over a preselected time period. Although CCPD was originally prescribed as a procedure that drained the patient's abdomen at the end of the sleep cycle leaving no fluid during the daytime, many if not most CCPD patients will leave the last dwell in place during the day; some patients require a manual exchange of dialysate as if the patient were on CAPD.

PD can provide a significant glucose load to the patient via the dialysate. The amount absorbed depends on the volume infused, the dwell time, the dialysate dextrose concentration, and the condition of the patient's peritoneal membrane.[30] The energy derived from the dialysate dextrose must be considered when formulating a nutrition care plan. Protein and amino acid losses via PD can be significant and typically range from 5 to 24 g/d.[31] Protein losses can be higher if therapy is complicated by peritonitis. PD is effective in removing electrolytes, trace elements, and vitamins, and is inefficient at removing medications.

Patients receiving PD can remain ambulatory, provide their own care, and have reduced dietary restriction because their waste products are constantly filtered. Patients with heart disease experience fewer complications with PD compared to HD because fluid shifts are not as rapid as those that occur with HD. Common complaints include bloating, abdominal fullness, and loss of appetite from the indwelling dialysate.

Continuous Renal Replacement Therapies

CRRTs are ideal for patients who are unable to tolerate standard HD.[32,33] Although HD remains the most common form of dialysis during AKI, CRRT has become the preferred method of dialysis for patients with AKI in some centers. Slow low efficiency dialysis (SLED) or continuous veno-venous HD (CVVH) may be appropriate. SLED is a modified HD treatment that uses low blood flow rates, low dialysate flow rates, and an extended dialysis time of usually 8 to 24 hours. SLED is an emerging technique because it can achieve adequate solute and volume removal while causing less hemodynamic instability than conventional HD but does not require special equipment other than standard HD equipment.[1]

Continuous arteriovenous hemofiltration, CVVH, and continuous veno-venous hemodiafiltration are forms of CRRT that are currently utilized for the therapy of AKI in the United States. Of these, CVVH is the most commonly used procedure. The "VV" types of CRRT rely upon a blood pump to drive blood flow for the therapy and the "AV" CRRT uses the energy from the patient's own arterial pressure to drive the blood flow. All of these therapies require a specialized filtration or diafiltration membrane that is highly permeable to fluid, electrolytes, minerals, and certain drugs. Because of this, solutes can be removed by convection. This can require large volumes of intravenous fluid to maintain adequate circulating blood volume. The filters are expensive, and patients require continuous anticoagulation; clotting of the extracorporeal circuit is a frequent occurrence. However, trained ICU staff can maintain the procedure, and the provision of enteral and parenteral feeding solutions is made easier because volume overload and electrolyte imbalance can be corrected over the entire procedure without having to make changes common to those needed for the provision of HD such as highly concentrated feeding solutions, electrolyte imbalances, and worsening metabolic acidosis between HD treatments. The decision to use a particular continuous form of HD or HF, SLED, or HD relies upon the experience and comfort of the attending physician and nursing staff with a particular form of RRT.

The effectiveness of SLED and CRRT makes it possible to provide nutrition support without the need to restrict protein or fluid to a great degree.[34] Patients with AKI can have increased protein needs because of the associated inflammatory response to the RF or other comorbid conditions.[25,26] CRRT allows increased protein to be given to patients.[35] The amount of dialysis delivered to a patient should be designed to remove the metabolic wastes created from catabolism and nutrition support. The nutrition regimen should never be designed to decrease the need for dialysis.

Nitrogen amounts lost during CRRT are dependent on the method used. However, the differences in amounts lost between methods are not significant.[36] Protein requirements for adults on CRRT are at least 1 g/kg/d and may be as high as 2.5 g/kg/d because small peptide and amino acid losses can be high.[34,37,38] However, the losses with SLED are minimally increased over those losses from standard HD. In one study, patients with AKI treated with CRRT had serum levels of amino acids that were below their normal range until the protein intake reached 2.5 g/kg/d.[39] Fluid losses can be as high as 20 L per day; therefore, fluid replacement is important for fluid balance.[34,38] Serum electrolytes need to be measured frequently throughout the therapy period.

Energy needs for patients receiving CRRT can be calculated as 1.3 times above their resting energy requirement or as 30 to 35 kcal/kg.[25,34,38] Dextrose-containing dialysate solutions have been used for CRRT and may also represent a significant calorie source.[34] Because CRRT may require up to 20 L of replacement fluid, the choice of replacement fluid can be significant. The dextrose load should be calculated and converted to carbohydrate calories, and this calorie load in the replacement fluid should be subtracted from the dextrose provided in the PN solution, or the enteral nutrition (EN) rate (or formula) should be adjusted to maintain a stable dextrose intake. The amount of glucose transferred across the dialysis or filtration membrane can range from 35% to 45% or higher depending on the dextrose concentration, dialysate flow rate, and the blood glucose concentration.[34] As an example, a 1 L/h dialysate flow at a concentration of 1.5% and a 40% uptake provides about 500 cal/d, as illustrated in the following equation.[34]

$$\text{L/h} \times 24 \text{ hrs} = 24 \text{ hrs} \times 15 \text{ g/L dextrose } (1.5\%) = 360 \text{ g} \times 0.4 \ (40\%) = 144 \text{ g} \times 3.4 \text{ kcal/g} = 490 \text{ kcal/day from the dialysate}$$

Use of dextrose-containing dialysate with a physiological concentration of dextrose (0.1% to 0.15%) or no dextrose may provide a better strategy to reduce calorie intake and minimize problems with glucose control.[34] CAPD fluids may also be used as CRRT dialysate solutions.[34] Wooley and colleagues provide a good review of available solutions.[34] The calories provided from both the dialysate and replacement fluid should be reduced from the total carbohydrate calories provided in PN or from EN feedings. The EN rate reduction can drop the protein intake, and additional protein powder replacement may be needed.

Glucose losses may occur in the ultrafiltrate fluids removed by CRRT. Glucose losses into the dialysate are equivalent to the serum blood glucose concentration they are dialyzed against.[39] These losses should be calculated as the PN solution dextrose concentrations or EN formula rates may need to be increased to compensate for the loss of the dextrose in the dialysate.

Standard adult doses of potassium, phosphorus, magnesium, and minerals may be required in patients on CRRT because of the large losses in the dialysate.[38,40] Premixed dialysate and replacement fluids are available to meet the electrolyte and fluid needs but not the mineral needs. Standard vitamin and mineral (trace element) packages should be provided to patients receiving CRRT to meet the recommended daily intake and the losses in the dialysate.[17,38]

Nutrition Assessment

Nutrition assessment is necessary to determine the appropriateness of the nutrition support regimen and response to therapy.[14,16] This topic is discussed in Chapter 9 and is reviewed in Table 29-5. The cause(s) of AKI/CKD and any associated complications should be noted. Medications must be evaluated to make certain that nephrotoxic agents are reduced or discontinued, and that renally cleared medications are appropriately adjusted. Current weight, change in weight, body mass index, and serum visceral protein concentrations like albumin and transferrin, C-reactive protein, creatinine, subjective global assessment (SGA), normalized protein equivalent to nitrogen appearance, and diet history are all useful in combination to establish the severity of malnutrition.[25,26] The combination of these measurements provides an assessment of visceral and somatic protein pools, body weight and hence fat mass, and nutrient intake.[25,26]

Serum albumin is recommended for routine measurement because there is a large body of literature that defines the normal serum albumin values, characterizes the nutritional and clinical factors affecting serum albumin concentrations, and demonstrates the relationship between serum albumin concentrations and outcome.[25,26] However, its usefulness is only certain when properly interpreted. In acute illnesses, the serum albumin will fall precipitously and will not reflect the patient's nutritional status. In patients with CKD, a slow fall or rise in the serum albu-

TABLE 29-5 Nutrition Assessment and Monitoring in Renal Failure

Medical history	Physical examination
	General appearance
Dietary history	Blood pressure
Interview	Fluid status
Diet recall	Skin turgor
	Urine output
Anthropometrics	Intake and output
Current weight	
Usual weight	Signs of nutrient deficiency
Dry weight	Muscle wasting
Height	
Medications	Diminished fat stores
	Chilosis
Nitrogen Status	Glossitis
Albumin	Poor wound healing
Urinary nitrogen	Rash
Appearance (UNA)[a]	
	Laboratory measures
Renal function	Electrolytes
BUN	Sodium
Creatinine	Potassium
	Chloride
Creatinin clearance[a]	Bicarbonate
	Minerals
	Calcium
	Phosphorus
	Magnesium
	Glucose
	Triglycerides/cholesterol
	Complete blood count

BUN, blood urea nitrogen; UNA, urea nitrogen appearance.
[a]See text for equation.

min may usually be interpreted as the development of protein malnutrition or improving protein nutrition, respectively.[25,26] The serum albumin can only be considered as a true marker of visceral protein metabolism when there is no evidence of any disorder that causes inflammation or a change in albumin metabolism (cirrhosis or nephritic syndrome). The transferrin concentration is best used to evaluate the state of circulating iron available for hematopoiesis and cannot be reliably interpreted as a marker of nutritional status except when there is no evidence of inflammation or iron deficiency. The C-reactive protein is useful in defining the presence of an inflammatory process that would have an adverse effect on a person's nutritional status. A normal C-reactive protein has no relationship to a normal nutritional status. The serum creatinine (in the absence of rhabdomyolysis or muscle injury) is reflective of the patient's skeletal muscle mass and can suggest long-standing malnutrition. The patient's age and sex must be factored into the interpretation of the serum creatinine. Normalized protein equivalent to nitrogen appearance is of little help outside the research arena and has little clinical use.

Body weight is useful because of the clear association between body weight and body fat mass and because body weight is correlated with clinical outcome.[25,26] Whenever possible, the patient's dry weight (without edema or ascites) should be used because it best represents the metabolically active lean tissue of an individual. Overweight and obese patients may need to use an adjusted dry weight when calculating Cr clearance to determine medication adjustments.[25,26] Finally, fluid status should be monitored with daily weight and intake and output records because most patients will require some degree of fluid restriction. SGA is recommended because it gives a comprehensive overview of nutritional intake and body composition, including a rough assessment of both muscle mass and fat mass, and because it is correlated with mortality rates.[25,26] The SGA is also easily calculated and requires no special tools or measurements.

Assessment of nutrient intake is essential for assessing the probability that a patient will develop PEW, for evaluating the contribution of inadequate nutrient intake to existing PEW, and for developing strategies to improve protein-energy nutritional status. Also, nutrient intake is correlated with clinical outcome.[25,26] A dietary history should be obtained because anorexia is common, and avoidance of certain foods may identify patients at risk for specific micronutrient deficiencies.

It is recommended that patients with AKI and patients with Stage V CKD be assessed for an inflammatory response because it can lead to weight loss and a depressed appetite, and is linked to increased mortalilty.[16,17] Acute-phase reactant protein (cytokines, C-reactive protein) as markers of inflammation may be useful measures for assessment, but more information is needed.[16]

Renal function should be assessed by the Cr and Cr index (release of muscle Cr as a function of body weight). An adult woman (in the absence of muscle injury) releases 15 to 20 mg Cr/kg body weight per 24 hours, while a similar adult man will release 20 to 25 mg/kg body weight of Cr per 24 hours. Old and frail individuals may release less, and body builders or those with a markedly increased muscle mass may release more. BUN and serum Cr are readily measured and are easy to monitor during the course of therapy. A low serum Cr suggests a low dietary protein intake and/or diminished skeletal muscle mass, and is associated with increased mortality rates.[25]

The Modification Diet in Renal Disease (MDRD) study developed a GFR formula that has less variability and is more accurate than other equations.[1,20] The MDRD formula factors in serum Cr, age, gender, ethnicity, BUN, and albumin. Some data suggest that the MDRD formula be modified for increased precision. The Cockcroft–Gault is also a useful equation that factors in age, weight, height, and gender.[20,41] The National Kidney Foundation (NKF) Kidney Disease Outcome Quality Initiative (www.kidney.org) provides both formula calculators for use. The serum Cr must be stable and unchanging for the calculation of either equation to be clinically relevant as an unstable Cr makes the calculation unreliable. The value of the MDRD and Cockcroft-Gault formulas lies in the fact that one can predict what alterations in renal function can be predicted by the result of the formula. For instance, it is not necessary to know that the GFR is 28 mL/minute or 24 mL/minute. The importance is that the GFR $<$ 30 mL/minute and that hyperkalemia, hyperphosphatemia, volume overload, medication clearance and metabolism, impaired 1-alpha hydroxylation of 25-OH vitamin D, secondary hyperparathyroidism, and a decreased clearance of insulin can be expected. It would also signal that planning for HD or PD as well as renal transplantation should begin. In a patient with AKI, the daily increase of the serum Cr means that the GFR is impaired such that the daily production of Cr cannot be cleared and the patient should be treated as if the GFR < 10 mL/minute.

Urea nitrogen appearance (UNA) is a measure of net protein degradation in patients with RF. This determination is based on the fact that urea is the major nitrogenous product of protein metabolism. The UNA is used to determine nitrogen balance because urinary nitrogen is usually very low (in patients with AKI or those with advanced CKD), and therefore cannot give a reliable measure of nitrogen metabolism. The UNA can be calculated as follows:

$$\text{UNA (g/d)} = \text{UUN} + \text{BUN} = \text{SUN}_f - \text{SUN}_i \times 0.60 \times \text{BW}_i + (\text{BW}_f - \text{BW}_i) \times \text{SUN}_f$$

where UUN is urinary urea nitrogen, BUN is blood urea nitrogen, SUN is serum urea nitrogen, BW is body weight (kg), 0.60 is the estimated fraction of body weight that represents body water, i is initial, and f is final values. All nitrogen measures are in g/d. This measure can be adjusted to represent total nitrogen appearance (TNA) as follows:

$$\text{TNA (g/d)} = 1.19\ \text{UNA} + 1.27$$

TNA attempts to account for all nitrogen output including urinary, fecal, change in BUN, and hemodialytic losses. There are no data on the efficacy of TNA with CRRT. This value can be converted to protein equivalents by dividing the result by 6.25. This difference between protein intake and TNA is a good measure of nitrogen economy in patients with RF. To promote a positive nitrogen balance in patients with AKI, protein intake should be adjusted according to catabolic rate, renal function, and dialysis losses.[16] However, positive nitrogen balance in AKI patients cannot be attained until the active, inflammatory disease processes have been controlled.

In CKD with GFR < 30 mL/min, several mechanisms controlling acid–base balance are ineffective. Patients develop an inability to normally secrete H1 in the distal tubule because of distal tubular damage and a decreased renal production of ammonia. Most patients also have a proximal tubule disorder resulting in mild bicarbonate wasting. Untreated metabolic acidosis worsens secondary hyperparathyroidism and causes skeletal muscle release and wasting of BCAAs.

Anemia is common in RF because of the associated decrease in erythropoietin production. Iron deficiency may occur because of blood loss associated with HD. Folate deficiency is rare, but vitamin B_{12} deficiency may be more common than previously thought.

Nutrition Requirements

Providing adequate calories, protein, and electrolytes to meet the needs of patients with CKD can both minimize the metabolic complications associated with their RF but also retard the progression of renal disease.[10,20,23] Table 29-6 lists the nutrition requirements for adults. Nutrition support should be considered for all normally nourished patients with CKD in whom oral intake is not anticipated for 5 to 7 days.

Energy

Energy needs for patients with AKI and CRF are similar to those of nonuremic patients (see Chapter 3). Typically, there is no appreciable increase in energy needs with RF alone.[15] Rather, it is the physiological stress of associated medical conditions and surgical interventions that increase the energy needs of patients with AKI or CKD. For patients with AKI, it is recommended that they receive 25 to 35 kcal/kg or 1.3 times their resting energy expenditure (REE).[34,37] For significantly underweight or obese patients, the European Society for Clinical Nutrition and Metabolism recommends a energy intake of 20 to 30 kcal/kg for enteral feeding adjusted to individual needs while for patients with AKI and stable CKD, 30 to 35 kcal/kg for PN is recommended.[17] For patients receiving CRRT, Kopple[9] suggests 35 to 38 total kcal/kg/d, while Seidner and colleagues[10] recommend a range of 30 to 40 total kcal/kg/d for most patients with CKD. Conditions such as severe sepsis, respiratory failure, and other hypercatabolic conditions may increase calorie requirements to 1.5 to 2 times the REE or 30 to 45 total kcal/kg/d.[40] Energy needs, in summary, for patients with AKI and CKD are similar to those of nonuremic patients and must be adjusted based on the severity of their illness, comorbid conditions, and type of dialysis.[13,40]

Indirect calorimetry is recommended for determining energy needs in patients with RF.[16] It is a noninvasive means for measuring the oxygen consumed compared to the carbon dioxide expired and then calculating the patient's resting metabolic rate.[42] Because indirect calorimetry has limited availability and may be expensive, equations are commonly used to calculate energy needs.[42] For either AKI or CKD, energy requirements can also be calculated using the Harris-Benedict equation for REE and an appropriate stress factor.[37] An adjusted weight should be used for patients over 120% of their ideal body weight. Patients with CKD receiving HD or CAPD may have PCM and may need additional calories for weight gain if they are underweight. Calorie distribution and fluid needs must be considered when determining an appropriate PN regimen or choosing an enteral tube feeding formula. Energy requirements are usually met by providing a balanced formula that provides protein (10% to 15% total calories), carbohydrate (55% to 70% total calories), and fat (20% to 30% total calories). Excessive lipid calories should be avoided to minimize risk of hypertriglyceridemia caused by diminished clearance rates in CKD. Fluid restriction is often necessary when RF is associated with oliguria or anuria. When nutrition support is provided via tube feeding, concentrated enteral formulas, which provide 1.5 to 2.0 kcal/mL, are generally preferred.

Energy delivery from RRT must be considered when deciding amounts to provide via enteral and parenteral solutions. PD can provide a significant number of calories with amounts being as great as 500 to 1000 kcal/d.[43] Figure 29-2 illustrates several methods that can be used for estimating calorie uptake from PD.[34] CRRT can be an indirect source of calories for patients with

TABLE 29-6 Adult Renal Failure Nutrition Requirements[10,13,16,17,21,34,37,38,40,45,51,53]

	Predialysis	PD	HD/CRRT	PN[a]
Energy	ARF:Harris-Benedict: or 35–50 kcal/kg	Stress factor 1.5–2.0	Same as predialysis or PD	Same as predialysis or PD
	CRF:Harris-Benedict: or 35–38 kcal/kg	Stress factor 1.1–1.2		
Protein	0.6–0.8 g/kg[a]	1.2–1.3 g/kg[a] Up to 1.5–1.8 g/kg	1.2–1.3 g/kg (HD)[a] Up to 1.5–1.8 g/kg (HD) > 1 g/kg (CRRT) Up to 2.5 g/kg (CRRT)	0.6–0.8 g/kg[a] Up to 2.5 g/kg
Fluid	As tolerated	As tolerated	As tolerated (CRRT) Urine output[b] 500 mL (HD)	As tolerated
Electrolytes				
Sodium	As tolerated	As tolerated	As tolerated (CRRT) 2 g/d (HD)	35–75 mEq/L
Potassium	As tolerated	3–4 g/d	2–3 g/d (HD)	10–40 mEq/L
Minerals				
Calcium	1.0–1.5 g/d	< 2000 mg/d	< 2000 mg/d (HD)	4.8–9 mEq/L
Phosphate	≤ 10 mg/kg/d	≤ 17 mg/kg/d	≤ 17 mg/kg/d (HD)	3–15 mM/L
Phosphorus restricted to 800–1000 mg/day for elevations of serum phosphorus or plasma PTH: Stage 3 and 4: Serum phosphorus > 4.6 mg/dL Stage 5: Serum phosphorus > 5.5 mg/dL OR Stage 3: Plasma intact PTH > 70 pmol/L Stage 4: Plasma intact PTH > 110 pmol/L Stage 5: Plasma intact PTH > 300 pmol/L				
Magnesium	DRI[c]	DRI[c]	DRI[c]	2–12 mEq/L
Vitamins	DRI[c]	DRI[c]	DRI[c]	Standard additive
Vitamin supplements		DRI with dialysis	DRI with dialysis	DRI with dialysis
Vitamin C	——	75–100 mg/d	75–100 mg/d	——
Pyridoxine	——	5–10 mg/d	——	——
Folic Acid	——	1 mg/d	1 mg/d	——
DHCC	As needed	As needed	As needed	As needed
Trace elements	DRI	DRI	DRI	Standard additive
Supplements				
Iron	As needed[d]	As needed[d]	As needed[d]	As needed[d]
Other				
Carnitine	——	As needed[e]	As needed[e]	——

ARF, acute renal failure; CRRT, continuous renal replacement therapy; DHCC, dihydroxycholecalciferol; DRI, dietary reference intake; HD, hemodialysis; PD, peritoneal dialysis; PN, parenteral nutrition; PTH, parathyroid hormone.
[a]Initial needs, increased needs with dialysis/stress/hypercatabolic states.
[b]Standard needs, adjust based on serum levels.
[c]Initially, adjust based on serum levels.
[d]For anemia, follow iron/ferritin status.
[e]Losses occur, but a standard dose has not been established.

FIGURE 29-2 Glucose Absorption Estimates

1. **Dwell time data – Wideroe**

Dwell time (hr)	% Glucose absorbed from dialysate
1	29 ± 4
4	74 ± 4
8	86 ± 3

Need glucose concentration and volume to determine dialysate glucose administered.

2. **Diagram estimate – Mactier**

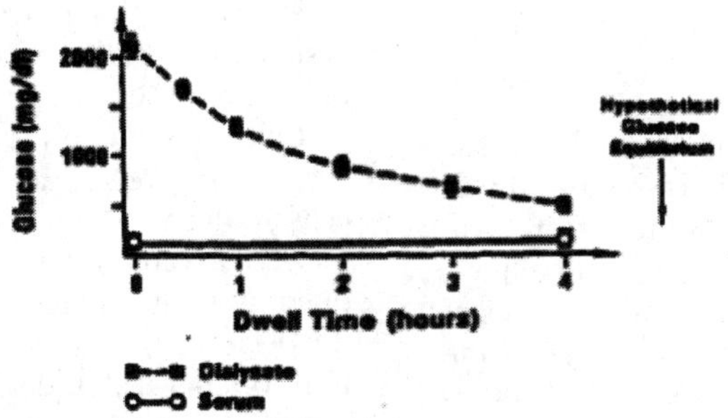

Intraperitoneal glucose concentrations (mean ± SEM) during four hour exchanges in 18 CAPD patients using 2L of 2.5% dextrose dialysis solution.

Percentage of glucose absorbed is based on identifying the dwell time and comparing glucose (mg/dL) level remaining to the starting glucose. The glucose lost represents glucose absorbed.

3. **Must reduce parenteral/enteral calorie intake by added dialysis calories to prevent overfeeding.**

Reprinted with permission from Macmillan Publishers Ltd: Wideroe TE, Sneby LC, Berg KJ, et al. Intraperitoneal insulin absorption during intermittent and continuous peritoneal dialysis. *Kidney International* 1983;23:22–28.

RF. Some CRRT solutions do contain a small amount of glucose, and a substantial glucose load can be delivered with replacement intravenous (IV) fluids (up to 20 L/d) given when fluid replacement is necessary. Hyperglycemia and inappropriate weight gain can occur if the glucose amount received during PD and CRRT is not considered. During HD, approximately 30 g of glucose is delivered during each HD dialysis session and usually is not considered when determining a nutrition support regimen.

Protein

Low-protein diets (0.6 to 0.8 g/kg) have traditionally been used in RF to reduce uremic symptoms, slow the progression of renal dysfunction, and obviate or delay the need for dialysis.[10,13,16,21] Although protein restriction can slow the progression of renal dysfunction in some subgroups of patients with CKD, there is no evidence that these diets provide any benefit in AKI. In fact, patients with AKI should be fed the amount of protein and calories needed by their overall condition. Very-low-protein diets, which only contain essential amino acids (EAAs) or a combination of EAA and keto-acids, have not been shown to provide any advantage over conventional protein restriction except in very small, limited studies of highly motivated patients and a single group of nephrologists. Patients with AKI and CRF and receiving dialysis need additional protein because of losses that occur through the dialysate.[10,21] Recommended protein requirements for patients receiving HD and PD are 1.2 to 1.3 g/kg.[10,16,21,37] The recommendations are outlined in Table 29-6. These are recommendations for well-nourished, stable, unstressed patients. Patients on CRRT should receive at least 1 g/kg/d of protein and may need as much as 2.5 g/kg/d.[16,34,37]

The use of amino acids designed for AKI has been controversial.[40] A preliminary study by Abel and colleagues in patients with AKI suggested that a parenteral solution of EAA and hypertonic dextrose could reduce the need for dialysis.[44] Lower serum concentrations of potassium and phosphorus in these patients suggested that protein synthesis was increased. A subsequent randomized controlled trial in hospitalized patients with AKI compared a similar formulation to hypertonic dextrose alone and found the EAA solution improved recovery of renal function, but not overall survival.[18] Following this study, Feinstein and colleagues compared a parenteral solution containing EAA to a mixture of EAA and nonessential amino acids and showed no difference in the rate or frequency of recovery from AKI or survival.[45] None of the patients was able to attain a positive nitrogen balance in this study, which provided up to 42 g of amino acids/d. A subsequent study with a mixture of EAA and amino acids that provided 82 g of amino acids/d was unable to demonstrate a positive nitrogen balance.[46] Others have shown no advantage of EAA over standard amino acids (SAAs) in AKI.[47] Formulations providing only EAA are not recommended.[40] Finally, BCAAs have demonstrated no advantage over SAA preparations in patients with AKI. Provision of these formulas for longer than 3 weeks and in larger amounts is not advised because serum essential and conditionally EAA imbalances may occur.[48,49] The nonprotein caloric intake may need to be as high as 150 to 250 kcal/g of nitrogen to promote protein anabolism. It is now recommended to provide standard mixed amino acid formulations for AKI patients.[16]

Fluid and Sodium Requirements

Fluid status must be closely monitored in all patients with RF. Urine, gastrointestinal (GI), and insensible losses should be considered when determining fluid requirements. Typical adults require 1200 to 2500 mL/d to maintain fluid balance. The need for fluid restriction often depends on the presence of oliguria or anuria. Patients who are anuric, defined as urine output of < 75 mL/d, are typically fluid restricted to 1000 to 1200 mL/d, which reflects usual insensible water losses/day.[2] Somewhat larger volumes of fluid may be tolerated in patients with oliguria, which is defined as urine output < 400 mL/d.[2] Concentrated EN or PN solutions are often required to meet these restrictions. Concentrated formulas may not be necessary in nonoliguric patients or those receiving RRT.[12,14] RF oliguria often leads to a decrease in urine sodium and potassium losses. In general, sodium or water should not be restricted in patients with nonoliguric AKI unless there is evidence of volume overload or hyponatremia. Patients with oliguric AKI will require sodium restriction once normovolemia has been attained. Water should be restricted only for patients with hyponatremia. Occasionally, fluid in excess of maintenance needs must be given to patients undergoing CRRT or during the diuretic phase of AKI. Fluid therapy adjustments should be determined by daily measurements of intake and output, weight, and serum sodium.

Electrolytes and Minerals

Patients with RF lose the ability to maintain normal serum concentrations of sodium, potassium, phosphate, and magnesium because of impaired excretion. Before nutrition support is instituted, tissue catabolism typically leads to elevated serum potassium, magnesium, and phosphate concentrations because the intracellular concentrations of these electrolytes are high. These electrolytes must be closely monitored during nutrition support and may need to be limited when providing enteral and parenteral solutions. If nutrition support occurs in the setting of protein anabolism, concentrations of these electrolytes may decline within the first few days of feeding (see Chapter 7). Electrolyte doses are predicated on the degree of anabolism and catabolism that must be considered when determining electrolyte requirements. In patients who are not severely malnourished or once feeding is stabilized in others, electrolyte requirements are generally low and dependent on renal and GI losses. Electrolytes (potassium, magnesium, calcium, phosphorus) should be adjusted based on the regular measurement of serum levels.[16]

RRT can be effective in clearing potassium, sodium, and magnesium. Certain dialyzer membranes will provide excellent phosphate clearance, but the effect is membrane dependent. Potassium can be added to both HD and PD solutions to maintain normal serum levels. With CRRT, electrolyte clearance may be high, and electrolyte supplementation may be necessary. Knowing the type of RRT used and the amount of fluid removed is useful in planning the solution volume, dextrose, and amino acid concentrations and additive amounts needed when formulating nutrient solutions. Table 29-6 lists the suggested ranges for electrolyte and mineral requirements at various stages of RF and types of RRT.

Calcium excretion is decreased in both AKI and CKD; however, blood levels are also affected by parathyroid hormone concentration and serum phosphate levels. Serum calcium does not increase because it becomes bound to phosphate, which is frequently elevated in RF. Serum calcium may decline slightly, but the decrease is great enough to result in increased parathyroid hormone levels. Under normal circumstances, an increase in serum parathyroid hormone levels leads to calcium release from bone, increased renal phosphate clearance, and increased conversion of 25-hydroxyvitamin D_3 to 1,25-dihydroxyvitamin D_3.[50] The active metabolite of vitamin D promotes calcium absorption from the gut. In CKD, renal phosphate clearance is suboptimal, and the activity of 1-a-hydroxylase is diminished. This leads to elevated serum phosphate concentrations and lower than expected levels of 1,25-dihydroxyvitamin D_3.

Derangements in mineral and bone metabolism common to CKD were found to be associated with increased morbidity and mortality. This prompted the development of *Clinical Practice Guidelines for Bone Metabolism and Disease in Chronic Kidney Disease* by the Kidney Disease Quality Outcomes Initiative.[51] The guidelines provide a framework for management of this complex problem. Recommendations are included for the evaluation of serum levels of phosphorus, calcium, and plasma; intact parathyroid hormone (PTH); management and/or treatment with vitamin D; phosphate binders; and dialysate bath. Serum levels of phosphorus, corrected calcium, and plasma PTH should be monitored with guideline recommendations implemented, where applicable, in patients with CKD requiring nutrition support.[17]

Guidelines for Phosphorus Evaluation and Management

The restriction of phosphorus to 800 to 1200 mg/d is based on either elevated serum phosphorus or plasma intact PTH levels. In Stage 3 and 4 CKD, phosphorus restriction is advised for patients with a serum phosphorus > 4.6 mg/dL and > 5.5 mg/dL for patients with Stage 5 CKD.[25,52] The phosphorus restriction is also advised for plasma intact PTH levels > 70 pg/mL for patients with Stage 3 CKD, > 110 pg/mL for patients with Stage 4 CKD, and > 300 pg/mL for patients with Stage 5 CKD. Further management of elevated serum phosphorus often includes calcium-, noncalcium-, or nonaluminum-based phosphate binders.[51,53] Calcium-based binders include calcium carbonate, calcium acetate, and calcium citrate. All of these agents are effective at reducing hyperphosphatemia while also being a good source of calcium for patients with CKD.[54] Calcium citrate should only be used in patients who are not taking or who are not exposed to aluminum salts including the use of aluminum cookware. Noncalcium, nonaluminum binders, such as magnesium carbonate and sevelamer, are also effective and are used in adults when there is a concern for soft-tissue calcification.[54]

Guidelines for Calcium Evaluation and Management

In CKD, the total amount of elemental calcium should not exceed 2500 mg/d, which includes both nutritional intake and medications (calcium-based binders). Hypercalcemia, as evidenced by a corrected calcium level > 10.2 for patients with Stage 5 CKD, may be treated by several measures, including decrease in total calcium provided (nutrition provision and medication adjustments), decrease or discontinuation of vitamin D preparations, and/or a decrease in calcium dialysate. Low calcium levels (< 8.4 mg/dL) should be corrected for those patients exhibiting clinical symptoms.[51,53]

Acid–Base Balance

Acidosis (see Chapter 7) occurs in RF because of loss of normal acid excretion or loss of bicarbonate.[12] Under normal circumstances, the body generates 1 mEq of acid per kg of body weight each day as a result of the metabolism of a normal diet. Inflammation with its associated catabolism coupled with an excessive dietary protein intake may lead to the development of a metabolic acidosis in patients with advanced CKD. This metabolic acidosis can lead to further protein breakdown, bone reabsorption, and a decrease in the responsiveness of adrenergic beta-receptors. Bicarbonate therapy is recommended for patients with CKD and patients with ESRD with a serum bicarbonate < 22 mEq/L or in acutely ill patients with a bicarbonate < 10 to 15 mEq/L.

Sodium bicarbonate can be given intravenously when the enteral route is not available. Bicarbonate forms an insoluble precipitate with calcium in PN solutions. Acetate is an acceptable salt to be used with PN solutions. A dialysate with a 40 mEq/L bicarbonate concentration is frequently used for HD. Oral citrate use in patients with CKD and ESRD is not recommended because it can markedly increase GI aluminum absorption and cause aluminum toxicity.[2]

Vitamins

Vitamin requirements are not well established for patients with AKI or CKD.[14] Generally, vitamins are supplemented in amounts that provide the dietary reference intake (DRI). Water-soluble vitamins are recommended for all dialysis patients.[37,40] On occasion, additional vitamins may be required depending on the patient's clinical condition and RRT use. Recommendations are outlined in Table 29-6.

Water-Soluble Vitamins

In the past, daily administration of water-soluble vitamins to patients with CKD was considered unnecessary because they are excreted by the kidney and were believed to be retained in CKD. However, it was soon learned that vitamin D and water-soluble vitamins are deficient in CKD. Although the exact requirements for water-soluble vitamins in RF are unknown, the DRI amounts for normal persons are recommended to be given daily to patients with CKD and ESRD. Water-soluble vitamins are not toxic, and there is an increase in clearance of these compounds with RRT. Requirements for these vitamins are met when adequate amounts of enteral tube feeding are given and with standard parenteral multiple vitamin preparations. A water-soluble vitamin supplement should be given to patients on renal-restricted diets. Additional vitamins may be needed in dialysis patients because of loss in the dialysate in combination with poor intake and altered metabolism. Vitamins A, D, and cyanocobalamin (B_{12}) are protein bound and are removed with HD.[55] Other water-soluble vitamins lost during HD include vitamin C, folic acid, thiamin (B_1), and pyridoxine (B_6).[56] CRRT vitamin requirements tend to mirror those needed in HD.

Vitamin C losses may be significant with suppression of white blood cell phagocytosis activity being observed in both HD and PD.[57,58] Amounts of 125 mg/d have been recommended for adults receiving RRT.[56,59] However, doses > 200 mg/d have led to elevated blood oxalate levels, which can result in deposition of oxalate in the heart, kidney, and blood vessels, and precipitate acute pseudogout.[40,59]

Some authors recommend folate supplementation because serum folate levels have been found to be low in patients with CKD receiving HD or CAPD, and the concentration of folate in HD and CAPD dialysis effluent has been found to be high. However, actual tissue levels may not be low because normal concentrations have been found in white and red blood cells.[60] Therefore, the need to supplement folic acid has remained controversial in renal disease. The elderly patient with AKI is at higher risk for folate deficiency.[13] If folate is measured, it should be measured as red blood cell folate, which is more representative of body stores.

Pyridoxine (B_6) has been studied extensively in HD. Normal levels have been reported in granulocytes and serum, but reduced enzyme activity suggests a functional deficiency.[55] Patients on CAPD have also been shown to have reduced enzyme activity. In addition, reduced pyridoxine (B_6) activity can lead to increased oxalate formation.[61] Pyridoxine supplementation of 5 mg/d or 50 mg three times a week has been advised in patients on CAPD, but this remains controversial. Elderly patients with AKI are at higher risk for a pyridoxine deficiency.[13]

Thiamin may be deficient in patients on HD; however, supplementation does not seem to improve enzyme activity in HD. Thiamin losses have been reported in CAPD.[62] Supplementation of riboflavin (B_2), biotin, niacin (B_3), and pantothenic acid does not seem necessary because these vitamins are not cleared by HD.[62] Similar data on these vitamins is not available for CAPD. Normal vitamin levels appear to be maintained in CAPD patients with AKI who received a standard water-soluble vitamin preparation and an appropriate diet.

Fat-Soluble Vitamins

Fat-soluble vitamin excesses or deficiencies should not pose a problem during AKI because of the short-term nature of this illness. Therefore, DRI guidelines should be followed for AKI. Standard enteral formulas and parenteral multiple vitamin preparations are adequate for most patients with AKI and CKD.[17] Vitamin K should be given in sufficient amounts each week as with any other patient on parenteral solutions.[8]

Patients with CKD often need 1,25-dihydroxyvitamin D_3, the most active metabolite of vitamin D metabolism, to maintain normal calcium homeostasis and prevent osteomalacia.[40,50] Active vitamin D therapy is used for the prevention or treatment of vitamin D insufficiency and vitamin D deficiency in CKD. Provision of vitamin D is integrated with serum calcium, phosphorus, and PTH levels. Indications for vitamin D therapy in CKD include serum levels of 25-dihydroxyvitamin D $<$ 30 ng/mL; indications for elevations in plasma intact PTH levels include $>$ 70 pg/mL for Stage 3 CKD, $>$ 110 pg/mL for Stage 4 CKD, and $>$ 300 pg/mL for Stage 5 CKD. Detailed discussion of bone disease management and algorithms for the integration of vitamin D dosing with corrected calcium levels, phosphorus levels, and plasma intact PTH levels are available within the Kidney Disease Quality Outcomes Initiative guideline document.[51]

Vitamin A status should be carefully monitored in patients with CKD, especially patients with ESRD on dialysis.[37] Supplements should not be provided if RRT is not used because excessive amounts can lead to toxicity.[37] If signs of hypervitaminosis A, such as visual disturbances, abnormal liver function tests, irritability, and fatigue occur, fat-soluble vitamins may need to be withheld.[13]

Trace Elements

Trace elements are reviewed in Chapter 8. Trace mineral requirements in RF are not well established.[14] Some trace elements (zinc, selenium, chromium, and iodine) are normally excreted by the kidneys.[63] Excess accumulation of trace elements is unlikely because losses also occur through the GI tract.[64] Commercially prepared enteral formulas and parenteral trace element solutions are generally well tolerated because they provide normal amounts of these substances. Because trace elements are protein-bound, one would imagine that supplementation would be required in RRT; however, this does not seem to be the case.[65] Of interest is recent application of inductively coupled plasma-mass spectrometry techniques in evaluations of Cu, Se, Zn, Mn, and Ni in a large group of patients on HD and age-matched controls. Patients on HD were found to have significantly lower concentrations of Se, Zn, and Mn and significantly higher Ni when compared to controls. Further research work employing these techniques may give insight on trace element imbalances and clinical monitoring needs.

Zinc

Low serum zinc levels have been demonstrated in patients receiving PD.[64] Low zinc levels are most likely the result of compartmental shifts from plasma to the intracellular space. Although patients with symptomatic zinc deficiency have reported improved taste acuity and improved appetite following supplementation, more information is required before routine zinc supplementation can be recommended prophylactically for all patients on PD.[13]

Trace Elements in Renal Replacement Therapy

Aluminum

Aluminum toxicity can occur in patients with Stage 4 and Stage 5 CKD with or without RRT.[13,51] Aluminum excess can lead to osteodystrophy, anemia, and encephalopathy. The best method for management of aluminum excess is to restrict its intake. The frequency of toxicity is lower now that dialysate solutions are commercially prepared with water devoid of aluminum, and PN solutions do not contain protein hydrolysates. Furthermore, aluminum-based phosphate binders have been replaced with calcium and noncalcium-based binders. One potential venue for aluminum accumulation is the use of PN vitamin preparations. Prudence in product selection and proper plasma monitoring of aluminum levels may be warranted. Awareness of diagnostic procedures to identify syndromes of aluminum toxicity is necessary. Detail of the features, causes, and considerations of therapy for aluminum toxicity may be found in the *Clinical Practice Guidelines for Bone Metabolism and Disease in Chronic Kidney Disease*.[51]

Iron

Many patients with CKD and ESRD have iron deficiency anemia because of decreased red blood cell survival, GI blood loss from angiodysplasia, bone marrow toxicity caused by elevated serum PTH levels, diminished oral intake, and losses through repeated laboratory testing of blood (may range from 30 to 90 mL/month). Iron status should be assessed by measuring serum iron, TIBC, iron saturation, and ferritin.[66,67] Ferritin levels must be interpreted with caution because many patients have chronic low-grade inflammation, which can cause falsely elevated values.[67,68] Serum transferrin is less reliable in patients with CKD because of metabolic abnormalities such as malnutrition and altered protein metabolism seen in RF.[69] DRI amounts of iron should be provided to patients with mild CRF. In ESRD, iron dosing should be sufficient to maintain adequate ferritin and iron saturation.[68,69] Iron is also necessary to ensure the effectiveness of erythropoietin (EPO), a hormone given to patients with CRF to improve red cell production and reduce anemia.[67,68] Iron supplementation is recommended if serum ferritin levels are $<$ 100 ng/dL. The goal of therapy is a serum ferritin level $>$ 100 ng/dL and a transferrin saturation $>$ 20%.[70] EPO will be ineffective with a serum ferritin level $<$ 100 ng/dL and a transferrin saturation $<$ 20%. Iron should be held if serum ferritin levels exceed 500 to 800 ng/dL.[67,69,70] Excess iron can exacerbate sepsis by potentiating the growth of certain bacteria and inhibiting neutrophil phagocytic activity. The goal of iron therapy in adults is to maintain the serum hemoglobin at 10 to 11 g/dL or hematocrit at 30% to 33%.[69,70] Iron supplementation frequently is not necessary for patients with AKI or for those receiving CRRT because they often receive blood transfusions during the critical phase of their illness.

HD may significantly affect iron status because of the blood loss in the dialyzer circuit and catheter, anticoagulant-related blood loss, and increased fragility of the red blood cells.[69,71] Patients with ESRD receiving PD may also require supplemental iron, although it does not seem to be lost in the PD dialysate.[67,69] Oral iron is generally preferred if tolerated because of the potential complications associated with intravenous iron. Iron sulfate and other iron salts are available as tablets or as a liquid for oral/enteral therapy. However, these patients frequently receive calcium salts, phosphate binders, proton pump inhibitors, and other medications that might impair iron absorption. If EPO is being used, oral iron usually cannot replete and maintain the body's iron stores of patients with CKD and on hemodialysis.[70,71] Iron dextran is given parenterally and may be used if oral therapy is not successful.[69] Intravenous iron dextran has the potential for inciting an anaphylactic reaction, and thus a test dose must always be given before regular dosing begins.[69] Newer forms of intravenous iron, such as iron sucrose and sodium ferric gluconate complex, are associated with less risk of life-threatening adverse reactions such as hypotension and anaphylaxis. However, multiple investigations report conflicting results. Chertow retrospectively reviewed 1981 adverse drug events reported to the U.S. Food and Drug Administration.[71] This study concluded that parenteral iron-related adverse drug events are rare (< 0.01%) overall. The adverse drug event rate was highest in the ferric gluconate (Ferrlecit™) and high-molecular-weight dextran formulation group as compared to low-molecular-weight iron dextran group such as InFed™. Injectable iron can be given during HD three times a week, intravenously or intramuscularly, at varying intervals.[67] Iron may need to be withheld when sepsis is suspected or documented because of its potential detrimental effect on the control of infection.[64,69]

Carnitine

Serum carnitine levels may be reduced in dialysis because carnitine seems to be lost in HD and PD.[40,72] Carnitine deficiency can lead to intradialytic hypotension, cardiomyopathy, skeletal muscle weakness, and anemia.[73] The mechanism by which carnitine deficiency contributes to anemia or hyporesponsiveness to EPO is unknown. Patients with CKD and on hemodialysis have shown improved exercise tolerance and well-being with carnitine supplementation.[74] Only intravenous carnitine is recommended for use for anemia treatment in patients with CKD and on HD.[73] Oral carnitine is not recommended for EPO-treated patients with CKD and on HD because of its limited bioavailability and lack of demonstrated efficacy.[71,75] The NKF recommends carnitine supplementation only in patients on HD who are unable to maintain a target hemoglobin of 11 to 12 g/dL or hematocrit of 33% to 36%, and who receive > 300 units per week of EPO and have adequate iron stores with no other known cause of anemia.[75] This recommendation has not been changed since hemoglobin targets for EPO therapy have been changed to 10 to 11 g/dL. The NKF recommendations would dose the carnitine at 20 mg/kg IV after each dialysis.

Nutrition Therapy

Oral Diets

A typical diet for a patient with RF generally restricts protein and phosphorus and sometimes sodium and potassium.[20] Restricted intake of meat, dairy, and egg products reduces protein, acid, and phosphorus intake. Phosphorus in adult oral diets should be restricted to 800 to 1200 mg/d. Potassium restriction includes limiting fruits and fruit juices, which are concentrated sources of potassium. Fluid restriction should be based on weight changes, fluid status, and urine output. Patients with a Cr clearance < 25 mL/min may benefit slightly from very-low-protein diets (0.28 g/kg/d), but this diet is difficult to follow and requires close monitoring for nutritional safety. In patients with a Cr clearance < 10 mL/min, a very-low-protein diet, as compared with a low-protein diet, did not significantly slow the progression of RF, but uremic symptoms were ameliorated.[76] Initially, in patients with CKD, protein intake is limited to 0.6 to 0.8 g/kg/d.[20] Intense nutrition intervention early in CKD reduces the risk of diabetes, hypertension, anemia, and dyslipidemias, and may delay the progression of renal dysfunction in some patients.[20]

Enteral Nutrition

Guidelines for nutritional support of patients with CKD receiving dialysis recommend a diet rich in protein (1.0 to 1.2 g/kg body weight/d) and low in phosphate (< 1200 to 1500 mg/d).[23] Diets high in energy and protein and standard enteral formulas tend to deliver a substantial amount of fluid, electrolytes, and phosphorus. Disease-specific formulas for enteral feeding including oral supplementation in patients with CKD were developed with a 2 kcal/mL energy provision and lower potassium, phosphorus, and sodium concentrations. A meta-analysis of 18 studies with a total of 541 patients was conducted to determine the potential benefits of EN in patients with CKD on dialysis.[23] Nutritional measures such as albumin, prealbumin, dietary intake, electrolyte status, and quality of life were evaluated. The use of supplemental oral intake did not affect electrolyte status. The study was unable to demonstrate an improvement in quality of life or clinical outcomes. Although the study group was too small to distinguish a difference between feeding with a disease-specific formula and a standard formula, an increased serum albumin and total dietary intake with the use of supplements was demonstrated.[23]

Disease-specific enteral formulas designed for patients with CKD and not on dialysis are usually not necessary for patients with CRRT. This is because the large volume of fluid and electrolytes removed by CRRT reduces the need for fluid restriction and increases the need for increased electrolyte supplementation. Because of the hypercatabolism seen with AKI, standard formulas may be a better option unless the patient is fluid restricted. Immune-enhancing formulas have been suggested for patients with AKI on CRRT but, because of the lack of controlled data, they are not recommended.[34] Patients who are receiving HD, PD, or CRRTs should not have their protein, energy, or fluid intake restricted, and these should be managed by increasing the amount of dialytic or filtration therapy delivered to the patient (Practice Scenario 29-1).

Practice Scenario 29-1

Question: What is the best approach to nutrition support in a hospitalized malnourished patient on HD?

Scenario: MR is a 66-year-old woman who has been admitted with a diagnosis of a left lower lobe pneumonia and acute respiratory failure with hypoxemia. She has been on HD for 6 years. Over the last 9 months, she has had multiple episodes of vascular access stenosis and clotting. This has resulted in the placement of central HD catheters while her vascular access has been revised. She has had four bacteremic episodes requiring intravenous antibiotics and has had recurring *Clostridium difficile* enterocolitis over this time. She has lost 10.2 kg body weight and now weighs 60 kg. Her last three monthly urea reduction ratios have been 55%, 50%, and 57% (adequate dialysis urea reduction ratio > 65%). The renal dietitian has documented inadequate energy and protein intake for the last 2 months. Her serum albumin has fallen from 3.5 g/dL 3 months ago to 2.2 g/dL today. Her oral intake over the last month has been one can of Glucerna™ daily and part of a tuna sandwich and some cookies daily. Physical examination shows loss of temporal, masseter, and interosseous muscles. She has little subcutaneous fat. She has an infected arteriovenous polytetrafluoroethylene graft in the right upper arm and a left subclavian HD catheter. Her abdomen is soft with good bowel sounds. Her BUN is 118 mg/dL, Cr is 3.4 mg/dL, calcium 7.8 mg/dL, potassium 3.2 mEq/L, and phosphorus 3.2 mg/dL. Her white blood cell count is elevated with a left shift, and blood cultures are positive at 12 hours for gram-positive cocci in pairs. She is placed on broad spectrum antibiotics. She is also committed to daily HD that represents a 25% increase over her outpatient procedures.

Intervention: The patient was started on a standard enteral formula via nasoenteric feeding tube with precautions taken to prevent refeeding syndrome.

Rationale: The patient has been malnourished for the past 3 months. This is a complication of chronic underdialysis and of recurrent inflammatory illness from vascular access thrombosis, infection, and repeated surgeries. The likelihood that diet stimulants will work or that she will take adequate oral supplements is quite unlikely. IDPN and PN are not indicated as she has a functional GI tract. An enteral tube should be placed as soon as her respiratory status is stabilized. Because she will receive daily dialysis, there is little concern for the need to have a concentrated feeding solution. She is at extremely high risk of the refeeding syndrome and the use of a "renal" formula is not needed.

1.2 g/kg × 60 kg = 78 g protein/day, 78/6.25 = 12.5 g N, 150 3 12.5 g N = 1870 kcal/day. As refeeding syndrome is highly likely, the enteral feeding should be started at a slow rate and increased every 12 hours until the goal rate is reached. Stat electrolytes, including phosphorus and calcium, should be obtained 6 hours after starting the enteral feeding and should be measured frequently thereafter. Before the enteral feeding is begun, she should receive enteral thiamine because her intake predisposes her to be thiamine deficient. She should also receive oral multivitamins. After stabilization of her medical, dialysis, and nutritional status, the enteral feeding should be changed to nocturnal or postprandial, and oral intake should be encouraged. Her diet should be liberalized to a totally select diet. She will require nutritional support for several weeks.

Parenteral Nutrition

If nutritional requirements cannot fully be met with EN or if the GI tract is nonfunctional, then PN should be used.[40] Fluid restriction requires concentration of both dextrose and SAA and a restriction of sodium chloride intake. Intravenous fat emulsion is commonly used daily to meet the patient's caloric needs while controlling the amount of fluid administered. Patients on HD are fluid restricted, but CRRT may allow liberalization of the fluid restriction and can simplify the PN formula. Overall intake and output, weight changes, and renal function should be assessed daily and fluids adjusted. Electrolytes should be adjusted based on the extent of the RF, status of RRT, and other medical conditions.[13,40] Water-soluble vitamins should be given, but fat-soluble vitamins with the exception of vitamin K1 should be restricted in short-term PN (< 8 weeks). Trace element supplementation is not needed in patients with AKI who receive blood products or in those in whom oral intake is restricted < 2 weeks. If needed, trace element solution should be given once every 1 to 2 weeks. There are no data to guide this recommendation, and each center may have its own supplementation guidelines. Specifically, selenium deficiency is to be avoided. Chromium, manganese, and copper deficiency are quite unlikely to occur in short-term PN (< 6 to 8 weeks) unless the patient remains hypercatabolic for an extended period of time (eg, burn patient with multiple débridements and grafts) (Practice Scenario 29-2).

Practice Scenario 29-2

Question: How would you formulate a PN solution for a hospitalized patient with nonoliguric AKI who is not going to be starting RRT?

Scenario: A 67-year-old man had recently undergone repair of an abdominal aortic aneurysm. He was admitted to the hospital 2 days before surgery with intense abdominal pain that was unrelated to meals or physical activity. On postoperative day 4, he developed respiratory failure requiring intubation for mechanical ventilation and intravenous vasopressor support. On postoperative day 5, his urine output rapidly declined, and he became oliguric with a continued increase in the serum Cr. The nutrition support team was consulted. He was eating normally until 2 days prior to admission, and he had little intake postoperatively. His height is 175.3 cm, weight 79.3 kg, usual weight 75 kg, and ideal weight 72 kg. On postoperative day 6, his abdomen was distended and tympanic to percussion, and bowel sounds were not audible on auscultation. An abdominal x-ray showed dilated loops of small and large bowel with air–fluid levels in the small bowel. Laboratory values were as follows: potassium = 5.2 mEq/L; BUN = 38 mg/dL; Cr = 4.6 mg/dL; and albumin = 2.3 g/dL. Other laboratory values are normal. The patient remained on nothing by mouth orders.

Intervention: This patient was started on PN. The PN was fluid restricted and supplemented for a patient that is not going to be started on dialysis immediately.

Answer: This patient should be started on nutritional support. In this case, PN because of a presumed small bowel obstruction or Ogilvie syndrome. In formulating a PN solution for a patient in AKI but not receiving dialysis, volume has to be restricted. This is done by limiting the amount of sodium salts used in the formula and by maximally concentrating the PN formula. Concentrated dextrose and 20% lipid emulsion should be used. Considering his insensible fluid losses and his nasogastric output, he should receive about 1800 mL/d. Because other intravenous medications and antibiotics account for 600 mL/d, the maximal PN volume is 1200 mL/d. The Harris-Benedict formula yields an REE of 1200 kcal, and adding a stress factor of 1.3 brings the total needs to approximately 2000 kcal/d. Patients with AKI who will not undergo dialysis require 0.6 to 0.8 g/kg/d of protein intake. His initial protein requirements would be 40 to 72 g/d. Because the PN fluid must be restricted to 1200 mL per day, concentrated sources of dextrose and amino acids should be used to compound this formulation. Standard amino acids should be provided.

In starting PN, half of the estimated energy needs would be provided on the first day in order to assess tolerance to the dextrose load. The initial prescription for this patient was 40 g of amino acids, 1000 kcal as a three-in-one solution with 70% of the nonprotein kcal as dextrose and 30% as lipid. If the patient were hyperglycemic, an argument could be made to increase the lipid calories to 50% of the total. With respiratory insufficiency, the increased lipids might assist because the respiratory quotient is 0.8 compared to the respiratory quotient of 1 for carbohydrate. Electrolytes should be provided based on the serum concentrations. If the serum sodium concentration is normal, then it is appropriate to add sodium chloride sufficient to mimic 0.45% saline solution or roughly 70 to 77 mEq/L. If the patient is hypernatremic, then less sodium chloride should be used; if the patient is hyponatremic, more sodium chloride should be used. The sodium chloride concentration in the PN must be adjusted daily based on daily measurements. Reduced amounts of phosphorus and magnesium should be provided because of the elevated Cr unless the patient is hypophosphatemic or hypomagnesemic. As this patient has had no intake for over 8 days, he is at risk for refeeding syndrome with hypophosphatemia and hypokalemia. In general, provision of phosphorus at 10 mM per 1000 kcal delivered is sufficient to begin PN. Again, phosphorus concentrations should be monitored daily and if the refeeding syndrome is a consideration.

Phosphorus should be checked 6 to 8 hours after the start of PN. Although the patient has mild hyperkalemia, potassium should not be held. Potassium should be administered at 10 to 20 mEq/1000 kcal supplied. In this case, it would be prudent to add 5 mEq/1000 kcal and to measure the potassium concentration 6 to 8 hours after starting the PN, especially if the refeeding syndrome is of concern. The PN regimen should include 10 mL/d standard multivitamin injection/week and TE should not be provided until the patient has been on PN > 2 weeks and has not had any blood products. As standard MVI is not indicated, individual water-soluble vitamins should be given (folic acid 1 to 2 mg, vitamin C 100 to 125 mg, thiamine 100 mg, a B-complex) and vitamin K1 1 to 2 mg/d. Serum glucose, electrolytes, calcium, phosphorus, and magnesium should be ordered 6 hours after the start of the PN and then measured regularly according to the findings. If the patient is hyperglycemic, regular insulin should be added to the PN and increased daily as needed. In general, 6 to 10 units/1000 kcal delivered represents a safe starting point for the addition of insulin.

Rationale: This patient would benefit from nutrition support because he has not had any nutrition for more than 8 days. Patients with severe injury without adequate oral intake for 5 to 7 days should receive either EN or PN. In this particular case, PN would be the best method of nutrition support because the patient has a nonfunctional GI tract. It was decided that RRT was not required at that time because the patient's BUN was well below 100 mg/dL, fluid accumulation was mild with an increase in weight of only 4 kg since admission, and electrolyte abnormalities were only slight. The PN should be planned without dialysis. The need to fluid restrict is based on assessment of his fluid status. In this case, this patient's weight is significantly increased from his preoperative weight because of accumulation of fluids administered during surgery and fluid retention from RF. His preoperative dry weight should be used to calculate estimated protein and energy requirements. Fluid restriction is common in AKI; in this case, intravenous fluids were to be restricted to no more than 1800 mL/d because this was less than GI, urinary, and insensible fluid losses. His calorie calculation would be based on the standard of the Harris-Benedict formula, which provides the basal calorie needs of 1200 kcal.[30] With Harris-Benedict adding a stress factor of 1.3 to 1, the estimate for total energy expenditure is 2000 to 2200 kcal/d. This is consistent with the American Society for Parenteral and Enteral Nutrition (A.S.P.E.N.) guidelines of 25 to 35 kcal/kg. Calorie needs in AKI are based not on the AKI per se but on the underlying medical condition when determining the stress factor. The activity factor in a hospitalized patient is 1.1 unless the patient is very active. For patients with AKI who will not need dialysis, 0.6 to 0.8 g of protein initially is recommended. This patient will need his full requirement (1.5 to 1.8 g/kg) but may have to be tapered up to that, based on tolerance. Based on A.S.P.E.N. standards, protein restriction is initially appropriate in patients not on dialysis with a goal of preventing or delaying dialysis while still meeting protein needs. As the patient stabilizes, the protein provided should be increased as tolerated and hopefully as renal function returns. SAAs should be provided.

Starting PN at half of the estimated energy needs facilitates evaluation of tolerance to the dextrose load. The initial prescription for this patient was 40 g of amino acids: 1100 kcal as a three-in-one solution with 70% of the nonprotein kcal as dextrose and 30% as lipid. Electrolytes should be provided based on the electrolyte serum level and current renal function. Additives should include sodium and calcium as needed. Typically in renal dysfunction, reduced amounts of potassium, phosphorus, and magnesium would be provided. Electrolytes should be adjusted based on serum Cr changes, renal function, and the amount of losses. Potassium supplementation was held because of the increased serum level. As the potassium level drops due to utilization, anabolism, and improving renal function additional potassium will be needed. A standard AKI PN regimen could include 10 mL/d standard multivitamin injection and standard trace element package daily to meet basic needs. His needs allowed only specific water-soluble vitamins to be given and trace elements were held. If the patient was being dialyzed then additional supplements may have been required.

Intradialytic Parenteral Nutrition

Intradialytic PN (IDPN) has been utilized for malnourished patients with inadequate oral intake when oral/enteral supplement was not effective and in whom standard PN was not felt to be indicated.[77] The goal of this therapy is to provide additional calories and protein to the malnourished patient on HD during HD as the volume of IDPN administered can be removed immediately by increasing the ultrafiltration rate during the dialysis procedure.[78] IDPN solutions typically range from ~350 to 1000 mL/dialysis.[78-80] IDPN is comprised of dextrose, amino acids, and use of fat emulsion.[78-80] This solution generally provides ~300 to 1200 kcal and 1.2 to 1.4 g of protein/kg per HD treatment.[78-80] The delivery of increased protein will necessitate changes to assure dialysis adequacy. Acidosis as a result of increased protein provision may occur and should be corrected if observed. Glucose monitoring before, during, and after IDPN is necessary, and the addition of short-acting insulin during therapy may be necessary. The protein and lipid calories generally prevent post-IDPN hypoglycemia as long as large amounts of exogenous insulin are avoided.

Lipids are used to provide an increase in caloric intake with minimal effect on volume delivery and hyperglycemia. Although there is concern about adverse effects of lipid delivery in dialysis patients because of preexisting hyperlipidemia, possible carnitine deficiency, and possible free fatty acid toxicity, clinically these have not been reported and do not seem to occur. Optimal solution composition of IDPN has not been defined. Clinical and physical monitoring are necessary for identification and correction of substrate intolerance, electrolyte imbalance, vitamin, and trace element deficiencies.[81]

Most information on the efficacy of IDPN is from small studies or anecdotal reports.[80,82] Some studies have demonstrated improved protein synthesis, reduced proteolysis, and improved energy metabolism, as well as increased serum albumin and weight gain.[78-80] The more malnourished the patient, the greater the improvement of albumin with using IDPN.[77] Nutritional improvements in one study did not extend to patients with behavioral health issues resulting in poor nutritional intake.[72] IDPN is not recommended for routine use at this time but rather should be reserved for those patients on HD who demonstrate malnutrition not amenable to oral or daily EN. It is an expensive therapy with multiple risks that has not clearly been shown to be associated with improved quality of life or survival. It is difficult to justify the use of IDPN except under very unusual circumstances. Proper attention to acute and chronic inflammatory states, impediments to oral intake of nutritious foods, adequate dialysis, medication side effects, and other states that can cause malnutrition, and the failure of EN must be considered. Failing this, daily PN should be considered as well before settling on IDPN.

References

1. Brady HR, Clarkson MR, Lieberthal W. Acute kidney injury. In: Brenner BM, ed. *The Kidney*. 8th ed. New York, NY; 2007:1215–1292.
2. Elderstein LER, Schrier RW. Acute kidney injury. In: Schrier RW, ed. *Renal and Electrolyte Disorders*. 6th ed. Philadelphia, PA: 2004: 401–455.
3. Formation of urine by the kidney. In: Guyton A, ed. *Basic Human Physiology*. Philadelphia, PA: Saunders; 1971:271–287.
4. Strejc JM. Considerations in the nutritional management of patients with acute kidney injury. *Hemodial Int*. 2005;9:135–142.
5. Bellomo R, Ronco C, Kellum JA, et al. Acute kidney injury - definition, outcome, measures, animal models, fluid therapy and information technology needs: the Second International Consensus Conference of the Acute Dialysis Quality Initiative (ADQI) Group. *Crit Care*. 2004;8:R204.
6. Thurau K. Pathophysiology of the acutely failing kidney. *Clin Exp Dial Apheresis*. 1983;7:9–24.
7. Star R. Treatment of acute kidney injury. *Kidney Int*. 1998;54: 1817–1831.
8. Wolk R, Stokowski R, Yorgin P. Nutrition support in the pediatric renal failure patient. In: Merritt RJ, et al., eds. *A.S.P.E.N. Nutrition Support Practice Manual*. Silver Spring, MD: American Society for Parenteral and Enteral Nutrition; 1998;18.1–18.13.
9. Kopple JD. Dietary protein and energy requirements in ESRD patients. *Am J Kidney Dis*. 1998;32:97S–104S.
10. Seidner D, Dweik R, Gupta B. Nutrition support in liver, pulmonary and renal disease. In: Shikora S, Blackburn G, eds. *Nutrition Support, Theory and Therapeutics*. New York, NY: Chapman & Hall; 1997:336–357.
11. Friedericksen DV, Van der Merwe L, Hattingh TL, Nel DG, Moosa MR. Acute kidney injury in the medical ICU still predictive of high mortality. *South Afr Med J*. 2009;99(12):873–875.
12. Caravaca F, Arrobas M, Pizarro J, Esparrago JF. Metabolic acidosis in advanced renal failure: differences between diabetic and nondiabetic patients. *Am J Kidney Dis*. 1999;33:892–898.
13. Morley JE. Nutrition and the kidney in the elderly patient in geriatric nephrology curriculum. *Am Soc Nephrology*. 2009;1–5.
14. Kopple JD. Nutritional therapy in kidney failure. *Nutrition Rev*. 1981;39:193–206.
15. Abel R. Nutritional support in patients with acute kidney injury. *J Am Col Nutr*. 1983;2:33–44.
16. Brown RO, Compher C. ASPEN clinical guidelines: nutrition support in adult acute and chronic renal failure. *J Parenter Enter Nutr*. 2010;34(4):366–377.
17. Cano N, Fiaccadori E, Tesinsky P, et al. ESPEN guidelines on enteral nutrition in acute kidney injury. *Clin Nutr*. 2006;25:295–310.
18. Abel RM, Beck CH, Abbott WM, et al. Improved survival from acute kidney injury after treatment with intravenous essential L-amino acids and glucose: results of a prospective, double-blind study. *N Engl J Med*. 1973;288:695–699.
19. National Kidney Foundation. Facts about CKD. 2000. www.kidney.org/kidney/disease. Accessed June 16, 2006.
20. Kent PS. Integrating clinical nutrition practice guidelines in chronic kidney disease. *Nutr Clin Pract*. 2005;20:213–217.
21. Walser M, Mitch WW, Maroni BJ, Kopple JD. Should protein intake be restricted in predialysis patients? *Kidney Int*. 1999;55: 771–777.
22. Bistrian BR. Role of the systemic inflammatory response syndrome in the development of protein-calorie malnutrition in ESRD. *Am J Kidney Dis*. 1998;32(6 suppl 4):S113–S117.
23. Stratton RJ, Bircher G, Fouque D, et al. Multinutrient oral supplements and tube feeding in maintenance dialysis: a systematic review and meta-analysis. *Am J Kid Dis*. 2005;46(3):387–405.
24. Stenvinkel P, Heimburger O, Paultre F, et al. Strong association between malnutrition, inflammation and atherosclerosis in chronic renal failure. *Kidney Int*. 1999;55:1899–1911.
25. Eknoyan G, Levin N. Nutrition in chronic renal failure from the National Kidney Foundation. *Am J Kid Dis*. 2000;35(6;Suppl 2): S9–S141.

26. Fouquel D, Kalantar-Zadeh K, Kopple J, et al. A proposed nomenclature and diagnostic criteria for protein–energy wasting in acute and chronic kidney disease. *Kidney Int.* 2008;73:391–398.
27. Carvana R, Keep D, Kozeny G, et al. Isolated ultrafiltration. In: Nissenson A, Fine R, eds. *Dialysis Therapy.* 2nd ed. Philadelphia, PA: Hanley & Belfus; 1993:104–107.
28. Wolfson M, Jones MR, Kopple JD. Amino acid losses during hemodialysis with infusion of amino acids and glucose. *Kidney Int.* 1982;21:500–506.
29. Schoenfeld P. Care of the patient on peritoneal dialysis. In: Cogan M, Schoenfeld P, eds. *Introduction to Dialysis.* 2nd ed. New York, NY: Churchill Livingstone; 1991:181–240.
30. Khanna R, Nolph K, Oreopoulos D. In: *The Essentials of Peritoneal Dialysis.* Boston, MA: Kluwer Academic Publishing; 1993:81,93–94.
31. Blumenkrantz MJ, Gahl GM, Kopple JD, et al. Protein loss during peritoneal dialysis. *Kidney Int.* 1981;19:593–602.
32. Uchino S, Kellum JA, Bellomo B, et al. Acute kidney injury in critically ill patients: a multinational, multicenter study. *JAMA.* 2005;294(7):813–818.
33. Bock KR. Renal replacement therapy in pediatric critical care medicine. *Curr Opin Pediatr.* 2005;17(3):368–371.
34. Wooley JA, Btaiche IF, Good KL. Metabolic and nutritional aspects of acute kidney injury in critically ill patients requiring continuous renal replacement therapy. *Nutr Clin Pract.* 2005;20:176–191.
35. Orlando Regional Healthcare. *Principles of Continuous Renal Replacement Therapy: Self-Training Manual*, Orlando, FL: Orlando Regional Healthcare, 2005.
36. Maxvold NJ, Smoyer WE, Custer JR, Bunchman TE. Amino acid loss and nitrogen balance in critically ill children with acute kidney injury: a prospective comparison between classic hemofiltration and hemofiltration with dialysis. *Crit Care Med.* 2000;28(4): 1161–1165.
37. A.S.P.E.N. Board of Directors. Guidelines for the use of parenteral and enteral nutrition in adult and pediatric patients. *J Parenter Enteral Nutr.* 2002;26(1):78SA–80SA.
38. Weisen P, Van Overmeire L, Delanaye P, et al. Nutrition disorders during acute kidney injury and renal replacement therapy. *J Parenter Enteral Nutr.* 2011;217–222.
39. Scheinkestel CD, Adams F, Mahony L, et al. Impact of increasing parenteral protein loads on amino acid levels and balance in critically ill anuric patients on continuous renal replacement therapy. *Nutrition.* 2003;19:733–740.
40. Druml W, Kerdorf HP. Parenteral nutrition in patients with renal failure—guidelines on parenteral nutrition. *German Medical Science.* 2009;7:1–11.
41. Cockcroft DW, Gault MH. Prediction of creatinine clearance from serum creatinine. *Nephron.* 1976;16:31–41.
42. Hipskind P, Glass C, Charlton D, Nowak D, Daasarathy S. Do handheld calorimeters have a role in assessment of nutrition needs in hospitalized patients? A systematic review of the literature. *Nutr Clin Pract.* 2011;26(4);426–433.
43. Manji S, Shikora S, McMahon M, et al. Peritoneal dialysis for acute kidney injury: overfeeding resulting from dextrose absorbed during dialysis. *Crit Care Med.* 1990;18:29–31.
44. Abel RM, Abbott WM, Fischer JE. Acute kidney injury: treatment without dialysis by total parenteral nutrition. *Arch Surg.* 1971; 103:513–514.
45. Feinstein E, Blumenkrantz M, Healy M, et al. Clinical and metabolic responses to parenteral nutrition in acute kidney injury: a controlled double-blind study. *Medicine.* 1981;60:124–137.
46. Feinstein EI, Kopple JD, Silberman H, Massry SG. Total parenteral nutrition with high or low nitrogen intakes in patients with acute kidney injury. *Kidney Int.* 1983;16(suppl):S319–S323.
47. Mirtallo JM, Schneider PJ, Mavko K, et al. A comparison of essential and general amino acid infusions in the nutritional support of patients with compromised renal function. *J Parenter Enteral Nutr.* 1982;6:109–113.
48. Kopple JD. The nutritional management of the patient with acute kidney injury. *J Parenter Enteral Nutr.* 1996;20:3–12.
49. Nakas H, Katayama T, Yokoyama S, et al. Complication of parenteral nutrition composed of essential amino acids and histidine in adults with renal failure. *J Parenter Enteral Nutr.* 1993; 17:86–90.
50. Ishimura E, Nishizawa Y, Inaba M, et al. Serum levels of 1,25 dihydroxyvitamin D, 24,25-dihydroxyvitamin D and 25-hydroxyvitamin D in nondialyzed patients with chronic renal failure. *Kidney Int.* 1999;55:1019–1027.
51. National Kidney Foundation. K/DOQI clinical practice guidelines for bone metabolism and disease in chronic kidney disease. *Am J Kidney Dis.* 2003;42(suppl 3):S1–S201.
52. Moore L. Implications for nutrition practice in the mineral-bone disorder of chronic kidney disease. *Nutr Clin Pract.* 2011;26(4); 391–400.
53. McCann L. Nutrient calculations. In: *Pocket Guide to Nutrition Assessment of the Renal Patient.* 3rd ed. New York, NY: National Kidney Foundation; 1998: 4–5.
54. National Kidney Foundation. Guideline 6: use of phosphate binders in CKD in KDOQI clinical practice guidelines for bone metabolism and disease in children with chronic kidney disease. 2011.
55. Blumberg A, Hanck A, Sander G. Vitamin nutrition in patients on continuous ambulatory peritoneal dialysis (CAPD). *Clin Nephrol.* 1983;20;244–250.
56. Makoff R, Gonick H. Renal failure and the concomitant derangement of micronutrient metabolism. *Nutr Clin Pract.* 1999;14: 238–246.
57. Ono K. The effect of vitamin C supplementation and withdrawal on the mortality and morbidity of regular hemodialysis patients. *Clin Nephrol.* 1989;31:31–34.
58. Pru C, Eaton J, Kjellstrand C. Vitamin C intoxication and hyperoxalemia in chronic hemodialysis patients. *Nephron.* 1985;39; 112–116.
59. Tarng DC, Wei YH, Huan TP, et al. Intravenous ascorbic acid as an adjuvant therapy for recombinant erythropoietin in hemodialysis patients with hyperferritinemia. *Kidney Int.* 1999;55:2477–2486.
60. Bamonti-Catena F, Buccianti G, Porcella A, et al. Folate measurements in patients on regular hemodialysis treatment. *Am J Kidney Dis.* 1999;33:492–497.
61. Marangella M, Vitale C, Petrarulo M, et al. Pathogenesis of severe hyperoxalaemia in Crohn's disease-related renal failure on maintenance haemodialysis: successful management with pyridoxine. *Nephrol Dial Transplant.* 1992;7:960–964.
62. Jagadha V, Deck J, Halliday W, Smyth H. Wernicke's encephalopathy in patients on peritoneal dialysis or hemodialysis. *Ann Neurol.* 1987;21:78–89.
63. Baumgartner TG. Trace elements in clinical nutrition. *Nutr Clin Pract.* 1993;8:251–263.
64. Fournier A, Corvazier M, Man W. Skin test sensitivity in zinc deficient patients in hemo- and peritoneal dialysis [abstract]. *Artif Organ.* 1989;13;296.
65. Hsieh YY, Shen WS, Lee LY, et al. Long-term changes in trace elements in patients undergoing chronic hemodialysis. *Biol Trace Elem Res.* 2006;109(2):115–121.
66. Nissenson A, Strobos J. Iron deficiency in patients with renal failure. *Kidney Int.* 1999;69:S18–S21.
67. Macdougall I. Strategies for iron supplementation: oral versus intravenous. *Kidney Int.* 1999;69:S61–S66.

68. Kaltwasser J, Gottschalk R. Erythropoietin and iron. *Kidney Int.* 1999;69:S49–S56.
69. Fishbane S. Iron treatment: impact of safety issues. *Am J Kidney Dis.* 1998;32(6):S152–S156.
70. National Kidney Foundation. Guidelines for anemia of chronic kidney disease. 2000. http://kidney.org/professionals/kdoqi/guide-lines_updates/ doqiupan_iii.html. Accessed June 16, 2006.
71. Chertow GM, Mason PD, Vaage-Nilsen O, Ahlmen J. On the relative safety of parenteral iron formulations. *Nephrol Dial Transplant.* 2004;19:1571–1575.
72. Feinstein E. Nutritional therapy in maintenance hemodialysis. In: Nissenson A, Fine R, eds. *Dialysis Therapy.* Philadelphia, PA: Hanley & Belfus; 1993:181–201.
73. Berns JS, Mosenkis A. Pharmacologic adjuvants to epoetin in the treatment of anemia in patients on hemodialysis. *Hemodial Inter.* 2005;9:7–22.
74. Bartel L, Hussey J, Elson C, et al. Depletion of heart and skeletal muscle carnitine in the normal rat by peritoneal dialysis. *Nutr Res.* 1981;1:261–266.
75. Schreiber B. Levocarnitine and dialysis: a review. *Nutr Clin Pract.* 2005:20:218–243.
76. Klahr MD, Levey AS, Beck GJ, et al. The effects of dietary protein restriction and blood pressure control on the progression of chronic renal disease. Modification of Diet in Renal Disease Study Group. *N Engl J Med.* 1994;330:877–884.
77. Ikizler TA. Protein and energy: recommended intake and nutrient supplementation in chronic dialysis patients. *Seminars Dialy.* 2004;17(6):471–478.
78. Cano N. Intradialytic parenteral nutrition: where do we go from here? *J Renal Nutr.* 2004;14:3–5.
79. Pupim LB, Flakoll PJ, Brouillette JR, et al. Intradialytic parenteral nutrition improves protein and energy homeostasis in chronic hemodialysis patients. *J Clin Invest.* 2002;110(4):483–492.
80. Charry N, Shalansky K. Efficacy of intradialytic parenteral nutrition in malnourished hemodialysis patients. *Am Soc Healthsystem Pharm.* 2002;59:1736–1741.
81. Moore E, Celano J. Challenges of providing nutrition support in the outpatient dialysis setting. *Nutr Clin Pract.* 2005; 20:202–212.
82. Orellana P, Juarez-Congelosi M, Goldstein SL. Intradialytic parenteral nutrition treatment and biochemical marker assessment for malnutrition in adolescent maintenance hemodialysis patients. *J Renal Nutr.* 2005;15(3):312–317.

30 Short Bowel Syndrome

Sherry Tarleton, RD, CNSC, and John K. DiBaise, MD, FACG

CONTENTS

Background . . . 512
Anatomic and Physiologic Considerations . . . 512
Intestinal Adaptation . . . 513
Nutritional Assessment . . . 513
Nutritional and Other Interventions . . . 514
Oral Diet . . . 514
Oral Fluids . . . 515
Enteral Nutrition . . . 517
Parenteral Fluids . . . 517
Parenteral Nutrition . . . 517
Intestinal Rehabilitation . . . 518
Medications . . . 518
Trophic Factors . . . 519
Surgery . . . 519
Complications and Monitoring . . . 520
Outcomes . . . 521
References . . . 521

Objectives

1. Describe symptoms, potential causes, and conditions associated with short bowel syndrome.
2. Become familiar with the medical and surgical management of short bowel syndrome and its complications.
3. Apply diet principles to better manage symptoms of short bowel syndrome.
4. Design and implement an appropriate nutrition support management plan in a short bowel patient.

Test Your Knowledge Questions

1. Which one of the following best reflects dietary modifications that may prevent the development of nephrolithiasis-related renal failure?
   A. A calcium-restricted diet with increased free water intake
   B. A low fat diet with adequate phosphorus repletion and increased free water intake
   C. A low fat and oxalate- and calcium-restricted diet.
   D. A low fat, oxalate-restricted diet, and adequate hydration.
2. Due to the malabsorptive process present in short bowel syndrome (SBS), patients are at a high risk for micronutrient deficiencies. Which one of the following is correct regarding the monitoring and repletion of micronutrients in SBS?
   A. As long as they are receiving parenteral nutrition, there is no reason to monitor micronutrients because the parenteral nutrition should satisfy all micronutrient needs.
   B. Micronutrients should be checked periodically. Micronutrients can usually be repleted via the oral route.
   C. Micronutrients should be checked on a monthly basis. Repletion should be administered in high doses both intravenously and orally.
   D. Micronutrients should be checked annually and all micronutrients should be repleted intravenously because this population is unable to absorb micronutrients administered orally.

3. Which of the following best describes how a clinician determines the most appropriate feeding route (eg, oral, enteral, parenteral, a combination) for a patient with SBS?
   A. All patients with SBS need to be on parenteral nutrition (PN) for the remainder of their lives; so as long as their energy and protein needs are met with PN, they can eat whatever they want for comfort.
   B. PN should always be discontinued as soon as oral and/or enteral nutrition is initiated to avoid the risk of PN-associated complications.
   C. The most appropriate nutrition regimen should be individualized according to the needs of the particular person.
   D. Insurance reimbursement plays the major role in deciding the feeding route.
4. Which one of the following characteristics of an initial enteral feeding regimen would be most appropriate for a patient with SBS?
   A. A fiber-free, calorie-dense formula administered via bolus infusion.
   B. A hydrolyzed, elemental formula that is high in medium-chain triglyceride oil.
   C. An isotonic, polymeric, fiber-containing formula administered via continuous gastric infusion.
   D. A semielemental, peptide-based formula administered nocturnally.

Test Your Knowledge Answers

1. The correct answer is **D**. Short bowel patients with fat malabsorption and an intact colon are at risk for oxalate kidney stones. Calcium normally binds to oxalate—a substance found naturally in many foods—in the colon, thus preventing its absorption. In the setting of fat malabsorption, calcium will bind to excess fat entering the colon, leaving the oxalates free to be absorbed into the bloodstream and excreted via the kidney, thus forming oxalate kidney stones. A low fat, oxalate-restricted diet plays a key role in the prevention of oxalate kidney stones. The use of a calcium supplement or consumption of food that is high in calcium may also help to bind the oxalate and facilitate its excretion in the feces.
2. The correct answer is **B**. Short bowel patients are at risk for micronutrient deficiencies, including vitamin, mineral, trace element, and essential fatty acid deficiencies. There are no formal guidelines regarding the monitoring and repletion of micronutrients in this setting. Nevertheless, micronutrients and an essential fatty acid profile should be checked at least annually and interventions for the repletion of deficient micronutrients should be made. Abnormal micronutrient levels should be monitored on a quarterly basis. Although some micronutrients can be increased in the parenteral nutrition (PN) solution, not all micronutrients will be able to be added to the PN solution due to formula stability issues or the nutrient may not come in single unit doses. Fortunately, it is possible to provide adequate micronutrient supplementation orally, although the regimen will need to be tailored to meet the increased needs. Some micronutrients are available for either intramuscular or intravenous administration.
3. The correct answer is **C**. There are many possible nutrition support options depending on the patient's bowel anatomy, length of time since surgery, current weight, labs, and hydration status. The most appropriate nutrition regimen should be individualized according to the needs of the particular person. As the adaptation process progresses and the patient becomes more stable, nutrition support may be decreased as tolerated.
4. The correct answer is **C**. When initiating enteral feedings in a short bowel patient, it is important that the formula be isotonic. Polymeric formulas are generally well tolerated. Gastric feeding may result in less diarrhea than small bowel feeding. The inclusion of soluble fiber may also be beneficial because it can slow gastric emptying, enhance adaptation, and provide an energy source in those patients who have a colon. Slow initiation of feedings administered via continuous gastric infusion as opposed to bolus administration may be better tolerated.

Background

Short bowel syndrome (SBS) is a malabsorptive syndrome resulting from extensive intestinal resection.[1,2] These patients frequently experience chronic diarrhea, dehydration, and macro- and micronutrient deficiencies often requiring enteral nutrition (EN) or parenteral nutrition (PN) support at home. Because of the wide range in small bowel length and the remarkable ability of the bowel to compensate for bowel resection, the definition of SBS should not be based solely on the length of remaining bowel; however, it generally does not become clinically apparent until about three-quarters of the small bowel has been removed. In adults, multiple resections for Crohn's disease and massive resections due to catastrophic mesenteric vascular events, radiation enteritis, adhesive obstruction, and trauma represent the more common causes of SBS.[3] Although considered rare, the prevalence of SBS is unclear. In the United States, the annual prevalence of home PN use has been estimated at about 120 per million, of whom approximately 25% had SBS.[4] These numbers likely underestimate the prevalence of SBS because they do not reflect patients with SBS who never required home PN or were able to be successfully weaned from PN.

Anatomic and Physiologic Considerations

Anatomic factors that affect the outcome of the SBS patient include not only the length, but also the region of the remaining small intestine and the presence of the colon. SBS includes one of the following bowel anatomies: jejuno-colic anastomosis, end-jejunostomy, or jejuno-ileocolonic anastomosis. Patients with a jejuno-colic anastomosis rarely have an ileocecal valve. Patients with a jejuno-ileal anastomosis have the best prognosis; however, this anatomy is also the least common. Patients with an end-jejunostomy are the most difficult to manage and are most likely to require permanent parenteral support.[5] An appreciation of the physiologic roles of the various regions of the gastrointestinal (GI) tract will aid in the understanding of the complications that may occur in the course of

SBS and the treatment suggestions discussed in the following sections.

A massive enterectomy is associated with gastric hypergastrinemia and hypersecretion that may last up to 12 months postoperatively.[6] This increases the volume of secretions entering the small bowel and lowers the pH of the secretions in the proximal gut, potentially aggravating fluid losses and leading to peptic complications and/or impairment in the function of digestive enzymes.[7]

The proximal 200 cm of the jejunum is the primary site of carbohydrate, protein, and water-soluble vitamin absorption.[8] Fat absorption occurs over a larger length of the small bowel, a length that increases as the amount of fat ingested increases. The junctions between jejunal epithelial cells are relatively large compared to other areas of the bowel, allowing the rapid flux of fluids and nutrients so that the jejunal contents can become iso-osmolar. As a result, the concentration of sodium in jejunostomy fluid is about 100 mEq per liter (range, 90 to 140). Sodium absorption in the jejunum can only occur against a concentration gradient, is dependent upon water fluxes, and is coupled to the absorption of glucose.[9] These factors become particularly important in the short bowel patient who only has the jejunum remaining.

In contrast to the jejunum, the ileum has tighter intercellular junctions.[9] This leads to less movement of water and sodium. The active transport of sodium chloride allows for significant fluid reabsorption and the ability to concentrate its contents. The ileum is also the primary site of carrier-mediated bile salt and B12 absorption and is the site of production of many GI hormones such as glucagonlike peptides 1 and 2 and peptide YY. These gut hormones are important for the control of bowel motility and intestinal epithelial growth.[10] Bile salts are necessary for the absorption of fat, and the bile salt pool is efficiently maintained through enterohepatic circulation. Following the resection of more than 100 cm of the distal ileum, the bile salt pool eventually becomes depleted leading to impaired micelle formation, decreasing solubilization of fat, and resulting in the malabsorption of fat. Although it is commonly believed that the ileocecal valve is beneficial in slowing transit and preventing the reflux of colonic contents into the small bowel, reports suggesting a benefit may in fact reflect the retention of a significant length of terminal ileum.[11]

The colon plays a vital role in fluid and electrolyte reabsorption with a capacity to absorb up to 6 L daily.[12] A complete loss of the colon often leads to problems with dehydration and electrolyte abnormalities for SBS patients. Enteroglucagon, neurotensin, and peptide YY are produced in the proximal colon (and ileum) and are responsible for the jejunal, ileal, and colonic brake phenomena that slows small intestinal transit in response to fat intake.[10,13] In addition to the resorptive capabilities of the colon, bacterial fermentation of malabsorbed carbohydrates to short-chain fatty acids (SCFAs) with subsequent absorption in the colon provides an additional energy source, up to 1000 kcal daily.[14]

Intestinal Adaptation

Intestinal adaptation refers to a process following intestinal resection in which the remaining bowel undergoes a variety of macroscopic and microscopic changes in response to a variety of stimuli including nutrients, gut peptides/hormones, and the remaining bowel, in order to increase its ability to absorb fluid and nutrients.[15] The majority of intestinal adaptation typically occurs within the first 2 years of a massive resection. Both structural (eg, increases in villus height, crypt cell depth, enterocyte number) and functional (eg, modifications of the brush border membrane fluidity, permeability, up- or downregulation of carrier-mediated transport, and a slowing in the rate of transit) intestinal changes can occur depending upon the extent and site of the intestine removed and the nutrient components of the diet.[16] The ileum is capable of both structural and functional adaptation, whereas the jejunum mainly adapts functionally.[17]

Nutritional Assessment

The assessment of the patient with SBS presents many challenges beginning with knowledge of the patient's remaining bowel anatomy. Knowledge of the remaining small bowel length can be useful to predict the clinical outcome and develop an individualized treatment plan. Information on the site of resection, remaining bowel length, condition of remaining bowel, presence of the colon, presence of the ileocecal valve, and presence and location of an ostomy should be obtained. The large range of small bowel length (300 to 800 cm) underscores the importance of being aware of the small bowel length *remaining* following a resection rather than the length of small bowel *removed*. When an operative report is unavailable or does not document the remaining bowel length, a barium contrast small bowel series may provide an estimate of bowel length and is useful to delineate other structural features such as the presence of bowel dilatation. Importantly, when considering small bowel length, measurements begin at the duodeno-jejunal flexure.[18]

A comprehensive nutritional assessment should be performed on all SBS patients. Information to be obtained should include a history pertinent to weight change, medication usage (including supplements), presence of GI and other symptoms that may affect oral intake or fluid loss, potential signs/symptoms of micronutrient deficiencies, and a physical assessment for signs of dehydration and malnutrition.[19]

Patients with SBS should be instructed on the measurement of daily input and output as periodic assessment of these parameters can help to guide fluid needs. A baseline assessment of fluid intake and urine and stool output for at least 24 hours should be obtained to determine the usual fluid and enteral balance (ie, oral fluid intake minus stool output). The blood urea nitrogen (BUN): creatinine ratio may also provide a measure of hydration status.[20] It is also important to obtain a food diary, preferably over a period of a few days, to determine the SBS patient's typical oral diet and daily energy intake.[21] A baseline assessment of electrolytes, including calcium, magnesium, and phosphorus and micronutrient levels, should be obtained at the initial clinic visit. In particular, levels of fat-soluble vitamins (A, D, E, K), vitamin B12, folate, iron studies, and zinc should be assessed. In some patients, a 72-hour fecal fat assessment may be needed to document malabsorption. Bone density should be assessed at baseline and monitored regularly (see the following). A serum parathyroid hormone (PTH) level is useful to identify those patients in need of more intensive management of their bone disease.[19]

Additional information that should be collected at baseline include pertinent past medical, psychiatric, and surgical history including comorbidities and the presence of bowel complications such as anastomotic strictures, chronic obstruction, and enterocutaneous fistulae and peritoneal drains. A nutrition support history should also be obtained, including information regarding the enteral and/or central access device, the formula used, the route and method of administration, and known prior complications. Finally, given the high level of motivation and adherence to the dietary, fluid, and medical treatments prescribed, it is useful to inquire about their education, motivation, support system, and potential economic or other barriers.[19]

Nutritional and Other Interventions

Following a massive intestinal resection, three distinct clinical stages have been described: acute, adaptation, and maintenance.[22] The patient's nutrition support needs will change depending on the stage. The *acute stage* is characterized by large fluid and electrolyte losses and generally occurs over the first few weeks following the resection. During this stage, the emphasis is on stabilizing the patient, including fluid and electrolytes. Once the patient's condition has stabilized, nutrition support is often commenced. In the *adaptation stage*, a shift of emphasis to nutritional support is the primary concern. This stage may last for up to 2 years and it is during this time that most adaptation and PN weaning occurs. Stage three is considered a homeostatic, *maintenance stage* where no further naturally occurring adaptive changes take place. The absorptive capacity of the GI tract reaches its maximum once the patient enters the maintenance phase. With aggressive management, PN weaning may still be successful during this stage despite the absence of additional intestinal adaptation.

Managing the SBS patient is complex, requiring a comprehensive, multidisciplinary approach and attention to detail. Specific dietary interventions combined with medical management and, occasionally, surgical strategies offer the potential of PN reduction and overall improved clinical outcome. Each of these areas is briefly discussed in the following sections.

Oral Diet

There is limited consensus on the importance of the oral diet in the management of SBS; nevertheless, clinical experience suggests an important role for diet in the successful management of these patients. The long-term success of an optimized diet requires extensive education and monitoring to maintain compliance and needs to be translated into foods and meal patterns that meet the individual's preferences and lifestyle.[23] The establishment of daily calorie and fluid intake goals for the patient followed by a careful follow-up and adjustments based on tolerance as determined by the development of symptoms, stool output, micronutrient levels, weight, and hydration status is critical. In general, most stable adult SBS patients absorb only about one-half to two-thirds as much energy as normal; thus, dietary intake must be increased by at least 50% from their estimated needs (ie, hyperphagic diet). The increased quantity of food tends to be best tolerated when consumed throughout the day in five to six meals.

Because patients with SBS are at risk for developing nutritional, fluid, and electrolyte disturbances, adherence to several basic dietary principles will help to enhance absorption and promote enteral autonomy (Table 30-1). Short bowel syndrome patients have been found to differ in their response to dietary manipulation depending upon the presence or absence of a colon. A diet high in complex carbohydrates (50% to 60%) and low in fat (20% to 30%) has been shown in studies involving small numbers of SBS patients to reduce fecal calorie loss and to increase overall energy and wet weight absorption in those patients with at least a portion of their colon present.[24,25] This diet also results in a reduction in steatorrhea, magnesium and calcium loss, and a reduction in oxalate absorption. Normally, dietary oxalate binds to calcium and is excreted in the stool; however, in the setting of fat malabsorption, calcium binds to fatty acids, leaving oxalate free to pass into the colon to be absorbed and then filtered by the kidney. In the kidney, oxalate binds to calcium, resulting in oxalate nephropathy. Therefore, oxalate restriction along with the inclusion of high calcium foods or calcium citrate supplementation is also important in those SBS patients with a colon in order to decrease the risk of oxalate nephropathy. In contrast, the high carbohydrate/low fat diet in SBS patients without a colon has not been found to result in improvement in absorption.[24,25] Indeed, it was found that a constant proportion of dietary fat is absorbed in the end-jejunostomy patient; therefore, more is absorbed when more is consumed.

Regardless of the bowel anatomy, the provision of complex macronutrients in the diet of SBS patients is preferred. Complex carbohydrates, including starches, reduce the osmotic load and may exert a positive effect on the adaptation process. In the intestine, starch is broken down more slowly than simple sugars, thus improving tolerance. Much like soluble fiber, some starches will be converted to SCFA by colonic bacterial fermentation and used as energy. Because the proximal jejunum is rarely resected in SBS patients, lactose is generally well tolerated[26] and should not be restricted unless the patient is clearly intolerant, because milk-based products provide an important source of calories and calcium. Concentrated sugars, fruit juices in particular, should be avoided because they generate a high osmotic load and potentiate stool output. Because nitrogen absorption is least affected by the decreased absorptive surface in SBS patients, no change in dietary protein is generally necessary and, specifically, the use of peptide-based diets in these patients is unnecessary. Medium-chain triglycerides (MCTs) are absorbed from both the small and large intestine, do not require digestion by pancreatic enzymes for their absorption, and may be useful as an alternative energy source in the presence of bile acid or pancreatic insufficiency.[27] However, MCTs are generally not well tolerated in the long term, have a slightly lower caloric density than long-chain triglycerides (LCTs) (8.3 versus 9 kcal per gram), do not contain essential fatty acids, exert a greater osmotic load in the small bowel, and have less stimulatory effect on adaptation compared to LCTs. The provision of essential fatty acids (ie, linoleic acid [an omega-6 fatty acid] and

TABLE 30-1 Diet Recommendations in Short Bowel Syndrome: Colon-in-Continuity Versus End-Jejunostomy

	Colon-in-Continuity	End-Jejunostomy	Additional Considerations
Calories	35–45 kcal/kg; may need up to 60 kcal/kg	35–45 kcal/kg; may need up to 60 kcal/kg	• Hyperphagia • 5–6 mini meals evenly spaced throughout the day
Carbohydrate	50%–60% of kcal	20–40% of kcal	• Limit simple sugars • Include complex carbohydrates (starches)
Protein	1.5–2.0 g/kg or 20%–30% of kcal	1.5–2.0 g/kg or 20%–30% of kcal	• High-quality lean protein
Fat	20%–30% of kcal	40%–60% of kcal	• May need 72 hour fecal fat test if going home on parenteral nutrition • Essential fatty acids as main component of oral fat intake • May consider MCT oil with fat malabsorption
Fiber	10–15 g per day (adjust per patient tolerance)	10–15 g per day (adjust per patient tolerance)	• Individuals with stool output > 3L daily should have 5–10 g of soluble fiber daily
Fluid	Isotonic/hypo-osmolar	Isotonic/high Na+ oral rehydration solutions	• Separate liquids from solids • Avoid simple sugars • Sip throughout the day • Commercial versus homemade ORS
Oxalate	Low oxalate diet	No restriction necessary	• Include high calcium food or calcium citrate supplement with meals to bind oxalate and alkalinize the urine
Lactose	Do not restrict if tolerated	Do not restrict if tolerated	• Dairy provides protein, calcium, and vitamin D
Sodium	Encourage liberal use of salt	Encourage liberal use of salt	• Do not restrict due to increased losses

MCT, medium-chain triglyceride; ORS, oral rehydration solution.

linolenic acid [an omega-3 fatty acid]), found in such substances as safflower and soybean oils, is important because deficiencies are common, particularly in the setting of low fat diets and fat malabsorption.[28] Polyunsaturated fats are a major source of essential fatty acids and should be encouraged to be used at each meal. Finally, soluble fiber supplementation may be useful given its potential effect on enhancing adaptation, slowing gastric emptying, and providing an additional energy source from its bacterial fermentation to SCFA[1,14]; it may, however, result in increased gas and bloating and increase stool output for the patient.

Oral Fluids

The optimal fluid components of the diet also depend on the remaining bowel anatomy (Table 30-2). The osmolality, sodium content, and glucose content of the fluid are important considerations because inappropriate fluids will exacerbate fluid losses in SBS. Osmolality refers to the concentration of particles, molecules, and ions in the fluid. If something is iso-osmolar, also referred to as isotonic, it will have the same concentration as blood and extracellular fluid (~300 mOsm per milliliter). Hyperosmolar fluids are concentrated and pull fluid from enterocytes in an attempt to dilute the concentration of the luminal contents, which then contribute to increased diarrhea. In contrast, hypo-osmolar fluids do not contain the sodium or glucose necessary to optimally facilitate absorption in an end-jejunostomy patient and may lead to dehydration if consumed in large amounts.

Fluid is normally secreted into the intestinal lumen during digestion. This fluid is typically iso-osmotic with blood due to the increased concentration of sodium. A healthy individual will secrete 20 to 30 g of sodium per day via intestinal secretions. Homeostasis occurs by reabsorption of the sodium by the intestine. Intestinal luminal sodium and glucose play important roles in promoting fluid absorption.[29] Glucose absorption is a two-stage process. In the first stage, active accumulation across the brush border membrane and into the enterocyte by sodium glucose cotransporter (SGLT1) occurs. In

TABLE 30-2 Tips to Improve Successful Use of an Oral Rehydration Solution (ORS)

Start slow. Start with 1 L per day and increase as tolerated.
Keep the ORS chilled.
Flavor with sugar-free sweeteners or low sodium broth.
Sip throughout the day.
Drink separately from food.
May be used as flushes or can be delivered continuously via an indwelling feeding tube.

TABLE 30-3 Fluid Recommendations in Short Bowel Syndrome: Colon-in-Continuity Versus End-Jejunostomy

Type of Fluid	Colon-in-Continuity	End-Jejunostomy	Examples of Fluid Type
Iso-osmolar (isotonic)	Those with less than 50% of a colon may benefit from ORS	ORS should be main source of hydration	• Gatorade or PowerAde • Milk • Diluted juice (at least 50% water) • Some enteral formulae ORS examples: • CeraLyte 70, 75, or 90 www.ceraproductsinc.com • Jianas Brothers (816) 421-2880 • Homemade versions
Hyperosmolar	Should be avoided	Should be avoided	Fruit juice, sugar-containing soda, Kool-Aid, Ensure, Boost, Carnation Instant Breakfast
Hypoosmolar	May be able to tolerate	Restrict to 4–6 oz per day	Water, sugar-free soda, Crystal Light, Sugar Free Kool-Aid, Decaf tea and coffee

ORS, oral rehydration solution.

the second stage, the downhill transport of glucose out of the enterocyte and into the blood across the basolateral membrane occurs by facilitated glucose transporter type 2 (GLUT2). The sodium gradient is maintained by the sodium–potassium pump in the basolateral membrane of the enterocyte. Glucose in the gut lumen stimulates sodium absorption across the small intestine, which is followed by anions and water. For each cycle of this transport, two sodium ions and one molecule of glucose/galactose are transported together across the cell membrane and hundreds of water molecules move into the epithelial cell.

Because of the regional differences in water and sodium handling described previously, those SBS patients without a colon generally require the use of a glucose-electrolyte oral rehydration solution (ORS) to enhance absorption and reduce secretion, whereas most of those patients with a colon can maintain adequate hydration without excessive fluid loss with hypotonic fluids.[30,31] An ORS will promote fluid absorption and help reduce diarrhea and optimize hydration status. One to 3 L of such fluid daily, sipped throughout the day, may be needed to maintain adequate hydration. There are commercial ORS products available as well as inexpensive, homemade recipes. Importantly, ORS products differ from commercial sports drinks in that the sodium content is considerably higher and the carbohydrate content is lower. The optimal sodium concentration of ORS to promote jejunal absorption is 90 to 120 mEq Na^+ per liter.[32,33] Because the high sodium concentration in ORS may be poorly palatable, suggestions on appropriate ways to improve the success of its use are described in Table 30-3. Practice Scenario 30-1 discusses the use of ORS in a clinical scenario.

Although fluid composition is less important in those with a colon, adequate dietary sodium should be provided.[34] Regardless of bowel anatomy, hyperosmolar fluids such as regular soda and fruit juices should be avoided, because they will aggravate stool losses. Clinical experience suggests that those patients who tend to experience bowel movements shortly after eating (ie, dumping) may benefit from avoiding drinking fluids during meals.[19]

Practice Scenario 30-1

Question: How can the hydration status of an SBS patient be optimized when it appears that he or she is already consuming an abundance of oral fluids?

Scenario: A 53-year-old woman was admitted to the hospital for dehydration. She has a complex past surgical history including pancolonic ulcerative colitis status after a total proctocolectomy with an ileal pouch anal anastomosis. Her course over the years has been complicated by the development of enterocutaneous fistulae and recurrent small bowel obstructions resulting in multiple additional operations, ultimately leaving her with less than 200 cm of small bowel and an end-jejunostomy. She has had about 20% unintentional weight loss since her last surgery (current BMI is 21 kg per square meter) and reports high volume ostomy output and low urine output. She has been advised to increase her fluid intake and to use oral nutritional supplements. Prior to admission, she collected 2 days of information regarding her fluid intake, urine output, and ostomy output: fluid intake was over 7 L per day, her ostomy output was about 3 L per day, and urine output was 200 mL per day.

Intervention: Upon admission, intravenous hydration was initiated, oral hypotonic fluids were restricted to 4 to 6 oz per day, and she was instructed on an appropriate short bowel diet and the use of an oral rehydration solution (ORS). After 72 hours, the intravenous hydration was discontinued and the patient sipped 2 L of ORS throughout the day. These maneuvers resulted in a decrease in ostomy output to less than 2 L per day and an increase in urine output to about 1 L per day.

Answer: Education regarding appropriate food and beverage choices is imperative in all patients with SBS. Limiting hypo-osmotic beverages and hyperosmotic food and beverages is important in order to optimize fluid and nutrient absorption and to minimize stool losses in this population. Despite the large volume of fluid and calories ingested by this patient, dehydration and weight loss occurred because of poor food and beverage choices.

Rationale: This patient had been consuming high sugar–containing fluids. Simple sugars should be limited in the diet of persons with SBS because of their osmotic effect. The osmotic effect refers to the process whereby a substrate load attracts water due to the body's compensatory mechanism to decrease the concentration, thereby resulting in diarrhea in certain clinical circumstances such as SBS. It is recommended that the intake of simple sugars be restricted in this setting. Hypo-osmotic "free" fluid intake may increase fluid loss for the short bowel patient without a colon, in particular. In this setting, the ingestion of free fluids results in net secretion of sodium into the intestinal lumen in an attempt to reach sodium balance. The secretion of fluid follows the sodium, resulting in increased luminal volume and increased stool output. An ORS, which is a high sodium/low sugar beverage, may be very helpful in promoting the net absorption of sodium and fluid across the bowel wall, thus limiting stool volume and improving hydration status and urine output. Commercial ORS products are available, as are inexpensive homemade recipes.

Enteral Nutrition

In patients with SBS, slow continuous infusion of enteral formula, either exclusively or in conjunction with oral feeding, following the postoperative period has recently been shown to significantly increase the net absorption of lipids, proteins, and energy compared with oral feeding alone.[35] EN may be initiated during the acute phase following extensive resection or later when attempts to wean PN have stalled. In the acute setting, the rate should be advanced slowly to avoid increased stool output and further aggravate fluid and electrolyte disturbances. Slow continuous infusion into the stomach rather than a bolus administration or infusion directly into the small bowel is advised in order to maximize intestinal transit time, improve nutrient contact time and absorption, and reduce diarrhea. Overnight feeding allows for the maximal use of the gut while enabling normal activities during the day. Use of a polymeric formula is generally well tolerated; however, a semielemental formula may be needed. Elemental formulas should be avoided because of their hypertonicity, expense, and lack of evidence supporting any benefits over the standard formula. Fiber-containing formulas may be advantageous in the SBS patient with an intact colon for reasons previously described.

Parenteral Fluids

Occasionally, parenteral fluids without macronutrients may be useful in those patients who require the fluid but not the calories. Parenteral fluids will be necessary if the stool output consistently exceeds fluid intake ("net secretors"). During the hot summer months, patients receiving PN overnight may require additional parenteral hydration during the day. This may also be needed in SBS patients who have successfully weaned from PN but who still require occasional parenteral fluid support. The intravenous fluid is commonly provided as a liter of normal saline infused over a couple of hours once daily as needed. Although the contents of the fluid may include only sodium chloride, occasionally dextrose, other electrolytes, vitamins, and bicarbonate may be added.

Parenteral Nutrition

Medicare criteria require that for PN to be covered in SBS, the resection has to have been performed within the 3 months prior to starting home parenteral nutrition (HPN) and that the residual small intestine measures less than 5 feet (150 cm) based on intraoperative or radiologic measurement.[36,37] If neither of these is the case, it becomes important to demonstrate malabsorption that is responsible for weight loss of at least 10% of body weight in the prior 3-month period and an albumin level of less than 3.5 g per deciliter. Two criteria can be used to demonstrate malabsorption, namely a fecal fat level of at least 50% of an intake of not less than 50 g per day during a 72-hour fecal fat collection, or stool losses in excess of 50% of an oral fluid intake of at least 2.5 to 3 L per day and a urine output of less than 1000 mL per day. Occasionally in SBS, there may be a benefit from a combination of both PN and EN to meet the nutritional needs and minimize the dependence on HPN. Typically, however, Medicare will not reimburse for both therapies. Practice Scenario 30-2 discusses the use of PN and EN in a patient scenario.

Although PN is associated with a number of factors that may result in a restriction of activities and may deleteriously impact daily life, with time and experience PN patients can modify their lifestyles to minimize the impact of this therapy. One example of such a modification is to cycle the PN over 10 to 14 hours overnight in order to allow the patient freedom from the infusion pump during the day. Programmable infusion pumps are used by most consumers. Portable pumps that can be carried in a backpack or tote are also available for the PN consumer who needs to infuse PN during the day. Furthermore, although clearly an extremely expensive therapy, the cost of PN tends to be offset by its lifesaving nature and the likelihood of recovery of intestinal function during the adaptation period. Patient support groups such as the Oley Foundation (www.oley.org) are important sources of information on practical topics (eg, body image, travel), education, and support and may reduce the risk of complications and enhance survival and the quality of life of the patient receiving either EN or PN support.

PN should be initiated and adjusted to meet the patient's fluid, electrolyte, energy, protein, and micronutrient needs. In situations of high ostomy output, increased fluid, potassium, magnesium, and zinc losses occur and need to be monitored and replaced appropriately. The amount of PN can be decreased when the patient demonstrates an ability to take oral nutrition without excessive stool or ostomy output with appropriate weight maintenance or gain. In calculating PN volume and content, changes in the patient's weight, energy levels, labs, stool or ostomy output, urine output, and complaints of thirst should be monitored. It should be recognized that the short bowel patient on PN remains at risk for micronutrient deficiencies and requires periodic monitoring and supplementation in addition to PN.[19,20]

Practice Scenario 30-2

Question: What is the most appropriate feeding route for a short bowel patient with severe malnutrition and failure to thrive who cannot or will not eat?

Scenario: A 20-year-old developmentally delayed woman was evaluated in the gastroenterology clinic for a failure to thrive. Anthropometric measurements are 160 cm, 31 kg, with a BMI of 12 kg per squared meter. She has a history of SBS following surgical resection of most of her small intestine due to complications occurring after an appendectomy 1 year ago, leaving her with approximately 80 cm of small intestine from the ligament of Treitz anastomosed to her ascending colon. She has been advised to eat a high calorie diet and include extra desserts and snacks to optimize weight gain; however, because of severe diarrhea, she has been avoiding all oral intake. Examination reveals a cachectic woman who appears much older than her stated age.

Intervention: She was admitted to the hospital where she was evaluated by the nutrition support service. PN was initiated along with the appropriate monitoring of electrolytes and hydration status. Both she and her family were educated on an appropriate short bowel diet and fluids. She was also begun on antidiarrheal and antisecretory agents, which decreased her stool output substantially. Nevertheless, she continued to refuse to eat for fear of worsening the diarrhea. It was decided by the team to also slowly initiate EN via gastrostomy tube.

Answer: PN is the most appropriate initial feeding route in this patient given the severity of her malnutrition and the severe diarrhea that has caused her to avoid oral nutritional intake. The addition of EN support may also be useful to facilitate bowel adaptation while the patient is avoiding oral intake and may eventually allow for an easier transition off the PN once the patient's overall condition has improved.

Rationale: PN may provide the entire energy, hydration, macronutrient, and micronutrient needs while the patient's bowel is undergoing adaptation and the oral diet and medical management program is being optimized. As the patient's symptoms and nutritional status improve, transitioning to an enteral and/or oral diet may allow for the eventual discontinuation of the PN support. In the scenario described, EN may be useful to facilitate bowel adaptation because the patient was refusing to eat. Bowel adaptation may occur over 2 or more years and the luminal nutrients provided by the EN are important for improving the mucosal structure and function. Concomitant EN support is unnecessary or can be discontinued if the patient is able to consume an adequate oral diet.

Intestinal Rehabilitation

Intestinal rehabilitation emphasizes strategies to reduce or eliminate the need for PN and intestinal transplantation.[38] The trade-off to the patient for not being on PN is the need to take several medications orally and to increase the amount of food and fluid ingested daily. Major lifestyle changes and increased out-of-pocket expenses are required on the part of the patient; consequently, patient education and ongoing support is important to enhance compliance with the care plan.

Table 30-4 lists a number of clinical factors considered useful in predicting the success of eliminating the use of PN in SBS patients.[39] It should be established from the outset whether the realistic goal is to reduce PN requirements or to completely eliminate PN. Diet, fluid intake, and medications (see the following) should be optimized before PN weaning begins. In addition, certain criteria should be met before reducing PN, including meeting the daily calorie and fluid intake goals established for the patient and frequent follow-up with subsequent reductions in PN based on tolerance as determined by the development of symptoms, stool and urine output, electrolyte and micronutrient levels, weight, and hydration status (Table 30-5).[20] Although an optimal interval for making PN reduction decisions has not been defined, once per week would seem appropriate while acknowledging that this needs to be individualized. PN reductions can be made by either decreasing the days that PN is infused per week or by decreasing the daily PN infusion volume equally throughout the week (eg, 10% reduction per day). Although the occasional patient may successfully discontinue PN without the gradual weaning strategy, this approach is not recommended for the SBS patient who has been receiving PN for an extended period of time.

Medications

Most medications are absorbed within the first 50 cm of the jejunum and can be used in patients with SBS; however, delayed-release medications should be avoided. The most important medications in the SBS patient are antimotility and antisecretory agents, which are frequently necessary to control stool losses. For reasons discussed previously, histamine type 2 receptor antagonists and proton pump inhibitors may be beneficial in reducing the volume of gastric secretions and the damaging effects of the excessive volume of low pH fluid on the upper gut mucosa and the function of digestive enzymes. Octreotide reduces the production of a variety of GI secretions and slows jejunal transit.[40] Open-label studies suggest a clinical

TABLE 30-4 Clinical Factors Predictive of Successful Weaning from Parenteral Nutrition

Length of the remaining bowel
Presence of a colon
Presence of an ileum/ileocecal valve
Absence of residual mucosal disease in the bowel
Degree to which intestinal adaptation has occurred
Patient age
Duration of time on parenteral nutrition
Nutritional status prior to attempted weaning parenteral nutrition
Fasting plasma citrulline level

TABLE 30-5 Criteria to Consider Before Weaning Parenteral Nutrition (PN)

Hydration: PN reductions should be considered only when the daily fluid intake goal is consistently achieved, urine output exceeds 1 L/day, and is at least 0.5 mL/kg/hr on nights without PN. If urine output cannot be easily measured, serum creatinine, blood urea nitrogen (BUN), urine sodium, and osmolarity can be used as surrogate measures of hydration.

Caloric goal: At least 80% of the caloric goal should be met in the absence of symptoms limiting oral intake.

Body weight: Patients should be able to maintain a stable body weight (ie, no more than 1.5 kg loss of body weight between PN reductions).

Labs: Stable serum electrolytes with or without supplementation.

Enteral balance (oral fluid intake minus stool output): Should be positive (at least 500 mL/day).

benefit of both short-acting and long-acting forms[41,42]; however, this beneficial effect is often short lasting and has not been shown to improve absorption or lead to the elimination of the need for PN. Due to an increased risk for cholelithiasis, expense, and the potential for octreotide to inhibit bowel adaptation, the use of this agent should be reserved for patients with large volume stool losses in whom fluid and electrolyte management is problematic and it should be avoided in the early adaptation stage.[43]

Antidiarrheals work mainly to reduce intestinal motility but also cause a slight reduction in intestinal secretion. Commonly used agents include loperamide, diphenoxylate, codeine, and a tincture of opium. The use of codeine and tincture of opium tends to be limited by their sedating effect, potential for addiction when used long-term, and cost. Loperamide and codeine may have a synergistic effect when used together.[44] Because loperamide enters the enterohepatic circulation, which is disrupted in SBS patients without an ileum, high doses are frequently needed. In the setting of SBS, these agents seem to be most effective when administered before meals and at bedtime. Clonidine, which can be administered transdermally, may also be useful to treat high output stool losses via its effects on intestinal motility and secretion.[45]

In an attempt to improve the depleted bile salt pool without aggravating stool losses, ox bile supplements and the synthetic conjugated bile acid, cholylsarcosine, have demonstrated improvements in fat absorption.[46,47] Unfortunately, these agents are not readily available for use at present. The use of bile acid sequestrants, such as cholestyramine, may actually worsen steatorrhea and fat-soluble vitamin losses in the SBS patient and should generally be avoided.[48] Pancreatic function is reduced in patients on PN only when there is no concomitant enteral/oral diet and, potentially, during the hypersecretory period if no antisecretory medications are being used. Although there may be concern about a mismatch of the timing of the mixing of ingested nutrients with pancreatic enzymes due to the alterations in anatomy and physiology, there is currently no evidence supporting the usefulness of pancreatic enzyme supplementation in SBS.

Trophic Factors

Trophic factors are pharmacologic agents developed with the intent to maximize intestinal absorption/adaptation with the goal of eliminating or at least minimizing the need for PN. Investigations in humans have focused on the use of trophic substances such as growth factors (eg, growth hormone [GH] and glucagonlike peptide-2 [GLP-2]) and nutrients (eg, glutamine). Glutamine is a "conditionally essential" amino acid that is a primary energy source for the enterocyte and has been shown to prevent mucosal atrophy and deterioration of gut permeability in patients receiving PN.[49] In a small, randomized, controlled, cross-over study in SBS, no difference in small bowel morphology, transit time, D-xylose absorption, or stool output was seen.[50] Nevertheless, a synergistic role of glutamine with GH has been suggested. In a recent prospective, randomized, controlled study of recombinant human GH and an optimized diet with or without glutamine in 41 PN-dependent SBS patients (most with colon-in-continuity), a significant reduction in PN requirements in all groups studied was seen at the end of the 4-week treatment period.[51] However, the extent of reduction was greatest in the group in which GH was administered in addition to the diet, and glutamine and the PN reduction remained significantly diminished in only the GH with the glutamine group 12 weeks later. An investigational GLP-2 analog was also shown in a very recent randomized, controlled study involving 81 SBS patients in which PN weaning was the primary end point to be safe, well tolerated, and significantly reduce PN requirements over the 6-month treatment period.[52] Although GH and glutamine are currently available for clinical use, the GLP-2 analog has yet to be U.S. Food and Drug Administration approved. The role of these agents in clinical practice remains to be defined.

Surgery

Because additional surgery is likely in many SBS patients, the goals of subsequent operations should be to preserve as much bowel as possible and maximize the function of the remaining bowel whenever possible. Examples of such operations include surgeries that restore intestinal continuity, relieve obstruction, repair a fistula, and eliminate diseased bowel. Autologous GI reconstruction refers to nontransplant surgical procedures that attempt to maximize the function of the SBS patient's existing intestine.[53] The choice of surgery is influenced by the existing bowel length, function, and caliber and can be divided into procedures that optimize function (eg, lengthen, taper) or slow transit (eg, reversed segment). These procedures should only be considered after the initial adaptive period and when the patient is stable and medical and dietary management has been maximized. Although there are encouraging results from case series, evidence of long-term success has not yet been documented.[54]

Intestinal transplantation may be considered in SBS patients with a lifelong need for PN when complications of PN such as liver disease, loss of venous access sites, or recurrent episodes of life-threatening catheter sepsis occur.[1,55] Small bowel transplantation (SBT) can be performed in isolation, in combination with liver transplantation, or in combination with transplantation of multiple organs. The outcome following intestinal transplantation has improved considerably with the development of more potent immunosuppressant medications and improvements in surgical techniques and postoperative care.[56] The SBT patient survival rates are beginning to approach those of liver transplant patients, particularly in those patients who are well enough to wait at home for their transplant.[56] Nevertheless, graft survival rates remain significantly lower than patient survival rates and a considerable percentage of patients with a functioning graft may still require PN.[56,57]

Complications and Monitoring

There are a number of problems related to the altered bowel anatomy that may complicate SBS (Table 30-6). Several of these complications have been described or referred to previously and several others will be discussed here. Although fluid and electrolyte problems are uncommon in the long-term home PN patient, they can still occur, particularly in patients with large enteric losses, and may result in difficult to replete hypokalemia, hypomagnesemia, and hypocalcemia. Patients with SBS should be instructed on the measurement of daily input and output because a periodic assessment of these parameters can help to guide fluid needs, with adequate hydration being based on a goal urine output of > 1 L per day and a urinary sodium concentration > 20 mEq per liter.[20] This becomes particularly useful in the patient who is being weaned from PN, as previously discussed. Serial weight measurements are also useful to track trends and serve as a warning of nutritional and/or hydrational compromise. Excessive urine output can be very disturbing to the SBS patient on PN, especially when occurring during nocturnal infusion, thus preventing a restful sleep. This is another reason to periodically monitor urine output and weight and review the PN formula. In this regard, a periodic assessment of the patient's overall functional status and quality of life is also recommended.

TABLE 30-6 Bowel-Related Complications in Short Bowel Syndrome

Malabsorptive diarrhea
Malnutrition
Fluid and electrolyte disturbances
Micronutrient deficiency
Essential fatty acid deficiency
Small bowel bacterial overgrowth
D-lactic acidosis
Oxalate nephropathy
Renal dysfunction
Metabolic bone disease
Acid peptic disease
Anastomotic ulceration/stricture
Bowel obstruction

Hypomagnesemia occurs as a consequence of secondary hyperaldosteronism, which results from the loss of the magnesium-absorbing gut, the binding of magnesium by unabsorbed fatty acids, and sodium/water depletion that increases urinary magnesium losses. This can become a difficult problem to correct orally.[1] Hypomagnesemia may lead to hypocalcemia as a result of impaired PTH release.[58] The correction of sodium depletion is critical in treating hypomagnesemia. Measurement of urinary sodium may assist in the assessment of sodium balance in some patients; a random urinary sodium concentration of < 10 mEq per liter is generally a good indicator of sodium depletion. Oral magnesium oxide can be administered in doses of 12 to 24 mEq per day and does not appear to increase stomal output, particularly when taken at night when intestinal transit is at its slowest. Finally, the oral administration of 1α-hydroxycholecalciferol may be useful because it can increase both intestinal absorption and renal absorption of magnesium.[59] If moderate to severe hypomagnesemia (< 1 mg per deciliter) persists, parenteral magnesium may be necessary. In stable SBS patients on PN, an assessment of electrolytes at least every 3 months is suggested.

Micronutrient monitoring and supplementation is important in all SBS patients and becomes necessary as PN is weaned. The frequency of monitoring will depend on the stage of PN weaning and the presence of existing or prior deficiencies.[20] In the stable SBS patient on or off PN, a semiannual assessment of micronutrients and essential fatty acids is advised. Because water-soluble vitamins are absorbed in the proximal small bowel, deficiencies in SBS patients are uncommon. In contrast, fat-soluble vitamin and essential fatty acid deficiencies are more commonly encountered. Supplemental zinc, and occasionally selenium, may be required in the presence of excessive stool losses. Iron supplementation is infrequently needed because it is absorbed in the upper GI tract, an uncommon site of resection in SBS patients. The lifetime administration of supplemental vitamin B12, usually administered subcutaneously on a monthly basis, is needed in those with more than 50 to 60 cm of the terminal ileum removed.[60]

A spectrum of metabolic bone disease including osteomalacia, osteoporosis, osteopenia, and secondary hyperparathyroidism may occur in SBS patients as a consequence of the effects of the PN, altered bowel anatomy, and other underlying patient factors. An assessment of bone density should be undertaken in all SBS patients regardless of the need of PN and repeated every 2 to 3 years, or annually in the osteoporotic. The identification of significant bone disease should lead to an assessment of calcium, phosphorus, magnesium, vitamin D (25-hydroxy vitamin D), and PTH status, and for the presence of metabolic acidosis. In patients receiving PN, an assessment of the PN formula and additives is warranted. The conventional management includes exercise, sunlight exposure, minimizing alcohol use, and eliminating tobacco use. Calcium, magnesium, and vitamin D replacement and the correction of metabolic acidosis should be provided as needed. Given the very poor bioavailability of bisphosphonates, only intravenous agents should be considered in the setting of SBS.[61]

The development of small intestinal bacterial overgrowth (SIBO) appears to be common in SBS patients and may affect their ability to successfully wean PN because of symptoms that impede oral intake and an exacerbation of malabsorption.[62]

The anatomic and physiologic changes that occur in SBS together with medications commonly used in these patients facilitate the development of SIBO. Oral broad-spectrum antimicrobial treatment is generally prescribed with success being judged by an improvement in symptoms, a reduction in stool output, and/or weight gain. The continuous use of low-dose antibiotics in SBS may be necessary. To reduce the risk of antibiotic resistance, a periodic rotation of the antibiotic used is advised in this situation.

Outcomes

Although SBS is clearly uncommon, it remains an important clinical problem due to its associated morbidity and mortality and the high costs involved in its care.[4] Quality of life has been shown to be worse in home PN patients, many of whom had SBS, compared to SBS patients not requiring PN.[63] With respect to survival, studies from France and the United States have demonstrated 2-year and 5-year survival rates for SBS at over 80% and 70%, respectively.[64,65] Furthermore, the study from France reported the PN dependency at 2 years of 49% and 45% at 5 years.[65] The length of the remaining bowel is closely linked to both the probability of regaining nutritional autonomy and survival.[34,66] Most SBS patients on PN will be able to discontinue PN within 2 years; those that are unable to wean PN completely during this time are unlikely to ever discontinue PN support.[34] In adult short bowel patients, a remnant small bowel length of < 100 cm was found to be highly predictive of permanent intestinal failure.[66] Survival was inversely correlated to the presence of an end-jejunostomy and a remnant small bowel length of < 50 cm. Cut-off values for remnant small bowel lengths separating transient from permanent intestinal failure/PN dependence were 100, 65, and 30 cm in end-jejunostomy, jejunocolic, and jejunoileocolic bowel anatomies, respectively. These results underscore the important contributions provided by the colon and distal ileum with regard to both weaning from PN and survival. Indeed, it has been suggested that, in terms of need for PN, the presence of at least half of the colon is equivalent to about 50 cm of small bowel.[67] Other factors shown to affect survival in SBS patients on or off PN include the patient's age, the primary disease process, comorbid diseases, the presence of chronic intestinal obstruction, and the experience of the team managing the patient.[5]

References

1. Buchman AL, Scolapio J, Fryer J. AGA technical review on short bowel syndrome and intestinal transplantation. *Gastroenterology.* 2003;124:1111–1134.
2. Vanderhoof JA, Langnas AN. Short-bowel syndrome in children and adults. *Gastroenterology.* 1997;113:1767–1778.
3. Dabney A, Thompson J, DiBaise J, et al. Short bowel syndrome after trauma. *Am J Surg.* 2004;188:792–795.
4. Howard L, Ament M, Fleming CR, et al. Current use and clinical outcome of home parenteral and enteral nutrition therapies in the United States. *Gastroenterology.* 1995;109:355–365.
5. Carbonnel F, Cosnes J, Chevret S, et al. The role of anatomic factors in nutritional autonomy after extensive small bowel resection. *J Parenter Enteral Nutr.* 1996;20:275–280.
6. Williams NS, Evans P, King RF. Gastric acid secretion and gastrin production in the short bowel syndrome. *Gut.* 1985;26:914–919.
7. Cortot A, Fleming CR, Malagelada JR. Improved nutrient absorption after cimetidine in short-bowel syndrome with gastric hypersecretion. *N Engl J Med.* 1979;11(300):79–80.
8. Borgstrom B, Daalq A, Lundh G, Sjovall J. Studies of intestinal digestion and absorption in the human. *J Clin Invest.* 1957;36: 1521–1536.
9. Fordtran JS, Rector FC Jr, Carter NW. The mechanisms of sodium absorption in the human small intestine. *J Clin Invest.* 1968;47: 884–900.
10. Nightingale JM, Kamm MA, van der Sijp JR, et al. Gastrointestinal hormones in short bowel syndrome. Peptide YY may be the 'colonic brake' to gastric emptying. *Gut.* 1996;39:267–272.
11. Fich A, Steadman CJ, Phillips SF, et al. Ileocolonic transit does not change after right hemicolectomy. *Gastroenterology.* 1992;103: 794–799.
12. Debongnie JC, Phillips SF. Capacity of the colon to absorb fluid. *Gastroenterology.* 1978;74:698–703.
13. Pironi L, Stanghellini V, Miglioli, et al. Fat-induced ileal brake in humans: a dose-dependent phenomenon correlated to plasma levels of peptide YY. *Gastroenterology.* 1993;105:733–739.
14. Nordgaard I, Hansen BS, Mortensen PB. Importance of colonic support for energy absorption as small bowel failure proceeds. *Am J Clin Nutr.* 1996;64:222–231.
15. Williamson RCN, Chir M. Intestinal adaptation: structural, functional and cytokinetic changes. *N Engl J Med.* 1978;298:1393–1402.
16. Thiesen A, Drozdowski L, Iordache C, et al. Adaptation following intestinal resection: mechanisms and signals. *Best Pract Res Clin Gastroenterol.* 2003;17:981–995.
17. Thompson JS, Ferguson DC. Effect of the distal remnant on ileal adaptation. *J Gastrointest Surg.* 2000;4:430–434.
18. Nightingale JM, Bartram CI, Lennard-Jones JE. Length of residual small bowel after partial resection: correlation between radiographic and surgical measurements. *Gastrointest Radiol.* 1991;16: 305–306.
19. Parrish CR. The clinician's guide to short bowel syndrome. *Pract Gastroenterol.* 2005;29(9)67–106.
20. DiBaise JK, Matarese LE, Messing B, Steiger E. Strategies for weaning parenteral nutrition in adult patients with short bowel syndrome. *J Clin Gastroenterol.* 2006; 40(Suppl):S94–S98.
21. Matarese LE, Steiger E. Dietary and medical management of short bowel syndrome in adult patients. *J Clin Gastroenterol.* 2006; 40(Suppl):S85–S93.
22. Pullan JM. Massive intestinal resection. *Proc R Soc Med.* 1959;52: 31–37.
23. Byrne TA, Veglia L, Camelio M, et al. Beyond the prescription: optimizing the diet of patients with short bowel syndrome. *Nutr Clin Pract.* 2000;15:306–311.
24. McIntyre PB, Fitchew M, Lennard-Jones JE. Patients with a high jejunostomy do not need a special diet. *Gastroenterology.* 1986;91: 25–33.
25. Norgaard I, Hansen BS, Mortensen PB. Colon as a digestive organ in patients with short bowel. *Lancet.* 1994;343:373–376.
26. Marteau P, Messing B, Arrigoni E, et al. Do short bowel patients need a lactose-free diet? *Nutrition.* 1997;13:13–16.
27. Jeppesen PB, Mortensen PB. The influence of a preserved colon on the absorption of medium chain fat in patients with small bowel resection. *Gut.* 1998;43:478–483.
28. Jeppesen PB, Howy CE, Mortensen PB. Deficiencies of essential fatty acids, vitamin A and E and changes in plasma lipoproteins in patients with reduced fat absorption or intestinal failure. *Eur J Clin Nutr.* 2000;54:632–642.

29. Lin R, Murtazina R, Cha B, et al. D-glucose acts via sodium/glucose cotransporter 1 to increase NHE3 in mouse jejunal brush border by a Na+/H+ exchange regulatory factor 2-dependent process. *Gastroenterology.* 2011;140:560–571.
30. Matarese LE, O'Keefe SJ, Kandil HM, et al. Short bowel syndrome: clinical guidelines for nutrition management. *Nutr Clin Pract.* 2005;20:493–502.
31. Kelly DG, Nadeau J. Oral rehydration solution: a "low-tech" oft neglected therapy. *Nutr Issues Gastroenterol.* 2004;28:51–62.
32. Sladen GE, Dawson AM. Inter-relationships between the absorptions of glucose, sodium and water by the normal human jejunum. *Clin Sci.* 1969;36:119–132.
33. Rodrigues CA, Lennard-Jones JE, Thompson DG, Farthing MJG. What is the ideal sodium concentration of oral rehydration solutions for short bowel patients. *Clin Sci.* 1988;74:69.
34. Nightingale JM, Lennard-Jones JE, Walker ER, Farthing MJ. Oral salt supplements to compensate for jejunostomy losses: comparison of sodium chloride capsules, glucose electrolyte solution, and glucose polymer electrolyte solution. *Gut.* 1992;33:759–761.
35. Joly F, Dray X, Corcos O, et al. Tube feeding improves intestinal absorption in short bowel syndrome patients. *Gastroenterology.* 2009;136:824–831.
36. Noridian Administrative Services LLC. TPN Decision Tree. https://www.noridianmedicare.com/dme/coverage/docs/trees/tpn_policy_decision_tree.pdf%3fd. Accessed June 25, 2011.
37. DiBaise JK, Scolapio JS. Home parenteral and enteral nutrition. *Gastroenterol Clin N Am.* 2007;36:123–144.
38. DiBaise JK, Young RJ, Vanderhoof JA. Intestinal rehabilitation and the short bowel syndrome: part 2. *Am J Gastroenterol.* 2004;99: 1823–1832.
39. Messing B, Crenn P, Beau P, et al. Long-term survival and parenteral nutrition dependence in adult patients with the short bowel syndrome. *Gastroenterology.* 1999;117:1043–1050.
40. Ladefofed K, Christensen KC, Hegnhoj J, Jarnum S. Effect of a long-acting somatostatin analogue SMS 201-995 on jejunostomy effluents in patients with severe short bowel syndrome. *Gut.* 1989;30:943–949.
41. Nehra V, Camilleri M, Burton D, et al. An open trial of octreotide long-acting release in the management of short bowel syndrome. *Am J Gastroenterol.* 2001;96:1494–1498.
42. O'Keefe SJD, Haymond MW, Bennet WM, et al. Long-acting somatostatin analogue therapy and protein metabolism in patients with jejunostomies. *Gastroenterology.* 1994;107:379–388.
43. Sukhotnik I, Khateeb K, Krausz MM, et al. Sandostatin impairs postresection intestinal adaptation in a rat model of short bowel syndrome. *Dig Dis Sci.* 2002;47:2095–2102.
44. King RF, Norton T, Hill GL. A double-blind crossover study of the effect of loperamide hydrochloride and codeine phosphate on ileostomy output. *Aust N Z J Surg.* 1982;52:121–124.
45. Buchman AL, Fryer J, Wallin A, et al. Clonidine reduces diarrhea and sodium loss in patients with proximal jejunostomy: a controlled study. *JPEN J Parenter Enteral Nutr.* 2006;30(6):487–491.
46. Little KH, Schiller LR, Bilhartz LE, Fordtran JS. Treatment of severe steatorrhea with ox bile in an ileectomy patient with residual colon. *Dig Dis Sci.* 1992;37:929–933.
47. Heydorn S, Jeppesen PB, Mortensen PB. Bile acid replacement therapy with cholylsarcosine for short-bowel syndrome. *Scand J Gastroenterol.* 1999;34:818–823.
48. Hoffman AF, Poley R. Role of bile acid malabsorption in pathogenesis of diarrhea and steatorrhea in patients with ileal resection. *Gastroenterology.* 1972;62:918–934.
49. van der Hulst RR, van Kreel BK, von Meyenfeldt MF, et al. Glutamine and the preservation of gut integrity. *Lancet.* 1993;341: 1363–1365.
50. Scolapio JS, McGreevy K, Tennyson GS, Burnett OL. Effect of glutamine in short-bowel syndrome. *Clin Nutr.* 2001;20:319–323.
51. Byrne TA, Wilmore DW, Iyer K, et al. Growth hormone, glutamine and an optimal diet reduces parenteral nutrition in patients with short bowel syndrome. A prospective, randomized, placebo-controlled, double-blind clinical trial. *Ann Surg.* 2005;242: 655–661.
52. Jeppesen PB, Gilroy R, Pertkiewicz M, et al. Randomised placebo-controlled trial of teduglutide in reducing parenteral nutrition and/or intravenous fluid requirements in patients with short bowel syndrome. *Gut.* 2011;60:902–914.
53. Thompson JS. Strategies for preserving intestinal length in the short bowel syndrome. *Dis Col Rectum.* 1987;30:208–213.
54. Sudan D, DiBaise J, Torres C, et al. A multidisciplinary approach to the treatment of intestinal failure. *J Gastrointest Surg.* 2005;9: 165–176.
55. Mazariegos GV, Steffick DE, Horslen S, et al. Intestine transplantation in the United States, 1999–2008. *Am J Transplant.* 2010; 10(4 Pt 2):1020–1034.
56. Grant D, Abu-Elmagd K, Reyes J, et al. 2003 report of the intestine transplant registry: a new era has dawned. *Ann Surg.* 2005;241: 607–613.
57. Rovera GM, Schoen RE, Goldbach B, et al. Intestinal and multivisceral transplantation: dynamics of nutritional management and functional autonomy. *J Parenter Enter Nutr.* 2003;27: 252–259.
58. Anast CS, Winnacker JL, Forte LR, Burns TW. Impaired release of parathyroid hormone in magnesium deficiency. *Clin Endocrinol Metab.* 1976;42:707–717.
59. Fukumoto S, Matsumoto T, Tanaka Y, et al. Renal magnesium wasting in a patient with short bowel syndrome with magnesium deficiency: effect of 1 alpha-hydroxyvitamin D3 treatment. *J Clin Endocrinol Metab.* 1987;65:1201–1204.
60. Booth CC. The effects of intestinal resection in man. *Postgrad Med J.* 1961;37:725–739.
61. Haderslev KV, Jiellesen L, Sorensen HA, et al. Effect of cyclical intravenous clodronate therapy on bone mineral density and markers of bone turnover in patients receiving home parenteral nutrition. *Am J Clin Nutr.* 2002;76:482–488.
62. DiBaise JK, Young RJ, Vanderhoof JA. Enteric microbial flora, bacterial overgrowth and short bowel syndrome. *Clin Gastroenterol Hepatol.* 2006;4:11–20.
63. Jeppesen PB, Langholz E, Mortensen PB. Quality of life in patients receiving home parenteral nutrition. *Gut.* 1999;44:844–852.
64. Scolapio JS, Fleming CR, Kelly DG, et al. Survival of home parenteral nutrition-treated patients: 20 years of experience at the Mayo Clinic. *Mayo Clin Proc.* 1999;74:217–222.
65. Messing B, Lemann M, Landais P, et al. Prognosis of patients with nonmalignant chronic intestinal failure receiving long-term home parenteral nutrition. *Gastroenterology.* 1995;108:1005–1010.
66. Jeppesen PB, Mortensen PB. Significance of a preserved colon for parenteral energy requirements in patients receiving home parenteral nutrition. *Scand J Gastroenterol.* 1998;33:1175–1179.
67. Nightingale JMD, Lennard-Jones JE, Gertner DJ, et al. Colonic preservation reduces the need for parenteral therapy, increases the incidence of renal stones but does not change the high prevalence of gallstones in patients with a short bowel. *Gut.* 1992;33: 1493–1497.

31 Solid Organ Transplantation

Jeanette M. Hasse, PhD, RD, LD, FADA, CNSC, and Laura E. Matarese, PhD, RD, LDN, FADA, CNSC

CONTENTS

Transplantation 524
Prevalence of Organ Transplantation 524
Indications for Organ Transplantation 524
Contraindications for Organ Transplantation 524
Immunosuppression 524
Phases of Transplantation 526
Pretransplant Phase 526
Acute Posttransplant Phase 527
Chronic Posttransplant Phase 528
Metabolic Aberrations Associated with Organ Transplantation 528
Glucose Alterations 528
Lipid Alterations 529
Protein Alterations 529
Determining Nutrition Status 529
Nutrient Requirements 529
Energy 529
Protein 530
Fluid 530
Micronutrients 530
Selecting a Nutrition Support Route 530
Transplant Complications 530
Nutrition Monitoring 533
Summary 534
References 534

Objectives

1. Identify indications and contraindications for organ transplantation.
2. Differentiate nutrition goals of the pre- and posttransplant phases.
3. Evaluate nutrition alterations associated with patients who have undergone organ transplantation.
4. Assess nutrition implications of immunosuppression.
5. Illustrate how posttransplant complications influence nutrient needs and options for the delivery of nutrition support.

Test Your Knowledge Questions

1. Which of the following is a contraindication for organ transplantation?
   A. Severe malnutrition
   B. End-stage organ failure
   C. Active infection
   D. History of substance abuse

2. Which of the following immunosuppressive agents is nephrotoxic and can cause hyperkalemia, hypomagnesemia, and hyperglycemia?
   A. Sirolimus
   B. Prednisone
   C. Tacrolimus
   D. Mycophenolate mofetil
3. Which of the following best describes nutrient requirements during the acute posttransplant phase?
   A. Moderate calories, high protein
   B. High calories, low protein
   C. Moderate calories, low protein
   D. High calories, high protein
4. Which of the following should be part of a nutrition care plan for a patient during an acute rejection episode that is being treated with high-dose corticosteroids?
   A. Provide increased amounts of dietary carbohydrate and monitor for signs of fluid overload.
   B. Provide increased amounts of dietary fat and monitor for signs of hyperlipidemia.
   C. Provide increased amounts of dietary carbohydrate and monitor for signs of azotemia.
   D. Provide increased amounts of dietary protein and monitor for signs of hyperglycemia.

Test Your Knowledge Answers

1. The correct answer is C. A significant, active infection such as pneumonia is likely to worsen after transplantation once immunosuppression is initiated. Malnutrition is a complication of serious organ failure; it is difficult to reverse without normal organ function. End-stage organ failure is not amenable to further medical or surgical treatment, but is an indication for transplantation. Finally, although active substance abuse is a contraindication for transplantation, transplantation may be considered if a candidate has demonstrated recovery.
2. The correct answer is C. In addition to these side effects, tacrolimus may also cause neurologic symptoms. Sirolimus may cause hyperlipidemia. Corticosteroids, such as prednisone, contribute to hyperglycemia but are not nephrotoxic and do not affect serum magnesium levels. The major nutrition-related side effect of mycophenolate mofetil is diarrhea.
3. The correct answer is A. Caloric needs are only moderately elevated after transplantation unless complications such as sepsis occur. Protein requirements are significantly elevated due to an increased catabolic rate caused by surgery, stress, and corticosteroids. Adequate micronutrients are required because stores may be depleted.
4. The correct answer is D. Because corticosteroids accelerate protein catabolic rate, it is essential to provide adequate protein to reduce nitrogen loss. Hyperglycemia is also a common side effect of high-dose corticosteroids. Hyperlipidemia is a long-term side effect of corticosteroids but is not usually a short-term complication.

Transplantation

Prevalence of Organ Transplantation

The field of organ transplantation continues to expand as the number of transplants performed increases each year, new medical advances are achieved, and the survival rate of recipients improves. Transplantation of organs such as the kidney, liver, pancreas, heart, lung, and intestine give recipients a second chance at life. According to the United Network of Organ Sharing (UNOS), the number of organ transplants increased from 15,001 in 1990 to 28,662 in 2010.[1] As of June 2011, there were 324 transplant centers in the United States and over 111,600 individuals waiting for transplants.[1] There is a limited supply of deceased donor organs, so the number of living donors has increased from 32% of donors in 1990 to 45% in 2010. Unfortunately, the number of individuals waiting for organ transplantation continues to exceed the number of those who undergo transplantation.

Indications for Organ Transplantation

Organ transplantation is indicated for individuals with decompensated end-stage organ failure. For recipients of liver, heart, and lung transplants, transplantation is lifesaving. Dialysis, insulin therapy, and parenteral nutrition (PN) are alternative treatments for patients with renal, pancreas, and intestinal failure. Some patients with these ailments may develop life-threatening complications such as loss of dialysis or PN intravenous (IV) access. For these patients, the benefits of transplantation must outweigh the risks of continuing medical therapy, the surgical procedure, and long-term immunosuppression. In addition, transplantation should be expected to result in a longer lifetime for a transplant recipient than for patients without a transplant.

Contraindications for Organ Transplantation

Not all individuals with organ failure are transplant candidates. Contraindications for transplantation include active or latent infection, sepsis, malignancy (some primary liver malignancies that are confined to the liver are acceptable for liver transplantation), multisystem organ failure, active substance abuse, advanced age, active psychiatric or psychological pathology, lack of any social support posttransplant, or other systemic illnesses with a poor prognosis.

Immunosuppression

The introduction of effective immunosuppressive drugs revolutionized the field of transplantation and allowed for prolonged patient and graft survival. There are multiple immunosuppressive medications that can be used in combination to prevent and treat rejection. Some side effects of these drugs may affect nutrient intake or use (Table 31-1).

TABLE 31-1 Immunosuppressive Medications, Nutrition Side Effects, and Interventions

Drug	Action	Nutrition Side Effects	Suggested Nutrition Therapy
Anti-thymocyte globulin (ATG), anti-lymphocyte globulin (ALG)	• Binds with lymphocytes, resulting in phagocytosis • Inhibits and destroys lymphocytes	• Fever and chills • Increased risk of infection, profound leukopenia, thrombocytopenia	• Provide nutrient-dense foods patient will eat • Monitor intake and ensure patient is receiving adequate nutrition
Basiliximab	• Acts against the IL-2R-alpha chain (CD25) on activated T-lymphocytes, and inhibits IL-2–mediated activation of lymphocytes	• None reported	
Corticosteroids	• Have anti-inflammatory properties • Inhibit cell-mediated and, to a lesser degree, humoral immunity • Inhibit lymphocyte proliferation • Inhibit lymphokine production	• Hyperglycemia • Sodium retention • Osteoporosis • Hyperphagia • Impaired wound healing and increased infection risk • Hypertension	• Monitor blood sugar and need for long-term carbohydrate-controlled diet and hypoglycemic agents • Avoid high-sodium foods • Ensure adequate calcium and vitamin D intake; consider need for bone-rebuilding medications • Behavior modification to prevent overeating • Ensure adequate protein intake; consider need for vitamin or mineral supplementation; achieve good glucose control • Avoid high-sodium foods, maintain a healthy weight
Cyclosporine	• Inhibits cell-mediated immunity; inhibits T-cell proliferation • Suppresses IL-2 production • Prevents γ-IFN release	• Hyperkalemia • Hypomagnesemia • Hypertension • Hyperglycemia • Hyperlipidemia	• Restrict high-potassium foods • Supplement with high-magnesium foods or supplements • Avoid high-sodium foods, maintain a healthy weight • Monitor blood sugar and need for long-term carbohydrate-controlled diet and hypoglycemic agents (see Chapter 34) • Limit fat and simple carbohydrate intake during long-term phase; maintain a healthy weight
Sirolimus	• Blocks the response of T- and B-cell activation by cytokines, which prevent cell-cycle progression and proliferation	• Hyperlipidemia • Gastrointestinal disorders (constipation, diarrhea, nausea/vomiting, dyspepsia)	• Limit fat and simple carbohydrate intake during long-term phase; maintain healthy weight • Monitor for adequate nutrient intake
Tacrolimus	• Suppresses T-cell–mediated immunity and IL-2 production	• Nausea, vomiting • Hyperkalemia • Hyperglycemia • Abdominal distress	• Try antiemetic medications; if vomiting does not subside, consider nutrition support • Avoid high-potassium foods • Monitor blood sugar and need for long-term carbohydrate-controlled diet and hypoglycemic agents • Monitor oral intake; consider alternate methods of nutrition support if intake is suboptimal
Mycophenolate mofetil, mycophenolic acid	• Inhibits DNA synthesis and mixed lymphocyte production • Inhibits antibody formation	• Diarrhea, nausea, vomiting	• Review drugs and substitute for those that may be causing diarrhea; make sure that patient is receiving adequate fluid to replace losses

IL, interleukin; IFN, interferon. Adapted with permission from Hasse JM. Solid organ transplantation. In: Matarese LE, Gottschlich MM, eds. *Contemporary Nutrition Support Practice: A Clinical Guide,* 2nd ed. Philadelphia, PA: WB Saunders; 2003:560–573.

Phases of Transplantation

There are three main phases of transplantation: pretransplant, acute posttransplant, and chronic posttransplant. Each phase is characterized by its own medical and nutrition goals.

Pretransplant Phase

The main goal of the pretransplant phase is to optimize the patient's condition to allow transplantation to be performed. One aspect of managing symptoms of end-stage organ failure is to provide appropriate medications to manage symptoms. Surgery or interventional procedures may be required; examples include placement of vascular shunts (to treat complications of portal hypertension) or ventricular assistance devices.

There are three major nutrition goals during the pretransplant phase. First, the patient's nutrition status must be maintained or improved. Many patients awaiting transplantation are malnourished.[2-3] Malnourished patients tend to have increased rates of posttransplant morbidity and mortality as well as increased hospital durations compared with well-nourished recipients.[2-5,7,12-14] Practice Scenario 31-1 highlights the cause and treatment of pretransplant malnutrition.

Pretransplant obesity also affects posttransplant outcomes. Obese kidney transplant recipients tend to have more wound complications compared with nonobese transplant recipients.[5-6] In kidney transplant recipients, some studies suggest that obesity is associated with delayed kidney graft function[7-8] or decreased graft survival.[21,27-29] However, other reports have not shown that obesity affects kidney graft survival.[16,18,20,24-26,28,30,10-11] In lung transplant recipients, obesity is also associated with an increased rate of posttransplant mortality.[15,12] In liver transplant recipients, obesity does not appear to affect graft function but may be associated with delayed wound healing, prolonged ventilatory requirements, and increased posttransplant infection rates.[13-14] One study that evaluated graft and patient survival in 23,675 liver transplants performed during a 9-year period from the UNOS database showed that obesity results in reduced long-term survival, mainly as a result of cardiovascular events.[15] Another study evaluating UNOS data in over 73,000 liver transplant patients concluded that body weight extremes (BMI <18.5 or ≥40 kg per square meter) affect survival.[16] Likewise, a study of 5978 lung transplant recipients concluded that being underweight or overweight affects patient outcomes.[17] However, in both obese kidney and liver transplant recipients, transplantation seems to confer a survival benefit when compared with waiting list mortality.[18,19] Recommendations are generally to encourage weight loss in obese patients waiting for a transplant, to closely evaluate cardiovascular status in obese patients before transplantation, and to consider corticosteroid-withdrawal strategies after transplantation to reduce weight gain.[20]

Second, appropriate nutrition therapy may help alleviate complications due to organ failure. For example, sodium restriction will help reduce fluid retention, potassium restriction treats hyperkalemia, and calcium and vitamin D supplementation may be necessary to prevent bone loss. Refer to Chapters on Pulmonary Failure, Liver Disease, Renal Disease, Short Bowel Syndrome, and Diabetes Mellitus (25, 27, 29, 30, 34) for specific guidelines on medical nutrition therapy for each disease state. See Practice Scenario 31-2 for an example of nutrition support required before small bowel transplantation.

A third pretransplant nutrition goal (often out of the control of the transplant team) is to provide nutrition to the donor. The effect of feeding is probably prominent in liver transplantation due to the liver's role in glycogen and ATP storage. With the increasing number of living donor transplants, nutrition may be important to the outcomes of living donor transplants. In at least one report,[21] short-term weight loss (mean of 5.9 ± 2% body weight) in nine living liver donors reduced the degree of steatosis (from 48.9 ± 25.6% to 20.0 ± 16.2% fat) allowing for successful liver donation. In a large retrospective study of the UNOS database evaluating outcomes from 23,303 patients, neither donor obesity nor moderate steatosis affected outcomes after liver transplantation.[22]

Practice Scenario 31-1

Question: What causes malnutrition pretransplant and how is it treated?

Scenario: A 55-year-old male with ischemic cardiomyopathy is awaiting heart transplantation. His condition deteriorates, requiring admission to a cardiac intensive care unit (ICU). He receives continuous IV infusions of milrinone and dobutamine. He is upgraded to Status IA (highest priority) for a heart transplant. The patient has experienced a loss of 15% of his usual body weight over a 4 to 6 month period due to anorexia and persistent nausea. However, he has recently gained 10 lb. due to fluid retention. His serum sodium level is132 mEq/L (normal range: 135 to 145 mEq/L) and his potassium level is 3.4 mEq/L (normal range: 3.5 to 5 mEq/L).

Intervention: A 2-g sodium diet is prescribed. A calorie count indicates that he is eating approximately 900 kcal and 40 g protein per day. His needs are estimated to be 2000 kcal and 85 g protein per day. High-calorie, high-protein oral supplements are ordered but he is unable to improve his oral intake. A nasointestinal tube is placed and a 2 kcal/mL formula is initiated at 20 mL per hour continuously. Serum levels of potassium, magnesium, and phosphorus are ordered daily.

Answer: The cause of malnutrition in a transplant candidate is multifactorial. It can be caused by reduced intake (due to anorexia, early satiety, nausea and vomiting, taste changes, poor dentition, limited food availability, severe diet restrictions), increased needs (due to acute or chronic illness), or malabsorption. In this case, the patient was unable to eat adequately despite providing additional food choices and supplements. A postpyloric feeding tube was chosen because of history of nausea and vomiting. A sodium restriction and concentrated tube feeding formula was chosen because of the fluid retention and mild hyponatremia. Because the patient was malnourished, refeeding syndrome was suspected, so the tube feeding was advanced slowly and electrolyte levels were supplemented if low.

Rationale: Patients with end-stage organ failure have many risk factors that can cause malnutrition. Early identification and treatment of these factors can help prevent nutrition deterioration. Aggressive nutrition interventions are warranted considering the adverse effect malnutrition can have on posttransplant outcomes.

Treatment of nutrition-related conditions (such as fluid retention, hyponatremia, and refeeding syndrome in this scenario) helps keep patients in an optimal condition for transplant.

Practice Scenario 31-2

Question: What is the nutrition goal during the preoperative phase of a patient undergoing intestinal transplantation?

Scenario: A 45-year-old male has short bowel syndrome secondary to small bowel volvulus with resulting ischemia necessitating resection of the majority of the intestine. He has 40 cm of remaining small bowel ending in a jejunostomy. He has been receiving PN for 16 months, and has had several line-related infections with multiple new lines replaced. He also has hepatitis C, PN-associated liver disease, cirrhosis, and severe jaundice. The pretransplant liver biopsy demonstrated steatohepatitis, hepatitis C, and portal pericellular and bridging fibrosis.

Physical Exam: Upon examination, the patient is severely jaundiced and exhibits moderate-to-severe muscle wasting and deficits of adipose tissue. There is no lymphadenopathy. The chest is clear to auscultation bilaterally. The abdomen shows splenomegaly. The liver is felt off the costal margin, and is irregular and slightly firm. There are normal bowel sounds. Extremities are without edema. His height is 182.9 cm and he weighs 67 kg upon referral. His serum laboratory values are as follows.

Laboratory test	Level (Normal level)
Total bilirubin	15.3 mg/dL (0.1–1.9)
Alanine aminotransferase (ALT)	559 IU/L (8–37)
Aspartate aminotransferase (AST)	438 IU/L (10–34)
Alkaline phosphatase	149 IU/L (44–147)
Gamma-glutamyl transpeptidase (GGT)	160 IU/L (0–51)
Albumin	3.4 g/dL (3.9–5.0)
Sodium	137 mEq/L (136–144)
Potassium	4.3 mEq/L (3.7–5.2)
Chloride	101 mEq/L (3.7–5.2)
Carbon dioxide	27 mmol/L (20–29)
Glucose	88 mg/dL (65–110)
Blood urea nitrogen (BUN)	27 mg/dL (7–20)

Intervention: The patient's ostomy output is >4 L per day. Four liters of PN were infused over 12 hours at night and an additional 2 L of normal saline are infused during the day. Dextrose and amino acids are supplied as 275 g and 100 g, respectively. The lipid component is dosed at 100 g per week. Vitamins and trace elements are customized based on measured serum values. The preoperative dual-energy X-ray absorptiometry test reveals osteoporosis, and IV bisphosphonates are started. Additional calcium and phosphorus is added to the PN solution.

Answer: The goal during the preoperative state is to optimize nutrition status, preserve or improve hepatic and renal function, and to keep the patient free from infection until organs become available.[40,41] As a result, the PN formula was designed to provide adequate hydration to preserve renal function, and the macronutrient portion of the PN was designed to minimize the deleterious effects on the liver. All micronutrients were corrected based on serum values.

Rationale: Following transplantation, recipients must take high doses of immunosuppressants and other nephrotoxic drugs. Therefore, it is important to prevent damage to the kidney in the preoperative phase. It is also important to minimize any damage to the liver so that the patient does not go into liver failure before the organs become available. In some cases, the liver damage may be able to be reversed and the patient may be able to be transplanted with an isolated small bowel.

Acute Posttransplant Phase

Immunosuppression must achieve a delicate balance to prevent rejection and infection. Most acute rejections occur within the first 3 months after transplantation. It is during this phase that infection is most common. For this reason, laboratory markers and physical signs of rejection and infection are monitored closely.

The main nutrition goals of the acute posttransplant phase are to establish adequate nutrient intake to replete lost nutrient stores, provide substrate to support the body's ability to fight infection, heal anastomoses and surgical wounds, and supply energy to allow a patient to participate in physical rehabilitation and activities of daily living.

There are some unique considerations for those patients undergoing small bowel transplants because it is the organ responsible for digestion and absorption that is being transplanted. The protocols for nutrition management used to achieve this transition vary among transplant centers. The nutrition aspects of care have changed over the years as the surgical techniques have evolved and experience has been gained in the care of these unique patients. Nutrient, fluid, and electrolyte requirements are met through a stepwise progression of transitions from PN to an oral diet. This transition occurs fairly rapidly after the surgery, but is individualized for each patient. PN is reinstituted in the early postoperative phase to support the patient until the allograft is functional. However, the PN prescription changes dramatically from the prescription used during the preoperative phase. The patient no longer requires the large volumes of PN that were necessary to maintain hydration before transplantation. Depending on the center, enteral nutrition is initiated by a nasogastric tube, a nasoduodenal tube, a gastrostomy tube, or a jejunostomy tube before PN is discontinued. Enteral feedings are generally started at full strength and slowly at 5 to 10 mL/hr. As the rate is advanced, the PN is gradually tapered.

The choice of enteral feeding formula remains somewhat controversial and will vary among centers. Because the lymphatics are disrupted at the time of procurement of the organs, it has been hypothesized that a low-fat, predigested, or elemental formula would be necessary to prevent chylous accumulation. However, there have been no data to suggest significant malabsorption of the intestinal allograft early after transplantation.[23] Although some centers use these elemental low-fat or fat-free formulas in the first month following a transplant, other centers use polymeric formulas containing whole, macronutrient components. Care should be given to the selection of a formula which is low in potassium because immunosuppression may result in hyperkalemia.

An oral diet is usually started within the first 2 weeks after transplantation as the allograft begins to function. Gastric emptying and the subsequent potential risk of aspiration are carefully monitored by an abdominal exam assessing for nausea or vomiting. As with the choice of enteral feeding, the use of a low-fat diet to reduce the risk of malabsorption and chylous ascites after an intestinal transplantation remains controversial and based solely on practice surveys during the early development of intestinal transplantation[24-25] Yet in each of these surveys, the reported risk of chylous ascites was low (<7%) and this early practice of limiting fat was based on minimizing the *potential* risk for this complication. Controlled trials to evaluate this theory are lacking. Spontaneous reconstitution of the lymphatic channels generally occurs within 1 month, thus indicating the self-limiting nature of fat malabsorption in the absence of chronic allograft damage.[26]

Chronic Posttransplant Phase

During the chronic posttransplant phase, ongoing monitoring for signs of rejection and infection should occur as well as monitoring for the recurrence of the primary disease that caused the organ failure. It is also common for patients to develop long-term problems with obesity, hypertension, hyperlipidemia, osteoporosis, and diabetes mellitus. The nutrition goal of this phase is, therefore, to prevent or treat these complications. See Practice Scenario 31-3 to understand some effects of the original pretransplant disease on posttransplant nutrition care.

Practice Scenario 31-3

Question: How does the pretransplant diagnosis affect posttransplant nutrition care?

Scenario: A 22-year-old male with a history of cystic fibrosis undergoes double lung transplant. He is 5′7″ tall and weighs 135 lb. The patient struggled before transplant to maintain his weight. The initial postoperative course is uneventful; the patient is extubated, and in a couple of days, his diet is advanced to a high-calorie, high-protein diet. Pancreatic enzymes are prescribed to be taken with meals. Because the patient has a history of fat-soluble vitamin deficiencies, serum levels of the vitamins are ordered. The serum vitamin A and D levels are low; the vitamin E level is within normal limits.

Intervention: A detailed diet history is obtained from the patient by the dietitian. The recall reveals he was eating between 3000 and 3400 kcal per day prior to admission to maintain his weight. Double meat portions and high-calorie, high-protein nutrition supplements between meals are ordered. Pancreatic enzymes are prescribed to be taken with meals. Vitamins A and D are supplemented along with a multivitamin.

Answer: Although a transplant may offer improved organ function, it does not necessarily "cure" other comorbid complications or nutrition complications after transplantation. The patient's cause for organ failure or other preexisting conditions will influence the nutrition care needed perioperatively because the conditions may not be corrected or cured by a transplant.

Rationale: In this scenario, lung transplantation improved the patient's lung function, but did not correct or cure his cystic fibrosis. The patient had malabsorption prior to the transplant, which would still be present after transplantation. In this scenario, using energy expenditure equations or even measuring REE is of limited value; predicting or measuring energy expenditure does not account for malabsorption, which is common among individuals with cystic fibrosis. It was important to resume the pancreatic enzymes to assist with absorption. Vitamin supplementation is recommended for transplant patients although special formulations or high-dose supplementation is required for patients who are vitamin deficient. Vitamin levels should be rechecked in a couple of months to determine if the current supplement can restore vitamin levels to normal.

Just as this patient had contended with complications of his original disease after transplantation, so do other organ transplant recipients. Some conditions, such as malnutrition, ascites, edema, etc. can resolve with time after transplantation, but patients will require appropriate therapy until they are resolved. Similarly, transplantation improves organ function but sometimes does not rid the patient of the original disease that caused the failure, so that failure could happen again after transplant. A few examples are viral hepatitis, autoimmune liver disease, nonalcoholic steatohepatitis (NASH), primary sclerosing cholangitis in liver transplant recipients, or hypertension and diabetes mellitus in renal transplant recipients.

Metabolic Aberrations Associated with Organ Transplantation

Physiologic stress associated with transplantation and the side effects of immunosuppressive agents causes changes in the metabolism of carbohydrates, lipids, and proteins.

Glucose Alterations

Hyperglycemia is the most common abnormality in glucose metabolism that occurs during the early posttransplant period. Causative factors include physiologic stress, infection, and medications. Corticosteroids increase serum glucose levels by inducing insulin resistance and influencing gluconeogenesis in the liver. In addition, corticosteroids decrease insulin receptor affinity in adipose tissue and muscle, and cause defects at the postreceptor level.[27] Cyclosporine and tacrolimus (calcineurin inhibitors) inhibit pancreatic islet cell function and insulin secretion as well as cause insulin resistance.[54] The rate of new-onset diabetes after transplantation is variable depending on the definition of diabetes, the organ transplant specified, and the time period after transplantation. However, according to a meta-analysis, the incidence of new-onset diabetes among all organ transplant recipients was 13.4%.[28] The rate of new-onset diabetes mellitus and the requirement for insulin was higher among patients receiving tacrolimus versus cyclosporine.[54,55]

Hyperglycemia in the postoperative period may be related to an increased risk of kidney transplant rejection. In a retrospective evaluation of 230 kidney transplant patients without diabetes mellitus receiving cyclosporine-based immunosuppression, patients with a serum glucose level >144 mg/dL had a 71% rate of acute rejection versus 42% in those with a glucose level <144 mg/dL.[29] Likewise, kidney transplant recipients with preexisting diabetes mellitus had an 11% rate of rejection if the 100-hour posttransplant glucose level was <201 mg/dL versus a 58% rejection rate when the glucose level was >201 mg/dL.[30]

The effect of postoperative hyperglycemia on outcomes in other organ transplant recipients has not been reported.

Likewise, there are no data showing the association between hyperglycemia and infection rates in the acute posttransplant period. However, it seems reasonable to use a treatment approach that aims for optimal glucose control. IV insulin drips may be used in the acute period when serum glucose levels are elevated. Treatment with long- and/or short-acting insulin may be required upon hospital discharge even in patients with no previous history of diabetes mellitus. However, as doses of immunosuppressant drugs are decreased and serum glucose levels improve, insulin doses may be decreased, converted to oral hypoglycemic agents, or discontinued.

Lipid Alterations

Hyperlipidemia is another common, long-term posttransplant problem affecting many patients who have undergone organ transplantation. Hyperlipidemia can be induced by cyclosporine and corticosteroids.[31] This effect is less when tacrolimus is used as the primary immunosuppressant. In addition, sirolimus appears to cause hyperlipidemia by altering the insulin-signaling pathway, thereby increasing adipose tissue lipase activity, decreasing lipoprotein lipase activity, or both.

Protein Alterations

Protein catabolic rate is accelerated after organ transplantation. The administration of corticosteroids is a main cause of increased protein oxidation. Protein losses from surgical drains, stomas, dialysis, and wounds also increase protein requirements. As corticosteroid doses are decreased or discontinued, the need for dietary protein may also decrease. Some transplant centers are using "steroid-free" immunosuppression regimens for certain transplant recipients. One could theorize that protein losses, and thus needs, would be lower with this type of regimen compared with catabolism associated with traditional steroid-containing treatment regimens. However, this has yet to be studied.

Determining Nutrition Status

The best approach to assessing a transplant patient's nutrition status is to use a combination of objective and subjective parameters. Objective parameters may lack validity, specificity, or interrater reliability in this population. Table 31-2 summarizes the benefits and drawbacks of using different types of nutrition assessment parameters to assess transplant recipients. Refer to Chapter 9 on Nutrition Screening and Assessment for a further discussion on nutrition assessment.

Nutrient Requirements

Energy

Organ transplant patients do not tend to be hypermetabolic unless secondary conditions such as sepsis are present. Factors that influence resting energy expenditure (REE) include gender, age, pretransplant nutrition status, and medical condition. Several studies have evaluated posttransplant energy needs; the time period during which indirect calorimetry was performed varied from the 2nd to the 28th day posttransplant. REE was 7% to 42% above predicted values.[32-33] Based on these studies, 1.3 to 1.5 times the calculated basal energy expenditure (BEE), or 30 to 35 kcal per kilogram, are recommended. Absorption capability should also be considered in the final calorie recommendation. This is especially true in the small bowel transplant recipients in whom the transplanted intestine may have variable absorption capacity depending on the health and the state of infection and rejection of the graft or in lung transplant recipients with cystic fibrosis.

TABLE 31-2 Benefits and Drawbacks of Nutritional Assessment Parameters When Assessing Organ Transplant Recipients

Parameter	Benefits	Drawbacks
Body weight	• Simple to perform • Reproducible • Low cost • Universal measurement	• Affected by body fluid changes
Anthropometric measurements	• Low cost • Portable	• Low interrater reliability • Influenced by a patient's fluid status • Low specificity
Serum protein values	• Reproducible • Easily available • Relatively low cost	• Affected by many nonnutritional factors (eg, fluid status, liver function, vitamin status, inflammation)
Urinary tests (eg, nitrogen balance, creatinine-height index)	• Relatively low cost	• Influenced by many nonnutritional factors (eg, renal and liver function, fluid status)
Immunocompetence tests (eg, skin test antigens, total lymphocyte count [TLC])	• Reproducible • Relatively low cost • TLC easily available	• Influenced by immunosuppressive drugs
Other tests such as bioelectrical impedance (BIA), dual energy X-ray absorptiometry (DXA)	• DXA considered highly accurate	• BIA affected by fluid status; BIA equation must be valid for population being evaluated • Increased cost • Unavailability or lack of daily clinical application (BIA, DXA)

Generally, 70% of nonprotein calories in nutrition support regimens are provided by carbohydrates. Because posttransplant hyperglycemia is prevalent, blood glucose levels should be treated as discussed in Chapters 23 and 34 on Critical Care and Sepsis and Diabetes Mellitus.

Lipids fulfill the remainder of nonprotein calories. Most enteral and parenteral products contain ω-6 fatty acids. However, ω-3 fatty acids are theorized to benefit transplant recipients by decreasing inflammatory response, enhancing transplant tolerance, and improving graft function.[34–35] Improved graft function has been observed in animals who receive fish oil versus vegetable oils along with cyclosporine immunosuppression following a renal transplantation.[67,68] ω-3 fatty acids have also been shown to improve survival in rats undergoing a heart transplantation.[65,69,70] In humans, fish oil has been shown to improve renal hemodynamics in liver transplant patients with cyclosporine immunosuppression.[75] The administration of 4 g per day of ω-3 fatty acids to a heart transplant patient with hyperlipidemia from rapamycin or everolimus resulted in a significant reduction in serum triglyceride levels.[36] Finally, renal transplant recipients have improved postrejection renal function recovery when treated with fish oil versus coconut oil.[73] One small pilot trial evaluated the use of an immune-enhancing formula (containing fish oil, arginine, and nucleic acids) in 15 liver transplant patients. Compared with historical controls, the experimental group had fewer infectious complications (33% of patients) versus 71% of control patients in the first 28 postoperative days.[37] A Cochrane review on fish oil and kidney transplantation concluded that fish oil may mildly improve cardiovascular risk factors, but there are not adequate data to support that fish oil reduces cardiovascular disease risk or improves renal function.[38] Larger clinical trials will be needed before the use of omega-3 fatty acids can be endorsed for regular use following a transplantation.

Protein

Protein requirements are directly related to corticosteroid dose; nutrition status; stress state; losses from drains, stomas, and wounds; and requirements for wound healing (see Chapter 21 on Wound Healing). Because corticosteroid doses are increased in the acute posttransplant phase and during rejection treatment, protein needs are higher in the acute phase (1.5 to 2 g per kg) versus the chronic posttransplant phase (1 g per kg). As mentioned earlier, some new antirejection regimens eliminate corticosteroids; theoretically, protein requirements would be lower than when regimens using corticosteroids are followed.

Fluid

Fluid requirements for transplant patients vary greatly depending upon volume status. Excess fluid administration and/or decreased urine output cause fluid overload. Renal insufficiency is common posttransplant due to nephrotoxic immunosuppressants. Diarrhea, chest tubes, wounds, surgical drains, nasogastric drainage, ostomy output, pancreatic secretions, and urine output are sources of fluid loss that increase fluid requirements.

Micronutrients

There are many causes of alterations in nutrient levels and posttransplant requirements. These are summarized in Table 31-3.

Selecting a Nutrition Support Route

Oral feeding is the preferred route of nutrition for organ transplant recipients. However, tube feeding and PN are needed occasionally as bridges to oral nutrition or during complications preventing an oral diet. Major indications for tube feeding or PN are discussed in Chapters 10 and 14 Overview of Enteral Nutrition and Overview of Parenteral Nutrition. An algorithm for nutrition support selection is featured in Figure 31-1. General nutrition support and monitoring guidelines for organ transplant recipients are highlighted in Table 31-4 and are also discussed in the European Society for Parenteral and Enteral Nutrition (E.S.P.E.N.) guidelines.[39] Tube feeding options for liver transplant recipients are summarized in Table 31-5.

Indications for PN in organ transplant patients include prolonged active gastrointestinal (GI) bleeding, an ileus, and a high-output intestinal fistula. In addition, PN is usually required initially after a small bowel transplantation and during periods of significant small bowel rejection or infection. When PN is required, there are several guidelines that can be considered when determining the appropriate PN formula. First, the volume of the PN is dependent on overall fluid needs, as discussed previously. If a patient is volume overloaded or has limited urine output, concentrated forms of amino acids, dextrose, and fat emulsions should be used. On the other hand, additional volume may be required for the intestinal transplant patient with a high ostomy output. Electrolyte and micronutrient content should be individualized based on laboratory values. As mentioned earlier, tight glucose control is desired and patients may require an IV insulin drip or insulin in the PN formulation if serum glucose levels are elevated.

Transplant Complications

There are many potential posttransplant complications that directly or indirectly affect nutrition. Examples include rejection, preservation injury, delayed graft function, infection, surgical complications, hyperglycemia, hypertension, renal insufficiency, and electrolyte abnormalities. There is a nutrition management component of many of these complications (Practice Scenario 31-4).

Practice Scenario 31-4

Question: What are common early posttransplant complications and how do they influence decisions about nutrition or nutrition support?

Scenario: A 56-year-old female undergoes liver transplantation for cirrhosis thought to be due to nonalcoholic steatohepatitis (NASH). The patient has a history of metabolic syndrome marked by obesity, hyperlipidemia, and diabetes mellitus. She had undergone gastric bypass several years earlier. Her current BMI is 32 kg/m^2.

She undergoes liver transplantation; her posttransplant course is unremarkable and she is discharged 7 days after her transplant. Two weeks later, the patient is readmitted to the hospital with elevated serum liver function tests. A liver biopsy is performed, which confirms acute rejection. The patient is treated with corticosteroids with the dose tapering down over 5 days. She complains of redness at the incision site. The wound appears infected and it is partially opened; a wound vacuum-assisted closure (VAC) is placed. Antibiotics are prescribed. The patient complains of nausea; she is eating only about half of her meals and is drinking ginger ale to reduce her nausea.

Intervention: When the corticosteroid taper is initiated, blood glucose levels are ordered to be measured at the bedside before meals and at bedtime. Despite the patient receiving her usual dose of long-acting insulin, the blood glucose levels are elevated, ranging between 180 and 240 mg/dL. Short-acting insulin is given on a sliding scale, and her long-acting insulin dose is increased. She is encouraged to avoid highly concentrated sweets such as the ginger ale. An antinausea medicine is prescribed on an as needed basis. A high-protein oral supplement is ordered and the patient is encouraged to eat the entrees at her meals.

Answer: Common posttransplant complications include rejection, infection, and technical/surgical complications. Each of these complications may require a change in the nutrition intervention either through nutrient needs, nutrient delivery, or adjunct therapy such as insulin therapy.

Rationale: Antirejection medications are needed to prevent and treat transplant rejection; antirejection medications have nutrition-related side effects (Table 31-1). Corticosteroids accelerate protein catabolic rate and nitrogen loss. The mechanism of how tacrolimus and corticosteroids cause hyperglycemia was discussed earlier in this chapter. Often, serum glucose levels increase after a transplantation as a response to immunosuppressive medications and postoperative stress. New onset diabetes mellitus after a transplantation can be transient as glucose levels often return to normal several weeks posttransplant and insulin therapy will not be required long term. Infection is a potential posttransplant complication often potentiated by immunosuppressive medications. Malnourished patients may be more likely to develop infections than well-nourished patients. On the other hand, severely obese patients tend to have increased rates of wound infections.[38-40] Antibiotics and antiviral and antifungal medications are usually given prophylactically during the early postoperative phase when immunosuppressive medications are at their highest doses. They are also administered when pathological organisms are identified in wounds, urine, blood, or other body fluids. These medications may adversely affect appetite and taste, and may cause nausea, vomiting, or diarrhea. These GI symptoms may preclude a patient from eating adequate amounts. In addition, if a wound VAC is used for a wound (whether infected or not), it will remove protein-containing body fluids, thus requiring protein supplementation.[42]

TABLE 31-3 Factors that Contribute to Vitamin and Mineral Abnormalities in Organ Transplant Patients

Factor (Transplanted Organ)	Nutrient Alterations
Alcoholism	• Vitamins A, B_6, and B_{12}; niacin; thiamin; folate; magnesium; and zinc levels are decreased
Antibiotics	• Vitamins E and K, and folate levels are decreased
Bile drainage (liver)	• Copper loss is increased; fat-soluble vitamins may be malabsorbed
Biliary obstruction, Wilson disease (liver)	• Copper levels are increased
Bleeding	• Iron loss is increased
Calcineurin inhibitors	• Magnesium loss is increased
Glucocorticoids	• Vitamin D and phosphorus levels are decreased • Urinary loss of calcium is increased
Hemochromatosis (liver)	• Iron stores are increased
Liver failure (liver)	• Ability to activate vitamin D is decreased • Vitamin K level is decreased
Ostomy loss (small bowel)/diarrhea	• Zinc loss is increased
Refeeding syndrome	• Magnesium, phosphorus, and potassium levels are decreased
Renal failure	• Vitamin D, calcium, and phosphorus metabolism is abnormal • Iron levels are decreased due to depressed erythropoietin • Vitamin A level is increased • Vitamin C, phosphorus, and potassium levels are decreased due to dialysis • Excretion of magnesium and zinc is decreased • Zinc may be decreased in dialysis patients
Steatorrhea	• Levels of vitamins A, D, E, and K are decreased • Calcium level is decreased
Wound	• Need for some vitamins (eg, A and C) and zinc may be increased to aid with healing

This article was published in Hasse JM, Roberts S. Transplantation. In: Rombeau JL, Rolandelli RH, eds. *Parenteral Nutrition*, 3rd ed. 529–561, Copyright W.B. Saunders Company (2001).

FIGURE 31-1 Nutrition Support Algorithm for Solid Organ Transplant Recipients

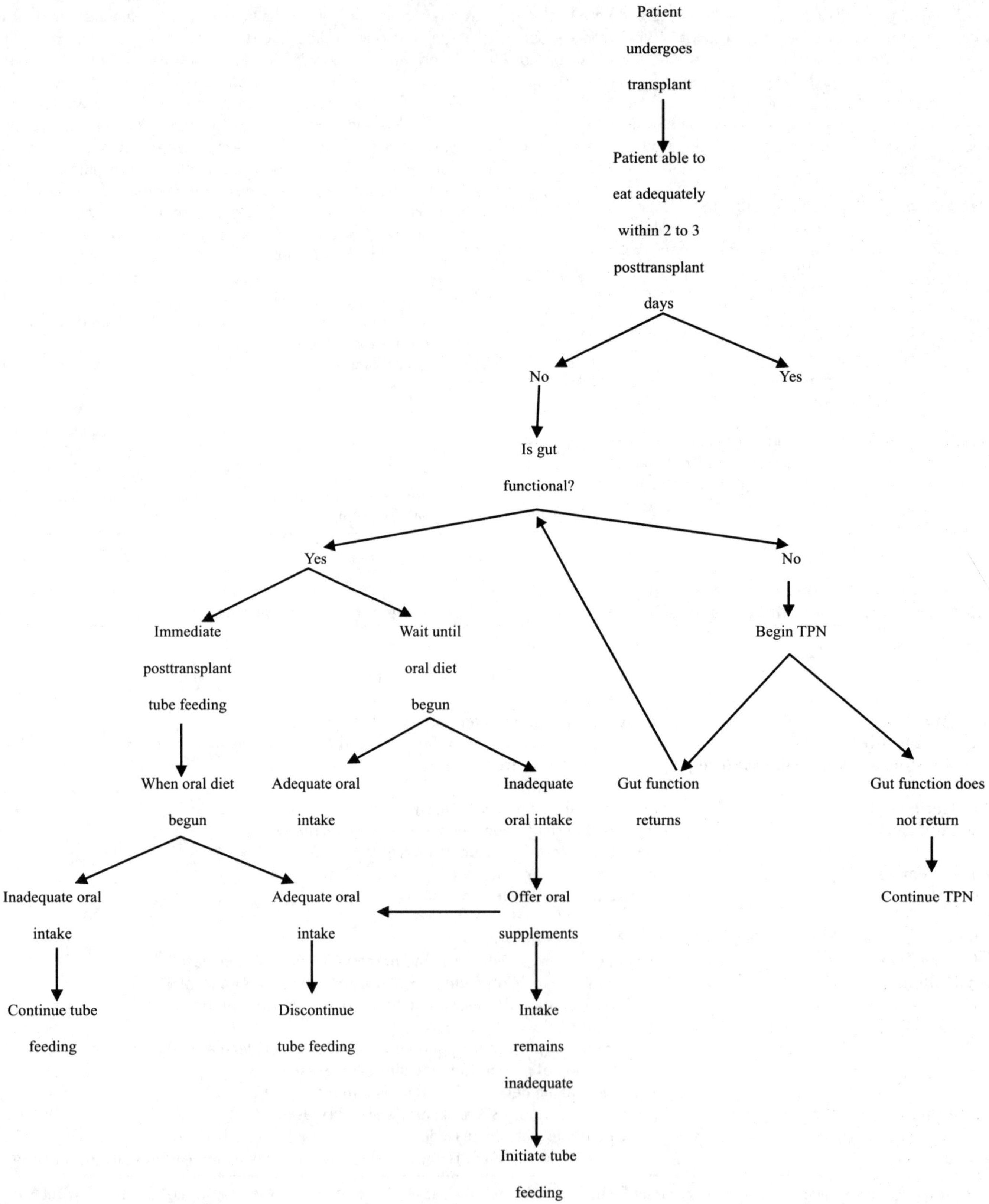

This article was published in Hasse JM, Roberts S. Transplantation. In: Rombeau JL, Rolandelli RH, eds. *Parenteral Nutrition*, 3rd ed. 529–561, Copyright W.B. Saunders Company (2001).

TABLE 31-4 General Guidelines for Nutrition Support Therapy and Monitoring for Organ Transplant Recipients

Route of Nutrition	Usual Recommendations	Monitoring
Oral	• Liquid diet – begin when patient is passing flatus	• Bowel sounds
	• General diet – begin when a patient begins to have bowel movements	• Intake and output, bowel movement record; nutrient intake study (calorie count)
	• Carbohydrate-controlled diet – when serum glucose level is elevated	• Laboratory values – glucose
	• Sodium-restricted diet – when fluid retention is severe	• Patient exam – edema, ascites • Laboratory values – sodium
	• Fluid restriction – when hyponatremia is present	• Nutrient intake study (calorie count)
Tube feeding	• Formula – Usually a polymeric, high-nitrogen formula – Diarrhea/constipation: high-fiber formula – Volume overload: concentrated formula – Impaired digestion: semielemental or polypeptide formula • Feeding schedule – change from a 24-hour infusion to a nocturnal schedule once the patient can eat 50% of needs	• Weight • Intake and output • Laboratory values – glucose, sodium, potassium, carbon dioxide, phosphorus, magnesium, calcium
PN	• Fluid – concentrate for decreased volume	• Weight, intake and output
	• Amino acids – 10% to 15% initial concentration	• Laboratory values – urea nitrogen, ammonia
	• Dextrose – 70% nonprotein calories	• Laboratory values – glucose
	• Lipid – 30% nonprotein calories	• Laboratory values – triglycerides
	• Electrolytes – according to laboratory values • Multiple vitamin infusion – daily • Trace elements – daily	• Laboratory values – sodium, potassium, phosphorus, magnesium, calcium
	• Insulin – if serum glucose is elevated	• Laboratory values – glucose

PN, parenteral nutrition. This article was published in the Journal of the American Dietetic Association, Vol 4, Hasse JM, Role of the dietitian in the nutritional management of adults post-liver transplantation, 473–476, Copyright American Dietetic Association (1991).

Nutrition Monitoring

Monitoring a patient's progress includes an evaluation of body weight, intake and output, and laboratory parameters (Table 31-4). In addition to these objective parameters, an evaluation of the patient's ability to ambulate, eat adequately, perform activities of daily living, and heal wounds are all signs of recovery and progress. Anthropometric measurements performed serially over time may provide information about body composition. Dual energy X-ray absorptiometry is an accurate method to determine body composition but is usually performed either to assess bone density or as part of a research protocol. Functional measurements such as handgrip strength may also provide insights into a patient's progress.

TABLE 31-5 Three Approaches to the Provision of Enteral Tube Feeding After Liver Transplantation[16]

Approach	Drawbacks
Place feeding tube after transplantation only after it is determined that oral intake will be delayed or is inadequate.	There is a delay in feeding patients. Needing to obtain tube feeding access can further delay the provision of nutrition. This is especially undesirable for patients who have severe complications or who are already malnourished.
Preselect patients who may benefit from tube feeding and place feeding tubes during surgery.	It is difficult to predict which patients will have posttransplant difficulties or delayed eating. If the selection is made based on nutrition status alone, those who are well nourished but have significant posttransplant complications will lack access for tube feeding,
Place feeding tubes in all patients during surgery and begin tube feeding within 12 to 24 hours of surgery.	Some patients will require tube feeding for only a short period of time (2 to 3 days) before oral intake is adequate. Some tubes can become dislodged and may require replacement if oral intake does not meet needs.

Summary

Organ transplantation is a medical therapy that can improve survival and quality of life in individuals with end-stage organ disease. The medical and surgical complexities influence nutrition status and nutrient delivery. Nutrition therapy varies with transplant type, nutrition status, stage of transplant, function of organ, and presence of complications. Tailoring nutrition therapy based on these characteristics can help improve transplant outcomes.

References

1. U.S. Department of Health and human Services. Organ Procurement and Transplantation Network. http://optn.transplant.hrsa.gov/data Accessed January 1, 2012.
2. Pikul J, Sharpe MD, Lowndes R, Ghent CN. Degree of preoperative malnutrition is predictive of postoperative morbidity and mortality in liver transplant recipients. *Transplantation.* 1994;57: 469–472.
3. Madill J, Maurer JR, deHoyas A. A comparison of preoperative and postoperative nutritional state of lung transplant recipients. *Transplantation.* 1993;56:347–350.
4. Allen JG, Arnaoutakis GJ, Weiss ES, et al. The impact of recipient body mass index on survival after lung transplantation. *J Heart Lung Transplant.* 2010;29(9):1026–1033.
5. Johnson DW, Isbel NM, Brown AM, et al. The effect of obesity on renal transplant outcomes. *Transplantation.* 2002;74:675–680.
6. Bennett WM, McEvoy KM, Henell KR, Valente JF, Douzdjian V. Morbid obesity does not preclude successful renal transplantation. *Clin Transplant.* 2004;18:89–93.
7. Moreso F, Seron D, Anunciada AI, et al. Recipient body surface area as a predictor of posttransplant renal allograft evolution. *Transplantation.* 1998;65:671–676.
8. Papalia T, Greco R, Lofaro D, et al. Impact of body mass index on graft loss in normal and overweight patients: retrospective analysis of 206 renal transplants. *Clin Transplant.* 2010;24(6): E241–246.
9. Meier-Kriesche H-U, Vaghela M, Thambuganipalle R, et al. The effect of body mass index on long-term renal allograft survival. *Transplantation.* 1999;68:1294–1297.
10. Modlin CS, Flechner SM, Gooormastic M, et al. Should obese patients lose weight before receiving a kidney transplant? *Transplantation.* 1997;64:599–604.
11. Howard RJ, Thai VB, Patton PR, et al. Obesity does not portend a bad outcome for kidney transplant recipients. *Transplantation.* 2002;73:53–55.
12. Madill J, Gutierrez C, Grossman J, et al. Nutritional assessment of the lung transplant patient: body mass index as a predictor of 90-day mortality following transplantation. *J Heart Lung Transplant.* 2001;20:288–296.
13. Testa G, Hasse JM, Jennings LW, et al. Morbid obesity is not an independent risk factor for liver transplantation. [Abstract]. *Transplantation.* 1998;66:S53.
14. Sawyer RB, Pelletier SJ, Pruett TL. Increased early morbidity and mortality with acceptable long-term function in severely obese patients undergoing liver transplantation. *Clin Transplant.* 1999; 13:126–130.
15. Nair S, Verma S, Thuluvath PJ. Obesity and its effect on survival in patients undergoing orthotopic liver transplantation in the United States. *Hepatology.* 2002;35:105–109.
16. Dick AA, Spitzer AL, Seifert CF, et al. Liver transplantation at the extremes of the body mass index. *Liver Transpl.* 2009;15(8):968–977.
17. Lederer DJ, Wilt JS, D'Ovidio F, et al. Obesity and underweight are associated with an increased risk of death after lung transplantation. *Am J Respir Crit Care Med.* 2009;180(9): 887–895.
18. Glanton CW, Kao T-C, Cruess D, Agodoa LYC, Abbott KC. Impact of renal transplantation on survival in end-stage renal disease patients with elevated body mass intake. *Kidney Int.* 2003;63:647–653.
19. Pelletier SJ, Maraschio MA, Schaubel DE, et al. Survival benefit of kidney and liver transplantation for obese patients on the waiting list. *Clin Transpl.* 2003:77–88.
20. Jindal RM, Zawada ET. Obesity and kidney transplantation. *Am J Kidney Dis.* 2004;43:943–952.
21. Hwang S, Lee S-G, Jang S-J, et al. The effect of donor weight reduction on hepatic steatosis for living donor liver transplantation. *Liver Transplant.* 2004;11:721–725.
22. Yoo HY, Molmenti E, Thuluvath PJ. The effect of donor body mass index on primary graft nonfunction, retransplantation rate, and early graft and patient survival after liver transplantation. *Liver Transpl.* 2003;9:72–78.
23. Kim J, Fryer J, Craig RM. Absorptive function following small intestinal transplantation. *Dig Dis Sci.* 1998;43:1925–1930.
24. Kaufman SS, Lyden ER, Brown CR, et al. Disaccharidase activities and fat assimilation in pediatric patients after intestinal transplantation. *Transplantation.* 2000;69:362–365.
25. Nour B, Reyes J, Tzakis A, et al. Intestinal transplantation with or without other abdominal organs: nutrition and dietary management of 50 patients. *Transplant Proc.* 1994; 26: 1432–1433.
26. Rovera G, Schoen R, Goldbach B, et al. Intestinal and multivisceral transplantation: dynamics of nutritional management and functional autonomy. *JPEN J Parenter Enteral Nutr.* 2003;27: 252–259.
27. Marchetti P. New-onset diabetes after liver transplantation: from pathogenesis to management. *Liver Transpl.* 2005;11(6): 612–620.
28. Heisel O, Heisel R, Balshaw R, Keown P. New onset diabetes mellitus in patients receiving calcineurin inhibitors: a systematic review and meta-analysis. *Am J Transplant.* 2004;4:583–595.
29. Thomas MC, Moran J, Mathew TH, Russ GR, Rao MM. Early perioperative hyperglycaemia and renal allograft rejection in patients without diabetes. *BMC Nephrology.* 2000;1:1.ROF.
30. Thomas MC, Mathew TH, Russ GR, Rao MM, Moran J. Early perioperative glycaemic control and allograft rejection in patients with diabetes mellitus: a pilot study. *Transplantation.* 2001;72: 1321–1324.
31. Charlton M. Obesity, hyperlipidemia, and metabolic syndrome. *Liver Transplantation.* 2009;15:S83–S89.
32. Hasse JM, Blue LS, Liepa GU, et al. Early enteral nutrition support in patients undergoing liver transplantation. *JPEN J Parenter Enteral Nutr.* 1995;19:437–443.
33. Plank LD, Metzger DJ, McCall JL, et al. Sequential changes in the metabolic response to orthotopic liver transplantation during the first year after surgery. *Ann Surg.* 2001;234:245–255.
34. Driscoll DF, Palombo JD, Bistrian BR. Nutritional and metabolic considerations of the adult liver transplant candidate and organ donor. *Nutrition.* 1995;11:255–263.
35. Badalamenti S, Salerno F, Lorenzano E, et al. Renal effects of dietary supplementation with fish oil in cyclosporine-treated liver transplant recipients. *Hepatology.* 1995;22:1695–1701.
36. Celik S, Doesch A, Erbel C, et al. Beneficial effect of omega-3 fatty acids on sirolimus- or everolimus-induced hypertriglyceridemia in heart transplant recipients. *Transplantation.* 2008; 86(2):245–250.

37. Plank LD, McCall JL, Gane EJ, et al. Pre- and postoperative immunonutrition in patients undergoing liver transplantation: a pilot study of safety and efficacy. *Clin Nutr.* 2005;24:388–396.
38. Lim AKH, Manley KJ, Roberts MA, Fraenkel MB. Fish oil for kidney transplant recipients. *Cochrane Database Syst Rev.* 2007;2: CD005282. DOI: 10.1002/14651858.CD005282.pub2
39. Weimann A, Braga M, Harsanyi L, et al. ESPEN Guidelines on Enteral Nutrition: surgery including organ transplantation. *Clin Nutr.* 2006;25(2):224–244.
40. Matarese LE, Costa G, Bond G, et al. Therapeutic efficacy of intestinal and multivisceral transplantation: survival and nutritional outcome. *Nutr Clin Pract.* 2007:22(5):474–481.
41. Matarese LE. Nutrition interventions before and after adult intestinal transplantation: the Pittsburgh experience. *Practical Gastroenterol.* 2010: XXXIV(11):11–26.
42. Hourigan LA, Linfoot JA, Chung KK, et al. Loss of protein, immunoglobulins, and electrolytes in exudates from negative pressure wound therapy. *Nutr Clin Pract.* 2010;25(5):510–516.

32 Human Immunodeficiency Virus (HIV) Infection

Peter J. Wasserman, RD, MA, Sorana Segal-Maurer, MD, and David S. Rubin, MD

CONTENTS

Background ... 537
Introduction ... 537
The Virus ... 538
Epidemiology of the HIV Pandemic ... 538
Diagnosis ... 539
Transmission ... 539
Immunopathogenesis ... 539
The Clinical Manifestation of Immunodeficiency ... 540
Antiretroviral Medications ... 540
Nutritional Metabolism in the Current cART Era ... 542
Wasting Syndrome/Disease ... 542
History ... 542
Epidemiology ... 542
Case Definition and Clinical Diagnosis ... 543
Wasting Disease Compared to Uncomplicated Starvation ... 543
Etiology and Pathogenesis of Wasting Disease ... 543
Clinical Encounter and Assessment ... 545
Nutrition-Focused Physical Examination ... 546
Medication Review ... 547
Social and Family History ... 547
Clinical Management ... 547
Orexigenic Agents ... 548
Anabolic–Androgenic Steroids ... 548
Recombinant Human Growth Hormone (rhGH) ... 550
Progressive Resistance and Aerobic Exercise ... 550
Thalidomide ... 550
Energy, Protein, and Electrolytes ... 550
Vitamin D ... 551
Omega-3 Fatty Acid Enrichment ... 551
Enteral Nutrition: Alimentation by Tube into the Upper Gastrointestinal Tract ... 551
Parenteral Nutrition: Intravenous Alimentation ... 551
Sarcopenia ... 552
Osteopenia and Osteoporosis ... 552
HIV-Associated Lipodystrophy Syndrome ... 553
Introduction ... 553
Epidemiology ... 553
Other Lipodystrophies ... 553
Etiology and Pathogenesis ... 553
Clinical Evaluation and Diagnosis ... 554
Clinical Management ... 555
Resistance and Aerobic Exercise ... 555
Thiazolidinediones ... 555
Metformin ... 555
Soft Tissue Fillers and Liposuction ... 555

Cardiovascular Disease ... 555
Background ... 555
Etiology ... 555
Clinical Evaluation ... 556
The Mediterranean Diet ... 556
HMG CoA Reductase Inhibitors (Statins) and Fibrates ... 556
Omega-3 Fatty Acids ... 556
Growth Hormone Releasing Factor Analog ... 556
References ... 557

Objectives

1. Describe the epidemiology of the human immunodeficiency virus (HIV) pandemic globally and within the United States.
2. Discuss the transmission, diagnosis, and treatment of HIV infection and acquired immunodeficiency syndrome (AIDS)/HIV disease.
3. Identify the abnormalities of nutritional metabolism associated with HIV infection in the current combination antiretroviral therapy (cART) era.
4. Evaluate diagnostic criteria, methodology, and treatment options for wasting syndrome, sarcopenia, dyslipidemia, osteopenia, and osteoporosis in patients with HIV infection.

Test Your Knowledge Questions

1. HIV infection is prevalent in:
   A. Men who have sex with men
   B. Urban heterosexuals in the lowest income strata
   C. Black and Hispanic/Latino Americans
   D. All of the above
2. The goal of antiretroviral therapy is to:
   A. Increase CD8+ T lymphocytes and decrease viral load
   B. Increase both CD4+ T lymphocytes and viral load
   C. Increase CD4+ T lymphocytes and neutrophils
   D. Increase CD4+ T lymphocytes and decrease viral load
3. _____ is /are predictive of the onset of wasting disease.
   A. Hypogonadism
   B. Hypermetabolism
   C. Decreased food intake
   D. All of the above
4. The central feature of HIV lipodystrophy is selective:
   A. Loss of specific fat depots
   B. Increases in specific fat depots
   C. Subcutaneous adipose tissue loss
   D. All of the above
5. Hypertriglyceridemia is a frequent finding in:
   A. Febrile HIV+ patients with septicemia
   B. HIV+ patients with abdominal obesity receiving cART
   C. Patients with HIV infection and wasting disease
   D. All of the above

Test Your Knowledge Answers

1. The correct answer is **D**. The HIV epidemic in the United States is geographically concentrated with marked ethnic/racial, social, and economic health disparities.
2. The correct answer is **D.** HIV infection leads to disease in the human host by depletion of CD4+ T-helper lymphocytes. Effective antiretroviral therapy suppresses viral replication. The level of viral replication is monitored clinically by quantitative polymerase chain reaction and reported as absolute and log copies per milliliter of serum sampled (viral load). This number should decline with viral suppression. HIV does not infect CD8-cytolytic T lymphocytes and neutrophils.
3. The correct answer **C.** Decreased food intake is predictive of the onset of wasting. Hypermetabolism may initially be compensated for by decreased activity or lethargy. Hypogonadism is not a uniform finding in all patients with involuntary weight loss or wasting.
4. The correct answer is **C.** Lipodystrophy is characterized by subcutaneous adipose tissue loss with visceral adipose tissue sparing or accumulation. Subcutaneous adipose tissue loss is often most evident in the face, buttocks, and lower extremities. Lipodystrophic patients may also demonstrate insulin resistance in association with the loss of subcutaneous adipose tissue.
5. The correct answer is **D.** Hypertriglyceridemia may occur in association with wasting disease, as a side effect of antiretroviral medications, in association with abdominal adiposity, or during febrile response to bacterial infection as a host defense mechanism.

Background

Introduction

Over 30 years ago, the first cases of AIDS in the United States were described in the Morbidity and Mortality Weekly Report.[1] HIV-related mortality rates rose steadily through the 1980s, peaking in 1995. During that period, median survival following an AIDS diagnosis was 18 to 36 months. In the 7 years following the introduction of combination antiretroviral therapy (cART), HIV-related mortality declined by 70%.[2] Currently, the Centers for Disease

Control and Prevention (CDC) estimates that over 1 million people are living with HIV or AIDS in the United States.[3] Median survival for newly diagnosed patients initiating therapy is now estimated in decades.[4,5] Formidable challenges remain: insufficient HIV testing, persisting health inequities including access to care and life years lost for patients in care, and community burden of disease.[4,5] One in five persons living with HIV is unaware of their infection and may unwittingly transmit the virus to others.[6] For many persons unaware of their HIV infection, diagnosis and linkage to care continues to occur at presentation for the treatment of opportunistic infection(s) and/or wasting disease. Patients in care with long-term controlled HIV infection are at greater risk for age-related comorbidities (including cardiovascular disease and osteoporosis/osteopenia) than the general population.[7,8]

The Virus

HIV, the causative agent of AIDS in humans, is a zoonotic retrovirus of the lentivirus family. Of the two types of HIV, type 1 is distributed throughout the world (pandemic) and type 2 is found in sub-Saharan Africa (in addition to HIV-1).[9] HIV-1 is believed to have crossed over to the human population from chimpanzees.[9] Of the three HIV-1 subgroups, group M accounts for most infections worldwide and has 10 identifiable clades or subtypes (A through H) based on genetic sequence diversity. Clade B virus predominates in Western Europe, North America, Haiti, and Brazil, whereas clade E predominates in Thailand. All clades are found in Africa. Molecular genetic tests currently used in North America may perform poorly on the non-clade B virus. Therapeutic response to various antiretrovirals may be different among different clades and between HIV-1 and HIV-2.

Epidemiology of the HIV Pandemic

The Joint United Nations Programme and World Health Organization estimate that 33.4 million people are infected with HIV worldwide.[10] Sub-Saharan Africa bears the greatest burden of disease with an estimated prevalence of 22.4 million cases (Table 32-1).[10]

Prevention programs targeting behavior change, condom use, voluntary HIV counseling and testing, and blood transfusion safety have been successful in lowering prevalence in several sub-Saharan countries.[11] Considerable progress in the provision of cART to those in need of treatment (WHO guidelines) has been made by national health services, the World Health Organization, the U.S. President's Emergency Plan for AIDS Relief, and nongovernmental organizations. However, less than 40% of those in need of treatment for HIV infection receive it.[10] Worldwide, the majority of those infected with HIV are expected to progress to AIDS and to succumb to opportunistic infections due to limited access to care in countries with poor public health infrastructure. High mortality rates in people during what would normally be their most productive years carry a significant and negative socioeconomic impact.

In the United States, over 1.1 million people are living with HIV infection. Annually, 56,000 new infections and 18,000 deaths occur (in people with HIV/AIDS), leading to a net increase of 40,000 HIV-infected people [5,11] Geographically, the burden of HIV infection is disproportionately borne by states in the South, Northeast, and West. Fifty-four percent of persons living with HIV/AIDS reside in 5 states and 90% reside in 23 states. Fifty-three percent of new HIV infections occur in men who have sex with men (MSM), 31% during heterosexual contact, 12% in association with injection drug use (IDU), and 4% in MSM who engage in IDU.[5] Health disparities are also evident in the ethnic/racial distribution of HIV acquisition: 45% are black, 35% are white/non-Hispanic, and 17% are Hispanic/Latino.[5] MSM, black, and Hispanic/Latino Americans are respectively 40, 8, and 3 times more likely to be HIV infected than white/non-Hispanic heterosexual Americans.[5]

However, HIV prevalence in heterosexuals residing in urban areas is 6 times higher in those of the lowest income strata versus the highest regardless of ethnicity.[12] This finding

TABLE 32-1 Regional HIV/AIDS Statistics, 2008

	Adults and Children Living with HIV	Newly Infected with HIV	Adult Prevalence (%)	AIDS Mortality
Sub-Saharan Africa	22.8 million	1.9 million	5.2	1.4 million
North Africa and Middle East	310,000	35,000	0.2	20,000
South and Southeast Africa	3.8 million	280,000	0.3	270,000
East Asia	850,000	75,000	<0.1	59,000
Oceania	59,000	3900	0.3	2000
Latin America	2.0 million	170,000	0.6	77,000
Caribbean	240,000	20,000	1.0	12,000
Eastern Europe and Central Asia	1.5 million	110,000	0.7	87,000
Western and Central Europe	850,000	30,000	0.3	13,000
North America	1.4 million	55,000	0.6	25,000
Total	33.4 million	2.7 million	0.8	2.1 million

Adapted with permission from AIDS Epidemic Update: Joint United Nations programme on HIV/AIDS & World Health Organization 2009.

suggests that ethnicity may be a surrogate marker for socioeconomic status in surveillance data sets, and that poverty is a major determinant of risk for HIV infection in the United States. In clinical practice, health history should include key socioeconomic factors (eg, educational attainment) to avoid unfounded assumptions about biology or "culture" based on ethnicity/race.

Diagnosis

A definitive diagnosis of HIV infection is made by enzyme immunoassay (EIA) or rapid HIV-1 antibody from serum, followed by a confirmatory western blot. Rapid point-of-care tests have been approved recently but still require serum confirmatory tests if positive. The diagnosis of acute or primary HIV infection before the formation of antibodies to HIV (or seroconversion) may be made by reverse-transcriptase polymerase chain reaction (RT-PCR) amplification of viral RNA (and/or proviral DNA), branched chain DNA (bDNA), or the detection of p24 antigen in peripheral blood. A diagnosis of AIDS may be made according to the CDC 1993 AIDS surveillance case definition (Table 32-2).[13]

TABLE 32-2 AIDS-Defining Events

Candidiasis of bronchi, trachea, or lungs or esophagus
Cervical cancer (invasive)
Coccidioidomycosis, disseminated
Cryptococcosis, extrapulmonary
Cryptosporidiosis, chronic intestinal (> 1-month duration)
Cytomegalovirus disease (other than liver, spleen, or lymph nodes)
Cytomegalovirus retinitis (with loss of vision)
Encephalopathy HIV-related
Herpes simplex: chronic ulcer(s) (> 1-month duration) or bronchitis, pneumonitis, or esophagitis
Histoplasmosis, disseminated
Isosporiasis, chronic intestinal (>1-month duration)
Kaposi sarcoma
Lymphoma: Burkitt, or immunoblastic, or primary of brain (primary central nervous system lymphoma)
Mycobacterium avium complex or disease caused by *M. kansasii*, disseminated
Disease caused by mycobacterium tuberculosis, any site (pulmonary or extrapulmonary)
Disease caused by mycobacterium, other species, or unidentified species, disseminated
Pneumocystis jiroveci (carinii) pneumonia
Pneumonia (recurrent)
Progressive multifocal leukoencephalopathy
Salmonella septicemia (recurrent)
Toxoplasmosis of the brain (encephalitis)
Wasting syndrome caused by HIV infection

Adapted from Centers for Disease Control and Prevention (CDC). 1993. Revised classification system for HIV-infection & expanded surveillance case definition for AIDS among adults & adolescents. *MMWR Morb Mortal Wkly Rep.* 1992/41:1–19.

TABLE 32-3 Modes of HIV Transmission

Route	Example
Percutaneous	Contaminated transfusion, intravenous drug use sharing of needles, contaminated surgical or dental instruments, or during an occupational exposure
Mucous membrane	Sexual contact (vaginal, anal, or oral), occupational (eg, eye splash)
Cutaneous contact of nonintact skin with large volume of infected fluids and/or for a prolonged duration	Occupational contact with abraded skin
Maternal–fetal	Intrauterine, intrapartum (ie, during labor), postpartum (ie, breast feeding)

Adapted from U.S. Department of Health and Human Services. Transmission facts. http://www.cdc.gov/hiv/pubs/facts/transmission.htm.

Transmission

HIV is found in all body fluids with the exception of urine or sweat. Transmission occurs when an uninfected host comes in contact with blood or blood-tinged body fluids (Table 32-3).[14] The mode of acquisition is denoted as the *risk factor* or transmission category. The most common form of HIV transmission worldwide is via heterosexual contact (however, in the United States, it remains male-to-male sexual contact).[5] The risk of transmission is increased when there is exposure to a large amount of the virus (high viral load), to a large amount of contaminated blood or body fluids, and/or if exposure is percutaneous or mucosal (or is of prolonged duration if cutaneous). The risk of sexual transmission is increased in the presence of sexually transmitted diseases (STDs), in uncircumcised men, and during receptive anal or receptive vaginal intercourse. The risk of maternal–fetal transmission is increased in the presence of high maternal viral load, the prolonged rupture of membranes, the presence of STD ulcerations in the birth canal and/or genitals, and with breast feeding. A much smaller proportion of transmission occurs by occupational exposure.

Immunopathogenesis

Acute HIV infection is marked by a rapid and severe loss of memory CD4+/CCR5+ T lymphocytes in gastrointestinal tissue.[15–17] Gut-associated lymphoid tissue (GALT) is a crucial component of the mucosal immune system and contains most of the body's memory CD4+ T lymphocytes.[18] Mucosal exposure to HIV leads to the epithelial production of inflammatory cytokines and diminished barrier integrity, allowing viral entry into the body.[19]

Upon its entry into the submucosal space, HIV is captured by follicular dendritic cells. These cells present multiple virions to CCR5+ CD4+ T cells residing in the gastrointestinal lamina propria, Peyer patches, and mesenteric lymph nodes. In turn, this leads to further activation of inflammatory pathways facilitating the productive infection of CCR5+ CD4+ T cells, cell death, and viral persistence in a subpopulation of latently infected resting T cells.[15,20,21] A minority population of CD4+ T cells do effect a virus-specific response during primary HIV infection.[22] However, the host immune response to HIV is ultimately overcome by viral evolution and other escape mechanisms.

GALT is the largest component of the mucosal immune system, contains most of the body's CCR5+ CD4+ T cells, and is the primary target tissue during acute HIV infection.[23] The density of target cells within the lamina propria and GALT allows HIV to propagate rapidly with severe and largely irreversible gut CCR5+ CD4+ T-cell loss occurring within days of HIV acquisition.[23–25] Early profound loss of CCR5+ CD4+ T cells is specific to the gut and precedes the loss of CD4+ T cells in systemic immune tissue (ie, blood, peripheral lymph nodes).[26] Fibrotic changes in Peyer's patch architecture leads to impaired immunocyte regeneration and is associated with sustained CD4+ T-cell depletion and blunted CCR5+ CD4+ T-cell reconstitution.[27] Blunting may occur in spite of patients receiving effective cART.[27]

Persisting polyclonal B-cell activation, increased CD 4+ and CD 8+ T-cell activation, and the expression of proinflammatory chemokines and cytokines mark chronic HIV infection of GALT.[28–31] Immune activation and inflammation are mediated directly and indirectly by HIV. Direct immune activation manifests as HIV-specific CD8+ T-cell cytolytic response, decreasing CD4+ T-cell response to ongoing HIV infection, and the activation of HIV-specific and nonspecific antibody-producing B cells, natural killer cells, and monocytes. Indirect immune activation occurs with the reactivation of other latent viruses (eg, cytomegalovirus).

Microbial translocation across the gut mucosa has been demonstrated by quantification of lipopolysaccharide and 16S rDNA (conserved DNA sequences common to gram-negative and gram-positive bacteria) in plasma from HIV-infected patients. An inverse relationship exists between blood CD4+ T-cell concentration and plasma lipopolysaccharide and 16S rDNA.[32,33] Microbial translocation is believed to participate in CD4+ T-cell activation in spite of a lack of overt bacteremia. Persistent immune activation ultimately leading to cell death is believed to contribute to systemic CD4+ T-cell depletion in chronic HIV infection.[34,35]

Patients initiating cART at low CD4 counts may experience a period of paradoxical clinical deterioration or immune reconstitution inflammatory syndrome (IRIS). This period of clinical deterioration is usually self-limited but can be life-threatening. IRIS is an inflammatory response caused by an enhanced antigen-specific immune response to a previously unseen (by the immune system) opportunistic or secondary infection. Clinical presentation may include lymphadenopathy, pulmonary infiltrates, headache, fever, and meningitis depending on the infective focus. In some instances, lymphadenopathy may lead to compartment syndromes requiring emergent treatment with anti-inflammatory agents (ie, corticosteroids). At greatest risk are patients initiating cART simultaneously or shortly following treatment for *Mycobacterium tuberculosis*, *Mycobacterium avium* complex, or *Cryptococcus neoformans*.

The Clinical Manifestation of Immunodeficiency

The natural history of HIV disease begins with an initial retroviral syndrome, a protracted flulike illness often accompanied by a rash, followed by CD4+ T-lymphocyte decline (rapidly over months or slowly over years). The progressive loss of CD4+ T lymphocytes leads to the deterioration of cell-mediated and humoral immunity. The risk of opportunistic or secondary infection or AIDS-defining malignances is driven by the CD4 count. For example, at a CD4 count of 200 to 500 cells/mm^3, patients may present with oral or vaginal candidiasis, reactivation of prior viral infections (ie, *Herpes simplex* or *Herpes zoster*) or bacterial infections (ie, *Staphylococcus aureus* or *Pseudomonas aeruginosa*). At CD4 counts less than 200 cells/mm^3, patients may present with opportunistic infections and AIDS-related malignancies. A diagnosis of AIDS is made whenever an HIV-infected person has a CD4 count less than 200 cells/mm^3 (or a CD4 cell percentage less than 14%) or is diagnosed with wasting syndrome or other AIDS-defining illness (Table 32-2). Wasting, hypogonadism or menstrual irregularities, nutrient malabsorption, and oropharyngeal candidiasis are prevalent in persons with AIDS. A presumptive diagnosis of *Candida* esophagitis may be made in patients experiencing dysphagia or odynophagia. Unlike oropharyngeal candidiasis, which usually responds rapidly to oral therapy, esophageal candidiasis may require intravenous antifungal therapy.

Antiretroviral Medications

The goal of antiretroviral therapy is to facilitate CD4+ T-lymphocyte reconstitution by the long-term suppression of viral replication. The ability of a particular antiretroviral regimen to suppress viral replication may be monitored by quantitative RT-PCR. Viral burden or viral load is reported as copies per milliliter or $\log_{10}$ copies per milliliter. Treatment-naïve patients initiating cART are expected to achieve a 2- to 3-log drop in viral load within 8 to 16 weeks. Viral burden is expected to remain below the threshold of detection by quantitative RT-PCR during cART. HIV specialist physicians usually monitor viral load by RT-PCR every 3 to 4 months in routine care.

Antiretrovirals are prescribed in combination (two or more classes) in an effort to prevent the emergence of resistant virus. A therapeutic adherence rate of 95% or better is associated with threefold lower all-cause mortality risk.[36] Achievement of a 95% adherence rate in practice means fewer than two missed doses per month. This level of therapeutic adherence is far greater than that required in the medical management of other chronic conditions.

There are six classes of U.S. Food and Drug Administration (FDA)-approved antiretroviral medications for the treatment of HIV infection (Table 32-4). The classes of FDA-approved

TABLE 32-4 Antiretroviral Medications[a]

Class/Generic Name	Brand Name	Capsule	Tablet	Liquid Form	Intravenous
Fixed-dose combination nonnucleoside, nucleoside, and nucleotide reverse transcriptase inhibitors					
Efavirenz/emtricitabine/tenofovir	**Atripla** (EFV/FTC/TDF)		X		
Rilpivirine/emtricitabine/tenofovir	**Complera** (RPV/FTC/TDF)		X		
Integrase inhibitors					
Raltegravir	**Isentress** (RAL)		X		
Coreceptor antagonist			(film coated or chewable)		
Maraviroc	**Selzentry** (MVC)		X		
Nucleoside/tide reverse transcriptase inhibitors (NRTI/NtRTI)[b]					
Abacavir /lamivudine	**Epzicom** (EPZ)		X		
Lamivudine/zidovudine	**Combivir** (CBV)		X		
Abacavir/lamivudine/zidovudine	**Trizivir** (TRZ)		X		
Emtricitabine/tenofovir	**Truvada** FTC/TDF		X Film coated		
Lamivudine	**Epivir** 3TC		X Film coated	X Flavored	
Zidovudine	**Retrovir** (AZT, ZDV)		X	X	X
Abacavir	**Ziagen** (ABC)		X	X	
Emtricitabine	**Emtriva** (FTC)	X		X	
Tenofovir	**Viread** (TDF)		X		
Didanosine	**Videx** (DDI)	X		Buffered	
	Videx EC	X		Powder	
Stavudine	**Zerit** d4T	X		X	
Protease inhibitors (PI)					
Darunavir	**Prezista** (DRV)		X		
Fosamprenavir	**Lexiva** (FPV)		X		
Indinavir	**Crixivan** (IDV)	X			
Saquinavir	**Invirase** (SQV)	X	X		
Lopinavir / low-dose ritonavir	**Kaletra** (LPV/r)		X	X	
Ritonavir	**Norvir** (RTV)	X	X	X	
Atazanavir	**Reyataz** (ATZ)	X			
Nelfinavir	**Viracept** NFV		X	X Oral powder	
Tipranavir	**Aptivus**	X			
Nonnucleoside reverse transcriptase inhibitors (NNRTI)					
Etravirine	**Intelence** (ETR)		X (may be dispersed in water)		
Delavirdine	**Rescriptor** (DLV)		X (may be dispersed in water)		
Efavirenz	**Sustiva** (EFV)		X		
Nevirapine	**Viramune** (NVP)		X	X	
Rilpivirine	**Edurant** (RPV)		X		
Fusion inhibitor (FI)					
Enfuvirtide	**Fuzeon** T-20 injection only				

[a]Monitor electrolytes (including bicarbonate levels), creatinine, transaminases, fasting glucose, and lipid panels in patients receiving cART.
[b]**Class warning** for **lactic acidosis,** consider in differential for nonspecific complaints of nausea, emesis, abdominal pain, fatigue, dyspnea, and weight loss. Routine screening not recommended.

antiretroviral medications are nucleoside reverse transcriptase inhibitors (NRTIs), nucleotide reverse transcriptase inhibitors (NtRTIs), nonnucleoside reverse transcriptase inhibitors (NNRTIs), protease inhibitors (PIs), fusion inhibitors, coreceptor antagonists, and integrase strand transfer inhibitors. Each class inhibits a specific stage of HIV interaction with cell-surface receptors, viral membrane-to-cell membrane fusion, or intracellular viral replication (Figure 32-1). Ritonavir is used as a pharmacologic booster for other protease inhibitors due to its inhibition of cytochrome 3A4 isoenzymes.

FIGURE 32-1 The HIV Replication Cycle

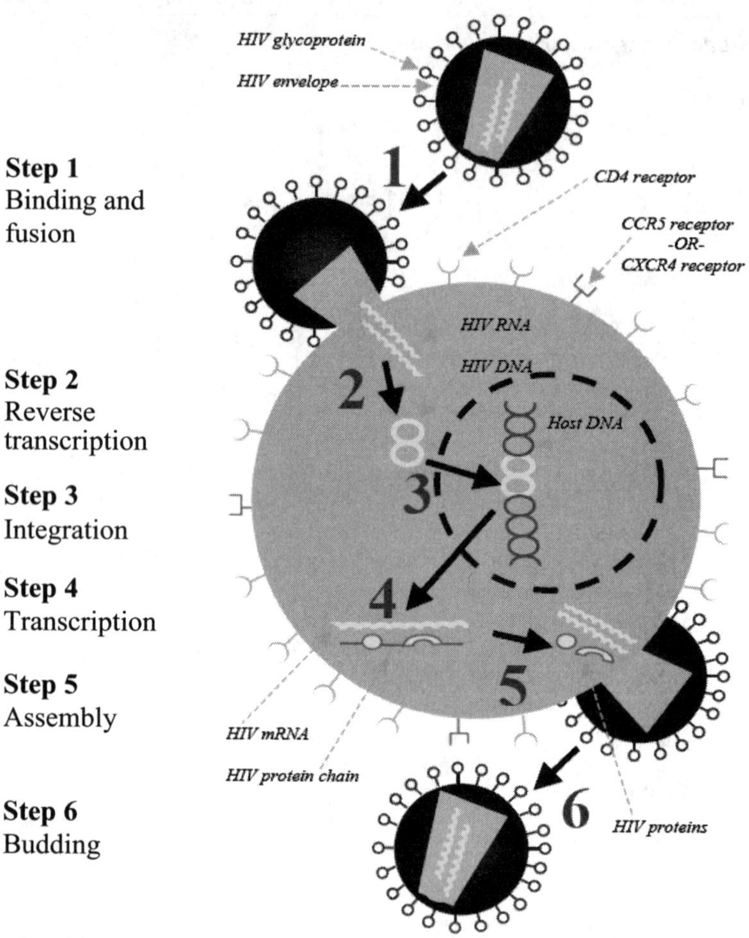

Adapted from The HIV Life Cycle. May 2005. AIDSinfo. http://www.aidsinfo.nih.gov/ContentFiles/HIVLifeCycle_FS_en.pdf.

Nutritional Metabolism in the Current cART Era

In the United States, more than 25% of persons living with HIV infection are over 50 years old, and 15% of incident HIV infections occur in this age group.[3] Seventy percent of people living with HIV/AIDS are men.[6] Increasingly, newly diagnosed persons with HIV/AIDS live in urban poverty areas and experience food and housing insecurity, as well as limited access to fresh foodstuffs.[12] These demographic data have profound implications for the nutritional care of persons with HIV infection.

Wasting disease was the prominent nutritional issue in patient management prior to the advent of cART. Although wasting disease still occurs, HIV infection has become a chronic condition for most patients. Noninfectious comorbidities (eg, cardiovascular disease, osteopenia/osteoporosis, sarcopenia) are now predominant in HIV medicine. They have a significant dietary component and are associated with aging.

Wasting Syndrome/Disease

History

Early in the HIV epidemic, wasting syndrome (disease) was often described in association with opportunistic infection and/or AIDS-related malignancies.[37] The CDC defined wasting syndrome in 1987 as an involuntary weight loss greater than 10% from baseline, chronic diarrhea or documented fever for more than 30 days, and associated weakness (asthenia). Before cART, the introduction of prophylaxis for *Pneumocystis carinii* (now known as *Pneumocystis jiroveci*) pneumonia (PCP) effectively diminished it as the predominant cause of AIDS-related morbidity and mortality, to be replaced by wasting syndrome. In spite of the widespread availability of cART, wasting continues to occur and it remains an AIDS-defining event associated with morbidity and mortality.[38]

Epidemiology

In the year 2002, investigators documented wasting incidence rates as high as 10.6/100 patient-years in HIV-infected women attending an urban clinic.[39] The prevalence of wasting syndrome was 22.1%.[39] The Nutrition for Healthy Living Cohort documented a 33.6% incidence of wasting in 2000. Of the patients in the cohort, 70% had CD4 counts of 200 cells/mm^3 or greater and 24% of patients had CD4 counts greater than 500 cells/mm^3.[40] Moyle et al.[41] reported that 66.1% of treatment-evaluable patients demonstrating wasting had baseline viral loads of less than 400 copies/mL. These findings suggest that wasting may not be solely linked to immunodeficiency or viral burden and that it may occur in the absence of opportunistic or secondary infection or other clinical disease.

The development of well-tolerated and more potent antiretrovirals over the last 6 years, along with the advent of fixed-dose combination tablets, has led to better medical outcomes. This has likely led to a reduction in the prevalence of wasting syndrome in HIV-infected patients receiving care in wealthy nations. However, no studies documenting a reduction in the prevalence of wasting syndrome in the current decade have been published. Recent publications document prevalent food insecurity in community-dwelling HIV-infected persons under care in North America.[42,43] In addition, a growing number of state AIDS Drug Assistance Programs (ADAP, a primarily federally funded program) in the United States have instituted waiting lists for the treatment of HIV infection. Structural inequalities, food insecurity, and a lack of access to antiretroviral therapy may manifest as wasting disease in individuals with HIV infection presenting for acute care.

Early in the HIV epidemic, investigators demonstrated that the degree of soft-tissue wasting was independently associated with when death ensued.[44] Weight loss or lower baseline body mass index (BMI) continue to be predictive of opportunistic infection, poor outcome, or mortality in spite of cART.[45,46] Loss of skeletal muscle and adipose tissue may lead to a patient's inability to execute the instrumental activities of daily living, ensuing social isolation, and depression, all of which may be obstacles to therapeutic adherence.

Case Definition and Clinical Diagnosis

The definition of wasting has undergone a number of changes in the years since the original 1987 CDC definition. Wasting is now defined by functional, physiologic, body weight–based parameters, mid-upper arm circumference, and other physical findings (Table 32-5). An evaluation of weight loss includes the degree of loss, whether it is acute or chronic, and medical and psychological context. Weight loss may be statistically but not medically significant. For example, an overweight patient may achieve weight loss after entry into care with attention to food quality and regularly scheduled aerobic and resistance exercise. Such loss would not warrant intervention. On the other hand, patient complaints of involuntary weight loss and diminished physical performance and well-being requires medical investigation and nutritional evaluation. In the classic investigation of semistarvation and refeeding, Keys et al.[47] found that physical performance began to decline after a weight loss of greater than 10% in healthy normal weight volunteers.

Analysis of body composition by the application of predictive equations to the measurement of body circumferences and skin folds, bioelectrical impedance analysis, imaging of lean body mass and fat mass by dual-energy X-ray absorptiometry (DEXA), or skeletal muscle and adipose tissue by magnetic resonance imaging (MRI) or computed tomography (CT) allow for the description of wasting disease and recovery at the tissue-system level. Mid-upper arm or thigh circumference and skin fold measurements correlate with body composition analysis by MRI and long-term clinical outcome.[48] This has led to an appreciation of the importance of anthropometric evaluation in the routine care of HIV-infected patients.

Wasting Disease Compared to Uncomplicated Starvation

Severe undernutrition and famine have long been known to influence human susceptibility to infection and to worsen the clinical course of infectious disease. Infectious disease may, in turn, blunt or prevent human physiologic adaptation to diminished nutrient intake. The human species evolved in an environment of intermittent food availability ("feast or famine"). During starvation, the endocrine system and major metabolic pathways mount an evolutionarily appropriate adaptive response. Skeletal muscle, organ, and adipose tissue are all subject to breakdown to yield substrate for energetic processes during starvation. Compensatory metabolic and constitutional changes occur in starvation in an attempt to minimize the loss of skeletal muscle and organ parenchyma. Decreases in the insulin-to-glucagon ratio are believed to mediate these changes, and basal metabolic rate is reduced in an effort to bring total energy expenditure into balance with the energetic value of food intake. Individuals may experience lethargy (a reduction of voluntary energy expenditure) and present with flat affect. Fat is preferentially used directly for energy (including brain keto acid use) and for the conversion of lactate and pyruvate to glucose (gluconeogenesis).[49,50] In muscle tissue, the use of fatty acids for energy reduces the breakdown of muscle fibers for the release of alanine, a primary gluconeogenic amino acid. This adaptation to preserve structural/functional proteins is known as nitrogen sparing. Death ensues from exhaustion of the two main energy depots (adipose tissue and skeletal muscle) and catabolism of organ parenchyma leading to organ system failure.

Etiology and Pathogenesis of Wasting Disease

The etiology of wasting disease in a given patient is multifactorial. Wasting may be an effect of HIV infection, which in turn worsens a patient's clinical course by increasing vulnerability to other infectious disease and decreasing capacity for self-care. Conversely, the lesions of opportunistic infection may in turn lead to wasting disease. Mechanisms may include food insecurity, decreased food intake and/or decreased nutrient assimilation due to disease process, abnormal metabolism, and/or endocrine dysfunction. The identification of causation determines the appropriate therapeutic intervention(s) (Table 32-6). The inability to mount a compensatory metabolic response to undernutrition due to viral effect on nutritional metabolism is what distinguishes the HIV-infected patient experiencing undernutrition from the uninfected patient experiencing the same. Maladaptive metabolic abnormalities in the HIV-infected patient experiencing undernutrition include increased resting energy expenditure (REE), inappropriate substrate use, and the futile cycling of lipids.

Chronic undernutrition may occur as a consequence of food insecurity in association with large-scale social forces: poverty or civil unrest, and/or the constitutional manifestations of AIDS, profound fatigue, and impaired physical or cognitive function. The inability to consistently acquire food and prepare meals (instrumental activities of daily living) may ensue from social, environmental, and/or biological causes. All of these factors singularly or in combination may affect nutriture, disease course, and medical outcomes. HIV-infected patients often present with a combination of these problems. Food insecurity is defined as limited or uncertain availability of nutritionally adequate, safe foods or the inability to acquire personally acceptable foods in socially acceptable ways.[51] Food insecurity may coexist with hunger or be experienced in the absence of hunger, and may contribute to wasting or obesity. The association with obesity, although counterintuitive, is likely due to reliance on inexpensive calorie-dense convenience foods (fast food or take out) and sugar-sweetened beverages.

Prolonged decrease in caloric intake is the proximate predictor and drive of wasting disease.[52] Decreased food intake may drive wasting in spite of compensatory lethargy, which attempts to bring total energy expenditure into balance with caloric intake.[52] Negative energy balance with catabolism ensues when the patient is no longer able to achieve a sufficient compensatory decrease in total energy expenditure. Depression in a patient may manifest as anorexia and involuntary weight loss. Anorexia due to systemic infection (eg, HIV viremia, bacteremia, disseminated opportunistic infection) is believed to ensue from the action of proinflammatory cytokines such as interleukin (IL)-6 on the central nervous system and viscera, mediating delayed gastric emptying and intestinal edema.

Compensatory lethargy may occur in wasting syndrome, but it is not accompanied by a decrease in basal metabolic rate or adaptive metabolic response to facilitate nitrogen sparing. Therapeutically, the difference lies in the effect of refeeding, which alone reverses starvation but not AIDS wasting.

In a seminal study, Grunfeld et al.[52] assessed REE and 28-day weight trend in a cohort of HIV-infected patients. REE increases of 11%, 25%, and 28% were documented in patients with HIV-infection (HIV+), AIDS, and AIDS with active secondary infection (AIDS-SI), respectively.[52] The difference in REE increase in patients with AIDS compared to patients with AIDS-SI was not statistically significant. The caloric value of *ad libitum* food and beverage intake in AIDS-SI patients was 17% less than REE, and they experienced weight loss during the study period.[52] The investigators demonstrated that decreased caloric intake (CI) or food intake was predictive of wasting, and that increased REE with a CI-to-REE ratio less than 1 were associated with wasting.[52] A number of other studies have documented similar results.[53] Clinically decreased food intake and the inability to mount a compensatory decrease in basal metabolic rate (quantified as REE) leads to accelerated weight loss and is the primary drive of wasting.

Dietary thermogenesis is the energy expended for nutrient absorption and assimilation. Patients with HIV infection experience both a temporal and quantitative change in diet-induced thermogenesis. In HIV infection, peak meal-induced thermogenesis occurs later, and the elevation is more prolonged. Patients with HIV infection and weight loss demonstrate greater increases than those with HIV infection alone.[54]

HIV-infected patients with wasting disease may demonstrate increases in hepatic *de novo* lipogenesis when compared to normotypic controls.[55] Approximately 30% of the caloric value of glucose is lost if lipogenesis precedes its oxidation instead of its direct use for energy. In a patient experiencing wasting, such a conversion would be energetically inappropriate and contrasts sharply with the use of lipids for gluconeogenesis in uncomplicated starvation. In a study of patients receiving nutritional supplementation orally, the accrual of lean body mass was inversely correlated with baseline *de novo* lipogenesis.[56] In AIDS patients, interferon alpha levels may be elevated and the peripheral tissue expression of lipoprotein lipase diminished, leading to a reduction in triglyceride clearance.[57,58] These findings demonstrate the effect of HIV *per se* (in the absence of suppressive therapy) and correlate with clinical hypertriglyceridemia in AIDS patients, and mark the futile cycling of lipids between peripheral and hepatic tissue. However, isolated hypertriglyceridemia is not uniformly associated with (or predictive of) wasting syndrome.[58] Nevertheless, it is important to check triglyceride levels in all HIV-infected patients when providing nutritional care and especially prior to the infusion of lipid-containing intravenous admixtures.

Increase in whole body protein turnover (synthesis and degradation) has been documented in HIV-infected patients and is consistent with a hypermetabolic state. The fraction of total protein synthesis accorded to skeletal muscle is similar in asymptomatic HIV-infected and uninfected individuals.[59] Muscle protein synthesis represents a decreased fraction of whole body protein synthesis in individuals demonstrating AIDS wasting.[59] This suggests a diminished ability to use amino acids for synthetic pathways in skeletal muscle and/or increased competition from oxidative (energy yielding) pathways or other tissue for amino acids (eg, hepatic or blood cell synthesis of immune effector proteins). In asymptomatic HIV-infected subjects, rates of amino acid oxidation were found to be elevated and were likely associated with predisposition toward skeletal muscle loss.[59] Conflicting data regarding skeletal muscle amino acid metabolism in HIV-infected patients may be due to the different experimental techniques employed in published studies.

Upregulation of autophagy is a cell-level response to nutrient and/or growth factor deprivation and is achieved by a common pathway in both viral infection and undernutrition.[60] Autophagy may also be an antiviral response in addition to promoting the survival of starved cells by intracellular digestion and recycling of cellular proteins, including virally encoded proteins, and lipids for nutritional purposes.[60]

The investigative and therapeutic administration of cytokines has been associated with anorexia, fatigue, and malaise. These responses are also seen in the innate immune response to acute infection. For example, the administration of tumor necrosis factor (TNF)-α to study animals led to decreased gastric emptying, increased intestinal edema, and worsening clinical anorexia.[61] Interestingly, the continued administration of TNF-α led to tolerance demonstrated by the animals' eventual resumption of oral intake.[61] In humans, the exact cause of anorexia is likely multifactorial, linked to cytokine milieu and not to a single factor. In AIDS wasting, unlike the acute phase response in febrile illness, patients have excess serum levels of TNF-α soluble receptor (cytokine antagonists and markers of immune activation).[62] As a result of this antagonism, the effect of TNF-α is blunted, underscoring that TNF-α is not the single major factor responsible for AIDS wasting.[62]

Regardless of cause, a detrimental clinical impact occurs when the patient is no longer able to achieve a compensatory decrease in total energy expenditure (leading to negative energy balance). The combination of an inability to maintain caloric intake and increased REE (hypermetabolism) drives wasting. Patients are at highest risk for wasting during episodes of opportunistic or secondary infection(s) and/or malignancy. The mechanical (eg, oral and esophageal disease) and psychological (eg, depression) causes of diminished food intake require evaluation and treatment as needed.

The incidence of opportunistic infection and malignancies of the gastrointestinal tract has declined with the widespread use of cART, but prevalence remains high in patients with immunodeficiency (CD4 count less than 200 cells/mm^3). Intestinal infection may be marked by maldigestion, malabsorption, and diarrhea. Infections of the small and large bowel may disseminate to other organ systems and further compromise nutrition. Malabsorption is characterized by decreased nutrient absorption accompanied by fecal water and electrolyte loss. Malabsorption may occur in association with structural changes in small intestinal villi or obstruction of the lymphatics. For example, infection with the protozoal gastrointestinal parasites *Cryptosporidium parvum* and *Enterocytozoon bieneusi* (microsporidia) results in partial atrophy of villi with diminished absorptive surface area (in spite of compensatory crypt hyperplasia). Moreover, immature enterocytes do not elaborate digestive and absorptive proteins, contributing to the loss of mucosal function. Infection with *Mycobacterium avium* complex results in extensive macrophage infiltration of the *lamina propria* and lymphatics, leading to obstruction. The resulting diarrhea (frequently defined as greater than or equal to four bowel movements per day) may lead patients to reduce food intake to reduce the frequency and urgency of bowel movements (thereby worsening wasting).

Both primary hypogonadism (testicular failure) and secondary hypogonadism (hypothalamic and/or pituitary failure) may occur in HIV-infected men.[63,64] In men with AIDS wasting syndrome loss of lean body mass (ascertained by DEXA), loss of skeletal muscle mass (calculated by measured urinary creatinine excretion on a meat-free diet), and decrease in exercise capacity were associated with low androgen levels.[65] Low testosterone levels were found in 19% of men in a cART era study.[66] The men were less than 90% of ideal body weight or demonstrated a greater than 10% loss from pre-illness weight.[66] Transient downregulation of testosterone synthesis may also occur during clinically active secondary or opportunistic infections.

Men with hypogonadism may present with complaints of depression, mood change or irritability, erectile dysfunction, decreased libido, decreased appetite, and a loss of muscle mass and/or weight (Practice Scenario 32-1). In the serum, testosterone is bound by sex hormone–binding globulin (SHBG). This protein may be increased in HIV infection, leading to decreased free (bioactive) testosterone levels while maintaining normal total testosterone levels. Therefore, hypogonadism is diagnosed on the basis of free, not total, testosterone. Free testosterone (and probably SHBG) levels should be routinely evaluated in male patients and blood drawn for its assay in the early morning. Evaluation is usually done during the convalescent phase of prolonged illness or routinely in outpatient care.

Women with wasting disease may also experience reduced serum testosterone levels. Testosterone testing has not been standardized for women. However, several successful clinical trials of treatment with exogenous testosterone have been reported.[67,68] Levels of free testosterone in eumenorrheic women may be affected by the phases of the menstrual cycle, and the optimal long-term replacement dosage of testosterone for women has not been determined.[65–67] This usage remains investigational.[67–69]

Patients with wasting syndrome may demonstrate acquired growth hormone (GH) resistance. Studies of undernutrition and wasting disease in HIV-infected patients have identified a role for insulin like growth factor-1 (IGF-1) in anabolism.[70,71] IGF-1 is produced by the liver in response to GH, and works with GH in a synergistic manner on target tissues. IGF-1 upregulates metabolism and/or cell proliferation depending on the level of cellular differentiation. For example, GH and IGF-1 have a trophic effect on muscle cells demonstrated by increased myocyte synthesis of myofibrillar protein during exposure. IGF-1 production is downregulated in undernutrition and severe chronic illness, functioning as an adaptive mechanism to free amino acids and other substrates for critical processes. Investigators have documented elevated GH levels with inappropriately low IGF-1 levels in cohorts of hypogonadal and eugonadal HIV-infected men demonstrating wasting.[71] These findings are consistent with acquired GH resistance at the level of the liver in profound undernutrition and wasting disease, and form the rationale for treatment with supraphysiologic doses of recombinant human growth hormone (rhGH).[72]

Practice Scenario 32-1

Question: A male patient presents to clinic 6 weeks after initiating cART complaining of an inability to gain weight and erectile dysfunction. What hormone deficiency would you have a high index of suspicion for and which medication might be associated with these complaints?

Scenario: A 46-year-old white male diagnosed with AIDS 3 months ago while hospitalized and treated for PJP and oral candidiasis presents to clinic complaining of erectile dysfunction, irritability, and an inability to gain weight.

Intervention: On evaluation, the patient was 6 ft (1.83 m) tall and weighed 145 lbs (65.9 kg). His weight was unchanged since discharge from the hospital (80.5% of his usual weight). BMI was 19.7; waist, 34 inches; hips, 38.75 inches; waist-to-hip ratio, 0.88; and mid-upper arm circumference and skin fold were less than the 10th percentile. BIA results revealed: phase angle, 4.9°; body cell mass, 55.5 lbs, 36%; fat mass, 19.7 lbs, 14. 4%; extracellular tissue-to-body cell mass ratio, 1.3. Laboratory results were significant for: CD4 150 cells/mL[3] (1.2%); CD4-to-CD8 ratio, 0.1; and HIV RT-PCR RNA less than 20 copies/mL (undetectable). A medication review revealed that he initiated cART with Atripla (fixed dose combination efavirenz, emtricitabine, tenofovir) daily. Other medications include: azithromycin 600 mg twice weekly and trimethoprim-sulfamethoxazole double strength tablet once daily for MAI and PJP prophylaxis, respectively. Food intake was excellent with a 24-hour dietary recall of approximately 2600 kcals/day with 95 g/day as protein.

Answer: The patient was not receiving megestrol acetate. Megestrol acetate is a synthetic progestin that may downregulate testosterone synthesis leading to erectile dysfunction and loss of lean body mass with prolonged receipt. An early morning blood draw was scheduled for a testosterone panel. Free testosterone was low on both initial and repeat panels. Testosterone replacement therapy was initiated with testosterone cream 5 g topical, daily to shoulders and upper arms.

Rationale: Irritability or mood changes, erectile dysfunction, and an inability to gain weight, particularly LBM, are suggestive of hypogonadism. Hypogonadism is a frequent finding in HIV-infected patients with wasting syndrome.[66] Testosterone replacement therapy in hypogonadal HIV-infected men has been shown to improve mood or the sense of well-being, improve sexual function, and augment muscle strength and lean body mass accrual.[193]

Clinical Encounter and Assessment

Clinical investigation of a complaint of wasting or involuntary weight loss should include evaluation for the degree and rapidity of the weight change (ie, acute versus chronic), depression, and ability to perform instrumental activities of daily living. It is often helpful to ask patients for a preillness photograph, when they last remember being at their usual weight, and the last time they engaged in enjoyable activities or hobbies (Figure 32-2).

In patients with a CD4 count less than 100 cells/mm^3, loss of appetite and weight may be the first signs of slowly progressive systemic opportunistic infections such as cytomegalovirus or *Mycobacterium avium* complex. In these patients, attention should be paid to weight loss decrement, presence of fever, and presence and location of abdominal pain. Complaints of diarrhea may be evaluated by determining the change from usual bowel movement pattern (frequency), consistency, amount or volume, and the presence of blood and/or mucus. For example, copious watery diarrhea may be associated with small bowel disease and mucus-containing small volume diarrhea with colonic disease.

Clinicians should be mindful of the social determinants of wasting disease. Food insecurity may be evaluated by using the U.S. Department of Agriculture food security questionnaire (6-item short form) or Radimer/Cornell questionnaire.[51,73] In many states, food stamps (Supplemental Nutrition Assistance Program) may be applied for online or by mail. The ability to shop for and prepare meals and access to supermarkets and kitchen facilities should also be evaluated. AIDS service organizations (ASOs) and dedicated government programs may provide home meal delivery, congregate meals, food pantries, or home attendants for shopping and cooking. Psychiatric counseling for depression and peer support groups may also be available through ASOs. However, patients frequently require an AIDS/HIV disease diagnosis and/or medical documentation of a medical condition that limits ambulation for home meal delivery or attendant care.

FIGURE 32-2 Wasting Treatment Strategies

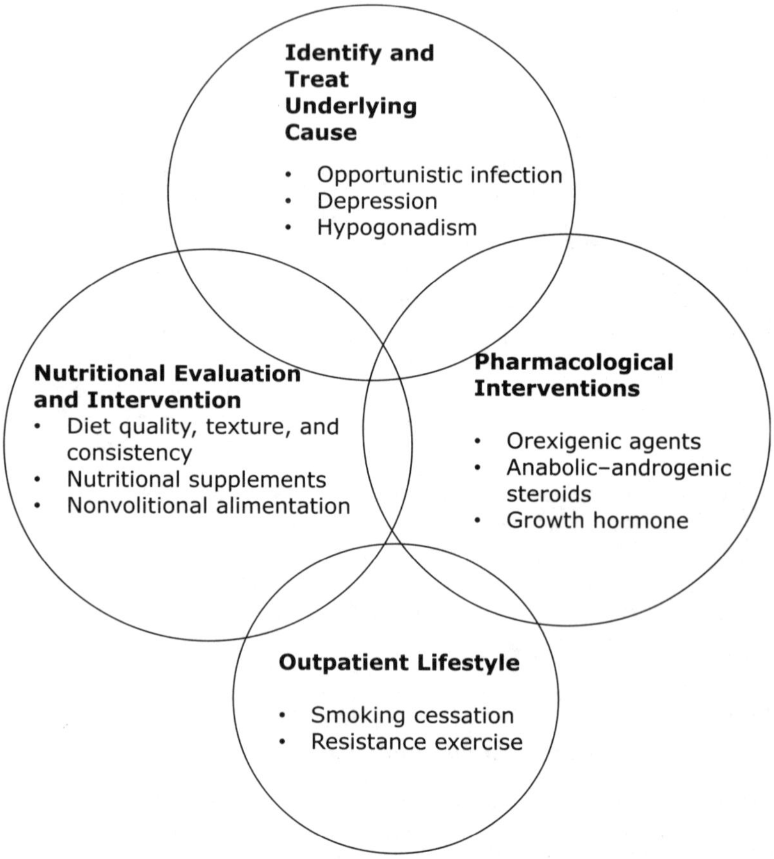

Nutrition-Focused Physical Examination

Patients with an HIV infection may present with wasting (involuntary loss of skeletal muscle and adipose tissue), sarcopenia (age-related loss of skeletal muscle with preservation or increase in adipose tissue), or lipodystrophy (focal or global loss of subcutaneous adipose tissue with the preservation of visceral adipose tissue and skeletal muscle). The nutrition-focused physical examination is essential in distinguishing between these clinical presentations.

Bilateral temporal wasting, periocular fat wasting, and the loss of Bichat's fat pad should be evaluated for during an examination of the head and neck. An oral examination should evaluate for missing dentition and oral mucosa ulcers (eg, aphthous or viral ulcers), malignancy (eg, Kaposi sarcoma), and fungal infections (eg, oral candidiasis), among others. Findings on inspection of the torso consistent with wasting include subclavicular muscle loss (with increased clavicle prominence), angular shoulders due to deltoid muscle loss (with increased acromion process prominence), and visible articulations of the ribs at the junction with the sternum. Waist circumference and the waist-to-hip ratio are often helpful in distinguishing wasting from lipodystrophy syndrome, because the patient with wasting is unlikely to experience isolated fat loss in the face, extremities, and buttocks without significant abdominal fat loss. The loss of appendicular skeletal muscle and subcutaneous fat mass may be evaluated for by measurement of mid-upper arm circumference and a skinfold using the National Health and Nutrition Examination Survey (NHANES) percentiles for reference ranges.[74] Skeletal muscle may also be clinically evaluated by having the patient press the tips of his or her forefinger and thumb together and observing the mass of the *interosseous dorsalis* or by placing the patient's leg at a right angle and observing muscle mass at the insertion of the *quadriceps femoris* and the *vastus medialis*.

Bioelectrical impedance analysis (BIA) indirectly measures body composition using a four-compartment model: lean body mass (LBM), which is divided into body cell mass (BCM) and extracellular (interstitial) mass (ECM); fat mass; and osseous tissue.[75] BCM by weight is primarily skeletal muscle. Phase angle is a geometrical expression of the resistance and capacitance components of this assay. Ott et al.[76] demonstrated that phase angles less than 5.6° and 4.8° were associated with diminished and

TABLE 32-5 Clinical Findings Consistent with Wasting Disease[a]

Subjective
Lethargy
Anorexia
Food insecurity
Loose fitting clothes
Physical Function
Difficulty or inability to stand without assistance
Vital signs
Unintentional weight loss[b]
$>$ 10%
$>$ 5% within 6 months
BMI
$<$ 18.5 or marked decline from usual BMI
Mid-upper arm circumference
$<$ 10th NHANES percentile
Physical findings
Head
Temporal wasting, periocular edema or fat loss, prominent zygomatic process
Torso
Subclavicular muscle loss, angular shoulders, visible articulations of ribs at junction with sternum
Sacral edema (in bed rest/bound patient)
Extremities
Diminished mass interosseous dorsalis when pressing thumb to forefinger
Diminished mass quadriceps femoris and vastus medialis when leg bent at right angle
Delayed mid-upper arm skin fold return, loss of turgor
Lower extremity edema

[a]Single findings may be consistent with wasting disease but not definitive per se.
[b]Note that individuals transitioning from highly structured environments providing regularly scheduled prepared meals and exercise programs to independent living may experience weight loss unrelated to disease processes (eg, the recently incarcerated).
BMI, body mass index; NHANES, National Health and Nutrition Examination Survey.

nonsurvival, respectively, in the absence of cART.[76] In addition, the ratio of ECM to BCM of 1.3 or greater was associated with nonsurvival in the absence of cART.[76] Serial BIA will describe weight loss or gain over time by soft tissue compartment, and will allow for the appreciation of each compartment's response to intervention(s) for wasting disease.

Medication Review

Medication review should include prescription and over-the-counter pharmaceuticals, as well as supplements and botanical (herbal) products. Certain botanical or supplemental products have negative drug interactions with cART (eg, garlic supplements, St. John's wort). Medications may require administration with a meal for absorption (eg, rilpivirine) or may interact with one another. Medications may also affect serum glucose, electrolyte, or lipid levels. Patients' routine meal composition and pattern should be identified and discussed. For example, a patient may think a cup of coffee and a donut or muffin are a meal, but this may not be adequate for drug absorption or the prevention of untoward gastrointestinal side effects with certain medications (eg, atovaquone or ritonavir-boosted protease inhibitor). Patients should be counseled that certain food stuffs negatively affect drug levels (eg, grapefruit). Patients receiving other medications, such as foscarnet, require close monitoring of serum calcium, magnesium, potassium, phosphorous, and glucose due to potential dose-related nephrotoxicity. Patients with lactose intolerance may experience diarrhea from pharmaceutical formulations with lactose as an excipient. Clinicians should be familiar with the information contained in medication package inserts, such as food effect, drug interactions and metabolism, excipients, and data on potential side effects.

Social and Family History

Social history should include social determinants of health (eg, educational attainment, housing, access to kitchen facilities and supermarkets). Health-related behaviors should also be evaluated and documented in the nutrition consultation. Tobacco, alcohol or other psychoactive substance use, and disordered sleeping habits may have quantitative and/or qualitative effects on food intake.[77] Prolonged bed rest and/or a lack of weight-bearing exercise may negatively impact a patient's skeletal muscle, bone mineral density, and food intake.[78]

Evaluation of family history (three generations for diabetes, cardiovascular disease events, bone fragility fractures, end-stage renal disease, cancer, etc.) may reveal potential intolerance of nutritional intervention or a requirement for additional testing. For example, a patient with a family history of diabetes may demonstrate glucose abnormalities while receiving megestrol acetate or rhGH. Patients with a family history of fragility fracture who have experienced wasting disease and low CD4 (additional risk factors) may be candidates for DEXA to evaluate for bone mineral density loss.

Clinical Management

Nutrition support of the wasted patient may include the following: the avoidance of food odors during periods of nausea, the alteration of foods (texture, consistency, acidity) to facilitate intake in the presence of oropharyngeal or esophageal lesions, ready-to-use therapeutic food, orexigenic agents, electrolyte management, and intravenous alimentation or feeding by intragastric tubes (Table 32-6). Nutrition should be focused on adequate nonprotein calorie and protein calorie intake, particularly during episodes of secondary or opportunistic infection, micronutrient adequacy, facilitating antimicrobial and/or antiretroviral absorption, and tolerance. Pharmaceutical agents are available for the creation of the sensation of hunger, physiologic hormone replacement, and to promote preferential accrual of skeletal muscle (Table 32-7).

TABLE 32-6 Components of Nutrition Support for Patients with Wasting Disease

Orexigenic agent
Address depression (social work, psychiatry, or chaplaincy consult)
Avoidance of food odors during periods of nausea (well-ventilated room and/or cold foods)
Supplementation to optimize nutrition intake
Alteration of food texture, consistency, acidity, or temperature to facilitate intake
Electrolyte and fluid management
Alteration of macronutrient content to facilitate drug absorption
Physiologic testosterone replacement therapy
Supraphysiologic recombinant human growth hormone or anabolic–androgenic steroid therapy (usually outpatient only)
Intravenous alimentation
Alimentation by gastric or enteric tube

Orexigenic Agents

Megestrol acetate (Megace or Megace ES oral suspension) is a synthetic progestin, related to progesterone, that has been shown to create the sensation of hunger and to promote weight gain in patients with AIDS wasting syndrome.[79] Investigators have documented gains of fat and lean body mass in HIV-infected patients receiving megestrol acetate.[79] As a progestational steroid, megestrol acetate downregulates testosterone synthesis and men may experience erectile dysfunction and/or acceleration of wasting when use is prolonged. Other documented side effects include hyperglycemia, thromboembolic events, and adrenal insufficiency (due to some glucocorticoid activity).[80] Dosages are megestrol acetate oral suspension 20 mL to deliver 800 mg daily or bioequivalent Megace ES 5 mL oral suspension to deliver 625 mg daily.

Dronabinol (delta-9-tetrahydrocannabinol or Marinol) is the active component of marijuana and is approved for the treatment of anorexia in patients with AIDS. Although not as potent as megestrol acetate, it does have mild antiemetic activity and a more benign side-effect profile.[81] It has not been shown to consistently increase food intake and to promote weight gain.[79,82] Potential side effects include psychotropic activity, drowsiness, and hypogonadism. Because of its long half-life, it may be dosed once daily at bedtime for those patients experiencing drowsiness as a side effect. The usual starting dosage is 2.5 mg orally twice daily or 5 mg orally once daily.

Anabolic–Androgenic Steroids

Lean body mass accrual has been documented in HIV-infected men with AIDS wasting syndrome receiving long-term testosterone replacement therapy.[83,84] Several preparations are available for physiologic testosterone replacement and include the transdermal patch, topical gel, or intramuscular injection. The testosterone patch (Androderm) is applied to the upper arm or buttocks to deliver 5 mg of testosterone daily. Transdermal delivery may also be achieved by topical gel (Testim or AndroGel). The dosage is 5 g of gel to deliver 5 mg of testosterone when applied daily. Patients should be counseled that topical testosterone may be transferable by contact. This is an important issue in those patients with female partners (especially pregnant ones) and/or in those in close contact with children. Testosterone esters (eg, testosterone enanthate, an unmodified 17β-ester depot formulation) are available for intramuscular (IM) injection. The usual dose is 200 mg IM every 2 weeks. Unlike daily dosing, this method results in perceptible peak and trough levels during the dosing interval instead of the steady-state physiologic levels obtained with the use of gel or patch.

Pharmacological dosing of testosterone to achieve anabolic–androgenic effect on muscle tissue has been investigated in eugonadal men and women with involuntary weight loss and/or wasting disease. Nandrolone decanoate (19-normethyl-testosterone 17β-ester) is a depot formulation available for long-acting IM delivery of testosterone. It is FDA approved for the treatment of anemia in chronic renal failure. Investigators have documented the association of its off-label use for AIDS wasting syndrome with increases in weight, lean body mass, and quality of life.[85–87] The usual dosage for the treatment of wasting syndrome is 100 to 200 mg IM every 2 weeks.

The treatment of women with androgenic–anabolic steroids has been shown to result in lean body mass accrual without a loss of adipose tissue, but remains investigational because of limited safety data.[88]

Oxandrolone (Oxandrin) is a 17α-methylated testosterone derivative for oral administration. Unlike nandrolone decanoate, it is approved for the treatment of weight loss caused by chronic infection. In a prospective randomized study, HIV-infected men who experienced a mean weight loss of 9% received Oxandrolone 20 mg administered orally once daily. Both arms of the study received testosterone enanthate (100 mg administered IM once weekly) to suppress endogenous testosterone production and participated in a supervised progressive resistance exercise program. The patients in the Oxandrolone arm demonstrated significantly greater increases in lean body mass and strength compared to patients in the control group.[89] Significant decreases in high-density lipoprotein (HDL) cholesterol were also documented in the Oxandrolone arm. Grunfeld et al.[90] document similar results in addition to the suppression of sex-hormone binding globulin, and total and free testosterone levels (subjects were not receiving IM testosterone).[90] Low-density lipoprotein cholesterol and transaminase levels were also significantly elevated in subjects receiving Oxandrolone.[90] Orally ingested 17α-methylated testosterone analogs are subject to first-pass hepatic metabolism, and long-term use has been associated with hepatotoxicity.[91] The identification of a single androgen receptor gene (and protein) suggests that, at bioequivalent dosages, all testosterone formulations have essentially the same physiologic effects.[92] Therefore, nonorally administered testosterone therapy may be preferred to minimize the potential for hepatotoxicity.

TABLE 32-7 Medications for the Treatment of Wasting Disease

	Orexigenic Agents			Physiologic Testosterone Replacement			Anabolic–Androgenic Steroids	
	Megestrol Acetate	Dronabinol	Growth Hormone	Testosterone Gels	Testosterone Patch	Testosterone Enonthate	Nandrolone Decanoate	Oxandrolone
FDA indication specific for AIDS wasting	Yes	Yes	Yes	No	No	No	No	No
Route of administration and dosage	Oral 800 mg daily (20 mL oral suspension)	Oral 2.5 mg twice daily before lunch and dinner	Subcutaneous injection 6 mg daily	Topical 5 g packet daily[a]	Topical 5mg patch daily[b]	Intramuscular injection 200 mg every other week[a]	Intramuscular injection 100–200 mg every other week[b]	Oral 20 mg daily[b]
Duration of clinical studies for AIDS wasting	12 weeks	6 weeks	12 weeks	Ongoing physiologic replacement	Ongoing physiologic replacement	At or above physiologic level during dosing interval	12 weeks	8 weeks
Mechanism of effect	Increase intake	Increase intake	Promote protein synthesis, nitrogen retention	Restore physiologic level, protein synthesis, nitrogen retention	Restore physiologic level, protein synthesis, nitrogen retention	Promote protein synthesis, nitrogen retention	Promote protein synthesis, nitrogen retention	Promote protein synthesis, nitrogen retention
Clinical effect	Increased appetite	Increased appetite	Increased lean body mass and decreased fat (visceral subcutaneous)	Increased lean body mass	Increased lean body mass	Increased lean body mass	Increased lean body mass	Increased lean body mass[d]
Major side effects[c] (see package insert for full information)	Hypogonadism Hyperglycemia Adrenal insufficiency	Dose-related euphoria, somnolence	Dose-related edema, insulin resistance, fat atrophy, arthralgias, myalgias	Application site reaction, acne, peripheral edema	Application site reaction, acne, peripheral edema	Gynecomastia acne, edema, excessive frequency and duration of penile erections	Testicular shrinkage, decreased HDL cholesterol, acne, virilizing effects in women are possible, edema	Decreased HDL cholesterol, hepatotoxicity, peliosis, hepatitis, reduced SHBG, virilizing effects in women are possible

[a]Male dosage.
[b]Male dosage. Female usage is investigational, see text for references.
[c]Testosterone at replacement dosages in hypogonadal males.
[d]Requires resistance exercise for effect.
HDL, high-density lipoprotein; SHBG, sex hormone–binding globulin.

Practice Scenario 32-2

Question: What clinical findings substantiate a diagnosis of wasting syndrome and plan for intravenous alimentation?

Scenario: A 43-year-old white male recently diagnosed with AIDS and treated for *Pneumocystis jiroveci* pneumonia in a community hospital presented to infectious disease clinic for further management. On the initial examination, he was noted to have orthostatic hypotension and was referred for admission to the hospital for IV hydration and management.

Intervention: In-house, the patient disclosed that he was experiencing watery diarrhea four or more times daily, occasionally accompanied by blood; periumbilical and left lower quadrant pain; and abdominal cramping. Symptoms worsened following meals. The patient also complained of odynophagia, anorexia, and a 20-lb weight loss over 6 months. He reported reducing food intake during the last month to avoid urgent bowel movements, which led to his occasionally soiling himself when away from home. Review of stool studies from his prior hospital admission for PJP was unremarkable except for the presence of white blood cells.

The patient was 5 ft 7 inches in height (1.7 m), weighed 125 lbs (56.8 kg, 76.2% of his usual weight of 74.5 kg), and had a BMI of 19.7. On the physical examination, he demonstrated temporal wasting, dry oral mucosa, no evidence of oral candidiasis or missing dentition, and marked subclavicular and deltoid muscle loss with visible contours of rib-to-sternum articulations (consistent with subcutaneous fat loss). Mid-upper arm circumference and skin folds were less than the 10th percentile. Lower extremities exhibited obvious pedal edema with diminished skeletal muscle mass at the insertions of the vastus medialis and quadriceps femoris.

The patient underwent endoscopy and colonoscopy. Visualization of the esophagus, small bowel, and colon revealed large shallow ulcers in the distal esophagus, a small ulcer in the antrum of the stomach, and several areas of erosion (loss of mucosal integrity), ulceration (deep lesions with necrotic tissue), and inflammation of the small bowel wall. Multiple areas of edema and erythema in addition to ulcers were visible in the transverse and right colon. Histology from all areas demonstrated characteristic basophilic nuclear inclusion bodies with narrow clear halos consistent with diffuse CMV enteritis/colitis, and distal esophagitis with gastric involvement. A 3-week course of intravenous foscarnet was ordered.

Answer: Diarrheal disease, involuntary weight loss, percentage usual weight, mid-upper arm circumference percentile, and BMI were consistent with wasting syndrome. Signs of wasting, obvious pedal edema, and diminished skeletal muscle mass indicated severity and clinical urgency. Orthostatic hypotension at presentation for care and documentation of extensive small bowel erosions, ulceration, and inflammation are consistent with intestinal secretory losses and diminished absorptive function. Severe disease and medical treatment plan (intravenous foscarnet for 21 days) suggest that the patient would benefit from intravenous alimentation.

Rationale: Repletion of lean body and fat mass, improved survival and functionality by Karnofsky score, and self-reported health feeling have been documented in patients with AIDS wasting syndrome with prominent malabsorption.[189-192] Rates of catheter-related bloodstream infection were low in spite of immunodeficiency in long-term prospective trials.[191]

Recombinant Human Growth Hormone (rhGH)

Patients with wasting syndrome receiving rhGH (somatropin or Serostim) at the supraphysiologic dose of 6 mg (0.1 mg/kg/d) administered subcutaneously once daily for 12 weeks demonstrated increases in LBM and positive nitrogen balance during treatment.[93] Side effects may include edema, arthralgias, and myalgias that can be addressed by lowering dietary sodium intake, dose reduction, and/or the use of nonsteroidal anti-inflammatory agents. Other significant side effects include hyperglycemia and carpal tunnel syndrome. The evaluation of candidates for treatment with rhGH should include serum glucose for hyperglycemia and family history for diabetes mellitus. A 2-hour 75 g oral glucose tolerance test may be considered prior to initiation of rhGH therapy in candidates with a family history of diabetes mellitus or other risk factors. It is important to note that patients lose body fat while receiving rhGH (an undesired effect in patients with significant peripheral lipoatrophy).

Progressive Resistance and Aerobic Exercise

Eugonadal men diagnosed with AIDS wasting syndrome demonstrated increases in lean body mass and HDL cholesterol at the completion of a 12-week supervised progressive resistance and aerobic exercise program.[94] An increase in cardioprotective HDL cholesterol may be of benefit to HIV-infected patients with wasting and low CD4+ T-cell count. CD4+ T-cell count less than 500 in HIV-infected outpatients is an independent risk factor for incident cardiovascular disease events.[95]

Thalidomide

Thalidomide is a potent teratogen originally marketed as a sedative. It is approved by the FDA for the treatment of *erythema nodosum leprosum* and is available under a restricted distribution program. Because of its immunomodulatory properties, clinical trials have been conducted in patients with AIDS wasting syndrome and in HIV-infected patients with aphthous stomatitis. Although it has been shown to be effective for the treatment of aphthous ulcers, its usage to promote the accrual of lean body mass should be considered investigational at this time. Side effects include somnolence, rash (which may be life threatening), and a significant risk of teratogenicity in pregnant women.[96]

Energy, Protein, and Electrolytes

Pharmacological intervention is of limited benefit in the absence of adequate alimentation (Practice Scenario 32-2). Alimentation may occur orally in response to hunger or appetite (volitional) or by feeding tube or intravenous infusion (nonvolitionally). The calculation of maintenance energy requirement includes basal metabolic rate and disease-related elevation, dietary thermogenesis, and voluntary activity. Additional energy for anabolism should be provided during nutritional rehabilitation at the convalescent stage. The Harris–Benedict predictive equation for basal metabolic rate is the most widely referenced in the literature and is useful when working without access to indirect calorimetry.[97] Refeeding should be initiated at less than the calculated energy requirement, slowly progressing toward goal intake over several days with patients' demonstration of tolerance.

Generally, HIV-infected patients have a higher protein requirement, which may be exacerbated during secondary or opportunistic infection due to increased synthesis of acute phase immunologic (eg, complement and immunoglobulins) and hemostatic proteins. High-nitrogen feeding (amino acids 1.5 to 1.8 g/kg of body weight) significantly improves nitrogen balance in patients with wasting syndrome receiving intravenous alimentation.[98] Investigators have also documented the maintenance of nutrient intake and decreased soft tissue catabolism in HIV-infected patients receiving nutrient-dense ready-to-use therapeutic foods by mouth.[99,100] Nutritional outcomes are improved when nutrition support is provided at earlier stages of wasting and with the initiation of cART.[101]

Patients with wasting disease may have profound electrolyte deficits and are at risk for refeeding syndrome. Sudden death due to arrhythmia and respiratory arrest during refeeding may occur when alimentation precipitates acute intravascular volume expansion, serum phosphate depletion, hypokalemia, and hypomagnesemia.[102] Electrolytes (eg, phosphorous, potassium, and magnesium) should be evaluated daily and replenished intravenously. Oral formulations of these electrolytes may be poorly tolerated due to dose-related cathartic effects (osmotic activity of these ions). Electrolyte normalization should commence prior to the provision of macronutrient-containing nutrition support. Patients with severe wasting or those with a history of chronic alcohol use may require a short course of intravenous thiamin before the initiation of refeeding. Orally administered cations (eg, calcium, magnesium, aluminum) may decrease the absorption of some antimicrobial agents (eg, azithromycin, levofloxacin), and coadministration should be avoided.

Sodium retention is a response to profound undernutrition and wasting disease. It may lead to a propensity to fluid overload during the early stages of refeeding. The syndrome of inappropriate antidiuretic hormone (SIADH) may occur in patients with central nervous system or lung disease. As a result, fluid balance, urinary output, and urine electrolytes should be monitored during nutrition support of these patients.

Vitamin D

Vitamin D deficiency and insufficiency are prevalent in HIV-infected and uninfected persons in the United States.[103,104] Risk factors for vitamin D deficiency include treatment with medications that may be prescribed for HIV-infected patients (eg, antimycobacterials, anticonvulsants, corticosteroids).[105,106] Severe vitamin D deficiency (< 25 nmol/L) has been associated with receipt of the nonnucleoside reverse transcriptase inhibitor efavirenz.[107] Vitamin D plays a crucial role in mediating the innate immune response to microbial pathogens.[108] Vitamin D deficiency is associated with current and past tuberculosis infections and latent tuberculosis infection.[108]

Hypovitaminosis D may manifest as lower extremity muscle weakness. Serum 25-[OH] vitamin D should be routinely assayed in patients and supplemented as needed. In the absence of a serum 25-[OH] vitamin D assay, lower extremity muscle weakness may be attributed solely to skeletal muscle loss in wasted patients in spite of hypovitaminosis D.

For those residing in North America, the Institute of Medicine recommended dietary allowance (RDA) and upper level intake for vitamin D are 600 and 4000 IU/d, respectively. Many experts recommend the maintenance of serum 25-[OH] vitamin D concentration at approximately 75 nmol/L (30 ng/mL).[109] Patients with profound vitamin D deficiency may require a loading dose of 50,000 IU weekly for 8 weeks prior to maintenance supplementation.[109]

Omega-3 Fatty Acid Enrichment

In patients with AIDS wasting without active secondary or opportunistic infection, investigators have documented the downregulation of hepatic triglyceride synthesis by dietary omega-3 fatty acid supplementation.[110] However, in a trial of arginine and omega-3 fatty acid–enriched formula compared to standard protein-energy dense formula, HIV-infected patients receiving the arginine/omega-3 formula did not demonstrate superior anthropometric or immunologic parameters.[110]

Enteral Nutrition: Alimentation by Tube into the Upper Gastrointestinal Tract

HIV-infected patients who are candidates for tube feeding include those with neurologic disease (eg, progressive multifocal leukoencephalopathy), oropharyngeal or esophageal lesions, profound anorexia with or without nausea, impaired gut function, and those who are unable to achieve significant volitional dietary intake. Intragastric feeding tubes are strongly preferred to minimize gastrointestinal side effects and to optimize medication absorption. Many antiretrovirals have food and pH requirements for absorption. The safety and benefit of nutrition by a gastrostomy tube in AIDS patients has been documented.[111] HIV-infected patients receiving nutrition by feeding tube demonstrated increases in both weight and body cell mass.[111,112] Medications administered by feeding tube should be evaluated for appropriate formulation or vehicle, the effect of coadministered drug excipients on their absorption (eg, buffers), and the effect of the excipients themselves (eg, lactose, oleic acid) on patient tolerance.

A potential complication of percutaneous endoscopic gastrostomy is "buried bumper" syndrome, in which the gastric bumper of the feeding tube migrates into or through the gastric wall, with accompanying severe complications. Loss of gastric wall mass in HIV-infected patients with wasting disease may contribute to risk for this complication, and severe abdominal pain in this setting requires endoscopic evaluation.

Parenteral Nutrition: Intravenous Alimentation

Patients with extensive small bowel disease, such as jejunoileitis, are candidates for intravenous alimentation (Practice Scenario 32-2). Patients frequently demonstrate panmalabsorption with the volume of diarrhea directly related to food intake by mouth. Opportunistic infections of the small bowel may lead to extensive small bowel erosion, ulceration, and edema or pseudo-obstruction, which precludes usage for alimentation. Marked improvements in functional status (Karnofsky index), subjective feeling of health, and increases in total body weight and lean body mass have been documented in HIV-infected patients with wasting syndrome receiving intravenous alimentation.[113,114] Profoundly immunodeficient HIV-infected patients with wasting syndrome receiving a 2-month course of home infusion demonstrated a low rate of catheter-related septicemia (0.26/100 patient days).[113]

Short-term infusion into a peripheral vein (peripheral parenteral nutrition) is particularly effective in wasted patients receiving antimicrobials known to cause electrolyte losses or limited tolerance of food by mouth. Peripheral infusion can deliver significant amounts of macronutrients per kilogram of body weight in these patients (with low body weight) while facilitating repletion and ongoing management of their electrolytes. Peripheral infusion of nutrition and provision of an oral diet are not mutually exclusive. We have observed a marked increase in appetite and oral intake subsequent to peripheral infusion of nutrients in wasted patients who initially present with profound electrolyte deficits and anorexia.

Sarcopenia

Sarcopenia refers to age-associated loss of skeletal muscle mass and function (Table 32-8). Its onset is antecedent to frailty. It is characterized at the tissue level by loss of muscle protein (contractile unit) content, selective loss of type 2 (fast twitch) motor units, and adipose and connective tissue infiltration. Functional limitation and a predisposition to falls and long bone fracture are believed to ensue from progressive sarcopenia.

Increased numbers of senescent cells and chronic low-grade inflammation characterize both aging and chronic HIV infection. Proinflammatory proteins secreted by senescent cells (the senescence-associated secretory phenotype) and chronically activated immunocytes are believed to be etiologic in age-related loss of organ system reserve capacity and functional decline.

In addition to chronic low-grade inflammation, sarcopenia has also been associated with several modifiable risk factors, including low serum testosterone in males, low 25-[OH] vitamin D, insulin resistance, lack of exercise (resistance and aerobic), alcohol use, protein undernutrition, and prolonged bed rest.

Preventive intervention and treatment for sarcopenia may target the modifiable risk factors associated with it. Mid-life handgrip strength and usual gait speed (timed walk) reflect total skeletal muscle function, and abnormalities are predictive of future disability.[115,116] These simple tests may be considered for clinical evaluation.

Osteopenia and Osteoporosis

Fragility fracture is the clinical consequence of osteoporosis (a fracture resulting from normal activity or a fall from less than standing height). Osteoporosis may be detected and diagnosed by DEXA scan of bone. Osteoporosis and osteopenia are defined by T score: a comparison of the bone density of a patient ≥ 50 years to that of a 25 to 35-year-old gender- and ethnicity-matched reference population. A T score of −2.5 standard deviations (SD) in a subject 50 or more years old is considered osteoporotic. A T score of −1.0 SD is considered osteopenia. These scores correlate with increased risk of fracture in community-dwelling men and women.

Triant et al.[8] documented an increased prevalence of hip, vertebral, and wrist fractures in HIV-infected persons versus those without known HIV infection receiving care in a large integrated health care system in the northeastern United States. Women experienced higher rates of vertebral and wrist fractures, whereas men experienced higher rates of vertebral, hip, and wrist fractures. The largest differences in fracture rates occurred in men less than 40 or over 60 years of age and women over 50 years of age.[8]

Investigators in the Netherlands recently documented a high baseline prevalence of osteopenia (45%) and osteoporosis (6%) in treatment-naïve young men with primary HIV infection (+ RT-PCR/- western blot).[117] Similarly, Duvivier et al.[118] documented a 31% baseline prevalence of osteopenia in young, treatment-naïve, primarily male patients initiating cART.[118] The high prevalence of osteopenia and osteoporosis in young men with primary HIV infection who are treatment-naïve is highly suggestive of an overlap in risk factors for HIV acquisition with those for osteoporosis.

TABLE 32-8 Sarcopenia Versus Wasting Disease

	Sarcopenia	Wasting Disease
Physiology	**Intrinsic** 1% SM loss/year > age 30	**Complication** of HIV/other infection or disease
Pathologic	Only at threshold level associated with loss function	**Always**
Onset	**Slow**, over decades	**Rapid**, usually in association with other complications
Weight loss	**Not always**	**Always**
Tissue depots	**Skeletal muscle loss** (adipose tissue may be preserved or increased)	**Lean body mass**, including skeletal muscle, **and adipose tissue lost**
Histopathology	**Selective loss type 2 muscle fibers**	**+/− type 2 muscle fiber loss/seen in HIV+ in absence of wasting**
Metabolic	**Decreased muscle protein synthesis prominent**	**Increased muscle protein catabolism prominent**

SM, Skeletal Muscle Mass

Patients may demonstrate loss of bone mineral density during the year following initiation of cART (regardless of antiretroviral regimen) followed by stabilization in spite of a higher rate of bone remodeling.[119,120] The documented loss is of a magnitude similar to that experienced by women during menopause, and stabilization led to an age-appropriate rate of bone mineral density loss.[119,120] Investigators have found that approximately 12% to 16% of HIV-infected patients will progress from normal bone mineral density to osteopenia or from osteopenia to osteoporosis.[121] Factors associated with clinical progression were male sex, current protease inhibitor–containing regimen, and/or duration of PI exposure.[115] Low weight (or BMI) are independently predictive of low bone mineral density in individuals with HIV infection.[122,123]

At the tissue level, studies suggest that HIV has a direct effect on osteoclast activity, leading to a higher rate of bone remodeling (turnover).[124] Elevated levels of proinflammatory cytokines may also upregulate osteoclast activity. Bone marrow–derived mesenchymal stem cells may differentiate into either osteoblasts or adipocytes (within the bone marrow). Mesenchymal stem cells exposed to sera from HIV-infected treatment-naïve patients *ex vivo* were driven down an adipogenic differentiation pathway.[125] This suggests exposure to HIV proteins may diminish the pool of osteoblast precursors or osteoblast function.[125]

Clinical and behavioral findings associated with bone mineral density loss and osteoporosis (secondary causes) include vitamin D deficiency, male hypogonadism, low calcium intake or high protein and/or sodium intake leading to urinary calcium losses, a lack of routine weight-bearing exercise, low protein intake in older persons, tobacco use, high alcohol intake, and glucocorticoid exposure. These modifiable risk factors are prevalent in patients under care for HIV infection.[103,126]

Nutritional interventions such as vitamin D and calcium supplementation, the evaluation of dietary protein intake, and sodium reduction are first-line therapies for osteopenia. A propensity to fall due to diminished hip, knee, and ankle musculature often leads to fractures in older patients. An affirmative answer to the question "Are you worried about falling?" is suggestive of need for strength and balance training.

Osteoporosis and osteopenia in HIV-infected patients likely result from an interplay of viral effect, a time limited but irreversible drop in bone mineral density with the initiation of cART, and an overrepresentation of traditional risk factors.

HIV-Associated Lipodystrophy Syndrome

Introduction

The central feature of lipodystrophy in HIV-infected patients is selective subcutaneous adipose tissue loss.[127,128] Visceral adipose tissue is spared.[127,128] The accumulation of visceral adipose tissue may occur in HIV-infected patients with a return to health following the initiation of cART or in otherwise healthy patients with well-suppressed virus. However, it is not compensatory and large cohort studies have demonstrated that HIV-infected men receiving cART have less abdominal adiposity than age- and ethnicity-matched controls.[127,128] Lipodystrophy has been strongly associated with first-generation nucleoside reverse transcriptase inhibitors (the thymidine analogs and the adenosine analog didanosine). Insulin resistance may accompany subcutaneous fat loss due to diminished levels of adipocyte-derived intercellular signaling molecules (adipocytokines) that enhance insulin sensitivity, and the increased release of proinflammatory cytokines (by macrophages within adipose tissue) that favor insulin resistance. The study of lipodystrophy has led to appreciation of subcutaneous adipose tissue as an endocrine organ with a pivotal regulatory role in nutritional metabolism as opposed to merely being a passive energy reservoir.[129]

Epidemiology

Prevalence estimates for lipodystrophy are complicated by the lack of a standard case definition.[130] The Fat Redistribution and Metabolic Change in HIV Infection study documented a 49% prevalence.[127] Incidence in North America, the European Union, the United Kingdom, and Australia have been declining since the later part of the last decade with decreased use of thymidine analogs (NRTIs). However, prevalence remains significant due to the persisting nature of subcutaneous adipocyte loss and the continued use of thymidine analogs in resource-constrained settings (eg, sub-Saharan Africa). Only partial, and usually subclinical, recovery of subcutaneous adipose tissue is achieved with discontinuance of thymidine analogs. However, progression is halted.

Other Lipodystrophies

Human lipodystrophic syndromes may occur in a hereditary or acquired manner and are not unique to HIV infection and its treatment.[131,132] They are characterized by partial or generalized subcutaneous adipose tissue loss. In the partial lipodystrophies (eg, Dunnigan variety familial partial lipodystrophy), insulin resistance and its complications are dependent on the extent of subcutaneous adipose tissue loss. Patients may also present with insulin resistance, triglyceride, and very low-density lipoprotein cholesterol (VLDL-C) elevations due to leptin deficiency and hepatosteatosis.[132]

Etiology and Pathogenesis

HIV-associated lipodystrophy may be viewed as subcutaneous adipose tissue–specific mitochondrial toxicity, with lethal and sublethal cellular injury, a loss of endocrine function, and depot-specific inflammatory change. Investigators have documented the disruption of several metabolic pathways within adipocytes, such as maturation, insulin signaling, glucose and free fatty acid uptake, and increased levels of apoptosis (cell death).[133]

Biopsies of adipose tissue from lipodystrophic patients have disclosed morphologic and biochemical abnormalities in association with inflammatory change.[133-134] Tellingly, specimens revealed a reduction in adipocyte mitochondrial DNA content.[135,136] Adipocytes were small and poorly differentiated and were characterized by a marked reduction in the expression of key functional proteins including insulin receptors and Glut 4-glucose transporter protein.[133-136] This cellular phenotype is consistent with clinical insulin resistance. Adipocytes obtained from lipodystrophic patients demonstrate decreased expression of the adipocyte-derived hormones adiponectin and leptin. Adiponectin is an insulin-sensitizing adipocytokine and deficiency may play a role in clinical insulin resistance.[137] Leptin plays a key role in mediating triglyceride oxidation. High serum free fatty acid levels may lead to insulin resistance by the inhibition of phosphorylation of insulin-related substrate-1 and insulin receptor tyrosine residues, leading to a disruption of intracellular insulin signalling.[138] Patients with severe generalized lipodystrophy, insulin resistance, and hepatic steatosis demonstrated marked improvements in glycemic control, and a reduction in hepatic triglyceride content when treated with leptin.[132]

Inhibition of mitochondrial DNA polymerase γ by NRTIs is believed to mediate adipocyte toxicity.[139] Mitochondria have multiple separate circularized genomes encoding respiratory chain proteins that are not encoded by nuclear chromosomal DNA. A dose reduction of respiratory chain proteins due to reduced mitochondrial DNA content may lead to mitochondrial dysfunction and adipocyte apoptosis (cell death).

The least *in vitro* inhibition DNA polymerase γ has been noted with abacavir, lamivudine, emtricitabine, and tenofovir.[140] This is consistent with the infrequency of peripheral lipoatrophy in treatment-naïve patients initiating cART with these agents and benefit documented in "switch studies" in treatment-experienced patients with lipoatrophy.[139]

Protease inhibitors may variably contribute to decreased glucose uptake due to reversible binding and inhibition of the Glut-4 glucose transporter.[141] Interaction between the protease inhibitor and Glut-4 is due to the drugs' aromatic peptide backbone, which also acts as substrate for HIV protease. Clinical effect is seen with the first-generation protease inhibitors indinavir and ritonavir (full dose as an antiretroviral not as a pharmacological booster).

Mitochondrial toxicity has also been associated with hepatic steatosis, mild hyperlactatemia, and rarely, with lactic acidosis.[142] Lactic acidosis is a potentially lethal complication usually encountered in obese female patients.[143] The prodrome of clinical lactic acidosis is nonspecific (eg, nausea, loss of appetite). Treatment includes the interruption of NRTIs and supplementation with thiamin and riboflavin to optimize mitochondrial function and biogenesis.

Clinical Evaluation and Diagnosis

Lipodystrophy is a clinical diagnosis based on physical findings. Subcutaneous adipose tissue loss may be focal or generalized (eg, facial only or facial and gluteal-femoral or head, trunk, and limbs). The most frequently affected areas are the face, buttocks and thighs, and lastly, the upper arms.

Several methods exist to evaluate adipose tissue depots, and regional distribution. Visual examination and anthropometric measurement are relied upon in clinical care. A relatively constant amount of adipose tissue is subcutaneous in the absence of disease or prolonged undernutrition. Limb adipocyte content is primarily subcutaneous. Serial measurement of mid-upper arm skinfold and circumference and hip circumference may be used to monitor subcutaneous fat. Waist circumference may be used to evaluate abdominal adiposity. Decreasing hip circumference demonstrated by serial measurement using the patient as his or her own historical control or elevated waist-to-hip ratio with a normal waist circumference are consistent with loss of gluteal–femoral subcutaneous adipose tissue. Gluteal–femoral adipose tissue loss may be associated with insulin resistance in HIV-infected patients.[144] Bioelectrical impedance analysis may also be used clinically. However, it assays total, not regional, adipose tissue. Loss of fat mass on serial BIA with the preservation of lean body mass in the absence of undernutrition may be consistent with lipodystrophy.

Facial adipose tissue loss is the most distressing stigmata of lipodystrophy for most patients. Facial lipoatrophy may be appreciated by noting a near total bilateral loss of Bichat's fat pads, manifesting as a visible subzygomatic notch, discernible zygomaticus major and minor muscles, and prominent nasolabial skin folds. On examination, the abdomen may be firm due to subcutaneous adipose tissue loss with relative sparing of omental and mesenteric adipocytes. Gluteal–femoral lipoatrophy may be appreciated by serial hip circumference measurements or current waist-to-hip ratio (less specific).[144] A decline in hip circumference from baseline or prior visit without a reduction in waist circumference is consistent with gluteal–femoral fat loss. A male waist-to-hip ratio greater than 0.94 or a female waist-to-hip ratio greater than 0.88 with a waist circumferences of less than 37 inches or 35 inches, respectively, are consistent with lipoatrophy. Waist and hip circumferences have opposite and independent associations. Gluteal–femoral subcutaneous adipose tissue is believed to be protective for insulin resistance and dyslipidemia.[145] Serial measurement of both should be included in routine outpatient care to monitor change over time.

Loss of subcutaneous fat in the extremities may be evaluated for by the measurement of mid-upper arm skinfold and circumference. NHANES percentiles may serve as reference ranges. Generally, a finding of less than the 10th percentile is consistent with peripheral lipoatrophy. Prominent vasculature ("cabeling") in the limbs is a frequent finding in lipoatrophy and is often accompanied by pseudomuscularity, which is marked by visible muscle insertions and contours.

Mesenteric and omental fat may be appreciated clinically by the measurement of waist circumference. A waist circumference of 37 inches or greater in either sex is independently associated with visceral abdominal adiposity.[146] Atypical expansion of adipose tissue depots may also occur in lipodystrophic patients. These include: dorsocervical fat pad enlargement ("buffalo hump"), submandibular fat accumulation with loss of facial contour ("moon facies"), and marked female breast hypertrophy with thoracic-level back pain.[147–149]

DEXA, CT, and MRI have been used extensively in research to determine regional and subcutaneous adipose tissue. Visceral and subcutaneous fat may be imaged by a single-slice CT or MRI. Values may be expressed in squared centimeters as subcutaneous adipose tissue (SAT) or visceral adipose tissue (VAT) absolute values or as ratios (eg, VAT-to-SAT, VAT-to-total adipose tissue). Total body fat and limb fat may be calculated by DEXA scan. DEXA may be used to determine the extent of peripheral lipoatrophy by examining the relationship of total fat-to-limb fat defined as a ratio.[150]

Insulin resistance may manifest as hyperinsulinemia with normal fasting glucose and HgbA1c. This may be evaluated for by fasting serum insulin and glucose levels for the determination of a homeostatic model assessment (HOMA) score or 2-hour 75 g oral glucose tolerance test with serum insulin levels and the calculation of insulin area under the curve.[151,152]

Clinical Management

Antiretroviral regimen change to replace thymidine analogs is an option for most patients. Genetic evaluation of the patient's virus for antiretroviral resistance is usually required prior to regimen changes. Studies of thymidine analog substitution with a guanosine analog (abacavir) or an adenosine analog (tenofovir) have demonstrated improvement in subcutaneous adipose tissue and dyslipidemia.[153,154] Improvements in lipoatrophy, although measurable, may take years to reach clinical significance.[153]

Resistance and Aerobic Exercise

Increases in trunk and limb muscle mass and cardiorespiratory fitness may be achieved through scheduled resistance and aerobic exercise.[155] Patients often find inexpensive devices such as resistance bands, aerobic exercise videotapes, and pedometers helpful. Community-dwelling patients should be encouraged to meet the CDC recommendations for aerobic and resistance exercise.[156]

Thiazolidinediones

Thiazolidinediones are insulin-sensitizing agents (peroxisome proliferator-activated receptor-gamma PPAR-γ agonists) indicated for the treatment of type 2 diabetes mellitus. Type 2 diabetic patients treated with these agents demonstrate increases in subcutaneous fat. Investigators have evaluated their use for the treatment of nondiabetic HIV-infected patients with peripheral lipoatrophy. Rosiglitazone was associated with improvements in peripheral subcutaneous adipose tissue and insulin sensitivity in HIV-infected patients with hyperinsulinemia and peripheral lipoatrophy.[157] A subsequent small study in HIV-infected patients with lipodystrophy also documented increases in subcutaneous adipose tissue, adiponectin levels, and insulin sensitivity.[158] However, patients in a larger study of rosiglitazone for the treatment of lipoatrophy did not demonstrate statistically significant improvement when compared to patients receiving placebo.[159] Whether clinically significant gains in subcutaneous adipose tissue can be achieved in nondiabetic patients with peripheral lipoatrophy remains under investigation. Thiazolidinediones are a reasonable treatment option for HIV-infected type 2 diabetics with peripheral lipoatrophy. Pioglitazone may have a more benign effect on lipid profiles than rosiglitazone and has not been associated with an increased coronary event risk.[160]

Metformin

Metformin is an insulin-sensitizing agent that decreases hepatic insulin resistance and glucose production. Use in HIV-infected individuals with visceral fat accumulation has been associated with decreases in visceral and subcutaneous adipose tissue, as well as improvement in insulin kinetics.[158,161,162] van Wiljk et al.[158] documented an improvement in flow-mediated vasodilation—an assessment of atherosclerotic process—in patients receiving metformin. Other investigators demonstrated a reduction in serum levels of tissue plasminogen activator tPA antigen and plasminogen activator inhibitor PAI-1 (inflammatory markers) with metformin therapy in insulin-resistant patients with lipodystrophy.[163]

Soft Tissue Fillers and Liposuction

Polylactic acid (Sculptra) and calcium hydroxylapatite (Radiesse) are soft tissue fillers administered by intradermal injection. A clinically significant effect has been demonstrated by patient self-assessment using a visual analog scale and by physician (and patient) evaluation using the Global Aesthetic Improvement Scale, respectively.[164–166] Both fillers are FDA approved for the treatment of HIV-associated facial lipoatrophy. Liposuction for dorsocervical fat accumulation is effective, but relapses are frequent and individual results vary.[165]

Cardiovascular Disease

Background

An increased rate of acute myocardial infarction has been observed in HIV-infected persons compared to uninfected persons of the same gender and similar age.[7] A higher rate of myocardial infarction than that predicted by the Framingham equation has been documented by the Data Collection on Adverse Events of Anti-HIV Drugs (D:A:D) Study Group, an international pharmacosurveillance consortium monitoring over 33,000 patients.[167] Excess risk of acute myocardial infarction is associated with direct HIV effect on atherosclerotic lesion burden (internal carotid intima-media thickness), lipid and lipoprotein metabolism, and inflammatory activity.[168–170]

Etiology

The natural history of an HIV infection is marked by proatherogenic lipid and lipoprotein changes. High-density lipoprotein cholesterol (HDL-C) is decreased early in HIV infection. Decline in HDL-C is followed by a latter small decrease in low-density lipoprotein cholesterol (LDL-C) with an increase in the small dense fraction. Small dense LDL-C is believed to more easily penetrate blood vessel walls where it undergoes oxidation and phagocytosis leading to atherosclerotic lesions. Progressive HIV disease (AIDS) may be accompanied by increases in serum triglyceride and VLDL-C. These proatherogenic changes in lipids and lipoproteins have been associated with increasing HIV-RNA levels (viral load) and decreasing CD 4+ T-cell count.[171]

Data from D:A:D suggests that specific antiretrovirals may also be associated with increased cardiovascular disease risk.[172] However, a study of CD4-guided intermittent antiretroviral therapy, to decrease cumulative drug toxicity, demonstrated an increase in cardiovascular disease events, and inflammatory and coagulation biomarkers in patients receiving intermittent therapy.[170] Antiretroviral therapy was clearly cardioprotective in spite of observational data from D:A:D, suggesting that some antiretrovirals may be slightly less so than others.[172] Two large studies in outpatient cohorts have also demonstrated that a low CD4 count is an independent risk factor for cardiovascular disease (CVD) events.[171,172]

Analysis of D:A:D data sets demonstrated stronger associations between traditional risk factors (male sex, higher BMI, older age, high total cholesterol, and tobacco use) and cardiovascular disease event risk than either cART exposure or duration.[173] Traditional risk factors and sedentary lifestyle may be overrepresented in HIV-infected cohorts under study. The effect of traditional risk factors is often prominent in patients receiving cART and is referred to as "return to health effect." Simply put, with the resolution of opportunistic infection(s) and constitutional symptoms subsequent to receiving cART, patients often demonstrate increases in weight, total, and LDL cholesterol. Increases represent patients' return to their baseline or premorbid weight, total and LDL cholesterol levels.

A negative impact of first-generation PIs on lipid metabolism was documented subsequent to their widespread use.[152] Associations with hepatic triglyceride accumulation, impaired triglyceride oxidation, impaired peripheral clearance of triglycerides, and an increase in serum VLDL-C were observed.[152] In vitro, the PIs ritonavir and saquinavir were shown to inhibit the proteasomal degradation of apolipoprotein B.[174] Fat loading of PI-treated hepatocyte cultures resulted in an increased secretion of VLDL-C. This finding was highly consistent with the tight clinical association of full-dose ritonavir (as an antiretroviral) and lopinavir-ritonavir with increases in triglycerides and VLDL cholesterol.[174]

Clinical Evaluation

The absolute risk for a cardiovascular disease event in an individual patient may be estimated using the Adult Treatment Panel III (ATP III).[175] Clinicians may elect more aggressive LDL-C goals due to data consistent with the underestimation of risk in HIV-infected patients by the Framingham equation.[167] An assay of high-sensitivity CRP and D-dimer may provide clinicians with additional information on a specific patient's risk for a CVD event.[176]

The Mediterranean Diet

The Mediterranean diet has demonstrated efficacy in primary and secondary prevention trials for cardiovascular disease and type 2 diabetes mellitus in individuals without known HIV infection.[177-179] A primary prevention trial of the Mediterranean diet documented reductions in hsCRP, improvement in markers of endothelial function, and improvement in insulin resistance.[180] Fiber intake has been inversely associated with insulin resistance and higher polyunsaturated fat intake was positively associated with insulin resistance in HIV-infected lipodystrophic patients.[181] In community-dwelling HIV-infected patients receiving cART, adherence to a Mediterranean diet was associated with better metabolic parameters and a lower risk for abdominal adiposity versus a typical Western diet.[182,183]

The Mediterranean diet is characterized by:

- A high intake of dark green leafy and other vegetables
- Fresh fruit as the typical daily dessert
- The use of whole grains for starches, and beans, nuts, seeds, and potatoes
- Olive oil as the principal source of fat
- Dairy products (principally cheese and yogurt)
- Fish two or more times a week
- Poultry consumed in moderate amounts
- Egg yolks limited to four per week
- Red meat consumed in low amounts
- Wine consumed in low-to-moderate amounts, normally with meals
- Low saturated fat ($\leq$ 7% to 8% of energy), with total fat ranging from $<$ 25% to $>$ 35% of energy

Clinicians should be mindful of the Institute of Medicine's guidelines for adult sodium intake (less than 1500 mg/day) and counsel patients accordingly.

HMG CoA Reductase Inhibitors (Statins) and Fibrates

The HIV Medical Association of the Infectious Disease Society of America and the Adult AIDS Clinical Trials Group issued guidelines for the management of dyslipidemia in HIV-infected adults receiving antiretroviral therapy.[184] Statins are recommended when elevated LDL and non-HDL cholesterol are the predominant findings. Generally, simvastatin and lovastatin are contraindicated in patients receiving PIs (in part due to the potential for CYP3A4- and OATP1B1-mediated interactions). In addition, pravastatin serum levels are increased by the protease inhibitor darunavir, and the concomitant use of these two drugs should be avoided. The lowest possible dosages of atorvastatin or rosuvastatin (with careful monitoring) are alternatives. Fibrates (gemfibrozil or fenofibrate) may be prescribed when hypertriglyceridemia is the predominant abnormality.

Omega-3 Fatty Acids

Lovaza is a pharmaceutical grade omega-3 fatty acid supplement approved for the treatment of hypertriglyceridemia in HIV-uninfected persons. A pilot study in HIV-infected patients (4 g daily orally) randomized to receive omega-3 fatty acid supplementation with diet and exercise counseling demonstrated statistically significant reductions in triglyceride levels at 1-month analysis.[185] Unfortunately, triglyceride reduction did not reach the ATP III goal of levels below 150 mg/dL and LDL cholesterol levels rose by 22% in the treatment group.[185] It should be noted that fibrates also increase LDL cholesterol levels. Of 26 subjects randomized to receive fish oil, 2 withdrew from the study because of unpleasant taste and nausea (historically associated with fish oil supplementation).[185] No significant change in platelet function was observed.[185]

Growth Hormone Releasing Factor Analog

Abdominal adiposity is associated with cardiovascular disease risk factors such as hypertriglyceridemia, insulin resistance, and low HDL cholesterol.[186] Findings suggestive of diminished pituitary growth hormone secretory stimulus in HIV-infected patients with abdominal adiposity mark the rationale for the clinical use of the growth hormone-releasing factor analog tesamorelin (Egrifta).[187] Tesamorelin markedly increases plasma levels of growth hormone and IGF-1. The safety and efficacy of tesamorelin (2 mg daily administered by subcutaneous injection) was evaluated in a 26-week trial (primary efficacy phase) with an additional 26-week rerandomized extension (safety) phase for those receiving active drug during the initial 26-week period.[188] Visceral adipose tissue was evaluated by waist circumference and CT. An evaluation of biochemical parameters included triglycerides, hemoglobin A1c (HgbA1c), and IGF-1.

At week 26, waist circumference decreased by 2.4 cm in the tesamorelin arm versus 0.8 cm in the placebo arm for an absolute between-group difference of 1.6 cm (1.5%).[188] Visceral adipose tissue assessed by CT decreased by 24 cm^2 (−13.1%) in the tesamorelin arm versus a 2 cm^2 increase in the placebo arm. Patients receiving tesamorelin demonstrated a mean 27 mg/dL decline in triglycerides and a 0.14 increase in HgbA1c.[188] A between-group absolute difference in HgbA1c was 0.12 for a 2.3% increase in the tesamorelin arm versus the placebo arm.[188] IGF-1 increased by 108 ng/mL (84.1%) in patients receiving tesamorelin versus no increase in the placebo arm.[188] The effects of tesamorelin are reversed after the cessation of treatment. Injection site reactions occurred in 25% of patients with 20% discontinuing therapy.[188]

Whether changes limited to the period during which patients are receiving the drug will lead to decreases in cardiovascular disease events is unknown. The increase in HgbA1c is an early signal that some patients may experience clinically significant abnormalities in glucose metabolism while receiving tesamorelin. IGF-1 is a potent mitogen, and it is unknown whether the 84% increase in IGF-1 levels in patients receiving tesamorelin will lead to negative events (eg, malignancy) with broader usage.

References

1. Centers for Disease Control. Kaposi's sarcoma and pneumocystis pneumonia among homosexual men—New York City and California. *MMWR Morb Mortal Wkly Rep.* 1981;30:305–308.
2. Kochanek KD, Murphy SL, Anderson RN, Scott C. Deaths: final data for 2002. *Natl Vital Stat Rep.* 2004;53:1–115.
3. Centers for Disease Control (CDC). *HIV/AIDS Surveillance Report,* 2005. Vol 17. Rev ed. Atlanta, GA: US DHHS, CDC;2007:1–54.
4. Harrison KM, Song R, Zhang X. Life expectancy after HIV diagnosis based national HIV surveillance data from 25 states, United States. *J Acquir Immune Defic Snydr.* 2010;53(1):124–130.
5. Mermin J. The Science and practice of HIV prevention in the United States. Centers for Disease Control and Prevention. Program and abstracts presented at: 18th Conference on Retroviruses and Opportunistic Infections; February 27–March 2, 2011; Boston, MA: Plenary 1.
6. Centers for Disease Control and Prevention (CDC). Prevalence and awareness of HIV infection among men who have sex with men—21 cities, United States, 2008. *MMWR Morb Mortal Wkly Rep.* 2010;59(37):1201–1207.
7. Triant VA, Lee H, Hadigan C, et al. Increased acute myocardial infarction rates and cardiovascular risk factors among patients with human immunodeficiency virus disease. *J Clin Endocrinol Metab.* 2007;92:2506–2512.
8. Triant A, Brown TT, Lee H, et al. Fracture prevalence among human immunodeficiency virus (HIV)-infected versus non-HIV-infected patients in a large U.S. healthcare system. *J Clin Endocrinol Metab.* 2008;93(9):3499–3504.
9. Gao F, Bailes E, Robertson DL, et al. Origin of HIV-1 in the chimpanzee Pan troglodytes. *Nature.* 1999;397: 436–441.
10. Joint United Nations Programme on HIV/AIDS. AIDS epidemic update: November 2009. http://data.unaids.org/pub/report/2009/jc1700_epi_update_2009_en.pdf. Accessed 12/8/2010.
11. Hall HI, Song R, Rhodes P, et al. Estimation of HIV incidence in the United States. *JAMA.* 2008;300:520–529.
12. Denning P, DiNenno E. Communities in crisis: Is there a generalized HIV epidemic in impoverished urban areas of the United States? Poster presented at: International Conference on AIDS; July 2010; Vienna, Austria.
13. Centers for Disease Control and Prevention (CDC). 1993 Revised classification system for HIV-infection & expanded surveillance case definition for AIDS among adults & adolescents. *MMWR Morb Mortal Wkly Rep.* 1992;41:1–19.
14. U.S. Department of Health and Human Services. Transmission facts. cdc.gov/hiv/pubs/facts/transmission.htm. Accessed 12/8/2010.
15. Li Q, Duan L, Estes JD, et al. Peak SIV replication in resting memory CD4+ T cells depletes gut lamina propria CD4+ T cells. *Nature.* 2005;434:1148–1152.
16. Uchiyama J, Kishi S, Yagita H, et al. Fas ligand-mediated depletion of CD4 and CD8 lymphocytes by monomeric HIV-1-glycoprotein 120. *Arch Virol.* 1997;142:1771–1785.
17. Picker LJ, Hagen SI, Lum R, et al. Insufficient production and tissue delivery of CD4+ memory T cells in rapidly progressive simian immunodeficiency virus infection. *J Exp Med.* 2004;200: 1299–1314.
18. Dion ML, Poulin JF, Bordi R, et al. Human immunodeficiency virus infection rapidly induces and maintains a substantial suppression of thymocyte proliferation. *Immunity.* 2004;6: 757–768.
19. Nazli A, Chan O, Dobson-Belaire WN, et al. Exposure to HIV-1 directly impairs mucosal epithelial barrier integrity allowing microbial translocation. *PloS Pathog.* 2010;6(4):1000852.doi: 10.1371.
20. Douek DC, Brenchley JM, Betts MR, et al. HIV preferentially infects HIV-specific CD4+ T-cells. *Nature.* 2002;417:95–98.
21. Zhang Z, Schuler T, Zupancic M, et al. Sexual transmission and propagation of SIV and HIV in resting and activated CD4+ T Cells. *Science.* 1999;286(5443):1353–1357.
22. Gloster SE, Newton P, Cornforth D, et al. Association of strong virus specific CD4 T cell responses with efficient natural control of primary HIV-1 infection. *AIDS.* 2004;18(5):749–755.
23. Mattapallil JJ, Douek DC, Hill B, et al. Massive infection and loss of memory CD4+ T cells in multiple tissues during acute SIV infection. *Nature.* 2005;434:1093–1097.
24. Brenchley JM, Schacker TW, Ruff LE, et al. CD4+ T cell depletion during all stages of HIV disease occurs predominantly in the gastrointestinal tract. *J Exp Med.* 2004;200:749–759.
25. Mehandru S, Poles MA, Tenner-Racz K, et al. Primary HIV-1 infection is associated with preferential depletion of CD4+ T lymphocytes from effector sites in the gastrointestinal tract. *J Exp Med.* 2004;200:761–770.
26. Veazey RS, DeMaria M, Chalifoux LV, et al. Gastrointestinal tract as a major site of CD4+ T cell depletion and viral replication in SIV infection. *Science.* 1998;17;280(5362):427–431.
27. Estes J, Baker JV, Brenchley JM, et al. Collagen deposition limits immune reconstitution in the gut. *J Infect Dis.* 2008;198(4): 456–464.

28. Eriksson K, Kilander A, Hagberg L, et al. Virus-specific antibody production and polyclonal B-cell activation in the intestinal mucosa of HIV-infected individuals. *AIDS*. 1995;9(7):695–700.
29. Levesque MC, Moody MA, Hwang KK, et al. Polyclonal B cell differentiation and loss of gastrointestinal tract germinal centers in the earliest stages of HIV-1 infection. *PLoS Med*. 2009;6(7):e1000107.
30. Olsson J, Poles M, Spetz AL, et al. Human immunodeficiency virus type 1 infection is associated with significant mucosal inflammation characterized by increased expression of CCR5, CXCR4, and beta chemokines. *J Infect Dis*. 2000;182(6):1625–1635.
31. McGowan I, Elliott J, Fuerst M, et al. Increased HIV-1 mucosal replication is associated with generalized mucosal cytokine activation. *J Acquir Immune Defic Syndr*. 2004;1;37(2):1228–1236.
32. Jiang W, Lederman MM, Hunt P, et al. Plasma levels of bacterial DNA correlate with immune activation and the magnitude of immune restoration in persons with antiretroviral-treated HIV infection. *J Infect Dis*. 2009;199(8):1177–1185.
33. Marchetti G, Bellistri GM, Borghi E, et al. Microbial translocation is associated with sustained failure in CD4+ T-cell reconstitution in HIV-infected patients on long-term highly active antiretroviral therapy. *AIDS*. 2008;22(15):2035–2038.
34. Brenchley JM, Price DA, Schacker TW, et al. Microbial translocation is a cause of systemic immune activation in chronic HIV infection. *Nat Med*. 2006;12(12):1365–1371.
35. Schacker TW, Nguyen PL, Beilman GJ, et al. Collagen deposition in HIV-1 infected lymphatic tissues and T cell homeostasis. *J Clin Invest*. 2002;110:1133–1139.
36. Lima VD, Harrigan R, Bangsberg DR, et al. The combined effect of modern highly active antiretroviral therapy regimens and adherence on mortality over time. *J Acquir Immune Defic Syndr*. 2009; 50(5):529–526.
37. Malebranche R, Arnoux E, Guerin JM, et al. Acquired immunodeficiency syndrome with severe gastrointestinal manifestations in Haiti. *Lancet*. 1983;2:873–878.
38. Siddiqui J, Phillips AL, Freedland ES, et al. Prevalence and cost of HIV-associated weight loss in a managed care population. *Curr Med Res Opin*. 2009;25(5):1307–1317.
39. Wasserman P, Segal-Maurer S, Rubin D. Significant prevalence of wasting among women on HAART 1997–2002 documented by bioelectrical impedance analysis. *Antiviral Ther*. 2002;7:L66.
40. Wanke CA, Silva M, Knox TA, et al. Weight loss and wasting remain common complications in individuals infected with human immunodeficiency virus in the era of highly active antiretroviral therapy. *Clin Infect Dis*. 2000;31:803–805.
41. Moyle GJ, Daar ES, Gertner JM, et al. Growth hormone improves lean body mass, physical performance, and quality of life in subjects with HIV-associated weight loss or wasting on highly active antiretroviral therapy. *J Acquir Immune Defic Syndr*. 2004;35:367–375.
42. Anema A, Weiser SD, Fernandes KA. High Prevalence of food insecurity among individuals receiving HAART in a resource-rich setting. *AIDS Care*. 2011;23(2):221–230.
43. Vogenthaler NS, Hadley C, Rodriguez AE, et al. Depressive symptoms and food insufficiency among HIV-infected crack users in Atlanta and Miami. *AIDS Behav*. 2011;15(7):1520–1526.
44. Kotler DP, Tierney AR, Wang J, Pierson RN Jr. Magnitude of body-cell-mass depletion and the timing of death from wasting in AIDS. *Am J Clin Nutr*. 1989;50:444–447.
45. Tang AM, Forrester J, Speigelman D, et al. Weight loss and survival in HIV-positive patients in the era of highly active antiretroviral therapy. *J Acquir Immune Defic Syndr*. 2002;31:230–236.
46. Zachariah R, Fitzgerald M, Massaquoi M, et al. Risk factors for high early mortality in patients on antiretroviral treatment in a rural district of Malawi. *AIDS*. 2006;20(18):2355–2360.
47. Keys A, Brozek J, Henschel A, et al. *The Biology of Human Starvation*. Minneapolis, MN: University of Minnesota Press: 1950.
48. Scherzer R, Heymsfield SB, Lee D, et al. Decreased limb muscle and increased central adiposity are associated with 5-year all-cause mortality in HIV infection. *AIDS*. 2011;25(11):1405–1414.
49. Elia M. Hunger disease. *Clin Nutr*. 2000;19:379–386.
50. Cahill GF Jr. Starvation in man. *N Engl J Med*. 1970;282:668–675.
51. Bickel G, Nord M, Price C, et al. *Guide to Measuring Household Food Security, Revised 2000*. Alexandria, VA: U.S. Department of Agriculture, Food and Nutrition; 2000.
52. Grunfeld C, Pang M, Shimizu L. Resting energy expenditure, caloric intake, and short term weight change in human immunodeficiency virus infection and the acquired immunodeficiency syndrome. *Am J Clin Nutr*. 1992;55:455–460.
53. Melchior JC, Salmon D, Rigaud D, et al. Resting energy expenditure is increased in stable, malnourished HIV-infected patients. *Am J Clin Nutr*. 1991;53:437–441.
54. Poizot-Martin I, Benourine K, Philibert P, et al. Diet-induced thermogenesis in HIV infection. *AIDS*. 1994;8:501–504.
55. Hellerstein MK, Grunfeld C, Wu K, et al. Increased de novo hepatic lipogenesis in human immunodeficiency virus infection. *J Clin Endocrinol Metab*. 1993;76:559–565.
56. Hoh R, Pelfini A, Neese RA, et al. De novo lipogenesis predicts short-term body composition response by bioelectrical impedance analysis to oral nutritional supplements in HIV-associated wasting. *Am J Clin Nutr*. 1998;68:154–163.
57. Grunfeld C, Kotler DP, Shigenaga JK, et al. Circulating interferon-alpha levels and hypertriglyceridemia in the acquired immunodeficiency syndrome. *Am J Med*. 1991;90(2):154–162.
58. Grunfeld C, Kotler DP, Hamadeh R, et al. Hypertriglyceridemia in the acquired immunodeficiency syndrome. *Am J Med*. 1989;86:27–31.
59. Yarasheski K, Zachweija J, Gischler J, et al. Increased plasma Gln and Leu Ra and inappropriately low muscle protein synthesis rate in AIDS wasting. *Am J Physiol*. 1998; 275(4 Pt 1):E577–E583.
60. Tallóczy Z, Jiang W, Virgin HW, et al. Regulation of starvation- and virus-induced autophagy by the eIF2alpha kinase signaling pathway. *Proc Natl Acad Sci USA*. 2002;99(1):190–195.
61. Patton JS, Peters PM, McCabe J, et al. Development of partial tolerance to the gastrointestinal effects of high doses of recombinant tumor necrosis factor-alpha in rodents. *J Clin Invest*. 1987;80: 1587–1596.
62. Thea DM, Reuven P, Khondi N, et al. Plasma cytokines, cytokine antagonists, and disease progression in African women infected with HIV-1. *Ann Intern Med*. 1996;124;757–762.
63. Croxson TS, Chapman WE, Miller LK, et al. Changes in the hypothalamic-pitutitary-gonadal-axis in human immunodeficiency virus-infected homosexual men. *J Clin Endocrinol Metab*. 1989;68: 317–321.
64. Dobs AS, Dempsey MA, Ladenson PW, Polk BF. Endocrine disorders in men infected with human immunodeficiency virus. *Am J Med*. 1988;84:611–616.
65. Grinspoon S, Corcoran C, Lee K, et al. Loss of lean body and muscle mass correlates with androgen levels in hypogonadal men with acquired immunodeficiency syndrome and wasting. *J Clin Endocrinol Metab*. 1996;81:4051–4058.
66. Rietschel P, Corcoran C, Stanley T, et al. Prevalence of hypogonadism among men with weight loss related to human immunodeficiency virus infection who were receiving highly active antiretroviral therapy. *Clin Infect Dis*. 2000;31:1240–1244.
67. Dolan S, Wilkie S, Aliabadi N, et al. Effects of testosterone administration in human immunodeficiency virus-infected women with low weight: a randomized placebo-controlled study. *Arch Intern Med*. 2004;164:897–904.

68. Miller K, Corcoran C, Armstrong C, et al. Transdermal testosterone administration in women with acquired immunodeficiency syndrome wasting: a pilot study. *J Clin Endocrinol Metab.* 1998;83: 2717–2725.
69. Javanbakht M, Singh AB, Mazer NA, et al. Pharmacokinetics of a novel testosterone matrix transdermal system in healthy, premenopausal women and women infected with the human immunodeficiency virus. *J Clin Endocrinol Metab.* 2000;85:2395–2401.
70. Smith WJ, Underwood LE, Clemmons DR. Effects of caloric restriction or protein restriction on insulin-like growth factor-1 (IGF-1) and IGF-binding proteins in children and adults. *J Clin Endocrinol Metab.* 1995;80:443–449.
71. Grinspoon S, Corcoran C, Stanley T, et al. Effects of androgen administration on the growth hormone-insulin-like growth factor 1 axis in men with acquired immunodeficiency syndrome wasting. *J Clin Endocrinol Metab.* 1998;83:4251–4256.
72. Scacchi M, Ida Pincelli A, Cavagnini F. Nutritional status in the neuroendocrine control of growth hormone secretion: the model of anorexia nervosa. *Front Neuroendocrinol.* 2003;24(3):200–224.
73. Weiser SD, Fernandes KA, Brandson EK, et al. The association between food insecurity and mortality among HIV-infected individuals on HAART. *J Acquir Immune Defic Syndr.* 2009;52(3): 342–349.
74. National Center for Health Statistics. National Health and Nutrition Examination Survey (NHANES). Centers for Disease Control and Prevention. U.S. Department of Health and Human Services (DHHS).
75. Lukaski HC, Bolonchuk WW, Hall CB, et al. Validation of tetrapolar bioelectrical impedance method to assess human body composition. *Appl Physiol.* 1986;60:1327–1332.
76. Ott M, Fischer H, Polat H, et al. Bioelectrical impedance analysis as a predictor of survival in patients with human immunodeficiency virus infection. *J Acquir Immuno Defic Syndr Hum Retrovirol.* 1995;9:20–25.
77. Hendricks K, Gorbach S. Nutrition issues in chronic drug users living with HIV infection. *Addict Sci Clin Pract.* 2009;5(1):16–23.
78. Ferrando AA, Tipton KD, Bamman MM, Wolfe RR. Resistance exercise maintains skeletal muscle protein synthesis during bed rest. *J Applied Physiol.*1997;82(3):807–810.
79. Mwamburi DM, Gerrior J, Wilson IB, et al. Comparing megestrol actetate therapy with oxandrolone therapy for HIV-related weight loss: similar results in 2 months. *Clin Infect Dis.* 2004;38:895–902.
80. Leinung M, Liporace R, Miller CH. Induction of adrenal suppression by megestrol acetate in patients with AIDS. *Ann Intern Med.* 1995;122:843–845.
81. Timpome JG, Wright DJ, Li N, et al. The safety and pharmacokinetics of single-agent and combination therapy with megestrol acetate and dronabinol for the treatment of HIV wasting syndrome. *AIDS Res Hum Retroviruses.* 1997;13:305–315.
82. Struwe M, Kaempfer SH, Geiger CJ, et al. Effect of dronabinol on nutritional status in HIV infection. *Ann Pharmacother.* 1993;27: 827–831.
83. Grinspoon S, Corcoran C, Anderson E, et al. Sustained anabolic effect of long-term androgen administration in men with AIDS wasting. *Clin Infect Dis.* 1999;28:634–636.
84. Bhashin S, Storer TW, Asbel-Sethi N, et al. Effects of testosterone replacement with a nongenital, transdermal system, Androderm, in human immunodeficiency virus-infected men with low testosterone levels. *J Clin Endocrinol Metab.* 1998;83:3155–3162.
85. Strawford A, Barbieri T, Neese R, et al. Effects of nandrolone decanoate therapy in borderline hypogonadal men with HIV-associated weight loss. *J Acquir Immune Defic Syndr Hum Retrovirol.* 1999;20:137–146.
86. Storer TW, Woodhouse LJ, Sattler F, et al. A randomized, placebo-controlled trial of nandrolone decanoate in HIV-infected men with mild to moderate weight loss with recombinant human growth hormone as active reference treatment. *J Clin Endocrinol Metab.* 2005;90:4474–4482.
87. Gold J, High HA, Li Y, et al. Safety and efficacy of treatment with nandrolone decanoate for treatment of wasting in patients with HIV infection. *AIDS.* 1996;10:745–752.
88. Mulligan K, Zackin R, Clark RA, et al. Effect of nandrolone decanoate therapy on weight and lean body mass in HIV-infected women with weight loss: a randomized double blind placebo-controlled, multicenter trial. *Arch Intern Med.* 2005;165:578–585.
89. Strawford A, Barbieri T, van Loan M, et al. Resistance exercise and supraphysiologic androgen therapy in eugonadal men with HIV-related weight loss; a randomized controlled trial. *JAMA.* 1999; 281:1282–1290.
90. Grunfeld C, Kotler DP, Dobs A, Bhasin S. Oxandrolone in the treatment of HIV-associated weight loss in men: a randomized, double-blind, placebo-controlled study. *J Acquir Immune Defic Syndr.* 2006;41(3):304–314.
91. Wasserman P, Segal-Maurer S, Rubin D. Low sex-hormone binding globulin and testosterone levels in association with erectile dysfunction among human immunodeficiency virus-infected men receiving testosterone and oxandrolone. *J Sex Med.* 2008; 5(1):241–247.
92. Lubahn D, Joseph DR, Sullivan PM, et al. Cloning of human androgen receptor complementary DNA and localization to the X chromosome. *Science.* 1988;240:327–330.
93. Schambelan M, Mulligan K, Grunfeld C, et al. Recombinant human growth hormone in patients with HIV-associated wasting: a randomized placebo controlled trial. *Ann Intern Med.* 1996;125:873–882.
94. Grinspoon S, Corcoran C, Parlman K, et al. Effects of testosterone and progressive resistance training in eugonadal men with AIDS wasting. *Ann Intern Med.* 2000;133:348–355.
95. Lichtenstein KA, Armon C, Buchacz K, et al. Low CD4+ T cell count is a rsk factor for cardiovascular disease events in the HIV outpatient study. *Clin Infect Dis.* 2010;51(4):435–437.
96. Reyes-Teran G, Sierra-Madero JG, Martinez del Cerro V, et al. Effects of thalidomide on HIV-associated wasting syndrome: a randomized double blind placebo-controlled clinical trial. *AIDS.* 1996;10:1501–1507.
97. Harris JA, Benedict FG. *A Biometric Study of Basal Metabolism in Man.* Vol 2. Washington, DC: Carnegie Institution of Washington; 1919.
98. Selberg O, Suttmann U, Melzer A, et al. Effect of increased protein intake and nutritional status on whole-body protein metabolism in AIDS patients with weight loss. *Metabolism.* 1995;44: 1159–1165.
99. Berneis K, Battegay M, Bassetti S, et al. Nutritional supplementation combined with dietary counseling diminish whole body protein catabolism in HIV infected patients. *Eur J Clin Invest.* 2000;1:87–94.
100. Fogaca H, Souza H, Carneiro AJ, et al. Effects of oral nutritional supplementation on the intestinal mucosa of patients with AIDS. *J Clin Gastroenterol.* 2000;30:77–80.
101. Ahoua L, Umutoni C, Huerga H, et al. Nutrition outcomes of HIV-infected malnourished adults treated with ready-to-use therapeutic food in sub-Saharan Africa: a longitudinal study. *J Int AIDS Soc.* 2011;14:2.
102. Nyirenda C, Zulu I, Kabagambe EK, et al. Acute hypophosphataemia in a patient starting antiretroviral therapy in Zambia – a new context for refeeding syndrome? *BMJ Case Rep.* 2009;doi:10.1136/bcr.07.2008.0469.

103. Wasserman P, Rubin DS. Highly prevalent vitamin D deficiency and insufficiency in an urban cohort of HIV-infected men under care. *AIDS Patient Care STDs.* 2010;24(4):223–227.
104. Adeyemi OM, Agniel D, French AL, et al. Vitamin D deficiency in HIV-infected and HIV-uninfected women in the United States. *J Acquir Immune Defic Syndr.* 2011;57(3):197–204.
105. Bolland MJ, Grey A, Horne AM, Thomas MT. Osteomalacia in an HIV-infected man receiving rifabutin, a cytochrome P450 enzyme inducer: a case report. *Ann Clin Microbiol Antimicrob.* 2008;7:3–7.
106. Hahn TJ, Hendrin BA, Scharp CR, Haddad JG. Effects of chronic anticonvulsant therapy on serum 25-hydroxycalciferol levels in adults. *N Engl J Med.* 1972;287:900–904.
107. Weltz T, Childs K, Ibrahim F, et al. Efavirenz is associated with severe vitamin D deficiency and increased alkaline phosphates. *AIDS.* 2010;24(12):1923–1928.
108. Gibney KB, Mihrshahi S, Torresi J, et al. The profile of health problems in African immigrants attending an infectious disease unit in Melbourne, Australia. *Am J Top Med Hyg.* 2009;80(5):805–811.
109. Ross CA, Manson JE, Abrams SA, et al. The 2011 report on dietary reference intakes for calcium and vitamin D from the Institute of Medicine: what clinicians need to know. *J Clin Endocrinol Metab.* 2011;96(1):53–58.
110. Pichard C, Sudre P, Karsegard V, et al. A randomized double-blind controlled study of oral nutritional supplementation with arginine and omega-3 fatty acids in HIV-infected patients. Swiss HIV Cohort Study. *AIDS.* 1998;12:53–63.
111. Ockenga J, Suttmann U, Selberg O, et al. Percutaneous endoscopic gastrostomy in AIDS and control patients: risks and outcomes. *Am J Gastoenterol.* 1996;91:1817–1822.
112. Kotler DP, Tierney AR, Ferraro R, et al. Enteral alimentation and repletion of body cell mass in malnourished patients with acquired immunodeficiency syndrome. *Am J Clin Nutr.* 1991;53:149–154.
113. Melchior JC, Chastang C, Gelas P, et al. Efficacy of 2-month total parenteral nutrition in AIDS patients: a controlled randomized prospective trial. *AIDS.* 1996;10:379–384.
114. Singer P, Rothkopf MM, Kvetan V, et al. Risks and benefits of home parenteral nutrition in acquired immunodeficiency syndrome. *J Parenter Enteral Nutr.* 1991;15:75–79.
115. Rantanen T, Guralnik JM, Foley D, et al. Midlife hand-grip strength as a predictor of old age disability. *JAMA.* 1999;281;(6):558–560.
116. Guralnik JM, Ferrucci L, Pieper CF, et al. Lower extremity function and subsequent disability: consistency across studies, predictive models, and value of gait speed alone compared to the short physical performance battery. *J Gerontol.* 2000;55A(4):M221–M231.
117. Grijsen ML, Vrouenraets SME, Steingrover R, et al. High prevalence of reduced bone mineral density in primary HIV-1 infected men. *AIDS.* 2010;24:2233–2238.
118. Duvivier C, Kolta S, Assoumou L, et al. Greater decrease in bone mineral density with protease inhibitor regimens compared with nonnucleoside reverse transcriptase inhibitor regimens in HIV-1 infected naive patients. *AIDS.* 2009;23(7):817–824.
119. Brown TT, McComsey GA, King MS, et al. Loss of bone mineral density after antiretroviral therapy initiation, independent of antiretroviral regimen. *J Acquir Immune Defic Syndr.* 2009;51(5):554–561.
120. Gallant JE, Staszewski S, Pozniak AL, et al. Efficacy and safety of tenofovir DF vs satavudine in combination therapy in antiretroviral-naïve patients. *JAMA.* 2004;292(2):191–201.
121. Bonjoch A, Figueras M, Estany C, et al. High prevalence of and progression to low bone mineral density in HIV-infected patients: a longitudinal cohort study. *AIDS.* 2010;24;2827–2833.
122. Arnsten JH, Freeman R, Howard AA, et al. Decreased bone mineral density and increased fracture risk in aging men with or at risk for HIV infection. *AIDS.* 2007;21:617–623.
123. Guillemi S, Harris M, Bondy GP, et al. Prevalence of bone mineral density abnormalities and related risk factors in an ambulatory HIV clinic population. *J Clin Densitom.* 2010;13(4):456–461.
124. Yin MT, McMahon DJ, Ferris DC, et al. Low bone mass and high bone turnover in postmenopausal human immunodeficiency virus infected women. *J Clin Endocrinol Metab.* 2010;95:620–629.
125. Cotter EJ, Chew N, Powderly WG, Doran PP. HIV type 1 alters mesenchymal stem cell differentiation potential and cell phenotype ex vivo. *AIDS Res Hum Retroviruses.* 2011;27(2):187–199.
126. Guaraldi G, Orlando G, Squillace N, et al. Prevalence of secondary causes of osteoporosis in HIV-infected individuals. Program and abstracts presented at: 8th International Workshop on Adverse Drug Reactions and Lipodystrophy in HIV; September 24–26, 2006; San Francisco, CA.
127. Bacchetti P, Gripshover B, Grunfeld C, et al. Fat distribution in men with HIV infection from the study of fat redistribution and metabolic change in HIV infection (FRAM). *J Acquir Immune Defic Syndr.* 2005;40:121–131.
128. Brown T, Wang Z, Chu H, et al. Longitudinal anthropometric changes in HIV-infected and HIV-uninfected men. *J Acquir Immune Defic Syndr.* 2006;43(3):356–362.
129. Kosmiski LA, Kuritzkes DR, Lichtenstein KA, Eckel R. Adipocyte-derived hormone levels in HIV lipodystrophy. *Antivir Ther.* 2003;8:9–15.
130. Carter VM, Hoy JF, Baily M, et al. The prevalence of lipodystrophy in an ambulant HIV-infected population: it all depends on the definition. *HIV Med.* 2001;2:174–180.
131. Abhimanyu G, Agarwal AK. Lipodystrophies: disorders of adipose tissue biology. *Biochim Biophys Acta.* 2009;1791(6):507–513.
132. Petersen KF, Oral EA, Dufour S, et al. Leptin reverses insulin resistance and hepatic steatosis in patients with lipodystrophy. *J Clin Invest.* 2002;109:1345–1350.
133. Hammond E, McKinnon E, Nolan D. Human immunodeficiency virus treatment-induced adipose tissue pathology and lipoatrophy: prevalence and metabolic consequences. *Clin Infect Dis.* 2010;51(5):591–599.
134. Bastard JP, Caron M, Vidal H, et al. Association between altered expression of adipogenic factor SREBP-1 in lipoatrophic adipose tissue from HIV-1 infected patients and abnormal adipocyte differentiation and insulin resistance. *Lancet.* 2002; 359:1026–1031.
135. Shikuma CM, Hu N, Milne C, et al. Mitochondrial DNA decrease in subcutaneous adipose tissue of HIV-infected individuals with peripheral lipoatrophy. *AIDS.* 2001;15:1801–1809.
136. Walker UA, Bickel M, Lutke Volksbeck SI, et al. Evidence of nucleoside analogue reverse transcriptase inhibitor-associated genetic and structural defects of mitochondria in adipose tissue of HIV infected patients. *J Acquir Immune Defic Syndr.* 2002;29:117–121.
137. Kosmiski L, Kuritizkes D, Lichtenstein K, Eckel R. Adipocyte-derived hormone levels in HIV lipodystrophy *Antivir Ther.* 2003;8:9–15.
138. Dresner A, Laurent D, Marcucci M, et al. Effects of free fatty acids on glucose transport and IRS-1-associated phosphatidylinositol 3-kinase activity. *J Clin Invest.* 1999;103:253–258.
139. Brinkman K, Smeitink JA, Romijn JA, Reiss P. Mitochondrial toxicity induced by nucleoside-analogue reverse-transcriptase is a key factor in the pathogenesis of antiretroviral-related-lipodystrophy. *Lancet.* 1999;354:1112–1115.

140. Moyle GJ, Sabin CA, Cartledge J, et al. A randomized comparative trial of tenofovir DF or abacavir as replacement for a thymidine analogue in persons with lipoatrophy. *AIDS*. 2006;20(16): 2043–2050.
141. Hertel J, Struthers H, Horj CB, Hruz PW. A structural basis for the acute effects of HIV protease inhibitors on GLUT4 intrinsic activity. *J Biol Chem*. 2004;279:55147–55152.
142. Chariot P, Drogou I, de Lacroix-Szmania I, et al. Zidovudine-induced mitochondrial disorder with massive liver steatosis, myopathy, lactic acidosis, and mitochondrial DNA depletion. *J Hepatol*. 1999;30:156–160.
143. Gerard Y, Maulin L, Yazdanpanah Y, et al. Symptomatic hyperlactatemia: an emerging complication of antiretroviral therapy. *AIDS*. 2000;14:2723–2730.
144. Snijder MB, Dekker JM, Visser M, et al. Larger thigh and hip circumferences are associated with better glucose tolerance: the Hoorn study. *Obes Res* 2003;11(1):104–111.
145. Seidell JC, Perusse L, Despres JP, Bouchard C. Waist and hip circumferences have independent and opposite effects on cardiovascular disease risk factors: the Quebec Family Study. *Am J Clin Nutr*. 2001;74(3):315–321.
146. Lemieux S, Prudhomme D, Bouchard C, et al. A single threshold value of waist girth identifies normal-weight and overweight subjects with excess visceral adipose tissue. *Am J. Clin Nutr*. 1996;64: 685–693.
147. Mallon PW, Wand H, Law M, et al. Buffalo hump seen in HIV-associated lipodystrophy is associated with hyperinsulinemia but not dyslipidemia. *J Acquir Immune Defic Syndr*. 2005;38: 156–162.
148. Gervasoni C, Ridolfo AL, Rovati L, et al. Maintenance of breast size reduction after mastoplasty and switch to a protease inhibitor-sparing regimen in an HIV-positive woman with highly active antiretroviral therapy-associated massive breast enlargement. *AIDS Patient Care STDS*. 2002;16:307–311.
149. Miller KK, Daly PA, Sentochk D, et al. Pseudo-Cushing's syndrome in human immunodeficiency virus-infected patients. *Clin Infect Dis*. 1998;27:68–72.
150. Miller J, Carr A, Emery S, et al. HIV lipodystrophy: prevalence, severity and correlates of risk in Australia. *HIV Med*. 2003;4: 293–301.
151. Carr A, Samaras K, Burton S, et al. A syndrome of peripheral lipodystrophy, hyperlipidaemia and insulin resistance in patients receiving HIV protease inhibitors. *AIDS*. 1998;12:F51–58.
152. Carr A, Samaras K, Thorisdottir A, et al. Diagnosis, prediction, and natural course of HIV-1 protease-inhibitor-associated lipodystrophy, hyperlipidemia, and diabetes mellitus: a cohort study. *Lancet*. 1999;353:2093–2099.
153. Martin A, Smith DE, Carr A, et al. Reversibility of lipoatrophy in HIV-infected patients 2 years after switching from a thymidine analogue to abacavir: the MITOX extension study. *AIDS*. 2004; 18:1029–1036.
154. Moyle GJ, Baldwin C, Langroudi B, et al. A 48-week, randomized, open-label comparison of three abacavir-based substitution approaches in the management of dyslipidemia and peripheral lipoatrophy. *J Acquir Immune Defic Syndr*. 2003;33:22–28.
155. Dolan SE, Frontera W, Librizzi J, et al. Effects of a supervised home-based aerobic and progressive resistance training regimen in women infected with human immunodeficiency virus: a randomized trial. *Arch Intern Med* 2006;166(11): 1225–1231.
156. Centers for Disease Control and Prevention. Physical Activity Guidelines for Americans. http://www.cdc.gov/physicalactivity/everyone/guidelines/adults.html. Accessed 12/10/2010.
157. Hadigan C, Yawetz S, Thomas A, et al. Metabolic effects of rosiglitazone in HIV lipodystrophy: a randomized, controlled trial. *Ann Intern Med*. 2004;140:786–794.
158. van Wijk JPH, de Koning EJP, Cabezas MC, et al. Comparison of rosiglitazone and metformin for treating HIV lipodystrophy: a randomized trial. *Ann Intern Med*. 2005;143:337–346.
159. Carr A, Workman C, Carey D, et al. No effect of rosiglitazone for treatment of HIV-1 lipoatrophy: randomised, double-blind, placebo-controlled trial. *Lancet*. 2004;363:429–438.
160. Goldberg RB, Kendall DM, Deeg MA, et al. A comparison of lipid and glycemic effects of pioglitazone and rosiglitazone in patients with type 2 diabetes and dyslipidemia. *Diabetes Care*. 2005;28: 1547–1554.
161. Hadigan C, Corcoran C, Basgoz N, et al. Metformin in the treatment of HIV lipodystrophy syndrome: a randomized controlled trial. *JAMA*. 2000;284:472–477.
162. Saint-Marc T, Tourine JL. Effects of metformin on resistance and central adiposity in patients receiving effective protease inhibitor therapy. *AIDS*. 1999;13:1000–1002.
163. Hadigan C, Meigs JB, Rabe J, et al. Increased PAI-1 and tPA antigen levels are reduced with metformin therapy in HIV-infected patients with fat redistribution and insulin resistance. *J Clin Endocrinol Metab*. 2001;86:939–943.
164. Lafaurie M, Dolivo M, Porcher R, et al. Treatment of facial lipoatrophy with intradermal injections of polylactic acid in HIV-infected patients. *J Acquir Immune Defic Syndr*. 2005;38:393–398.
165. Jones D. HIV facial lipoatrophy: causes and treatment options. *Dermatol Surg*. 2005;31:1519–1529.
166. Silvers SL, Eviatar JA, Pappas AL. Prospective, open-label, 18-month trial of calcium hydroxylapatite (Radiesse) for facial soft-tissue augmentation in patients with human immunodeficiency virus associated lipoatrophy: one-year durability. *Plast Reconstr Surg*. 2006;118(3 suppl):34S–45S.
167. Friis-Moller N, Thiebaut R, Reiss P, et al. Predicting the risk of cardiovascular disease in HIV-infected patients: the data collection on adverse effects of anti-HIV drugs study. Eur *J Cardiovasc Prev*. 2010;17(5):491–501.
168. Grunfeld C, Delaney JAC, Wanke C, et al. Preclinical atherosclerosis due to HIV infection: carotid intima-medial thickness measurements from the FRAM study. *AIDS*. 2009;23: 1841–1849.
169. Grunfeld C, Pang M, Doerrler W, et al. Lipids, lipoproteins, triglyceride clearance, and cytokines, in human immunodeficiency virus and acquired immunodeficiency syndrome. *J Clin Endocrinol Metab*. 1992;74:1045–1052.
170. Kuller LH, Tracy R, Belloso W, et al. Inflammatory and coagulation biomarkers and mortality in patients with HIV infection. *PloS Med*. 2008;5(10):e203.
171. Lichtenstein KA, Armon C, Buchacz K, et al. Low CD4+ T cell count is a risk factor for cardiovascular disease events in the HIV outpatient study. *Clin Infect Dis*. 2010;51(4):435–447.
172. Worm SW, Sabin C, Weber R, et al. Risk of myocardial infarction in patients with HIV infection exposed to specific individual antiretroviral drugs from the 3 major drug classes: the data collection on adverse events of anti-HIV drugs (D:A:D) study. *J Infect Dis*. 2010;201:318–330.
173. Friis-Mollner N, Reiss P, Sabin CA, et al. Class of antiretroviral drug and risk of myocardial infarction. *N Engl J Med*. 2007; 356(17):1723–1735.
174. Liang JS, Distler O, Cooper DA, et al. HIV protease inhibitors protect apolipoprotein B from degradation by the proteasome: a potential mechanism for protease inhibitor-induced hyperlipidemia. *Nat Med*. 2001;7:1327–1331.

175. Grundy SM, Cleeman JI, Merz CN, et al. Implications of recent clinical trials for the National Cholesterol Education Program Adult Treatment Panel III guidelines. *Circulation.* 2004;110(2):227–239.
176. Woodward M, Rumley A, Welsh P, MacMahon S, Lowe G. A comparison of the associations between seven hemostatic or inflammatory variables and coronary heart disease. *J Thromb Haemost.* 2007;5:1795–1800.
177. deLongeril M, Salen P, Martin J, et al. Mediterranean diet, traditional risk factors, and the rate of cardiovascular complications after myocardial infarction: final report of the Lyon diet heart study. *Circulation.* 1999;99:779–785.
178. Buckland G, Gonzalez CA, Aqudo A, et al. Adherence to the Mediterranean diet and risk of coronary heart disease in the Spanish EPIC Cohort Study. *Am J Epidemiol* 2009;170(12):1518–1529
179. Martinez-Gonzalez MA, de la Fuente-Arrillaga C, Nunez-Cordoba JM, et al. Adherence to Mediterranean diet and risk of developing diabetes: prospective cohort study. *BMJ.* 2008;336(7657): 1348–1351.
180. Esposito K, Marfella R, Citotola M, et al. Effect of a Mediterranean-style diet on endothelial dysfunction and markers of vascular inflammation in the metabolic syndrome: a randomized trial. *JAMA.* 2004;292:1440–1446.
181. Hadigan C, Jeste S, Anderson EJ, et al. Modifiable dietary habits and their relation to metabolic abnormalities in men and women with human immunodeficiency virus infection and fat redistribution. *Clin Infect Dis.* 2001;33:710–717.
182. Tsiodras S, Poulia KA, Yannakoulia M. Adherence to Mediterranean diet is favorably associated with metabolic parameters in HIV-positive patients with the highly active antiretroviral therapy-induced metabolic syndrome and lipodystrophy. *Metabolism.* 2009;58(6):854–859.
183. Turcinov D, Stanley C, Rutherford GW, et al. Adherence to the Mediterranean diet is associated with a lower risk of body-shape changes in Croatian patients treated with combination antiretroviral therapy. *Eur J Epidemiol.* 2009;24(5):267–274.
184. Dube MP, Stein JH, Aberg JA, et al. Guidelines for the management of dyslipdemia in human immunodeficiency virus (HIV)-infected adults receiving antiretroviral therapy: recommendations of the HIV Medical Association of the Infectious Disease Society of America and the Adult AIDS Clinical Trials Group. *Clin Infect Dis.* 2003; 37(5):613–627.
185. Wohl DA, Hsiao-chaun T, Busby M, et al. Randomized study of the safety and efficacy of fish oil (omega-3 fatty acid) supplementation with dietary and exercise counseling for the treatment of antiretroviral therapy-associated hypertriglyceridemia. *Clin Infect Dis.* 2005;41:1498–1504.
186. Liu J, Fox CS, Hickson DA, et al. Impact of abdominal visceral and subcutaneous adipose tissue on cardiometabolic risk factors: the Jackson Heart Study. *J Clin Endocrinol Metab.* 2010;95(12): 5419–5426.
187. Reitschel P, Hadigan C, Corcoran C, et al. Assessment of growth hormone dynamics in immunodeficiency virus-related lipodystrophy. *J Clin Endocrinol Metab.* 2001;86:504–510.
188. Falutz J, Allas S, Kotler D, et al. A placebo controlled, dose ranging study of growth hormone releasing factor in HIV-infected patients with abdominal fat accumulation. *AIDS.* 2005;19: 1279–1287.
189. Kotler DP, Tierney AR, Culpepper-Morgan JA, et al. Effect of total parenteral nutrition on body composition in patients with acquired immunodeficiency syndrome. *J Parenteral Enteral Nutr.* 1990;14(5):454–458.
190. Vietri Nicholas J, Skidmore PJ, Dooley DP. Esophageal ulceration due to cytomegalovirus infection in a patient with acute retroviral syndrome. *Clin Infect Dis.* 2002;34(1):e14–15.
191. Melchior JC, Chastang C, Gelas P, et al. Efficacy of 2-month total parenteral nutrition in AIDS patients: a controlled randomized prospective trial. The French multicenter total parenteral nutrition cooperative group study. *AIDS.* 1996;10(4):379–384.
192. Melchior JC, Gelas P, Carbonnel F, et al. Improved survival by home total parenteral nutrition in AIDS patients: follow-up of a controlled randomized prospective trial. *AIDS.* 1998;12(2): 336–337.
193. Wang C, Swerdloff RS, Iranmanesh A, et al. Transdermal testosterone gel improves sexual function, mood, muscle strength, and body composition parameters in hypogonadal men. *J Clin Endocrinol Metab.* 2000;85:2839–2853.

33 Cancer

Robin B. Mendelsohn, MD, and Mark A. Schattner, MD

CONTENTS

Background . . . 564
Trends and Impact of Cancer . . . 564
Prevalence of Malnutrition in Patients with Cancer . . . 564
Significance of Malnutrition in Patients with Cancer . . . 565
Etiology of Malnutrition in Patients with Cancer . . . 565
Metabolic Alterations . . . 565
Energy Expenditure . . . 565
Carbohydrate Metabolism . . . 565
Protein Metabolism . . . 565
Lipid Metabolism . . . 565
Mediators of Altered Metabolism . . . 566
Impaired Caloric Intake, Maldigestion, and Malnutrition . . . 566
Changes of Taste and Food . . . 566
Learned Food Aversions . . . 566
Depression . . . 566
Disturbances of the Gastrointestinal Tract . . . 567
Nutritional Therapies . . . 567
Oral Dietary Therapy . . . 567
Enteral Nutrition . . . 568
Indications . . . 568
Enteral Access and Formula . . . 568
Home Enteral Nutrition . . . 569
Total Parenteral Nutrition . . . 569
Indications . . . 569
Home Total Parenteral Nutrition . . . 569
Pharmacotherapy . . . 569
Hormones . . . 569
Appetite Stimulants . . . 570
Cytokine Inhibitors . . . 571
Drugs to Relieve Symptoms . . . 572
Effect of Nutrition on Tumor Growth . . . 572
Nutrition Management of Patients with Specific Cancers . . . 572
Nutrition Support in Patients with Cancer of the Head and Neck . . . 572
Nutrition Support in Patients with Cancer of the Esophagus . . . 573
Nutrition Support in Patients with Cancer of the Stomach . . . 573
Nutrition Support in Patients with Cancer of the Pancreas . . . 574
Nutrition Support in Patients with Cancer of the Colon and Rectum . . . 574
Nutrition Support in Patients with Gynecologic Cancers . . . 575
Nutrition Support in Patients Undergoing Hematopoietic Stem Cell Transplantation . . . 575
Nutrition Support During Palliative Care . . . 576
References . . . 577

Objectives

1. Discuss the etiology and significance of malnutrition in cancer patients.
2. Identify the options and indications for the various therapies used for the treatment of cancer and malnutrition.
3. Understand the techniques that are available and appropriate for nutrition support of cancer patients under varying circumstances.

Test Your Knowledge Questions

1. Which of the following is true about the mechanisms of weight loss in cancer patients?
   A. Because of the tumor itself, cancer patients have increased energy expenditure and nitrogen loss resulting in weight loss.
   B. Like in simple starvation, protein catabolism slowly decreases in an attempt to preserve lean body mass.
   C. Cancer patients have a decreased cytokine response to the tumor itself.
   D. As opposed to simple starvation, cancer patients have an increase in glucose turnover.
2. Enteral nutrition (EN) is appropriate in which of the following patients?
   A. A well-nourished patient with colon cancer undergoing chemotherapy
   B. A severely malnourished gastric cancer patient with nausea and vomiting
   C. A moderately malnourished patient with head and neck cancer with dysphagia
   D. A well-nourished recipient of a hematopoietic stem cell transplant
3. Which of the following is true regarding a patient with newly diagnosed pancreatic cancer awaiting chemotherapy?
   A. A nutrition assessment should be performed
   B. Enteral nutrition should be initiated because the patient will likely need nutrition support during chemotherapy
   C. Parenteral nutrition should be initiated because that patient will likely need nutrition support during chemotherapy
   D. If the decision is made to undergo surgery, the patient should receive parenteral nutrition

Test Your Knowledge Answers

1. The correct answer is **D**. The mechanism of weight loss in cancer patients is multifactorial. Though it was originally thought that the cancer itself led to increased energy expenditure and nitrogen loss, it is now known that this response it not consistent and is widely variable. In cancer patients with weight loss there is increased glucose turnover, which is in stark contrast to patients with simple starvation who have decreased glucose turnover. Whereas in simple starvation, where protein catabolism slowly decreases in an attempt to preserve lean body mass, in cancer this is lost and protein turnover actually increases with the progression of disease and weight loss. The presence of increased circulating cytokines, changes in hormones and neuropeptide levels, as well as tumor-derived products, are all potential causes for weight loss in cancer patients.
2. The correct answer is **C**. Enteral nutrition is indicated in patients undergoing anticancer therapies who are malnourished and who have a functional gastrointestinal tract. Nutritional support is not routinely indicated in patients undergoing treatment who are not malnourished. The patient with gastric cancer with nausea and vomiting has symptoms of gastric outlet obstruction and would require a further evaluation prior to initiating enteral nutrition.
3. The correct answer is **A**. As per the American Society for Parenteral and Enteral Nutrition (A.S.P.E.N.) guidelines, patients with cancer are nutritionally at risk and should undergo a nutrition screening to identify those who require formal nutrition assessment. Neither enteral nutrition nor parenteral nutrition is indicated routinely in patients undergoing a treatment who are not malnourished. The role of surgery perioperatively is controversial, and not usually recommended in patients who are not malnourished.

Background

Trends and Impact of Cancer

Cancer is a tremendous public health issue in the United States. It was estimated that in 2011, over 1.5 million people would be diagnosed with cancer, and over 570,000 people would die from their disease.[1] The lifetime risk of a person developing cancer is 1 in 2. Cancer accounts for nearly one quarter of all deaths in the United States annually, second only to heart disease. Though the cancer death rate has been declining steadily, there has been a slow increase in cancer deaths since 2007, which is attributed to the growth and aging of the American population.[1]

The financial costs of cancer are enormous, both to the patients themselves and to society at large. The National Institutes of Health (NIH) estimated that in 2008, total cancer care cost $228.1 billion, with $93.2 billion in direct medical care, which is about 20% higher than heart disease. Compared to other causes of death, cancer represents the largest toll on the national economy due to years of life and productivity lost. And, as the American population continues to grow and age, this economic burden will undoubtedly continue to increase.[2]

Prevalence of Malnutrition in Patients with Cancer

The true prevalence of malnutrition in patients with cancer is difficult to determine due to the absence of a standard for nutrition screening in cancer patients and a lack of agreement on the validity of these measures. Recently, an International Guideline Committee was formed to develop a consensus definition for malnutrition in adults and decided to use an etiology-based approach focusing on the inflammatory response.[3] They proposed the following: "Starvation-related malnutrition" refers to chronic starvation without inflammation, "chronic disease-related malnutrition" refers to inflammation that is chronic and of mild-to-moderate degree, and "acute disease or injury-related malnutrition" refers to when inflammation is acute and of severe degree. Most studies, however, use weight loss as the primary indicator of malnutrition and involuntary weight loss greater than 10% as evidence of significant malnutrition.

In a large multicenter cooperative study of patients with 12 types of cancer, DeWys et al.[4] reported that over half of cancer patients present with weight loss at the time of diagnosis. The extent of weight loss varied, with the lowest frequency of weight loss (31% to 40%) in patients with sarcomas, breast, and hematologic cancers; intermediate frequency (54% to 64%) in patients with colon, prostate, and lung cancers; and highest frequency (over 80%) in patients with pancreas and gastric cancers. Multiple other subsequent studies have shown similar results and have demonstrated that malnutrition is not only affected by tumor type, location, grade, and stage, but also by the anticancer therapy and patient characteristics including age, gender, and comorbidities, namely diabetes and intestinal disorders.[4] Furthermore, they indicate that since the majority of cancer patients present with weight loss this underscores the importance of an early assessment of nutritional status in these patients.

Significance of Malnutrition in Patients with Cancer

In their multicenter, cooperative study described above, DeWys et al. showed that patients receiving chemotherapy who presented with weight loss had decreased performance status and survival when compared with those without weight loss.[4] In cancer patients, malnutrition is associated with longer length of hospital stay, increased cost, increased morbidity and mortality, and has been shown to make anticancer treatments less effective leading to longer duration of treatment.[5]

Etiology of Malnutrition in Patients with Cancer

The etiology of malnutrition and weight loss in cancer patients is multifactorial. Cancer not only causes widespread cellular and metabolic alterations, which affect metabolism, but also leads to impaired caloric intake and maldigestion. In addition, the cancer therapies themselves can have significant side effects resulting in gastrointestinal dysfunction.

Metabolic Alterations

Energy Expenditure

The initial belief was that cancer itself led to increased energy expenditure and nitrogen loss, resulting in weight loss. Further studies, however, revealed that this response is not consistent and have found resting energy expenditures to be widely variable. An association with age, sex, height, weight, nutrition intake, nutrition status, or extent of tumor was not found. Tumor type, however, was predictive with gastric, pancreatic, and biliary cancer patients being the most hypermetabolic.[6]

Carbohydrate Metabolism

Many cancer patients exhibit glucose intolerance, thought to be due to increased endogenous glucose production, increased resistance to both exogenous and endogenous insulin, and inadequate insulin release. Other factors, including bed rest, weight loss, and sepsis, may also contribute to hyperglycemia as they do in other diseases.

This increase in glucose turnover and weight loss is in stark contrast to those patients with simple starvation who have decreased glucose turnover and weight loss.[7]

An increase in wasteful metabolic cycles, such as the Cori cycle, likely also contributes to altered glucose metabolism in cancer patients. Tumor cells produce lactate, which is used as a substrate for gluconeogenesis in the Cori cycle and reconverted to glucose. For each cycle, there is a net loss of four high energy phosphate bonds leading to a large amount of energy wasted in this futile cycle. Though initial studies showed that the increase in the Cori cycle had a large contribution to increased energy expenditure in patients with metastatic disease and weight loss, subsequent studies showed that an increase in the Cori cycle has only a minor role in the alterations of glucose metabolism.[8] There is ongoing research identifying other futile cycles.

Protein Metabolism

Cancer patients also have increased protein turnover thought to be due to increased hepatic protein synthesis, increased muscle protein degradation, and impaired protein synthesis. Whereas in simple starvation where protein catabolism slowly decreases in an attempt to preserve lean body mass, in cancer this is lost and protein turnover actually increases with the progression of disease and weight loss.[8]

Increased protein breakdown in cancer patients is due to at least three different proteolytic pathways: (1) lysosomal energy-dependent proteolysis (including cysteine proteases cathepsins B, H, and L, and aspartate proteases cathepsin D), which is mainly responsible for cell receptor and extracellular protein degradation; (2) calcium-dependent proteases (including calpains I and II), which are mainly involved in tissue injury, autolysis, and necrosis; and (3) the ubiquitin–proteasome dependent pathway, which is adenosine triphosphate (ATP) dependent and works with the calpain system to break down myofilaments. The ubiquitin–proteasome pathway is the most extensively studied and thought to be the predominant mechanism of protein breakdown, especially in patients with $> 10\%$ weight loss.[8]

Lipid Metabolism

The depletion of adipose tissue and lipid stores due to increased lipolysis is seen in cancer patients with weight loss. Compared with normal subjects and cancer patients without weight loss, cancer patients with weight loss have an increased turnover of both free fatty acids and glycerol. Increased lipolysis has been attributed to multiple causes including poor oral intake, stress response to illness leading to adrenal medullary stimulation and increased circulating catecholamine levels, insulin resistance, and the release of lipolytic factors produced by the tumor itself or by myeloid tissue cells.[8] One factor, the lipid mobilizing factor, had been well characterized and extensively studied (see Mediators of Altered Metabolism, which follows).

Mediators of Altered Metabolism

Recent data demonstrate that various mediators including glycoproteins, proinflammatory cytokines, and neuropeptides induce a systemic inflammatory response leading to the metabolic derangements delineated previously.

Glycoproteins

Two glycoproteins, proteolysis-inducing factor (PIF) and lipid-mobilizing factor (LMF), have been found to be important mediators of the cachexia seen in many patients with cancers.

Proteolysis-Inducing Factor

PIF, a 24 kDa molecular mass sulfated glycoprotein, is produced by human tumors and was found in the urine of cancer patients (namely pancreatic, lung, breast, ovary, rectum, colon, and liver) who were losing weight, but not in the urine of cancer patients who were maintaining their weight. In fact, PIF expression directly correlates with the severity of weight loss. There are multiple mechanisms by which PIF induces weight loss. PIF has a direct effect on skeletal muscle by decreasing protein synthesis and increasing protein degradation by upregulating the ubiquitin-proteasome–dependent pathway. PIF also increases the expression of proinflammatory cytokines (ie, interleukin [IL]-6 and 8), which independently cause weight loss and induce the shedding of syndecans (transmembrane proteoglycans), which have been shown to be related to increased metastases and mortality.[7–8]

Lipid-Mobilizing Factor

LMF is a glycoprotein produced by a variety of tumors that is identical to the plasma protein zinc-alpha2-glycoprotein (ZAG) and causes an increase in lipolysis. LMF/ZAG has been shown to increase lipid mobilization and substrate use by increasing mitochondrial oxidative pathways in adipose tissue. In animal studies, LMF has been shown to lead to decreased body fat and weight independent of caloric intake. Moreover, the degree of LMF activity has been demonstrated to correlate with the degree of weight loss and tumor burden.[7–8]

Proinflammatory Cytokines

Tumor Necrosis Factor Alpha

Animal studies have shown tumor necrosis factor (TNF)-α to be a significant mediator of weight loss by inducing the enzyme lipoprotein lipase, which hydrolyzes fatty acids from plasma lipoproteins, stimulating lipolysis, and suppressing transcription. Human studies, however, are less consistent. Why there is this discrepancy is unclear. Some hypotheses include differences in measuring techniques, fluctuations in TNF-α serum levels, or the short half-life of TNF-α. Lastly, some have proposed that perhaps TNF-α has a direct local effect before circulating through the bloodstream.[7–8]

Interleukin 1, Interleukin 6, and Interferon Gamma

Animal models have shown IL-1, IL-6, and interferon gamma (IFN-γ) to be important mediators in weight loss of cancer patients. Human studies, however, have been inconsistent.[7–8]

Neuropeptides

Neuropeptide Y (NPY) is a 36 amino acid neuropeptide found in the hypothalamus. In starvation, NPY levels rise and stimulate feeding and decrease energy expenditure in order to restore energy balance. In cancer, however, this is lost, and animal studies have shown that NPY levels are inappropriately low and do not have orexigenic effects. Data from human studies are very limited.[7–8]

Cancer cachexia may also be partly due to orexigenic (appetite stimulating) neuropeptides such as NPY and anorexigenic-stimulating neuropeptides such as pro-opiomelanocortin (POMC).[8] Alpha melanocyte stimulating hormone (α-MSH), a product of POMC, induces anorexia by binding to two different melanocortin receptors (Mc3r and Mc4r) in the hypothalamus. Studies in rats showed that blocking this binding reverses cancer anorexia in animals with cancer. Why tumors cause an upregulation in α-MSH is not clear, but it is likely that cytokines (ie, IL-1, IL-6, TNF-α) are involved.[7–8]

Impaired Caloric Intake, Maldigestion, and Malabsorption

Changes of Taste and Appetite

Many cancer patients complain of decreased taste and appetite, which is hypothesized to be due to the proinflammatory cytokines and neuropeptides described previously.[7] In addition, cancer treatments, including chemotherapy, radiation, and surgery, can lead to alterations in taste, and these changes may persist for months after the completion of therapy.

Learned Food Aversions

Cancer patients who receive chemotherapy or radiation may develop food aversions. In their classic study, Bernstein et al.[10] tested children who were given chemotherapy associated with nausea and vomiting for a learned food aversion. Their study had three groups: one group undergoing gastrointestinal (GI) toxic chemotherapy, who were given a novel ice cream flavor; one group undergoing GI toxic chemotherapy, who were not given ice cream; and a control group who were not undergoing chemotherapy and were given ice cream. When tested later for aversions to this novel ice cream flavor, controls chose it three times more frequently than the experimental group, indicating a learned aversion. Similar findings have been reported in adults. The risk of developing a learned food aversion is directly related to the GI toxicity of the therapy.

Depression

Studies have reported up to 58% of cancer patients as having depressive symptoms and up to 38% as having major depression.[9] The mechanism is likely multifactorial due to both the stress of the diagnosis and treatment as well as neurohumoral changes induced by the tumor. Similar to patients without cancer, depression is associated with impaired oral intake and malnutrition in patients with cancer. A recent meta-analysis showed that depression predicted mortality in cancer patients.[10]

Disturbances of the Gastrointestinal Tract

GI malignancies, namely esophageal, gastric, intestinal, and pancreatic, frequently cause direct mechanical obstruction by the primary tumor. In addition, peritoneal disease can cause both mechanical obstruction and intestinal dysfunction without frank obstruction. Although acute obstruction presents with symptoms that require immediate medical attention, malignant obstruction develops slowly over time and causes a progressive decrease in food intake leading to weight loss. Recurrent episodes of intestinal obstruction are very common in cancer patients and can lead to significant decreases in quality of life.

In addition, cancer patients can also suffer from altered intestinal motility due to a multitude of causes. Firstly, tumors themselves can induce an immune-mediated destruction of components of the enteric nerve plexus, resulting in a paraneoplastic syndrome of gastroparesis and intestinal pseudo-obstruction. Secondly, prolonged postoperative ileus is common after a surgical resection for cancer. Thirdly, patients treated with radiation therapy can have both acute and chronic effects on GI motility. Finally, medications, especially chemotherapeutic agents and narcotics, can alter GI motility. As with frank obstruction, disturbances in motility result in impaired oral intake and weight loss. The severity of dysmotility is also directly correlated with the degree of malnutrition.[5,11]

Malabsorption

Cancer patients may have malabsorption due to a multitude of reasons. The theory initially was that the cancer itself altered intestinal mucosa, resulting in malabsorption.[12] Subsequent studies, however, showed this altered intestinal mucosa in patients without cancer but with malabsorption, indicating that these mucosal changes are likely due to malabsorption as opposed to the cancer. Many chemotherapeutic agents cause diarrhea. Studies in both children and adults have shown that certain chemotherapeutic agents can lead to malabsorption. Radiation can also cause direct toxicity to the GI mucosa, leading to radiation enteritis and colitis. In fact, one review of patients with radiation enteritis who were dependent on parenteral nutrition (PN) found that malabsorption was the primary cause of intestinal failure in about 10% of patients.[13] Surgical resection of both the small and the large bowel is associated with malabsorption. Patients who undergo pancreatic resections for pancreatic cancer often suffer from exocrine pancreatic insufficiency and malabsorption. Rarely, radiation therapy can cause pancreatic insufficiency.[14]

Fistulae, either due to direct tumor invasion, surgery, or radiation, cause a bypass of bowel, leading to malabsorption. Up to 85% of fistulae occur in the postoperative setting, most commonly after a cancer operation.[15] Cancer, chemotherapy, and radiation all hinder spontaneous fistulae healing. The degree of malabsorption depends on the site and extent of the bypass. The most significant malabsorption is seen in gastrocolic (between the stomach and the colon), enterocolic (between the small intestine and the large intestine), enteroenteric (between the small intestine and the small intestine), and enterocutaneous (between the small bowel and the skin) fistulae. Managing the nutrition of these patients is difficult, and must focus on replacing the ongoing loss of fluids, electrolytes, and minerals.

Additionally, small bowel bacterial overgrowth (SIBO) may also contribute to malabsorption by damaging enterocytes. In these patients, SIBO is usually due to an anatomic abnormality such as a fistulae, strictures, and surgical resections, most notably surgically created blind loops, ileocecal resections (bacteria migrate from the colon to the small intestine), and gastric resections (lose protective barrier from gastric acid). Multiple studies have confirmed that the majority of postgastrectomy patients have SIBO.[16]

Lastly, malabsorption may be due to a protein-losing enteropathy, which has been associated with multiple malignancies including gastric cancer, lymphoma, and melanoma, and is also a rare complication of chemotherapy and radiation therapy.

Nutritional Therapies

There are four major modalities for nutritional therapy in the cancer patient: oral dietary therapy, enteral nutrition (EN), PN, and pharmacologic therapy.

Studies have shown that screening cancer patients using validated screening tools, such as the patient-generated subjective global assessment (PGSGA), the subjective global assessment (SGA), and the nutrition risk assessment (NRA), will identify those who are malnourished. Studies using the validated nutrition assessments have shown that identifying and appropriately treating moderately or severely malnourished patients decreases morbidity and mortality. Although the data supporting the direct effects of screening for malnutrition in cancer patients are lacking, the data showing the clear detrimental effects of weight loss as described previously are strong. A.S.P.E.N. therefore recommends that every cancer patient undergo formal nutrition screening.[17] Further studies are needed to evaluate the efficacy of nutrition screening in improving outcomes.

Oral Dietary Therapy

Simple oral interventions in cancer patients focus on modifying the regular diet in order to maintain nutritional intake despite GI symptoms to regain weight or to minimize weight loss. Such interventions include modifying the amount of food (eg, small, frequent meals), adding additional food (eg, snacks, high caloric density foods, oral nutritional supplements), or changing the type of food (eg, liquids, mechanical soft diet). Most practitioners opt to try this strategy first because it is easy and noninvasive.

Dietary modifications are most appropriately based on the nature of GI impairment. For instance, to avoid symptoms of dumping syndrome, patients who have undergone a gastrectomy should eat small, frequent meals with calorically dense foods and avoid insoluble fiber and simple carbohydrates. Similarly, patients with partial small bowel obstruction or dysmotility should eat small, frequent meals with calorically dense food and minimal amounts of fiber. Patients with radiation enteritis should avoid fiber and lactose products. Those with short bowel syndrome should eat small, frequent meals; avoid fiber, lactose, and simple sugars; and should drink liquids separately from meals.[13]

If the issue is merely poor intake of calories due to the many reasons described previously, there are multiple oral supplements available. Many refer these patients to a dietitian for advice about meal plans and supplements. The data behind this, however, are inconclusive. Early studies found individualized nutritional counseling not to be beneficial. More recent studies, however, suggest that nutritional counseling may improve oral intake, weight loss, and quality of life.[18]

When oral intake is compromised because of difficulty with certain types of food, changing the consistency of food may help. For instance, patients with head and neck cancer often develop dysphagia. They should be referred to a speech and swallow specialist. Soft foods like puddings and pureed foods can often be safely swallowed, whereas thin liquids are associated with an increased frequency of aspiration. Once it has been determined what consistency of foods a patient can safely swallow, a dietitian can develop a meal plan to provide adequate nutrition.[13]

Enteral Nutrition

EN is used when oral supplementation fails, but the GI tract remains functional. Tubes placed through the nose or percutaneously into the stomach or jejunum can help overcome some of the most common causes of poor nutrition intake in cancer patients.

Indications

There are little data to support additional nutrition support in cancer patients undergoing chemotherapy, radiation, or surgery who are not malnourished.

The randomized, controlled studies conducted looking at EN compared to standard oral diet in cancer patients who are not malnourished undergoing major operations failed to show a difference in morbidity and mortality. One study looked at preoperative EN in patients with percutaneous biliary drains undergoing surgery that did show a small reduction in morbidity and mortality in the EN group, but they did not clearly report the cancer status of all the patients, and four patients received both EN and PN.[19] Therefore, A.S.P.E.N. guidelines recommend that nutrition support should not be routinely used in cancer patients undergoing surgery.[19]

Similarly, data from randomized trials examining the efficacy of EN given as an adjuvant therapy in patients receiving chemotherapy for a variety of cancers have failed to demonstrate a clear benefit in terms of survival or response to treatment. Therefore, the routine use of EN support in patients receiving chemotherapy or undergoing operations for cancer cannot be justified and is not recommended by A.S.P.E.N.[19]

Studies done investigating whether patients undergoing radiation for cancer should routinely receive nutritional support are sparse and have failed to show a change in morbidity or mortality.[19]

EN, however, is indicated in patients undergoing anticancer therapies who are malnourished and anticipated to be unable to ingest adequate nutrition for a prolonged period of time.[19] EN is recommended for malnourished patients given that studies have shown that EN improves certain parameters such as weight and nitrogen balance and the known deleterious effects of malnutrition. Because of this, A.S.P.E.N. recommends nutrition in moderately to severely malnourished patients beginning 7 to 14 days preoperatively after the risks of nutrition support and delaying the procedure are weighed against the benefits.[19] EN is preferred over PN because it is more physiologic, simpler, safer, and cheaper.

Enteral Access and Formula

The decision to initiate enteral feeding must also take into account the mode of enteral access (see Chapter 12). The options include tubes placed through the nose or percutaneously into the stomach or jejunum ending in the stomach or jejunum.[20]

If the duration of enteral support is estimated to be short term, transnasal tubes are the best option. If, however, a patient will require EN for a longer period of time, the placement of a percutaneous feeding tube should be considered. In general, gastrostomies are preferred because feeding through the stomach is more physiologic and allows for the use of hypertonic nutrient formulas and bolus infusions. In the case of gastric outlet obstruction, gastroparesis, proximal fistula or leak, or suspicion of aspiration of gastric contents, a jejunostomy is indicated.[22]

After the placement of the enteral device, the next decision is the type of enteral formula to choose (see Chapter 11). Over the last decade, immune-enhancing formulas have been developed, hoping to offer some benefit to cancer patients. Four major nutrients, arginine, glutamine, omega-3 fatty acids, and polyribonucleotides, have been of particular interest and have been shown to alter immune response. In 1990, Cerra et al.[23] demonstrated that an enteral formula supplemented with these nutrients could alter the outcome of in vitro tests of immune response in intensive care unit (ICU) patients.[21] This inspired multiple clinical trials, mostly in surgical patients, investigating the effects of this formula on cancer patients, and continues to be an active area of research. Earlier studies looked at perioperative cancer patients receiving EN with a mixture of immune modulators and found improved immune parameters, a decrease in infectious complications, and improved clinical outcomes. A meta-analysis of six randomized trials of standard EN versus immune-modulating EN in patients with cancer demonstrated that supplementing the patient with immune-modulating formula was associated with a decrease in infections and length of stay, but did not have an effect on survival.[22] Fewer studies have been done on single nutrient enhanced formulas. Studies with arginine and head and neck cancer patients undergoing surgery have shown fewer infections and shorter lengths of stay, suggesting a survival benefit. The consensus recommendations made by the U.S. Summit on Immune-Enhancing Enteral Therapy are that malnourished patients undergoing GI or major head and neck surgery would benefit from 5 to 7 days of immune-enriched enteral feedings preoperatively.[23] A.S.P.E.N. echoes these recommendations and suggests that immune-enhancing enteral formulas containing mixtures of arginine, nucleic acids, and essential fatty acids may be beneficial in malnourished cancer patients undergoing major operations.[19]

Home Enteral Nutrition

Because many patients receive outpatient treatment and often require treatment for prolonged periods of time, home enteral nutrition (HEN) has become a part of nutrition supplementation. Though clinical outcomes of these patients are largely dependent on the underlying cancer, many patients do benefit from HEN. Complications are low, with an overall complication rate of less than 0.4 per patient per year.[24] Quality of life has not been well studied in patients with cancer receiving HEN. The mere presence of a feeding tube is associated with a reduced quality of life, but it is thought that this is not because of the feeding tube itself, but the underlying disease and malnutrition that led to the tube. A recent study showed that a specialized nutrition support team reduces morbidity and the cost of HEN, which would help improve quality of life.[25]

Total Parenteral Nutrition

There is evidence that PN improves nutritional indices such as body weight, total body fat, and replenishes specific minerals, trace elements, and vitamins of patients undergoing chemotherapy.[26] In addition, studies have shown that PN may have a stimulatory effect on tumor cell cycle kinetics.[27,28] Some hypothesized that PN may help improve tumor response to cell cycle–specific chemotherapy. PN, however, does not alter many of the metabolic derangements encountered in the cancer patient. Despite PN, cancer patients still have increased glucose oxidation and turnover, muscle proteolysis, increased lipolysis, and overall loss of body nitrogen.[19]

Indications

The majority of studies conducted with PN in the perioperative period also did not show a decrease in morbidity and mortality, and in fact some show an increase in morbidity and mortality in the PN group. The largest prospective randomized trial investigating the role of PN perioperatively was the Veterans Administration (VA) Cooperative Study, in which 395 patients with cancer and benign disease were randomized to receive 7 to 15 days of preoperative PN and 3 days of postoperative PN, or oral feeding plus intravenous fluids.[29] They demonstrated a clear benefit to PN in severely malnourished patients, no clear benefit in moderately malnourished patients, and clear harm in mildly or nonmalnourished patients. There were a few studies that did show a benefit to PN, but they had faulty designs and heterogeneous groups, including both nourished and malnourished patients. There have also been studies comparing EN and PN in the surgical patient that showed no differences between the groups.[19]

PN given during chemotherapy as a preventive measure has also not been shown to decrease toxicity, improve tumor response, or decrease mortality. Most of these studies were small and poorly designed. Nonetheless, because no benefit was shown, and there can be harm from the nutritional therapy, it is not recommended as a routine adjunctive treatment to chemotherapy.[19]

A few randomized studies have examined the use of PN in patients receiving radiotherapy treatment. These studies did not show any clear benefit from the routine administration of PN.[19]

There are circumstances, however, in which nutritional support with PN should be considered. For instance, A.S.P.E.N recommends PN in patients who are receiving anticancer treatment who are malnourished, anticipated to be unable to ingest or absorb adequate nutrition for a prolonged period of time, and who are not candidates for EN.[19] There are other indications, such as those undergoing hematopoietic stem cell transplantation, which will be discussed in the following section.

Home Total Parenteral Nutrition

In a select group of patients, long-term PN given at home may be lifesaving. Research has proven that cancer patients who have had severe GI injury, such as massive intestinal resection or severe radiation enteritis, and in whom the cancer has been cured or is well controlled benefit from long-term PN at home.[30] Home PN offers very little benefit in patients with widely metastatic disease and a poor prognosis.[31] In terminally ill patients, PN should be avoided. The concern that such patients should not be "starved to death" is not a justification for PN. A noncontrolled study of terminally ill cancer patients hospitalized at a long-term care facility suggests that these patients did not experience hunger or thirst, and that in those who experienced such symptoms, small amounts of food alleviated the symptoms.[32]

Pharmacotherapy

A variety of nutrients and medications, including hormones, appetite stimulants, and cytokine antagonists, have been used to help improve the appetite or counter metabolic abnormalities that cause inefficient nutrient use in patients with continued anorexia or unresponsive weight loss.

Hormones

Animal studies have shown that growth hormones, both IGF-I alone or IGF-I with insulin, help curtail weight loss in cancer-bearing rodents. In clinical trials, however, these agents led to modest weight gain but no other benefits and no improvement in quality of life.[33]

Ghrelin, a potent orexigenic peptide hormone produced by the stomach, has been shown to increase appetite and caloric intake in normal individuals and in animal models of cancer cachexia. It was therefore hypothesized that ghrelin may be an effective treatment for cancer-induced cachexia. One small randomized study showed that IV ghrelin led to a marked increase in energy and caloric intake and reported no side effects.[34] There was concern that its use would be limited by its promotion of cellular proliferation and invasion of certain types of cancer, but a recent randomized, placebo-controlled, double-blind, double cross-over study demonstrated that ghrelin was safe and well tolerated, but unfortunately did not show any change in nutritional intake.[35] Clearly, more studies are needed.

Melatonin, the major product of the pineal gland, has been found to have anticancer and anticachectic effects possibly mediated by the inhibition of TNF production. There is promising data that show melatonin given 20 mg per day orally leads to less weight loss and greater survival rates.[35] Again, further studies are needed before melatonin can be recommended.

Appetite Stimulants

Corticosteroids

Glucocorticoids are widely used for appetite stimulation. The mechanism of action has not been elucidated, but is likely related to anti-inflammatory and euphoric effects that are thought to be mediated by alterations in IL-6 levels. Randomized, controlled studies demonstrate that steroids improve appetite and quality of life compared with placebo, but this effect is short lived (less than 4 weeks), and long-term use is associated with negative nitrogen balance, net calcium loss, glucose intolerance, and immunosuppression.[35]

Successful corticosteroid use for the treatment of anorexia and other supportive care symptoms in patients with a very short life expectancy has been reported.[36] Fifty home hospice patients with advanced cancer were studied after corticosteroid therapy was initiated for the treatment of symptoms such as weakness, anorexia, headache, drowsiness, nausea and vomiting, dyspnea, and confusion. Significant improvements occurred in all symptom categories except drowsiness. The most frequently used agent was dexamethasone with a mean daily dose of 7 mg and a range of 4 to 16 mg per day.

In general, the risk of adverse effects, such as muscle wasting and immunosuppression, outweigh any nutritional advantage with the long-term use of corticosteroids. However, terminal patients with poor performance status could be considered potential candidates for corticosteroid intervention because the positive pharmacologic effects on other symptoms associated with end-stage cancer may outweigh the risks associated with the negative adverse effects.

Anabolic Steroids

Although anabolic agents are not known to affect cytokine activity, they are used in an attempt to stimulate muscle anabolism. Multiple studies have reported anabolic agent use in other clinical conditions or diseases such as HIV infection or burns, but there are very few published investigations that characterize use in patients with cancer cachexia.[35] A large prospective study directly compared an anabolic corticosteroid (fluoxymesterone) to a progestational agent (megestrol acetate) and a corticosteroid (dexamethasone) for the treatment of cancer anorexia and cachexia.[37] They found that fluoxymesterone was less effective and had more side effects than megestrol acetate and dexamethasone.

Oxandrolone is an oral anabolic androgenic steroid approved by the U.S. Food and Drug Administration (FDA) for promoting weight gain in patients after extensive surgery, chronic infections, or severe trauma, as well as in patients who are unable to gain or maintain normal weight for no apparent physiologic reason, and for counteracting the protein catabolism associated with long-term use of corticosteroids. Oxandrolone has been studied more extensively in patients with HIV and burns than in cancer, and has resulted in increased body weight and body cell mass in HIV patients and improved muscle protein metabolism and decreased hospital stays in burn patients. Very few studies have reported on the use of oxandrolone in cancer patients, but its use has been promoted for several years.[35] A recent phase III study using oxandrolone 10 mg twice a day in patients with cancer cachexia demonstrated an increase in lean body mass, but was unable to show an effect on weight loss or quality of life.[38] More research is needed before oxandrolone can be recommended for weight loss in cancer patients. Oxandrolone is contraindicated in cancers that could be promoted by testosterone, such as prostate or testicular cancer. Oxandrolone interacts with warfarin and may result in large increases in the International Normalized Ratio (INR) or prothrombin time. The warfarin dose may need to be decreased significantly to avoid the risk of bleeding.[39]

Progestagens

Currently, progestagens (medroxyprogesterone acetate and megestrol acetate) are considered to be the best treatment available for cancer-associated cachexia.[40] These agents improve appetite and ameliorate weight loss in numerous studies of patients with cancer and cachexia, with maximal weight gain generally seen within 8 weeks. Improvement in quality of life has been demonstrated in several large prospective studies in patients with cancer cachexia treated with megestrol acetate, but a survival benefit has not been shown.[35] A recent Cochrane Database review[43] found a benefit of megestrol acetate with regard to appetite improvement and weight gain, but could not analyze quality of life due to differences in the studies. The mechanism behind these effects is not completely understood, but may be related to glucocorticoid activity. These agents also induce the release of NPY from the hypothalamus and downregulate the synthesis and release of proinflammatory cytokines. Although the change in weight is thought to largely be due to increased adipose tissue and edema, emerging evidence indicates that megestrol acetate has antiproteolytic properties through inhibition of the ATP-ubiquitin–dependent proteolytic pathway.[41] Megestrol acetate is generally well tolerated and has fewer side effects than dexamethasone but can exacerbate underlying diabetes mellitus and rarely leads to adrenal suppression. It may also be associated with a small increase in the risk of deep venous thrombosis, edema, and impotence in men.

Cannabinoids

Cannabinoids have been investigated in cancer patients for antiemetic and appetite-stimulant properties. Dronabinol is the synthetic oral form of tetrahydrocannabinol (THC), which is the active agent in marijuana thought to be responsible for these effects. A recent multicenter, phase III, randomized, double-blind, placebo-controlled clinical trial from the Cannabis-In-Cachexia-Study-Group found no difference in patients' appetite or quality of life between dronabinol and placebo.[42] Another randomized trial of 469 patients with advanced cancer and cachexia compared dronabinol to megestrol acetate and demonstrated megestrol acetate to be superior for appetite improvement and weight gain.[43] Furthermore, combination therapy with both agents was not superior to treatment with megestrol acetate alone. The mechanism of action of dronabinol is not completely understood, but is likely mediated by cannabinoid receptor–related processes. Adverse effects include dizziness, ataxia, and confusion. Based on the inconsistent evidence of clinical use in cancer patients, the routine use of dronabinol as an appetite stimulant is not recommended.[35]

Cyproheptadine

Cyproheptadine is a potent histamine and serotonin antagonist that competes with histamine for H1-receptor sites on effector cells in the GI tract, in blood vessels, and in the respiratory tract. It has been shown to increase the appetite among patients with anorexia nervosa and wasting due to tuberculosis. In a prospective randomized, placebo-controlled trial involving 295 patients with advanced cancer, cyproheptadine at a dose of 8 mg orally three times a day resulted in a small subjective improvement in appetite but did not prevent weight loss.[44] However, in patients with diarrhea and weight loss due to the carcinoid syndrome, cyproheptadine can result in significant weight gain.[45] This is most likely due to a direct blockade of the excess serotonin and histamine produced by the tumor. Sedation is a frequent adverse effect reported with the use of cyproheptadine, which may limit its usefulness in advanced cancer patients by potentially worsening mental status. The routine use of cyproheptadine as an appetite stimulant is not recommended.[46]

Hydrazine Sulfate

Hydrazine sulfate is a gluconeogenesis inhibitor thought to alter metabolic abnormalities in protein and glucose metabolism described in cancer patients with cachexia. A prospective, placebo-controlled trial of hydrazine sulfate in 65 patients with advanced non–small cell lung cancer showed that hydrazine sulfate at a dose of 60 mg orally three times a day was associated with significantly greater caloric intake and serum albumin maintenance.[47] Several subsequent larger studies, however, have not shown any benefit. Hydrazine sulfate therefore cannot be recommended for the treatment of cancer cachexia outside of research protocols at this time.[35]

Olanzapine

Olanzapine is a thienobenzodiazepine atypical antipsychotic that blocks multiple neurotransmitters, including dopamine at D1, D2, D3, and D4 brain receptors; serotonin at 5-HT_{2a}, 5-HT_{2c}, 5-HT_3, and 5-HT_6 receptors; catecholamines at α1 adrenergic receptors; acetylcholine at muscarinic receptors; and histamine at H1 receptor dopaminergic and serotonin activities. Increased appetite and weight gain have been reported in non–tumor-bearing patients receiving olanzapine and is thought to be caused by a blockade of serotonin 5-HT_2 and 5HT_3 receptors. Additional mechanisms have been proposed.[48] A recent randomized study found that the combination of olanzapine and megestrol acetate resulted in more weight gain, appetite improvement, and increased quality of life in patients with advanced GI or lung cancer than megestrol acetate alone.[49] However, further clinical data are needed before olanzapine can be recommended for routine use as an appetite stimulant in cancer patients.

Mirtazapine

Mirtazapine is a tetracyclic antidepressant that antagonizes presynaptic α2–adrenergic receptors resulting in increased norepinephrine and serotonin release. Mirtazapine also antagonizes serotonin 5-HT_2 and 5HT_3 receptors.[51] Mirtazapine has been investigated for its effects on pain, quality of life, nausea, anxiety, insomnia, appetite, and weight gain in patients with advanced cancer. In a recent open-label single-institution phase II trial, mirtazapine (15 to 30 mg by mouth daily) was given to nondepressed patients with cancer-related cachexia or anorexia and found improved appetite and quality of life.[50] Mirtazapine may be a promising agent for the treatment of cancer-related cachexia, but its role as an appetite stimulant needs further study before routine use can be recommended.

Cytokine Inhibitors

Because cytokines play such a pivotal role in the development of cachexia in cancer patients, cytokine inhibitors have the potential to be potent agents in the treatment of malnutrition in cancer. In murine models of cancer cachexia, monoclonal antibodies against TNF, IL-6, and IFN-γ resulted in improved oral intake and decreased protein and fat loss. Clinical trials with cytokine inhibitors are more limited. Thalidomide (α-N-phthalimidoglutaramide) has been shown to suppress TNF-α production in monocytes in vitro, to normalize elevated TNF-α levels in vivo, and to prevent weight loss in patients with AIDS and tuberculosis. In a recent randomized, placebo-controlled trial, 50 patients with pancreatic cancer and cachexia were randomized to thalidomide 200 mg daily or placebo for 24 weeks.[51] They reported that thalidomide was well tolerated and effective at attenuating loss of weight and lean body mass. More studies are needed before thalidomide can be recommended.

Pentoxifylline, an orally available methylxanthine derivative used in the treatment of peripheral vascular disease, is a phosphodiesterase inhibitor that inhibits TNF-α synthesis by decreasing gene transcription. Animal models demonstrate that pentoxifylline inhibits the production of TNF-α. However, a prospective randomized, double-blind, placebo-controlled trial involving 70 patients with advanced cancer cachexia did not show any improvement in appetite or weight gain and patients frequently reported GI side effects.[52] Larger studies are necessary to elucidate the role pentoxifylline plays in cancer cachexia.

The omega-3 fatty acids EPA and docosahexaenoic acid (DHA), provided by fish oils, have been investigated in patients with cancer-related anorexia and weight loss. Laboratory and clinical studies have shown that EPA has several potential anticachectic effects, including: (1) the attenuation of protein degradation induced by proteolysis-inducing factor, (2) the prevention of excess hepatic protein turnover, (3) the inhibition of IL-6 production, and (4) the inhibition of tumor-derived lipid-mobilizing factor. Initial uncontrolled trials of fish oil provided alone or as a part of a liquid nutritional supplement in pancreatic cancer patients with cachexia reported positive effects on weight gain and performance status. However, recent controlled trials have reported less favorable results. In a recent large, randomized, placebo-controlled study, 518 patients with advanced GI and lung cancer with weight loss were randomized to EPA at a dose of 2 or 4 g daily or placebo for 8 weeks.[53] Their results indicated no statistically significant benefit from single agent EPA in the treatment of cancer cachexia and recommended that future studies should concentrate on other agents or combination regimens. Furthermore, a recent meta-analysis based on five trials concluded that there were not sufficient data to determine if oral EPA is superior to placebo.[54] There are some data, however, that illustrate that EPA-enriched oral nutrition is beneficial for cancer cachexia.[19]

Drugs to Relieve Symptoms

Medications to relieve cancer- or treatment-related symptoms that impair oral intake are a critical aspect of nutritional support. For example, optimal antiemetic therapy can now adequately control acute and delayed emesis. Unfortunately though, the incidence of chemotherapy-induced nausea and vomiting is greatly underestimated by doctors and nurses. Therefore, a careful history and review of systems is essential in these patients.

As described previously, studies have reported up to 58% of cancer patients as having depressive symptoms and up to 38% as having major depression.[11] Some studies have shown pharmacotherapy for depression using selective serotonin reuptake inhibitors or tricyclic antidepressants to be effective in cancer patients, but a recent systematic review concluded that there are limited data in this area and more adequately powered studies are necessary before making recommendations.[55] Pain control is an important component of symptomatic management in cancer patients and can lead to improved appetite and nutrition status.

Effect of Nutrition on Tumor Growth

Animal studies have suggested a concern that nutrition support may enhance tumor growth. Glucose and essential nutrients as well as the influence of hormones and growth factors, which are stimulated in response to nutrition support, may promote tumor growth. The data in humans are conflicting. A recent review looked at five randomized clinical trials, five comparative nonrandomized clinical trials, three comparative nonrandomized trials, and four trials with patients who were controls for themselves and found that increased tumor growth was not observed in control patients without nutritional support.

Tumor growth was reported in 7 out of 12 studies in patients receiving nutritional support.[56] Though nutritional support may stimulate tumor growth, it is a reasonable intervention in cancer patients in the setting of moderate-to-severe malnutrition and intolerance of adequate oral or enteral nutrition.[19]

Nutritional Management of Patients with Specific Cancers

Nutrition Support in Patients with Cancer of the Head and Neck

This group includes patients with cancer of the lip, oral cavity, tongue, salivary glands, pharynx, larynx, nasal cavity, ear, and skull base. In the United States, it is estimated that there will be 39,400 new cases of head and neck cancer in 2011.[1] These patients are often malnourished at the time of diagnosis due to the location of the tumor and its effect on swallowing. This is compounded by the fact that many patients also have a history of alcohol and tobacco use, which predisposes them to malnutrition. Up to 57% of patients with cancer of the head and neck have significant weight loss prior to beginning treatment, and 75% to 80% of patients will experience weight loss during the treatment period.[57] In addition, the vast majority of patients will experience acute toxicity related to treatment.

Prophylactic placement of a percutaneous endoscopic gastrostomy (PEG) feeding tube, either before the initiation of radiation or at the time of surgical resection, in head and neck cancer patients has been shown in many studies to result in a lower rate of hospitalization for dehydration, a higher therapy completion rate, and weight gain or maintenance, leading to decreased unscheduled treatment interruptions. Retrospective studies have shown that patients fed via nasogastric tubes had more persistent dysphagia than those fed via PEG. Some have suggested that patients who receive all of their nutrition via PEG may forget how to swallow. A recent review concluded that there is not sufficient evidence to determine the optimal method of enteral feeding for patients with head and neck cancer undergoing treatment and that larger, randomized studies are necessary.[58]

For malnourished patients undergoing tumor resection, 7 to 10 days of preoperative EN support is associated with a reduction in morbidity and improved quality of life. Factors that have been shown to predict the need for perioperative enteral support include recent heavy alcohol use, tongue base involvement and surgery, pharyngectomy, composite resection, reconstruction with a myocutaneous flap, radiation therapy, tumor size, and moderately to poorly differentiated histology.[59] In patients with inoperable cancer, EN during palliative radiation successfully maintained nutritional status and allowed more patients to return to their regular activities than those patients receiving only oral nutrition.[60] Most patients with head and neck cancer will regain their ability to eat and can have the PEG tube removed. However, a significant minority will have prolonged dependence on enteral feeding. In these patients, complete EN can be safely provided via a PEG tube or a low-profile gastrostomy device indefinitely with few complications.

Nutrition Support in Patients with Cancer of the Esophagus

Over the past few decades, the incidence of adenocarcinoma of the esophagus has increased in the United States and other Western countries, whereas the incidence of esophageal squamous cell carcinoma has remained largely unchanged.[61] It is estimated that, in 2011, there will be approximately 17,000 new cases of esophageal cancer diagnosed in the United States.[1] Dysphagia is almost universal in patients with cancer of the esophagus and is associated with an average weight loss of 10 kg at presentation.[62] The majority of patients with esophageal cancer will present with or develop malnutrition. In a recent study of 1000 cancer patients being treated as outpatients, those with esophageal cancer had the highest percentage of weight loss of all the primary tumors investigated.[63] Patients with esophageal cancer who present with weight loss have been shown to have an overall decreased survival.

Treatment for esophageal cancer includes resection, chemotherapy, radiation therapy, and frequently, a combination of these modalities. All of these therapies may impair oral intake and compound malnutrition. Radiation therapy can cause esophagitis and strictures, whereas chemotherapy can lead to odynophagia from esophagitis and mucositis. An esophagectomy requires a bilateral vagotomy, and delayed gastric emptying is often seen even after a pyloroplasty. Options for the palliation of malignant dysphagia include dilation, placement of a self-expanding metal stent (SEMS), ablation therapy, chemotherapy/radiation, and surgery. The choice of modality depends on the location of the disease, the stage of the tumor, the functional status of the patient, and physician expertise. Dilation is usually not considered a primary modality because its relief is temporary and most patients require repeat dilation within 1 to 2 weeks. SEMS has evolved as a common intervention for malignant dysphagia because it is a relatively easy procedure, is associated with minimal morbidity and mortality, and provides rapid palliation of dysphagia. Ablation therapies, including laser treatment, argon plasma coagulation, chemical injection of ethanol, and photodynamic therapy are not widely available and are also associated with relatively high reintervention rates. There are no data to support that chemotherapy and radiation provide better palliation than SEMS or that it is associated with higher morbidity. Surgery is associated with a very high morbidity and mortality rate and is therefore not usually recommended for palliation.[64] In addition, anastomotic leaks and strictures occur, which prevent oral intake. Though these complications hinder oral intake and lead to malnutrition, the remaining GI tract is usually functional. EN via gastrostomy or jejunostomy is therefore an effective method of nutritional support in these patients (Practice Scenario 33-1).

Feeding tubes can also be placed for nutritional support in these patients. Direct percutaneous endoscopic jejunostomy (dPEJ) is ideal, but PEG tubes can be placed if needed.[65] There have been four randomized, controlled studies and one historical study comparing EN with PN in esophageal cancer patients and most showed no differences between the two groups. One study did suggest that PN was more effective than EN in promoting weight gain. Nonetheless, EN is the preferential choice given it is more physiologic, less costly, and has fewer complications.[66]

Practice Scenario 33-1

Question: What is the intervention of choice for the palliation of dysphagia associated with newly diagnosed esophageal cancer?

Scenario: A 55-year-old man with history of tobacco and alcohol use presented to his primary care physician with dysphagia for 2 months that initially began with dysphagia to solids, and then progressed to liquids. He experienced a 10-pound weight loss. He denied any odynophagia, hoarseness, shortness of breath, abdominal pain, nausea, vomiting, or changes in his bowel habits. His physician referred him to a gastroenterologist who performed an endoscopy and found a large, friable, partially obstructing mass in the distal esophagus; biopsies were positive for adenocarcinoma. He then underwent an endoscopic ultrasound for staging and was found to have a stage III:T3N1M0 lesion (stage III, metastatic disease; T3, tumor invasion into the adventitia; N1, regional lymph node involvement; M0, no distant metastases).

Intervention: The patient underwent an endoscopic placement of a SEMS, resumed a mechanical soft diet, and was able to obtain adequate nutrition and gain weight.

Answer: SEMS is the treatment of choice for the palliation of malignant dysphagia if feasible.

Rationale: Although dilation and ablative techniques are options, they only provide temporary relief and the patient would likely require frequent reinterventions. Given the high morbidity and mortality associated with surgery, a palliative esophagectomy is not recommended. SEMS is preferable over a PEG tube because, although a PEG will provide him with adequate nutrition, it would not relieve his dysphagia and may also delay treatment.[67]

Nutrition Support in Patients with Cancer of the Stomach

Although the rate of gastric cancer continues to decline worldwide, it remains one of the most common causes of cancer-related mortality.[1] Despite advances in endoscopic techniques for early gastric cancer, surgery remains the mainstay of treatment. Long-term survival after surgery has improved substantially over the last few decades because of improved developments in diagnosis, management, surgical techniques, and adjuvant chemotherapy. Following a total or subtotal gastrectomy, patients may complain of early satiety. Patients may also suffer from postgastrectomy syndromes, such as dumping syndrome, which can lead to a decreased quality of life. There are two types of dumping syndrome: early and late. Symptoms of early dumping syndrome occur within 15 to 30 minutes following ingestion of a meal and are characterized by postprandial diaphoresis, tachycardia, faintness, diarrhea, and cramping. Because these patients are lacking a gastric reservoir, there is a rapid inflow of a hypertonic diet into the small intestine, leading to excessive secretion of GI hormones and resulting in these symptoms. Late dumping syndrome, on the other hand, occurs within 2 to 3 hours after a meal and is characterized by symptoms of hypoglycemia, including dizziness and sweating. This set of symptoms and signs is related to catecholamine discharge mediated by a heightened insulin response and hypoglycemia due to the rapid entry of the meal into the upper small bowel. A recent large-scale study interviewed 1153 patients who underwent a gastrectomy for gastric cancer and found that substantially more patients suffered from early dumping syndrome than late dumping syndrome.[67] They also found that factors that decreased the rate of early dumping syndrome included reduced weight loss, old age, and type of surgical procedure (pylorus preserving gastrectomy, distal gastrectomy with Roux-en-Y reconstruction, and distal gastrectomy with Billroth I).

This syndrome may be intense enough to discourage food consumption. The first intervention in these patients is initiating an antidumping diet, which involves eating small, frequent meals with calorically dense foods while avoiding insoluble fiber and simple carbohydrates. When dietary measures fail, the next step would be pharmacologic therapy. One option is adding acarbose and an α-glycosidase hydrolase inhibitor, which interferes with the absorption of carbohydrates in the small intestine. Four small studies suggest that giving acarbose 50 to 100 mg three times a day improved glucose tolerance, decreased the release of GI hormones, and reduced hypoglycemia, leading to an improvement in dumping symptoms. These target only the symptoms of late dumping, and patients often complain of bloating and flatulence. Another option is octreotide. Multiple studies have shown somatostatin analogs to be the most effective treatment of dumping syndrome, and favor using the slow-release preparation. Treatment refractory patients may need continuous enteral feeding through a dPEJ. If all this fails, surgery is the last option.[68]

Furthermore, these patients may suffer from fat malabsorption secondary to bacterial overgrowth and impaired timing of the release of pancreatic enzymes. Clinical trials of supplements of pancreatic enzymes have had mixed results, although they may be tried in a patient with steatorrhea. The absorption of iron, calcium, and fat-soluble vitamins may also be impaired. Deficiencies of iron, calcium, and fat-soluble vitamins may also develop. Treatment is with the oral administration of iron plus ascorbic acid and by supplements containing both water-soluble and fat-soluble vitamins. Parenteral supplementation of B12 is needed because the loss of gastric acidity, intrinsic factor, and R protein inhibits cobalamin availability.[13]

Nutrition Support in Patients with Cancer of the Pancreas

In 2011, the estimated incidence of pancreatic cancer in the United States was 40,000 and the estimated death rate was about 38,000.[1] Prognosis remains very poor and, therefore, mortality rates almost mimic incidence rates. Most patients present with symptoms at the time of diagnosis, and the most common clinical presentations are progressive weight loss and anorexia, mid-abdominal pain, and jaundice. In a prospective study of patients with unresectable pancreatic cancer, all patients had experienced weight loss by the time of presentation with a median loss of 14% of preillness weight.[69] Moreover, pancreatic duct obstruction may result in pancreatic insufficiency, and common bile duct or ampulla of Vater obstruction may result in bile insufficiency, leading to maldigestion, malabsorption, and the exacerbation of weight loss.[70]

The only chance for cure is surgery, and about 20% of patients are thought to be resectable. Because the majority of resectable tumors are in the head of the pancreas, the surgery of choice is a pancreaticoduodenectomy (PD) in which in the standard operative procedure the distal half of the stomach is removed, the pancreas is transected (usually at the neck but by varying amounts and, rarely, the entire gland may be removed), the entire duodenum, and a few centimeters of the jejunum distal to the ligament of Treitz are resected. McLeod et al.[74] analyzed the nutritional status of 25 patients who were alive and free of disease more than 6 months after a PD. Though most patients remained well-nourished, 5 developed steatorrhea and 10 developed diabetes mellitus. Nonetheless, the authors concluded that full nutritional recovery is possible after a PD. There is conflicting evidence regarding whether modification of the standard PD, in which the stomach and pylorus are spared, offers any long-term nutritional benefit. The role of nutrition perioperatively is also controversial. A systematic review of perioperative nutritional supplementation in patients undergoing PD showed that most patients are nutritionally depleted at the time of surgery and that EN was superior to PN for nutrition support.[71]

The majority of patients, however, are found to be unresectable at the time of diagnosis or recur shortly after surgery. These patients can suffer from partial or complete gastric outlet obstruction from direct tumor effect, intestinal dysmotility from intra-abdominal metastasis, and pancreatic exocrine insufficiency. The oral diet should consist of small, calorically dense meals and sufficient pancreatic enzyme supplementation. Unfortunately, these often fail to help restore nutritional status. SEMS has been shown to be a safe and effective therapy for the palliation of gastric outlet obstruction in these patients and has multiple advantages to surgery including increased clinical success, shorter time from procedure to starting oral intake, reduced morbidity, lower incidence of delayed gastric emptying, shorter hospital stay, and lower cost.[72] A recent study demonstrated that peritoneal disease was not a contraindication to enteral stenting in these patients unless there are signs of multifocal obstruction.[73] Those patients deemed candidates for treatment may benefit from dPEJ placement and continuous infusion of EN.

Nutrition Support in Patients with Cancer of the Colon and Rectum

Despite the use of colonoscopies, colon cancer is the third most common cause of cancer and the third most common cause of cancer-related mortality in the United States.[1] Patients with colon cancer usually present with little or no weight loss.

Surgical therapy involves the removal of the segment of colon containing the tumor. More extensive resections (usually a total proctocolectomy) are performed in patients with underlying ulcerative colitis or hereditary colon cancer syndromes.

Resection of the right colon with the ileocecal valve and a portion of the terminal ileum may be associated with watery diarrhea due to multiple reasons, including the loss of the breaking effect of the ileocecal valve, entry of increased amounts of bile salts into the colon with stimulation of water excretion into the colonic lumen (choleretic diarrhea), and impaired water and sodium absorption due to some loss of surface area in the colon. Cholestyramine binds bile salts and often markedly attenuates the diarrhea. Resections of the left colon or rectum rarely have a significant impact on nutritional status. Patients with colon cancer typically maintain a good nutritional status and do not require specialized nutrition support.

Nutrition Support in Patients with Gynecologic Cancers

Gynecologic malignancies, most commonly ovarian cancer, and their multimodal therapies may be associated with severe malnutrition.

Patients with ovarian cancer commonly develop an intestinal obstruction during the course of their illness. Surgery can be considered but is associated with significant perioperative mortality and reobstruction rates. A recent meta-analysis found only low quality evidence comparing surgery and medical management.[74] They did not feel there was sufficient evidence to yield a conclusion, but did state that the evidence supporting prolonged survival after surgery was weak. The alternative for these women is placement of a gastrostomy tube (ie, PEG) for drainage and the palliation of symptoms. Drainage PEG tubes can be successfully placed in 89% of patients with a low (4%) complication rate.[75] Though these will successfully elevate symptoms, the issue of malnutrition will not be solved.

The use of PN in these patients remains controversial. A study from Memorial Sloan-Kettering Cancer Center (MSKCC) examined 21 patients with malignant bowel obstruction from ovarian cancer who had drainage PEGs and were receiving chemotherapy. Eleven patients also received PN support. Those patients who were given PN had significantly longer survival.[76] Though the use of home PN in patients has not been shown to improve survival or quality of life, in a small subgroup of patients with a good performance status, PN has been shown to improve nutritional status and quality of life.[77] The decision to administer PN in these patients must be an individualized one in order to carefully select who may benefit from PN.

Nutrition Support in Patients Undergoing Hematopoietic Stem Cell Transplantation

Hematopoietic stem cell transplantation (HSCT) is an increasingly used treatment for a variety of disorders, including hematologic malignancies. The process includes the IV infusion of hematopoietic stem cells from a suitable donor into the patient who has received a defined conditioning regimen before the infusion of cells. An autologous transplant is the infusion of the patient's own stem cells, which were harvested before conditioning therapy. The infusion of stem cells from a histocompatible donor is an allogeneic transplant. The least common type of HSCT is a syngeneic transplant where stem cells are harvested from an identical monozygous twin. Conventional HSCT recipients undergo a toxic pretransplant conditioning regimen, which includes high doses of chemotherapy that may or may not include total body irradiation (TBI). The side effects of this regimen can include GI toxicities (eg, nausea, vomiting, anorexia, dysgeusia, mucositis, diarrhea, xerostomia, viscous saliva), infections, organ dysfunction (eg, veno-occlusive disease, acute renal failure, respiratory failure, cardiac toxicity), and acute graft-versus-host disease (GVHD). Because of these potential and prevalent complications in the early posttransplant period, all patients undergoing HSCT are at nutritional risk. Recently, nonmyeloablative HSCT (NMHSCT), often referred to as a mini-transplant, has been employed to reduce the toxicity associated with the transplant regimen and to use the immunologic effect of GVHD in an attempt to enhance tumor cell kill by a graft-versus-tumor interaction. This type of transplant is commonly used in older patients, in those who have failed a conventional HSCT, or who have preexisting organ dysfunction. Although the early posttransplant side effects are not as extreme, patients undergoing NMHSCT are still at nutritional risk because of the prevalence of GVHD[19] (Practice Scenario 33-2).

A complete nutritional assessment (see Chapter 9) should be performed on all HSCT patients before transplant. Unfortunately, the ideal nutritional assessment measurements for HSCT patients have not been defined; however, weight loss has been associated with a higher risk of nonrelapse mortality in adult HSCT patients. A.S.P.E.N. guidelines indicate that nutrition support is appropriate in patients undergoing hematopoietic cell transplantation who are malnourished and who are anticipated to be unable to ingest and/or absorb adequate nutrients for a prolonged period of time, defined as 7 to 14 days.[19] The studies comparing EN and PN in this cohort show that PN is associated with increased morbidity, increased diarrhea, increased hyperglycemia, and delayed time to engraftment, but less weight loss and less loss of body fat. Therefore, if PN is chosen, it should be discontinued after engraftment or when the patient is able to consume adequate calories through EN or an oral diet. EN should be chosen in patients with a functional GI tract.[19]

Energy needs will vary with the individual and the type of transplantation, but usually, energy requirements are estimated at 1.5 × basal energy expenditure (BEE), or approximately 30 to 35 kcal per kilogram. Protein intake should be aimed at 1.5 g per kilogram during the first 1 to 3 months after transplantation. Fluid needs must be tailored to the individual with careful documentation of the blood products, PN, oral intake, IV medications, and fluids. Intake should be balanced against output.[78] Because volume overload is not uncommon in the HSCT patient, it should be monitored, and the restriction of fluid and possibly sodium may be required.

Because glutamine is known to help heal and maintain tissues, especially in the GI tract, oral glutamine has been investigated for the treatment of chemotherapy and radiation-induced mucositis. Although there is some evidence that oral glutamine may help reduce the duration of mucositis, data are conflicting, and a recent Cochrane review concluded that there is no benefit for oral glutamine supplementation in the prevention of mucositis.[79] In addition, multiple studies have investigated whether glutamine-enriched EN and PN are beneficial in patients undergoing HSCT. Glutamine-enriched EN has not been shown to reduce morbidity and mortality in HSCT patients. PN-enriched glutamine has been shown to improve nitrogen balance, decrease the length of stay, and decrease morbidity. Therefore, A.S.P.E.N. concludes that parenteral glutamine may benefit patients undergoing HSCT, but there is no role for oral glutamine. At the present time, though, parenteral glutamine is not commercially available in the United States.[19]

Low microbial diets varying in their degree of sterility are used for HSCT patients. Most HSCT centers restrict foods with high bacterial content to minimize the introduction of pathogenic organisms into the GI tract, but the degree of modification is highly variable. Many centers have adopted a more liberal low microbial diet that allows well-washed fruits and vegetable and only excludes extremely high-risk foods, such as unpasteurized dairy products, raw or undercooked meats, herbal products, aged cheeses, and unwashed, damaged, or moldy fruits and vegetables. Educating patients and families about safe food handling practices and high-risk foods to avoid is recommended. Autologous graft patients usually follow these diets for 3 months posttransplant; allogeneic patients may require a year or more if they remain on immunosuppressive therapy.[19] A general multivitamin and mineral supplement without iron is appropriate.

Besides the well-known GI complications associated with HSCT, a number of other complications in the posttransplant period can negatively affect nutritional status, including infections, organ failure, veno-occlusive disease, and GVHD. GVHD occurs when the immunocompetent donor T cells recognize the HSCT recipient (or host) as foreign and mount an immune reaction. GVHD sets in motion a cascade of events designed to eradicate the foreign bodies or tissues of the recipient, resulting in tissue destruction. The impact of nutrition support on the incidence of GVHD is unclear. There are also no data on the benefit of nutrition support in GVHD, but based on the degree of malnutrition, it is appropriate to institute nutrition support in patients who develop moderate-to-severe GVHD with poor oral intake and/or significant malabsorption. Given most of these patients have severe GI symptoms, many recommend patients remain nothing by mouth to avoid further damage to the GI mucosa. However, this could lead to gut atrophy and further GI dysfunction. One study showed that EN was safe in patients with GI GVHD.[80] Moreover, the incidence of GI GVHD seems to decrease with increased oral protein intake. Nonetheless, there are insufficient data to make recommendations for oral nutrition or prophylactic PEG placement in patients with GI GVHD. PN is usually the modality of choice. Again, because of infectious complications, this should be discontinued as soon as patients are able to take in effective calories orally or by EN.[19]

Practice Scenario 33-2

Question: When is nutrition support indicated in patients with GVHD?

Scenario: A 50-year-old man presented with a 1 month history of fever, weight loss, bone pain, and easy bruising. His primary care physician checked routine blood work, and he was found to have pancytopenia, with a low white blood cell count, low hemoglobin, and low platelets. A bone marrow biopsy was performed, which confirmed the diagnosis of acute myelogenous leukemia (AML). He was initiated on induction chemotherapy, but unfortunately did not respond. His brother was found to be a Human Leukocyte Antigen (HLA) match, so he subsequently underwent an allogeneic HSCT 2 months later. His posttransplant course was complicated by severe mucositis, necessitating PN support. His mucositis slowly improved, and he was tolerating an oral diet by day +14 and PN was discontinued. He engrafted on day +21. On day +45, he developed nausea, vomiting, and profuse diarrhea with an inability to tolerate oral intake. His weight was 58 kg. An abdominal X-ray was negative for obstruction, and stool studies were negative for infection. He subsequently underwent a colonoscopy and upper endoscopy that confirmed severe GVHD of the GI tract.

Intervention: He was initiated on treatment of GVHD and PN with a total of 2000 kcal (35 kcal per kilogram) with 90 g (1.5 g per kilogram) of protein. After 3 weeks, he was able to tolerate oral intake and PN was discontinued.

Answer: Nutrition support is indicated in patients with moderate-to-severe GVHD with poor oral intake and/or malabsorption.

Rationale: Data supporting the use of nutrition support in patients with GVHD are sparse. There are no data investigating whether nutrition support actually leads to the resolution of GVHD. However, given that GVHD results in profound and prolonged nutritional compromise, it is appropriate to offer nutritional support in these patients.[19]

Nutrition Support during Palliative Care

EN and PN use in patients with advanced incurable cancer is controversial and raises multiple ethical issues. Before the initiation of nutrition support in an advanced cancer patient, the clinician must consider the patient's and/or family's wishes, potential risks and benefits, and estimated survival (see Chapter 39).

The primary objective for initiating nutrition support in advanced cancer patients is to conserve or restore the best possible quality of life and to control any nutrition-related symptoms that cause discomfort or distress. Most patients with advanced cancer do not benefit from nutrition intervention as defined by improved nutrition status, increased survival, or improved quality of life. The adverse effects caused by nutrition support may actually worsen the patient's quality of life and the overall palliative care of the patient. However, certain patient groups with advanced cancer and good performance status have demonstrated favorable response to EN or PN such as those with inoperable, malignant bowel obstruction, those with minimal symptoms from disease involving major organs such as brain, liver, or lungs, and those with relatively indolent disease progression.[19]

In general, nutrition support is not usually indicated in patients with a prognosis of survival less than 3 months, although accurately predicting survival is frequently difficult. Good performance status, such as a Karnofsky Performance Scale Index greater than 50, is also associated with better outcomes for palliative nutrition support.[19] Other issues that should be considered before determining suitability for home nutrition such as home environment, caregivers, and financial support are similar to those for patients without cancer (see Chapter 38).

In general, cachexia, anorexia, or dehydration at the end of life is not uncomfortable. These patients should be instructed to eat and drink as desired, and restrictive diets should be discontinued. Sips of water, ice chips, and glycerin swabs can be used to palliate symptoms of thirst, dry mouth, and mucositis. All unnecessary medications should be discontinued, especially those that may exacerbate these symptoms (ie, anticholinergic medications).[13] The clinician should guide the patient and family in making decisions regarding goals of therapy, a timeline for reevaluating goals, and criteria for withdrawal of nutrition support.

References

1. Cancer facts and figures. American Cancer Society Web site. www.cancer.org. Accessed July 12, 2011.
2. John R, Ross H. *The Global Economic Cost of Cancer*. Atlanta, GA: American Cancer Society; 2010.
3. Jensen GL, Mirtallo J, Compher C, et al. Adult starvation and disease-related malnutrition: A proposal for etiology-based diagnosis in the clinical practice setting from the International Consensus Guideline Committee. *JPEN J Parenter Enteral Nutr*. 2010;34:156–159.
4. Argilés JM. Cancer-associated malnutrition. *Eur J Oncol Nurs*. 2005;9(Suppl 2):S39–50.
5. De Luis DA, Izaola O, Cuellar L, et al. Nutritional assessment: predictive variables at hospital admission related with length of stay. *Ann Nutr Metab*. 2006;50:394–398.
6. Falconer JS, Fearon KC, Plester CE, et al. Cytokines, the acute-phase response, and resting energy expenditure in cachectic patients with pancreatic cancer. *Ann Surg*. 1994;219(4):325–331.
7. Tisdale MJ. Mechanisms of cancer cachexia. *Physiol Rev*. 2009 Apr;89(2):381–410.
8. Davis MP, Dreicer R, Walsh D, et al. Appetite and cancer-associated anorexia: a review. *J Clin Oncol*. 2004;22:1510–1517.
9. Massie MJ. Prevalence of depression in patients with cancer. *J Natl Cancer Inst Monogr*. 2004;32:57–71.
10. Schneider S, Moyer A. Depression as a predictor of disease progression and mortality in cancer patients: a meta-analysis. *Cancer*. 2010;116(13):3304.
11. Schattner M, Shike M. Nutrition support of the patients with cancer. In: Shils ME, Shike M, eds. *Modern Nutrition in Health and Disease*. Philadelphia, PA: Lippincott Williams & Wilkins; 2006: 1290–1313.
12. Creamer B. Malignancy and the small-intestinal mucosa. *Br Med J*. 1964;5422:1435–1436.
13. Scolapio JS, Ukleja A, Burnes JU, Kelly DG. Outcome of patients with radiation enteritis treated with home parenteral nutrition. *Am J Gastroenterol*. 2002;97(3):662–666.
14. Dookeran KA, Thompson MM, Allum WH. Pancreatic insufficiency secondary to abdominal radiotherapy. *Eur J Surg Oncol*. 1993;19(1):95–96.
15. Falconi M, Pederzoli P. The relevance of gastrointestinal fistulae in clinical practice: a review. *Gut*. 2001;49(Suppl 4):iv2–10.
16. Paik CN, Choi MG, Lim CH, et al. The role of small intestinal bacterial overgrowth in postgastrectomy patients. *Neurogastroenterol Motil*. 2011;23(5):e191–196.
17. August DA, Huhmann MB. A.S.P.E.N. clinical guidelines: nutrition support therapy during adult anticancer treatment and in hematopoietic cell transplantation. *JPEN J Parenter Enteral Nutr*. 2009;33(5):472–500.
18. Ravasco P, Monteiro-Grillo I, Vidal PM, et al. Dietary counseling improves patient outcomes: a prospective, randomized, controlled trial in colorectal cancer patients undergoing radiotherapy. *J Clin Oncol*. 2005;23:1431–1438.
19. Foschi D, Cavagna G, Callioni F, Morandi E, Rovati V. Hyperalimentation of jaundiced patients on percutaneous transhepatic biliary drainage. *Br J Surg*. 1986;73(9):716–719.
20. Schattner M. Enteral nutritional support of the patient with cancer: route and role. *J Clin Gastroenterol*. 2003;36(4):297–302.
21. Cerra FB, Lehman S, Konstantinides N, et al. Effect of enteral nutrients on in vitro tests of immune function in ICU patients: a preliminary report. *Nutrition*. 1990;6:84–87.
22. Heys SD, Walker LG, Smith I, et al. Enteral nutritional supplementation with key nutrients in patients with critical illness and cancer. *Ann Surg*. 1999;229:467–477.
23. Moore FA. Effects of immune-enhancing diets on infectious morbidity and multiple organ failure. *JPEN J Parenter Enteral Nutr*. 2001;25(2 suppl):S36–S42.
24. Schattner M, Barrera R, Nygard S, et al. Outcome of home enteral nutrition in patients with malignant dysphagia. *Nutr Clin Pract*. 2001;16:292–295.
25. Klek S, Szybinski P, Sierzega M, et al. Commercial enteral formulas and nutrition support teams improve the outcome of home enteral tube feeding. *JPEN J Parenter Enteral Nutr*. 2011;35(3): 380–385.
26. Shike M, Russel DM, Detsky A, et al. Changes in body composition in patients with small cell lung cancer. The effect of total parenteral nutrition as an adjunct to chemotherapy. *Ann Intern Med*. 1984;101:303–309.
27. Baron PL, Lawrence W, Chan WM, et al. Effects of parenteral nutrition on cell cycle kinetics of head and neck cancer. *Arch Surg*. 1986;121:1282–1286.
28. Bozzetti F, Gavazzi C, Cozzaglio L, et al. Total parenteral nutrition and tumor growth in malnourished patients with gastric cancer. *Tumori*. 1999;85(3):163–166.
29. Veterans Affairs Total Parenteral Nutrition Cooperative Study Group. Perioperative total parenteral nutrition in surgical patients. *N Engl J Med*. 1991;325:525–532.
30. Howard L, Ament M, Fleming R, et al. Current use and clinical outcome of home parenteral and enteral nutrition therapies in the United States. *Gastroenterology*. 1995;109:355–365.
31. Koretz RL. Should patients with cancer be offered nutritional support: does the benefit outweigh the burden? *Eur J Gastroenterol Hepatol*. 2007;19(5):379–382.
32. McCann RM, Hall WJ, Groth-Junker A. Comfort care for terminally ill patients. *JAMA*. 1994;272:1263–1266.
33. Coss CC, Bohl CE, Dalton JT. Cancer cachexia therapy: a key weapon in the fight against cancer. *Curr Opin Clin Nutr Metab Care*. 2011;14(3):268–273.
34. Neary NM, Small CJ, Wren AM, et al. Ghrelin increases energy intake in cancer patients with impaired appetite: acute, randomized, placebo-controlled trial. *J Clin Endocrinol Metab*. 2004; 89(6):2832–2836.
35. Strasser F, Lutz TA, Maeder MT, et al. Safety, tolerability and pharmacokinetics of intravenous ghrelin for cancer-related anorexia/cachexia: a randomised, placebo-controlled, double-blind, double-crossover study. *Br J Cancer*. 2008;98(2):300–308.
36. Mercadante S, Fulfaro F, Casuccio A. The use of corticosteroids in home palliative care. *Support Care Cancer*. 2001;9:386–389.
37. Loprinzi CL, Kugler JW, Sloan JA, et al. Randomized comparison of megestrol acetate versus dexamethasone versus fluoxymesterone for the treatment of cancer anorexia/cachexia. *J Clin Oncol*. 1999;17(10):3299–3306.

38. Lesser GJ, Case D, Ottery. A phase III randomized study comparing the effects of oxandrolone (Ox) and megestrol acetate (Meg) on lean body mass (LBM), weight (wt) and quality of life (QOL) in patients with solid tumors and weight loss receiving chemotherapy. *J Clin Oncol.* 2008;26(May 20 Suppl).
39. U.S. Food and Drug Administration. Safety: Oxandrin (oxandrolone, USP). http://www.fda.gov/Safety/MedWatch/SafetyInformation/SafetyAlertsforHumanMedicalProducts/ucm155484.htm. Accessed July 10, 2011.
40. Mantovani G, Madeddu C. Cancer cachexia: medical management. *Support Care Cancer.* 2009 Aug 18. [Epub ahead of print]
41. Busquets S, Serpe R, Sirisi S, et al. Megestrol acetate: its impact on muscle protein metabolism supports its use in cancer cachexia. *Clin Nutr.* 2010 Dec;29(6):733–737.
42. Cannabis-In-Cachexia-Study-Group, Strasser F, Luftner D, et al. Comparison of orally administered cannabis extract and delta-9-tetrahydrocannabinol in treating patients with cancer-related anorexia-cachexia syndrome: a multicenter, phase III, randomized, double-blind, placebo-controlled clinical trial from the Cannabis-In-Cachexia-Study-Group. *J Clin Oncol.* 2006;24(21): 3394–3400.
43. Jatoi A, Windschitl HE, Loprinzi CL, et al. Dronabinol versus megestrol acetate versus combination therapy for cancer-associated anorexia: a North Central Cancer Treatment Group study. *J Clin Oncol.* 2002;20(2):567–573.
44. Kardinal CG, Loprinzi CL, Schaid DJ, et al. A controlled trial of cyproheptadine in cancer patients with anorexia and/or cachexia. *Cancer.* 1990;65(12):2657–2662.
45. Moertel CG, Kvols LK, Rubin J. A study of cyproheptadine in the treatment of metastatic carcinoid tumor and the malignant carcinoid syndrome. *Cancer.* 1991;67(1):33–36.
46. Mattox TW. Treatment of unintentional weight loss in patients with cancer. *Nutr Clin Pract.* 2005;20:400–410.
47. Chlebowski RT, Bulcavage L, Grosvenor M, et al. Hydrazine sulfate influence on nutritional status and survival in non-small-cell lung cancer. *J Clin Oncol.* 1990;8(1):9–15.
48. Davis MP, Khawam E, Pozuelo L, Lagman R. Management of symptoms associated with advanced cancer: olanzapine and mirtazapine. *Expert Rev Anticancer Ther.* 2002;2:365–376.
49. Navari RM, Brenner MC. Treatment of cancer-related anorexia with olanzapine and megestrol acetate: a randomized trial. *Support Care Cancer.* 2010;18(8):951–956.
50. Riechelmann RP, Burman D, Tannock IF, et al. Phase II trial of mirtazapine for cancer-related cachexia and anorexia. *Am J Hosp Palliat Care.* 2010;27(2):106–110.
51. Gordon JN, Trebble TM, Ellis RD, et al. Thalidomide in the treatment of cancer cachexia: a randomised placebo controlled trial. *Gut.* 2005;54(4):447–448.
52. Goldberg RM, Loprinzi CL, Mailliard JA, et al. Pentoxifylline for treatment of cancer anorexia and cachexia? A randomized, double-blind, placebo-controlled trial. *J Clin Oncol.* 1995;13(11): 2856–2859.
53. Fearon KC, Barber MD, Moses AG. Double-blind, placebo-controlled, randomized study of eicosapentaenoic acid diets in patients with cancer cachexia. *J Clin Oncol.* 2006;24(21): 3401–3407.
54. Dewey A, Baughan C, Dean T, Higgins B, Johnson I. Eicosapentaenoic acid (EPA, an omega-3 fatty acid from fish oils) for the treatment of cancer cachexia. *Cochrane Database Syst Rev.* 2007; 24(1):CD004597.
55. Rodin G, Lloyd N, Katz M, et al. The treatment of depression in cancer patients: a systematic review. *Support Care Cancer.* 2007; 15(2):123–136.
56. Bozzetti F, Mori V. Nutritional support and tumour growth in humans: a narrative review of the literature. *Clin Nutr.* 2009;28(3): 226–230.
57. Munshi A, Pandey MB, Durga T, al. Weight loss during radiotherapy for head and neck malignancies: what factors impact it? *Nutr Cancer.* 2003;47(2):136–140.
58. Locher JL, Bonner JA, Carroll WR, et al. Prophylactic percutaneous endoscopic gastrostomy tube placement in treatment of head and neck cancer: a comprehensive review and call for evidence-based medicine. *JPEN J Parenter Enteral Nutr.* 2011;35(3): 365–374
59. Schweinfurth JM, Boger GN, Feustel PJ. Preoperative risk assessment for gastrostomy tube placement in head and neck cancer patients. *Head Neck.* 2001;23(5):376–382.
60. Daly JM, Hearne B, Dunaj J, et al. Nutritional rehabilitation in patients with advanced head and neck cancer receiving radiation therapy. *Am J Surg.* 1984;148(4):514–520.
61. Tougeron D, Richer JP, Silvain CJ. Management of esophageal adenocarcinoma. *Visc Surg.* 2011 Jun 27. [Epub ahead of print]
62. Goodwin WJ, Byers PM. Nutritional management of the head and neck cancer patient. *Med Clin North Am.* 1993;77:597–610.
63. Bozzetti F. Screening the nutritional status in oncology: A preliminary report on 1,000 outpatients. *Support Care Cancer.* 2009;17: 279–284.
64. Javle M, Ailawadhi S, Yang GY, et al. Palliation of malignant dysphagia in esophageal cancer: a literature-based review. *J Support Oncol.* 2006;4(8):365–373.
65. Stockeld D, Fagerberg J, Granstrom L, et al. Percutaneous endoscopic gastrostomy for nutrition in patients with oesophageal cancer. *Eur J Surg.* 2001;167(11):839–844.
66. Bozzetti F. Nutritional support in patients with oesophageal cancer. *Support Care Cancer.* 2010;18(Suppl 2):S41–S50.
67. Mine S, Sano T, Tsutsumi K, et al. Large-scale investigation into dumping syndrome after gastrectomy for gastric cancer. *J Am Coll Surg.* 2010 Nov;211(5):628–636.
68. Tack J, Arts J, Caenepeel P, et al. Pathophysiology, diagnosis and management of postoperative dumping syndrome. *Nat Rev Gastroenterol Hepatol.* 2009;6(10):583–590.
69. Wigmore S, Plester C, Richardson R, Fearon K. Changes in nutritional status associated with unresectable pancreatic cancer. *Br J Cancer.* 1997;75(1):106–109.
70. Gupta R, Ihmaidat H. Nutritional effects of oesophageal, gastric and pancreatic carcinoma. *Eur J Surg Oncol.* 2003;29(8):634–643.
71. Goonetilleke KS, Siriwardena AK. Systematic review of peri-operative nutritional supplementation in patients undergoing pancreaticoduodenectomy. *JOP.* 2006;7(1):5–13.
72. Shaw JM, Bornman PC, Krige JE, et al. Self-expanding metal stents as an alternative to surgical bypass for malignant gastric outlet obstruction. *Br J Surg.* 2010;97(6):872–876.
73. Mendelsohn RB, Gerdes H, Markowitz AJ, et al. Carcinomatosis is not a contraindication to enteral stenting in selected patients with malignant gastric outlet obstruction. *Gastrointest Endosc.* 2011; 73(6):1135–1140.
74. Kucukmetin A, Naik R, Galaal K, et al. Palliative surgery versus medical management for bowel obstruction in ovarian cancer. *Cochrane Database Syst Rev.* 2010;(7):CD007792.
75. Herman LL, Hoskins WJ, Shike M. Percutaneous endoscopic gastrostomy for decompression of the stomach and small bowel. *Gastrointest Endosc.* 1992;38(3):314–318.
76. Abu-Rustum NR, Barakat RR, Venkatraman E, Spriggs D. Chemotherapy and total parenteral nutrition for advanced ovarian cancer with bowel obstruction. *Gynecol Oncol.* 1997;64: 493–495.

77. Cozzaglio L, Balsola F, Costentino F, et al. Outcome of cancer patients receiving home parenteral nutrition. Italian Society of Parenteral and Enteral Nutrition. *JPEN J Parenter Enteral Nutr.* 1997;21(6):339–342.
78. Lipkin AC, Lenssen P, Dickson BJ. Nutrition issues in hematopoietic stem cell transplantation: state of the art. *Nutr Clin Prac.* 2005;20:423–439.
79. Worthington HV, Clarkson JE, Bryan G, et al. Interventions for preventing oral mucositis for patients with cancer receiving treatment. *Cochrane Database Syst Rev.* 2011;13(4).
80. Imataki O, Nakatani S, Hasegawa T, et al. Nutritional support for patients suffering from intestinal graft-versus-host disease after allogeneic hematopoietic stem cell transplantation. *Am J Hematol.* 2006;81(10):747–752.

34 Nutritional and Medical Management of Diabetes Mellitus in Hospitalized Patients

Laura Newton, MA, RD, and W. Timothy Garvey, MD

CONTENTS

Introduction 581
Diagnosis, Classification, and Pathophysiology 582
Diagnosis 582
Classification and Pathophysiology 582
Type 1 Diabetes Mellitus 582
Type 2 Diabetes Mellitus 583
Gestational Diabetes Mellitus 583
Prediabetic Conditions 583
Stress-Induced Hyperglycemia 584
Hyperglycemia and Diabetes Complications 585
Measurement of Glycemia 585
Fasting Glucose 585
Postprandial Glucose 585
Hemoglobin A1c 585
Glycemic Variability 585
Glycemic Control and Diabetes Complications 585
Glycemic Targets in Hospitalized Patients 586
Hyperglycemia and Outcomes in Hospitalized Patients 586
Glycemic Target Recommendations 586
Hypoglycemia 587
Medications for Control of Diabetes in Hospitalized Patients 587
Oral Agents and Insulin 587
Intravenous Insulin Therapy 588
Subcutaneous Insulin Injections 590
Subcutaneous Insulin Preparations 590
Sliding-Scale Insulin Therapy 590
Basal-Bolus Insulin Therapy 591
Estimation of the Total Daily Insulin Dose 591
The 1500 Rule and 1800 Rule 592
Nutrition Assessment 592
Calorie Needs 593
Protein Needs 593
Electrolytes 593
Oral Diet 593
Gastroparesis 594
Enteral Feeding 594
Enteral Nutrition 594
Delivery of Enteral Nutrition 595

Insulin Therapy during Enteral Feeding. 596
Continuous Enteral Feeding 596
Intermittent Enteral Feeding 596
Diabetes-Specific Formulas and Insulin Therapy. 597
Parental Feeding 598
Parenteral Nutrition 598
Monitoring. 598
Insulin Therapy during Parenteral Nutrition. 598
Nutrition and Diabetes Treatment during Transitions from Intensive Care Unit to Floor and Floor to Home 599
Acknowledgments 600
References 600

Objectives

1. Describe the diagnosis, classification, and pathophysiology of diabetes mellitus.
2. Discuss the complications of uncontrolled hyperglycemia, particularly in hospitalized patients.
3. Describe the recommended glycemic targets for hospitalized patients.
4. Discuss the medications used for control of diabetes in hospitalized patients.
5. Review the management of diabetic patients receiving enteral nutrition (EN) or parenteral nutrition (PN).

Test Your Knowledge Questions

1. A hospitalized patient with a history of type 2 diabetes is on a sliding-scale insulin regimen and no other sources of insulin or antihyperglycemic agents. Glucose monitoring occurs four times per day (before each meal and at bedtime). Yesterday, the four measurements were 195 mg/dl (breakfast), 155 mg/dl (lunch), 79 mg/dl (supper), and 143 mg/dl (bedtime). Regular insulin is given in response to the elevated glucose levels according to the hospital's sliding-scale regimen, and it was held at dinner for glucose < 90 mg/dl. The proper course of action is to:
   A. Continue current sliding-scale insulin regimen
   B. Institute basal-bolus insulin therapy
   C. Add an oral antihyperglycemic agent
   D. Initiate an insulin drip
2. What is the recommendation for optimal glucose range for the majority of critically ill patients receiving intravenous (IV) insulin therapy?
   A. 80 to 110 mg/dl
   B. 110 to 140 mg/dl
   C. 140 to 180 mg/dl
   D. 180 to 220 mg/dl
3. If a patient with severe diabetic gastroparesis requires enteral feeding, which of the following methods should be used to initiate enteral feeding?
   A. Continuous enteral feeding through a gastric tube
   B. Intermittent or bolus feeding through a gastric tube
   C. Continuous feeding through a jejunal tube
   D. Intermittent or bolus feeding through a jejunal tube

Test Your Knowledge Answers

1 The correct answer is **B**. Utilizing basal-bolus insulin therapy will control fasting glucose with basal insulin and doses of rapid-acting or regular insulin for mealtimes or correction.[1] This is a more proactive approach than simply reacting to glucose levels. The sliding-scale insulin approach alone can predispose the patient to wide fluctuations in glucose levels. Prolonged therapy with sliding-scale insulin as the sole insulin regimen is not recommended and may potentially lead to complications including hypoglycemia. Insulin drips are typically only administered in the intensive care unit (ICU) setting due to the frequent monitoring and time involved. Oral antihyperglycemics are not appropriate for most hospitalized patients due to the inconsistency of nutrition consumption at regular intervals.

2. The correct answer is **C**. Once IV insulin therapy has been started, the current recommendation by American Association of Clinical Endocrinologists (AACE) and the American Diabetes Association (ADA) is that the glucose level should be maintained between 140 and 180 mg/dl.[1] Increased benefits may be appreciated at the lower end of this range and lower glucose targets may be appropriate for some patients; however, targets < 110 mg/dl are not recommended due to the risk of hypoglycemia. Institutions should have in place an insulin infusion protocol that emphasizes safety and efficacy.

3. The correct answer is **C**. Dietary modifications, adequate glucose control, and medications should first be employed to control and treat diabetic gastroparesis. If these measures are unsuccessful and a patient is unable to take sufficient nutrition orally, a jejunal feeding tube can deliver nutrition and medications, if necessary, beyond the site of gastric stasis. Continuous feeding over intermittent or bolus feeding is preferred until tolerance is established with jejunal feeding due to the potential for diarrhea or "dumping syndrome" to occur from rapid infusion of a large volume directly into the small intestine (see Chapter 13).

Introduction

Diabetes mellitus is a group of disorders characterized by abnormal glucose metabolism. It affects 25.8 million people or 8.3% of the U.S. population.[2] Diabetes is the leading cause of kidney failure, new cases of blindness, and nontraumatic lower-limb amputations in the United States. In 2010, 1.9 million people over the age of 20 were newly diagnosed with diabetes.[2] Medical costs for those with diabetes are 2.3 times higher than expenditures for those without diabetes. Factoring in the costs of undiagnosed diabetes, prediabetes, and gestational diabetes, the total cost of diabetes in the United States in 2007 was $218 billion.[2]

Adequate glycemic control is a major focus for health care providers. Optimal control in the outpatient setting is associated with a decrease in the micro- and macrovascular complications of diabetes, and, in critically ill, hospitalized patients, studies demonstrate that careful glucose control can reduce mortality, shorten the length of stay, decrease days on mechanical ventilation, and result in fewer infectious complications. During critical illness, hyperglycemia and insulin resistance is exacerbated in patients with diabetes and is also commonly observed in patients without a preexisting history of diabetes (ie, "stress hyperglycemia").

Due to the adverse impact of diabetes and hyperglycemia on clinical outcomes, this chapter will review the classification and diagnosis of diabetes, the underlying pathophysiology, approaches for glycemic control, and nutrition support recommendations, with an emphasis on the challenges associated with the care of hospitalized patients.

Diagnosis, Classification, and Pathophysiology

Diagnosis

The diagnosis of Diabetes Mellitus is based on measurements of blood glucose at levels of hyperglycemia that have been shown to place patients at risk for vascular complications. These thresholds have traditionally involved glucose determinations under fasting conditions, during oral glucose tolerance tests (OGTT), or random measurements. However, recently a criterion for the diagnostic use of hemoglobin A1c (HbA1c) has been added, primarily to identify patients who have diabetes on the basis of elevated 2-hour OGTT glucose levels who may have gone undiagnosed due to the failure of health professionals to perform OGTTs on a more widespread basis.[3] The diagnostic criteria for diabetes are shown in Table 34-1. Symptoms of uncontrolled diabetes include excessive thirst, polyuria and nocturia, fatigue, blurred vision, and unintended weight loss.

Classification and Pathophysiology

A classification scheme for the group of metabolic diseases known as diabetes mellitus has been established by the ADA.[4] This classification broadly discriminates between diseases caused by primary dysfunction of insulin-producing pancreatic β-cells and diseases characterized by a combination of insulin resistance and an impairment in insulin secretion that renders insulin secretory capacity unable to fully compensate for the prevailing degree of insulin resistance. It should be noted that individuals may not always clearly fit in one type or class of diabetes. Furthermore, individuals with no history of diabetes may develop acute hyperglycemia or diabetes under conditions of severe stress as in critically ill patients hospitalized due to infection, sepsis, trauma, or cardiovascular event, or as a result of certain medications that can impair insulin action or secretion. The major types of diabetes encountered clinically are described in the following.

Type 1 Diabetes Mellitus

Formerly known as insulin-dependent diabetes mellitus or juvenile-onset diabetes, type 1 diabetes mellitus (T1DM) is due to deficient insulin secretion resulting from autoimmune destruction of pancreatic β-cells. While often presenting in children and adolescents, it can occur at any age. The rate of β-cell destruction is variable, with some patients presenting with acute hyperglycemia and ketoacidosis, while others may preserve some insulin secretion for years before becoming dependent on exogenous insulin therapy. Patients with T1DM are also vulnerable to other autoimmune disorders such as celiac sprue, autoimmune thyroid disease, Addison disease, and others. An example of delayed onset disease is Latent Autoimmune Diabetes of Adults (LADA). LADA generally presents in adults > 40 years of age as a result of slowly progressive autoimmune destruction of β cells and a slow decline in insulin secretion, with evidence of prediabetes for multiple years prior to the diagnosis of overt diabetes.

Once severe or absolute insulin deficiency is established, these patients require insulin to sustain life and to prevent the development of diabetic ketoacidosis. Upon hospitalization, patients with T1DM must be administered insulin throughout each 24-hour period without cessation (eg, using basal long-acting insulin injections or continuous IV insulin therapy). In diabetic ketoacidosis, the lack of insulin leads to severe

TABLE 34-1 Diagnostic Criteria for Categories of Glucose Tolerance

	Fasting Glucose	Two-hour Glucose during OGTT	HbA1c	Random Glucose
Diabetes	≥ 126 mg/dl (7.0 mmol/L)	≥ 200 mg/dl (11.1 mmol/L)	≥ 6.5%	≥ 200 mg/dl (11.1 mmol/L) with symptoms
Prediabetes	Impaired fasting glucose: 100–125 mg/dl (5.6–6.9 mmol/L)	Impaired glucose tolerance: 140–199 mg/dl (7.8–11.0 mmol/L)	5.7–6.4%	
Normoglycemic	< 100 mg/dl (5.6 mmol/L)	< 140 mg/dl (7.8 mmol/L)	< 5.7%	

HbA1c, hemoglobin A1c; OGTT, oral glucose tolerance test.

hyperglycemia, polyuria and dehydration, and release of fatty acids that are metabolized to ketoacids. Treatment involves aggressive volume repletion beginning with normal saline, continuous IV insulin therapy, and potassium repletion, together with a search for comorbid precipitating events or disease processes.

Type 2 Diabetes Mellitus

Formerly known as non–insulin-dependent diabetes or adult-onset diabetes, type 2 diabetes mellitus (T2DM) is due to the combination of insulin resistance and impaired insulin secretion that is unable to compensate for the prevailing degree of insulin resistance. A total of 90% to 95% of all patients with diabetes have T2DM. Insulin resistance occurs early in life, and it may be exacerbated by the development of obesity, particularly abdominal obesity. This places metabolic stress on β-cells, which hypersecrete insulin to maintain glucose homeostasis. T2DM results when insulin secretory capacity begins to fail, creating a state of relative insulin deficiency that can no longer compensate for insulin resistance. Risk factors for developing T2DM include increasing age, obesity, lack of physical activity, and a positive family history indicative of a substantial genetic basis for the disease.

Three major metabolic defects generate and sustain hyperglycemia in T2DM. The first is impaired β-cell insulin secretion due largely to a functional defect in glucose:section coupling and also due to a moderate decrease in β-cell mass. Fasting insulin levels are usually elevated, although not to the degree that would be commensurate with the hyperglycemia (a state of relative insulin deficiency), and peak insulin responses to glucose or meals is decreased in magnitude and delayed in time. Second, rates of hepatic glucose production are elevated and correlate well with fasting glucose levels. Hepatic glucose output rates are elevated as a result of increased gluconeogenesis due in part to hepatic insulin resistance, increased flux of metabolic substrates to the liver, and high levels of glucoregulatory hormones such as glucagon. Finally, skeletal muscle, which mediates the bulk of insulin-mediated glucose uptake, is insulin resistant due to intrinsic defects in insulin action. These three major defects, present in varying degrees in essentially all patients with T2DM, act in concert to produce hyperglycemia. Medical therapy for diabetes acts to reverse one or more of these metabolic abnormalities in order to achieve glycemic control.

In T2DM, hyperglycemic hyperosmolar syndrome can result when glucose levels rise above 600 mg/dl accompanied by severe dehydration, without the development of pronounced ketoacidosis. The usual setting is an elderly patient, without access to free water or with an impaired thirst mechanism, who stops taking diabetes medications or develops an intercurrent illness (eg, urinary tract infection, pneumonia, stroke, psychotropic medications). The hyperosmolar state produces varying degrees of obtundation or even coma. The mortality in patients with hyperglycemic hyperosmolar syndrome is as high as 15% primarily due to the precipitating illness and the fact that most patients are elderly.[5] Treatment involves rehydration and gradual reduction in hyperglycemia using continuous IV insulin therapy, as well as treatment of intercurrent illness.

Gestational Diabetes Mellitus

The term Gestational Diabetes Mellitus (GDM) has been used for women with the onset or identification of abnormal glucose tolerance during pregnancy. In 2010, the International Association of Diabetes and Pregnancy Study Groups, an international consensus group with representatives from multiple obstetrical and diabetes organizations, including the ADA, recommended a change to this terminology.[6] In this system, diabetes diagnosed during pregnancy is classified as either overt diabetes or GDM. Patients with overt diabetes have more pronounced degrees of hyperglycemia and are considered to likely have had preexisting diabetes prior to pregnancy that had not been diagnosed. Patients with overt diabetes of pregnancy meet the standard criteria for diabetes during pregnancy (Table 34-1) and should be treated in a manner similar to pregnant patients with preexisting diabetes. Patients with GDM have more modest glucose elevations; even so, the degree of glucose intolerance is serious in that it is associated with increased rates of macrosomia, preeclampsia, cesarean section, and poor maternal-fetal outcomes. Because ambient glucose concentrations are normally reduced during pregnancy, the glycemic criteria for GDM are lower than that for diabetes outside of pregnancy. GDM is usually detected at 24 to 28 weeks of gestation when a random screening OGTT is conducted; if the screening test is abnormal, this is followed by a full fasting 2-hour or 3-hour OGTT for diagnosis. The diagnostic criteria for screening and diagnosis of GDM are delineated in Table 34-2.

Prediabetic Conditions

There are two prediabetic conditions that identify individuals at high future risk for the development of T2DM, as well as cardiovascular disease events. These conditions also place individuals at higher risk of glucocorticoid-induced hyperglycemia and stress hyperglycemia upon hospitalization. The first is termed prediabetes, which encompasses those with increased glucose levels that are higher than the normal range but do not yet meet criteria for diabetes. Prediabetes can be diagnosed on the basis of impaired fasting glucose, impaired glucose tolerance defined by the 2-hour post-OGTT glucose value, or by an elevation in HbA1c, as shown in Table 34-1. The second prediabetic condition is metabolic syndrome, which is defined by a cluster of risk factors mechanistically related to insulin resistance, including abdominal obesity, dyslipidemia, glucose intolerance, elevated blood pressures, and systemic inflammation. The underlying pathophysiological processes in the metabolic syndrome confer risk for both diabetes and cardiovascular disease, which has given rise to the term cardiometabolic disease. The most common diagnostic criteria for the metabolic syndrome are those advocated by the Adult Treatment Panel III of the National Cholesterol Program; other criteria have been established by the International Diabetes Federation and the World Health Organization, as shown in Table 34-3. The treatment for these prediabetic conditions is lifestyle intervention consisting of diet and exercise with a goal to achieve and sustain 5% to 10% weight loss. One of the traits used to identify metabolic syndrome is impaired fasting glucose; thus, patients can meet criteria for both metabolic syndrome and prediabetes. Patients found to exhibit

TABLE 34-2 Diagnostic Criteria for Gestational Diabetes Mellitus

GDM *IADPSG Criteria*	GDM *ACOG Criteria*		Overt Diabetes in Pregnancy
Diagnosis	**Screening**	**Diagnosis**	**Diagnosis**
24–28 weeks Fasting OGTT (75 g; 2 hours)	24–28 weeks Random OGTT (50 g; 1 hour)	24–28 weeks Fasting OGTT (100 g; 3 hours) Two or more abnormal values	Anytime during pregnancy
One or more abnormal values	1-hour value		
Fasting glucose ≥ 92 mg/dl (5.1 mmol/L) 1-hour glucose≥ 180 mg/dl (10.0 mmol/L) 2-hour glucose≥ 153 mg/dl (8.5 mmol/L)	1-hour glucose 130–140 mg/dl (7.2–7.8 mmol/L)	Fasting glucose≥ 95 mg/dl (5.1 mmol/L) 1-hour glucose ≥ 180 mg/dl (10.0 mmol/L) 2-hour glucose ≥ 155 mg/dl (8.5 mmol/L) 3-hour glucose ≥ 140 mg/dl (7.8 mmol/L)	Fasting glucose ≥ 126 mg/d (7.0 mmol/L) 2-hour post OGTT ≥ 200 mg/dl (11.1 mmol/L) Random glucose ≥ 200 mg/dl (11.1 mmol/L)

ACOG, American Congress of Obstetricians and Gynecologists; GDM, gestational diabetes mellitus; IADPSG, International Association of Diabetes and Pregnancy Study Groups; OGTT, oral glucose tolerance test.

metabolic syndrome traits together with prediabetes on the basis of impaired fasting glucose and/or impaired glucose tolerance should be targeted for aggressive lifestyle interventions and perhaps diabetic oral agents (eg, metformin), according to consensus statements by the ADA[7] and the AACE.[8]

Stress-Induced Hyperglycemia

Hyperglycemia associated with critical illness is often called stress hyperglycemia or stress diabetes. It can occur in patients without a history or diagnosis of diabetes, and it can accompany a variety of disease conditions such as myocardial infarction, shock, sepsis, trauma, burns, and cerebrovascular accidents. Prior to 2001, stress-induced hyperglycemia was considered to represent glucose in the range of 180 to 200 mg/dL. However, in the latest consensus statement on inpatient glycemic control, the AACE and ADA define hyperglycemia as any blood glucose level in excess of 110 mg/dl.[9,10] Multiple factors can contribute to the development of stress hyperglycemia. Severe physiological stress is accompanied by

TABLE 34-3 Diagnostic Criteria for Metabolic Syndrome

	Adult Treatment Panel III Criteria	International Diabetes Foundation Criteria	World Health Organization Criteria
Risk Factor/Trait	**Any three out of the five risk factors**	**Abnormal waist + two risk factors**	**IFG or IGT + two risk factors**
Waist circumference	≥ 40 in (102 cm) in males ≥ 35 in (85 cm) in females	Region specific (eg, ≥ 90 cm in males and ≥ 80 cm in females among south Asians)	Body mass index > 30 Waist/hip > 0.90 men and > 0.85 women
Fasting triglycerides	≥ 150 mg/dl (> 1.7 mmol/L)	≥ 150 mg/dl (> 1.7 mmol/L)	≥ 150 mg/dl (> 1.7 mmol/L)
HDL cholesterol	< 40 mg/dl in males (< 1.04 mmol/L); < 50 mg/dl in females (< 1.29 mmol/L)	< 40 mg/dl in males (< 1.04 mmol/L); < 50 mg/dl in females (< 1.29 mmol/L)	< 35 mg/dl in males (<0.9 mmol/L); < 39 mg/dl in females (< 1.0 mmol/L)
Blood pressure	Systolic ≥ 130 and/or diastolic ≥ 85 mm Hg and/or use of medication for hypertension	Systolic ≥ 130 and/or diastolic ≥ 85 mm Hg and/or use of medication for hypertension	Systolic ≥ 140 and/or diastolic ≥ 90 mm Hg and/or use of medication for hypertension
Fasting glucose	≥ 100 mg/dl (5.6 mmol/L) and/or use of medication for hyperglycemia	≥ 100 mg/dl (5.6 mmol/L) and/or use of medication for hyperglycemia	IFG: Fasting ≥ 100 mg/dl (5.6 mmol/L) and/or IGT: 2-hour 140–199 mg/dl (7.8–11.0 mmol/L)
Microalbuminuria			≥ 20 μg/min ≥ 30 mg/g creatinine

HDL, high-density lipoprotein; IFG, impaired fasting glucose; IGT, impaired glucose tolerance.

increased production of counterregulatory hormones such as glucocorticoids and catecholamines, which raise blood glucose levels by promoting hepatic gluconeogenesis and glycogenolysis. Stress also triggers a systemic inflammatory response with increased production of proinflammatory cytokines such as interleukin-1, interleukin-6, and tumor necrosis factor, which also act to augment gluconeogenesis and worsen insulin resistance. Exogenous sources of glucose such as nutritional support and dextrose-containing solutions can compound the problem as well as medications such as corticosteroids, beta blockers, and thiazide diuretics. Insulin resistance, in particular, is a prominent contributor to stress hyperglycemia, and hyperinsulinemia has been found to correlate with illness severity and mortality.[11,12]

The presence of stress hyperglycemia is associated with increased length of hospital stay and high rates of morbidity and mortality, which, in some studies, can exceed rates observed in patients with an antecedent known diagnosis of T2DM.[13] Thus, new hyperglycemia in patients admitted to general hospital wards and to the ICU is a strong marker for poor clinical outcomes and increased mortality. For this reason, all hospitalized patients should be screened for hyperglycemia, and, when detected, stress hyperglycemia should be aggressively managed as is the case in patients with antecedent diabetes.

Hyperglycemia and Diabetes Complications

Measurement of Glycemia

The measures used to assess and manage hyperglycemia in diabetic patients include the following:

Fasting Glucose

High fasting glucose levels contribute a major portion to HbA1c elevations in patients with poor glycemic control. The extent of fasting hyperglycemia is highly correlated with elevated rates of hepatic glucose production, and it is an important parameter used to titrate doses of basal insulin.

Postprandial Glucose

Another measurement used is postprandial glucose, which is assessed 2 hours after a meal or an OGTT. Postprandial glucose elevations have a greater influence on HbA1c levels when diabetes is better controlled (when HbA1c values are closer to target), and the 2-hour post-OGTT glucose is a strong risk factor for cardiovascular disease. The glucose value at 2 hours, as well as the glucose level immediately preceding the next meal, are used to titrate doses of rapid-acting or short-acting insulin (ie, the nutritional component of insulin therapy) subsequently given prior to that meal.

Hemoglobin A1c

The HbA1c level is a chronic measure of glycemia that integrates ambient glucose levels over a 1- to 2-month period. It is highly correlated with the development of microvascular disease complications, and it is the most useful indicator of overall treatment efficacy. The ADA recommends a therapeutic target of < 7%, and a value of ≥ 8% is a call to action requiring a meaningful change in therapy.[3] It is helpful to obtain HbA1c when hyperglycemic patients are admitted to the hospital. If the HbA1c is normal on admission in a hyperglycemic patient who is not on any diabetes medications, this is consistent with stress hyperglycemia. In addition, the extent of the HbA1c is helpful is selecting optimal diabetes treatment regimens upon discharge from the hospital.

Glycemic Variability

A factor gaining increasing attention in glycemic management, particularly in critically ill patients, is that of glucose variability. Glucose variability refers to the magnitude in fluctuations in glucose levels over time. This measure has been given impetus with the increasing use of continuous glucose monitoring devices, some of which are programmed to provide a measure of the "mean amplitude of glycemic variations." However, such a measure can be computed using frequent home glucose measurements or frequent glucose measurements in the ICU or on the hospital floor. Glycemic variability has been linked with increased risk of hypoglycemia as well as oxidative stress and damage to vascular endothelium. In one retrospective ICU study, mortality increased from 5.9% to 30.1% from the lowest to highest levels of glucose variability in critically ill adult patients.[14] Even among patients in a euglycemic range of 70 to 99 mg/dl, mortality increased fivefold in those with higher glucose variability. These findings have been confirmed in other studies, even when a strict glucose control protocol was implemented.[15,16] Therefore, achieving low glucose variability appears to be an important independent contributor to a positive patient outcome.

Glycemic Control and Diabetes Complications

Hyperglycemia promotes the vascular complications of diabetes. This includes microvascular disease responsible for retinopathy, nephropathy, and neuropathy, as well as the macrovascular complications of coronary artery, cerebrovascular, and peripheral vascular diseases. As the HbA1c rises above 6.5% to 7%, there is a progressive increase in the risk of retinopathy and nephropathy, and high fasting and 2-hour post-OGTT glucose are risk factors for cardiovascular disease events. Conversely, randomized clinical trials clearly show that intensive glycemic control effectively prevents microvascular disease complications. Prevention of macrovascular disease is controversial. However, intensive therapy has been noted to produce lower rates of cardiovascular disease events in both T1DM (Diabetes Control and Complications Trial/-Epidemiology of Diabetes Interventions and Complications trial) and T2DM (United Kingdom Prospective Diabetes Study) when initiated in earlier stages of diabetes with follow-up over longer duration of time, in contrast with more short-term studies in patients with advanced disease that fail to demonstrate benefits of intensive therapy (Action to Control Cardiovascular Risk in Diabetes, Action in Diabetes to Prevent Vascular Disease, Veterans Affairs Diabetes Trial). Based on a large body of supportive evidence, the ADA has recommended control of glycemia below 7% HbA1C to prevent diabetes vascular complications when this can be safely achieved.[3]

The mechanisms that produce vascular disease from hyperglycemia are operative in the vessel wall. Hyperglycemia leads to uncontrolled influx of glucose into non–insulin-dependent cells, including endothelial cells, which results in endothelial dysfunction and defects in vascular autoregulation. In the retina, endothelial dysfunction results in decreased retinal blood flow, increased vascular permeability of retinal capillaries, the production of growth factors (eg, vascular endothelial growth factor), and proliferation of vessels with eventual vitreous hemorrhage. Systemically, there are defects in nitric oxide–mediated vasodilatation and an increase in vascular reactivity. Hyperglycemia augments cellular oxidative stress and reactive oxygen species generation, which activate Nuclear Factor-KappaB and proinflammatory gene expression. This results in the production of cytokines (interleukin-1, interleukin-6, tumor necrosis factor-α), which can mediate tissue injury and worsen insulin resistance. In large vessels, cytokines promote the margination and entry of macrophages into the vascular wall, which then phagocytose oxidized low-density lipoprotein, followed by conversion into foam cells and fatty streaks, the initiating lesions for atherosclerosis.

Additional adverse effects of hyperglycemia that are relevant to hospitalized patients pertain to the immune response, wound healing, and volume and electrolyte status. Hyperglycemia at levels > 180 mg/dl impairs the immunological response by inducing abnormalities in granulocyte adhesion, chemotaxis, phagocytosis, and the intracellular killing of bacteria. These functions can be improved, along with the clinical risk of infection, when glycemia is controlled below 180 mg/dl.[17,18] In granulocytes, the respiratory burst and superoxide anion production responsible for bacteriocidal activity is impaired during hyperglycemia, but it can be normalized following glycemic control. Hyperglycemia also impairs wound healing via a multifactorial process that includes induced defects in fibroblast function, angiogenesis, and collagen production, poor capillary perfusion, nonenzymatic glycation of tissue proteins, and increased protein catabolism. Finally, hyperglycemia results in glycosuria and an osmotic diuresis, resulting in the loss of water and electrolytes such as potassium, sodium, and magnesium. Electrolyte abnormalities can be accentuated during rehydration, and the correction of hyperglycemia with fluid shifts between the intracellular and extracellular compartments accompanies net influx of potassium into cells.

Glycemic Targets in Hospitalized Patients

Hyperglycemia and Outcomes in Hospitalized Patients

There is a large literature proving that hyperglycemia, regardless of its cause, is associated with increased morbidity and mortality in hospitalized patients. Hyperglycemia results in deleterious outcomes in both critically-ill and non-critically-ill patients, and increases resources utilization resulting in higher hospital costs and length of stay.[18-20] The presence of hyperglycemia in patients being administered PN dramatically increases the mortality rate,[21] and one reason is the 5-fold higher risk of catheter infections due to hyperglycemia, particularly those involving *Candida albicans*.[22,23] Hyperglycemia has been reported to increase risk of infection, sepsis and shock, poor wound healing, congestive heart failure, stroke, myocardial infarction, renal failure, transplant rejection, time on ventilators, and length of ICU stay after patients are admitted to the hospital, and to portend poor outcomes for patients admitted to the hospital for multiple disease processes including trauma, myocardial infarction, organ transplantation, pneumonia, chronic obstructive pulmonary disease, and various surgical procedures.[12,16,24-26] Importantly, as discussed below, good glycemic control can reverse or prevent these complications of hyperglycemia in hospitalized patients.

Glycemic Target Recommendations

Strong evidence that intensive glucose control could improve patient outcomes in hospitalized patients was provided by the landmark Leuven trials, which demonstrated that glucose targets of 80 to 110 mg/dl were associated with reduced morbidity and mortality in surgical ICU patients[19] and in medical ICU patients[20] who remained in intensive care for > 3 days, when compared with a standard care glucose target of 180 to 200 mg/dl. Other randomized control trials from 2001 to 2005 and related meta-analyses[21] similarly supported intensive glucose control in critically ill patients, and, in mid-decade, expert advisory bodies such as the AACE[22] and the ADA recommended glycemic goals of 80 to 110 mg/dl in the ICU, and pre-meal glucose of 90 to 110 mg/dl and postprandial glucose of < 180 mg/dl in stable hospitalized patients. However, in the latter part of the decade (2005 to 2010), randomized control trials and related meta-analyses[23] failed to document the benefits of these tight targets, including the large Normoglycaemia in Intensive Care Evaluation and Survival Using Glucose Algorithm Regulation study.[24] These latter trials demonstrated either no improvement in mortality or an increase in mortality correlated with higher rates of hypoglycemia in the intensive treatment arm versus less intensive therapy aiming for glucose targets of approximately 140 to 180 mg/dl. As a result, AACE and ADA in a joint statement[25] have revised recommendations for glycemic targets as shown in Table 34-4. To summarize these recommendations, in the critically ill, IV insulin therapy should be initiated for glucose > 180 mg/dl. Once insulin therapy is initiated, the blood glucose should be kept in a range from 140 to 180 mg/dl in the majority of critically ill patients. More stringent goals (110 to 140 mg/dl) may be appropriate for some patients as long as this can be accomplished without significant hypoglycemia. IV insulin infusion should be administered through a protocol that defines variable-rate adjustments in the insulin infusion based on glucose fluctuations. In noncritically ill patients, pre-meal blood glucose target should be < 140 mg/dl and random blood glucose (including postprandial) should be < 180 mg/dl. In non-ICU patients with diabetes or hyperglycemia, scheduled subcutaneous insulin is preferred for achieving and maintaining glucose control. The components of the subcutaneous insulin regimen should include (1) basal, (2) nutritional, and (3) correctional or supplemental components (ie, the basal-bolus approach). The AACE/ADA Consensus Statement discouraged the use of prolonged therapy with sliding-scale insulin as the sole regimen. Antihypoglycemic

TABLE 34-4 AACE/ADA Consensus Statement on Glycemic Targets and Treatment for Inpatient Glycemic Control[10]

	Critically Ill	Noncritically Ill
Glycemic targets	• Maintain glucose 140–180 mg/dl • Glucose < 140 mg/dl may be appropriate in some patients • Glucose < 110 mg/dl is not recommended	• Premeal glucose < 140 mg/dl • Random glucose < 180 mg/dl • Reassess therapy for premeal glucose < 100 mg/dl • Change therapy for premeal glucose < 70 mg/dl
Recommended Treatment	• Initiate IV insulin infusion for any glucose ≥ 180 mg/dl	• Scheduled subcutaneous insulin therapy with components: ✓ Basal ✓ Nutritional ✓ Correctional • Preference for rapid-acting insulins • Prolonged use of sliding scale as sole therapy is discouraged

AACE, American Association of Clinical Endocrinologists; ADA, American Diabetes Association; IV, intravenous.

oral agents were considered not appropriate in most hospitalized patients who require therapy for hyperglycemia.

The recommendation of less stringent glycemic targets should in no way be interpreted to mean that careful and judicious glycemic control is not indicated. The adherence to the glycemic targets in Table 34-4 should be carefully enforced. The explanations for inconsistent trial results assessing optimal glycemic targets from 2001 to 2005 compared with 2005 to present are not clear, although differences in glucose measurements, patient selection, glycemic variability, quality of hospital algorithms and policies, use of nutrient support, and the capability of the health care team to intensively use insulin without high risk of hypoglycemia have all been suggested. In making the statement that glucose targets of 110 to 140 mg/dl may be appropriate in some critically ill patients, AACE/ADA are giving deference to a substantial literature showing that hyperglycemia is linked to higher morbidity rates and hospital costs, and that lowering glucose acts to improve these outcomes. On the other hand, hypoglycemia also adversely affects outcomes and can be associated with increased mortality. Thus, we believe the current recommendations (Table 34-4) should be followed based on current knowledge, and that the health care team should consider lower glycemic goals (110 to 140 mg/dl) when this can be safely achieved.

Hypoglycemia

Hypoglycemia is a serious complication in hospitalized patients being treated for hyperglycemia. A large retrospective cohort study demonstrated that hypoglycemia in T2DM patients was associated witha 7% increase in mortality, higher inpatient charges, longer hospital stay, and a 58% likelihood of discharge to a skilled nursing facility than in matched T2DM patients who did not experience hypoglycemia.[26] Another study reported that the prevalence of hypoglycemia defined as glucose ≤ 50 mg/dl was linearly related to inpatient mortality, postdischarge mortality, and hospital length of stay.[27] Clinical situations that place patients at risk of hypoglycemia include changes in nutritional status such as an order for nothing by mouth (NPO), discontinuation of enteral or PN, change in clinical status such as the development of sepsis, prolonged use of sliding-scale insulin regimens, failure of clinical team to make adjustments in insulin based on glucose measurements, poor timing of meals with insulin injections and glucose testing, transfer to different patient care teams, inpatient use of oral agents, and errors in the writing and filling of medication orders. Certain patient characteristics confer higher risk of hypoglycemia such as advanced age, malnutrition, renal impairment, liver failure, and previous history of severe hypoglycemic episodes, gastroparesis, or autonomic neuropathy.

To prevent hypoglycemia, protocols for the identification and treatment of hypoglycemia need to be developed by all hospitals, and designed for execution by nursing staff. These protocols should prompt a review of the treatment regimen and potential changes in therapy for glucose < 70 mg/dl. Glucose < 60 mg/dl should prompt measured intervention according to the hospital's approved hypoglycemia response algorithm, and glucose < 40 mg/dl should also trigger an immediate call to the physician. In conscious patients capable of oral intake, glucose tablets (total 15 to 20 g) is the preferred treatment (repeat in 15 minutes if point-of-care glucose measurement shows continuing hypoglycemia), together with a small mixed meal or snack. Other sources of providing approximately 15 g of carbohydrate can substitute for the glucose tablets (4 oz. of apple juice). If the patient is NPO, establish IV access and administer approximately 15 g of carbohydrate IV, which equates to 30 mL of a 50% dextrose solution. If the full 50 mL ampoule of the 50% dextrose is pushed, the patient will often experience overshoot hyperglycemia. If IV access is not promptly available, glucagon 1 mg can be injected intramuscularly. If the patient is not responsive, administer 25 g dextrose (50 mL of a 50% dextrose solution) by IV push and follow glucose levels carefully.

Medications for Control of Diabetes in Hospitalized Patients

Oral Agents and Insulin

In the outpatient setting, patients with diabetes are ideally placed on a lifestyle intervention program consisting of dietary recommendations and regular exercise as medically tolerated, with a goal to achieve and sustain 5% to 10% weight loss in patients who are overweight or obese. Patients with T1DM are treated with basal (long-acting) insulin and bolus (rapid-acting) insulin at mealtimes with the dose determined in part by carbohydrate counting. T2DM is a progressive disease initially requiring a single oral agent and then combination therapy with multiple drugs and/or insulin to maintain glycemic control targets over the duration of the disease. Diabetes medications can be categorized based on their ability to ameliorate one of the three main defects that cause hyperglycemia, namely, impaired insulin secretion, elevated hepatic glucose output, and peripheral insulin resistance. Drugs that enhance insulin secretion can do so in an obligatory fashion regardless of ambient glucose or enhance secretory responses only when glucose levels rise above normal. Obligatory insulin secretagogues entail higher risk of hypoglycemia and include sulfonylureas (glyburide, glimepiride, and glipizide) and meglitinides (repaglinide and nateglinide). Drugs that enhance insulin secretion under conditions of rising glucose include incretin axis drugs, glucagon-like peptide-1 (GLP-1) analogues (exenatide and liraglutide), and dipeptidyl peptidase-4 inhibitors that inhibit degradation of endogenously produced GLP-1 (sitagliptin, saxagliptin, and linagliptin). Drugs that act primarily to restrain hepatic glucose production include long-acting insulin and metformin, the most widely used oral agent worldwide. Finally, the thiazolidinedione class of oral agents lowers glucose by enhancing insulin sensitivity (pioglitazone and rosiglitazone). There is one additional category of glucose-lowering medications that cause the gut to more slowly absorb carbohydrates either by inhibiting enzymatic digestion by alpha-glucosidases (acarbose and miglitol) or by slowing gastric emptying (pramlintide).

In hospitalized patients, insulin is the preferred drug for controlling hyperglycemia. This particularly applies to acutely ill patients and in the ICU setting. Insulin is the only drug with the combined features of (1) rapid onset of action, (2) flexible titration capacity to adjust to changing needs for greater or lesser glucose-lowering effect, (3) ability to rapidly alter dosing schedule to adjust to variable nutrient intake, (4) wide dosing schedule with essentially no maximal dose, (5) multiple options for route of administration (subcutaneous, IV, intramuscular), and (6) lack of drug-drug interactions. Oral agents, on the other hand, have slower onset, are less flexible regarding dose alterations that adjust to clinical needs, confer untoward effects, and can interfere with administration of other drugs and radiographic procedures employing iodinated dyes (eg, metformin). In general, patients should be withdrawn from oral agents and treated with insulin upon admission to the hospital. The categories of insulin preparations available for use in hospitalized patients are described in Table 34-5.

Intravenous Insulin Therapy

Continuous infusion of IV insulin is the optimal approach for controlling hyperglycemia in critically ill patients. In particular, the literature supports the use of IV insulin therapy to improve outcomes for treating diabetic ketoacidosis and hyperglycemic hyperosmolar syndrome; controlling hyperglycemia during pre-, intra-, and postoperative care; organ transplantation; high-dose glucocorticoid therapy; cardiogenic shock; NPO status (eg, pancreatitis); during PN; and critical care illness.[28] In these settings, IV insulin provides a rapid therapeutic effect and flexibility to adjust to rapidly changing needs for glycemic control. Human regular U-100 insulin is most commonly used for IV insulin therapy; rapid-acting insulins (aspart, glulisine) are also approved for IV infusion but offer no advantages over regular insulin when administered by the IV route. Generally, IV insulin therapy is reserved for ICUs or in special medical wards staffed by experienced and trained personnel using tested protocols; otherwise, IV insulin infusions may place patients at undue risk of hypoglycemia in the absence of adequate nursing and physician resources. Thus, IV insulin therapy is best conducted in venues where hospitals have implemented related protocols and policies, whether for critical, perioperative, or noncritical care, with attention to training and staffing, coordination, safety, and quality assurance as overseen by a multidisciplinary oversight committee.

To initiate IV insulin, a dose of insulin should be given IV push (5 to 10 units) for glucose values over 150 mg/dl to prime a rapid escalation in insulin levels. When the glucose is < 150 mg/dl, the insulin infusion can be initiated without the IV push. Because IV insulin has a half-life of < 6 minutes, the effects of the IV push will be short lived, and it should be followed up immediately with continuous infusion at 0.5 to 2 units/hour. Insulin-resistant patients may require the higher infusion rate of 2 units/hour or higher, and suggested initial infusion rates are shown in Table 34-6. The important point is to monitor the patient's glucose level carefully and adjust the insulin infusion rate accordingly. Insulin is generally placed in saline or half-normal saline (although other IV solutions can be used) at a concentration of 1 unit per 1 to 10 mL IV solution and infused using calibrated electronic volumetric pumps. Insulin infusion via a dedicated line and pump enables the health care team to vary the infusion rate independent of other IV solutions, including PN. It is a standard practice to flush 50 mL of the IV insulin solution through the tubing before connecting to the IV access catheter in order to occupy adherence sites for insulin on polyvinyl chloride tubing.

Upon initiation of continuous IV infusion, the glucose should be checked every hour for up to 6 hours until glucose levels are stabilized at the target level, at which point the frequency of glucose testing can be extended to once every 2 to 3 hours. The infusion rate of 0.5 to 2 units/hour may need to be increased or decreased depending on the glycemic response. In patients that are NPO, this insulin infusion rate is primarily acting to restrain hepatic glucose production at a level that maintains the targeted glucose range, and is analogous to basal insulin (see following discussion). Upon initiation of PN or continuous enteral feeding, the insulin infusion will need to be increased because, in addition to inhibition of hepatic glucose output, additional insulin is needed for glucose disposal and nutrient metabolism (ie, the nutritional component of insulin therapy). In many patients, this will require approximately a doubling of the insulin infusion rate over the level needed while NPO (Table 34-6) during continuous infusion of PN or enteral feeding at an isocaloric level.

TABLE 34-5 Insulin Preparations Available for Intravenous and Subcutaneous Bolus and Basal Applications

	Class	Name	Brand	Maker	Onset	Peak	Duration	Comments
Intravenous		Human regular (U-100)	Humulin R	Lilly	Immediate	Immediate	< 10 minutes	No differences in rapid-acting and regular given intravenously
		Aspart	Novolog	NovoNordisk				
		Glulisine	Apidra	Sanofi				
Bolus (subcutaneous)	Rapid acting	Lispro	Humalog	Lilly	5–15 minutes	30–90 minutes	< 5 hours	At mealtime; pump indication/CSII
		Aspart	Novolog	NovoNordisk	5–15 minutes	30–90 minutes	< 5 hours	
		Glulisine	Apidra	Sanofi	5–15 minutes	30–90 minutes	< 5 hours	
	Short acting	Human regular (U-100)	Humulin R	Lilly	30–60 minutes	2–4 hours	5–8 hours	15–45 minutes prior to meal
			Novolin R	NovoNordisk	30–60 minutes	2–4 hours	5–8 hours	
Basal (subcutaneous)	Intermediate acting	Human NPH	Humulin N	Lilly	2–4 hours	4–10 hours	10–18 hours	Once or twice a day
			Novolin N	NovoNordisk	2–4 hours	4–10 hours	10–18 hours	
		Human regular (U-500)	Humulin R (U-500)	Lilly	2–4 hours	4–10 hours	10–16 hours	Similar to NPH; use tuberculin syringe
	Long acting	Glargine	Lantus	Sanofi	2–4 hours	None	24 hours	Usually once a day
		Detemir	Levemir	NovoNordisk	3–6 hours	None	18–24 hours	
Mixed (subcutaneous)	Premixed	Human NPH/ regular	Humulin 70/30	Lilly	30–60 minutes	Dual	10–18 hours	All mixed insulins have dual peaks reflecting the combination of rapid-/short- and intermediate-/long-acting insulins; does not allow independent manipulation of insulin components; usually twice a day
			Novolin 70/30	NovoNordisk	30–60 minutes	Dual	10–18 hours	
			Humulin 50/50	Lilly	30–60 minutes	Dual	10–18 hours	
		Lispro protamine/ Lispro	Humalog Mix 75/25	Lilly	5–15 minutes	Dual	10–18 hours	
		Lispro protamine/ Lispro	Humalog Mix 50/50	Lilly	5–15 minutes	Dual	10–18 hours	
		Aspart protamine/ Aspart	Novolog Mix 70/30	NovoNordisk	5–15 minutes	Dual	10–18 hours	

CSII, continuous subcutaneous insulin infusion; NPH, neutral protamine Hagedorn.
Note: All insulins available in vial as well as pen or cartridge except Human regular U-500 in vial only.

TABLE 34-6 Estimations for Initiation of Intravenous Insulin Therapy

	Nothing by Mouth (Units per Hour)	During Isocaloric Feeding (Units per Hour)
Type 1 diabetes mellitus	0.5–1.0	1–2
Type 2 diabetes mellitus	1–2	2–5
Insulin-resistant type 2 diabetes mellitus or high-dose glucocorticoids	2–4	4–10

An infusion rate of 10 units/hour provides for a maximal biological effect of insulin in the vast majority of patients, so this rate should only be exceeded on rare occasions. When PN or enteral feeding is discontinued for an "off" cycle or for diagnostic tests, the insulin infusion rate can be decreased to the level needed while NPO (basal), although it is important to consider that the biological effects of the higher insulin infusion rate will only gradually dissipate over the next 30 to 60 minutes. Therefore, the insulin infusion rate should be diminished 30 to 60 minutes prior to the discontinuation of PN or enteral feeding. Again, it is important that insulin infusion rates be individualized to patient needs based on careful glucose monitoring. Many hospitals use algorithms for IV insulin therapy that can be executed by nursing staff in a manner that assures ongoing communication between nurses and physicians.[28] Ideally, these algorithms will allow for timely correction of hyperglycemia, corrective increments and decrements in the insulin infusion rate based on the rate of decline or rise in glucose levels, adjustments for various patterns and strategies for nutrient intake, and a plan for reacting to hypoglycemia or a rapid decline in glycemia.

Subcutaneous Insulin Injections

Subcutaneous Insulin Preparations

Subcutaneous injections are generally used to control hyperglycemia in noncritically ill patients who are consuming meals or who are on bolus enteral feeding schedules. The insulin preparations approved for use in the hospital setting are similar to those used in outpatients. As shown in Table 34-5, subcutaneous insulin preparations can be categorized as basal insulins, including neutral protamine Hagedorn (NPH), glargine, detemir, and human regular U-500. Basal insulin is injected once or twice a day, and is designed to achieve a steady state level of hyperinsulinemia, with a small or absent peak following injection, with the main purpose of controlling hepatic glucose output. Because the liver continuously produces glucose under fasting conditions, and does so at elevated rates in hyperglycemic patients, basal insulin administration is needed even in patients who are not eating or receiving PN or enteral feeding. The second category includes bolus insulins that are given to achieve a peak after meals to coincide with rising postprandial glucose. These insulins represent the nutritional component of subcutaneous insulin therapy and are intended to lower plasma glucose by promoting tissue glucose uptake and nutrient metabolism following meals, as would occur physiologically with endogenous insulin secretory responses. Bolus insulins include rapid-acting insulin (lispro, aspart, glulisine), with onset in 5 to 15 minutes, peak at 30 to 90 minutes, and duration of approximately 4 hours, and short-acting insulin (human regular), with onset in 30 to 60 minutes, peak at 2 to 4 hours, and duration of 5 to 8 hours. Basal and bolus insulins are used in conjunction to physiologically provide both a chronic level of insulinemia over 24 hours regardless of nutrient intake (basal) together with acute insulin peaks following meals (nutritional). Rapid-acting and short-acting insulins can be used for the correctional component of therapy when an extra dose must be added to the prescheduled bolus when the premeal glucose is elevated. The third category is comprised of premixed insulins that combine both basal and bolus insulins in a single preparation. Premixed insulins simplify administration for the patient but have the disadvantage that the fixed dose ratios do not allow independent alterations in doses of basal versus bolus insulin as needed for improving glycemic control. For this latter reason, it is generally advantageous to use basal and bolus insulins separately, as opposed to premixed formulations, in hospitalized patients.

Sliding-Scale Insulin Therapy

There are two principal approaches to the use of subcutaneous insulin injections: sliding scale and basal-bolus. The "sliding-scale" approach employs rapid-acting or regular insulin administered subcutaneously at intervals. Insulin injections are given according to a preset schedule, and the dose is based on the glucose level measured just prior to time of the new injection according to a sliding scale that indicates the number of units to be injected. The timing of the glucose measurements and insulin injections is usually every 6 hours, which is appropriate for regular insulin given that this matches the duration of action of subcutaneous regular insulin. A rational interval for rapid-acting insulin is every 4 hours, which equates with the duration of action; even so, rapid-acting insulin is sometimes scheduled every 6 hours leaving the patient without any effect of exogenous insulin for 1 or 2 hours leading up to the next glucose measurement. The sliding-scale approach is reactionary in that the insulin dose is always driven by the current glucose measurement. Sliding-scale insulin is administered without any schedule for basal insulin and without set doses to be given at meals; the one important factor that drives the insulin dose at each interval is the current glucose level. Once the glucose value declines below a certain level, insulin is usually withheld until the next interval measurement, leaving the patient without any exogenous insulin to restrain ongoing hepatic glucose production. By its nature, the sliding-scale approach can predispose to wide fluctuations in glucose levels as a consequence of withholding insulin doses and due to reactionary dosing based on the current glucose level. Nevertheless, the sliding-scale approach is widely used and perpetuated in our teaching hospitals. AACE and the ADA recommend against prolonged use of sliding scales as the sole approach to insulin therapy.[10]

Basal-Bolus Insulin Therapy

The preferred approach for subcutaneous insulin administration is basal-bolus. As the name implies, this approach includes basal insulin administration to control fasting glucose combined with scheduled doses of rapid-acting or regular insulin given for bolus at meal times. The ADA and AACE both recommend that patients receive the total daily dose of insulin as three components: basal insulin, a nutritional component before meals, and a correctional component to be added to the meal dose when premeal glucose levels exceed the targeted level.

Estimation of the Total Daily Insulin Dose

In applying this to hospitalized patients, the first objective is to estimate the total daily insulin requirements, and Figure 34-1 illustrates several ways to do this based on the information in hand. First, the total daily insulin dose can be estimated from the number of units required to control glycemia in the outpatient setting in insulin-treated diabetics. Second, in patients who have been managed with IV insulin therapy, the total daily dose for subcutaneous insulin can be estimated as approximately 70% of the dose used IV to control glycemia over 24 hours.[29] Third, formulas based on body weight can be used to estimate the total daily insulin dose (T1DM: 0.3 to 0.5 units/kg/day; T2DM: 0.5 to 0.8 units/kg/day; very-insulin-resistant T2DM and high-dose glucocorticoids: 0.9 to 1.5 units/kg/day). It is important to consider, however, that insulin requirements are determined by additional factors other than body mass index. Therefore, these formulas provide a reasonable starting estimation for total daily insulin dose that often must be altered based on careful monitoring of blood glucose. Fourth, the total daily insulin dose can be estimated by reverse calculation using the 1500 Rule or the 1800 Rule (see following discussion). This is done by noting the

FIGURE 34-1 Approach to Initiation of Subcutaneous Basal-Bolus Insulin Therapy in Hospitalized Patients: Basal, Nutritional, and Correctional Components

Estimate Total Daily Dose

- If treated with insulin as outpatient, use outpatient dose if well controlled.
- ~70% of total daily IV insulin requirement in ICU during TPN or enteral feeding
- T2DM: 0.5 to 0.8 units/kg/day; T1DM: 0.3 to 0.5 units/kg/day; T2DM very resistant: 0.9-1.5 units/kg/day

Estimate Basal Dose
Basal Component

- Total daily dose ÷ 2 = basal insulin dose
- If basal insulin is glargine or detemir, give once a day (e.g., at bedtime)
- If basal insulin is NPH, split dose in two and give 2 doses daily

Estimate Bolus Dose
Nutritional Component

- Total daily dose ÷ 2 = the sum of all bolus doses
- Dose before each meal is total daily dose ÷ 6 assuming 3 isocaloric meals daily
- If bolus insulin is rapid-acting, give 5 to 15 min prior to meal
- If bolus insulin is human regular, give 30 min before meal

Monitoring

Measure glucose 4 times daily before each of 3 meals and evening snack

Correctional Doses
Correctional Component

- Add units of rapid- or short-acting insulin to scheduled pre-meal bolus dose
- 3 dosing schedules for patients exhibiting low, medium, and high requirement

Glucose (mg/dl)	Low Dose	Medium	High Dose
<60	Follow hypoglycemia protocol		
60 – 149	No correctional dose		
150 – 199	1	1	2
200 – 249	2	3	4
250 – 299	3	5	7
300 – 349	4	7	10
350 – 400	5	9	13
>400	Call physician		

ICU, intensive care unit; IV, intravenous; NPH, neutral protamine Hagedorn; T1DM, type 1 diabetes mellitus; T2DM, type 2 diabetes mellitus; TPN, total parenteral nutrition.

Reprinted from Endocrine Practice, Vol. 12, DeSantis AJ, Schmeltz LR, Schmidt K, et al., Inpatient management of hyperglycemia: the Northwestern experience, 491–505, Copyright 2006, with permission from the American Association of Clinical Endocrinologists.

magnitude of a decline in glucose following an injection of regular or rapid-acting glucose, and calculating the sensitivity factor as delta glucose decline (mg/dl) divided by the number of insulin units. If the glucose fell by 80 mg/dl (eg, from 200 to 120 mg/dl) following an injection of five units, the sensitivity factor is 80 ÷ 5 = 16, which is the decline in glucose (mg/dl) produced by one unit of insulin. If regular insulin was used, divide 1500 by the sensitivity factor to estimate the total daily insulin dose, which is the 1500 Rule (1,500 ÷ 16 = 94 units). If rapid-acting insulin was used, divide 1800 by the sensitivity factor, which is the 1800 Rule (1,800 ÷ 16 = 112 units).

After estimating the total daily insulin dose, begin by administering half of the estimated total daily dose as basal insulin (once a day glargine or detemir, or twice a day NPH). Basal insulin should not be held even if the patient is NPO because its main purpose is to control hepatic glucose production, which occurs throughout the 24 hour period. Administer the other half of the total daily dose as the sum of all bolus doses (nutritional) to be given at meal times (human regular or lispro, aspart, or glulisine). Assuming three isocaloric meals per day, this would amount to one-sixth of the total daily dose (or one-third of the total bolus insulin) given at each meal. The patient is monitored with four glucose measurements before each meal and before the bedtime snack. The basal dose can be titrated upward or downward based of the fasting morning glucose, and each of the three premeal bolus doses are titrated to the glucose measured prior to the next meal. In addition to basal and bolus doses, a correctional dose of rapid-acting or short-acting insulin is added to each scheduled premeal dose based on glucose level elevations above 150 mg/dl, as suggested in Figure 34-1. The basal-bolus approach is more physiological in mimicking patterns of basal and meal-related insulin secretion in normal humans, and is proactive in arriving at total daily insulin doses and diurnal patterns of insulin needed for effective glycemic control. In contrast, sliding-scale insulin administration is reactionary, nonphysiological, and essentially equates only to the correctional component of insulin administered in the basal-bolus treatment approach. A critical aspect of basal-bolus insulin therapy is the inclusion of long-acting insulin, which is designed to inhibit hepatic glucose output throughout each 24-hour period. There are only two randomized clinical trials comparing basal-bolus with sliding scale in hospitalized patients both performed by the same investigator group, one in medical inpatients[30] and the other in surgical inpatients.[31] Both studies demonstrated that basal-bolus results in improved glycemic control (with an average reduction in glucose of 20 to 30 mg/dl) and reduced hospital complications, without any difference in the frequency of hypoglycemia (glucose < 40 mg/dl), when compared with sliding scale. Other studies have documented the shortcomings of sliding scale,[32] including an increase in higher rates of mortality.[33] For these reasons, the ADA and AACE have recommended that the basal-bolus approach be employed for subcutaneous insulin therapy in hospitalized patients.[10]

The 1500 Rule and 1800 Rule

The determination of correctional dose algorithms has been refined by formulas that estimate each patient's insulin "sensitivity factor" in order to construct a patient-specific insulin dosing regimen. The most commonly employed are the 1500 Rule and the 1800 Rule, and variations of these rules are sometimes used by hospitals to establish algorithms that guide insulin therapy. The 1500 Rule estimates the point drop in glucose (mg/dl) for every one unit of regular insulin; the 1800 Rule estimates the decrement in glucose for every one unit of rapid-acting insulin (lispro, aspart, glulisine). To calculate the sensitivity factor for regular insulin, divide 1500 by the total daily insulin dose. For example, if the total daily insulin requirement is 60 units, then the sensitivity factor is 25 (1500 ÷ 60), which indicates that one unit of regular insulin will result is a decline of 25 mg/dl in the blood glucose level. Therefore, if the premeal glucose is 195 mg/dl and the target is 120 mg/dl, then three units of regular insulin (ie, 75 mg/dl ÷ 25) will reduce the glucose level by the 75 mg/dl needed to reach target, and should be added to the scheduled insulin dose for that meal to bring the glucose into an acceptable range leading up to the next meal. If rapid-acting insulin was being used for bolus, then the sensitivity factor is 30 (1800 ÷ 60), indicating that one unit of rapid-acting insulin is predicted to reduce blood glucose by 30 mg/dl. For a premeal glucose of 195 mg/dl where 120 mg/dl is the target, 2.5 units of rapid-acting insulin (ie, 75 mg/dl ÷ 30) should be added to the scheduled insulin dose for that meal. These rules can be used to construct insulin dosing algorithms for sliding scales or correctional doses of rapid- or short-acting insulin in the context of basal-bolus therapy.

Nutrition Assessment

A thorough nutrition assessment should be conducted in patients with diabetes or hyperglycemia. The dietary history should aid in the identification of patients at risk for nutrient deficiencies and evaluate for changes in body weight and appetite; nausea, vomiting, and diarrhea; use of supplements such as vitamins, minerals, or herbs; and problems chewing or swallowing. Close attention should be paid to the diabetes medical history including glucose control, self-monitoring practices, adherence to diet and lifestyle modifications, medications that could affect glucose levels or gastrointestinal function, and diabetes complications, as well as an assessment of the patient's educational status as pertains to diabetes. Regarding medications, use of oral hypoglycemic agents, insulin, or both should be noted as well as the doses and schedule of administration. A comprehensive physical examination should pay meticulous notice to skin integrity as patients with long-standing diabetes are particularly at risk for skin breakdown and poor wound healing.

In acutely ill patients, serum protein levels are affected by the acute-phase response to injury, infection, or inflammation. Hepatic reprioritization occurs resulting in decreased synthesis of negative acute-phase proteins such as albumin, prealbumin, and transferrin and an increase in positive acute-phase proteins such as C-reactive protein.[34] Serum protein levels in critically ill patients with diabetes should be interpreted cautiously and used more as a marker of severity of illness rather than nutrition status. Renal function should be evaluated as diabetic nephropathy can alter some of the laboratory values often used in nutrition assessment such as prealbumin, retinol-binding protein, and transferrin. Both prealbumin and retinol-binding protein are degraded in the kidney; therefore, levels may be increased in those diabetic patients with kidney disease. However, following trends in these levels over time in single patients can still provide valuable information regarding changes in nutritional status.

Calorie Needs

Accurate determination of energy needs is necessary to avoid the complications of over- or underfeeding. Indirect calorimetry is the gold standard for measuring energy expenditure but is not always available or may deliver unreliable information in certain clinical situations. In the absence of indirect calorimetry, predictive equations may serve as a starting point for assessing caloric needs. Multiple equations exist including simplistic formulas, such as 25 to 30 kcal/kg/body weight, which is a commonly used predictor of energy requirements, to the Harris-Benedict equation, to more complex formulas involving body temperature, presence of trauma, or burns, etc.[35] While these may provide an acceptable starting point in formulating the nutrition regimen, given the high degree in variability across clinical situations and populations, predictive equations should be used with caution while continuously evaluating the patient's response to nutrition therapy and adjusting nutrition support accordingly.

Many patients with T2DM may be obese, which further complicates estimation of calorie needs. A number of predictive equations account and adjust for obesity and others do not.[35] Several organizations promote permissive hypocaloric feeding for those with a body mass index ≥ 30, defined as 60% to 70% of target energy requirements, 11 to 14 kcal/kg actual body weight, or 22 to 25 kcal/kg ideal body weight.[36] While insulin sensitivity may be improved with some degree of weight loss, it should be noted that failure to receive more than 25% of estimated caloric needs is associated with a greater incidence of nosocomial infections.[37]

Avoidance of overfeeding calories for patients with diabetes or hyperglycemia is crucial as excess caloric intake can contribute to hyperglycemia and poor outcomes associated with hyperglycemia. Other sources of caloric intake, such as propofol (administered in a 10% lipid solution at 1.1 kcal/mL), other medication solutions, or IV fluids containing dextrose, should be accounted for when determining the calories to be provided by nutrition support. The overall goal of nutrition therapy is to provide adequate nutrition to meet the needs of hyperglycemic patients while maintaining glucose levels as normal as possible.

Protein Needs

Protein needs of patients with diabetes or hyperglycemia may vary depending on the level of stress and degree of malnutrition. Normal protein requirements for stable diabetics are the same as for patients without diabetes: 0.8 gm/kg/day or 15% to 20% of daily energy intake.[38] Needs may increase up to 2.0 gm/kg during stress or illness. For critically ill obese patients, particularly if receiving hypocaloric nutrition, protein needs should be provided in a range ≥ 2.0 gm/kg ideal body weight.[36]

In patients with diabetes without nephropathy, normal protein intake of 15% to 20% of calories does not appear to be associated with the development of diabetic nephropathy, but the long-term effects of higher protein intake have not been determined.[38] However, protein requirements deserve careful attention in those patients with diabetic nephropathy. In patients with micro- or macroalbuminuria, a reduced protein intake of 1 g or less/kg body weight is associated with a slowing in the decline of renal function is some (but not all) studies, and has been shown to improve glomerular filtration rate and urinary albumin excretion rate in the later stages of chronic kidney disease.[38] Therefore, protein intake at 1.0 g/kg body weight has been recommended in patients with diabetic nephropathy. Protein intake should not be restricted in the critically ill patient in the hopes of avoiding dialysis in those with renal disease.

Electrolytes

As insulin facilitates glucose entry into cells, hypophosphatemia and hypokalemia can develop from intercellular shift of phosphorus and potassium. These electrolytes may need to be supplemented until levels are stabilized. Hyperglycemia contributes to a hyperosmolarity that results in the movement of fluid from the intracellular to the extracellular compartment, causing a dilutional decrease in serum sodium level. The serum sodium concentration has been calculated to fall by 1 meq/L for every 62 mg/dL (3.5 mmol/L) rise in the serum glucose concentration.[39] As hyperglycemia is corrected, the serum sodium level rises as insulin drives glucose and water into the intracellular compartment. Fluid and electrolytes should be monitored closely and supplemented as needed to maintain adequate urine output and normal serum electrolyte levels.

Oral Diet

With regard to an oral diet for outpatients with diabetes, the ADA offers a high level of flexibility regarding carbohydrate intake to accommodate personal and ethnic food preferences, while emphasizing fat composition enriched in monounsaturated and polyunsaturated fats.[38,40–42] The recommended daily allowance for carbohydrate intake is 130 g average minimum requirement[43]; however, patients with diabetes may increase dietary carbohydrates up to 60% to 70% of calories. Monitoring carbohydrate by carbohydrate counting, exchanges, or estimation, and adjusting medical therapy accordingly, is the key strategy in maintaining optimal glucose control. As is the case for patients without diabetes, the recommendation for fiber intake is 14 g fiber per 1000 calories consumed, or 25 to 30 grams/day, in patients with diabetes. Very high fiber intakes (approximately 50 g/day) may reduce hyperglycemia in some patients; however, the palatability and feasibility of such intake is questionable. The goal with regard to fat intake in diabetes is to limit saturated fat intake to < 7% of total calories and to minimize transfatty acids. Dietary cholesterol should be limited to < 200 mg/day. Protein intake at 15% to 20% of daily calories is advised. For overweight and obese patients, weight loss of 5% to 10% of body weight is recommended, and both low-carbohydrate and low-fat calorie-restricted diets have been found to be effective in the short-term for weight loss (up to 2 years).[38] For patients with T1DM and T2DM, medical nutrition therapy involving multiple visits with a registered dietitian that involves the nutrition care process of nutrition assessment, nutrition diagnosis, nutrition interventions, and nutrition monitoring and evaluation will help achieve optimal glycemic control.[38,40–42]

In hospitalized patients with diabetes, a consistent carbohydrate meal planning system is often utilized that focuses on the total grams of carbohydrate consumed as a key strategy for achieving optimal glucose control.[38,40,42] The diet order does not detail a specific calorie level but rather specifies the amount of carbohydrate at each meal or snack. This may be stated in terms of grams of carbohydrate or carbohydrate exchange servings per meal. Typically, a consistent carbohydrate meal plan provides between 1800 to 2000 calories per day with three to five carbohydrate servings per meal, with a single carbohydrate serving consisting of approximately 15 g of carbohydrate. Utilization of this type of meal planning also assists nursing in determining the amount of rapid-acting or short-acting insulin to administer at mealtime for the nutritional component of basal-bolus therapy. Factors such as overweight/obesity, nutritional status, injury, infection, or fever can predominate as the major determinants of calories per se. In some instances, the use of oral supplements may be necessary or desired to help meet the patient's nutritional requirements, and diabetes-specific nutrition supplements are available that limit carbohydrate content and result in lower glucose values following ingestion.

In long-term health care facilities, the ADA also recommends a meal-planning system that emphasizes consistency in the timing and carbohydrate content of meals, rather than calorie goals, because undernutrition and inadequate intake are common in some institutionalized populations.[38] In these settings, medications can be adjusted to control glucose rather than restrict food intake or selection as nursing home residents have been found to eat better on less restrictive diets.

Gastroparesis

Gastroparesis, or delayed gastric emptying, produces the symptoms of nausea, vomiting, early satiety, bloating, and weight loss. Symptoms may wax and wane over time and can vary in terms of degree of severity. Although gastroparesis has classically been associated with advanced T1DM with poor glucose control, it is also a common complication in T2DM. The pathogenesis of diabetic gastroparesis is multifactorial with abnormalities noted in several aspects of gastric motility including disturbances of gastric emptying, gastric accommodation, contraction, and antral motor function.[44] These abnormalities are primarily due to autonomic dysfunction. Delayed gastric emptying may also be aggravated by medications, especially opioids.

The management of gastroparesis involves supportive measures (hydration and nutrition) and optimizing glucose control. Because dietary fat delays gastric emptying and fiber is poorly digested, dietary modifications include a low-fat and low-fiber diet, as well as small frequent meals. Patients should chew food well and remain upright for 1 to 2 hours after a meal. In some instances, liquid meals or pureed/blenderized foods may be indicated as long as they are nutritionally complete, as liquids empty from the stomach faster than solid foods. Supplementation of fluids and electrolytes may be necessary if recurrent vomiting has occurred. For these patients, close assessment of hydration, electrolyte, and acid-base status is indicated. Certain medications such as metoclopramide or erythromycin may be used to enhance gastric motility.[36,44] Other treatments that have been used in severe cases to improve motility include implanted gastric neurostimulators (gastric pacemakers) and botulinum toxin.

EN through a jejunostomy tube may be necessary if oral intake is insufficient or poorly tolerated. As jejunal feeding bypasses the need for gastric emptying, the formula does not necessarily need to be low in fat. Formula selection should be based on the patient's individual needs, glucose control, and the ability to tolerate the required volume of formula infused. One method often employed is for the patient to receive EN continuously at night and permitted oral intake during the day as tolerated. PN is rarely indicated for diabetic gastroparesis and should not be initiated unless other methods of nutrition support and pharmacotherapy have failed.

Enteral Feeding

Enteral Nutrition

EN via tube feeding is the preferred route of feeding the patient with diabetes or hyperglycemia if unable to take an oral diet. EN is associated with fewer complications than PN, particularly with regard to metabolic abnormalities, infection risk, and glucose control.[45] The ADA states that the nutritional needs for patients requiring tube feeding can be met using either a standard or diabetes-specific enteral formulas.[38] Diabetes-specific formulas are designed specifically for patients with diabetes and/or hyperglycemia, and generally contain less carbohydrate, more fiber, and more fat than standard formulas, while protein content and micronutrient composition are similar. Diabetes-specific formulas are characterized in Table 34-7.

Carbohydrate sources in enteral formulas typically consist of cornstarch, fiber, fructose, and oligosaccharides. In some diabetes-specific formulas, carbohydrates have been chemically modified to resist rapid enzymatic digestion and absorption, and converted to slowly digested carbohydrates such as isomaltulose and sucromalt. Both of these have a low glycemic index, and studies have found that ingestion of these resulted in a slower digestion and absorption rate and thus reduced postprandial glycemic responses.[46–49] The amount and source of fat in diabetes-specific formulas also varies from standard formulas. Sources of fat in standard enteral products typically derive from corn, safflower, sunflower, and soybean oils, which are rich sources of omega-6 fatty acids, and this raises the concern of a potential immunosuppressive effect if taken in large amounts. In some diabetes-specific formulas, monounsaturated fatty acids and omega-3 fatty acids are emphasized as a fat source to counter the immunosuppressive effect of omega-6 fatty acids. In addition, enrichment of mono- and polyunsaturated fatty acids in diabetes-specific formulas, when

TABLE 34-7 Nutritional Composition of Diabetes-Specific Enteral Formulas

Enteral Formula[a]	Caloric Density	Percent Carbohydrate Calories Sources of Carbohydrate	Percent Protein Calories	Percent Fat Calories Sources of Fat	Fiber (gm/L)
Glucerna® 1.0	1.0 kcal/mL	34.3% Corn maltodextrin, soy fiber, fructose	16.7%	49% High oleic safflower oil, canola oil, soy lecithin	14.4
Glucerna® 1.2	1.2 kcal/mL	35% Corn maltodextrin, isomaltulose, fructose, sucromalt, short-chain fructo-oligo-saccharides, oat fiber, soy fiber	20%	45% High oleic safflower oil, canola oil, soy lecithin, marine oil	16.1
Glucerna® 1.5	1.5 kcal/mL	33% Corn maltodextrin, isomaltulose, fructose, sucromalt, short-chain fructo-oligo-saccharides, oat fiber, soy fiber	22%	45% High oleic safflower oil, canola oil, soy lecithin	16.1
Nutren® Glytrol®	1.0 kcal/mL	40% Maltodextrin, modified cornstarch, gum Arabic, oligo-fructose, inulin	18%	42% Canola oil, high oleic safflower oil, medium chain triglycerides, soy lecithin, monoglycerides	15.2
Diabetisource® A/C	1.2 kcal/mL	36% Corn syrup, fructose, tapioca dextrin, partially hydrolyzed guar gum, pea puree, green bean puree, peach puree	20%	44% Canola oil, refined menhaden oil	15

[a]Information obtained from product websites. Accessed March 3, 2012.

substituted for saturated fatty acids, can exert favorable effects on insulin sensitivity and circulating lipid and lipoproteins. An increase in the fiber content may also assist with glucose control by improving insulin sensitivity as well as the glycemic index. Soluble fiber can delay gastric emptying and decrease intestinal transit time, although this effect may not always be desirable as in the case of a patient with gastroparesis.

A systematic review and meta-analysis involving 7 studies of EN and 16 studies of oral supplements comparing isocaloric diabetes-specific formulas to standard formulas found that use of the diabetes-specific formulas resulted in lower postprandial glucose levels.[47] One study by Pohl et al. randomized patients with T2DM and neurological disorders requiring long-term tube feeding to a standard or diabetes-specific formula; they observed lower fasting glucose and HbA1c together with a reduction in the daily insulin requirement in patients receiving the diabetes-specific formula.[48] Another study compared standard and diabetes-specific formulas when used as a meal replacement in ambulatory patients with T2DM and also in hospitalized patients receiving continuous enteral feeding while being monitored by continuous glucose monitoring; in these protocols, the diabetes-specific formula led to lower glucose values and reduced glucose variability while reducing requirements for regular insulin.[49]

A concern regarding the use of diabetes-specific formulas in critically ill patients is that the higher fat content may further delay gastric emptying in patients with gastroparesis or poor gastric emptying, whether due to diabetic autonomic neuropathy, hemodynamic compromise, or medications affecting gastric motility. Placement of the postpyloric enteral feeding tube may improve tolerance in patients with poor gastric emptying. Further research should be conducted to evaluate these outcomes as well as the economic impact assessing formula costs versus potential benefits resulting from improvements in glycemia and reduced insulin requirements.

Delivery of Enteral Nutrition

Gastric feeding administered via intermittent or bolus feedings may be used in stable patients without abnormalities involving gastric emptying.[36] Adequate delivery of gastric contents into the intestine should be assured by checking for residual contents prior to the next tube feeding. If the gastric route is not tolerated, a feeding tube should be placed into the small intestine. For most hospitalized patients, continuous tube feeding will result in improved tolerance over intermittent or bolus feedings, especially for critically ill patients. Continuous tube feedings should be started at full strength at a modest rate

(20 mL/hr) and the infusion rate advanced as tolerated (10 to 20 mL/hr increment increase every 12 hours), while glucose control is monitored and maintained.

Patients receiving EN should be closely monitored for hyperglycemia and hypoglycemia, gastrointestinal tolerance, adequacy of caloric intake, and salt and volume status by relying on physical examination (eg, skin assessment) and laboratory values. For patients receiving continuous EN, glucose monitoring every 4 to 6 hours is recommended.[10] Electrolyte status should be closely monitored as hypokalemia and hypophosphatemia can result from redistribution into cells along with glucose. Patients may need increasing insulin doses as enteral feedings are advanced until an optimal insulin schedule on isocaloric intake can be determined. As discussed below, these changes will primarily involve the nutritional bolus component of subcutaneous insulin therapy (rapid- or short-acting insulin) as opposed to the basal component. Those who did not initially require insulin before enteral feedings may subsequently need insulin to control blood glucose at target levels.

Insulin Therapy during Enteral Nutrition

Insulin should be used to treat diabetes and hyperglycemia during enteral feeding. The optimal pattern of insulin administration will vary depending on whether the enteral feeding is by continuous infusion or by intermittent tube feedings, and whether diabetes-specific versus standard EN formulas are being used.

Continuous Enteral Feeding

With continuous enteral infusion at a fixed rate, the patient will require a level of steady state hyperinsulinemia that is appropriate for the rate at which carbohydrates are being continuously absorbed. In addition, the insulin regimen should be able to accommodate increments in the continuous enteral infusion rate while still maintaining good glycemic control. Finally, the insulin protocol should be able to allow for discontinuations of enteral feeding (eg, diagnostic tests, clinical events) and for off cycles during the 24-hour period when enteral feeding is withdrawn (eg, continuous enteral feeding for 16 hours then off for 8 hours). Continuous IV insulin infusion best meets these requirements in ICUs or hospital venues where trained staff and hospital algorithms for managing IV insulin infusion therapy are in place. Table 34-6 suggests ranges of infusion rates for initiating IV insulin therapy in patients with T1DM and T2DM while receiving continuous isocaloric enteral feeding. The IV infusion rate is then titrated on the basis of hourly glucose to achieve the glucose target at any given rate of continuous enteral formula infusion. During off cycles or when enteral feedings need to be discontinued, the insulin infusion rate can be decreased to the basal level needed to maintain the patient at the target glucose level while NPO. Because it will take 30 to 60 minutes for the biological effects of the higher insulin infusion rate to deactivate, the insulin infusion rate should be decreased to the basal level approximately 30 to 60 minutes prior to the discontinuation of enteral feeding. An alternative way to manage discontinuations of enteral feeding is to maintain a dextrose infusion at a "keep open" rate (ie, 5 to 10 mL/hour) at all times, and then increase the rate of dextrose infusion to prevent hypoglycemia when EN is stopped. Increasing the infusion rate of a 5% dextrose solution to 30 to 40 mL/hr should suffice for this purpose. Glucose levels should be monitored at intervals during both off and on cycles of continuous enteral feeding.

If the hospital unit does not have the capacity for IV insulin therapy, diabetes and hyperglycemia can be controlled using subcutaneous insulin during continuous enteral feeding. One study compared a basal-bolus regimen consisting of glargine and human regular insulin with sliding-scale human regular insulin and observed equivalent degrees of glycemic control in enterally fed patients; however, more than half of the sliding-scale patients required the addition of NPH insulin for persisting hyperglycemia, which essentially converted this treatment group to a basal-bolus treatment category.[50] We favor a basal-bolus approach where one-half of the total daily insulin dose is given as long-acting (glargine or detemir at bedtime) or as intermediate-acting insulin (NPH twice a day), and one-half of the total daily dose is given as regular insulin divided into four equal doses with each dose given every 6 hours. An alternative way to estimate regular insulin doses is to divide the total daily carbohydrate intake in grams by 10, and to divide that number by 4 to determine the number of units of regular insulin to be given every 6 hours. An off cycle can be scheduled 6 hours following the last dose of regular insulin, and regular insulin is held until the enteral feeding infusion is resumed. In addition to basal-bolus therapy, other potential approaches for subcutaneous insulin treatment include the following.

1. Use of NPH insulin given at higher doses to provide both basal and nutritional insulin components. With this approach, one should be careful to avoid hypoglycemia during off cycles or when the enteral feeding is discontinued. Glargine or detemir should not be used in this setting because their longer duration of action could cause hypoglycemia if the feeding is interrupted. The administration of NPH can be supplemented with a sliding-scale employing short-acting insulin.
2. Short-acting insulin (human regular) given every 6 hours or rapid-acting insulin given every 4 hours using a sliding-scale approach with glucose values checked every 6 or 4 hours, respectively. This approach fails to provide the basal component of insulin therapy when interruptions of enteral feeding necessitate withholding of the short-acting or rapid-acting insulin, and can then result in loss of glucose control.
3. Mixed insulins (70/30 or 50/50 long-acting/short- or rapid-acting) given in equal doses at 6-hour intervals. The use of these fixed-dose regimens do not allow for independent adjustment of the basal (long- or intermediate-acting) and nutritional (short- or rapid-acting) components of insulin therapy.

Intermittent Enteral Feeding

Enteral tube feedings administered intermittently is well suited to basal-bolus insulin therapy and can be managed similar to patients eating discrete meals. Often, tube feedings are delivered more frequently than regular meals, and rapid-acting insulin can be useful for bolus insulin therapy in this setting. For example, tube feedings spaced every 4 hours approximates the duration of action of rapid-acting insulins. In this instance, one-sixth of the bolus insulin component (or one-twelfth of the total daily insulin dose) is given prior to each tube feeding and titrated to a glucose measurement leading up to the time of the next tube feeding. For tube feedings given every 6 hours, the human regular insulin becomes the optimal bolus insulin preparation given its duration of action that approximates 6 hours. Rapid- or short-acting insulin is held during periods when tube feedings are discontinued, and long- or intermediate-acting insulin (representing approximately one-half of the total daily insulin dose) is used to provide the basal insulin component throughout the day (Practice Scenario 34-1).

Practice Scenario 34-1

Question: What is the optimal management for a patient with type 2 diabetes requiring enteral feeding?

Scenario: A 66-year-old female was admitted to the hospital after a cerebrovascular accident. Her previous medical history includes hypertension and type 2 diabetes for which she was managed with glargine 15 units at night and aspart 10 units prior to each meal. Review of medical records from her primary care doctor revealed acceptable glucose control with most recent HgbA1C of 6.3%. A fiberoptic endoscopic evaluation of swallowing study demonstrated profound dysphagia with all consistencies of liquids and solids. A percutaneous endoscopic gastrostomy tube was placed to administer EN, and she was made NPO. Her initial tube feeding order was 200 mL every 6 hours of a diabetes-specific enteral formula providing 1.5 kcal/mL with caloric distribution of 33% carbohydrate, 22% protein, and 45% fat. She received a free water flush after each feeding and medication administration. The volume of bolus feedings was increased over 2 days to a volume of 400 mL every 6 hours. Her home insulin regimen was reinstated with 15 units glargine at night and 10 units aspart prior to each bolus feeding. She tolerated the enteral feeding without problems (no diarrhea, constipation, nausea, vomiting, or abdominal discomfort), although she was frustrated with her inability to swallow oral food and liquids. Swallowing therapy was continued as she was transferred to an inpatient rehabilitation hospital for ongoing care. Postprandial glucose levels (after tube feeding bolus) ranged from 150 to 200 mg/dl while fasting/prefeeding levels were 150 to 170 mg/dl. Her weight was 60 kg.

Intervention: Tube feedings were decreased to 350 mL every 6 hours to decrease caloric intake and glargine was increased to 20 units each night.

Answer: Her fasting/premeal glucose levels suggest that her basal insulin requirements were not being met, therefore the glargine was increased. The enteral feeding regimen of 400 mL every 6 hours was excessive, providing 2400 kcal (40 kcal/kg). As she was stable medically, the decision was made to decrease the caloric intake. The total volume was reduced to 300 mL every 6 hours to provide 1800 calories (30 kcal/kg); the frequency of boluses was maintained to accommodate her therapy schedule and to not be as disruptive during the overnight hours. As the formula was higher in fat than most standard enteral formulas, close attention to her gastrointestinal tolerance was assessed as well as plans for assessment of lipid status if she was to remain on enteral feeding long-term. Because her caloric intake was being decreased to both prevent overfeeding and lower postmeal glucose, the current doses of aspart were continued along with continued glucose monitoring to assess for changes if needed.

Rationale: Nutritional needs for patients with diabetes can be met with either a standard or lower-carbohydrate enteral formula.[47] While diabetes-specific enteral formulas have been shown to lower postprandial rise in glucose levels and peak glucose levels compared to standard formulas, long-term effects and improved outcomes such as length of stay and infection risk have not been conducted and/or confirmed. Clinical judgment and overall cost-benefit analysis should be included in the selection of enteral formulas to use. Avoidance of overfeeding calories is crucial for all patients, particularly those with diabetes or hyperglycemia, as elevated glucose levels have been associated with an increased risk of infections and other complications. Noncritically ill hospitalized patients are often best managed with a subcutaneous regimen of scheduled insulin, with basal, nutritional, and correctional components.[10] For patients not receiving continuous enteral nutrition, the schedule for monitoring glucose levels should be frequent enough to detect hyperglycemia during or after feedings.[10]

Diabetes-Specific Formulas and Insulin Therapy

The previous discussion pertains to insulin therapy for patients being administered standard enteral formulas. If diabetes-specific formulas are used in enteral feeding protocols, the need for lower insulin requirements should be anticipated. As discussed in the section on EN, diabetes-specific formulas result in lower glycemic excursions and serum insulin concentrations when compared with standard formulas in patients being fed by tube feeding. In a review and meta-analysis by Elia et al.,[47] four trials were identified showing a reduction in total daily insulin doses of 26% to 71% using diabetes-specific formulas compared with standard formulas. In another study of patients with T2DM on continuous enteral feeding (16 hours on/8 hours off), the diabetes-specific formula led to a 26% decrease in insulin, lower mean glucose levels, and a reduction in glucose variability as determined using continuous glucose monitoring.[49] Therefore, in basal-bolus insulin therapy, a rational approach is to reduce bolus doses (ie, the nutritional component) by 30% to 50% when initiating therapy, followed by empiric titration based on glucose monitoring. The use of diabetes-specific formulas should not be expected to result in the need for marked changes in the basal insulin component. When enteral feedings are given intermittently, the dose of short- or rapid-acting insulin to be injected before the next bolus feeding could also be estimated as the number of carbohydrates in grams divided by 10.

Parenteral Feeding

Parenteral Nutrition

If contraindications to enteral feeding exist, PN may be necessary to provide adequate nutrition intake. Optimal glucose control is vital for the patient with diabetes or hyperglycemia receiving PN. Studies of hospitalized patients, including those critically and noncritically ill, found that hyperglycemia associated with PN is a risk factor for the development of infections, renal and cardiac dysfunction, and increased mortality.[50,51] The macronutrient composition of PN can exacerbate hyperglycemia because carbohydrate is provided in the form of dextrose. Ideally, carbohydrate should be provided in the amount necessary to spare the use of protein for energy while avoiding hyperglycemia. Minimum requirements for carbohydrate delivery are 1 mg dextrose/kg/min and a maximum 4 to 7 mg/kg/min. For adult patients with diabetes mellitus or stress hyperglycemia, PN should begin with 100 to 150 g/day of dextrose or a 10% to 15% final dextrose concentration administered over 24 hours to avoid hyperglycemia and the possibility of refeeding syndrome in patients at high risk.[52] Over the next 1 to 3 days, the patient should be stabilized regarding good glycemic control and attention to electrolyte levels. At that point, the dextrose dose in PN can be advanced to the recommended maximum in critically ill patients or those with diabetes, which is 4 mg/kg/min.[53,54] Equations for calculating the dextrose infusion rate to achieve target level of administration and avoid excessive dextrose in PN are found in Table 34-8.

For all ICU patients starting PN, mild permissive underfeeding is initially recommended, defined as 80% of energy requirements.[53] The rationale behind this is to reduce the risk of hyperglycemia and/or to prevent the refeeding syndrome. One prospective randomized trial found that administration of a lower-calorie PN formulation (20 kcal/kg) versus a standard formulation (30 kcal/kg) resulted in fewer episodes of hyperglycemia and lower insulin requirements.[54] PN with a higher percentage of calories from fat may help control glucose levels. However, the source of lipid in PN is primarily triglyceride containing long-chain fatty acids, which, in high amounts, may induce hyperlipidemia and cholestasis as well as immunosuppression. The recommended maximal dose of lipid emulsion infusion is approximately 1.0 to 1.3 g/kg/day.[53] For obese patients (body mass index ≥ 30), caloric targets should be 60% to 70% of estimated needs.[53] Adequate protein is necessary for wound healing, fighting infection, and promoting anabolism. For those patients receiving PN at a rate that is less than calculated energy requirements, up to 2 gm protein/kg ideal body weight as amino acids may be indicated.

Monitoring

Blood glucose should be monitored carefully in capillary blood (ie, fingerstick) using a calibrated glucometer, in venous blood, or in arterial blood if access is available. Point-of-care measurements should be performed using carefully calibrated glucometers. Glucose should be monitored every 2 to 6 hours, depending on facility protocols, insulin requirements, and general clinical condition. At the initiation of IV insulin therapy, glucose checks every hour may be warranted until the optimal insulin infusion rate is established. Approaches to insulin therapy are discussed below. Standard protocols for monitoring all aspects of PN should be employed as discussed in the chapter on PN (see Chapter 14). In particular, magnesium, phosphorus, and potassium requirements increase as patients convert from a catabolic to anabolic state, and circulating levels can be diminished by carbohydrate infusion and insulin therapy. For these reasons, special attention to electrolytes, magnesium, and phosphorus is warranted, and supplementation of these minerals may be needed for the first few days of PN. PN should not be advanced in total calories, particularly regarding calories from dextrose, until glucose control and electrolyte levels are stable.

Hypoglycemia may occur if the PN is abruptly discontinued, whether or not the patient is receiving insulin; this is known as "rebound hypoglycemia." If it is necessary to interrupt PN, 10% dextrose can be infused at the same rate until PN resumes. A situation in which this may occur is if a new bag of PN infusion is unavailable or its delivery to the bedside has been delayed. Another method to avoid rebound hypoglycemia with PN is to taper the infusion over the last 1 to 2 hours prior to discontinuation.

Insulin Therapy during Parenteral Nutrition

Hyperglycemia is a common complication of PN. The risk of PN-associated hyperglycemia increases with age, severity of illness, rate of dextrose infusion, and antecedent diagnosis of diabetes.[28] In patients with diabetes not previously treated with insulin, 77% required insulin to control hyperglycemia during PN and insulin doses averaged 100 units/day.[55] Moreover, PN-induced hyperglycemia is independently associated with increased mortality and hospital complications such as pneumonia and acute renal failure.[56] One factor contributing to the hyperglycemia is that the IV infusion of carbohydrate bypasses the gut's entero-incretin axis and fails to stimulate the release of gut incretin peptides (GLP-1 and gastric inhibitory peptide), which enhance endogenous insulin secretory responses as would occur with enteral feeding. This leads to higher levels of glycemia that require insulin therapy for control.

The optimal approach is IV insulin therapy where the infusion rate of regular insulin can be regulated by a volumetric pump using a dedicated line. This permits alterations in the insulin infusion rate independent of the rate of PN infusion. IV insulin therapy can be used to reduce hyperglycemia to target levels within 24 hours in the majority of patients. Ongoing management of glycemia can continue with the variable rate insulin infusion. If there is a need to discontinue the dedicated IV insulin catheter, 80% of the IV regular insulin dose required for glycemic control established using the variable rate can be added to the bag of PN. From that point forward, the insulin infusion line can be discontinued, although the amount of insulin added to the PN may still require day-to-day adjustments. Institutions should have approved protocols in place for using continuous IV insulin infusion that employs frequent glucose monitoring. In the ICU setting, continuous insulin infusion has demonstrated to be the most effective method for achieving glycemic goals.[28]

Not all hospital venues may have the capacity for IV insulin therapy. In these instances, it is commonplace for insulin to be added initially to the PN as first-line insulin therapy without a separate variable rate infusion line. A disadvantage is that the incremental additions of insulin to the PN can require several days to arrive at the effective insulin dose that maintains patients at target. One approach for initially estimating the amount of insulin to add to PN is to provide 0.05 to 0.1 units of regular insulin per gram of dextrose in the PN solution (eg, 15% dextrose is 150 g/L so add 150 × 0.1 units = 15 units of regular insulin to PN). This amount can be increased as needed in response to blood glucose levels, and it is usually accompanied by the need for supplemental subcutaneous regular insulin for glycemic control administered via sliding scale. The amount of insulin added to the bag of PN is typically increased each day by adding two-thirds of the previous day's subcutaneous insulin requirement to the PN, or by increasing the amount of added insulin by 0.05 units of regular insulin per gram of carbohydrate. If glucose values remain > 180 mg/dl even after insulin has been increased to 0.2 units/g carbohydrate in the PN, and despite the use of correctional subcutaneous insulin, the initiation of continuous IV insulin therapy should strongly be considered. Once the effective dose is identified, the addition of insulin to PN is an effective way to manage associated hyperglycemia. For stable patients or home-care patients on PN, insulin can added to the formulation before administration, and patients can use correctional subcutaneous insulin injections based on fingerstick glucose determinations as required to maintain optimal glucose control (Practice Scenario 34-2).

Practice Scenario 34-2

Question: How is glycemic control maintained in a patient receiving PN?

Scenario: A 65-year-old male was admitted to the ICU due to severe abdominal pain, fever, and hypotension. He was recently diagnosed with adenocarcinoma of the colon and started chemotherapy 4 days prior to admission. He has a history of T2DM that he controlled fairly well through his diet (last reported HbA1c 7.8%, 4 months prior to admission). The family reported he had been experiencing nausea and vomiting for 3 days prior to admission and a weight loss of 20 pounds over the past 2 months due to abdominal pain and intermittent nausea and vomiting. An abdominal x-ray revealed a small bowel obstruction, and blood cultures were positive for *Klebsiella pneumonia*. He was started on antibiotics, IV fluids, and pressors for resuscitation. A nasogastric tube was placed for decompression and he was ordered NPO. On hospital day 3, he was started on PN providing 1000 calories and 100 g dextrose. In the ICU, his initial blood glucose levels were persistently > 200, prompting institution of continuous IV insulin therapy for glycemic control. Thereafter, levels were maintained around 150 to 160 mg/dl. The PN was increased over the next 2 days to provide 1800 calories, 90 g protein, 300 g carbohydrate, and 42 g fat. By day 5, he was stable off pressors, the insulin drip was discontinued, and he was transferred to the floor. PN was continued due to the persistent small bowel obstruction, and he remained NPO. On day 6, he was treated with a sliding scale of regular insulin with doses given at 6-hour intervals; the total amount of regular insulin given was 36 units. His glucose levels increased to 190 to 220 mg/dl. On admission, his weight was 65 kg. On day 3, 5, and 7, it was 69 kg, 68 kg, and 68 kg, respectively.

Intervention: The total amount of insulin he received the previous day through the insulin drip is calculated at 36 units, and two-thirds that amount (ie, 24 units) is placed in the new PN order for the next day as the sliding scale is continued.

Answer: Glycemic control can be managed in patients receiving PN by a continuous IV infusion, a subcutaneous insulin regimen, or adding insulin to the PN formula. In this case, the patient was transferred out of the ICU and glucose could no longer be maintained with an insulin drip. Therefore, insulin was added to the PN solution and additional needs met if necessary through subcutaneous injections using a sliding scale. Caloric goals for this patient were initially estimated at 25 to 30 kcal/kg (1625 to 1950 kcal), using admission weight because any weight gain above that level was likely from fluid resuscitation. Starting PN at 1000 calories and 100 g dextrose was chosen to reduce the risk of hyperglycemia, and because he was also at increased risk of the refeeding syndrome due to the degree of weight loss and decreased intake prior to admission. As glucose and electrolyte levels remained stable, the PN order was increased to the goal amount.

Rationale: Regarding the use of PN itself, it is appropriate early in this patient's hospital course due to his small bowel obstruction, which precluded enteral feeding, and the 12.5% weight loss he experienced prior to admission. American Society for Parenteral and Enteral Nutrition (A.S.P.E.N.) recommendations are that, if EN is not feasible and the patient has evidence of protein-calorie malnutrition, it is suitable to start PN as soon as possible after admission and adequate resuscitation.[36] For glycemic control, a continuous IV insulin infusion is typically only administered in the ICU setting due to the frequent monitoring and need for trained staff. Once the insulin drip is operative, insulin should not also be placed in the PN solution due to the risk of hypoglycemia. For patients not being treated with an IV insulin infusion, insulin can be added to the PN solution or provided through scheduled subcutaneous administration with basal, nutritional, and correctional components.[10] Another important factor in achieving glycemic control in patients receiving PN is to avoid excess dextrose infusion and overfeeding (Table 34-8). For this reason, limiting initial carbohydrate to 100 to 150 g dextrose is appropriate to reduce the risk of PN-induced hyperglycemia in patients with elevated glucose levels.[52] The dextrose infusion for patients with diabetes should be limited to < 4 mg/kg/min, which, for this patient, would calculate to be a maximum of 374 g dextrose per day.[53] Patients with diabetes or hyperglycemia requiring PN require frequent monitoring of glucose levels as well as close attention paid to total carbohydrate, caloric intake, and electrolytes.

Nutrition and Diabetes Treatment during Transitions from Intensive Care Unit to Floor and Floor to Home

The transition from IV insulin therapy to subcutaneous insulin therapy, both in the ICU and in the process of moving to the general hospital floor, is frequently accompanied by deterioration in glycemic control. Two aspects are of critical importance in an effective transition. First, it will be important to estimate the total

TABLE 34-8 Equations for Calculating Dextrose Infusion Rates in Parenteral Nutrition

To determine maximal carbohydrate to be placed in a formula prescription over 24 hours:

1. To calculate the daily maximum dextrose for a critically ill patient:

   4 mg/kg/min × weight (kg) × 1440 (minutes/24 hours) ÷ 1000 = dextrose g/day

   Example: Calculate the maximum amount of dextrose a 70-kg critically ill patient should receive: 4 mg/kg/min × 70 kg × 1440 minutes ÷ 1000 = 403 g dextrose/day

To determine if current PN formula is being infused at a rate that does not exceed the maximum:

2. To calculate the dextrose infusion rate to be used in PN:

   Grams of dextrose/day in PN ÷ weight (kg) ÷ 1440 (minutes/24 hours) × 1000 = dextrose infusion rate as mg/kg/min

   Example: Patient is receiving 500 g dextrose per day in PN. Does this rate exceed maximum of 4 mg/kg/min in a 70-kg patient?

   500 g dextrose/day in PN ÷ 70 kg ÷ 1440 minutes × 1000 = 5.0 mg/kg/min

   Therefore, current PN exceeds maximum for carbohydrate in PN and should be decreased to provide a rate of < 4 mg/kg/min determined using formula 1.

PN, parenteral nutrition.

daily dose of subcutaneous insulin based on the IV insulin requirements during IV insulin therapy. A retrospective analysis by Weant and Ladha found that a total daily subcutaneous insulin dose equal to 60% to 78% of the 24-hour IV insulin dose achieved glucose levels within a 80 to 150 mg/dl target range 70% of the time.[29] Therefore, while variability exists, 70% of the IV dose requirement is a rational estimation of the total daily subcutaneous insulin dose. The basal-bolus regimen can then be established with 50% of total daily dose given as basal and 50% administered in bolus injections as described previously. In patients on advancing diet, full isocaloric meals will not be consumed at mealtimes, and the bolus doses (nutritional component) should be decreased accordingly without substantial alteration in the basal insulin dose. Based on carbohydrate counting principles, one unit of rapid- or short-acting insulin could be given for every 10 grams or so of carbohydrate in the meal to be consumed. The bolus insulin doses at meals can be advanced with the diet such that full bolus doses can be anticipated, which equals 50% of the estimated total daily insulin dose, when the patient advances to regular isocaloric meals. A critical aspect often neglected in hospitals is the need to give regular insulin 30 minutes before the meal, and rapid-acting insulin 5 to 15 minutes before the meal, to consistently achieve full therapeutic effectiveness. The second important aspect for the ICU to floor transition is to begin subcutaneous injections prior to the discontinuation of continuous IV insulin infusion in the ICU. Specifically, the basal dose of long- or intermediate-acting insulin should be given 2 to 3 hours prior to discontinuing the IV insulin infusion. In addition, the patient should not miss the bolus insulin injection prior to the next meal, even if the dose must be decreased in patients on advancing diets.

A second critical transition occurs at discharge from the hospital. Poorly controlled diabetes following discharge is associated with a marked increase in rates of rehospitalization,[57] and The Joint Commission has targeted postdischarge diabetes management as a national goal for patient safety.[58] It is important to begin diabetes education in the hospital and to arrange for a clear hierarchy of follow-up care and communication prior to discharge. The patient should understand the dietary prescription, know how to perform home glucose monitoring, and how to take medications including insulin. The patient should have a clear understanding of what actions to take at different home glucose levels, and how to respond to hypoglycemia. Discharge planning should include follow-up appointments and contacts for medical advice prior to the first appointments, as well as prescriptions and access to all medications, glucometers and strips, and insulin syringes as needed. HbA1c should be measured, preferably upon admission, to help establish diagnosis of diabetes or stress diabetes and guide selection of discharge medications. The AACE has made cogent recommendations for discharge therapy based on the HbA1c,[59] as follows: if HbA1c < 7% in patients with previous diagnosis of diabetes, discharge on therapeutic regimen that anteceded the hospitalization; if HbA1c is 7% to 8%, increase dose of previous oral agents or add another oral agent or add basal insulin at bedtime; if HbA1c is > 8%, add basal insulin at bedtime if patient is already on oral agent(s); if HbA1c is > 9%, consider discharge on basal-bolus regimen continuing doses established in the hospital.

Acknowledgments

The authors acknowledge research support from the National Institutes of Health (DK-038764, DK-083562) and the Merit Review program of the Department of Veterans Affairs. We also gratefully acknowledge the support of the University of Alabama and Birmingham (UAB) Center for Clinical and Translational Science (UL1 RR025777), the UAB Nutrition and Obesity Research Center (P30-DK56336), and the UAB Diabetes Research and Training Center (P60-DK079626). We are also grateful to the UAB Nutrition Consult Service comprised of faculty and fellows in the Department of Nutrition Sciences and to our patients.

References

1. American Diabetes Association. Executive summary: standards of medical care in diabetes – 2011. *DiabetesCare.* 2011;34(Suppl 1):S4–S10.
2. Centers for Disease Control and Prevention. *National Diabetes Fact Sheet: National Estimates and General Information on Diabetes and Prediabetes in the United States, 2011*. Atlanta, GA: U.S. Department of Health and Human Services; 2011.
3. American Diabetes Association. Standards of medical care in diabetes-2011. *Diabetes Care.* 2011;34(Suppl 1):S11–S61.

4. American Diabetes Association. Diagnosis and classification of diabetes mellitus. *Diabetes Care.* 2011;34(Suppl 1):S62–S69.
5. American Diabetes Association. Hyperglycemic crisis in diabetes. *Diabetes Care.* 2004;27(Suppl 1):S94–S102.
6. American Diabetes Association. Diagnosis and classification of diabetes mellitus. *Diabetes Care.* 2010;33(Suppl 1):S62–S69.
7. Nathan DM, Davidson MB, DeFronzo RA, et al., American Diabetes Association. Impaired fasting glucose and impaired glucose tolerance: implications for care. *Diabetes Care.* 2007;30:753–759.
8. Garber AJ, Handelsman Y, Einhorn D, et al. Diagnosis and management of prediabetes in the continuum of hyperglycemia: when do the risks of diabetes begin? A consensus statement from the American College of Endocrinology and the American Association of Clinical Endocrinologists. *Endocrine Practice.* 2008;14:933–946.
9. Van den Berghe G, Wouters P, Weekers F, et al. Intensive insulin therapy in critically ill patients. *N Engl J Med.* 2001;345:1359–1367.
10. Moghissi ES, Korytkowski MT, DiNardo M, et al., American Association of Clinical Endocrinologists; American Diabetes Association. American Association of Clinical Endocrinologists and American Diabetes Association consensus statement on inpatient glycemic control. *Endocr Pract.* 2009;15(4):353–369.
11. Das S, Misra B, Roul L, et al. Insulin resistance and beta cell function as prognostic indicator in multi-organ dysfunction syndrome. *Met Syndr Relat Disord.* 2009;7:47–51.
12. Mizock BA. Alterations in fuel metabolism in critical illness hyperglycemia. *Best Pract Res Clin Endocrinol Metab.* 2001;15:533–551.
13. Umpierrez GE, Isaacs SD, Bazargan N, et al. Hyperglycemia: an independent risk marker of in-hospital mortality in patients with undiagnosed diabetes. *J Clin Endocrinol Metab.* 2002;87:978–982.
14. Krinsley JS. Glycemic variability: a strong independent predictor of mortality in critically ill patients. *Crit Care Med.* 2008;36(11): 3008–3013.
15. Hermanides MD, Vriesendorp TM, et al. Glucose variability is associated with intensive care unit mortality. *Crit Care Med.* 2010;38(3):838–842.
16. Dossett LA, Cao H, Mowery NT, et al. Blood glucose variability is associated with mortality in the surgical intensive care unit. *Am Surg.* 2008;74(8):679–685.
17. McMahon MM, Bistrian BR. Host defenses and susceptibility to infection in patients with diabetes mellitus. *Infect Dis Clin North Amer.* 1995;9:1–9.
18. Pomposelli JJ, Baxter JK, Babineau TJ, et al. Early post-operative glucose control predicts nosocomial infection rate in diabetic patients. *J Parent Enteral Nutr.* 1998;22:77–81.
19. Van den Berghe G, Wouters P, Weekers F, et al. Intensive insulin therapy in critically ill patients. *N Eng J Med.* 2001;345:1359–1367.
20. Van den Berghe G, Wilmer A, Hermans G, et al. Intensive insulin therapy in the medical ICU. *N Engl J Med.* 2006;354:449–461.
21. Pittas AG, Siegel RD, Lau J. Insulin therapy for critically ill hospitalized patients: a meta-analysis of randomized controlled trials. *Arch Intern Med.* 2004;164(18):2005–2011.
22. Garber AJ, Moghissi ES, Bransome ED Jr, et al., American College of Endocrinology Task Force on Inpatient Diabetes Metabolic Control. American College of Endocrinology position statement on inpatient diabetes and metabolic control. *Endocr Pract.* 2004;10(Suppl 2):4–9.
23. Kansagara D, Fu R, Freeman M, et al. Intensive insulin therapy in hospitalized patients: a systematic review. *Ann Intern Med.* 2011; 154(4):268–282.
24. Finfer S, Chittock DR, Su SY, et al. Intensive versus conventional glucose control in critically ill patients. *N Engl J Med.* 2009;360: 1283–1297.
25. Moghissi ES, Korytkowski MT, DiNardo M, et al. American Association of Clinical Endocrinologists and the American Diabetes Association consensus statemnent on inpatient glycemic control. *Diabetes Care.* 2009;6:1119–1131.
26. Curkendall SM, Natoli JL, Alexander CM, et al. Economic and clinical impact of inpatient diabetic hypoglycemia. *Endocr Pract.* 2009;15:302–312.
27. Turchin A, Matheny ME, Shubina M, et al. Hypoglycemia and clinical outcomes in patients with diabetes hospitalized in the general ward. *Diabetes Care.* 2009;32:1153–1157.
28. Clement S, Braithwaite SS, Magee MF, et al. Management of diabetes and hyperglycemia in hospitals. *Diabetes Care.* 2004;27: 553–591.
29. Weant KA, Ladha A. Conversion for continuous insulin infusions to subcutaneous insulin in critically-ill patients. *Ann Pharmacother.* 2009;43:629–634.
30. Umpierrez GE, Smiley D, Zisman A, et al. Randomized study of basal-bolus insulin therapy in the inpatient management of patients with type 2 diabetes (RABBIT 2 trial). *Diabetes Care.* 2007;30:2181–2186.
31. Umpierrez GE, Smiley D, Jacobs S, et al. Randomized study of basal-bolus insulin therapy in the inpatient management of patients with type 2 diabetes undergoing general surgery (RABBIT 2 surgery). *Diabetes Care.* 2011;34:256–261.
32. Golightly LK, Jones MA, Hamamura DH, et al. Management of diabetes mellitus in hospitalized patients: efficacy and effectiveness of sliding scale therapy. *Pharmacother.* 2006;26:1421–1432.
33. Becker T, Moldoveanu A, Cukierman T, et al. Clinical outcomes associated with the use of subcutaneous insulin-by-glucose sliding scales to manage hyperglycemia in hospitalized patients with pneumonia. *Diabetes Res Clin Pract.* 2007;78:392–397.
34. Gabay C, Kushner I. Acute-phase proteins and other systemic responses to inflammation. *N Engl J Med.* 1999;340:448–454.
35. Frankenfield DC, Coleman A, Alam S, et al. Analysis of estimation methods for resting metabolic rate in critically ill adults. *J Parenter Enteral Nutr.* 2009;33(1):27–36.
36. McClave SA, Martindale RG, Vanek VW, et al., American Society for Parenteral and Enteral Nutrition (A.S.P.E.N.) Board of Directors, American College of Critical Care Medicine, Society of Critical Care Medicine. Guidelines for the provision and assessment of nutrition support therapy in the adult critically ill patient: Society of Critical Care Medicine (SCCM) and American Society for Parenteral and Enteral Nutrition (A.S.P.E.N.). *J Parenter Enteral Nutr.* 2009;33(1):277–316.
37. Rubinson L, Diette GB, Song X, et al. Low caloric intake is associated with nosocomial bloodstream infections in patients in the medical intensive care unit. *Crit Care Med.* 2004;32:350–357.
38. American Diabetes Association, Bantle JP, Wylie-Rosett J, Albright AL, et al. Nutrition Recommendations and interventions for diabetes: a position statement of the American Diabetes Association. *Diabetes Care.* 2008;31(Suppl 1):S61–S78.
39. Katz MA. Hyperglycemia-induced hyponatremia—calculation of expected serum sodium depression. *N Engl J Med.* 1973;289: 843–844.
40. Franz MJ, Powers MA, Leontos C, et al. The evidence for medical nutrition therapy for type 1 and type 2 diabetes in adults. *J Am Diet Assoc.* 2010;110(12):1852–1889.
41. Franz MJ, Bantle JP, Beebe CA, et al. Evidence-based nutrition principles and recommendations for the treatment and prevention of diabetes and related complications. *Diabetes Care.* 2002;25:148–198.
42. Boucher JL, Swift CS, Franz MJ, et al. Inpatient management of diabetes and hyperglycemia: implications for nutrition practice and the food and nutrition professional. *J Amer Diet Assoc.* 2007;107(1):105–111.

43. Institute of Medicine. *Dietary Reference Intakes: Energy, Carbohydrate, Fiber, Fat, Fatty Acids, Cholesterol, Protein, and Amino Acids.* Washington, DC: National Academies Press; 2002.
44. Vittal H, Farrugia G, Gomez G, et al. Mechanisms of disease: the pathological basis of gastroparesis—a review of experimental and clinical studies. *Nat Clin Pract Gastroenterol Hepatol.* 2007;4:336–346.
45. Ukleja A, Romano M. Complications of parenteral nutrition. *Gastroenterol Clin North Am.* 2007;36:23–46.
46. Vanschoonbeek K, Lansink M, venLaere KM, et al. Slowly digestible carbohydrate sources can be used to attenuate the postprandial glycemic response to the ingestion of diabetes-specific enteral formulas. *Diabetes Educ.* 2009;35(4):631–640.
47. Elia M, Ceriello A, Laube H, et al. Enteral nutrition support and use of diabetes-specific formulas for patients with diabetes. *Diabetes Care.* 2005;28:2267–2279.
48. Pohl M, Mayr P, Mertl-Roetzer M, et al. Glycemic control in patients with type 2 diabetes mellitus with a disease-specific enteral formula: stage 2 of a randomized, controlled multicenter trial. *J Parenter Enteral Nutr.* 2009;33(1):37–49.
49. Alish, CA, Garvey WT, Maki KC, et al. A diabetes-specific enteral formula improves glycemic variability in patients with type 2 diabetes. *Diabetes Technol Ther.* 2010;12(6):419–425.
50. Cheung NW, Napier B, Zaccaria C, et al. Hyperglycemia is associated with adverse outcomes in patients receiving parenteral nutrition. *Diabetes Care.* 2005;28(10):2367–2371.
51. Pasquel FJ, Spiegelman R, McCauley M, et al. Hyperglycemia during parenteral nutrition: an important marker of poor outcome and mortality in hospitalized patients. *Diabetes Care.* 2010;33(4):739–741.
52. McCowen KC, Malhotra A, Bistrain BR. Stress-induced hyperglycemia. *Crit Care Clin.* 2001;17:107–124.
53. American Society for Parenteral and Enteral Nutrition Board of Directors and the Clinical Guidelines Task Force. Guidelines for the use of parenteral and enteral nutrition in adult and pediatric patients. *J Parenter Enteral Nutr.* 2002;26(suppl):1SA–138SA. Errata 2002;26:144.
54. Ahrens CL, Barletta JF, Kanji S, et al. Effect of low-calorie parenteral nutrition on the incidence and severity of hyperglycemia in surgical patients: a randomized, controlled trial. *Crit Care Med.* 2005;33(11):2507–2512.
55. Hirsch IB, Paauw DS. Diabetes management in special situations. *Endocrinol Metab Clin North Amer.* 1997;26:631–645.
56. Kumar PR, Crotty P, Raman M. Hyperglycemia in hospitalized patients receiving parental nutrition is associated with increased morbidity and mortality: a review. *Gastroenterol Res Pract.* 2011; Epub 2010 Aug 3.
57. Robbins JM, Webb DA. Diagnosing diabetes and preventing rehospitalizations: the urban diabetes study. *Med Care.* 2006;44:292–296.
58. Kimmel B, Sullivan MM, Rushakoff RJ. Survey on transition from inpatient to outpatient for patients on insulin: what really goes on at home? *Endocr Pract.* 2010;29:1–23.
59. American Association of Clinical Endocrinologists. *Protocols/Order Sets.* http://resources.aace.com/protocols.asp. Accessed March 3, 2012.

35 Obesity

Ryan T. Hurt, MD, PhD, and Thomas H. Frazier, MD

CONTENTS

Introduction 604
Defining Obesity 604
Obesity Epidemiology 604
Obesity Genetics 605
Environmental Factors 606
Obesity Neuroendocrine Pathophysiology 606
Comorbidities of Obesity 607
The Ambulatory Obese Patient 607
Initial Clinical Evaluation 607
Weight Loss Methods 608
Dieting 608
Physical Activity 609
Behavioral Treatment 609
Pharmacological Treatment 610
Bariatric Surgery 610
Nutrition Assessment of Bariatric Surgery Patients 611
Preoperative Nutrition Assessment 611
Postoperative Nutrition Assessment 611
Early Postoperative Nutrition Care 611
Nutritional Deficiencies 612
The Critically Ill Obese Patient 612
Effect of Obesity on Intensive Care Unit Mortality 612
Impact of Obesity on Critical Care 613
Obesity and Intensive Care Unit Nutritional Assessment 613
Initial Nutritional Assessment 613
Determining Energy Expenditure in Obesity 614
High-Protein Hypocaloric Feeding 614
Protein Requirements 614
The Impact of Obesity on the Delivery of Nutrition 614
Enteral Access 614
Monitoring the Delivery of Nutrition in the Critically Ill Obese Patient 615
Practicality of Enteral Nutrition Delivery 615
References 615

Objectives

1. Define the current classification of overweight and obesity for adults.
2. Determine the treatment options for obese patients in the ambulatory setting.
3. Discuss the role of nutritional support in bariatric surgery patients.
4. Discuss the complexity of nutritional support in obese patients in the intensive care unit (ICU).
5. Determine the optimal enteral nutritional support for obese patients in the ICU.

Test Your Knowledge Questions

1. Which of the following statements regarding the current World Health Organization (WHO) and National Institutes of Health (NIH) classification of overweight and obesity are true?
   A. Overweight is defined as a body mass index (BMI) of 25 to 29.9 kg/m^2, and obesity is defined as BMI $\geq$ 30 kg/m^2.
   B. Obesity is defined as $\geq$ 120% ideal body weight (IBW).
   C. Obesity is defined as body fat $\geq$ 20% of body weight for men and $\geq$ 30% for women.
   D. Obesity is defined as a BMI $>$ 25 kg/m^2, and morbid obesity is defined as a BMI $>$ 30 kg/m^2.
2. Which of the following is a criterion for selecting patients to undergo gastric bypass surgery?
   A. BMI $\geq$ 35 kg/m^2 and no history of substance abuse or psychiatric disorders
   B. BMI $\geq$ 35 kg/m^2 and obesity-associated comorbidities
   C. BMI $\geq$ 30 kg/m^2 and obesity-associated comorbidities
   D. BMI $\geq$ 30 kg/m^2 and inability to achieve weight control with low-calorie diets
3. What is the enteral feeding strategy based on energy requirements for obese patients according to the most recent American Society for Parenteral and Enteral Nutrition (A.S.P.E.N.) and Society of Critical Care Medicine Guidelines?
   A. Hypocaloric with normal protein
   B. Hypocaloric with low protein
   C. Hypocaloric with high protein
   D. Hypercaloric with high protein
4. What is the most accurate way of determining energy requirements for obese patients in the ICU requiring enteral nutrition (EN) support?
   A. The Harris-Benedict equation
   B. Indirect calorimetry (IC)
   C. The Mifflin equation
   D. The Penn State equation

Test Your Knowledge Answers

1. The correct answer is **A**. Overweight and obesity in adults are now classified by use of the BMI, in contrast to prior use of IBW or percent body fat. Use of the BMI is encouraged because it provides a standardized method for expressing weight relatively independent of height, and correlates reasonably well with body fat as well as mortality. Although BMI does not always accurately reflect excess body fat (ie, when ascites or edema is present), it represents a simple and reproducible method for categorizing weight.
2. The correct answer is **B**. Patients are candidates for gastric bypass surgery if BMI $\geq$ 40 kg/m^2, or if BMI is $\geq$ 35 kg/m^2 along with weight-related comorbidities, and if more conservative efforts have not resulted in adequate weight control. Weight-related comorbid conditions need not be present for consideration of surgery; indeed, some advocates of surgical treatment suggest that surgery is best performed before lasting health problems or surgical risks are present. Those with active bulimia, active substance abuse, or major disturbances of thought or mood should be evaluated carefully and treatment instituted before surgery.
3. The correct answer is **C**. High-protein hypocaloric feeding has been recommended (Grade D) by the most recent guidelines from the Society of Critical Care Medicine and A.S.P.E.N. The guidelines suggest that for obese patients (BMI $>$ 30 kg/m^2), the goal of the EN regimen should not exceed 60% to 70% of target energy requirements. Protein requirements for patients with class I and II obesity may be estimated by the equation 2.0 g/kg IBW/d, and for patients with Class III, 2.5 g/kg IBW/d.
4. The correct answer is **B**. While the use of predictive equations (Harris-Benedict, Penn State, and Mifflin) have been widely utilized for predicting resting metabolic rate, most predictive equations were validated in patients without extremes of weight or age. Overestimation of total energy requirements when using actual body weight (ABW) and underestimation when using the IBW leads to inadvertent overfeeding and underfeeding, respectively. Attempting to account for altered body composition with these equations by using corrections for ABW has led to even more confusion. For these reasons, when available, IC should be used for determining the energy requirements of the critically ill obese patient.

Introduction

Obesity is becoming the leading cause of preventable death in the United States. The incidence of obesity in adults in the United States has doubled over the past 30 years. Approximately 70% of adults in the United States are considered overweight or obese.[1,2] A conservative estimate would place the overall health care burden for obesity at approximately 150 billion U.S. dollars per year.[2,3] In addition, it is quickly emerging as a global epidemic that is having worldwide health consequences. Obesity has over 60 associated comorbid medical conditions including 12 different types of cancer.[4] These associated medical conditions, such as type 2 diabetes mellitus, hypertension, coronary artery disease, nonalcoholic fatty liver disease (NAFLD), and obstructive sleep apnea, can complicate management in both the ambulatory and the ICU settings for obese patients. Both clinical settings present unique challenges for nutriton specialists treating obesity and its associated comorbidities.

Defining Obesity

The WHO and NIH classify obesity using the BMI. The recommended classifications are as follows: underweight BMI $\leq$ 18.49 kg/m^2, normal weight BMI $\geq$ 18.5 to 24.9 kg/m^2, overweight BMI $\geq$ 25.0 to 29.9 kg/m^2, obesity class I BMI $\geq$ 30 to 34.9 kg/m^2, obesity class II BMI $\geq$ 35 to 39.9 kg/m^2, and obesity class III BMI $\geq$ 40 kg/m^2.[5] Furthermore, class III obesity has been referred to as morbid, severe, extreme, and super obesity (Table 35-1).

Obesity Epidemiology

The number of overweight and obese adults has steadily increased in the past 30 years.[2,6,7] U.S. adults classified as obese or overweight has risen from 45% in 1962 to 66% in 2004.[2,6,7]

TABLE 35-1 Classifications for Obesity by BMI

- Underweight: BMI < 18. 5 kg/m²
- Normal weight: BMI ≥ 18.5 to 24.9 kg/m²
- Overweight: BMI ≥ 25.0 to 29.9 kg/m²
- Obesity: BMI ≥ 30 kg/m²
- Severe obesity: BMI ≥ 40
- Super obesity: BMI ≥ 50
- Obesity class I: BMI of 30.0 to 34.9 kg/m²
- Obesity class II: BMI of 35.0 to 39.9 kg/m²
- Obesity class III: BMI ≥ 40 kg/m²

The recommended classifications for body mass index as adopted by the World Health Organization, National Institutes of Health, and numerous professional societies. Class III obesity is often referred to as severe, extreme, or morbid obesity.

The number of overweight (but not obese) individuals has remained relatively stable over the same time period.[2] There was a rapid rise in the prevalence of obesity between 1980 and 2004 (15% to 33% of the population), doubling the prevalence in only 25 years.[2] There is some data to suggest that the increasing prevalence of overweight and obesity has leveled off in the past few years.[6] This could lead to the conclusion that the epidemic is stabilizing. However, one needs to consider that with 67% of the adult population being classified as overweight or obese, there is a limited number of individuals left to be afflicted. Furthermore, recent animal and human evidence involving the genetics of obesity suggest that a proportion of the population may be resistant to obesity and its related complications.[8,9]

Despite the overall leveling off of the overall prevalence of obesity, there has been a disproportionate increase in obesity class III. The percentage of adults classified with obesity class III (BMI ≥ 40 kg/m²) increased from 0.9% in 1960 to 5.1% in 2004.[2] Within the obesity class III, the percentage of individuals with a BMI ≥ 50 are increasing at greater rate than all other obesity groups. There are now approximately 1.5 million adults in the United States with a BMI ≥ 50 kg/m².

Obesity is not just a problem limited to the United States but clearly is a global epidemic. The WHO has recognized the increased worldwide prevalence of obesity and the global implications caused by this trend. Obesity and overweight are among the top 10 leading causes of global mortality.[10] The majority of countries in North America, Central America, South America, Western Europe, the Middle East, and Eastern Europe report a combined prevalence of overweight (BMI ≥ 25.0 to 29.9 kg/m²) and obesity (BMI ≥ 30 kg/m²) at 40% or greater of the population aged 45 to 59 years.[11] Asian countries have reported lower rates of obesity using the WHO classification, but the use of BMI to make this classification may be problematic due to cultural and ethnic variability in the relationship between BMI and the amount of body fat as well as adipose distribution.[12] In these Asian countries, rates of type 2 diabetes mellitus and cardiovascular disease are increased at BMIs less than the WHO cutoff for overweight (BMI ≥ 25 kg/m²), which is most likely due to proportionate increases in body fat percentage compared to other ethnicities and races.[13,14]

Obesity Genetics

The variation in prevalence of obesity observed between different races suggests a genetic role. There are many diseases and medical conditions that are complex and involve interplay between genetic, developmental, environmental, and behavioral factors. The most commonly recognized heterogeneous disease is cancer. There are many different types of cancer, different environmental influences, various mechanisms of action, and variable response to a wide range of treatments. Like cancer, obesity is a complex heterogeneous disease that is associated with many conditions and involves numerous subtypes. Obese individuals have combinations of associated conditions such as diabetes, atherosclerosis, hypertension, hyperlipidemia, and obstructive sleep apnea, to name only a few. Where obese individuals carry the extra adiposity, such as around the abdomen, hips, buttocks, and organs, is highly variable. Some obese individuals have strong food cravings while others do not, suggesting differences in the neuroendocrine control over appetite regulation.[15,16] It is this complex, heterogeneous nature of obesity that makes finding treatments difficult and often frustating for health care professionals and patients alike. Interactions between gene environment and gene behavior are critical to understanding the heterogeneity of obesity and developing potential targeted therapies.[17,18]

There are a number of rare monogenic causes of obesity including 25 genetic syndromes such as Prader Willi and Alstrom, which have obesity as a central feature of the disorder.[19] Furthermore, there are a number of mutations in genes that cause nonsyndromic monogenic forms of obesity.[19,20] These mutations are located in genes which affect leptin (*LEP*) and leptin receptors (*LEPR*) and hypothalamic *POMC* and melanocortin-4 receptor gene (*MC4R*).[20] Mutations in these genes have been well studied in rodent models, and the phenotypes compared to humans are similar in the majority of cases.[19] Leptin defeciency has had successful directed therapy, specifically recombinant leptin.[20] In children treated with recombinant leptin, food ingestion ceased to be the focus of daily activity, and weight loss was significant. These monogenic diseases are only a small fraction of the obesity cases with most involving variation in multiple genes (polygenic).[21]

Polygenic obesity is the result of a group of a gene variants (alleles) that have an influence on body weight.[21] These polygenic variants presumably account for the vast majority of cases of obesity.[21] There are over 30 polygenic variants currently recognized as potential contributors to weight regulation.[22,23] Recent advances in molecular techniques have provided the tools to perform genome wide association studies (GWASs). These GWASs have a greater ability to detect these polygenic variants and advances in chip technology have made high density single nucleotide polymorphism GWASs possible.[21,22] The first two gene variants to be discovered using GWAS were the *MC4R* and fat mass– and obesity-associated gene (*FTO*).[24,25] A recent GWAS evaluated the combined contribution of *MC4R* and *FTO* in a European population and found the combined polymorphisms were additive in obesity and type 2 diabetes mellitus.[24] A recent

GWAS using single nucleotide polymorphisms of 249,796 subjects correlated with BMI confirmed 14 previous known loci and 18 new loci associated with elevated BMI.[23] There are undoubtedly many genes that have not yet been identified.

Environmental Factors

Genetics alone cannot explain the recent obesity epidemic. Our "obesogenic" environment provides increased opportunities for obtaining low-cost, energy-dense foods and decreased opportunity and need for physical activity. Rather than simply the increased access to food explaining the obesity epidemic, it is likely more to do with the access to energy-dense foods, which has contributed to the increased obesity rates observed over the past 30 years. The genetic predisposition toward obesity combined with the exposure to energy-dense foods could be one of the major driving factors of our current obesity epidemic.[26] Numerous factors have lead to increased availability of energy-dense foods and decreased opportunity for physical activity. A recent large prospective cohort analysis (120,877 patients) over 4 years found that on average participants gained 3.35 pounds. This 4-year weight gain was most associated with intake of potato chips, potatoes, fries, processed meats, and sugar-sweetened beverages based on daily servings. Vegetables, fruits, nuts, whole grains, and yogurt and increased physical activity were inversely associated with weight gain.[27] Energy-dense foods, such as potato chips, potatoes, fries, processed meats, and sugar-sweetened beverages, provide empty calories with little nutritional value. Food additives such as high fructose corn syrup and trans-fatty acids have been linked with obesity-associated conditions such as metabolic syndrome, dyslipidemia, and NAFLD.[28–32] There is much debate about the role of these additives in the development of the obesity epidemic, and clinicians should focus on overall reduction of fats and excess sugars from diets.[33–44]

The other major component of the obesogenic environment is decreased physical activity. Self-reported levels of physical activity were compared to weight change after 10 years.[45] Individuals who reported low physical activity at the follow-up (10 years) were more likely to have had a major weight gain (> 13 kg) than other individuals who reported medium or high levels of physical activity.[45] A prospective study measured 24-hour energy expenditure and subsequent weight gain in 95 adult subjects.[46] Subjects with low 24-hour energy expenditure (200 kcal below predicted values) were four times more likely to gain significant weight (≥ 7.5 kg) than subjects with high 24-hour energy expenditure (200 kcal above predicted values) over a 2-year period.[46] These studies support the notion that the recent obesogenic environment (including energy-dense food and decreased physical activity) combined with the genetic predisposition to develop obesity have been major factors in the obesity epidemic.

Obesity Neuroendocrine Pathophysiology

The pathophysiology of obesity is complex due in large part to the heterogeneous nature of the disease. The laws of thermodynamics as applied to obesity dictate that energy intake be increased over energy expenditure to increase body fat. However, solely depending on this explanation for obesity does not account for the complex interplay between the central nervous system (CNS) and metabolically active organs that allow humans to regulate energy intake and expenditure. A recent prospective study of 50 obese nondiabetic adults participating in a low-calorie diet program over 10 weeks highlights this point.[47] At baseline, 10 weeks (after the diet was complete), and 62 weeks, serum levels of a number of adipokines (leptin, ghrelin, peptide YY, cholecystokinin [CCK]) and insulin were measured. After the initial average weight loss of 13.5 kg, there was a shift in the neuroendocrine response from these adipokines and insulin that would promote hunger. This neuroendocrine respone persisted at 62 weeks and corresponded with increased subjective hunger scores. In addition, subjects gained an average of 5 kg at 62 weeks. The authors concluded that weight relapse had a strong neuroendocrine basis and was not the result of simply resuming bad habits.[47] In addition to the neuroendocrine response, obesity-induced inflammation and its metablic consequences (eg, NAFLD, type 2 diabetes mellitus, dyslipidemia, etc.) further complicates our understanding of obesity and its treatment and consequences.

The CNS recieves information from several regulatory loops that help control energy balance.[15,16] The brain gets information about metabolic need from the most metabolically active tissues including adipose, liver, stomach, muscle, and bone. Furthermore, the CNS gets information about current energy availability in the environment through our sensory organs and primarily through the stomach, small intestine, pancreas, and liver.

Central controls influence food intake, and energy expenditure can be divided into satiation/satiety signals and "adiposity" hormones.[16] Satiaiton/satiety signals such as CCK, ghrelin, peptide YY, and glucagon-like peptide-1 (GLP-1) result in feelings of fullness, which contribute to cessation of food intake (satiation) and/or suppression of appetite after meal intake (satiety).[16] "Adiposity" hormones are secreted not in response to a meal, but instead as a result of the amount of adipose tissue present in the host organism. Both satiety/satiation signals and adiposity hormones represent a complex messaging system between the CNS and peripheral nervous system that influence energy homeostasis and intake. In addition to the aforementioned mechanisms, many of these molecules (eg, leptin) are also important to the maladaptive obesity-induced inflammation and its resultant complications.[48]

As macronutrients are consumed, a number of these satiety/satiation signals result in a message delivered to the CNS. CCK is secreted from I cells (mucosal epitheilal cells in the small intestine) in response to fat and protein as they pass into the duodenum. CCK then influences a number of gastrointestinal mechanisms such as motility, gastic acid secretion, pancreatic enzyme secretion, and contraction of the gallbladder.[49] Satiation signaling, however, is produced by CCK through a paracrine mechanism via vagal sensory nerves.[50] These signals are relayed to the dorsalmedial hindbrain and result in CCK-induced satiation.[51]

Another satiation signal, peptide YY, is released by intestinal L cells lining the distal small intestine and colon.[52] Peptide YY is released in response to meals and serum levels rise rapidly even before the meal reaches the distal small intestine or colon, suggesting an indirect neuronal reflex.[53,54] Subsequent sustained circulating levels of peptide YY is thought to be by direct stimulation of L cells by dietary fat.[55] The anorexigenic activity of peptide YY has been attributed to the expression of neuropeptide Y_2 receptors in neurons of the arcuate nucleus in the hypothalamus.[52,56] In addition, peptite YY can decrease motility and influence electrolyte absorption in the colon.[57]

In opposition to CCK and peptide YY, ghrelin is a potent orexigen that stimulates food intake.[58] In response to fasting, specific endocrine cells in the stomach and duodenum release ghrelin, which appears to have several actions including acting directly on receptors in the hypothalamus to increase hunger. Actions in the hypothalamus then result in compensatory stimulation of appetite.[58,59] Another major effect of ghrelin is its stimulation of growth hormone release.[60] Following diet and exercise-induced weight loss, serum concentrations of ghrelin increase.[61,62] These compensatory changes may partially explain the difficulty in maintaining long-term weight loss.

Intestinal I cells located predominantly in the ileum and colon are triggered to produce GLP-1. While our understanding of this process is not complete, there appears to be neural, nutrient, and endocrine control of GLP-1 release.[63] The peripheral actions of GLP-1 are numerous and include stimulation of insulin release, glucagon secretion inhibition, inhibition of gastrointestinal motility and secretions, anorectic actions, and others. Central actions of GLP-1 include reducing food intake via caloric homeostatic circuits in the hypothalamus and eliciting symptoms of stress in the amygdala.[64–67] The satiation actions of GLP-1 stemming from the variety of aforementioned mechanisms has been seen in both animal models and human studies.[64,68,69] These actions are further demonstrated with long-acting GLP-1 pharmacotherapy for diabetes mellitus, which results in not only improvement in glucose control, but can also result in meaningful weight loss.[70] Several other satiation/satiety signalling molecules, such as glicentin, GLP-2, glucagon, and enterostatin, have recently been described.[15] While satiation signals are dependant on the intake of nutrients, "adiposity" signals are directly related to the amount of body fat present in the host organism.[15] As a result of these contrasting control mechanisms, satiation signalling is a phasic response while "adiposity" signaling is a tonic phenomenon. Both insulin and leptin are classically recognized as "adiposity" signals.[15] Pancreatic beta cells and white adipose tissue release insulin and leptin, respectively, in response to the amount of body fat present. These hormones then act centrally on the hypothalamus to influence energy homeostasis resulting in decreased food intake and weight loss. Confounding the use of hormones like leptin for the treatment of obesity is the development of resistance, as well as their multiple, often intolerable actions that are not directly related to weight loss.[15] In addition to controlling appetite, leptin also plays a role in both innate and adaptive inflammatory responses. Leptin has been shown to increase the production of proinflammatory cytokines from macrophages.[48] The neuroendocrine pathophysiology is complex, incompletely understood, and further complicated when the over 60 recognized obesity-associated conditions are considered.

Comorbidities of Obesity

There are a large number of diseases and comorbid conditions associated with obesity. These associated conditions are responsible for the increased morbidity and mortality in obese individuals.[44,71,72] Numerous large epidemiologic studies have found that obesity is associated with increased all-cause mortality.[71,72] Obesity is associated with cause-specific mortality including ischemic heart disease, diabetes, and respiratory disease.[73] In the Prospective Studies Collaboration, 57 prospective studies with approximately 900,000 subjects were analyzed for all-cause and cause-specific mortality according to BMI.[73] All-cause mortality was increased by appromiately 30% in obese subjects compared to normal-weight individuals.[73] Cause-specific mortality for increased BMI included 40% for vascular mortality; 60% to 120% for diabetic, renal, and hepatic mortality; and 20% for respiratory causes.[73] Obesity class I subjects had a reduction of median survival by 2 to 4 years. Obesity class III subjects had a reduction of median survival by 8 to 10 years, which is a similar reduction of median survival observed in smokers.[73] Furthermore, there are at least 12 types of cancers that are associated with obesity including postmenopausal breast cancer, colon, esophageal, and renal.[72]

The Ambulatory Obese Patient

Initial Clinical Evaluation

The initial steps in diagnosing and treating an overweight or obese patient are to calculate BMI, measure waist circumference, and classify the patient's status. Further assessment of obesity should address the presence of comorbid conditions such as cardiovascular disease, hypertension, dyslipidemia, and sleep apnea, as well as tobacco abuse. Patients who are classified as obese, or as overweight with increased waist circumference ($>$ 89 cm for women, $>$102 cm for men) and have two or more risk factors for cardiovascular disease or diabetes, are candidates for weight loss. Overweight patients without associated risk are also candidates for weight loss if they are motivated, while those who are not motivated to lose weight can be counseled to maintain weight. Motivation is important to assess because patients sometimes request obesity treatment because of family or health care provider concern rather than self-motivation.

The goal of obesity treatment is to achieve and sustain weight loss and to reduce health risk. A reasonable initial goal is loss of 10% of initial weight over 6 months. The rationale for this recommendation is based on multiple trials of weight loss, which demonstrate that an average loss of 6% to 8% is achieved over approximately 6 months, after which loss becomes more difficult.[74] Greater amounts of initial weight loss are possible, but they are less likely to be sustained. After a 10% loss is achieved, efforts should be focused on maintenance of lost weight. If more than 10% weight loss is desired, after a 6-month period of weight maintenance motivated patients can then restart losing weight.

Many patients will have weight loss goals higher than 10% and may want to achieve their goal in less than 6 months. These goals are often unrealistic and may lead to failed attempts at long-term weight loss. Patients should be counseled about the benefits of smaller amounts of weight loss that are realistic to maintain. Modest weight loss (eg, 5% to 15%) improves glucose tolerance, decreases fasting blood sugar and hyperinsulinemia, improves serum lipid concentrations, reduces blood pressure, and improves sleep apnea.[75–78] Slow weight loss is more likely to promote development of skills that improve long-term weight maintenance, while rapid weight loss is less likely to be maintained. Repeated cycles of weight loss and gain are associated with negative health and psychological effects and lost effort, time, and expense of repeated loss and gain further justify modest loss and maintenance.[74,79] Furthermore, recidivism and cycling of weight loss with weight gain may alter body composition, ultimately decreasing lean body mass and increasing body fat mass.

Weight Loss Methods

An essential part of weight loss is negative energy balance: energy expenditure exceeds energy intake. Thus, effective weight loss strategies must address decreasing intake of food, increasing the output of energy, or both. There are a number of other factors that are involved in effective weight loss, including behavioral factors. Combining behavior strategies with decreased intake of food and increased activity will lead to the most effective weight loss strategy. This combined strategy is called lifestyle intervention and has been used successfully in patients with diabetes and obese patients.[80–82]

Dieting

Diets popularly promoted for weight loss number in the hundreds or more, and Americans spend close to $40 billion annually on weight loss products.[83] No specific body weight reduction strategy has consistently been shown to both safely reduce weight and to result in long-term maintenance for most participants. Negative energy balance induced by decreases in intake will reduce weight regardless of the composition of the diet, and differences in lost weight and body composition between diets are generally small compared to the overall effect of reducing intake.[84] In a recent study, 811 overweight and obese subjects were randomized to one of four caloric reduction strategies that varied in percentages of energy derived from fat, protein, and carbohydrates for 2 years. After 6 months, participants' weight loss was not different in the groups. The average weight loss at 2 years was 4 kg, and measurements of satiety, hunger, and satisfaction with the diet were the same for the four groups.[84] This study emphasizes the importance of reduced calorie consumption to help create a negative energy balance regardless of diet strategy and macronutrient composition used.

Energy intake to a lower limit of 800 kcal/d is considered a low-calorie diet, while intake below that level is considered a very-low-calorie diet. Weight loss on a low-calorie diet is typically 0.5 to 1 kg/wk, although the relationship between level of energy intake and actual weight lost depends on a number of factors, including the degree of obesity, level of activity, gender, and age. Most obese patients will lose weight when consuming between 1000 and 1500 kcal/d.[85] The ideal macronutrient composition and meal pattern of a low-calorie diet remains controversial. Limiting dietary fat without also decreasing energy intake is unlikely to achieve weight loss. There is no scientific evidence to warrant recommendation that low calorie diets routinely be very low in fat (< 20% of energy), very low in carbohydrate (< 100 g/d), or very high in protein (> 130 g/d). There have been a number of studies demonstrating minor differences in weight loss in contrasting diets (variable carbohydrate and fat content) at 6 months, but no significant weight differences at 12 to 24 months.[86,87]

Diets can be structured around portion size, calories or fat, or by use of other constructs. Structuring a diet and lifestyle plan must be a joint effort between patient and clinician. An inflexible, clinician-driven plan that is not developed with consideration of the patient's lifestyle and intellectual capacity may result in short-term loss but is unlikely to be effective long-term. Low-calorie diets offer the advantage of sustainability over longer periods of time and can be adapted to a wide range of lifestyles. Low-calorie diets based on commonly consumed foods are advantageous to specialized or commercial diets because they are less expensive and easily obtained. However, commercial plans and prepared foods may offer structure and convenience, decrease the need for planning, and limit choice in high-risk situations. Energy intake on a low-calorie diet is theoretically at a level where food consumed can provide adequate micronutrients without need for supplementation. However, consumption of micronutrient-rich foods may vary, and because micronutrient reference intakes are not established for those who are consuming hypocaloric diets, it is reasonable to recommend a standard multivitamin. Calcium supplementation may be necessary for individuals consuming few dairy products. Medical monitoring of patients on low-calorie diets is minimal because the rate of weight loss and diet quality do not predispose to serious complications. Patients on medications for hypertension, diabetes, and other conditions should be monitored to assess the need for medication adjustments with reduced energy intake and weight loss.

Very-low-calorie diets typically contain 400 to 800 kcal/d, but below 800 kcal/d little additional weight is lost perhaps because of diminished compliance and/or from decreased resting energy expenditure. Protein intake usually ranges from 70 to 100 g/d. Very-low-calorie diets can be based on liquid products or on consumption of lean meat, fish, or poultry supplemented with micronutrients. Weight losses are in the range of 2 kg/wk. Weight lost by very-low-calorie diets is more rapid and can be greater over time than that achieved by low-calorie diets. Long-term maintenance of weight lost by very-low-calorie diets has not been superior to that of low-calorie diets,[88] although a meta-analysis suggested that there may be modest long-term advantage following very-low-calorie diets.[89] Medical monitoring (preferably weekly and not less frequently than every 2 weeks) is necessary because of risks of electrolyte abnormalities, dehydration, gallstone formation, cardiac arrhythmia, and other complications.[88]

Because low-calorie diets promote a similar longer-term outcome without the health risks and necessary monitoring of very-low-calorie diets, low-calorie diets are preferred for most patients. There are, however, several circumstances in which a very-low-calorie diet might be considered. Poorly controlled comorbid conditions may respond favorably to a period of rapid weight loss. Patients who are unable to achieve weight goals on a low-calorie-diet may benefit from a very-low-calorie diet, perhaps because of the increased structure of the diet and frequency of clinical monitoring, which both promote compliance. Weight loss before semielective or elective surgery is often recommended to reduce postoperative morbidity, and a very-low-calorie diet can be considered if a 10% reduction over 6 months is not inconsistent with need for surgery.[90–92]

Physical Activity

Physical activity expends energy, promotes a sense of well-being, maintains or increases lean body mass, and improves several obesity-related comorbid conditions. However, increasing physical activity is unlikely to result in significant weight loss without a concomitant decrease in energy intake. A meta-analysis of weight loss trials suggests that when exercise is added to hypocaloric diets, there has not been significantly more weight lost than with diet alone.[93] However, exercising during weight loss does promote preservation of lean mass.[94]

Probably the greatest role increased physical activity plays in obese patients undergoing lifestyle intervention is the prevention of weight gain after successful weight loss from dieting and the maintenance of lean body mass. A meta-analysis examined the role of exercise, exercise plus diet, and diet alone on weight gain.[95] Over the course of 15 weeks, weight loss in the exercise only group was 2.9 kg, compared to the diet only group who experienced weight loss of 10.7 kg. The weight loss that occurred by combining diet with exercise was not significantly different from that seen with diet alone. At 1-year follow-up, however, the diet plus exercise group (mean 8.6 ± 0.8 kg total weight lost) had maintained the weight loss better than the diet only group (6.6 ± 0.5 kg).[95] Other studies have confirmed that use of exercise alone usually incurs only a small amount of weight loss and that its more important role is maintaining the weight loss after a successful diet program.[96,97]

A plea for patients to increase activity without specific objectives is often met with little and short-lived success. Thus, a realistic and detailed exercise prescription is often useful. It is important to start very slowly, with consideration of the patient's existing capacity for activity. For example, those with a BMI exceeding 40 kg/m^2 may have severely limited capacities and may experience fatigue dyspnea or joint pain after walking very short distances. For such persons, increasing the frequency of small amounts of physical activity, frequent breaks, and finding creative ways to promote movement are necessary. Creative exercise regimens include chair exercises, water aerobics, and walking in the shallow end of a pool, all of which facilitate exercise among those with pain in weight-bearing joints.

Structured exercise programs offer education, some degree of supervision, and a social environment. However, time constraints, cost, and other factors often discourage patients from participation in structured programs. Two recent trials have evaluated the effects of structured exercise compared to increases in lifestyle-based activity and have reported that both interventions were associated with comparable beneficial effects on blood pressure, blood lipids, and fitness.[98,99] Thus, patients who do not participate in structured exercise should be encouraged to incorporate increase physical activity during lifestyle intervention.

Behavioral Treatment

Eating and exercising are ultimately behaviors. Many patients have excellent knowledge of good dietary choices and the need for activity, and yet cannot put this knowledge into practice. Several trials have demonstrated that behavioral treatment increases efficacy of dietary as well as pharmacological interventions.[80,100] The first step in behavioral treatment is to set realistic goals for the proposed lifestyle intervention (eg, 5% to 10% of initial weight in the first year). A specific date for the initiation of lifestyle intervention should be set. Helping the patient realize that his or her excessive weight has been gained over a period of years in most cases and will take extended time and commitment to lose may help prevent unrealistic weight loss expectations. Despite these discussions at the beginning of lifestyle intervention, many patients still have unrealistic expectations. In a trial of sibutramine, 53 obese subjects were told they could expect to lose 5% to 15% of initial weight in the first year.[101] Despite being told this, subjects expected to lose 28% of initial weight, and this unrealistic weight loss expectation persisted during the trial. Patients who do not meet their expectations during lifestyle intervention may often be frustrated and discouraged from future interventions.

Subsequent behavioral treatment focuses on several key issues including self-monitoring, stimulus control, and relapse prevention.[81] Self-monitoring is necessary to identify maladaptive behaviors and to elevate the patient's level of consciousness about behaviors. The use of food diaries and activity records should be part of behavioral treatment. Patients should record everything they eat, noting the calories and situations in which they are eating. There are numerous applications for cellular phones that make these tasks simple. Stimulus control refers to identifying and restructuring environmental factors (such as television, phones, and reading materials) leading to maladaptive behavior and providing alternative responses to these stimuli. Patients should be encouraged to turn off the television and phone during meal time. Placing fresh fruits, vegetables, and low-calorie foods in prominent positions such as the front of the refrigerator or counter can help control stimuli that contribute to overeating. Relapse control entails development of strategies to prevent relapse or limit the extent of relapse when it occurs. Frequent reinforcement of the lifestyle intervention and encouragement from the clinician can help when relapse occurs.[81]

A recent randomized controlled trial of 390 obese adults demonstrated that enhanced lifestyle intervention helped approximately one-third of the subjects maintain meaningful weight loss at 2 years.[102] The enhanced lifestyle consisted of quarterly primary care physician visits combined with brief monthly sessions with lifestyle coaches who instructed participants about behavioral weight control. In addition, patients were given meal replacements or weight loss medications (orlistat or sibutramine). Enhanced lifestyle counseling was superior to usual care in both short- and long-term weight loss. Behavioral treatment can be provided to individual patients (as in the previous example) or in groups, the latter of which may be more cost-effective and provide additional social support.

Pharmacological Treatment

All individuals should initially attempt to decrease weight by nonpharmacological means. Those who do not achieve weight goals may then be considered for addition of medication to diet and lifestyle changes. Drug therapy can be considered in those with a BMI ≥ 30 kg/m² or in those with existing comorbid conditions and BMI ≥ 27 kg/m².[103] These criteria reflect the increased risk of weight-related disease associated with these levels of BMI.

Medications currently available for the treatment of obesity have been shown to have a favorable impact on loss of weight and to assist in maintenance of lost weight. The benefits of medications on weight change include greater average losses, greater maintenance of lost weight, and increased proportions of patients able to achieve weight losses of 5%, 10%, or ≥ 15% of initial weight. Drug use may augment weight loss in partial responders to dietary and lifestyle intervention, or rend responders from otherwise nonresponders. Medications do not generally alter weight loss goals, which remain at 5% to 10% of initial weight. Patients need to understand that medications will serve only as an adjunct to dietary and lifestyle changes.

Currently the only long-term (≥ 12 weeks) pharmacotherapy approved by the U.S. Food and Drug Administration (FDA) for weight loss is orlistat. Orlistat is a gastrointestinal lipase inhibitor that prevents absorption of dietary triglycerides and eventual utilization of free fatty acids. This causes gastrointestinal side effects such as flatus, loose stools, and fecal incontinence, which can lead to poor patient compliance. Orlistat is available in both prescription and over-the-counter formulas. There have been five randomized, double-blinded, placebo trials that demonstrated long-term effects (2 to 4 years) on weight loss in obese subjects.[104-108] A recent meta-analysis demonstrated an average weight loss of 2.89 kg at 12 months compared to placebo.[109] The other long-term weight loss drug sibutramine was removed from the market in 2010 because of cardiovascular concerns.[110] Because of poor tolerance and the cost is often not covered by insurance, the overall impact of orlistat on weight loss is minimal.

Phentermine has been approved for short-term weight loss (≤ 12 weeks) and was half of the medication phentermine-fenfluramine, which was removed from the market because of cardiovascular side effects. Unlike fenfluramine, phentermine has not been shown to damage heart valves.[103] Phentermine is an adrenergic agent that promotes weight loss by activation of the sympathetic nervous system to increase resting energy expenditure and decrease food intake. This sympathetic activation can lead to tachycardia and high blood pressure, and use in patients with cardiovascular conditions including hypertension should be cautioned. A recent meta-analysis demonstrated a 3.6 kg weight loss at 6 months for phentermine compared to placebo.[109]

A number of other pharmacological agents have been shown to be associated with significant weight loss when used for other indications. The antidepressants bupropion and fluoxetine have been shown to have modest but significant weight loss. When bupropion is combined with naltrexone, weight loss is greater than the single agents alone.[111] This combination has not been FDA approved for weight loss in obesity. Metformin, exenatide, pramlintide, and liraglutide are associated with weight loss in obese patients with type 2 diabetes mellitus.[103] The seizure medications topiramate and zonisamide have been associated with mild to moderate weight loss.[103] There are a number of dietary supplements given in pharmacological doses (pharmaconutrition) that have been associated with weight loss. Some examples include green tea, L-carnitine, L-arginine, L-leucine, soy and whey protein, and St. John's wort.[48,112,113] Because most of these agents have not been shown to produce long-term meaningful (greater than 5% of baseline) weight loss, and long-term safety has not been assessed, we do not recommend their routine use in the ambulatory obese patient. Nutrition specialists should review all supplements used for weight loss, counsel the patient on potential risks, and dispel the purported claims of such agents.

Bariatric Surgery

To be considered for bariatric surgery, patients must have a BMI > 40 kg/m², or have a BMI > 35 kg/m² and suffer from one or more severe obesity-associated comorbidities such as type 2 diabetes mellitus, obstructive sleep apnea, cardiomyopathy, NAFLD, or severe joint disease (Table 35-2).[114,115] This guideline was given a grade A recommendation in the recent perioperative guidelines approved by the American Association of Clinical Endocrinologists, The Obesity Society, and the American Society for Metabolic and Bariatric Surgery.[115] In early 2011, the FDA approved expanding the indication for laparoscopic adjustable gastric band (LAGB) to patients with a BMI between 30 to 35 kg/m² and at the highest risk of obesity-related complications, although medical societies have not given recommendations as of yet. In addition, all potential candidates should have demonstrated repeated failure to control weight by medical means including supervised lifestyle intervention programs. Patients should be acceptable surgical candidates and well informed of the risks of surgery.

Surgical treatment for intractable extreme obesity has dramatically increased in frequency. Since its inception over five

TABLE 35-2 Indications and Contraindications of Surgical Management of Obesity.[114]

Indications for Surgical Management of Obesity

- Be well motivated
- Failed numerous lifestyle interventions for weight loss
- Appropriate Surgical Candidate
- BMI >40 kg/m²
- or have a BMI >35 kg/m² with comorbidities such as DM2, OSA, cardiomyopathy

Contraindications for Surgical Management of Obesity

- Binge eating disorders
- Untreated depression
- Inability to comply with postoperative care
- Inappropriate surgical candidate (including severe cardiovascular disease)

decades ago, a number of surgical procedures have been developed to promote weight loss. The choice of which procedure is best for patients should be based on risk and full disclosure to the patient. Most bariatric surgery is now performed laparoscopically to minimize wound complications, postoperative pain, and recovery time. The most commonly performed procedures are the Roux-en-Y-gastric bypass (RYGB) and the LAGB.[115]

The LAGB is a gastric restrictive procedure that produces early satiety and limits food intake.[115] The band is positioned on the upper stomach, just below the gastroesophageal junction, where it limits food intake by constricting the stomach to a shape similar to an hourglass. The upper chamber is a 15- to 20-mL gastric pouch. Short-term complications (overall complication rate $< 10\%$) are rare but include band slippage, erosion, balloon failure, port malposition, and band infections.[116] LAGB is associated with better weight loss maintenance than lifestyle intervention alone.[115] A recent study evaluated the long-term complications with LAGB in 317 obese adults.[117] The failure rate increased from 13.2% at 18 months to 36.9% at 7 years. Approximately 22% of patients required major reoperation (band removal) at some point during the 7-year study.[117] In addition, only 43% of patients had weight loss of $> 50\%$ during 7 years.[117]

The RYGB is the most common type of bariatric surgery in the United States (approximately 80%).[115] The weight loss associated with RYGB is greater than that achieved by restrictive procedures such as LAGB. In RYGB, the upper portion of the stomach is transected and small proximal gastric pouch is created. The gastric pouch is connected to a proximal jejunum segment (Roux-en-Y), bypassing the rest of the stomach, duodenum, and a portion of the jejunum.[115] Thus, weight loss is accomplished by both restriction and malabsorption. The standard Roux-en-Y limb is approximately 100 cm. The RYGB limits food intake and can induce some nutrient malabsorption. The longer the Roux limbs (as in distal RYGB), the greater the potential for macronutrient malabsorption.[118] RYGB is associated with increased initial hospitalization, perioperative complications, and increased mortality (0.06% for LAGB; 0.17% for RYGB) compared to LAGB.[119]

The biliopancreatic diversion (BPD) also causes weight loss by a combination of gastric restriction and malabsorption.[115] A subtotal gastrectomy is performed and a proximal gastric pouch is created (200 to 500 mL). There is a common channel created using the distal small intestine, which is anastomosed to the gastric remnant and the ileum. This common channel is where the majority of macronutrients and micronutrients are absorbed, thus BPD is a more malabsorptive process. BPD bypasses more bowel and therefore is a more malabsorptive procedure than RYGB. These factors have limited BPD as an option for weight loss. Side effects include steatorrhea, flatus, and metabolic bone disease.[120]

Nutrition Assessment of Bariatric Surgery Patients

Preoperative Nutrition Assessment

Nutrition specialists are often a part of a multidisciplinary team whose goal is to provide comprehensive care to obese patients before and after bariatric surgery. The *NIH Consensus Statement on Bariatric Surgery* recommended utilizing a team approach including physician obesity specialist, bariatric surgeon, psychologist, primary care physician, and nutrition specialist.[121] The preoperative evaluation should include a comprehensive medical history, physical examination, and appropriate laboratory testing.[115] Patient commitment for compliance with follow-up appointments and medical requirements following surgery should be assessed. Patients with uncontrolled severe psychiatric illness or current alcohol or drug abuse should be excluded.[115]

The nutrition specialist should perform a preoperative nutritional assessment including patient's weight history, previous weight loss strategies, alcohol intake, vitamin and supplement use, physical activity, and motivation to make long-term lifestyle modification.[122] The lifestyle modification program should include losing 5% to 10% of preoperative weight in the months prior to surgery. Some studies have shown that patients who lose 5% to 10% of preoperative weight are less likely to have surgical complications, have shorter hospital stays, have reduced need for conversion to open surgical technique, and have improved long-term weight loss.[123–125] A preoperative anesthesia evaluation should follow current guidelines and identify those at increased cardiovascular risk.[126]

Postoperative Nutrition Assessment

Early Postoperative Nutrition Care

Nutrition specialists who are part of a bariatric surgery team should be involved in the postoperative nutrition assessment. In general, bariatric patients are advanced to clear liquids on postoperative day 1. In RYGB and BPD, patients will often undergo a swallow test to evaluate for leaks prior to starting on liquid diet. On postoperative day 3, patients are advanced to full liquids that are protein-rich, noncarbonated, and low in sugar ($\leq$ 15 g per serving).[115] On postoperative days 3 to 10, patients should consume a minimum of 48 to 64 fluid ounces per day ($\geq$ 24 to 32 ounces of clear liquids plus 24 to 32 ounces of full liquids). Potential full liquids include nonfat milk, Lactaid milk, soy milk, light yogurt blended, or plain nonfat yogurt blended. Clear liquids can be increased at 2 to 4 weeks postoperatively to 48 to 64 or more ounces, and full liquids should be replaced with low-fat, high-protein pureed soft solid foods such as eggs, ground lean meats, low-fat cottage cheese, yogurt, and moist fish.[115,125] During this period, patients should be encouraged to eat four to six small meals per day of these protein sources without fluids (waiting 30 minutes after the meals to resume fluid intake) chewing thoroughly prior to swallowing.[115,125] Goal protein should be 60 to 80 g per day and should be consumed first. During weeks 4 to 6 postoperatively, if patients have tolerated the protein foods, then well-cooked soft vegetables or fruit may be added after daily protein goals are met. Fluids are maintained at 48 to 64 oz of clear, noncarbonated, caffeine-free, noncaloric liquids. For week 7 postoperatively and beyond, daily caloric needs should be based on height, weight, and age. A healthy balanced diet of low-fat protein, well-cooked vegetables, fruits, and whole grains should be consumed as part of three meals with two snacks. Rice, bread, and pasta should be avoided until protein goals are met.[115] Fluids should be continued at 48 to 64 oz of clear noncarbonated, caffeine-free, noncaloric liquids. Follow-up with nutrition specialists should be recommended if patients are having difficulty maintaining dietary goals or regain weight.

There are a number of nutritional complications that can arise following bariatric surgery. Vomiting frequently occurs in LAGB patients but is less common in RYGB or BPD patients. Usually, vomiting is due to eating habits such as eating too quickly, not chewing food well enough, or overeating.[127] If vomiting persists despite correcting eating habits, it should be evaluated by the clinician. A rare cause of nausea and vomiting following bariatric surgery is part of the syndrome of acute postgastric reduction surgery neuropathy. Acute postgastric reduction surgery neuropathy is a polynutritional (vitamin B_{12} and/or thiamine deficiency), multisystem disorder characterized by protracted postoperative vomiting, hyporeflexia, and muscular weakness.[128] Stenosis and ulcers (frequently due to nonsteroidal anti-inflammatory drug use) are rare causes of vomiting in RYGB and BPD, and in LAGB patients it can be related to the band being too tight or having eroded.[127] Dumping syndrome is common in the first few months after RYGB because of the inability of the pylorus to regulate gastric emptying of simple carbohydrates. Dumping can occur early (10 to 30 minutes after eating) causing nausea, bloating, abdominal cramps, or explosive diarrhea, or it can occur late (1 to 3 hours after eating) causing flushing, dizziness, or lightheadedness.[125] Most patients experience early dumping, and it responds to reduction of carbohydrate intake, smaller portion sizes, and avoidance of liquids for at least 30 minutes following meals.[125] Other long-term complications that are associated with rapid weight loss following surgery include gallstone formation and NAFLD.

Nutritional Deficiencies

Bariatric surgery can lead to profound protein, macronutrient, and micronutrient deficiencies despite adhering to strict dietary programs.[115] Familiarity of the types of bariatric surgery allow the clinician to anticipate potential nutrition deficiencies that may occur following surgery.[127] Nutritional deficiencies are usually more severe in malabsorptive surgical procedures such as RYGB and BPD.[129] Current recommendations for routine vitamin/mineral supplementation in RYGB and BPD include a standard adult or prenatal multivitamin twice a day, calcium citrate, vitamin D_3, vitamin B_{12}, folic acid, and elemental iron (Table 35-3). LAGB patients should take a multivitamin twice a day, calcium citrate, and vitamin D_3, but do not require routine folic acid, vitamin B_{12}, or iron supplements.[115,125] Fat-soluble deficiencies such as vitamins A, E, and K are rare in RYGB patients who routinely take two multivitamins; however, they are common in BPD patients and replacement may be needed.

The current recommended biochemical surveillance of nutritional status for malabsorptive surgical procedures depend on the surgical procedure (Table 35-4). BPD patients should have the recommended biochemical surveillance every 3 months following surgery during the first year and every 3 to 6 months thereafter. RYGB patients should be followed every 3 to 6 months during the first year and then annually thereafter. Depending on symptoms, bariatric patients should have biochemical evaluation when clinically indicated outside the surveillance schedule.

TABLE 35-3 Nutrient Supplementation after Bariatric Surgery (adapted from Mechanick et al.[115])

Supplement	Dose
Multivitamin	Two daily
Calcium citrate	1200–2000 mg daily
Vitamin D	400–800 IU daily
Folic acid	400 μg daily
Elemental iron (menstruating women)	40–65 mg daily
Vitamin B_{12}	≥ 350 μg po daily or 1000 μg im monthly or 3000 μg im every 6 months

im, intramuscularly; po, by mouth.

TABLE 35-4 Recommended Routine Biochemical Surveillance of Nutritional Status after Bariatric Surgery

BPD	RYGB
CBC	CBC
Electrolytes + glucose	Electrolytes + glucose
Iron studies + ferritin	Iron studies + ferritin
Liver function (ALT, AST)	Liver function (ALT, AST)
Lipid profile	Lipid profile
Vitamin B_{12}	Vitamin B_{12}
25-hydroxyvitamin D	25-hydroxyvitamin D
Intact PTH	Intact PTH (optional)
Thiamine	Thiamine (optional)
Folate	Folate (optional)
Albumin + prealbumin	
Vitamin E	
Vitamin K + INR	
24-hour calcium	
Zinc	
Selenium	

ALT, alanine aminotransferase; AST, aspartate aminotransferase; BPD, biliopancreatic diversion; CBC, complete blood count; INR, international normalized ratio; PTH, parathyroid hormone; RYGB, Roux-en-Y-gastric bypass. Adapted by permission from Macmillan Publishers Ltd. Mechanick JI, Kushner RF, Sugerman HJ, et al. American Association of Clinical Endocrinologists, The Obesity Society, and American Society for Metabolic & Bariatric Surgery medical guidelines for clinical practice for the perioperative nutritional, metabolic, and nonsurgical support of the bariatric surgery patient. *Obesity (Silver Spring)*. Apr 2009;17 Suppl 1:S1-70.

The Critically Ill Obese Patient

Effect of Obesity on Intensive Care Unit Mortality

Obesity in general is associated with increased all-cause mortality.[71,130,131] Furthermore, obesity is also associated with increased cause-specific mortality, as mentioned previously.[73]

However, despite an association with higher Acute Physiology and Chronic Health Evaluation (APACHE) II scores and the increased all-cause and cause-specific mortality, in the ICU, obesity has been associated with improved outcomes. This observation has been made in a number of clinical studies including three meta-analyses.[132–134] The reason for improved ICU outcomes is not clear and appears to be counterintuitive.

A meta-analysis on the effect of obesity in critically ill patients (14 included studies) demonstrated no difference overall in ICU mortality between lean and obese patients. However, ICU length of stay and duration of mechanical ventilation were significantly longer in obese patients compared to nonobese controls.[132] Improved survival was observed in patients with class I and class II obesity, compared to their lean counterparts.[132] A second meta-analysis, which evaluated 22 studies, concluded that there was no significant difference in ICU or hospital mortality between obese patients and normal-weight controls.[133] There were no differences in ICU length of stay or duration of mechanical ventilation. A third meta-analysis found that individuals with a BMI in a range of 30 to 40 kg/m^2 had a lower mortality rate compared to normal-weight controls.[134] ICU length of stay was significantly increased for patients who were underweight or had class III obesity when compared to normal-weight individuals.[134]

There are several potential explanations for the "ICU conundrum." The use of the BMI may not be the best estimate of obesity-associated ICU mortality. For patients with obesity class I and II, waist circumference and presence of central adiposity (which are predictors of visceral adiposity) may be a better anthropometric measure of risk. A recent prospective study in two general ICUs evaluated mortality in obese subjects comparing abdominal adiposity.[135] Subjects with increased abdominal adiposity had higher APACHE II scores and increased mortality compared to obese controls without central adiposity (44% versus 25%, respectively, $p < 0.01$). Furthermore, after adjustment for age and APACHE II scores, abdominal obesity was associated with an increased risk of mortality. BMI > 30 kg/m^2 was not an independent risk factor for increased mortality.[135]

Another limitation to making conclusions about the effect of obesity on mortality based on these meta-analyses is that the three studies failed to differentiate the type of ICU (trauma or surgical versus medical) to which patients were admitted. There appears to be a discrepancy in clinical outcomes between the trauma ICU studies and medical or mixed ICU studies. Those studies with a higher percentage of trauma patients demonstrate an increased hospital or ICU mortality in obese patients compared to normal-weight subjects.[132] Medical ICU studies have shown the opposite trend or no significant differences in mortality.[133] These are different patient populations with different pathophysiological consequences, and thus obesity may impact outcomes differently.[136] The best explanation for the "ICU conundrum" may be that the overall curve for mortality across all categories of BMI is U-shaped. Mortality may be lowest for patients who are overweight or class I or II obesity. Mortality in turn may be higher for underweight individuals (BMI < 20 kg/m^2) and patients with class III obesity.

Impact of Obesity on Critical Care

Regardless of differences in mortality, the presence of obesity in the critically ill patient can present unique challenges to the overall management. The presence of any of the more than 60 comorbidities make assessment and treatment of obese patients difficult, requiring very individualized management. Intubation can oftentimes be difficult because of the large neck circumference and as indicated by the Mallampati score (standard anestheisa airway assessment), especially in obese class III patients.[137] Futhermore, obese class III patients have severely reduced functional residual capacity and heavy noncompliant chest walls, making mechanical ventilation difficult.[138] Placement of central venous and arterial catheters for monitoring and vascular access can be extremely difficult because of the lack of defined anatomical landmarks. Repositioning and mobilizing obese ICU patients is difficult but essential in preventing skin breakdown. Obese patients need specialized beds, lifts, and dedicated teams to move them, to ensure that both staff and patient are protected from injury.

Obesity and Intensive Care Unit Nutritional Assessment

Initial Nutritional Assessment

With the rising prevalence of obesity in the ICU population, health care providers must be prepared to address the specific nutritional needs of these patients. Performance of the initial focused nutritional assessment of the critically ill obese patient should include a detailed history, physical examination, and determination of energy/protein requirements. Although obese patients may have different metabolic responses to stress (obesity-associated inflammation, hyperglycemia, and dyslipidemia) compared to lean patients, it is important to note that the basic principles of ICU care, such as the need for and benefit from early EN, are much the same as in their lean counterparts.[26,139] However, the ability of the health care team to deliver these needs is often adversely affected by the physical and functional limitations induced by obesity.[140] Obese patients admitted to the ICU should have a detailed nutritional assessment performed by a nutrition specialist.

Nutrition assessment of the critically ill obese patient includes evaluating the presence of preexisting protein-calorie malnutrition or micronutrient deficiencies, oral intake prior to hospitalization, recent weight change, and the details of any obesity-related surgeries. In addition, presence, treatment, and control of any preexisting or evolving comorbidities, such as obstructive sleep apnea, cardiovascular disease, type 2 diabetes mellitus, and NAFLD, must be addressed. Finally, recent use of any weight loss pharmacotherapies, including complementary and alternative medicines, should be ascertained.

A thorough physical exam in the obese patient must include accurate measures of BMI and initial and subsequent body weights, which are crucial in determining a patient's protein and energy requirements. Usual body weight and IBW should be determined. Abnormalities discovered on a complete skin examination, such as acanthosis nigricans, can provide clues to undiagnosed or poorly controlled comorbidities, such as insulin resistance. A record of any skin wounds upon admission to the ICU and throughout the course of hospitalization should be recorded as obese patients are likely to have more complex wound injuries and related complications.[141] Finally, because central adiposity often better reflects visceral fat deposition and obesity-induced inflammation, determination of waist-to-hip ratio and waist circumference should be obtained in class I and II obesity.[130,135,142–144]

Determining Energy Expenditure in Obesity

The optimal way to predict energy and protein requirements for the critically ill obese patient remains a topic of much debate and controversy. While the use of predictive equations, such as the Harris-Benedict, have been widely utilized for predicting resting metabolic rate, the evidence of their accuracy in critically ill patients is lacking.[145,146] In addition, most predictive equations were validated in patients without extremes of weight or age. Overestimation of total energy requirements when using ABW and underestimation when using the IBW leads to inadvertent overfeeding and underfeeding, respectively.[141] Attempting to account for altered body composition with these equations by using corrections for adjusted body weight has led to even more confusion.

For these reasons, when available, IC should be used for determining the energy requirements of the critically ill obese patient. When IC is not available, predictive equations such as the Mifflin equation[147–149] or the Penn State 1998 equation[150] can be used. Alternatively, estimating energy requirements with simpler weight-based equations has also been utilized.[141,151,152] With these equations, nutrition specialists must be aware of the frequent inaccuracies that may occur and apply clinical judgment to assess the appropriateness of nutrition therapy derived from their use.

High-Protein Hypocaloric Feeding

Numerous negative observations resulting from "hyperalimentation" in the 1970s have led to the idea of a possible benefit of hypocaloric feeding in obesity. Such observations include the fact that the metabolic rate may not be markedly increased in patients with critical illness, that weight gain during nutrition support in critical illness usually involves an increase in fat mass out of proportion to lean body mass, that provision of glucose in excess of needs causes increased lipogenesis and fatty liver, and that hyperglycemia increases the risk of infectious complications. For example, a controlled trial of preoperative nutrition in which patients received 1000 kcal above the metabolic rate actually increased infectious complications.[153]

It is important to distinguish high-protein hypocaloric feeding (providing adequate or increased protein while delivering lower calories) from permissive underfeeding (delivering inadequate amounts of all macronutrients). High-protein hypocaloric feeding is thought to maintain nitrogen balance and lean body mass while facilitating the mobilization of adipose tissue for fuel utilization. Six studies have examined high-protein hypocaloric nutrition in critically ill obese patients.[154–157] Some major findings of these studies include lower insulin requirements, decreased ICU stay, decreased number of days receiving antibiotics, improved wound healing, better closure of fistulas, and a trend toward reduced duration of mechanical ventilation in subjects receiving high-protein hypocaloric feeding strategies. Only one of these studies involved EN.[154] It is important to note that none of these studies demonstrated inferior outcomes when compared to eucaloric feeding.[158] Further randomized controlled studies are needed to evaluate major outcomes, such as mortality, in the ICU.

High-protein hypocaloric feeding has been recommended (Grade D) by the most recent guidelines for the Provision and Assessment of Nutrition Support Therapy in the Adult Critically Ill Patient, from the Society of Critical Care Medicine and A.S.P.E.N.[159] The guidelines suggest that for all classes of obesity where BMI is > 30 kg/m^2, the goal of the EN regimen should not exceed 60% to 70% of target energy requirements, a number that can be determined by the simplistic weight-based equations 11 to 14 kcal/kg ABW/d or 22 to 25 kcal/kg IBW/d.[139,159] For obese patients, the dose of parenteral nutrition with regard to protein and caloric provision should follow the same recommendations as that given for EN.[159]

Protein Requirements

Protein requirements for patients with class I and II obesity may be estimated by the equation 2.0 g/kg IBW/d, and for patients with Class III, 2.5 g/kg IBW/d.[159,160] A 24-hour urine collection for urinary urea nitrogen may be collected and used to subsequently adjust the prescription for protein delivery.[154] Given the dynamic changes that can occur in the ICU and the inaccuracy of predictive measures, nutrition specialists should routinely monitor nitrogen balance and cumulative protein balance throughout a patient's hospital course.

The Impact of Obesity on the Delivery of Nutrition

Enteral Access

Obesity is associated with increased abdominal pressure, which promotes gastroesophageal reflux and aspiration.[161,162] Comorbidities such as diabetes mellitus and its associated enteric neuropathy are more prevalent in obesity. Delayed gastric emptying and poor tolerance to gastric feeding as a result of diabetic gastroparesis can further complicate enteral access. Limitations in weight for fluoroscopy tables may preclude or complicate feeding tube placement that requires imaging for guidance and/or confirmation. For these reasons, selective postpyloric feeding and use of prokinetics may be needed more frequently in the critically ill obese patient.

Placement of a percutaneous endoscopic gastrostomy tube may be relatively contraindicated in morbidly obese patients.[141] Surgical and endoscopic placement of percutaneous endoscopic gastrostomy tubes in this population are associated with increased rates of complications, including postprocedure ileus, wound infection, and possibly mortality.[163,164] Because a large pannus increases risk for displacement of the percutaneous endoscopic gastrostomy tube, the authors recommend efforts to secure the stomach against the abdominal wall should be made with multiple T-fasteners; movement of the pannus may be further reduced by using an abdominal binder.

Monitoring the Delivery of Nutrition in the Critically Ill Obese Patient

Obese patients may be more prone to increased morbidity in the ICU compared to lean patients.[140] The level of enteral feeding within the gastrointestinal tract, the appropriate access device, and whether simultaneous gastric decompression of the stomach is required should be determined in all critically ill patients, a practice that should occur regardless of the presence or absence of obesity. Likewise, all critically ill patients should be fully resuscitated prior to initiating EN in order to reduce the likelihood for bowel ischemia.[159]

Serial performance of IC may be needed to reassess changing caloric requirements as the patient's clinical condition improves or deteriorates. Cumulative caloric balance should be followed to confirm that patients are maintained at 60% to 70% of expenditure throughout the provision of the nutrition regimen. Monitoring nitrogen balance periodically with serial 24-hour collections of urinary urea nitrogen assists in confirming the adequacy of protein provision.[165] In high-protein hypocaloric feeding, excess protein load should also be monitored with measurements of blood urea nitrogen, creatinine, and daily physical assessments for asterixis.

Because fluid status can be difficult to assess in patients with morbid obesity, strict records of intake/output should be followed to assure delivery of the nutrition regimen. Volume-based feeds may help in assuring delivery of the prescribed EN. Patients should be monitored to maintain moderate glucose control, keeping glucose levels < 180 mg/dL (10 mmol/L).[159] See Practice Scenario 35-1 for an example of the use of enteral nutrition in a critically ill obese patient.

Practice Scenario 35-1

Question: What are the EN recommendations for a critically ill obese trauma patient?

Scenario: A 46-year-old obese (BMI 36 kg/m^2, ABW 121 kg, IBW 81 kg, height 183 cm) man with a past history of NAFLD is admitted to the trauma service following a motor vehicle accident; he required mechanical ventilation. The trauma team predicts that the patient will require at least 1 week of mechanical ventilation and consult the nutrition support service for recommendations for EN.

Intervention: A physical exam was performed and history obtained from the family. The trauma team placed nasoenteric feeding tube and IC was performed to determine the energy requirements. Energy expenditure measured by IC was 2985 kcal/day. Protein requirements were estimated by the equation for obesity class II.

Answer: Obese patients should receive a high-protein hypocaloric feeding regimen via a nasoenteric feeding tube (that allows for concurrent nasogastric decompression, which may be required). The feeding should provide 162 g/day of protein (IBW 81 kg × 2.0 g/kg IBW/day). Goal calorie delivery should be approximately 2089 kcal/day (70% of resting energy expenditure 2985 as estimated by the IC).

Rationale: High-protein hypocaloric feeding has been recommended (Grade D) by the most recent guidelines for the Provision and Assessment of Nutrition Support Therapy in the Adult Critically Ill Patient, from the Society of Critical Care Medicine and A.S.P.E.N. The guidelines suggest that for BMI that is >30 kg/m^2, the goal of the EN regimen should not exceed 60% to 70% of target energy requirements.[159] Predicting protein requirements can be performed with simplistic weight-based equations. Protein requirements for patients with class I and II obesity may be estimated by the equation 2.0 g/kg IBW/d, and for patients with Class III, 2.5 g/kg IBW/d.[159,160]

Practicality of Enteral Nutrition Delivery

The availability of tube feeding formulations suited for achieving the recommendations of high-protein hypocaloric feeding for obese patients in the ICU is evolving. The addition of various protein modules to current formulations represents the best available method of meeting these recommendations. A number of practical issues arise in attempting to add the large amount of protein powder required to achieve 2.0 to 2.5 g/kg IBW/d (while remaining hypocaloric) to available enteral formulas. More often than not, an excessive volume of fluid is required for the protein powder to be dissolved, and the consistency of such a mixture is often unsuitable for delivery through smaller caliber enteral tubes. The addition of such quantities of protein several times per day requires a large amount of time and effort from an already overworked ICU nursing staff. These issues in practicality frequently lead to inadequate delivery of protein and underscore the need for an enteral formula specifically designed to meet these recommendations.

References

1. Ogden CL, Carroll MD, Flegal KM. Epidemiologic trends in overweight and obesity. *Endocrinol Metab Clin North Am.* 2003;32(4):741–760, vii.
2. Ogden CL, Yanovski SZ, Carroll MD, Flegal KM. The epidemiology of obesity. *Gastroenterol.* 2007;132(6):2087–2102.
3. Finkelstein EA, Ruhm CJ, Kosa KM. Economic causes and consequences of obesity. *Annu Rev Public Health.* 2005;26:239–257.
4. Calle EE, Rodriguez C, Walker-Thurmond K, Thun MJ. Overweight, obesity, and mortality from cancer in a prospectively studied cohort of U.S. adults. *N Engl J Med.* 2003;348(17):1625–1638.
5. Kuczmarski RJ, Flegal KM. Criteria for definition of overweight in transition: background and recommendations for the United States. *Am J Clin Nutr.* 2000;72(5):1074–1081.
6. Ogden CL, Carroll MD, McDowell MA, Flegal KM. Obesity among adults in the United States—no statistically significant change since 2003-2004. *NCHS Data Brief.* 2007;1:1–8.
7. Ogden CL, Kuczmarski RJ, Flegal KM, et al. Centers for Disease Control and Prevention 2000 growth charts for the United States: improvements to the 1977 National Center for Health Statistics version. *Pediatrics.* 2002;109(1):45–60.
8. Choi JW, Wang X, Joo JI, et al. Plasma proteome analysis in diet-induced obesity-prone and obesity-resistant rats. *Proteomics.* 2010;10(24):4386–4400.
9. Fawcett KA, Barroso I. The genetics of obesity: FTO leads the way. *Trends Genet.* 2010;26(6):266–274.
10. Lopez AD, Mathers CD, Ezzati M, Jamison DT, Murray CJ. Global and regional burden of disease and risk factors, 2001: systematic analysis of population health data. *Lancet.* 2006;367(9524):1747–1757.

11. James PT. Obesity: the worldwide epidemic. *Clin. Dermatol.* 2004;22(4):276–280.
12. Goh VH, Tain CF, Tong TY, Mok HP, Wong MT. Are BMI and other anthropometric measures appropriate as indices for obesity? A study in an Asian population. *J Lipid Res.* 2004;45(10):1892–1898.
13. WHO Expert Consultation. Appropriate body-mass index for Asian populations and its implications for policy and intervention strategies. *Lancet.* 2004;363(9403):157–163.
14. Stevens J, Nowicki EM. Body mass index and mortality in Asian populations: implications for obesity cut-points. *Nutr Rev.* 2003;61(3):104–107.
15. Woods SC, D'Alessio DA. Central control of body weight and appetite. *J Clin Endocrinol Metab.* 2008;93(11 Suppl 1):S37–S50.
16. Woods SC, Seeley RJ, Cota D. Regulation of food intake through hypothalamic signaling networks involving mTOR. *Annu Rev Nutr.* 2008;28:295–311.
17. Agurs-Collins T, Bouchard C. Gene-nutrition and gene-physical activity interactions in the etiology of obesity. Introduction. *Obesity (Silver Spring).* 2008;16(Suppl 3):S2–S4.
18. Bouchard C. Gene-environment interactions in the etiology of obesity: defining the fundamentals. *Obesity (Silver Spring).* 2008; 16(Suppl 3):S5–S10.
19. Chung WK, Leibel RL. Considerations regarding the genetics of obesity. *Obesity (Silver Spring).* 2008;16(Suppl 3):S33–S39.
20. Farooqi S, O'Rahilly S. Genetics of obesity in humans. *Endocr Rev.* 2006;27(7):710718.
21. Hinney A, Hebebrand J. Polygenic obesity in humans. *Obes Facts.* 2008;1(1):35–42.
22. Hinney A, Vogel CI, Hebebrand J. From monogenic to polygenic obesity: recent advances. *Eur Child Adolesc Psychiatry.* 2010;19(3): 297–310.
23. Speliotes EK, Willer CJ, Berndt SI, et al. Association analyses of 249,796 individuals reveal 18 new loci associated with body mass index. *Nat Genet.* 2010;42(11):937–948.
24. Cauchi S, Stutzmann F, Cavalcanti-Proenca C, et al. Combined effects of MC4R and FTO common genetic variants on obesity in European general populations. *J Mol Med.* 2009;87(5):537–546.
25. Stutzmann F, Cauchi S, Durand E, et al. Common genetic variation near MC4R is associated with eating behaviour patterns in European populations. *Int J Obes (Lond).* 2009;33(3):373–378.
26. Hurt RT, Frazier TH, McClave SA, Kaplan LM. Obesity epidemic: overview, pathophysiology, and the intensive care unit conundrum. *J Parenter Enteral Nutr.* 2011;35(5 Suppl):4S–13S.
27. Mozaffarian D, Hao T, Rimm EB, Willett WC, Hu FB. Changes in diet and lifestyle and long-term weight gain in women and men. *N Engl J Med.* 2011;364(25):2392–2404.
28. Bantle JP. Dietary fructose and metabolic syndrome and diabetes. *J Nutr.* 2009;139(6):1263S–1268S.
29. Bantle JP, Raatz SK, Thomas W, Georgopoulos A. Effects of dietary fructose on plasma lipids in healthy subjects. *Am J Clin Nutr.* 2000;72(5):1128–1134.
30. Bray GA, Nielsen SJ, Popkin BM. Consumption of high-fructose corn syrup in beverages may play a role in the epidemic of obesity. *Am J Clin Nutr.* 2004;79(4):537–543.
31. Vos MB, McClain CJ. Fructose takes a toll. *Hepatology.* 2009;50(4): 1004–1006.
32. Vos MB, Weber MB, Welsh J, et al. Fructose and oxidized low-density lipoprotein in pediatric nonalcoholic fatty liver disease: a pilot study. *Arch Pediatr Adolesc Med.* 2009;163(7):674–675.
33. Bray GA. The epidemic of obesity and changes in food intake: the fluoride hypothesis. *Physiol Behav.* 2004;82(1):115–121.
34. Choi HK, Curhan G. Soft drinks, fructose consumption, and the risk of gout in men: prospective cohort study. *BMJ.* 2008;336(7639): 309–312.
35. Vos MB, Kimmons JE, Gillespie C, Welsh J, Blanck HM. Dietary fructose consumption among US children and adults: the Third National Health and Nutrition Examination Survey. *Medscape J Med.* 2008;10(7):160.
36. Stender S, Dyerberg J. Influence of trans fatty acids on health. *Ann Nutr Metab.* 2004;48(2):61–66.
37. Stender S, Dyerberg J, Astrup A. High levels of industrially produced trans fat in popular fast foods. *N Engl J Med.* 2006;354(15): 1650–1652.
38. Stender S, Dyerberg J, Astrup A. Fast food: unfriendly and unhealthy. *Int J Obes (Lond).* 2007;31(6):887–890.
39. Stender S, Dyerberg J, Bysted A, Leth T, Astrup A. A trans world journey. *Atheroscler Suppl.* 2006;7(2):47–52.
40. Dansinger M. Ban trans fats in 2007. *Med Gen Med.* 2006;8(4):58.
41. Mozaffarian D, Katan MB, Ascherio A, Stampfer MJ, Willett WC. Trans fatty acids and cardiovascular disease. *N Engl J Med.* 2006; 354(15):1601–1613.
42. Mozaffarian D, Willett WC. Trans fatty acids and cardiovascular risk: a unique cardiometabolic imprint? *Curr Atheroscler Rep.* 2007;9(6):486–493.
43. Pietinen P, Ascherio A, Korhonen P, et al. Intake of fatty acids and risk of coronary heart disease in a cohort of Finnish men. The Alpha-Tocopherol, Beta-Carotene Cancer Prevention Study. *Am J Epidemiol.* 1997;145(10):876–887.
44. Hurt RT, Kulisek C, Buchanan LA, McClave SA. The obesity epidemic: challenges, health initiatives, and implications for gastroenterologists. *Gastroenterol Hepatol.* 2010;6(12):780–792.
45. Williamson DF, Madans J, Anda RF, Kleinman JC, Kahn HS, Byers T. Recreational physical activity and ten-year weight change in a US national cohort. *Int J Obes Relat Metab Disord.* 1993;17(5):279–286.
46. Ravussin E, Lillioja S, Knowler WC, et al. Reduced rate of energy expenditure as a risk factor for body-weight gain. *N Engl J Med.* 1988;318(8):467–472.
47. Sumithran P, Prendergast LA, Delbridge E, et al. Long-term persistence of hormonal adaptations to weight loss. *N Engl J Med.* 2011;365(17):1597–1604.
48. Cave MC, Hurt RT, Frazier TH, et al. Obesity, inflammation, and the potential application of pharmaconutrition. *Nutr Clin Pract.* 2008;23(1):16–34.
49. Chandra R, Liddle RA. Cholecystokinin. *Curr Opin Endocrinol Diabetes Obes.* 2007;14(1):63–67.
50. Lorenz DN, Goldman SA. Vagal mediation of the cholecystokinin satiety effect in rats. *Physiol Behav.* 1982;29(4):599–604.
51. Edwards GL, Ladenheim EE, Ritter RC. Dorsomedial hindbrain participation in cholecystokinin-induced satiety. *Am J Physiol.* 1986;251(5 Pt 2):R971–R977.
52. Kirchner H, Tong J, Tschop MH, Pfluger PT. Ghrelin and PYY in the regulation of energy balance and metabolism: lessons from mouse mutants. *Am J Physiol Endocrinol Metab.* 2010;298(5):E909–E919.
53. le Roux CW, Batterham RL, Aylwin SJ, et al. Attenuated peptide YY release in obese subjects is associated with reduced satiety. *Endocrinol.* 2006;147(1):3–8.
54. Renshaw D, Batterham RL. Peptide YY: a potential therapy for obesity. *Curr Drug Targets.* 2005;6(2):171–179.
55. Onaga T, Zabielski R, Kato S. Multiple regulation of peptide YY secretion in the digestive tract. *Peptides.* 2002;23(2):279–290.
56. Batterham RL, Bloom SR. The gut hormone peptide YY regulates appetite. *Ann N Y Acad Sci.* 2003;994:162–168.
57. Liu CD, Aloia T, Adrian TE, et al. Peptide YY: a potential proabsorptive hormone for the treatment of malabsorptive disorders. *Am Surg.* 1996;62(3):232–236.
58. Wiedmer P, Nogueiras R, Broglio F, D'Alessio D, Tschop MH. Ghrelin, obesity and diabetes. *Nat Clin Pract Endocrinol Metab.* 2007;3(10):705–712.

59. Asakawa A, Inui A, Kaga T, et al. Ghrelin is an appetite-stimulatory signal from stomach with structural resemblance to motilin. *Gastroenterol.* 2001;120(2):337–345.
60. Kreitschmann-Andermahr I, Suarez P, Jennings R, Evers N, Brabant G. GH/IGF-I regulation in obesity—mechanisms and practical consequences in children and adults. *Horm Res Paediatr.* 2010; 73(3):153–160.
61. Cummings DE, Weigle DS, Frayo RS, et al. Plasma ghrelin levels after diet-induced weight loss or gastric bypass surgery. *N Engl J Med.* 2002;346(21):1623–1630.
62. Foster-Schubert KE, McTiernan A, Frayo RS, et al. Human plasma ghrelin levels increase during a one-year exercise program. *J Clin Endocrinol Metab.* 2005;90(2):820–825.
63. Dube PE, Brubaker PL. Nutrient, neural and endocrine control of glucagon-like peptide secretion. *Horm Metab Res.* 2004;36 (11-12):755–760.
64. Gutzwiller JP, Drewe J, Goke B, et al. Glucagon-like peptide-1 promotes satiety and reduces food intake in patients with diabetes mellitus type 2. *Am J Physiol.* 1999;276(5 Pt 2):R1541–R1544.
65. Kinzig KP, D'Alessio DA, Seeley RJ. The diverse roles of specific GLP-1 receptors in the control of food intake and the response to visceral illness. *J Neurosci.* 2002;22(23):10470–10476.
66. Larsen PJ, Tang-Christensen M, Holst JJ, Orskov C. Distribution of glucagon-like peptide-1 and other preproglucagon-derived peptides in the rat hypothalamus and brainstem. *Neuroscience.* 1997;77(1):257–270.
67. Larsen PJ, Tang-Christensen M, Jessop DS. Central administration of glucagon-like peptide-1 activates hypothalamic neuroendocrine neurons in the rat. *Endocrinol.* 1997;138(10): 4445–4455.
68. McMahon LR, Wellman PJ. Decreased intake of a liquid diet in nonfood-deprived rats following intra-PVN injections of GLP-1 (7-36) amide. *Pharmacol Biochem Behav.* 1997;58(3):673–677.
69. Naslund E, Bogefors J, Skogar S, et al. GLP-1 slows solid gastric emptying and inhibits insulin, glucagon, and PYY release in humans. *Am J Physiol.* 1999;277(3 Pt 2):R910–R916.
70. Mafong DD, Henry RR. Exenatide as a treatment for diabetes and obesity: implications for cardiovascular risk reduction. *Curr Atheroscler Rep.* 2008;10(1):55–60.
71. Adams KF, Schatzkin A, Harris TB, et al. Overweight, obesity, and mortality in a large prospective cohort of persons 50 to 71 years old. *N Engl J Med.* 2006;355(8):763–778.
72. Pischon T, Nothlings U, Boeing H. Obesity and cancer. *Proc Nutr Soc.* 2008;67(2):128–145.
73. Whitlock G, Lewington S, Sherliker P, et al. Body-mass index and cause-specific mortality in 900,000 adults: collaborative analyses of 57 prospective studies. *Lancet.* 2009;373(9669):1083–1096.
74. Kiernan M, Winkleby MA. Identifying patients for weight-loss treatment: an empirical evaluation of the NHLBI obesity education initiative expert panel treatment recommendations. *Arch Intern Med.* 2000;160(14):2169–2176.
75. Kelley DE. The regulation of glucose uptake and oxidation during exercise. *Int J Obes Relat Metab Disord.* 1995;19(Suppl 4): S14–S17.
76. Wadden TA, Anderson DA, Foster GD. Two-year changes in lipids and lipoproteins associated with the maintenance of a 5% to 10% reduction in initial weight: some findings and some questions. *Obes Res.* 1999;7(2):170–178.
77. McCarron DA, Reusser ME. Body weight and blood pressure regulation. *Am J Clin Nutr.* 1996;63(3 Suppl):423S–425S.
78. Strobel RJ, Rosen RC. Obesity and weight loss in obstructive sleep apnea: a critical review. *Sleep.* 1996;19(2):104–115.
79. Weight cycling. National Task Force on the Prevention and Treatment of Obesity. *JAMA.* 1994;272(15):1196–1202.
80. Wadden TA, Berkowitz RI, Womble LG, et al. Randomized trial of lifestyle modification and pharmacotherapy for obesity. *N Engl J Med.* 2005;353(20):2111–2120.
81. Wadden TA, Crerand CE, Brock J. Behavioral treatment of obesity. *Psychiatr Clin North Am.* 2005;28(1):151–170, ix.
82. Rubin RR, Fujimoto WY, Marrero DG, et al. The Diabetes Prevention Program: recruitment methods and results. *Control Clin Trials.* 2002;23(2):157–171.
83. Kruger J, Galuska DA, Serdula MK, Jones DA. Attempting to lose weight: specific practices among U.S. adults. *Am J Prev Med.* 2004;26(5):402–406.
84. Sacks FM, Bray GA, Carey VJ, et al. Comparison of weight-loss diets with different compositions of fat, protein, and carbohydrates. *N Engl J Med.* 2009;360(9):859–873.
85. National Institutes of Health. Clinical guidelines on the identification, evaluation, and treatment of overweight and obesity in adults—the evidence report. *Obes Res.* 1998;6(Suppl 2):51S–209S.
86. Stern L, Iqbal N, Seshadri P, et al. The effects of low-carbohydrate versus conventional weight loss diets in severely obese adults: one-year follow-up of a randomized trial. *Ann Intern Med.* 2004; 140(10):778–785.
87. Foster GD, Wyatt HR, Hill JO, et al. A randomized trial of a low-carbohydrate diet for obesity. *N Engl J Med.* 2003;348(21): 2082–2090.
88. National Task Force on the Prevention and Treatment of Obesity, National Institutes of Health. Very low-calorie diets. *JAMA.* 1993;270(8):967–974.
89. Anderson JW, Konz EC, Frederich RC, Wood CL. Long-term weight-loss maintenance: a meta-analysis of US studies. *Am J Clin Nutr.* 2001;74(5):579–584.
90. Benotti PN, Still CD, Wood GC, et al. Preoperative weight loss before bariatric surgery. *Arch Surg.* 2009;144(12):1150–1155.
91. Wiezer M, Jansen I, Thorell A. Preoperative weight loss: a component of the preoperative program in bariatric surgery. *Obes Surg.* 2010;20(1):130; author reply 131.
92. Solomon H, Liu GY, Alami R, Morton J, Curet MJ. Benefits to patients choosing preoperative weight loss in gastric bypass surgery: new results of a randomized trial. *J Am Coll Surg.* 2009; 208(2):241–245.
93. Ballor DL, Keesey RE. A meta-analysis of the factors affecting exercise-induced changes in body mass, fat mass and fat-free mass in males and females. *Int J Obes.* 1991;15(11):717–726.
94. Ballor DL, Poehlman ET. Exercise-training enhances fat-free mass preservation during diet-induced weight loss: a meta-analytical finding. *Int J Obes Relat Metab Disord.* 1994;18(1):35–40.
95. Miller WC, Koceja DM, Hamilton EJ. A meta-analysis of the past 25 years of weight loss research using diet, exercise or diet plus exercise intervention. *Int J Obes Relat Metab Disord.* 1997;21(10): 941–947.
96. Slentz CA, Duscha BD, Johnson JL, et al. Effects of the amount of exercise on body weight, body composition, and measures of central obesity: STRRIDE—a randomized controlled study. *Arch Intern Med.* 2004;164(1):31–39.
97. Curioni CC, Lourenco PM. Long-term weight loss after diet and exercise: a systematic review. *Int J Obes (Lond).* 2005;29(10): 1168–1174.
98. Andersen RE, Wadden TA, Bartlett SJ, Zemel B, Verde TJ, Franckowiak SC. Effects of lifestyle activity vs structured aerobic exercise in obese women: a randomized trial. *JAMA.* 1999;281(4): 335–340.
99. Dunn AL, Marcus BH, Kampert JB, Garcia ME, Kohl HW 3rd, Blair SN. Comparison of lifestyle and structured interventions to increase physical activity and cardiorespiratory fitness: a randomized trial. *JAMA.* 1999;281(4):327–334.

100. Phelan S, Wadden TA. Combining behavioral and pharmacological treatments for obesity. *Obes Res.* 2002;10(6):560–574.
101. Wadden TA, Womble LG, Sarwer DB, Berkowitz RI, Clark VL, Foster GD. Great expectations: "I'm losing 25% of my weight no matter what you say." *J Consult Clin Psychol.* 2003;71(6):1084–1089.
102. Wadden TA, Volger S, Sarwer DB, et al. A two-year randomized trial of obesity treatment in primary care practice. *N Engl J Med.* 2011;365(21):1969–1979.
103. Kaplan LM. Pharmacologic therapies for obesity. *Gastroenterol Clin North Am.* 2010;39(1):69–79.
104. Davidson MH, Hauptman J, DiGirolamo M, et al. Weight control and risk factor reduction in obese subjects treated for 2 years with orlistat: a randomized controlled trial. *JAMA.* 1999;281(3):235–242.
105. Hauptman J, Lucas C, Boldrin MN, Collins H, Segal KR. Orlistat in the long-term treatment of obesity in primary care settings. *Arch Fam Med.* 2000;9(2):160–167.
106. Rossner S, Sjostrom L, Noack R, Meinders AE, Noseda G. Weight loss, weight maintenance, and improved cardiovascular risk factors after 2 years treatment with orlistat for obesity. European Orlistat Obesity Study Group. *Obes Res.* 2000;8(1):49–61.
107. Sjostrom L, Rissanen A, Andersen T, et al. Randomised placebo-controlled trial of orlistat for weight loss and prevention of weight regain in obese patients. European Multicentre Orlistat Study Group. *Lancet.* 1998;352(9123):167–172.
108. Torgerson JS, Hauptman J, Boldrin MN, Sjostrom L. XENical in the prevention of diabetes in obese subjects (XENDOS) study: a randomized study of orlistat as an adjunct to lifestyle changes for the prevention of type 2 diabetes in obese patients. *Diabetes Care.* 2004;27(1):155–161.
109. Li Z, Maglione M, Tu W, et al. Meta-analysis: pharmacologic treatment of obesity. *Ann Intern Med.* 2005;142(7):532–546.
110. Sibutramine (Meridia) withdrawn. *Med Lett Drugs Ther.* 2010;52(1350):88.
111. Greenway FL, Fujioka K, Plodkowski RA, et al. Effect of naltrexone plus bupropion on weight loss in overweight and obese adults (COR-I): a multicentre, randomised, double-blind, placebo-controlled, phase 3 trial. *Lancet.* 2010;376(9741):595–605.
112. Blanck HM, Serdula MK, Gillespie C, et al. Use of nonprescription dietary supplements for weight loss is common among Americans. *J Am Diet Assoc.* 2007;107(3):441–447.
113. Saper RB, Eisenberg DM, Phillips RS. Common dietary supplements for weight loss. *Am Fam Physician.* 2004;70(9):1731–1738.
114. NIH conference. Gastrointestinal surgery for severe obesity. Consensus Development Conference Panel. *Ann Intern Med.* 1991;115(12):956–961.
115. Mechanick JI, Kushner RF, Sugerman HJ, et al. American Association of Clinical Endocrinologists, The Obesity Society, and American Society for Metabolic & Bariatric Surgery medical guidelines for clinical practice for the perioperative nutritional, metabolic, and nonsurgical support of the bariatric surgery patient. *Obesity (Silver Spring).* 2009;17(Suppl 1):S1–S70, v.
116. Buchwald H, Avidor Y, Braunwald E, et al. Bariatric surgery: a systematic review and meta-analysis. *JAMA.* 2004;292(14):1724–1737.
117. Suter M, Calmes JM, Paroz A, Giusti V. A 10-year experience with laparoscopic gastric banding for morbid obesity: high long-term complication and failure rates. *Obes Surg.* 2006;16(7):829–835.
118. Brolin RE, LaMarca LB, Kenler HA, Cody RP. Malabsorptive gastric bypass in patients with superobesity. *J Gastrointest Surg.* 2002;6(2):195–203; discussion 204–205.
119. Tice JA, Karliner L, Walsh J, Petersen AJ, Feldman MD. Gastric banding or bypass? A systematic review comparing the two most popular bariatric procedures. *Am J Med.* 2008;121(10):885–893.
120. Prachand VN, Ward M, Alverdy JC. Duodenal switch provides superior resolution of metabolic comorbidities independent of weight loss in the super-obese (BMI > or = 50 kg/m^2) compared with gastric bypass. *J Gastrointest Surg.* 2010;14(2):211–220.
121. NIH conference. Gastrointestinal surgery for severe obesity. Consensus Development Conference Panel. *Ann Intern Med.* 1991;115(12):956–961.
122. Cunningham E. What is the registered dietitian's role in the preoperative assessment of a client contemplating bariatric surgery? *J Am Diet Assoc.* 2006;106(1):163.
123. Alvarado R, Alami RS, Hsu G, et al. The impact of preoperative weight loss in patients undergoing laparoscopic Roux-en-Y gastric bypass. *Obes Surg.* 2005;15(9):1282–1286.
124. Still CD, Benotti P, Wood GC, et al. Outcomes of preoperative weight loss in high-risk patients undergoing gastric bypass surgery. *Arch Surg.* 2007;142(10):994–998; discussion 999.
125. Kulick D, Hark L, Deen D. The bariatric surgery patient: a growing role for registered dietitians. *J Am Diet Assoc.* Apr 2010;110(4):593–599.
126. Fleisher LA, Beckman JA, Brown KA, et al. ACC/AHA 2007 guidelines on perioperative cardiovascular evaluation and care for noncardiac surgery: a report of the American College of Cardiology/American Heart Association Task Force on Practice Guidelines (Writing Committee to Revise the 2002 Guidelines on Perioperative Cardiovascular Evaluation for Noncardiac Surgery): developed in collaboration with the American Society of Echocardiography, American Society of Nuclear Cardiology, Heart Rhythm Society, Society of Cardiovascular Anesthesiologists, Society for Cardiovascular Angiography and Interventions, Society for Vascular Medicine and Biology, and Society for Vascular Surgery. *Circulation.* 2007;116(17):e418–e499.
127. McMahon MM, Sarr MG, Clark MM, et al. Clinical management after bariatric surgery: value of a multidisciplinary approach. *Mayo Clin Proc.* 2006;81(10 Suppl):S34–S45.
128. Chang CG, Adams-Huet B, Provost DA. Acute post-gastric reduction surgery (APGARS) neuropathy. *Obes Surg.* 2004;14(2):182–189.
129. Davies DJ, Baxter JM, Baxter JN. Nutritional deficiencies after bariatric surgery. *Obes Surg.* 2007;17(9):1150–1158.
130. McTigue K, Larson JC, Valoski A, et al. Mortality and cardiac and vascular outcomes in extremely obese women. *JAMA.* 2006;296(1):79–86.
131. Pischon T, Boeing H, Hoffmann K, et al. General and abdominal adiposity and risk of death in Europe. *N Engl J Med.* 2008;359(20):2105–2120.
132. Akinnusi ME, Pineda LA, El Solh AA. Effect of obesity on intensive care morbidity and mortality: a meta-analysis. *Crit Care Med.* 2008;36(1):151–158.
133. Hogue CW Jr, Stearns JD, Colantuoni E, et al. The impact of obesity on outcomes after critical illness: a meta-analysis. *Intensive Care Med.* 2009;35(7):1152–1170.
134. Oliveros H, Villamor E. Obesity and mortality in critically ill adults: a systematic review and meta-analysis. *Obesity (Silver Spring).* 2008;16(3):515–521.
135. Paolini JB, Mancini J, Genestal M, et al. Predictive value of abdominal obesity vs. body mass index for determining risk of intensive care unit mortality. *Crit Care Med.* 2010;38(5):1308–1314.
136. Matheson PJ, Hurt RT, Franklin GA, McClain CJ, Garrison RN. Obesity-induced hepatic hypoperfusion primes for hepatic dysfunction after resuscitated hemorrhagic shock. *Surgery.* 2009;146(4):739–747; discussion 747–748.
137. Brodsky JB, Lemmens HJ, Brock-Utne JG, Vierra M, Saidman LJ. Morbid obesity and tracheal intubation. *Anesth Analg.* 2002;94(3):732–736; table of contents.

138. Ladosky W, Botelho MA, Albuquerque JP Jr. Chest mechanics in morbidly obese non-hypoventilated patients. *Respir Med.* 2001;95(4):281–286.
139. McClave SA, Kushner R, Van Way CW 3rd, et al. Nutrition therapy of the severely obese, critically ill patient: summation of conclusions and recommendations. *J Parenter Enteral Nutr.* 2011;35(5 Suppl):88S–96S.
140. Kiraly L, Hurt RT, Van Way CW 3rd. The outcomes of obese patients in critical care. *J Parenter Enteral Nutr.* 2011;35(5 Suppl): 29S–35S.
141. Port AM, Apovian C. Metabolic support of the obese intensive care unit patient: a current perspective. *Curr Opin Clin Nutr Metab Care.* 2010;13(2):184–191.
142. Schneider HJ, Friedrich N, Klotsche J, et al. The predictive value of different measures of obesity for incident cardiovascular events and mortality. *J Clin Endocrinol Metab.* 2010;95(4):1777–1785.
143. Testa G, Cacciatore F, Galizia G, et al. Waist circumference but not body mass index predicts long-term mortality in elderly subjects with chronic heart failure. *J Am Geriatr Soc.* 2010;58(8): 1433–1440.
144. Welborn TA, Dhaliwal SS. Preferred clinical measures of central obesity for predicting mortality. *Eur J Clin Nutr.* 2007;61(12): 1373–1379.
145. Walker RN, Heuberger RA. Predictive equations for energy needs for the critically ill. *Respir Care.* 2009;54(4):509–521.
146. Boullata J, Williams J, Cottrell F, Hudson L, Compher C. Accurate determination of energy needs in hospitalized patients. *J Am Diet Assoc.* 2007;107(3):393–401.
147. Frankenfield D, Roth-Yousey L, Compher C. Comparison of predictive equations for resting metabolic rate in healthy nonobese and obese adults: a systematic review. *J Am Diet Assoc.* 2005; 105(5):775–789.
148. Carrasco F, Papapietro K, Csendes A, et al. Changes in resting energy expenditure and body composition after weight loss following Roux-en-Y gastric bypass. *Obes Surg.* 2007;17(5):608–616.
149. Dobratz JR, Sibley SD, Beckman TR, et al. Predicting energy expenditure in extremely obese women. *J Parenter Enteral Nutr.* 2007;31(3):217–227.
150. Anderegg BA, Worrall C, Barbour E, Simpson KN, Delegge M. Comparison of resting energy expenditure prediction methods with measured resting energy expenditure in obese, hospitalized adults. *J Parenter Enteral Nutr.* 2009;33(2):168–175.
151. Stucky CC, Moncure M, Hise M, Gossage CM, Northrop D. How accurate are resting energy expenditure prediction equations in obese trauma and burn patients? *J Parenter Enteral Nutr.* 2008; 32(4):420–426.
152. Zauner A, Schneeweiss B, Kneidinger N, Lindner G, Zauner C. Weight-adjusted resting energy expenditure is not constant in critically ill patients. *Intensive Care Med.* 2006;32(3):428–434.
153. Jeejeebhoy KN. Permissive underfeeding of the critically ill patient. *Nutr Clin Pract.* 2004;19(5):477–480.
154. Dickerson RN, Boschert KJ, Kudsk KA, Brown RO. Hypocaloric enteral tube feeding in critically ill obese patients. *Nutrition.* 2002;18(3):241–246.
155. Dickerson RN, Rosato EF, Mullen JL. Net protein anabolism with hypocaloric parenteral nutrition in obese stressed patients. *Am J Clin Nutr.* 1986;44(6):747–755.
156. Burge JC, Goon A, Choban PS, Flancbaum L. Efficacy of hypocaloric total parenteral nutrition in hospitalized obese patients: a prospective, double-blind randomized trial. *J Parenter Enteral Nutr.* 1994;18(3):203–207.
157. Choban PS, Burge JC, Scales D, Flancbaum L. Hypoenergetic nutrition support in hospitalized obese patients: a simplified method for clinical application. *Am J Clin Nutr.* 1997;66(3): 546–550.
158. Joffe A, Wood K. Obesity in critical care. *Curr Opin Anaesthesiol.* 2007;20(2):113–118.
159. McClave SA, Martindale RG, Vanek VW, et al. Guidelines for the Provision and Assessment of Nutrition Support Therapy in the Adult Critically Ill Patient: Society of Critical Care Medicine (SCCM) and American Society for Parenteral and Enteral Nutrition (A.S.P.E.N.). *J Parenter Enteral Nutr.* 2009;33(3): 277–316.
160. Choban PS, Dickerson RN. Morbid obesity and nutrition support: is bigger different? *Nutr Clin Pract.* 2005;20(4):480–487.
161. Honiden S, McArdle JR. Obesity in the intensive care unit. *Clin Chest Med.* 2009;30(3):581–599, x.
162. Pieracci FM, Hydo L, Pomp A, Eachempati SR, Shou J, Barie PS. The relationship between body mass index and postoperative mortality from critical illness. *Obes Surg.* 2008;18(5):501–507.
163. Alexander JW. Wound infections in the morbidly obese. *Obes Surg.* 2005;15(9):1276–1277.
164. Calton WC, Martindale RG, Gooden SM. Complications of percutaneous endoscopic gastrostomy. *Military Medicine.* 1992;157(7): 358–360.
165. Dickerson RN. Hypocaloric feeding of obese patients in the intensive care unit. *Curr Opin Clin Nutr Metab Care.* 2005;8(2): 189–196.

36 Nutrition Support for Older Adults

Charles Mueller, PhD, RD, CNSD, and Rena Zelig, MS, RD, CSG

CONTENTS

Background ... 621
Sarcopenia ... 622
Frailty ... 622
Advanced Dementia ... 623
Nutrition Screening and Assessment ... 623
Nutrient Requirements ... 624
Dietary Interventions ... 625
Nutrition Support ... 625
References ... 627

Objectives

1. Review the theoretical and known causes of aging.
2. Describe and differentiate the conditions of sarcopenia, frailty, and advanced dementia.
3. Distinguish the roles of nutrition (dietary) interventions and nutrition support interventions used in health care for older adults.

Test Your Knowledge Questions

1. Which of the following are thought to contribute the most to the process of aging?
   A. Antagonistic pleiotropy
   B. Mutation theory
   C. The genome
   D. All of the above
2. Of the following, which is the best currently known nutrition intervention to minimize negative outcomes associated with sarcopenia?
   A. Protein supplementation
   B. Amino acid supplementation
   C. Protein adequacy
   D. Omega-3 fatty acid adequacy
3. What is the most reasonable justification to initiate enteral (tube) feeding in an individual with advanced dementia?
   A. Decreased morbidity
   B. Specific and limited goal
   C. Improved mortality
   D. Improved quality of life
4. Which of the following nutrition support interventions has demonstrated the best outcomes in frail community-dwelling older adults and in postoperative orthopedic surgery populations?
   A. Oral nutritional supplement
   B. Intravenous hydration
   C. Enteral (tube) feeding
   D. Parenteral nutrition

Test Your Knowledge Answers

1. The correct answer is **D**. Antagonistic pleiotropy, mutation theory, and the genome all have a role in aging. In mutation theory, genes that decrease infancy survival are selected against, whereas dangerous late life mutant genes are not selected against and are passed on in younger adulthood, thus the importance of the genome. Pleiotropic genes helpful in early life are potentially harmful in late life (eg, hormones that increase fertility early cause cancer later in life). These genes are also not selected against, but rather passed on, and accumulate.
2. The correct answer is **C**. Adequacy of protein intake appears to be the most important nutritional factor in preserving lean body mass in the elderly. The type of protein, essential amino acid supplementation, and omega-3 fatty acid supplementation may all have roles in preventing sarcopenia.
3. The correct answer is **B**. Enteral (tube) feeding has not been shown to be an effective intervention to decrease mortality, improve morbid outcome, or improve quality of life in patients with advanced dementia. However, according to the American Dietetic Association Position on Ethical and Legal Issues in Nutrition, Hydration, and Feeding, a specific and realistically achievable goal may be a reason to initiate tube feeding in an older adult with advanced dementia.
4. The correct answer is **A**. Oral nutrition supplements have demonstrated the best outcome in frail community-dwelling older adults and in postorthopedic surgery populations. Enteral (tube) feeding, parenteral nutrition, and intravenous hydration have demonstrated limited success in achieving positive outcomes in older adults.

Background

The number of adults aged 65 years and older worldwide is projected to increase from approximately 420 million in 2000 to 973 million in 2030.[1] In the United States, those older than 65 years in 2000 numbered 35 million and are projected to increase to 70 million by 2030.[2,3] This chapter focuses on nutritional issues in older adults with an emphasis on nutrition support. Older adults probably comprise one of the largest homogeneous patient groups using nutrition support, particularly enteral nutrition (EN). In 1995, approximately 121,000 percutaneous endoscopic gastrostomies (PEGs) were placed in elderly patients for use in both acute- and long-term care settings.[4] More recently, 1.6% (6464) of all U.S. Department of Veterans Affairs dementia patients (413,627) received a PEG over a 12-year time frame.[5] Parenteral nutrition (PN) use is obscure, and the authors identified one article dating back to 1997 that identified limited resources for central line and intravenous (IV) therapies available in nursing facilities within the Boston area.[6] Of 100 nursing facilities surveyed in 1996, 79 had IV programs and 54 facilities managed central venous catheters.[6]

The health care problems most associated with morbidity and mortality in older adults such as heart disease, stroke, cancer, influenza, and pneumonia are similar to those of younger adults. Medical conditions more unique to older adults include bronchitis, urinary tract infections, rheumatoid, and osteoarthritis, dementia, and pressure ulcers. Refer to Chapter 21 for a detailed discussion of pressure ulcers. Additional problems include decreased mobility, incontinence, impaired vision and hearing, and malnutrition. Malnutrition has multiple causes as suggested by and listed in Table 36-1. Chapter 9 discusses the etiologies of malnutrition.

The process of aging can be attributed in part to senescence, described as the irreversible process of cellular aging causing decreased function, morbidity, and even death. Almost all organ-system senescence contributes to malnutrition. A review of organ system senescence is beyond the scope of this chapter and can be reviewed in detail elsewhere.[7] A number of theories have been proposed to explain senescence and the aging process on the cellular level including free radical (damage), protein error, genomic ability to resist the aforementioned, and evolutionary causation embodied by mutation theory and antagonistic pleiotropy. Free radical theory proposes that reactive oxygen species, although essential to normal cellular function, also induce cellular damage, for example by uncoupling proteins that are vital for cellular health. Mitochondria are the single most active site of oxidative damage, losing their efficiency in oxidative phosphorylation reactions (decreased production of adenosine triphosphate).[8] Genomic ability to resist free radical damage suggests variable inherited capacity to mount free radical protection.[9] Mutation theory suggests that mutant genes that decrease infancy survival will be selected against whereas dangerous late life mutant genes will not be selected against (and will be passed on in younger adulthood.) Pleiotropic genes helpful in early life may not be helpful in late life (eg, hormones that increase fertility early cause cancer later in life). These antagonistic pleiotropic genes are not selected against and are passed on and also accumulate.[10]

Given the inevitable outcome of aging, treatment goals for older adults focus less on definitive treatment of disease than on maximizing functional status, that is to say, the innate ability to function at a given point in time to the extent to which the environment supports that ability. Often, the environment is altered to improve the functional status of an individual. Thus, in addition to successfully treating a condition, maximizing functional status and quality of life are primary outcomes in geriatric

TABLE 36-1 Causes of Malnutrition in the Elderly

Chronic disease
Poor oral health
Loss of taste and smell loss
Polypharmacy
Social isolation
Dementia
Obesity
Sarcopenia/frailty
Loss of functional capacity: inability to procure, prepare, and consume food

health care, including nutritional interventions.[11] This chapter will focus on issues related to functional decline including sarcopenia, frailty, dementia, and the use of nutritional interventions and particularly nutrition support to prevent functional decline and associated poor outcome.

Sarcopenia, frailty, dementia, and related functional decline compromise ability to procure and prepare food, leading to perhaps unintended weight loss. Such adults are also more likely to encounter chewing and swallowing difficulty and diminished hydration (compounded by age-associated loss of thirst sensation). The net result is an increased risk for malnutrition, exacerbated sarcopenia, frailty,[12] and eventually, disability, institutional placement, and mortalilty.[13] This chapter will also focus on the nutritional assessment of older adults including nutrient requirements, particularly among those with sarcopenia, frailty, and dementia.

Sarcopenia

Sarcopenia is the decline in skeletal muscle mass, strength, and function associated with age.[14–16] It can predict disability when a decrease in muscle mass, aside from an absolute decrease in mass, is adjusted for height and fat mass.[17] Sarcopenia is associated with elevated inflammatory cytokines and low albumin concentrations in the serum characteristic of inflammatory metabolism, which are also common in the muscle wasting diseases associated with cachexia.[18–20] Multiple factors, including myofiber degeneration caused by myocyte apoptosis mediated by mitochondrial DNA mutations, oxidative stress, endocrinosenescence, and inflammatory mediators, appear to be the mechanisms of sarcopenia. However, the precise relationships among these factors are not clear, including interactions with nutritional status.[17,21–23]

The principal intervention for sarcopenia is resistance training, although many older people may not be able or willing to undertake an exercise program.[24,25] Although there is evidence that (higher) protein intake in community-dwelling elderly is associated with slower loss of skeletal muscle mass,[26] the primary role of nutrition in the management of sarcopenia is the adequate intake of energy, protein, and essential nutrients.[27,28] The type of protein,[29] essential amino acid content,[30] and omega-3 fatty acids[31] may also have roles in the management of sarcopenia.

Resistance training appears to reverse skeletal muscle inability to accumulate protein, perhaps by reversing age-related insensitivity to insulinlike growth factor 1 (IGF-1).[32] Dietary protein supplementation above adequate levels does not enhance the effect of resistance training on retaining or improving skeletal muscle mass and function.[28] However, whey protein stimulated postprandial muscle protein synthesis more effectively than did casein and casein hydrolysate in older men, which was attributed to a combination of faster digestion and absorption kinetics and higher leucine content of whey.[29] Essential amino acid supplementation resulted in improved lean body mass at 6 and 18 months in a randomized (treatment versus placebo) older adult population with sarcopenia[33] and improved muscle protein fractional synthesis rate and increased lean body mass, but not strength at 3 months in another clinical trial with older women.[34] Omega-3 fatty acid supplementation stimulated muscle protein synthesis (compared to a corn oil control) in older adults, although subjects in the study did not have sarcopenia.[31]

Frailty

Loss of muscle mass and strength (ie, sarcopenia) is a hallmark of frailty. The most widely cited index used to establish frailty proposes a diagnosis of frailty if three or more of the following exist in an individual: unintentional weight loss (10 pounds in the last year), self-reported exhaustion, weakness (grip strength), slow walking speed, and low physical activity.[35] Older adults with at least three of these characteristics are at increased risk for adverse clinical outcomes. Although inflammation (and chronic disease) probably plays a causative role in frailty,[36] oxidative stress and organ system senescence also play a role. In this view of causation, frailty is the result of an aggregate of abnormalities rather than a single cause.[37]

Somewhat similar to sarcopenia, nutritional inadequacy appears to play a role in frailty. However, nutritional interventions have not improved outcomes associated with frailty, although individual nutrients appear to have a potential role in the treatment of frailty. Low daily intake of energy; protein; vitamins D, E, and C; and folate were significantly and independently associated with frailty in an older adult European cohort,[38] and high Mini Nutritional Assessment (MNA) scores were inversely associated with a neuropsychiatric score in a population of older adults with dementia living at home.[39] A review of clinical trials[40] that included community-dwelling frail older adults found no evidence for the effectiveness of nutritional interventions on disability measures. In the same review, three of eight physical exercise intervention trials reported a positive outcome for disability.[40] More recently, a 3-month multicomponent exercise program increased lean body mass and strength in a small sample of obese frail older adults, and diet and exercise together produced the best results in the preservation of lean body mass and improvement in strength, gait, and balance.[41]

Data from the Third National Health and Nutrition Examination Survey indicated that serum 25-hydroxyvitamin D (25-(OH)D) levels less than 15 ng/mL were associated with increased risk for frailty after adjusting for the season of the year and latitude to account for sunlight exposure.[42] Serum 25-(OH)D levels below 20 ng/mL and above 30 ng/mL were associated with the greatest odds for frailty in older women.[43] A similar study of elderly men found the odds for frailty increased with serum 25-(OH)D levels less than 20 ng/mL.[44]

Vitamin D, along with carotenoids, creatine, dehydroepiandrosterone and b-hydroxy-b-methylbutyrate (HMB) have been identified as potentially therapies to treat frailty in older adults,[45] although few clinical trials in frail, sarcopenic, older subjects have been published. One recent study randomized bedridden nursing home subjects receiving EN to either HMB supplement ($n = 40$) or control ($n = 39$) and found higher blood urea nitrogen (BUN) levels in the control group and lower urinary urea nitrogen excretion in the HMB group at 2 to 4 weeks.[46] The investigators concluded that HMB supplementation may reduce muscle breakdown in the population.

Advanced Dementia

Dementia often accompanies frailty, but it can occur earlier in old age. It is particularly relevant to nutrition support because it comprises one the largest homogeneous populations using EN in the United States.[5] Advanced dementia is a state of chronic, progressive, usually irreversible deterioration of cognition, which eventually renders patients mute, dysphagic, unable to walk, and unable to perform activities of daily living. Other features include an inability to recognize family members, minimal verbal communication, total functional dependence, incontinence of urine and stool, and inability to ambulate independently. Dementia is caused by primary neurodegenerative diseases (such as Alzheimer disease or Parkinson disease), alcoholism, or vascular disease.[47] Advanced dementia patients have a 6-month mortality rate of 25% and a median survival of 1.3 years, which is a life expectancy similar to that of commonly recognized end-of-life conditions such as end-stage congestive heart failure. An 18-month prospective study found 86% of an advanced dementia cohort had eating problems and that survival was poor after the onset of this problem.[48]

A frequent inability to meet nutritional requirements orally makes older adults with advanced dementia potential candidates for nutrition support, usually EN because gastrointestinal function remains intact. Deficiency of a number of nutrients, including vitamins B12, B6, folate, and omega-3 fatty acids, has been associated with dementia, including Alzheimer dementia. A systematic review concluded that evidence is not yet sufficient to draw definitive conclusions on the associations of these vitamins and omega-3 fatty acids with dementia or cognitive decline.[49] Needless to say, the use of EN in elderly adults with advanced dementia is controversial despite the relative common practice. A Cochrane Database evaluation[50] of the outcome of tube feeding in older adults with advanced dementia did not identify any randomized controlled trials to use in the evaluation. Among controlled observational studies, there was no evidence that EN increases survival, improves nutritional status, or decreases the prevalence of pressure ulcers. However, none of the studies evaluated quality of life.[50] The Academy of Nutrition and Dietetics (formerly the American Dietetic Association) allows that EN use may be appropriate for advanced dementia patients who have specific and limited goals.[51] Such a goal might be improvement in physical function, which did improve among patients with advanced dementia who received adequate EN support according to a 6-month review of their medical records.[52] Enteral (tube) feeding would seem to be a prerequisite for any functional improvement in those who cannot meet nutritional requirements orally.

Nutrition Screening and Assessment

Nutrition screening (identifying those at risk for malnutrition and in need of more extensive assessment and intervention) and nutrition assessment of older adults can be obscured by physiologic and metabolic abnormalities associated with chronic disease, inflammation, sarcopenia, frailty, and diminished functional status.[53] In 2010, a consensus group proposed new definitions for malnutrition that accommodate the contributions of inflammatory metabolism in the pathogenesis of malnutrition.[54] These definitions are discussed in Chapter 9. Issues related to the procurement and preparation of food (food security) common among older adults, which apart from inflammatory complications can produce starvation-related malnutrition, further complicate the causes of malnutrition and subsequent intervention.[55] An assessment of functional capacity can assist in evaluating an older individual's ability to provide for their food security. Activities of daily living and instrumental activities of daily living are two commonly used tools for assessing the ability of an individual to both eat independently and procure and prepare food.[56] Table 36-2 summarizes the elements of these two assessment tools.

The most effective tools to assist screening the nutritional assessment of older adults not only capture anthropometric and clinical status, but also the functional ability to maintain or achieve adequate intake. With the possible exception of a thorough assessment by a qualified clinician, evidence suggests that the Mini Nutritional Assessment is the most valid assessment tool for malnutrition in ambulatory older adults and those residing in long-term care facilities.[57] The Nutrition Risk Screening-2002 (a screening tool) accomplishes the same, albeit identifying older adults at a risk for malnutrition in acute-care settings.[57]

Medicare- and Medicaid-certified long-term care facilities mandate the use of the Minimum Data Set (MDS), the clinical assessment tool that is the basis for the Resident Assessment Instrument. The MDS assesses all aspects of clinical status and facilitates problem identification, clinical interventions, and care plans for long-term care residents. As part of this assessment, the MDS solicits the individual resident's perception of their health, well-being, and activity preferences. The nutrition assessment component consists of items including swallowing status, current height and weight, weight history, current nutrition intervention(s), and the percent of required intake by the artificial (nutrition support) route if applicable.[58]

TABLE 36-2 Elements of the Functional Assessment of the Older Adult[a]

Activities of daily living (physical self-maintenance scale)
Toileting
Feeding
Grooming
Ambulation
Bathing
Instrumental activities of daily living
Ability to use the telephone
Shopping
Food preparation
Housekeeping
Laundry
Mode of transportation
Responsibility for own medication
Ability to handle finance

[a]Developed from reference 53.

Nutrient Requirements

Nutritional requirements (to achieve nutrient adequacy) in older adults are generally the same as in younger adults with some modifications associated with physiologic and functional decline (ie, organ/system senescence, sarcopenia, chronic disease, and diminished physical activity). Generally, older adults have slightly decreased requirements for fluid and energy, slightly increased requirements for protein, and increased requirements for vitamin B6, vitamin D, and calcium. Table 36-3 summarizes these nutrient requirements. In general, older adults require less fluid (although fluid status often requires a close attention due to a decrease in thirst sensitivity) and less energy than younger adults due to decreased muscle mass and daily activity. Older adults are particularly prone to unintended weight loss,[59] which can be due to inadequate intake (starvation-related malnutrition) and/or chronic disease (chronic disease–related malnutrition), sarcopenia, organ/system senescence, or frailty, which may be a combination of the previous four problems. Adequacy of fluid and energy, and perhaps a higher protein intake than that for younger adults, are the principal nutritional priorities in older adults. As with all patients and particularly older adults, nutritional requirements will vary considerably depending on the individual clinical condition and circumstances.

Fluid requirements are complicated by endocrinosenescence and the inability of the aging kidney to concentrate urine and conserve fluid in conditions of dehydration. In addition, older adults do not respond to thirst cues as well as younger adults.[60,61] Therefore, although the absolute requirement for fluid may be less than in younger adults, the decreased ability to conserve fluid focuses on the need to meet the minimal requirement; see Table 36-3 and Practice Scenario 36-1. Decrease in basal energy requirements for older adults is due mostly to a decline in lean body mass, but also, to a degree, a decrease in lean body mass (protein) turnover.[62,63] A further reduction in total daily energy requirement is due to decreased activity. If energy intake is not adjusted as requirements decrease, weight gain can result and contribute to even more of a reduction in activity. In fact, sarcopenic obesity and subsequent frailty is an increasing phenomenon among the elderly and is associated with an increased incidence of obesity in younger adults.[41] Energy requirements for all older adults should be estimated after a thorough evaluation of an individual's clinical status, activity level, and body habitus. Carbohydrate and fat requirements are similar to those of younger adults, although because gastrointestinal irregularities occur more frequently in older adults, most experts advise a dietary fiber intake of 25 to 35 g/day.[64]

The Dietary Reference Intake of protein for all adults (19 years and older), including older men and women, is 0.8 g/kg/day.[65] However, most experts recommend slightly higher intakes based on nitrogen balance studies and, more recently, concerns related to sarcopenia and the risk for chronic disease conditions (inflammatory metabolism) associated with old age.[26,66,67] Nitrogen balance studies over time (to allow the quantification of muscle mass change and potential equilibration of intake and nitrogen loss) have demonstrated that 0.8 g/kg dietary protein may be inadequate to maintain muscle mass and strength in older men and women.[66] A 3-year prospective study of protein intake and lean body mass loss in community dwelling older men and women concluded that those in the highest quintile of protein intake lost the least amount of lean body mass over 3 years. Mean protein intake at the highest quintile was 1.2 g/kg.[26] Others have suggested that higher rates of nonmuscle protein turnover (eg, hepatic acute-phase proteins associated with inflammatory metabolic adaptation) justify slightly higher protein requirements (1.0 to 1.3 g/kg) in frail older adults.[67]

The micronutrient requirements for vitamins D and B6 and calcium are higher in older rather than in younger adults. Vitamin D in particular has been recently noted for a potential role in frailty, as previously discussed,[42–44] and its requirement may be even greater than the suggested Dietary Reference Intake (Table 36-3). Vitamin B6 requirements are also higher in older adults because of evidence of changes in the vitamin's metabolism and bioavailability associated with age.[68] The suggested Dietary Reference Intake for calcium is also higher in older adults of both genders. The need in women is perhaps greater due to the higher risk for osteoporosis, but the risk for calcium abnormalities in general is higher in older adults. Most older adults cannot achieve the recommended intake (1200 mg/day) without supplementation.[69] The Dietary Reference Intake for B12 is not increased for older adults; however, older adults are more likely than younger adults to be deficient,[70] perhaps due to malabsorptive disorders related to aging and also the prolonged use of proton pump inhibitors and metformin.[71] However, the association between anemia and B12 deficiency in older adults is not conclusive[72] and the administration of B12 has not reduced adverse cardiovascular outcomes or altered cognitive decline in those with mild to moderate Alzheimer disease.[71] The relationship between neurologic function and B12 supplementation is being investigated.[70]

TABLE 36-3 Nutritional Requirements

Fluid	30 mL/kg (1500 mL/day minimum)[a]
Energy	20–30 mL/kg
Protein	1.0–1.2 g/kg
Dietary fiber	25–35 g/day
Vitamin D[a]	15 μg, 600 IU per day (age 51–70); 20 μg, 800 IU per day (> age 70)
Vitamin B6[b]	1.5 mg/day (females > age 51); 1.7 mg/day (males > age 51)
Calcium[b]	1200 mg/day (females > age 51) 1000 mg/day (males age 51–70); 1200 mg/day (males > age 70)

[a]Chernoff, R. Carbohydrate, fat, and fluid requirements in older adults. In: Chernoff R, ed. *Geriatric Nutrition*. 3rd ed. Sudbury, MA: Jones & Bartlett Publishers; 2006.
[b]Nutrients with higher Dietary Reference Intake than for adults ≤ 50 years.

Practice Scenario 36-1

Question: How can fluid requirements be met in a stroke patient with dysphagia?

Scenario: An 85-year-old male is admitted to a skilled nursing facility for rehabilitation after being hospitalized with a primary diagnosis of a cerebrovascular accident (CVA). He presented with right-sided weakness, aphasia, and dysphagia, and requires assistance with all activities of daily living. A speech language pathologist (SLP) has worked with the patient for 2 weeks and upgraded his diet from puree consistency (National Dysphagia Diet level 1) with spoon-thick liquids to a mechanically altered consistency (National Dysphagia Diet level 2) with nectar-thickened liquids. Although he continues to receive speech therapy, the SLP does not believe that he will progress to tolerating thin liquids in the near future. Nectar-thickened liquids are readily available in the facility as juices, milk, water, and coffee, but the patient does not like the consistency of the thickened liquids and is only consuming approximately 700 mL daily. On physical exam, his skin is warm and dry and the turgor indicates tenting. He is missing half of his teeth, his oral mucosa is dry, and the condition of his oral cavity is fair. Blood pressure is 96/62 mm Hg. Nonnormal recent lab values indicate an elevated blood urea nitrogen (BUN) of 32 mg/dL and a creatinine of 1.1 mg/dL with a normal glomerular filtration rate (GFR).[60] He is 70 inches tall and his current weight is 170 pounds. The family reports a weight loss of 10 pounds since he suffered the CVA a month ago.

Intervention: The Frazier Free Water Protocol was implemented and the nursing staff was instructed to provide frequent aggressive oral hygiene care (brushing and rinsing with hydrogen peroxide, suction as needed) three times a day.

Answer: By implementing the Frazier Free Water Protocol, fluid requirements can be met in a CVA patient with dysphagia who does not display sufficient oral intake of thickened liquids.

Rationale: The patient was showing signs and symptoms of dehydration as evidenced by his dry skin and oral mucosa, tenting of the skin, and elevated serum BUN. His fluid consumption, which totaled approximately 700 mL, was meeting less than 30% of his estimated fluid needs (approximately 2450 mL based on the provision of 30 mL/kg actual body weight). Liberalizing and upgrading his diet to allow thin liquids would increase aspiration risk, so the diet order for thickened liquids was continued with the addition of the Frazier Free Water Protocol. Frequent and aggressive oral hygiene care minimizes pulmonary exposure to pathogenic bacteria from the saliva in the oral cavity. The Frazier Free Water Protocol is suggested as an example of a protocol that can be implemented in acute care or skilled nursing facility settings to minimize dehydration and the occurrence of pulmonary pathology.

Frazier Free Water Protocol Guidelines[a]

- Water intake is unrestricted prior to a meal, and allowed 30 minutes after a meal
- The period of time following the meal allows for spontaneous swallows and gravity to clear pooled solid or thickened liquid residues
- Aggressive oral care is provided to patients who are unable to clean their own teeth and mouths
- Implement oral care protocol by training staff, patient, and family member
  - Twice daily brushing
  - Suctioning of oral secretions as needed to decrease bacterial load
  - Keep oral mucosa moist
  - Allow frequent and convenient cleansing
  - Three times per day oral rinse with 1.5% H_2O_2 (> 3% is harmful and < 1% has no benefit); dilute with water not normal saline

[a]Frazier Rehab Institute. Water Protocol. http://www.jhsmh.org/Health-Services/Rehab-Services-Frazier-Rehab/Specialties/Frazier-Water-Protocol.aspx. Accessed June 13, 2011.

Dietary Interventions

Nutrition care and intervention for older adults ranges from healthy diet to EN and PN support, the latter of which are the focus of this chapter. The first intervention item in Figure 36-1 is a healthy diet, which can be characterized as a diet comprised of relatively high amounts of vegetables, fruits, whole grains, poultry, fish, and low fat dairy products. Such a diet has been associated with superior nutritional status, quality of life, and survival in older community-dwelling adults as compared to diets with relatively high amounts of high fat dairy products, sweets, and desserts.[73]

A healthy diet and the ability to procure and prepare it requires the availability of the food items, the ability to obtain them, and the ability to prepare and consume them. Community-dwelling older adults are at particular risk for food insecurity, defined as the ability to maintain consistent access to nutritious food.[74] Home-delivered meals are one intervention that can address this problem.[75] However, the challenge to clinicians and public health professionals is to address issues associated with food insecurity with those that are problematic to older adults including sarcopenia, obesity, frailty, dementia, and food safety, among others.[55]

In acute and particularly long-term care settings, dietary interventions should be guided by an individual nutrition assessment. In general, liberalized diets have been advocated to both improve a patient's quality of life and preserve nutritional status, particularly in older frail adults. Therapeutic diets may be less palatable and acceptable to older individuals, thus compromising intake. In addition, participation by older adults in the content of their diet facilitates pleasure in eating and also can improve their perceived quality of life.[76] The decision to liberalize a dietary restriction should be made by a qualified clinician because of a potential for adverse outcomes.[77] Restorative dining (Figure 36-1) refers to improving or maintaining the ability of an older adult to eat independently, to rehabilitate the individual who cannot eat independently to a level where he or she requires minimal assistance, or to enable the caregiver to provide assistance for those who cannot eat entirely independently.[78]

Nutrition Support

The most comprehensive evidence-based guidelines on the use of EN and PN for older adults come from the European Society for Parenteral and Enteral Nutrition (ESPEN).[79,80] In these guidelines, EN support refers to both oral nutritional supplements (ONS) and enteral (tube) feeding, and PN refers to

FIGURE 36-1 Nutritional Interventions in the Elderly

Healthy diet (including procurement and preparation)
Individualized diet
Restorative dining
Provide for food preferences
Adjust medications
Socialization during meals
Change food consistency/texture
Provide eating aids
Provide nutritional supplement
Comfort feeding
Enteral and parenteral nutrition

central and peripheral vein administration of fluid and nutrients as well as the subcutaneous administration of fluid and electrolytes (hypodermoclysis). ONS is recommended for older adults with multiple morbidities, for the frail, and for those following orthopedic surgical procedures. Tube feeding is recommended in those with neurologic dysphagia and is not indicated in final disease states, including advanced dementia. When patients cannot meet nutrition requirements enterally, PN is a safe and effective alternative and should not be withheld as a treatment due to older age. Its use should be measured against clinically feasible chances of survival, including increased susceptibility to glycemic, fluid, electrolyte, and micronutrient complications due to older age. Hypodermoclysis is a potential intervention for moderate dehydration. Both hydration and PN are appropriate in terminal illness when consistent with the goals of palliative treatment.[79,80]

ONS interventions have the best evidence for improving nutritional status regardless of diagnosis particularly when instituted sooner rather than later in the progression of frailty, sarcopenia, or muscle atrophy from bed rest.[79] ONS and assisted oral feeding can be costly and can consume staff time; however, the initiation of tube feeding should not to be considered as an alternative. ONS may promote rehabilitation in older women after a hip fracture.[81] A Cochrane review found some evidence for the effectiveness of ONS in preventing postoperative complications in hip fracture populations but found little evidence of improved mortality.[82]

Tube feeding in older adults is most frequently accomplished via PEG.[5,34,83] Less frequently, nasoenteric feeding tubes or bridles are used, although most experts recommend PEGs for patient comfort, ease of use, and long-term durability. The most frequent reason for tube feeding in older adults is neurologic dysphagia, principally from the same causes of advanced dementia diseases such as Alzheimer disease, Parkinson disease, alcoholism, or vascular disease, although acute vascular events (eg, stroke), as in Practice Scenario 36-1, do not necessarily produce dysphagia. In cases where rehabilitation is a realistic goal, tube feeding to provide adequate nutrition is a prerequisite for recovery or functional improvement.[52,79] There is no evidence that tube feeding improves survival in cases of severe or advanced disease, including conditions that feature dementia. Unless a specific and limited goal is realistically attainable, as suggested by the American Dietetic Association Guidelines, tube feeding in advanced dementia is equivalent to tube feeding in end-stage disease and is therefore not indicated.[51,79] Although some experts have emphasized that the risks of tube feeding provide concern for its use in older adults,[84] this has not been the experience of others who have documented only very minor and infrequent complications.[52,85] Rather, a lack of a beneficial outcome[50] is the basis for concern for the use of tube feeding in older adults with advanced disease.

Comfort feeding (Figure 36-1) is suggested medical record terminology for those who wish to forgo tube feeding and to prevent the interpretation of forgoing artificial nutrition and hydration as equivalent to not feeding. A "comfort feeding only" order indicates steps are to be taken to feed a patient with care, perhaps by hand.[86] Practice Scenario 36-2 addresses this issue, individualized nutrition care, and the liberalization of therapeutic dietary restrictions.

When older adults cannot meet nutritional requirements via the enteral route, parenteral PN is an option. PN is safe when managed correctly, although the clinical chances for improvement and the increased likelihood of complications in elderly patients should be considered in the decision to implement PN.[80] As previously mentioned, PN usage data in older adults is obscure. Anecdotally, reticence to use PN is perhaps due to clinicians' perceptions that the risks (at the end of life) outweigh the benefits. In addition, the fragility of skin and veins, the required expertise in management and compounding solutions, and the cost may moderate its use. PN is infused through peripheral catheters, peripherally inserted central catheters, or central catheters (usually tunneled catheters for long-term administration). Chapter 16 addresses PN access in detail. Peripheral delivery with the catheter tip in a peripheral vein is discouraged by the authors based on the clinical opinion that the fragility of peripheral veins and the need for a frequent change of site causes understandable distress to older patients, although advances in peripheral catheters (polyurethane and silicon catheters, including midline catheters), which can remain in place longer than the standard peripheral catheter, are noted in the ESPEN guidelines.[80] However, if PN is indicated, short-term infusion is perhaps clinically meaningless and every effort should be made to accommodate patient comfort.

Older adults are more susceptible to metabolic complications on PN because of insulin resistance and often impaired cardiac and renal function. They are also more likely than younger adults to have micronutrient deficiencies. The repletion of depleted lean body mass is slower than in younger adults.[80]

Hypodermoclysis is as effective as IV rehydration for older adults with mild or moderate dehydration. It may cause fewer complications, cost less, offer greater patient comfort, and take less nursing time to administer than IV rehydration.[87] It is beginning to gain favor in American long-term health care settings, although it is a more common practice in Europe.[88]

Neither the ESPEN guidelines[79,80] nor the American Society for Parenteral and Enteral Nutrition (A.S.P.E.N.) ethics position[89] recommend the use of EN or PN in end-stage disease or terminal illness, including advanced stages of dementia and neurologic conditions, such as persistent vegetative state. Chapter 39 reviews this issue and related ethical considerations in detail.

Practice Scenario 36-2

Question: What is an alternative approach to artificial nutrition and hydration in a patient with advanced dementia?

Scenario: A 93-year-old female is to be discharged home, status posthospitalization for a hip fracture. Her prior medical history includes dementia, depression, hypertension, hyperlipidemia, and osteoporosis. The patient, family, and primary physician decided against surgery. The patient's dementia has progressed and she has a do not resuscitate order. She has a living will stating that she does not wish to use artificial nutrition and hydration when she can no longer meet her fluid and nutrient requirements. She is 5 feet tall and her current weight is 95 pounds. Six months prior she weighed 120 pounds. She has fallen several times in the past 2 months, the most current resulting in the hip fracture. She now requires total assistance with her activities of daily living, including eating, because she has difficulty cutting up her food.

Laboratory data: Sodium (Na), 142 mmol/L; potassium (K), 3.9 mmol/L; blood urea nitrogen (BUN), 33 mg/dL; creatinine (Cr), 1.1 mg/dL; glucose (Glu), 100 mg/dL; calcium (Ca), 7.7 mg/dL; albumin (Alb), 2.6 g/dL; serum osmolality, 310 mOsm/Kg.

Her discharge medications include donepezil, citalopram, enoxaparin, metoprolol, valsartan, ezetimibe, and docusate sodium. A nutrition-focused physical examination reveals that her teeth are in poor condition with many missing, and that she has bitemporal wasting but no edema. Her skin assessment indicates a stage II pressure ulcer on her sacrum. Blood pressure is 105/75. During her hospitalization, her meal consumption was documented as 25% to 50% of her energy requirement. Following the advice of their doctor, the family avoids cooking for her with salt and restricts foods that are high in cholesterol, but report that since they started to do so they have noticed that her intake has declined and that her weight loss has accelerated.

Intervention: The patient was discharged on a regular diet. The family was instructed to encourage and assist her at meals as needed, and to provide her with her food preferences as six small nutrient-dense meals or snacks made up of finger foods throughout the day. An oral nutritional supplement was also recommended to help meet calorie, protein, and fluid needs.

Answer: Alternate approaches to artificial nutrition and hydration in a patient with advanced dementia include: the liberalization of therapeutic diet, the provision of oral nutritional supplements, the provision of small frequent nutrient-dense meals and snacks throughout the day as finger foods when possible, and the assistance as needed with meals.

Rationale: Therapeutic diets are part of disease treatment; however, when oral intake is inadequate, such diets may contribute to unintentional weight loss. The patient's blood pressure is managed medically and dietary control of hypercholesterolemia is not a priority in a 93-year-old woman. Thus, her diet can be liberalized to facilitate adequate intake.[a] In patients with Alzheimer disease, an individualized meal plan should emphasize food preferences, nutrient density, supplements, and feeding assistance.[a] Use of finger foods helps maintain independence at meals and enhances meal time enjoyment.[b] Palliative care is the clinical priority for this patient, and dietary restrictions can be liberalized as long as foods and beverages provided can be safely consumed.[a,b]

References

1. Centers for Disease Control and Prevention. Public health and aging: trends in aging–United States and worldwide. *JAMA.* 2003;289(11):1371–1373.
2. Liu CK, Fielding RA. Exercise as an intervention for frailty. *Clin Geriatr Med.* 2011;27(1):101–110.
3. U.S. Census Bureau. International Database. Table 094. Midyear Population, by Age and Sex. http://www.census.gov/population/www/projections/natdet-D1A.html. Accessed November 21, 2011.
4. Grant MD, Rudberg MA, Brody JA. Gastrostomy placement and mortality among hospitalized Medicare beneficiaries. *JAMA.* 1998;279(24):1973–1976.
5. Braun UK, Rabeneck L, McCullough LB, et al. Decreasing use of percutaneous endoscopic gastrostomy tube feeding for veterans with dementia–racial differences remain. *J Am Geriatr Soc.* 2005; 53(2):242–248.
6. Weinberg AD, Pals JK, Wei JY. The utilization of intravenous therapy programs in community long-term care nursing facilities. *J Nutr Health Aging.* 1997;1(3):161–166.
7. Chernoff R. *Geriatric Nutrition.* 3rd ed. Sudbury, MA: Jones & Bartlett Publishers; 2006.
8. Harper ME, Bevilacqua L, Hagopian K, Weindruch R, Ramsey JJ. Ageing, oxidative stress, and mitochondrial uncoupling. *Acta Physiol Scand.* 2004;182(4):321–331.
9. Knight JA. The biochemistry of aging. *Adv Clin Chem.* 2000; 35:1–62.
10. Gavrilov LA, Gavrilova NS. Evolutionary theories of aging and longevity. *ScientificWorldJournal* 2002;2:339–356.

[a]Dorner B, Friedrich EK, Posthauer ME. Position of the American Dietetic Association: Individualized nutrition approaches for older adults in healthcare communities. *J Am Diet Assoc.* 2010;110(10):1549–1553.
[b]O'Sullivan Maillet J. Position of the American Dietetic Association: Ethical and legal issues in nutrition, hydration, and feeding. *J Am Diet Assoc.* 2008;108(5):873–882.

11. Kane RL, Ouslander JG, Abrass IB. Clinical implications of the aging process. In: Kane RL, Ouslander JG, Abrass IB, eds. *Essentials of Clinical Geriatrics*. 5th ed. Heightown, NJ: McGraw-Hill; 2004: 3–18.
12. Bartali B, Frongillo EA, Bandinelli S, et al. Low nutrient intake is an essential component of frailty in older persons. *J Gerontol A Biol Med Sci*. 2006;61(6):589–593.
13. Topinkova E. Aging, disability and frailty. *Ann Nutr Metab*. 2008; 52(Suppl 1):6–11.
14. Waters DL, Baumgartner RN, Garry PJ, Vellas B. Advantages of dietary, exercise-related, and therapeutic interventions to prevent and treat sarcopenia in adult patients: an update. *Clin Interv Aging*. 2010;5:259–270.
15. Cruz-Jenthoft AJ, Baeyens JP, Bauer JM, et al. European Working Group on Sarcopenia in Older People. Sarcopenia: European consensus on definition and diagnosis: report of the European Working Group on Sarcopenia in Older People. *Age Ageing*. 2010; 39(4):412–423.
16. Fielding RA, Vellas B, Evans WJ, et al. Sarcopenia: an undiagnosed condition in older adults. Current consensus definition: prevalence, etiology, and consequences. International working group on sarcopenia. *J Am Med Dir Assoc*. 2011;12(4):249–256.
17. Delmonico MJ, Harris TB, Lee JS, et al. Alternative definitions of sarcopenia, lower extremity performance, and functional impairment with aging in older men and women. *Am Geratr Soc*. 2007; 55:769–774.
18. Visser M, Kritchevsky SB, Newman AB, et al. Lower serum albumin concentration and change in muscle mass: the Health Aging and Body Composition Study. *Am J Clin Nutr*. 2005;82:531–537.
19. Argiles JM, Busquets S, Felipe A, Lopez-Soriano FJ. Muscle wasting in cancer and ageing: cachexia versus sarcopenia. *Adv Gerontol*. 2006;18:39–54.
20. Thomas DR. Loss of skeletal muscle mass in aging: examining the relationship of starvation, sarcopenia, and cachexia. *Clin Nutr*. 2007;26:389–399.
21. Marzetti E, Leeuwenburgh C. Skeletal muscle apoptosis, sarcopenia, and frailty at old age. *Exp Gerontol*. 2006;41:1234–1238.
22. Hiona A, Leeuwenburgh C. The role of mitochondrial DNA mutations in aging and sarcopenia: implications for the mitochondrial vicious cycle theory at old age. *Exp Gerontol*. 2008;43(1):24–33.
23. Lee CE, McArdle A, Griffiths RD. The role of hormones, cytokines and heat shock proteins during age-related muscle loss. *Clin Nutr*. 2007;26:524–534.
24. Mangione KK, Miller AH, Naughton IV. Cochrane review: Improving physical function and performance with progressive resistance strength training in older adults. *Phys Ther*. 2010;90(12): 1711–1715.
25. Burton LA, Sumukadas D. Optimal management of sarcopenia. *Clin Interv Aging*. 2010;5:217–228.
26. Houston DK, Nicklas BJ, Ding J, et al. Dietary protein intake is associated with lean mass change in older, community-dwelling adults: the Health, Aging, and Body Composition (Health ABC) Study. *Am J Clin Nutr*. 2008;87(1):150–155.
27. Paddon-Jones D, Short KR, Campbell WW, Volpi E, Wolfe RR. Role of dietary protein in the sarcopenia of aging. *Am J Clin Nutr*. 2008;87(5):1562S–1566S.
28. Campbell WW. Synergistic use of higher–protein diets or nutritional supplements with resistance training to counter sarcopenia. *Nutr Rev*. 2007;65(9);416–422.
29. Pennings B, Boire Y, Senden JM, et al. Whey protein stimulates postprandial protein accretion more effectively than do casein and casein hydrolysate in older men. *Am J Clin Nutr*. 2011;93(5): 997–1005.
30. Morley JE, Argiles JM, Evans WJ, et al. Nutritional recommendations for the management of sarcopenia. *J Am Med Dir Assoc*. 2010;11(6):391–396.
31. Smith GI, Atherton P, Reeds DN, et al. Dietary omega-3 fatty acid supplementation increases the rate of muscle protein synthesis in older adults: a randomized controlled trial. *Am J Clin Nutr*. 2011; 93(2):402–412.
32. Adamo ML, Farrar RP. Resistance training, and IGF involvement in the maintenance of muscle mass during the aging process. *Ageing Res Rev*. 2006;5(3):310–331.
33. Solerte SB. Gassaruso C, Bonacasa R, et al. Nutritional supplements with oral amino acid mixtures increases whole-body lean mass and insulin sensitivity in elderly subjects with sarcopenia. *Am J Cardiol*. 2008;101(11A):69E–77E.
34. Dillon EL, Sheffield-Moore M, Paddon-Jones D, et al. Amino acid supplementation increases lean body mass, basal muscle protein synthesis, and insulin-like growth factor-1 expression in older women. *J Clin Endocrinol Metab*. 2009;94(5):1630–1637.
35. Fried LP, Tangen CM, Watson J, et al. Frailty in older adults: evidence for a phenotype. *J Gerontol A Biol Sci Med Sci*. 2001;56; M146–M157.
36. Hubbard RE, O'Mahony MS, Calver BL, Woodhouse KW. Nutrition, inflammation, and leptin levels in aging and frailty. *J Am Geriatr Soc*. 2008;56(2):279–284.
37. Hubbard RE, Woodhouse KW. Frailty, inflammation and the elderly. *Biogerontology*. 2010;11(5):635–641.
38. Bartali B, Frongillo EA, Bandinelli S, et al. Low nutrient intake is an essential component of frailty in older persons. *J Gerontol A Biol Sci Med Sci*. 2006;61(6):589–593.
39. Isaia G, Mondino S, Germinara C, et al. Malnutrition in an elderly demented population living at home. *Arch Gerontol Geriatr*. 2011;53(3):249–251.
40. Daniels R, van Rossum E, de Witte L, Kempen GI, van den Heuvel W. Interventions to prevent disability in frail community–dwelling elderly: a systematic review. *BMC Health Serv Res*. 2008; 8:278.
41. Villareal DT, Smith GI, Sinacore DR, Shah K, Mittendorfer B. Regular multicomponent exercise increases physical fitness and muscle protein anabolism in frail, obese, older adults. *Obesity*. 2011; 19(2);312–318.
42. Wilhelm-Leen ER, Hall YN, DeBoer IH, Chertow GM. Vitamin D deficiency and frailty in older Americans. *J Intern Med*. 2010; 268(2):171–180.
43. Ensrud KE, Ewsing SK, Fredman L, et al. Circulating 25–hydroxyvitamin D levels and frailty status in older women. *J Clin Endocrinol Metab*. 2010;95(12):5266–5273.
44. Ensrud KE, Blackwell TL, Cauley JA, et al. Circulating 25–hydroxyvitamin D levels and frailty in older men: the osteoporotic fractures in men study. *J Am Geriatr Soc*. 2011;59(1):101–106.
45. Cherniack EP, Florex HJ, Troen BR. Emerging therapies to treat frailty syndrome in the elderly. *Altern Med Rev*. 2007:12(3): 246–258.
46. Hsieh LC, Chow CJ, Chang WC, Liu TH, Chang CK. Effect of beta-hydroxy-beta-methylbutyrate on protein metabolism in bed-ridden elderly receiving tube feeding. *Asia Pac J Clin Nutr*. 2010; 19(2):200–208.
47. Beers MH, ed. *The Merck Manual*, 18th ed. Whitehouse Station, NJ: Merck & Co., Inc.; 2006:1811–1821.
48. Mitchell SL, Teno JM, Kiely DK, et al. The clinical course of advanced dementia. *N Engl J Med*. 2009;361(16):1529–1537.
49. Dangour AD, Whitehouse PJ, Rafferty K, et al. B vitamins and fatty acids in the prevention and treatment of Alzheimer's disease and dementia: a systematic review. *J Alzheimers Dis*. 2010;22(1):205–224.

50. Sampson EL, Candy B, Jones L. Enteral tube feeding for older people with advanced dementia. *Cochrane Database Syst Rev.* 2009; 15(2):CD007209.
51. O'Sullivan Maillet J. Position of the American Dietetic Association: ethical and legal issues in nutrition, hydration, and feeding. *J Am Diet Assoc.* 2008;108(5):873–882.
52. Mueller C, Gilbride J, Nestle M. Enteral nutrition support in elderly residents of long-term care facilities. *Top Clin Nutr.* 2003; 18(1):13–20.
53. Mueller C. Inflammation, old age, and nutrition assessment. *Top Clin Nutr.* 2008;23(2):131–138.
54. Jensen GL, Mirtallo J, Compher C, et al. Adult starvation and disease-related malnutrition: a proposal for etiology-based diagnosis in the clinical practice setting from the International Consensus Guideline Committee. *JPEN J Parenter Enteral Nutr.* 2010;34(2):156–159.
55. Johnson MA, Dwyer JT, Jensen GL, et al. Challenges and new opportunities for clinical nutrition interventions in the aged. *J Nutr.* 2011;141(3):535–541.
56. Lawton MP. The functional assessment of elderly people. *Am J Geriatr.* 1971;19(6):465–481.
57. Sieber CC. Nutritional screening tools--how does the MNA compare? Proceedings of the session held in Chicago May 2–3, 2006 (15 Years of Mini Nutritional Assessment). *J Nutr Health Aging.* 2006;10(6):488–492.
58. Centers for Medicare & Medicaid Services. Appendix F: Item matrix. In: *MDS 3.0 RAI Manual.* http://www.cms.gov/NursingHomeQualityInits/downloads/MDS30ItemSubsetsV1.zip. Accessed June 6, 2011.
59. Dorner B. Friedrich EK, Posthuarer ME. Practice Paper of the American Dietetic Association: Individualized nutrition approaches for older adults in healthcare communities. *J Am Diet Assoc.* 2010; 110(10):1554–1563.
60. Naitoh M, Burrell LM. Thirst in elderly subjects. *J Nutr Health Aging.* 1998;2(3):172–177.
61. Rolls BJ, Phillips PA. Aging and disturbances of thirst and fluid balance. *Nutr Rev.* 1990;48(3):137–144.
62. Zurlo F, Larson K, Bogardus C, et al. Skeletal muscle metabolism is a major determinant of resting energy expenditure. *J Clin Invest.* 1990;86(5):1423–1427
63. Welle S, Nair KS. Relationship of resting metabolic rate to body composition and protein turnover. *Am J Physiol.* 1990;258(6 pt 1): E990–E998.
64. Chernoff R. Carbohydrate, fat and fluid requirements in older adults. In: Chernoff R, ed. *Geriatric Nutrition.* 3rd ed. Sudbury, MA: Jones & Bartlett Publishers; 2006:23–30.
65. Institute of Medicine of the National Academies. *Dietary Reference Intakes for Energy, Carbohydrate, Fiber, Fat, Fatty Acids, Cholesterol, Protein, and Amino Acids (Macronutrients).* Washington, DC: National Academies Press; 2002/2005.
66. Campbell WW, Carnell NS, Thalacker AE. Protein metabolism and requirements. In: Chernoff R, ed. *Geriatric Nutrition.* 3rd ed. Sudbury, MA: Jones & Bartlett Publishers; 2006:15–22.
67. Morais JA, Chevalier S, Gougeon R. Protein turnover and requirements in the healthy and frail elderly. *J Nutr Health Aging.* 2006;10(4):272–283.
68. Suter PM. Vitamin metabolism and requirements in the elderly: Selected aspects. In: Chernoff R, ed. *Geriatric Nutrition.* 3rd ed. Sudbury, MA: Jones & Bartlett Publishers; 2006:31–76.
69. Lindeman RD. Mineral requirements. In: Chernoff R, ed. *Geriatric Nutrition.* 3rd ed. Sudbury, MA: Jones & Bartlett Publishers; 2006: 77–93.
70. Dangour AD, Allen E, Clarke R, et al. A randomized controlled trial investigating the effect of vitamin B12 supplementation on neurological function in healthy older adults: the Older People and Enhanced Neurological function (OPEN) study protocol. *Nutr J.* 2011;10:22.
71. Langan RC, Zawistoski KJ. Update on vitamin B12 deficiency. *Am Fam Physician.* 2011;83(12):1425–1430.
72. den Elzen WP, van der Weele GM, Gussekloo J, Westendorp RG, Assendelft WJ. Subnormal vitamin B12 concentrations and anaemia in older people: a systematic review. *BMC Geriatr.* 2010; 10:42.
73. Anderson AL, Harris TB, Tylavsky FA, et al. Dietary patterns and survival of older adults. *J Am Diet Assoc.* 2011;11(1):84–91.
74. Franklin B, Jones A, Love D, et al. Exploring mediators of food insecurity and obesity: A review of recent literature. *J Community Health.* 2012;37(1):253–264.
75. Frongillo EA, Wolfe WS. Impact of participation in home-delivered meals on nutrient intake, dietary patterns, and food insecurity of older persons in New York state. *J Nutr Elder.* 2010;(3): 293–310.
76. Dorner B, Niedert KC, Welch PK. Position of the American Dietetic Association: Liberalized diets for adults in long-term care. *J Am Diet Assoc.* 2002;102(9):1316–1323.
77. Arcand J, Ivanov J, Sasson IJ, et al. A high-sodium diet is associated with acute decompensated heart failure in ambulatory heart failure patients: a prospective follow-up study. *Am J Clin Nutr.* 2011;93(2):332–337.
78. Robinson G, Leif BJ. *Nutrition Management & Restorative Dining for Older Adults.* Chicago, IL: Consultant Dietitians in Healthcare Facilities/The American Dietetic Association; 2001:117–119.
79. Volkert D, Berner YN, Berry E, et al. ESPEN Guidelines on enteral nutrition: Geriatrics. *Clin Nutr.* 2006;25(2):330–360.
80. Sobotka L, Schneider SM, Berner YN, et al. ESPEN Guidelines on parenteral nutrition: Geriatrics. *Clin Nutr.* 2009;28(4): 461–466.
81. Akner G, Cederholm T. Treatment of protein-energy malnutrition in chronic nonmalignant disorders. *Am J Clin Nutr.* 2001;74(1):6–24.
82. Avenell A, Handoll HH. Nutritional supplementation for hip fracture aftercare in older people. *Cochrane Database Syst Rev.* 2006;(4):CD001880. doi:10.1136/ebn.10.2.56.
83. Dorner B, Posthauer ME, Friedrich EK, Robinson GE. Enteral nutrition for older adults in nursing facilities. *Nutr Clin Pract.* 2011;26(3):261–272.
84. Finucane TE, Christmas C, Travis K. Tube feeding in patients with advanced dementia. A review of the evidence. *JAMA.* 1999; 282(14):1365–1367.
85. Freeman C, Ricevuto A DeLegge MH. Enteral nutrition in patients with dementia. *Curr Opin Gastroenterol.* 2010;26(2): 156–159.
86. Palecek EJ, Teno JM, Casarett DJ, et al. Comfort feeding only: a proposal to bring clarity to decision-making regarding difficulty with eating for persons with advanced dementia. *J Am Geriatr Soc.* 2010;58(3):580–584.
87. Pershad J. A systematic data review of the cost of rehydration therapy. *Appl Health Econ Policy.* 2010;(8):203–214.
88. Martin CM. Hypodemoclysis: renewed interest in an old technique. *Consult Pharm.* 2010;25(4):209–212.
89. Barrocas A, Geppert C, Durfee SM, et al. A.S.P.E.N. ethics position paper. *Nutr Clin Prac.* 2010;25(6):672–679.

37 Chylothorax and Chylous Ascites

Thomas H. Frazier, MD, David A. Spain, MD, FACS, and Stephen A. McClave, MD

CONTENTS

Background . . . 631
Lymphatic System . . . 631
Anatomy . . . 631
Physiology . . . 631
Chylothorax . . . 632
Definition . . . 632
Etiology . . . 632
Chylous Ascites . . . 632
Definition . . . 632
Etiology . . . 633
Nutritional/Immunological Effects of Sustained Chyle Leak . . . 633
Nutrition Management . . . 634
References . . . 636

Objectives

1. Describe the anatomy and function of the lymphatic system.
2. Recognize the common clinical scenarios of chylothorax and chylous ascites.
3. Define the metabolic/nutrition consequences of a chyle leak.
4. Develop an appropriate nutrition regimen for a chyle leak and outline how to document efficacy.

Test Your Knowledge Questions

1. The primary purpose of chyle is the absorption of:
   A. Long-chain triglycerides (LCTs)
   B. Medium-chain triglycerides (MCTs)
   C. Carbohydrates
   D. Aromatic amino acids
2. Which of the following fluid and electrolyte abnormalities or vitamin deficiencies are common among patients with lymphatic injury and a chyle leak?
   A. Hypernatremia
   B. Hypervolemia
   C. Folate deficiency
   D. Vitamin D deficiency
3. Conservative medical management in a patient with an identified lymphatic injury and a chyle leak might include which of the following?
   A. High-fat oral diet
   B. Elemental enteral feeding formula
   C. Pancreatic enzymes
   D. Albumin infusion

4. Evidence that medical management has failed and that surgical intervention should be considered for a lymphatic injury and chyle leak would include which of the following?
   A. High output (> 500 mL/d) of chylous effluent for > 2 days
   B. Continued output of chylous effluent of any volume for > 14 days
   C. Development of hypocalcemia
   D. Development of hypoalbuminemia

Test Your Knowledge Answers

1. The correct answer is **A.** The primary purpose of chyle is the absorption and transportation of LCTs in the intestines. Chyle is formed in the lacteals of the intestine during digestion in response to the presence of intraluminal fat. The chyle binds with LCTs to form chylomicrons, which are then absorbed and transported by the intestinal lymphatics to the bloodstream. MCTs are absorbed directly as are carbohydrate and amino acids.[1]
2. The correct answer is **D.** Patients with a lymphatic injury and a chyle leak may sustain profound losses of fluid volume, electrolytes, and vitamins. The most typical finding is hyponatremia and a mild metabolic acidosis. Patients may sustain enough fluid losses to develop intravascular volume depletion. Hypoproteinemia and hypoalbuminemia reduce osmotic pressure in the vascular space and extravasation of fluid complicates the hypovolemia further. Patients are also at significant risk for deficiencies of the fat-soluble vitamins (see Chapter 8), which include vitamins A, D, E, and K. Vitamin D deficiency in particular may be one of the more common vitamin deficiencies in these patients and may result in clinical hypocalcemia.[2] Patients are not necessarily at risk for deficiency of water-soluble vitamins, such as folate.
3. The correct answer is **B.** It is appropriate to give patients with a lymphatic injury and chyle leak a trial period of medical management at the time of initial diagnosis to help close the leak. This may involve either a low-fat diet taken by mouth or an elemental enteral feeding formula comprised of individual amino acids and carbohydrate (which is nearly fat-free) infused through a feeding tube. The oral diet often may be supplemented by MCTs, which are absorbed directly across the mucosa of the small bowel and into the portal vein, and do not require transport through lymphatics for absorption. Further conservative medical management may also include parenteral nutrition (PN) with or without octreotide therapy. Octreotide, a somatostatin analog, may be synergistic with the PN in reducing lymphatic flow and helping to seal the leak. Although patients may develop hypoproteinemia and hypoalbuminemia because of excessive losses of protein through the chyle leak, albumin infusions are expensive and have not been shown to change patient outcome. Therefore, albumin infusions are discouraged.
4. The correct answer is **B.** Once the diagnosis of a lymphatic injury and a chyle leak is made, and patients are placed on conservative medical management, several parameters must be followed to evaluate response to therapy. High output of chylous effluent of > 500 mL/d for > 5 days or a persistent leak of any volume for > 2 weeks despite conservative therapy is an indication that the medical management has failed to seal the leak, and surgical intervention should be considered.[2,3] Likewise, development of a clinical complication such as sepsis (see Chapter 23) may be indicative of immune suppression resulting from the chyle leak and an indication that conservative medical therapy has not been successful. Development of hypoproteinemia and hypoalbuminemia in the absence of other complications is fairly common in this patient population and should not be indications for surgical intervention.

Background

Chyle is the fat-containing, creamy white fluid that forms in the lacteals of the intestine during digestion. It is composed primarily of lymphatic fluid and chylomicrons. Chyle is transported through the lymphatics and enters the venous circulation via the thoracic duct. Approximately 70% of the ingested dietary fat passes through this system. In addition, the lymphatic system plays an important role in absorption of fat-soluble vitamins and the reabsorption of proteins lost through capillary leakage. Thus, injuries to the lymphatic system resulting in a chyle extravasation into the pleural and/or peritoneal space may have profound effects on the nutritional status of patients.

Lymphatic System

Anatomy

Variations in lymphatic anatomy are common. In approximately half the population, the cisterna chyli is formed by the confluence of three lymphatic trunks: two lumbar trunks from each of the lower extremities and one intestinal trunk (Figure 37-1). This confluence usually occurs to the right of the posteromedial portion of the aorta at the level of the renal arteries (L2 vertebrae) and produces a duct that ascends superiorly. In the remaining patients, a retroperitoneal lymphatic plexus condenses into a duct at the diaphragm. In either case, the formed duct enters the chest through the aortic hiatus as the thoracic duct. The thoracic duct ascends the right hemithorax in the posterior mediastinum. At the level of the fourth or fifth thoracic vertebrae, it passes to the left chest and proceeds superiorly. The duct enters the neck anterior to the left subclavian artery and empties into the venous system at the confluence of the left subclavian vein and internal jugular vein.

Physiology

One of the primary purposes of the intestinal lymphatic system is the transport of ingested fats. Lymph flow in the fasting state may be as low as 1 mL/min, but the flow increases to > 200 mL/min following a high-fat meal. Between 50% and 90% of thoracic duct lymph drainage is derived from the

FIGURE 37-1 Anatomy of the Thoratic Duct and Lymphatic System

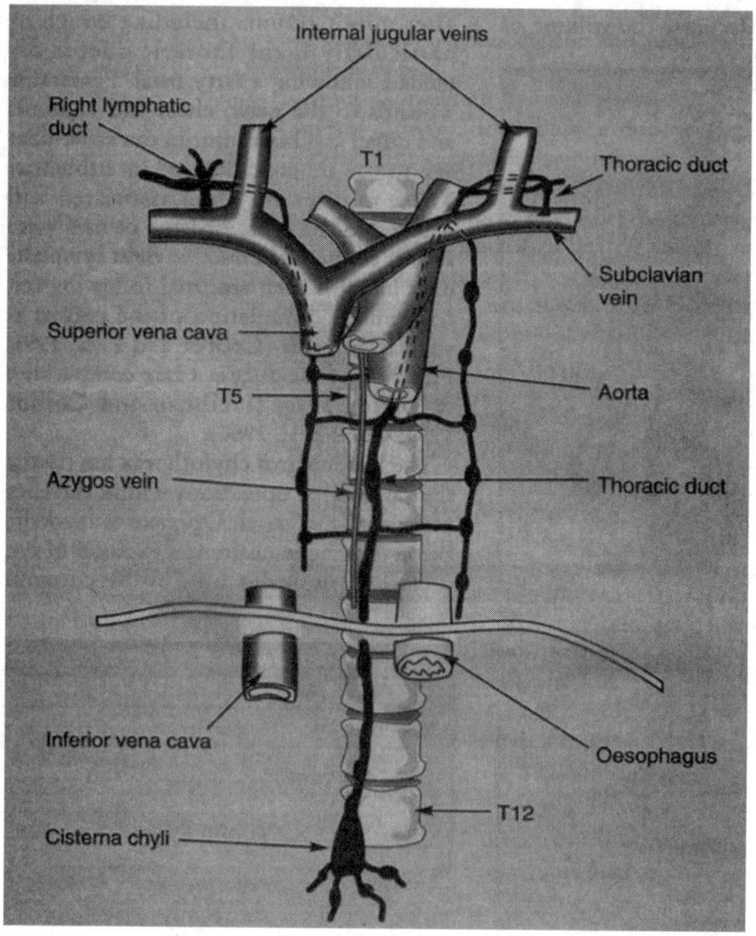

Reprinted with permission from Paes ML, Powell H. Chylothorax: an update. *Br J Hosp Med.* 1994;51:483–490.

abdomen. LCTs are absorbed and transported by the intestinal lymphatics to the bloodstream as chylomicrons. MCTs are absorbed directly into the portal circulation and, therefore, do not stimulate increased lymphatic flow (see Chapter 5). Following a meal, it takes approximately 2 to 3 hours for the fat to be absorbed from the small intestine.

Chylothorax

Definition

Chylothorax is characterized by the accumulation of chyle within the pleural space. Most patients present with symptoms consistent with a pleural effusion, which is then confirmed with a chest radiograph. Thoracentesis reveals the typical milky, white fluid. Biochemical studies of the fluid are most often used to confirm the diagnosis. Fluid analysis usually documents a high protein and lipid content with elevated triglycerides and low cholesterol (Table 37-1).[1,4]

Etiology

The most common causes of primary chylothorax are malignancies, while secondary chylothorax is usually related to surgery and/or trauma (Table 37-2).[3] The chyle leak usually results from a direct injury to the thoracic duct or from failure to ligate major lymphatic branches.[5] The majority of postoperative cases are seen following esophagectomy or surgery involving the right pulmonary hilum. Thus, most patients have a right-sided chylothorax. However, operations at or above where the thoracic duct crosses the midline may result in either bilateral effusions or left-sided collections. This can be confused with volume overload. Most postoperative patients present early with chylous drainage from the chest tube. Occasionally, patients will present weeks later, returning to the hospital some time after discharge with a symptomatic pleural effusion.[5] Thoracentesis at that time will confirm the diagnosis. Chyle can be difficult to discern from purulent fluid, and diagnosis should also be confirmed by biochemical testing of the effluent.

Chylothorax may also occur as the direct result of a lymphatic abnormality (ie, primary or spontaneous chylothorax). The more common causes of spontaneous chylothorax are lymphatic obstruction and lymphangiectasis. Lymphatic obstruction is usually caused by malignancy, involving either a lymphoma or mediastinal lymph node metastasis. If a patient presents with spontaneous chylothorax (ie, not after an operation), an aggressive investigation for malignancy should be undertaken.[3] If no obvious cause for the chylothorax is found, bipedal lymphangiography has been used to identify lymphatic abnormalities,[3] although this is largely being replaced by lymphoscintigraphy.[1] Occasionally, chylothorax may be seen in a patient with cirrhosis and chylous ascites.

Chylous Ascites

Definition

Similar to chylothorax, chylous ascites is an uncommon condition that is caused by disruption or obstruction of the abdominal lymphatics. Most patients present with symptomatic ascites, such as abdominal distention, increasing abdominal girth, and dyspnea. Postoperative patients who develop chylous ascites frequently present with increased abdominal

TABLE 37-1 Biochemical Characteristics of Chyle

Total lipid content 0.4 to 4.0 g/dL
Triglycerides 150 to 1100 mg/dL (or more)
Cholesterol < 220 mg/dL
Lymphocytes 400 to 7000 cells $\times 10^8$/dL
Total protein > 3 g/dL
pH alkaline

TABLE 37-2 Etiologies of Chylothorax

Amyloidosis
Congenital chylothorax
Coronary artery bypass grafting
Coughing (violent) following a heavy meal
Malignancies
Neck surgery, complications of radical dissection
Spontaneous accumulation
Thoracic cage compression (particularly during cardiopulmonary resuscitation)
Thoracic duct trauma from thoracotomy tubes
Thoracic surgery, including procedures involving the esophagus, lungs, and heart
Thrombosis of the left subclavian vein from an indwelling catheter
Tuberculosis and other infectious processes
Vomiting (violent) following a heavy meal

girth following the initiation of an oral diet, usually around postoperative day 5. The resumption of diet, especially one containing fats, leads to increased lymph flow and the subsequent accumulation of ascites. Chylous ascites should also be suspected in any patient with known abdominal malignancy that develops abdominal distention.

Etiology

The most common cause of chylous ascites in adults is malignant obstruction, which carries a poor prognosis because of the extent of the underlying disease (Table 37-3). Malignancies associated with chylous ascites include lymphomas and carcinomatosis, which are often secondary to ovarian, gastric, or colonic primaries. Chylous ascites may also occur after abdominal surgery. Operations can lead to lymphatic injury, such as abdominal aortic surgery involving dissection in the retroperitoneum at or near the cisterna chyli. These patients have a favorable prognosis and usually respond to conservative management.[6,7] Chylous ascites may also occur in patients with cirrhosis or spontaneous bacterial peritonitis. A fluid wave may be found on physical examination, but this may be difficult to appreciate in an early postoperative patient. Ultrasound examination will confirm the presence of ascites. The diagnosis is confirmed by paracentesis with return of milky, chylous fluid. Similar to chylothorax, this fluid will have a high protein and high lipid content (which is comprised of high triglyceride concentrations but low cholesterol).[6]

TABLE 37-3 Etiologies of Chylous Ascites

Malignancies
Lymphoma
Carcinomatosis (ovarian, colon, gastric primary)
Postoperative
Abdominal aortic injury
Retroperitoneal lymphadenectomy
Liver transplantation
Cirrhosis
Spontaneous bacterial peritonitis
Congenital abnormalities of the lymphatic system
Tuberculosis and other infectious processes

Nutritional/Immunological Effects of Sustained Chyle Leak

Patients who have sustained a lymphatic injury, but for routine purposes are kept on nothing by mouth orders after an operation, may demonstrate a period of asymptomatic chyle leak. Continued fasting prolongs this period and may lead to delay in making the diagnosis of a chyle leak. Adverse clinical effects depend on the amount or magnitude of the leak, the rate and duration of flow, the size of the cavity, and ultimately the clinical and dietary management of the patient.[2] Local effects may result from the leak of chyle into the pleural cavity, and range from compression of the ipsilateral lung to mediastinal shift with compression of the contralateral lung and impairment of cardiac function.[2] The greatest morbidity, however, stems from alterations in protein and fat metabolism, compromise of immunologic function, and deterioration in nutritional status.

Because normal chyle flow can range up to 4 L/d (10 to 100 mL/kg/d), a sustained chyle leak can result in hypovolemia, electrolyte imbalances, anemia, and hemodynamic instability.[2] Fluid losses alone can be as high as 2.5 L/d.[3] Patients may demonstrate a metabolic acidosis because the pH of chyle is usually > 7 (Table 37-1). The most common electrolyte disturbances include hyponatremia and hypocalcemia.[2]

Prolonged chyle loss may deplete body protein and reserves of fat and vitamins. The lipid content of chyle ranges from 0.4 to 4.0 g/dL and is characterized by a high-triglyceride, low-cholesterol concentration. Patients with lymphatic injury are at risk for vitamin deficiencies (see Chapter 8), particularly the fat-soluble vitamins A, D, E, and K. Hypoproteinemia may result because of losses in chyle of albumin, fibrinogen, immunoglobulin, and enzymes such as amylase, lipase, and alanine aminotranferase.[2] Protein loss is greater when lymphatic injury involves chylothorax than when it involves chylous ascites. In patients with both clinical manifestations, the protein concentration in the pleural effusion is twice that of the ascites.[1] The degree of protein loss may be related to etiology because the chyle effluent in cirrhotic patients with chylothorax has a lower concentration of protein, lactate dehydrogenase, cholesterol, and leukocytes than that seen in patients with chylothorax due to other causes.[1] The protein depletion may result in transcapillary fluid shifts and may compound problems of fluid management and maintenance of intravascular volume.[2] Ironically, the continued loss of protein and fat substrate is accompanied by increased metabolic demand because of the hypermetabolism associated with surgery, trauma, and sepsis[2] (see Chapters 23 and 24).

Adverse immunological effects result from the loss of cellular protein in the chyle leak. Lymphocytes (over 90% of which are T cells) comprise the bulk (95%) of the cellular content of chyle.[2] Thus, a sustained chyle loss depletes the T-cell population and impairs cell-mediated immunity. Humoral immunity is also affected because a compensatory increase in B-lymphocytes occurs. While complement levels and granulocyte function remain normal, patients with sustained chyle leak tend to be anergic, lymphopenic, hypoalbuminemic, and have decreased serum levels of antibody and gamma-globulins. The end result is an overall increased risk of bacterial and viral sepsis.[2]

Nutrition Management

The management of chylothorax and chylous ascites is controversial. The debate focuses on whether patients with a lymphatic injury should receive immediate surgical repair or should instead receive conservative treatment with medical management. More recent evidence also supports the use of lymphangiography in the identification of chylous injuries and also in their treatment.[8] The choice of these options in therapy seems to be related to the virulence of the underlying disorder, surgical risk, and the amount/flow of chyle.[6]

The general principles of conservative medical management for chyle leak include draining of the pleural cavity or peritoneal space, reducing chyle flow, treating the underlying cause, providing adequate nutritional support, and in the case of chylothorax, obliterating the pleural space with pleurodesis.[2,3] While conservative therapy is appropriate for the more healthy, stable patient, it should probably be provided for no longer than 2 weeks.[2,3]

A number of clinical landmarks have been identified to indicate the point at which patients managed by conservative therapy should progress to surgical intervention. Excessive chyle leak (defined in adults by > than 500 mL/d or in children by > 10 mL/kg/d or > 100 mL/d for each year of age) for > 5 days or a persistent leak of any volume for > 2 weeks may indicate the need for surgery.[2,3] In one study, mean chyle output in patients with successful conservative management was 6.7 mL/kg/d at day 5. Those who failed and required reoperation had an average drainage of 23.5 mL/kg/d.[5] Loculated chylothorax with fibrin clots, incarcerated lung, failure to expand a compressed lung, or the development of nutritional, metabolic, or infectious complications may indicate the need to progress from conservative management to more aggressive surgical therapy.

Nutrition management should be started as soon as the chyle leak is suspected and the diagnosis is established.[2] Again, some controversy exists as to whether patients should be placed directly on PN (see Chapter 14) or should be kept on a high-protein, nearly fat-free diet fortified with MCTs (given orally or infused through a nasoenteric tube). Although one investigator described an algorithm in which PN would be used first (citing the advantage of rapid correction of fluid and electrolyte imbalances),[7] most investigators recommend assessing the patient's response to an elemental low-fat diet first before going to PN.[2,6,9] Neither form of nutritional therapy seems to be more effective than the other in reducing the absolute amount of chyle output.[9]

The oral diet in the patient with a chyle leak should be high in protein and should contain little or no long-chain fatty acids (< 10 g per day). Long-chain fatty acids require transport from the gut through the lacteals, to the thoracic duct, and on into the venous system. MCTs may be metabolized in the intestinal wall and transported directly into the portal circulation.[2,3] Elemental enteral formulas (see Chapter 11), which comprise individual amino acids and contain < 2% to 3% of its total caloric content as long-chain fatty acids, are ideal for these patients. The MCT oil is added as a substitute for the long-chain dietary fat. These formulas usually require infusion through a nasoenteric tube because they are not palatable. Compared with normal oral diets, such high-protein, elemental MCT diets have been shown to better reduce the quantity and duration of chyle loss, to ameliorate symptoms, and reduce morbidity (while the underlying disease process is being treated), and to lead to spontaneous closure of the chyle leak.[3] In the long-term, such a diet could lead to an essential fatty acid (linoleic acid) deficiency, but this is less likely to occur in adults if conservative therapy is continued for a maximum of only 2 weeks. Another drawback of these formulae is the tendency to cause diarrhea.

Use of PN (see Chapter 14) may be required for those patients who cannot tolerate the restricted oral diet, for patients in whom diet manipulation fails to close the chyle leak, or where the underlying disorder requires more aggressive nutrition therapy.[6] PN has also been suggested in patients with large losses of chyle output and patients who have undergone foregut reconstructive surgery.[2] Fasting the patient who has been placed on PN decreases blood flow to the splanchnic circulation. The reduction in intestinal blood flow results in secondary reduction in lymph flow because of the Starling principle.[10] The end result is that chyle flow decreases from a postprandial state as high as 225 mL/min to a fasting state as low as 0.93 mL/min.[7] Often, patients placed on PN may be given clear liquids without any demonstrable increase in chyle flow.[9,11]

In patients who fail to respond to PN therapy alone, octreotide may be added to further reduce gastrointestinal secretions and splanchnic blood flow. Octreotide, a somatostatin analog, may be given as a subcutaneous injection (100 mcg twice a day) or by continuous infusion.[10] Octreotide by itself may markedly reduce lymphorrhea after injury. When given together with PN, octreotide may lead to rapid cessation of the chyle leak in as little as 2 days. Once the chyle leak abates, the octreotide should be withdrawn over 2 to 4 days.[12]

Throughout the period of conservative therapy and nutrition support, fluid and electrolytes should be monitored closely with particular attention to serum calcium, sodium, and potassium concentrations (see Chapter 7). Patients should be monitored for deficiency of fat-soluble vitamins, and patients may need to be supplemented with vitamin D. Maintaining intravascular volume is important and may be particularly difficult in the face of hypoproteinemia and hypoalbuminemia. While some investigators advocate replacing proteins, coagulation factors, and immunoglobulins that are lost,[12] it is not advisable to provide intravenous albumin infusions routinely. Patients with lymphatic injury are at increased risk for nosocomial infection because of a number of risk factors, including compromise of cellular immunity, deterioration of nutritional status, generalized organ dysfunction, and the presence of indwelling foreign bodies (such as a chest tube).[2] While some investigators go as far as to suggest barrier nursing with isolation rooms,[2] most patients with lymphatic injury may be managed simply by maintaining meticulously sterile procedures, performing cultures at any sign of infection, and avoiding unnecessary antibiotics.

Once there is cessation of the chyle leak, food intake may be reintroduced and/or restrictions removed. Patients on clear liquids may be advanced to a low-fat diet.[10] Some investigators advocate testing patients with a high-fat meal before removing the chest tube to confirm that the lymphatic leak has been sealed. Failure to stop the chyle leak after 2 weeks of conservative therapy may be an indication to proceed with surgical intervention. Practice Scenario 37-1 discusses the nutritional management of a patient with a chylothorax, and Practice Scenario 37-2 discusses the nutritional management of a patient with chylous ascites.

Practice Scenario 37-1

Question: What are the options for nutritional management of chylous effusions?

Scenario: A 27-year-old Caucasian female is referred for heart–lung bypass surgery for worsening congenital cyanotic heart disease. Her physical examination reveals jugular venous distention and 2+ lower extremity edema. Pulmonary exam is significant for bibasilar crackles. She had no palpable adenopathy. The remainder of her physical examination was unremarkable. Laboratory testing revealed a serum albumin of 3.2 g/dL (normal 3.5 to 5.0), transferrin of 203 mg/dL (normal 215 to 365), a total lymphocyte count of 1500 cells × 10^8/dL, and an otherwise normal white blood cell differential count. After heart-lung bypass, the patient is subsequently extubated and advanced to a postoperative diet. After bilateral chest tubes are removed, the patient is discharged to home.

She now returns to the hospital several weeks later complaining of fatigue and dyspnea with exertion. The patient is afebrile with a normal white blood cell count. At that time, laboratory testing revealed a serum albumin of 2.6 g/dL (normal 3.5 to 5.0) and transferrin of 195 mg/dL (normal 215 to 365). A chest radiograph revealed bilateral pleural effusions. Over the next few days, the patient experiences no improvement in her symptoms and her effusions worsen despite aggressive diuresis. An echocardiogram reveals an ejection fraction of 50%. Bilateral thoracentesis was performed, and several hundred milliliters of milky-appearing fluid was removed from each hemithorax. Fluid analysis confirms the diagnosis of chylous fluid (total lipid content: 22 g/L; triglycerides: 856 mg/dL; cholesterol: 102 mg/dL; white blood cell count: 1150 cells × 10^8/dL, 95% were lymphocytes; ≠ protein, ≠ triglycerides, ≠ cholesterol).

Intervention: A nasoenteric tube is placed, and the patient is given an elemental enteral formula. Bilateral chest tubes are placed to ensure adequate external drainage. Initial drainage from the chest tubes is 400 to 500 mL/d for the first 6 days, but over the next several days, the chest tube drainage decreased to approximately 100 mL/d and then both stopped. The patient is subsequently discharged home on low-fat, MCT diet by mouth with her chest tubes removed. The patient's diet is liberated 2 weeks later with no return in effusions.

Answer: Nutritional management of this patient's chylothorax involved elemental enteral formula via nasoenteric tube. Alternatives include an oral, high-protein, nearly fat-free diet fortified with MCT or PN with or without octreotide. It is important to note that in order to avoid an essential fatty acid deficiency, these diets should be used no longer than 2 weeks.

Rationale: Following a high-fat meal, lymph flow is > 200 mL/min (compared to 1 mL/min in the fasting state). The goal of nutritional management in patients with chylous effusions is to reduce the quantity and duration of chyle loss thereby leading to spontaneous closure of the chyle leak. Dietary modifications can also ameliorate symptoms and reduce morbidity.[3] Compared with normal oral diets, high-protein, elemental MCT diets have been shown to better reduce the quantity and duration of chyle loss. Elemental formulas are ideal for this condition because fats usually comprise only 2% to 3% of total calories.

Practice Scenario 37-2

Question: What is the nutritional management for a patient being treated for chylous ascites with conservative medical management?

Scenario: A 62-year-old African American man is referred for elective repair of an abdominal aortic aneurysm. He has a past medical history of atherosclerotic coronary artery disease, hypertension, and a past history of a myocardial infarction. He is a former smoker. Physical examination on admission reveals a well-developed, well-nourished man in no acute distress. His lungs are clear to auscultation and percussion; cardiac examination showed a regular rate and rhythm, normal S^1 and S^2, and no murmurs or gallops. His abdominal exam is unremarkable aside from a 5 to 6 cm pulsatile mass to the left of the midline in the periumbilical region.

At surgery, a 6-cm infrarenal abdominal aortic aneurysm is identified and repaired with a Dacron graft. No other abnormalities were found, and there was no obvious chyle leak at the time of surgery. His immediate postoperative course is unremarkable and on postoperative day 5, the patient is started on clear liquids without complication. The patient was subsequently advanced to a regular diet on postoperative day 6.

On postoperative day 8, the patient is now complaining of increasing abdominal discomfort. On physical examination, his abdomen is distended with a fluid wave and shifting dullness consistent with new onset ascites. The patient was otherwise stable, and there was no change in his hematocrit. An ultrasound confirms the presence of ascites. A paracentesis was performed, which returned 600 mL of a white, milky, odorless fluid. Fluid analysis reveals the following:

White blood cell count	26,000 cells × 10^8/dL
Differential	92% lymphocytes
Total protein	6.2 g/dL
Cholesterol	110 mg/dL (with serum cholesterol of 156 mg/dL)
Amylase	22 IU/L
Triglyceride	1086 mg/dL (with a serum triglyceride of 163 mg/dL)
Cytology	negative
Culture × 2	negative

Intervention: The patient is placed on an oral low-fat diet fortified with MCT oil. Over the next 6 days, the patient continues with ascites despite large-volume therapeutic paracentesis. In addition, the patient is dizzy on standing, and his serum sodium and ionized calcium are 128 mEq/L and 4.0 mg/dl (normal 4.56 to 5.40 mg/dl), respectively. He is given volume resuscitation with normal saline for his hypovolemia and hyponatremia. His calcium is corrected and he is given vitamin D supplementation.

Answer: Fluid/electrolyte abnormalities and deficiencies of fat-soluble vitamins (in particular, vitamin D) are the most likely problems that may be anticipated. Maintaining intravascular volume is important and may be particularly difficult in the face of hypoproteinemia and hypoalbuminemia.

Rationale: Normal chyle flow can range up to 4 L/d (10 to 100 mL/kg/d). Thus, a sustained chyle leak can result in hypovolemia, electrolyte imbalances, anemia, and hemodynamic instability.[2] Fluid losses alone can be as high as 2.5 L/d.[3] Patients may demonstrate a metabolic acidosis because the pH of chyle is usually > 7 (Table 37-1). The most common electrolyte disturbances include hyponatremia and hypocalcemia.[2] Prolonged chyle loss may deplete body protein and reserves of fat and vitamins, particularly the fat-soluble vitamins A, D, E, and K.

References

1. Romero S, Martin C, Hernandez L, et al. Chylothorax in cirrhosis of the liver—analysis of its frequency and clinical characteristics. *Chest*. 1998;114:154–159.
2. Merrigan BA, Winter DC, O'Sullivan GC. Chylothorax. *Br J Surg*. 1997;84:15–20.
3. Browse NL, Allen DR, Wilson NM. Management of chylothorax. *Br J Surg*. 1997;84:1711–1716.
4. Seriff NS, Cohen ML, Samuel P, Schulster PL. Chylothorax—diagnosis by lipoprotein electrophoresis of serum and pleural fluid. *Thorax*. 1997;32:98–100.
5. Doerr CH, Allen MS, Nichols FC III, Ryu JH. Etiology of chylothorax in 203 patients. *Mayo Clin Proc*. 2005;80:867–870.
6. Alban CJ, Littooy FN, Freeark RJ. Postoperative chylous ascites: diagnosis and treatment: a series report and literature review. *Arch Surg*. 1990;125:270–273.
7. Pabst TS, McIntyre KE, Schilling JD, et al. Management of chyloperitoneum after abdominal aortic surgery. *Am J Surg*. 1993;166:194–199.
8. Matsumoto T, Yamagami T, Kato T, et al. The effectiveness of lymphangiography as a treatment method for various chyle leakages. *Br J Radiol*. 2009;82(976):286–290.
9. Petrasek AJ, Ameli FM. Conservative management of chylous ascites complicating aortic surgery: a case report. *Can J Surg*. 1996;39:499–501.
10. Shapiro AMJ, Bain VG, Sigalet DL, Kneteman NM. Rapid resolution of chylous ascites after liver transplantation using somatostatin analog and total parenteral nutrition. *Transplantation*. 1996;61:1410–1411.
11. Dougenis D, Walker WS, Cameron EWJ, Walbaum PR. Management of chylothorax complicating extensive esophageal resection. *Surg Gynecol Obstet*. 1992;174:501–506.
12. Rimensberger PC, Muller-Schenker B, Kalangos A, Beghetti M. Treatment of a persistent postoperative chylothorax with somatostatin. *Ann Thorac Surg*. 1998;66:253–254.

PART IV

MANAGEMENT AND PROFESSIONAL ISSUES

38. **Home Nutrition Support** 639
Marion Winkler, PhD, RD, CNSC
Elizabeth Hagan, RN, CNSC, BSN
Jorge E. Albina, MD

39. **Ethics and Law** 656
Cynthia M.A. Geppert, MD, MA, PhD, MPH, FAPM, DAAPM
Albert Barrocas, MD, FACS
Denise Baird Schwartz, MS, RD, FADA, CNSC

40. **Quality Improvement** 677
Naomi E. Cahill, RD, MSc

41. **Application of Research, Derivation of Guidelines, and Evidence-Based Practice** 693
Kelly A. Tappenden, PhD, RD

38 Home Nutrition Support

Marion Winkler, PhD, RD, CNSC, Elizabeth Hagan, RN, CNSC, BSN, and Jorge E. Albina, MD

CONTENTS

Overview ... 640
Advantages and Benefits of Home Nutrition Support ... 640
Patient Selection and Indications for Home Nutrition Support ... 640
Discharge Planning ... 642
Reimbursement Eligibility Criteria ... 642
Safety Evaluation ... 643
Needs Assessment ... 645
Selection of Home Care and Infusion Provider Services ... 646
Nutrition Care Plan ... 646
Short- and Long-Term Goals ... 646
Route and Access for Home Nutrition Support ... 646
Nutrient Requirements ... 646
Administration Schedule ... 647
Prevention of Rehospitalization ... 647
Patient Education ... 647
Educational Materials ... 648
Learning Assessment ... 648
Teaching and Evaluation Strategies ... 648
Clinical Monitoring in the Home ... 649
Prevention of Complications ... 650
Role of Nutrition Support Clinicians ... 651
Quality of Life, Outcomes Management, and Resources ... 652
Tools to Monitor Quality of Life ... 652
Improving Care and Tracking Outcomes ... 652
Patient Support ... 653
Summary ... 653
References ... 653

Objectives

1. Describe the process for establishing a safe and appropriate discharge plan for the patient beginning home enteral nutrition (EN) or parenteral nutrition (PN).
2. List the elements involved in developing treatment goals for home nutrition support.
3. Identify teaching strategies for effective patient education.
4. Summarize the role of nutrition support clinicians in caring for patients receiving home EN or PN.
5. Review monitoring protocols and interpret clinical data to prevent complications of home EN or PN.

Test Your Knowledge Questions

1. Medicare coverage for home PN is possible with adequate documentation in which of the following conditions?
   A. Anorexia nervosa
   B. Massive small bowel resection resulting in short bowel syndrome with < 150 cm bowel remaining

   C. Six weeks of bowel rest for severe pancreatitis
   D. Swallowing disorder with history of aspiration pneumonia
2. Which of the following is a primary reason for administering home EN or PN as a cyclic infusion?
   A. To reduce the number of nursing visits
   B. To avoid electrolyte imbalances
   C. To enhance metabolism of nutrients
   D. To provide a more normal lifestyle
3. Success of home nutrition support is dependent on which of the following strategies?
   A. Facilitating insurance reimbursement for nutrition support
   B. Providing one-on-one care to the patient at home
   C. Educating the patient and/or caregiver in managing EN or PN at home
   D. Providing comfort to the families caring for the patient
4. Which of the following should clinicians do to support their patients in dealing with life-long dependency on home nutrition support?
   A. Include the patient in decision making regarding choice of access device and administration schedule.
   B. Recognize symptoms of depression and refer for additional evaluation and care.
   C. Promote the benefit of patient support groups.
   D. All of the above.

Test Your Knowledge Answers

1. The correct answer is **B**. Coverage for home PN under Medicare is available for patients who have undergone massive small bowel resection leaving 150 cm or less residual bowel. Operative notes must include documentation of intestinal length. Patients with anorexia nervosa would not meet Medicare criteria for permanent severe pathology of the alimentary tract. A patient requiring bowel rest for 6 weeks for severe acute pancreatitis may have an appropriate clinical indication for home PN; however, under Medicare, bowel rest must be required for 3 months or longer and the patient must have evidence that EN is contraindicated. A patient who has a swallowing disorder with or without evidence of aspiration pneumonia would be a candidate for EN.
2. The correct answer is **D**. The primary reason to administer home nutrition support using a cyclic or overnight infusion is to allow the patient freedom during the day and to improve quality of life. Cyclic infusions are appropriate if a patient is able to tolerate the volume over a shorter period of time as evidenced by frequency of urination, blood glucose control, and absence of gastrointestinal (GI) symptoms such as bloating, cramping, or diarrhea for EN.
3. The correct answer is **C**. Home nutrition support requires use of complex technical equipment. Ensuring willingness and ability to safely manage this equipment as well as all related procedures will prevent complications. Short-term goals for the new home nutrition support patient/caregiver are optimizing organization and safety of the home environment and identification of risks related to potential complications. Long-term goals are to promote independence, compliance, and prevent hospital readmission.
4. The correct answer is **D**. Patients who receive long-term home EN or PN are at high risk for developing depression, social isolation, and poor quality of life. Patients and their caregivers should have an active role in determining the appropriate access device and infusion therapy plan to fit their lifestyle. Home care professionals should help patients to adapt and cope with the required lifestyle adjustments by painting a realistic picture of what will occur at home, providing education on skilled procedures and complexity of the technology, and designing a care plan consistent with the patients' desired goals. Patients should be introduced to the many organizations that provide important outreach services, educational materials, and emotional support.

Overview

Home-based care provides skilled health-related services in a familiar and comfortable environment with support from family members and trained health care professionals. According to the 2010 statistics of the National Association for Home Care and Hospice[1] approximately 12 million people in the United States required some form of home health care delivered by more than 33,000 providers. Annual spending for home health care in 2009 was estimated at $72.2 billion. Medicare is the largest single payer of home care services, accounting for nearly 41% of the total expenditures for home health and hospice.

The diagnosis-related group (DRG) for nutrition and miscellaneous metabolic disorders (DRG 296) was among the 10 most common DRGs of Medicare beneficiaries discharged to home health care in 2000 to 2004.[1] Home nutrition support allows many patients with chronic diseases to be managed successfully outside the hospital for the correction of nutritional disorders. The discharge of the first patient on home PN in 1968 established a model for other "high-tech" home infusion therapies. While there are no current available statistics for home EN or PN utilization in the United States, earlier citations estimate the prevalence of home EN and home PN as 415 per 100,000 population and 120 per 100,000, respectively.[2]

Advantages and Benefits of Home Nutrition Support

The advantages of home EN and PN relate to survival, economic, and quality-of-life (QOL) outcomes.[2–4] Home care services are cost-effective when compared to typical per day charges in a hospital or skilled nursing facility.[1] Technological advances for home care now allow patients to avoid prolonged hospital stays or repeated hospitalizations for nutrition therapies. Home infusion enables patients and their family members to take an active role in the nutrition therapy.

Patient Selection and Indications for Home Nutrition Support

Standards of practice from the American Society for Parenteral and Enteral Nutrition (A.S.P.E.N.) specify that home nutrition support should be used in adult patients who cannot meet

TABLE 38-1 Indications for Home Enteral Nutrition

- Mechanical gastrointestinal tract dysfunction
- Motility disorders
- Malabsorptive syndromes
- Malignancies of the head and neck and digestive system
- Dysphagia and swallowing disorders
- Acute and progressive neurologic conditions
- Hyperemesis gravidarum
- Failure to thrive
- Inborn errors of metabolism

TABLE 38-2 Indications for Home Parenteral Nutrition

- Intestinal failure or dysfunction
- Short bowel syndrome
- Malabsorptive disorders
- Chronic bowel obstruction
- Crohn's disease
- Radiation enteritis
- Intestinal and pancreatic fistulae
- Pancreatitis
- Severe, life-threatening malnutrition

their nutrient requirements orally and who are able to receive the therapy safely outside of an acute care facility.[5] Prior to the initiation of home nutrition support, candidates should have stabilization of their primary disease and clinical condition. Clinical indications for home EN and PN encompass more disease states than those specified as reimbursement-eligible under the Medicare coverage guidelines and by other public or private insurers. Tables 38-1 and 38-2 list indications for home EN and PN. The *International Classification of Diseases, Ninth Edition* (ICD-9), codes for common diagnoses related to the need for EN and PN are listed in Table 38-3.

Clinicians should evaluate the risks and benefits of home nutrition support on an individual basis along with relevant cultural and religious values and patient and family preferences.[6] In some situations, the burden of home nutrition support management may outweigh the benefits. Whether or not

TABLE 38-3 *International Classification of Diseases, Ninth Edition*, Codes for Common Diagnoses Related to Home Enteral and Parenteral Nutrition

Code	Anatomic Conditions	Code	Intestinal Disease and Malabsorptive Disorders
145.9	Carcinoma of the mouth	157	Cancer of the pancreas
141.9	Carcinoma of the tongue	277.0	Cystic fibrosis
151.9	Carcinoma of the stomach	555.0	Regional enteritis
195.0	Carcinoma of the head, face, neck	555.9	Crohn's disease
230.0	Carcinoma of the oral cavity	557	Acute vascular insufficiency of intestine (ischemia)
230.1	Carcinoma of the esophagus	557.9	Acute vascular insufficiency of intestine (pain)
230.2	Carcinoma of the larynx	560.9	Unspecified intestinal obstruction
230.7	Carcinoma of the intestine	564.2	Postvagotomy
530.3	Esophageal stricture or stenosis	569.9	Intestinal disorder
530.84	Tracheoesophageal fistula	577.0	Acute pancreatitis
537.3	Duodenal obstruction	577.1	Chronic pancreatitis
537.4	Gastrojejunocolic fistula	579.30	Short bowel syndrome
569.81	Intestinal fistula	579.4	Pancreatic steatorrhea
802.2	Mandible fracture	579.8	Malabsorption: other specified intestinal
		579.9	Malabsorption: unspecified
		787.91	Diarrhea
Code	**Motility Disorders**	**Code**	**Nutritional Disorders**
478.3	Vocal cord paralysis	263	Malnutrition
507	Aspiration pneumonia	263.9	Malnutrition: protein-calorie
530.81	Esophageal reflux	272.9	Lipid metabolism
536.3	Gastroparesis	275.2	Magnesium disorder
536.9	Unspecified functional disorder of the intestine	275.41	Hypocalcemia
560.9	Pyloric obstruction	276.5	Dehydration
564.2	Postgastrectomy dumping syndrome	276.9	Fluid and electrolyte imbalances
643	Hyperemesis gravidarum	278	Morbid obesity
787.2	Dysphagia	280.1	Iron deficiency anemia (diet)
		285.9	Anemia: unspecified
		783.2	Abnormal weight loss

gastrostomy feedings in patients with advanced dementia affords a survival benefit is controversial.[6-10] A careful evaluation of whether the patient is expected to recover, for example following a stroke or traumatic brain injury, or have a limited life expectancy, as in the case of severe functional and cognitive impairment in advanced dementia, may help identify appropriate candidates for home EN. Objective predictors for the need for EN following stroke include a wet voice after swallowing water, National Institutes of Health stroke scale score, abnormal laryngeal elevation, abnormal gag reflex, incomplete oral labial closure, and coughing during or after swallowing.[11] Similarly, the benefits and burdens associated with the use of artificial nutrition and hydration in the terminally ill patient with end stage disease should be carefully evaluated.[6,12] In these situations, it is important to consider that loss of the desire to eat and drink is a natural part of the dying process.[13]

Discharge Planning

Patients receiving home nutrition support usually are discharged from an acute care or rehabilitation care facility; however, a small percentage of patients may initiate nutrition support in the home.[14] It is never too early to begin the discharge planning process. Table 38-4 lists how hospital personnel can facilitate the transition to home. In addition to nutritional needs, factors that should be assessed as part of the discharge planning process include financial and insurance considerations, home safety evaluation, and a physical and psychological needs assessment.

Reimbursement Eligibility Criteria

Investigation into the patient's individual insurance coverage is second only to the decision that nutrition support is needed after hospital discharge. Understanding the reimbursement process includes knowledge of restrictions or limitations for services, equipment, and supplies. In situations of limited, pending, or no insurance coverage, discharge may be delayed until sufficient home health benefits are available.

TABLE 38-4 How Hospital Personnel Can Facilitate Discharge

- Obtain required diagnostic tests and procedures to demonstrate medical necessity and verify insurance coverage
- Establish feeding access
- Determine tolerance to the formula
- Explain risks and benefits of home nutrition support
- Assess the ability to perform activities of daily living, enteral and parenteral nutrition–related tasks
- Conduct psychosocial assessment
- Identify caregiver
- Identify all necessary home infusion therapies
- Identify who will write the home enteral or parenteral nutrition orders after discharge
- Establish the type and amount of communication desired by the physician and nutrition support team after discharge

Insurance coverage for home EN and PN varies by type of program as well as individual plans. Government programs (eg, Medicare and Medicaid) have strict coverage criteria and require detailed history, tests, and nutritional data to determine eligibility. Coverage policies and reimbursement for EN and PN also vary with private payers and managed care organizations and frequently require preauthorization or precertification. Most require that the therapy be medically necessary and the sole source of nutrition. Many insurance policies establish their own criteria for EN and PN, while others follow the guidelines for coverage set forth by Medicare.[15] Case-by-case review is often required. Regardless of the type of insurance, it is also important to determine whether the patient has home health benefits of sufficient scope for a therapy that may be needed indefinitely. Supplemental insurance may provide additional home nursing visits or care for non–nutrition-related needs such as wound care, tracheostomy care, ostomy care, or disease and medication management.

EN and PN are primarily covered under the "prosthetic device" benefit under the Medicare Part B program.[15] This provision requires a permanent dysfunction of a body organ. For EN or PN to be reimbursed by Medicare, the therapy requirements must fit into a defined benefit category and be "reasonable and necessary for the diagnosis or treatment of illness or injury or to improve the functioning of a malformed body part."[15] For either therapy, there must be "provision of sufficient nutrients to maintain weight and strength commensurate with the patient's overall health status," and the condition must have a "permanent impairment of long and indefinite duration" of at least 3 months.[15] Medicare Part D technically pays for PN for all situations that are not covered under Part B; however, Part D does not pay for the equipment, supplies, or professional services associated with the provision of PN or any other Part D–covered infusion therapy.[16]

Table 38-5 outlines key elements for eligibility and documentation of medical necessity for home EN. Eligible conditions typically include anatomic disorders such as obstruction due to head and neck cancer or reconstructive surgery as well as those resulting from a motility disorder such as severe dysphagia following a stroke or gastroparesis (Practice Scenario 38-1). EN is not covered for individuals who have a functional GI tract and whose need for EN is due to anorexia or nausea associated with end-stage disease. Under Medicare guidelines, standard polymeric formulas are considered appropriate for the majority of patients requiring home EN. Additional documentation of medical necessity is required for specialty products. Clinicians should be aware that not all formulas within a Medicare coverage category are clinically equivalent or interchangeable even though they may be reimbursed at the same rate. If coverage requirements are met, administration supplies and equipment (replacement feeding tubes, tube anchoring devices) are covered, but quantity and frequency are specified. Enteral infusion pumps are covered only with documentation that gravity feeding is not tolerated or contraindicated for situations such as reflux, aspiration, dumping syndrome, glycemic control, circulatory overload, slow infusion rate, or jejunal feeding.

TABLE 38-5 Key Elements for Documentation of Medical Necessity for Home Enteral Nutrition

- Condition will require enteral nutrition for > 3 months
- Condition involves permanent nonfunction or disease of the gastrointestinal tract or impaired digestion or absorption (anatomic disorders; motility disorders)
- Adequate nutrition is not possible by dietary adjustment or oral nutrition supplementation
- Diagnosis (*International Classification of Diseases, Ninth Edition*, code) pertinent to need for enteral nutrition (Table 38-3)
- Radiographic evidence of obstruction
- Motility studies
- Swallowing studies
- Operative notes
- Weight and weight history
- Nutritional assessment
- Justification for specialty enteral formulation, if applicable
- Caloric prescription expressed in calories/kg/day (usually between 20 and 35)
- Site of feeding tube
- If feeding pump requested, evidence that gravity feeding causes reflux, aspiration, severe diarrhea or dumping syndrome or blood glucose fluctuations, circulatory overload, or need for jejunostomy feeding

Table 38-6 lists the requirements for eligibility and documentation of PN. Because of the requirement for permanent dysfunction of the alimentary tract for payment of PN under Medicare, conditions such as swallowing disorders, psychological disorders, anorexia, dyspnea of severe pulmonary or cardiac disease, medication side effects, or renal failure are not routinely covered.[15] The PN prescription must also meet specified calorie, protein, and lipid guidelines. Infusion pumps and supplies are covered for patients who meet PN eligibility criteria. Generally, Medicare does not pay for nursing care for administration of feedings; however, there is limited coverage for teaching the patient and family how to administer infusions.

Practice Scenario 38-1

Question: What clinical documentation is necessary to support eligibility for reimbursement under Medicare for a patient who has a swallowing disorder and requires home EN?

Scenario: A 70-year-old male with a complicated medical history was hospitalized with bilateral cerebral infarcts, left upper and right lower extremity paralysis, and aspiration pneumonia. On physical examination, he was alert, oriented, and not short of breath. His nostrils and oral cavity were clear and neurocranial nerves II to XII were intact. His voice was hoarse, he produced a poor cough, and he was witnessed choking with oral intake. A speech-language pathologist evaluated him and conducted a bedside swallow study. Findings included an inability to initiate a dry swallow, regurgitation with trials of puree and thin liquids, coughing, choking, and an absent pharyngeal swallow. A percutaneous endoscopic gastrostomy (PEG) tube was placed for an anticipated prolonged course of therapy. The patient agreed to the discharge plan that included going home with his wife who would provide care of the PEG tube and administration of tube feedings with the assistance of a daughter who lived nearby. The patient and caregiver's education needs were identified and a care plan was developed. An intermittent feeding schedule was designed to accommodate the patient's lifestyle and caregiver considerations. The patient has Medicare as his primary insurance. Visiting nurse services were arranged for training and monitoring of EN. A durable medical equipment company was contacted to provide the EN formula, equipment, and supplies. The durable medical equipment provider requested documentation of the medical necessity for EN and for the infusion pump.

Intervention: The hospital-based nutrition support team, working in collaboration with the discharge planner, provided documentation that the patient's condition involved dysphagia and that adequate nutrition was not safe by oral means. Diagnostic studies to document dysphagia and aspiration pneumonia along with the dietitian's nutritional assessment was submitted to the durable medical equipment company as documentation of medical necessity.

Answer: EN products are covered under the prosthetic device benefit under the Medicare Part B program. Required documentation for medical necessity includes a diagnosis pertinent to the need for EN (dysphagia), history and physical examination (bilateral cerebral infarcts, left upper and right lower extremity paralysis, aspiration pneumonia, hoarse voice, poor cough, choking with oral intake), swallowing study (speech-language pathologist notes), diagnostic tests (chest x-ray demonstrating aspiration pneumonia), nutrition assessment (weight and weight history, pertinent laboratory results), and documentation from clinician that a pump is required because of known aspiration.

Rationale: Documentation of medical necessity includes evidence that the patient's diagnosis and clinical condition fit into a defined Medicare benefit category and the therapy is reasonable and necessary for the diagnosis or treatment of illness or injury or to improve the functioning of a malformed body part. In this case, the patient was unable to swallow or eat food due to dysphagia with evidence of aspiration pneumonia. Medical necessity was demonstrated by inclusion of the speech-language pathologist's swallow evaluation recommending nonoral nutrition and radiographic evidence of aspiration pneumonia. The medical necessity for a pump was met with preexisting diagnosis of aspiration pneumonia.

Safety Evaluation

Once it is determined that the criteria for medical necessity and benefit coverage are met, the next step is to evaluate the safety of the home environment and manageability of necessary equipment. The following questions should be explored to determine the safety of the home environment[5]:

1. Is the neighborhood accessible to the home health care provider for delivery and professional visits?
2. Is the environment clean with reliable utilities (sanitary water, electricity, refrigeration, storage space, electrical outlets, telephone)?

TABLE 38-6 Key Elements for Documentation of Medical Necessity for Home Parenteral Nutrition[15]

- Condition will require parenteral nutrition > 3 months
- Condition is severe enough that patient cannot maintain weight and strength on oral intake or a combination of oral or enteral nutrition
- Diagnosis (*International Classification of Diseases, Ninth Edition*, code) pertinent to need for parenteral nutrition (Table 38-3)
- Weight and weight history
- Serum albumin within 1 week of home parenteral nutrition
- Specific disease criteria and supporting documentation

  Massive small bowel resection within 3 months leaving less than 5 feet of small bowel beyond the ligament of Treitz
  - Operative report with evidence of 5 feet or less of small bowel
  - Radiographic reports

  Short bowel syndrome with net gastrointestinal fluid and electrolyte malabsorption on an oral diet of 2.5 to 3 L/day, enteral losses exceeding 50% of the oral/enteral intake, and urine output of 1 L/day
  - Operative report indicating extent of resection
  - Radiographic reports
  - Motility studies
  - Intake and output records demonstrating net fluid loss
  - Signs of dehydration and electrolyte imbalance
  - Results of 72-hour fecal fat test
  - List of medications used to control diarrhea
  - Documentation of nutrient modification and/or failed tube trial

  Severe exacerbation of regional enteritis requiring bowel rest for at least 3 months
  - Operative report
  - Pathology report
  - Radiographic reports
  - Indication for bowel rest

  Pancreatitis with or without pseudocyst requiring bowel rest for at least 3 months
  - Operative report
  - Radiographic report
  - Indication for bowel rest

  Enterocutaneous fistula requiring bowel rest for at least 3 months where feeding distal to the fistula is not possible
  - Operative report
  - Radiographic report
  - Motility studies
  - Contraindication to enteral nutrition
  - Evidence of inability to place tube distal to fistula

  Complete mechanical small bowel obstruction where surgery is not an option
  - Operative report that confirms obstruction
  - Radiographic report that confirms obstruction
  - Evidence of inability to place tube distal to obstruction

  Severe fat malabsorption and malnutrition where fecal fat exceeds 50% of oral/enteral intake on a diet of a least 50 grams of fat per day as measured by a 72-hour fecal fat test
  - Fecal fat test
  - Operative report
  - Radiographic report
  - Pharmacologic approaches tried
  - Evidence of enteral nutrition failure
  - Nutrition assessment with evidence of malnutrition defined as > 10% weight loss over 3 months or less and serum albumin of 3.4 g/dL or lower

  Severe motility disorder that is unresponsive to prokinetic medication
  - Radiographic report
  - Motility studies
  - Medications attempted to improve motility
  - Result of tube trial or contraindication to tube feeding
  - Nutrition assessment with evidence of malnutrition defined as > 10% weight loss over 3 months or less and serum albumin of 3.4 g/dL or lower

3. Can the patient move safely around the house and to the bathroom (stairs, carpeting)?
4. Is the patient/caregiver willing and able to learn the home infusion procedures and operation of the equipment?
5. Is the caregiver willing and able to provide additional needed assistance for care within the home?
6. Is the patient/caregiver able to learn to recognize problems and contact help from the home health care provider or emergency services?
7. Is laboratory monitoring available as frequently as needed to prevent fluid and electrolyte complications?

Needs Assessment

Assessment for home care suitability includes evaluation of the skilled nursing needs, performance of activities of daily living, medication management, wound and skin care, and the patient's ability to recognize when to seek medical attention. When beginning home nutrition support, the patient and caregiver additionally should be assessed for their ability to learn to reliably monitor weight, hydration status, and blood or urine glucose, recognize early signs of infection, and care of the EN or PN access device and site.

Patients and caregivers should be prepared for the necessary time commitment for administration of EN or PN (Practice Scenario 38-2). While this will become easier with repetition, initially the responsibility may be overwhelming. Reassurance and patience on the part of the home health care professionals will inspire confidence. While leaving an institutional environment usually indicates health improvement, this new responsibility adds to the stress of illness. As with any chronic health condition, depression can be the downfall of successful therapy. Depression is a common response to chronic illness and may increase risk of home nutrition support–related complications. Signs of depression should prompt referral for additional evaluation and care.

Home nutrition support requires use of complex technical equipment. When possible, demonstration of the equipment prior to discharge will provide both an opportunity for teaching and insight into the patient's and caregiver's ability to learn. If mastering the use of equipment and learning procedures is not possible in the acute care or rehabilitation setting, extra teaching time should be allotted for the initial home visits. Ensuring willingness and ability to safely manage special equipment and procedures will prevent complications and hospital readmission.[17] Extra time spent for one-on-one teaching care and management of nutrition support results in increased patient satisfaction and compliance.[18]

Social changes due to loss of job, family role, disconnection from friends, and limitation in physical stamina all contribute to stress on hospital discharge. Culture and religious beliefs may also influence health-related practices and should be considered in the overall patient assessment. The patient's perception of health and illness will affect behaviors, tolerance of discomfort, knowledge of options, and expectations of change and outcome. Ensuring appropriate follow-up in the form of appointments and telephone numbers of providers may be beneficial. Providing information on available local or national organizations for peer support and education has been shown to improve outcomes associated with home nutrition support.[19]

Practice Scenario 38-2

Question: How do you evaluate a patient's ability to learn skills and procedures associated with safe and effective home care therapy?

Scenario: A 62-year-old female with Crohn's disease was identified as a potential home PN candidate after multiple admissions for dehydration. Training for home PN began in the hospital several days before discharge. The home care clinician demonstrated the various procedures for home PN using the actual equipment on models with vascular access devices. The patient was able to correctly return demonstrate use of sterile gloves, needle and syringe, and priming of intravenous tubing. Because of her desire to maintain independence, all education was focused on the patient. After discharge, the home care nurse reports that the patient is having difficulty performing the techniques of the infusion protocol and is not likely to be safe alone.

Intervention: A caregiver is identified and with the patient's approval, home care teaching continues. The home care nurse is able to negotiate that the patient and caregiver have different roles and each learn and manage separate aspects of PN procedures.

Answer: The transition from hospital to home can be an overwhelming experience for any patient, especially for one who needs to become independent in self-care. Despite being technically capable of performing tasks, the reality of the responsibility and necessary time commitment for home nutrition support procedures can only be effectively evaluated in the real home setting. The home care clinician is in a key position to assess education needs and abilities, family dynamics, and identify alternate caregivers among the patient's family and friends. A patient's anxiety and fear about the home care experience can be lessened by painting a realistic picture of what will occur at home and adequately portraying the complexity of the technology. Conducting a thorough patient assessment helps identify the patient's emotional and experiential readiness to learn. Establishing a teaching plan with short- and long-term objectives helps to prioritize the learning steps. Engaging the patient in active participation by demonstrating each procedure and requesting a return demonstration enhances training. Use of checklists, illustrations, and other materials matched to the patient's style of learning, intelligence, and comprehension improves the teaching and learning experiences. The instructor should encourage the patient to ask questions, address individual concerns, and provide encouragement.

Rationale: The patient may have the cognitive and physical ability to learn but learning may be influenced by the emotional and experiential readiness to learn. Recognition that the patient lives alone, has minimal support systems, and a substantial medical history with frequent hospitalizations is essential for the development of a realistic care plan. Although patients are trained in many aspects of home PN management before they leave the hospital, they should be reassured that additional training and retraining will occur upon arrival home.

Selection of Home Care and Infusion Provider Services

A variety of organizations may participate in the delivery and management of home care nutrition services including durable medical equipment companies, home infusion providers, and nursing care agencies. Home care providers specializing in nutrition support are available to assist with the transition from the hospital to home. These agencies will either provide all home care needs or coordinate with another community agency for home nursing visits and medical equipment, nutrition formulations, and supplies. A predischarge teaching visit provides insight for the patient as to what he or she is expected to learn and a chance for the home care clinician to assess the patient's receptiveness and ability to manage at home. Because home nutrition support often is delivered as an overnight or 24-hour infusion, the home care provider needs to be readily available by telephone and have capability for home visits at any hour of day or night if needed.

Nutrition Care Plan

Short- and Long-Term Goals

Short-term goals are to provide patient education and ensure safety. Patients and caregivers should be provided with information about how to contact all home care providers, reasons to call for help, how to decrease risk, and how to promote comfort. Long-term goals are to promote independence and prevent rehospitalization. Independence is achieved through comprehensive patient and family education addressing care of the enteral or vascular access device, troubleshooting high-tech equipment, and restrictions in diet or activity. Optimizing the organization and safety of the home environment will decrease therapy-related anxiety, facilitate learning, and promote independence.

Barriers to achieving short- and long-term nutrition support goals can be overcome with intensive patient and family teaching, assessment of compliance, and monitoring for early signs and symptoms of problems. Identifying and communicating areas of individual patient risks will assist the members of the health care team who are managing the patient to anticipate special needs. Any information regarding safety, community resources, and ways to improve the ability to manage within the home environment will promote good QOL and reduce complications. Well-educated home EN and PN patients will experience less stress.

Route and Access for Home Nutrition Support

Decisions about the route and access device for infusion of home EN or PN should be made early in the discharge planning process. The access device chosen should be one that the patient/caregiver can safely manage and minimizes risk of complications (see Chapters 12 and 16). Information on device insertion date, style, location, length, patency, and site condition should be made available to the home care provider.

Long-term enteral access devices include percutaneous gastrostomy or jejunostomy tubes. These may be placed as an endoscopic, laparoscopic, radiologic, or open surgical procedure. The device should be positioned so that it does not interfere with daily activities such as bathing and clothing changes. The external tubing should be anchored securely to the skin to minimize irritation during movement. Gastric feeding is preferred over small bowel feeding for several practical reasons. Compared to jejunal, gastric tubes are easier to place and replace, and are larger gauge with lower incidence of occlusion. Gastric feedings can be administered as bolus feedings at meal times or spaced throughout the day. In cases of gastroparesis, ileus, gastric outlet obstruction, or significant gastric reflux, small bowel feedings are a good alternative. If needed, a combination gastrojejunostomy tube can be considered in order to simultaneously provide gastric decompression and small bowel feeding.

Long-term PN requires a central venous access device. Central venous catheter placement is defined by the final catheter tip location in the superior or inferior vena cava. Home PN catheters may be placed into either a large peripheral vein, such as the basilic or cephalic, or into the subclavian or internal jugular vein. The catheter is then advanced to the distal portion of the superior vena cava. A peripherally inserted central catheter is readily placed, replaced, or removed, and is a low risk for insertion complications. Subclavian or internal jugular catheters are either tunneled or implanted. Tunneled catheters, known as Hickman, Broviac, or Groshong catheters, enter the vein and are then tunneled subcutaneously to exit lower on the chest wall. The purpose of the tunnel is to decrease the risks of infection and accidental removal.

An implanted device, or port, is a disk with a self-sealing silicone septum and rigid titanium or plastic base. It is surgically placed into a subcutaneous pocket and connected to a catheter that is inserted into a vein using a medical wire and advanced into the central venous system. The most common location of an implanted port is on the chest wall, but in some situations the upper arm may be the site of choice. Because the entire port is under the skin, no nursing care is needed and unrestricted bathing is permitted after the incision heals. The port is accessed using a specially designed right angle, tapered needle with a side opening known as a Huber needle. Tunneled or implanted devices on the chest wall are usually not visible under clothing and allow full range of arm and hand movement.

External or tunneled catheters require regular, direct nursing care or patient/caregiver training for proper catheter and site care. Catheter dressings and tubing should be clean and dry at all times. Implanted ports require professional care or training for needle placement, site care, and catheter flushing.

Nutrient Requirements

Nutrient requirements are developed following a nutrition assessment (see Chapter 10). Energy requirements are determined by predictive equations or measured using indirect calorimetry, if available. Nutrient and total fluid requirements should be determined considering whether the EN or PN therapy is providing total or partial nutrition support. Goals of therapy should be determined with the patient and caregiver, and individualized based on assessment of nutritional status, body composition, and performance status and function, while taking into account any preexisting nutritional deficits. The overall goals of nutrition therapy are to restore macro- and micronutrients, replete and maintain normal serum electrolyte levels, maintain euglycemia, and improve or maintain lean body mass, performance status, and function. In situations where a patient's body weight is either above or below preferred, a weight maximum or minimum goal may be set.

Patients who are either on nothing by mouth status or have abnormal fluid losses will likely need additional fluid or water. For the home EN patient, water can either be delivered through the routine tube flushes (by dividing the desired daily volume between the flushes), additional water boluses, or by diluting the enteral formula. For the home PN patient, the PN volume is based on the desired total daily fluid volume, inclusive of fluid losses. A period of evaluation to assess tolerance of EN or PN as well as achieving fluid and electrolyte stability is invaluable for determining the home nutrition support prescription. Good tolerance includes achieving normal blood glucose and acceptable urine output. Careful supervision of changes to the formula in the inpatient setting may minimize changes and maximize uncomplicated delivery in the home setting for what may be an indeterminate period of time.

Administration Schedule

The patient and caregiver's preferences should be carefully considered when determining the infusion cycle. Gastric feedings may be delivered as either bolus or continuous infusion. The number of bolus feedings typically is three to five times per day, but some patients may tolerate less or require more. Gastric residuals should be checked every 4 to 8 hours as the rate of infusion is advanced for continuous feeds or prior to each scheduled bolus feeding. Small bowel feedings require controlled delivery through an electronic pump for continuous feeding. Based on individual patient situations, continuous feeding may be delivered over < 24 hours if EN is supplementing an oral diet or to allow the patient to have time off the pump and to resume a more normal lifestyle. An ambulatory, battery-operated pump allows movement within the home as well as the ability to go out of the home with the infusion, if needed. A cycled schedule may be used to infuse over 8 to 14 hours per day to allow freedom from connections. This decision is based on total volume of feeding, demonstrated tolerance of high infusion rate (GI symptoms), and the patient's or caregiver's ability to manage the equipment.

PN always requires controlled pump delivery. While most PN regimes begin as a 24-hour infusion, decreasing the number of hours of infusion allows for freedom to resume normal activities. By increasing the flow rate, the total infusion time is decreased. This is referred to as a cyclic infusion. The fluid tolerance can be assessed by monitoring urine volume and frequency. The convenience of a shorter infusion cycle is balanced against the higher volume delivered over a shorter period of time. The cycle should include a tapered rate at the end of the infusion to minimize risk of hypoglycemia.[20] The tapers typically include 1 hour at the beginning and 1 to 2 hours at the end of the infusion. Careful monitoring of blood glucose is needed as the infusion rate is increased. Maximum glucose utilization rate is 4 to 7 mg/kg/minute. The generally accepted rate of glucose infusion is 5 mg/kg/minute.[21] To derive grams of dextrose per day, the formula for this calculation is:

$$\text{Weight (kg)} \times \text{desired glucose infusion rate} \times \text{minutes per day}/1000$$

For a 60-kg female to infuse at 5 mg/kg/minute for 12 hours, the grams of dextrose per day equals the following:

$$60\ \text{kg} \times 5\ \text{mg} \times 770\ \text{minutes}/1000 = 231\ \text{grams.}$$

More rapid infusion rates may cause hyperglycemia. Blood glucose checks should be scheduled within the first 2 hours, 4 to 6 hours later, and at the end of the cycle. Insulin therapy should be initiated and advanced cautiously, and blood glucose monitoring continued until acceptable blood glucose levels are achieved. Regimens for home insulin administration may be either a sliding scale or addition of regular insulin to the PN solution. Diabetics may have basal insulin requirements met by insulin in the PN solution, while breakthrough elevations in blood glucose are covered with subcutaneous injections.

Prevention of Rehospitalization

Because hospital readmission is discouraging, disruptive, and costly, prevention and/or early intervention are key. While clearly not all complications can be prevented, there are known strategies that minimize risk.[22] Reasons for complications within the first 90 days of home nutrition support include inadequate training, patient and caregiver noncompliance, prescription error, health care worker error, and equipment malfunction.[23]

Early recognition of the signs and symptoms of complications promotes early treatment intervention. Regular measurement of weight and awareness of output are essential for early detection of dehydration or volume overload. If possible, patients leaving an inpatient facility should be provided with the equipment to measure urine output as well as instructions for use.

A standardized protocol for diagnosis and management of common complications facilitates obtaining the vital information the home care clinician needs for treatment decisions. One example is the use of standing orders to obtain blood cultures and complete blood count in the event of fever $> 101.5°F$.

Community resources provide peer support in order to enhance independence and promote a sense of well-being.[24] Patients who participate in peer support groups report less depression, anxiety, worry, and rehospitalizations, and increased self-care and satisfaction with the care by their health care professionals.[19]

Patient Education

The goal of patient education is to provide needed information to enable patients to be responsible for their own therapy. Patients are sent home with complex care requiring skilled procedures such as dressing changes, catheter access, feeding tube flushes, and medication administration. Education is the foundation for success and avoids procedure and therapy-related complications.[25] Empowering patients with verbal and written references to recognize signs and symptoms will enable appropriate action in the event of serious complications such as fever, thirst, cramping, or bleeding. When available, involvement of a significant other in education sessions will provide a backup, second set of hands, and reinforcement for administration of nutrition support.

Educational Materials

According to the National Assessment of Health Literacy in the United States, at least one-third of Americans have limited reading comprehension.[26] In order to meet the recommended reading grade level of fifth to sixth, all words should be familiar, less than three syllables, and medical and technical terms should be limited or avoided altogether.[27] If complex or medical language is used, this should be explained using familiar words. Despite the availability of methods to calculate health literacy, the Institute of Medicine reported that more than 300 studies found printed health-related materials exceed the average reading ability of Americans.[28]

Printed patient education material should be selected on the basis of content and complexity. The written style should be simple, casual, and conversational. Additionally, materials should bridge language barriers or be printed in the patient's primary language. Content should be relevant to the specific type of nutrition support as well as age and culture of patient. All information should be accurate and reflect current standards of practice.[29] The most important information should be highlighted or otherwise easy to locate. Key points should be repeated as a means of reinforcement. Terms used should be consistent throughout the document. Although medical equipment may be identified by the manufacturer's names or abbreviations, only one term should be used within an educational guide.

All steps for any skilled procedures should be organized, precise, and easy to read. The more complex or detailed the content, the more difficult it is for most people to understand and retain the information. Active verbs are preferred when listing directions. Any excess wording should be minimized to present the important points in a concise manner. Keep steps simple and avoid too much information. Table 38-7 provides suggested content for printed education materials.

The use of lists and graphic illustrations help clarify written text, emphasize skills presented, and provide cues for future reference. Drawings and photographs illustrate important points of information. All illustrations should focus on patient action and be simple, realistic, and relevant.[30] Attractive and friendly illustrations will keep the patient's attention and add motivation to read the information.[31] Use of mnemonics will reinforce learning new concepts.

Learning Assessment

Engaging the patient and family in the belief that the nutrition support is valuable will improve the patient's health and facilitate the desire to learn. Patients can be motivated by the desire to achieve a particular goal or outcome expected from home nutrition support. The instructor can influence the patient's attitude by conveying enthusiasm and providing encouragement that the outcome will be successful. When learning a new skill, motivation to continue comes from positive reinforcement. When a person succeeds at a task, he or she is usually motivated to continue learning. Other helpful strategies are to create a friendly environment and to convey respect for patient needs, desires, and limitations.

A patient's readiness to learn is affected by physical or emotional conditions. Physical limitations such as pain, fatigue, and immobility will need to be taken into account when scheduling teaching sessions. Emotional anxiety or stress apart from the task of learning the necessary skills for delivery of nutrition support will interfere with learning concentration. A one-on-one session conducted in a private and quiet environment may enhance learning readiness. Teaching sessions should be scheduled at the patient's convenience and during a time of day free from other family obligations. Accommodations will need to be made to address physical limitations such as impaired dexterity, mobility, vision, or hearing.

After an initial demonstration, the patient or family should be asked to use return demonstration of the required procedure to assess learning. For new learners, this will most likely require repeated demonstration. The goal is to have the patient become independent with the home nutrition support in order to improve QOL and make living with home EN or PN as normal as possible.[32]

TABLE 38-7 Components of Patient-Specific Education for Home Nutrition Support

- Why the therapy is being recommended
- How the type of nutrition support is expected to work in the body
- Step by step directions for skilled procedures
- Common pitfalls to avoid
- Signs and symptoms of complications
- Telephone numbers of all health care providers

Teaching and Evaluation Strategies

High-tech home care equipment both contributes to nutrition support delivery and at the same time imposes significant constraints on patients' lives.[33,34] A patient's perception of how this technology impacts his or her private and social life will influence acceptance.[35] Factors such as motor noise, light, misunderstood digital messages, alarms, and tubing attachment are physical barriers to acceptance. Fear of exposure to illness, anxiety over equipment malfunction, and altered body image interfere with usual family and social activities.[36] Use of appropriate technology and proper education on the use of equipment will increase compliance and acceptance of home therapy.[37]

The objective of the initial home visit is to teach or reinforce correct technique for EN or PN infusion. The home care nurse can also use this training period to assess knowledge and explain reasons behind the procedures and techniques. Issues such as storage of supplies, refrigeration of formulas, and disposal of medical waste can be addressed efficiently within the home. Corrections to the patient's technique can be made immediately while observing the patient and caregiver within the home environment. Selection of an appropriate work area with adequate lighting, proper hand hygiene, use of clean or disposable toweling, and restriction of pets are issues that should be addressed. Preparation of PN may require the patient/caregiver to demonstrate competence in the use of needles and syringes. Management of a vascular access device may require sterile technique for flushing or dressing changes. The goals of this visit and ongoing teaching are for the patient and caregiver to demonstrate understanding of the procedures and techniques and to be comfortable in the care of EN or PN equipment, access devices, and site.

Subsequent home visit objectives are to ensure adherence to the regimen and compliance with procedure and handling techniques. Repetition of demonstration of procedures should be consistent and careful. Follow-up home visits provide reassurance to the patient and caregiver that continued assistance and support is available. Using a printed guide of steps for new procedures adds readily available reference that will reduce procedure-related anxiety and promote confidence as the patient works toward independence. Every effort should be made to anticipate and respond to the patient's physical and emotional needs through interdisciplinary communication amongst the prescribing physician, members of the nutrition support team (if applicable), the home infusion provider, and home nursing agencies.

Consistent reassessment at regular intervals can be readily accomplished through telephone contact. Focused questions should target known issues or problems. Special needs can also be addressed on an individual and ongoing basis to eliminate barriers to achieving goals of therapy. Developing a relationship with the patient and family will initially reduce therapy-related anxiety and result in increased satisfaction and enhanced compliance with nutrition support–related procedures. Table 38-8 describes strategies for relationship building.

TABLE 38-8 Strategies for Building Patient Trust

- Consistently reinforcing goals
- Making regular and frequent contact
- Providing encouragement
- Demonstrating respect for others and their concerns
- Expressing understanding of circumstances
- Anticipating needs
- Dealing with limitations
- Ensuring services are available for all needs

Clinical Monitoring in the Home

Home care visits are used to obtain the patient's vital signs, record weight, assess hydration status, note any pertinent physical examination findings, observe and assess the enteral or vascular access device site, review medication use, and if applicable evaluate readiness to transition to oral nutrition.

Easily obtained, objective physical assessment criteria are blood pressure, pulse, temperature, and weight. Keeping a record of these in the home facilitates communication among various home care providers. Additionally, this record can be brought to office visits or referenced during telephone calls to the primary care provider. Dehydration can be recognized by blood pressure and pulse changes, especially when measured both as lying and standing positions (orthostatic vital sign measurement). Elevations of temperature and pulse may be early signs of infection. Rapid weight loss or gain reflect change in fluid status and should be assessed in the context of other symptoms of fluid retention (edema, shortness of breath) or dehydration (low urine output, dry mouth). Recording of output (emesis, urine, and stool) can be difficult in the home and should be limited to special situations requiring evaluation of formula volume, significant electrolyte imbalance, or as a means to prevent rehospitalization. Patients/caregivers should be educated about reporting significant changes in character or volume of outputs.

Observation of the enteral or vascular access device site should be done at each home visit. Early signs and symptoms of infectious problems may be recognized by visual inspection of the insertion site, dressing, and surrounding skin for inflammation. Signs of mechanical malfunction of the device include leaking, difficulty flushing, or frequent pump alarm. Pain or swelling may indicate vascular access catheter damage and subcutaneous infiltration.

Adequacy and tolerance of therapy is assessed through functional status, physical examination, and laboratory values. Functional status is how well a patient performs activities of daily living. These include ambulation, bathing, dressing, and meal preparation. Level of independence with household chores, hobbies, and recreational activities are other performance indicators. Physical examination will reveal changes in weight, anthropometrics, or signs of nutrient deficiencies.

All laboratory results should be documented at "baseline" on discharge or at the beginning of home nutrition support and then regularly throughout the course of therapy (Practice Scenario 38-3). Suggested collection of laboratory parameters includes glucose, blood urea nitrogen, and creatinine, and electrolytes on a weekly basis for 4 weeks or until stable. Additionally, complete blood count, serum proteins, liver function, triglycerides, vitamins, minerals, and trace elements should be monitored after 1 month. Ongoing quarterly follow-up should include all these parameters, unless there is a change in clinical condition necessitating more frequent monitoring on an individual, case-by-case basis.[5] Table 38-9 lists laboratory parameters and frequency of assessment for PN. In order to facilitate processing and correct billing, it is helpful to inform the laboratory of the diagnosis, clinical condition, or ICD-9 codes that correlate with the requested diagnostic test (Table 38-3). Table 38-10 provides examples of clinical monitoring parameters for EN.

TABLE 38-9 Laboratory Monitoring for Home Parenteral Nutrition[a]

	New Patients			Stable Patients
Parameter	**Baseline**	**Weeks 1, 2, and 3**	**Week 4**	**Every 3 months prior to office visit**
Glucose, blood urea nitrogen, creatinine, electrolytes, calcium, magnesium, phosphorus	X	X	X	X
CBC with differential and reticulocyte count	X	X	X	X
Total bilirubin, direct bilirubin, AST, ALT, LDH, alkaline phosphatase, triglycerides	X		X	X
Serum proteins	X		X	X
Vitamin B_{12}, RBC folate, iron indices, trace elements, vitamin D 25-OH	X		X	X

ALT, alanine aminotransferase; AST, aspartate aminotransferase; CBC, complete blood count; LDH, lactate dehydrogenase; RBC, red blood cell.
[a]Adapted from Rhode Island Hospital Nutritional Support Service.

Practice Scenario 38-3

Question: What is the appropriate clinical monitoring plan to ensure a successful transition from the hospital to home for a newly discharged home PN therapy patient?

Scenario: A 59-year-old woman suffered a mesenteric thrombosis resulting in loss of all but 60 cm of small bowel, an end jejunostomy, and a mucous fistula. PN was initiated in the hospital and after an extended hospitalization the patient was discharged home with a large volume PN solution designed to provide total daily fluid requirements and meet energy and nutrient goals. The patient advanced to an oral diet appropriate for short bowel syndrome and was receiving medication to decrease gastric hypersecretion, slow motility, and reduce ostomy output. The macro- and micronutrient component of her PN solution was established during hospitalization and she was stable on the regimen prior to discharge. The patient discharge instructions included weight, measuring urine output volume, and blood work weekly for the first 4 weeks.

Intervention: Laboratory data was obtained within 48 hours prior to discharge and initiation of PN at home as specified in the A.S.P.E.N. standards of practice for home care patients.[5] A protocol specified the frequency of laboratory testing (complete blood count, chemistries, liver function tests, iron studies, trace elements) particularly for potential signs of dehydration. Home visits were scheduled to provide education on how to monitor weight, intake and output, temperature, access device site inspection, psychosocial assessment, and functional status, and who to contact for reports and problems.

Answer: According to the A.S.P.E.N. standards for specialized nutrition support of home care patients,[5] the process of patient monitoring must assure that the nutrition goals are achieved and that risk of complications due to nutrition therapy are reduced. Laboratory parameters are assessed at baseline, at least weekly for 1 to 4 weeks, monthly for 3 months, then at 6-month intervals unless there is a change in clinical condition necessitating more frequent monitoring on an individual, case-by-case basis. Review of systems and inspection of the access device and site should occur at each home care visit. Periodic review of the patient's acceptance of the therapy, compliance with procedures, psychosocial adjustment, and general well-being is necessary.

Rationale: The patient's nutrition status is monitored and documented regularly, and includes observation for signs and symptoms of intolerance to therapy, evaluation of weight change, evaluation of hydration status, review of systems and physical examination, periodic review of biochemical and other pertinent laboratory data, assessment for clinical signs of nutrient deficiencies or excesses, assessment of other disease states that may affect the nutrition therapy, potential for nutrition therapy and medication interactions, evaluation of functional status and performance, inspection of access device and site, and patient compliance with techniques and procedures. Ongoing review of the appropriateness of the nutrition therapy and need for continued nutrition support is conducted. Additionally, there is periodic review of the psychosocial status of the patient and caregiver as well as reassessment of the patient's home environment. Patients who are eating or will be transitioning to food or EN require monitoring of fluid, nutrient, and oral intake as well as monitoring of urine, stool, and other GI losses or output.

Prevention of Complications

Complications related to nutrition support can be summarized as mechanical, infectious, or metabolic.[3] Mechanical complications include occlusion, leakage, malposition or accidental removal of the access device, or equipment failure or malfunction. Infectious complications relate to the access device, exit site, and surrounding skin. Metabolic complications include blood glucose or fluid and electrolyte abnormalities, GI intolerance, organ system dysfunction, and

TABLE 38-10 Clinical Monitoring of Home Enteral Nutrition

- Medical progress
- Weight
- Hydration
- Elimination
- Laboratory values as clinically indicated
- Enteral nutrition tolerance
- Medication and water administration
- Drug-nutrient interaction
- Access device and site care
- Medical equipment and supplies
- Achievement of nutrition goals
- Readiness to transition to oral diet including ability to chew and swallow safely, and need for modification of food consistency and texture

vitamin, mineral, and trace element deficiencies or toxicities (see Chapters 10 and 17).

Home EN is relatively safe and complications can usually be avoided or corrected.[3,5,38] Frequent tube surveillance, proper skin care, prevention of excessive traction on the tube, and routine tube flushing with water can prevent mechanical complications associated with the feeding tube. GI intolerance may occur in patients receiving home EN.[3] A thorough evaluation of the potential causes of diarrhea should be undertaken before prescribing antidiarrheal agents, as diarrhea may be related to new medications, infection, underlying disease, preparation and sanitation of the formula, change in rate or method of administration, or presence or absence of fiber. Patients on home EN may also experience constipation that may be due to hydration, activity, medications, or laxative use. Complaints of nausea, bloating, or abdominal distention should be evaluated for change in clinical condition, medications, or method of feeding administration. Periodic evaluation of routine serum chemistries is necessary for monitoring metabolic complications associated with fluid, electrolyte, or mineral abnormalities.

In patients receiving home PN, catheter infection is the most common complication of PN therapy and the most common reason for hospital readmission.[39,40] Signs and symptoms of a catheter-related bloodstream infection may include fever, lethargy, chills, rigors, elevated leukocytes, and hyperglycemia. Redness, tenderness, or discharge from the skin site may indicate catheter exit site infection. Immediate evaluation and intervention is necessary for suspected or actual infection.[41] If a patient experiences a catheter-related bloodstream infection, follow-up monitoring should include a home visit for reassessment of the patient and/or caregiver's compliance with procedures. This visit serves as a review of proper handling of EN or PN access and equipment as well as an opportunity for evaluation of the home environment.

Catheter occlusion may occur because of a kink in the catheter or from thrombus or precipitation of PN components. Diagnostic studies may be indicated when catheter flushing or aspiration is difficult. Patients requiring long-term home PN and those who have had multiple catheters are at increased risk of catheter-related venous thrombosis, and some patients may require anticoagulation therapy for prevention.[42]

Abnormal liver function is not uncommon in patients requiring long-term home PN.[43] The mechanism for liver dysfunction is not completely understood and is thought to be multifactorial.[3] Potential causes of PN-associated liver dysfunction include overfeeding, excessive intravenous fat dosage, lack of enteral stimulation, infection, choline deficiency, and aluminum toxicity.[44] If signs of cholestasis occur, ultrasonography should be obtained to rule out extrahepatic causes. The PN solution should routinely be evaluated to be sure the patient is not receiving excessive calories or excess lipids.[45] Cycling of the PN infusion if the patient is receiving continuous therapy may be beneficial. Every attempt should also be made to encourage oral intake or transition to or inclusion of EN.

Metabolic bone disease is seen in patients receiving long-term home PN.[46] The cause of osteopenia and osteoporosis is also multifactorial and may include preexisting disease, malabsorption, use of steroids, inactivity, mineral deficiency (calcium, phosphorus, magnesium), or vitamin D deficiency or excess.[47] Annual bone mineral density testing should be obtained.

Micronutrient deficiencies are less common in patients receiving long-term PN because of routine addition of multivitamin and trace element additives to the PN formulation.[48] Patients should be monitored for iron deficiency because iron is not routinely added to PN. Monitoring of serum levels of trace elements should be conducted biannually to prevent deficiency and toxicity. Because serum values are not always representative of deficiency and toxicity, patients should be examined for physical signs.

Role of Nutrition Support Clinicians

Continuity of care and communication within and among all organizations participating in the care of the patient receiving home EN or PN should be frequent, structured, in depth, and ongoing.[5] The home care provider should coordinate needs for EN or PN with other professional services providing wound care, ostomy care, respiratory care, physical therapy, or home health aide services.

Frequently, the hospital-based nutrition support team or home infusion provider takes responsibility for monitoring safe delivery of EN or PN; however, these activities should be coordinated with the patient's primary care physician (if he or she is not the prescribing physician) and all other medical specialists. It is not uncommon for a patient who is receiving home EN or PN to receive regular follow-up care from a gastroenterologist, endocrinologist, or an oncologist. A psychologist or psychiatrist may also be involved for treatment of anxiety or depression. Regular communication with the primary care physician is essential for new or ongoing cardiac, respiratory, renal, or neurological concerns. Collaboration by all specialists including the home nutrition support team or provider can be achieved through active communication and documentation.

The A.S.P.E.N. home care standards recommend interdisciplinary collaboration by the referring physician, nutrition support practitioners, and home care provider.[5] Ideally, a physician with expertise in home EN and PN is available for the management of the patient's nutritional care plan, interpretation of diagnostic testing, and evaluation of changes in medical condition. The roles and responsibilities and required competencies of the home care pharmacist, nurse, and dietitian are detailed in the A.S.P.E.N. discipline-specific standards of professional practice and may overlap depending on the availability of each professional in the home care setting.[49–52]

The home care pharmacist has an essential role in evaluating the nutrition therapy prescription, compounding of PN formulations, evaluating drug-nutrient interactions, dispensing medical supplies and equipment, and monitoring laboratory results. The home care nurse has an active role in teaching the patient and caregiver, conducting in-home patient physical and psychosocial assessment, performing dressing changes and access site care, collecting blood or other specimens, medication oversight, evaluating compliance, and monitoring the response to nutrition support.

The home care dietitian assists in the development of the nutrition care plan; recommends nutrition therapy based on energy, macro-, and micronutrient requirements; performs and evaluates the nutrition-focused physical examination; assesses adequacy and appropriateness of nutrient delivery and intake; and monitors the transition to tube feeding and/or oral diet. A process for timely communication among the physician, nutrition support practitioners, home care provider, patient, caregiver, and any other health care professionals is essential.

Quality of Life, Outcomes Management, and Resources

Tools to Monitor Quality of Life

QOL is a multidimensional concept that includes evaluation of physical health status, psychological well-being, social and cognitive function, and illness and treatment. Because expectations regarding health and the ability to cope with limitations and disability can greatly affect a person's perception of health and satisfaction with life, people with the same objective health status may have very different QOL. The World Health Organization defines QOL as "An individual's perception of their position in life in the context of the culture and value system in which they live and in relation to their goals, expectations, standards, and concerns."[53] Good QOL is generally accepted as a "state of complete physical, mental, and social well-being and not merely the absence of disease."[53] QOL may also be defined as the subjective perception of satisfaction or happiness with life in domains of importance to an individual. Home PN-dependent adults define QOL as "how much one enjoys life, being happy and satisfied with life, and being able to do what you want to do when you want to do it."[54]

There is no gold standard measure of QOL, and until recently there has been no validated therapy-specific instrument for home nutrition support. Consequently, most published studies use generic measures of health status or disease-specific questionnaires to study the QOL of home EN and PN patients.[55,56] Published research demonstrates poor QOL in patients receiving home EN and PN that is influenced by age, self-esteem, drug and narcotic usage, depression, coping skills, family and peer support systems, financial insecurity, and underlying disease.[55–59] Qualitative reviews of home EN- and PN-dependent adults identify disturbed social life, inability to eat normally, diarrhea, pain, polyuria, sleep disruption, and a need for psychosocial support as factors influencing QOL.[54,60–65] Despite technological inconveniences associated with infusion therapy, patients do recognize and report the benefit of being kept alive with home EN or PN.[54,57,65]

Baxter and colleagues[66] designed the first patient-based treatment-specific QOL questionnaire for home PN (HPN-QOL). The instrument includes eight functional scales (general health, travel, physical function, coping, ability to eat and drink, employment, sexual function, emotional function), two home PN items, and nine symptom scales (body image, weight, immobility, fatigue, sleep pattern, GI symptoms, pain, presence of stoma, financial issues). The HPN-QOL differentiates between QOL affected by home PN therapy versus the underlying illness or disease. While this tool still requires validation in the United States, benefits of using a therapy-specific QOL instrument for individual patient care include providing information for therapy management and identifying problems requiring intervention.[66]

Clinicians and patients should discuss QOL at routine intervals whether a validated instrument is used or not. We know from studies and discussion with individuals requiring long-term home EN or PN that it is important to know that one can live a "normal" life even with home EN or PN dependency.[54,65] Patients have a strong desire for information to help them better understand the prognosis of their condition and the rationale for the therapy.[67–70] Because these individuals face potentially long-term therapies requiring substantial lifestyle adaptations with known risks and complications, a frank and open conversation about goals and expectations is necessary. Open communication between clinician and patient can help identify how a patient defines QOL and what makes QOL poor or good. When introducing these therapies, paint a realistic picture of what will occur at home and adequately portray the complexity of the technology.[34] Continue to dialogue with the patient to help him or her adapt and adequately cope with the lifestyle adjustments associated with home EN or PN.

Improving Care and Tracking Outcomes

Tracking outcomes can easily identify how well nutrition support is provided and the benefit to the patient in terms of avoidance of complications, improved nutritional parameters, and enhanced performance status and function.[71] A.S.P.E.N. has launched a new system to maintain a prospective, longitudinal nutrition therapy patient registry in order to improve patient outcomes. The registry is a comprehensive, web-based tool that allows clinicians to enter patient data, measure and analyze results, benchmark outcomes, and publish findings. In the initial phase, the registry will maintain data on patients receiving home PN; in subsequent phases, it will expand to include other populations and therapies. For more information visit the website at www.nutritioncare.org/sustain/.

Patient Support

Many organizations provide important outreach services, free educational materials, and emotional support to patients, families, and caregivers.[34,72] The Oley Foundation (www.Oley.org), established in 1983, is a national, nonprofit education, self-help, and research organization for consumers of home EN and PN. Networking occurs through communication with volunteer regional coordinators who provide inspiration, support, and information via a toll-free hotline. Some of the educational resources available through the Oley Foundation include a video library, equipment and formula exchange, bimonthly newsletters with articles about medical advances and personal experiences, the My HPN online education modules (Take Charge, Catheter-Associated Infection, Fluid Balance, Glucose Control), and an annual summer conference. An important resource is an Internet link to other national and international organizations related to home EN and PN, GI societies, disease- and condition-specific societies and foundations, home care agencies, equipment and products, infection control and safety, insurance and disability benefits, discount and free prescription services, government agencies, and parenting and caregiver resources. Table 38-11 lists selected online social media that provides an additional opportunity for networking between home EN and PN patients and their families.

TABLE 38-11 Selected Online Social Media for Networking Among Home Enteral Nutrition and Home Parenteral Nutrition Consumers

www.inspire.com/groups/oley-foundation	The Oley Foundation Support Community connects patients, families, friends, and caregivers for support and inspiration.
www.copingwell.com/copingwell	A self-help manual for adults living with home enteral nutrition to learn to cope more effectively with the therapy-related challenges they face.
www.feedingtubeawareness.com	A parent organization whose mission is to share information about the day-to-day life caring for infants and young children with feeding tubes.
www.shortbowelfoundation.org	A nationally based foundation providing education, support, and advocacy services to patients, families, and health care providers who deal with short bowel syndrome or similar medical conditions.
Living Life on Total Parenteral Nutrition (TPN)—Facebook https://www.facebook.com/groups/299634454491/?ref=ts&__adt=2&__att=iframe	A place for parents of children on total parenteral nutrition or a place for anyone who lives on total parenteral nutrition to share tips and ideas, or to vent if one is struggling with total parenteral nutrition–related issues.

Summary

Home care involves more than simply transferring nutrition support from the hospital to the home. Home care providers need to be prepared to teach therapy-related skills and provide education to ensure the technology used is safe and effective. Ongoing clinical monitoring is essential to prevent complications and promote successful achievement of nutritional outcomes, as well as patient satisfaction and comfort. Multidisciplinary collaboration between the prescribing physician, hospital-based nutrition support team, home infusion provider, and home care nursing agencies along with the patient and caregiver is necessary for successful transition from inpatient setting to home.

References

1. The National Association for Home Care. *Basic Statistics About Home Care*. Updated 2010. www.nahc.org. Accessed May 1, 2011.
2. Howard L, Ament M, Fleming CR, et al. Current use and clinical outcome of home parenteral and enteral nutrition therapies in the United States. *Gastroenterol*. 1995;109:355–365.
3. DiBaise JK, Scolapio JS. Home parenteral and enteral nutrition. *Gastroenterol Clin N Am*. 2007;36:123–144.
4. Howard L. Home parenteral nutrition: survival, cost, and quality of life. *Gastroenterol*. 2006;130:S52–S59.
5. Kovacevich DS, Frederick A, Kelly D, et al. Standards for specialized nutrition support: home care patients. *Nutr Clin Pract*. 2005;20: 579–590.
6. Barrocas A, Geppert C, Durfee S, et al. A.S.P.E.N. ethics position paper. *Nutr Clin Pract*. 2010;25:672–679.
7. Finucane TE, Christmas C, Travis K. Tube feeding in patients with advanced dementia: a review of the evidence. *JAMA*. 1999;282: 1365–1370.
8. Gillick MR. Rethinking the role of tube feeding in patients with advanced dementia. *N Engl J Med*. 2000;342:206–210.
9. Sampson EL, Candy B, Jones L. Enteral tube feeding for older people with advanced dementia. *Cochrane Database Syst Rev*. 2009: CD007209.
10. Teno JM, Mitchell SL, Kuo SK, et al. Decision-making and outcomes of feeding tube insertion: a five state study. *J Am Geriatr Soc*. 2011;49:881–886.
11. Wojner AW, Alexandrov AV. Predictors of tube feeding in acute stroke patients with dysphagia. *AACN Clin Issues*. 2000;11(4): 531–540.
12. Monturo C. The artificial nutrition debate: Still an issue ... after all these years. *Nutr Clin Pract*. 2009;24:206–213.
13. Palecek EJ, Teno JM, Casarett DJ, et al. Comfort feeding only: a proposal to bring clarity to decision-making regarding difficulty with eating for persons with advanced dementia. *J Am Geriatr Soc*. 2010;58:580–584.
14. Newton AF, DeLegge MH. Home initiation of parenteral nutrition. *Nutr Clin Pract*. 2007;22:57–65.
15. Medicare Coverage Issues Manual. *Department of Health and Human Services (DHHS), Healthcare Financing Administration (HCFA), 65-10, Enteral and Parenteral Nutritional Therapy Covered as Prosthetic Device*. http://cms.hhs.gov. Accessed May 1, 2011.

16. Medicare Parts B/D Coverage Issues. www.cms.gov/pharmacy/downloads/partsbdcoverageissues.pdf. Accessed October 10, 2011.
17. Bonifacio R, Alfonsi L, Santarpia L, et al. Clinical outcome of long-term home parenteral nutrition in non-oncological patients: a report from two specialised centres. *Intern Emerg Med.* 2007;2:188–195.
18. Shepperd S, Doll H, Angus RM, et al. Avoiding hospital admission through provision of hospital care at home: a systematic review and meta analysis of individual patient data. *CMAJ.* 2009;180:175–182.
19. Smith CE, Curtas S, Werkowitch M, et al. Home parenteral nutrition: does affiliation with a national support and educational organization improve patient outcomes? *J Parenter Enteral Nutr.* 2002;26:159–163.
20. Metheny NM. Parenteral nutrition. In: Metheny NM, ed. *Fluid & Electrolyte Balance: Nursing Considerations*. Sudbury, MA: Jones & Bartlett Learning, LLC, 2012:169–178.
21. A.S.P.E.N. Board of Directors and the Clinical Guidelines Task Force. Guidelines for the use of parenteral and enteral nutrition in adult and pediatric patients. *J Parenter Enteral Nutr.* 2002; 26(Suppl):1SA–138SA. Errata 2002;26:144.
22. Smith CE, Curtas S, Kleinbeck SVM, et al. Clinical trial of interactive and videotaped educational interventions reduce infection, reactive depression, and rehospitalizations for sepsis in patients on home parenteral nutrition. *J Parenter Enteral Nutr.* 2003;27:137–145.
23. de Burgoa LJ, Seidner D, Hamilton C, et al. Examination of factors that lead to complications for new home parenteral nutrition patients. *J Infusion Nurs.* 2006;29:74–80.
24. Dakof GA, Taylor SE. Victim's perceptions of social support: What is helpful from whom? *J Pers Soc Psychol.* 1990;58:80–89.
25. Cox JA, Westbrook LJO. Home infusion therapy. Essential characteristics of a successful education process - a grounded theory study. *J Infusion Nurs.* 2005;28:99–107.
26. National Center for Education Statistics. *National Assessment of Adult Literacy of America's Adults in the 21st Century, NCES Pub. No. 2006470.* Washington, DC: National Center for Education Statistics. http://nces.ed.gov/naal/pdf/2006470.pdf. Accessed May 1, 2011.
27. Sand-Jecklin K. The impact of medical terminology on readability of patient education materials. *J Community Health Nurs.* 2007;24:119–129.
28. Nielsen-Bohlman L, Panzer AM, Hamlin B, et al., eds. *Health Literacy: A Prescription to End Confusion*. Washington DC: National Academies Press; 2004.
29. Clayton LH. Strategies for selecting effective patient nutrition education materials. *Nutr Clin Pract.* 2010;25:436–442.
30. Doak LG, Doak CC, Meade CD. Strategies to improve cancer education materials. *Oncol Nurs Forum.* 1996;23:1305–1312.
31. Doak C, Doak L, Root J. *Teaching Patients with Low Literacy Levels*. 2nd ed. Philadelphia: Lippincott; 1996.
32. Gifford H, DeLegge M, Epperson LA. Education methods and techniques for training home parenteral nutrition patients. *Nutr Clin Pract.* 2010; 25:443–450.
33. Marden SF. Technology dependence and health-related quality of life: a model. *J Adv Nurs.* 2005;50:187–195.
34. Winkler MF, Ross VM, Piamjariyakul U, et al. Technology dependence in home care: impact on patients and their family caregivers. *Nutr Clin Pract.* 2006;21:544–556.
35. Lehoux P. Patients' perspectives on high-tech home care: a qualitative inquiry into the user-friendliness of four technologies. *BMC Health Serv Res.* 2004;4:28–36.
36. Lehoux P, Saint-Arnaud J, Richard L. The use of technology at home: what patient manuals say and sell vs. what patients face and fear. *Sociol Health Illn.* 2004;26;617–644.
37. Huisman-de Waal G, van Achterberg T, Jansen J, et al. "High-tech" home care: overview of professional care in patients on home parenteral nutrition and implications for nursing care. *J Clin Nurs.* 2011;20:2125–2134.
38. Siepler J. Principles and strategies for monitoring home parenteral nutrition. *Nutr Clin Pract.* 2007;22:340–350.
39. Bozzetti F, Mariani L, Bertinet DB, et al. Central venous catheter complications in 447 patients on home parenteral nutrition: an analysis of over 100,000 catheter days. *Clin Nutr.* 2002;21:475–485.
40. Ghabril MS, Aranda-Michel J, Scolapio JS. Metabolic and catheter complications of parenteral nutrition. *Curr Gastroenterol Rep.* 2004;6:327–334.
41. Mermel LA, Farr BM, Sherertz RJ, et al. Guidelines for the management of intravascular catheter-related infections. *Clin Infect Dis.* 2011;32:1249–1272.
42. Steiger E. Dysfunction and thrombotic complications of vascular access devices. *J Parenter Enteral Nutr.* 2006;20:S70–S72.
43. Dray X, Joly F, Reijasse D, et al. Incidence, risk factors, and complications of cholelithiasis in patients with home parenteral nutrition. *J Am Coll Surg.* 2007;204:13–21.
44. Cavicchi M, Beau P, Crenn P, et al. Prevalence of liver disease and contributing factors in patients receiving home parenteral nutrition for permanent intestinal failure. *Ann Intern Med.* 2000;132:525–532.
45. Fulford A, Scolapio JS, Aranda-Michel J. Parenteral nutrition-associated hepatotoxicity. *Nutr Clin Pract.* 2004;19:274–283.
46. Seidner DL. Parenteral nutrition-associated metabolic bone disease. *J Parenter Enteral Nutr.* 2002;26(5 suppl):S37–S42.
47. Pironi L, Tjellesen L, DeFrancesco A, et al. Bone mineral density in patients on home parenteral nutrition: a follow-up study. *Clin Nutr.* 2004;23:1288–1302.
48. Howard L, Ashley C, Lyon D, et al. Autopsy tissue trace elements in 8 long-term parenteral nutrition patients who received the current U.S. Food and Drug Administration formulation. *J Parenter Enteral Nutr.* 2007;31:388–396.
49. Seashore JH, McMahon MM, Wolfson M, et al. Standards of practice for nutrition support physicians. *Nutr Clin Pract.* 2003;18:270–275.
50. Rollins C, Durfee SM, Holcombe BJ, et al. Standards of practice for nutrition support pharmacists. *Nutr Clin Pract.* 2008;23:189–194.
51. American Society for Parenteral and Enteral Nutrition Board of Directors and Nurses Standards Revision Task Force, DiMaria-Ghalili RA, Bankheard R, et al. Standards of practice for nutrition support nurses. *Nutr Clin Pract.* 2007;22:458–465.
52. Russell M, Stieber M, Brantley S, et al. American Society for Parenteral and Enteral Nutrition (A.S.P.E.N.) and American Dietetic Association (ADA): standards of practice and standards of professional performance for registered dietitians (generalist, specialty, and advanced) in nutrition support. *Nutr Clin Pract.* 2007;22:558–586.
53. Orley J. The World Health Organization (WHO) quality of life project. In: Trimble MR, Dodson WE, eds. *Epilepsy and Quality of Life.* New York: Raven, 1994:99–133.
54. Winkler MF, Hagan E, Wetle T, et al. An exploration of quality of life and the experience of living with home parenteral nutrition. *J Parenter Enteral Nutr.* 2010;34:395–407.
55. Baxter JP, Fayers PM, McKinlay AW. A review of the instruments used to assess the quality of life of adult patients with chronic intestinal failure receiving parenteral nutrition at home. *Br J Nutr.* 2005;94:633–638.
56. Winkler MF. Quality of life in adult home parenteral nutrition patients. *J Parenter Enteral Nutr.* 2005;29:162–170.

57. Baxter JP, Fayers PM, McKinlay AW. A review of the quality of life of adult patients treated with long-term parenteral nutrition. *Clin Nutr*. 2006;25:543–554.
58. Fortune DG, Varden J, Parker S, et al. Illness beliefs of patients on home parenteral nutrition (HPN) and their relation to emotional distress. *Clin Nutr*. 2005;24:896–903.
59. Persoon A, Huisman-de Waal G, Naber TA, et al. Impact of home parenteral nutrition on daily life - a review. *Clin Nutr*. 2005;24: 304–313.
60. Silver HJ. The lived experience of home total parenteral nutrition: an online qualitative inquiry with adults, children, and mothers. *Nutr Clin Pract*. 2004;19:297–304.
61. Brotherton AM, Judd PA. Quality of life in adult enteral tube feeding patients. *J Hum Nutr Diet*. 2007;20:513–525.
62. Brotherton A, Abbott J. Clinical decision making and the provision of information in PEG feeding: an exploration of patients and their carers' perceptions. *J Hum Nutr Diet*. 2009;22:302–309.
63. Walker A. In the absence of food: a case of rhythmic loss and spoiled identity for patients with percutaneous endoscopic gastrostomy feeding tubes. *Food, Culture and Soc*. 2005;8:161–180.
64. Huisman-de Waal G, Naber T, Schoonhoven L, et al. Problems experienced by patients receiving parenteral nutrition at home: results of an open interview study. *J Parenter Enteral Nutr*. 2006;30: 215–221.
65. Thompson CW, Durrant L, Barusch A, et al. Fostering coping skills and resilience in home enteral nutrition (HEN) consumers. *Nutr Clin Pract*. 2006;21:557–565.
66. Baxter JP, Fayers PM, McKinlay AW. The clinical and psychometric validation of a questionnaire to assess the quality of life of adult patients treated with long-term parenteral nutrition. *J Parenter Enteral Nutr*. 2010;34:131–142.
67. Mansilla ME. Benefits from artificial nutritional support: a testimonial. *Nutrition*. 2003;19:78–80.
68. Kindle R. Life with Fred: 12 years of home parenteral nutrition. *Nutr Clin Pract*. 2003;18:235–237.
69. Ireton-Jones C, Lang RK, Gravenstein ME, et al. Home nutrition support from the patient's perspective: the real reality story! *Nutr Clin Pract*. 2006;21:542–543.
70. Fairman J, Compher C, Morris J, et al. Living long with short bowel syndrome: a historical case of twenty-nine years of living with home parenteral nutrition. *J Parenter Enteral Nutr*. 2007;31: 127–134.
71. Ireton-Jones C, DeLegge M. Home parenteral nutrition registry: a five-year retrospective evaluation of outcomes of patients receiving home parenteral nutrition support. *Nutrition*. 2005;21: 156–160.
72. Kovacevich DS. Parenteral and enteral nutrition support groups. *Nutr Clin Pract*. 2003;18:238–239.

39 Ethics and Law

Cynthia M.A. Geppert, MD, MA, PhD, MPH, FAPM, DAAPM, Albert Barrocas, MD, FACS, and Denise Baird Schwartz, MS, RD, FADA, CNSC

CONTENTS

Background 657
The "Can" of Nutrition Support Technology 657
Artificial Nutrition and Hydration in Palliative Care 658
Artificial Nutrition and Hydration in Advanced Dementia 659
The Vegetative State 659
The "Should" of Bioethics 661
Ethical Theory 661
Key Ethico-Legal Concepts 662
Informed Consent 662
Decisional Capacity 662
Surrogate Decision Making 662
Standards of Surrogate Decision Making 662
Withholding versus Withdrawing Treatment 663
Futility/Quality of Life 663
Empirical Ethics Research 663
General Ethical Analysis of Artificial Nutrition and Hydration 664
Cultural Values and Religious Beliefs 664
Judaism 664
Catholicism 665
Conscience Clauses 666
The "Must" of the Law 666
Precedent Cases: Cruzan, Quinlan, and Schiavo 668
Advance Directives 668
Resolving Ethical Conflicts Around Artificial Nutrition and Hydration: Crucial Conversations 669
Role of Nutrition Support Professionals in Ethical Decision Making for Artificial Nutrition and Hydration 670
Translating Ethical Decision Making for Artificial Nutrition and Hydration into Clinical Practice 671
Summary 671
References 675

Objectives

1. Apply ethics principles and reasoning to the resolution of ethical and legal dilemmas encountered in clinical nutrition practice.
2. Critically analyze clinical ethics arguments related to the use of artificial nutrition and hydration for patients in a persistent vegetative state (PVS), with advanced dementia, or at the end of life.
3. Differentiate and incorporate scientific, clinical, ethical, and legal considerations in nutrition support decisions.
4. Reflect sensitivity to cultural values and religious beliefs in approaching ethical issues related to nutrition support.

Test Your Knowledge Questions

1. Which of the following is a potential benefit of feeding tube placement in advanced dementia?
   A. Prevention of aspiration pneumonia
   B. Facilitation of nursing home placement
   C. Prolonging survival
   D. Preventing or healing of pressure ulcers
2. Which of the following best expresses the position of the 2004 Papal allocution regarding the use of artificial nutrition and hydration (ANH)?
   A. ANH is obligatory for patients with terminal illness and in a PVS.
   B. ANH is obligatory for patients in a PVS and with advanced dementia.
   C. ANH is obligatory for patients in a PVS, with terminal illness, and with advanced dementia.
   D. ANH is obligatory for patients in a PVS.
3. Which of the following is accurate concerning the withholding or withdrawing of ANH in patients who are at the end of life?
   A. When ANH is withheld or withdrawn from patients at the end of life, they die from hunger and starvation.
   B. When ANH is withheld or withdrawn from patients at the end of life, they die from dehydration and thirst.
   C. ANH can ethically be withheld or withdrawn from a patient at the end of life.
   D. ANH can ethically be withheld from a patient at the end of life, but not withdrawn.

Test Your Knowledge Answers

1. The correct answer is **B**. This question examines many of the common misunderstandings about feeding tube placement in patients with dementia. A 2009 Cochrane review demonstrated that feeding tubes do not diminish the incidence of aspiration pneumonia in patients with advanced dementia,[1] nor do feeding tubes prevent the development of pressure ulcers or result in the healing of extant ulcers. This is because feeding tubes do not in general improve nutritional status. In addition, restraints are often needed when feeding tubes are placed in patients with advanced dementia, which increases the risk of developing pressure sores.
2. The correct answer is **D**. This chapter explains the considerable controversy among Roman Catholic theologians and ethicists on the meaning and implications of the Papal allocution for the use of ANH. However, the official papal position as of this writing is that ANH is ordinary medical treatment that should be provided for patients in a PVS and as such is morally obligatory. The papal position, as stated in the allocution of Pope John Paul II issued in 2004, only pertained to the use of ANH in PVS, not in advanced dementia or terminal illness.[2]
3. The correct answer is **C**. Both families and health care professionals often find the withdrawal of treatment more difficult emotionally than the withholding of treatment including ANH. But legally and ethically, there is no material difference between the withdrawal or withholding of ANH at the request of a competent patient or an authorized surrogate. Families and patients often fear that the patient will die from painful starvation or thirst, but it is the underlying terminal disease process that actually is responsible for the patient's death, not a lack of food and water. Palliative care experts have shown that any discomfort patients experience from thirst or hunger can usually be alleviated through meticulous mouth care, the use of ice chips, and allowing patients small bites of whatever foods they desire.[3]

Background

Healthcare professionals confront clinical dilemmas at the intersection of law, ethics, culture, and technology on a daily basis. Technology provides the physiological support to keep selected organs functioning, albeit often in a dysfunctional fashion. It is often associated with burdens, risks, and discomfort, particularly in individuals with disease states or conditions in whom these interventions may be considered to be low yield or "futile." As individuals, family members, and professionals, we are often conflicted by the challenges presented, the available technology contrasted with our obligations to the individual, as well as our conformity to our state and federal law. One of the authors has styled this milieu of technology as what can be done, ethics as what should be done, and law as what must be done, as "the troubling trichotomy."[4] In nutrition support therapy, these moral conflicts most often involve ANH.

ANH is a truly double-edged treatment: it can enable a patient with head and neck cancer to have adequate nutrition necessary for successful chemotherapy; it may also permit an elderly patient with end-stage dementia to survive for years in a nursing home bereft and burdened.[5] Patients and families in theory have a right to informed consent or refusal of ANH, and yet practically few express their wishes with a clarity and consistency sufficient to guide health care decision making or increasingly satisfy the dictates of the law.[6]

In this chapter, we review the primary ethical principles and arguments, the most important legal precedents and rulings, and the empirical evidence regarding the clinical benefits and risks regarding ANH in three common and controversial clinical conditions: advanced dementia, terminal illness, and PVS. The Schiavo case underscored that what many professionals thought was a solid congruence among the three poles of the trichotomy regarding the use of ANH actually contained far more structural weakness that broke upon fracture lines of religion and politics.[7]

The subsequent sections of this chapter are intended to guide nutrition support professionals through the issues that encompass the troubling trichotomy.[8]

The "Can" of Nutrition Support Technology

Modern medical history is a story of exponential technological innovation and scientific discovery that outstrips the growth of jurisprudence and ethical analysis regarding these new developments, creating unprecedented dilemmas. The introduction of total parental nutrition in 1968 marked the beginning of an explosion of therapeutic and technical options in the delivery of ANH. As the technology has evolved, it has become apparent from the evidence reviewed in this chapter that the provision of ANH in advanced disease states may in some circumstances be legal but not truly ethical.

Artifical Nutrition and Hydration in Palliative Care

The central ethical question to be asked about the use of ANH at the end of life is whether it is palliative or painful to not have access to food and water when dying. Two common sense moral intuitions create a distressing contradiction in which health care professionals, families, and patients alike are caught. This concept is illustrated in Practice Scenario 39-1. The first is that patients who are terminally ill often experience a decreased hunger and thirst drive. Physiologically, it is absolutely true that patients with end-stage disease processes such as cancer or heart failure will become dehydrated and malnourished. The philosophical issue is whether this causes suffering. Some person's instinctual answer is of course it does and anyone who has this response will naturally be repulsed by the inhumanity and cruelty of the idea of depriving sick and dying loved ones of the basic necessity of food and water. But hospice and palliative care professionals have long clinically recognized that dying patients stop eating and drinking as a matter of course and comfort.[9] The literature now documents, and the science now explains, these observations regarding what is technically known as "terminal or palliative dehydration."

Zerwekh introduced this concept into the nutrition support literature in a series of pioneering articles beginning in the 1980s.[10] Zerwekh reported detrimental effects of intravenous hydration on the terminal patient including increased gastrointestinal fluids, causing vomiting and the need for nasogastric suctioning, respiratory distress with choking and drowning sensations from fluid retention in the lungs, peripheral edema, and increased urine production (if the kidneys have not shut down), leading to a requirement for catheterization in a patient too weak to ambulate.[11] These symptoms bring discomfort to the patient near death and emotional distress to loved ones observing the decline.

Conversely, the state of dehydration in such a patient results in relief from choking and drowning sensations with less coughing and congestion as pulmonary secretions are lessened; decreased urine output with less need for catheterization; fewer bed-wetting episodes; decreased gastrointestinal fluid with fewer bouts of vomiting, bloating, and diarrhea; decreased peripheral edema; and no need for restraints to prevent patients from dislodging their tubes or intravenous lines. Because many other researchers have confirmed Zerwekh's findings and theory, palliative care has shifted from the acute care standard of universal hydration to one of universal nonhydration.[3] Several theories have been advanced for the ameliorative effect of terminal dehydration. The analgesic theory proposes that starvation boosts the production of ketones having an anesthetic effect. Synergistically, dehydration may increase the production of endogenous opioids.[12]

Patients experiencing terminal dehydration cannot readily distinguish dry mouth from thirst, and research shows that most discomfort is surprisingly the result of the former, not the latter.[9,13] Often, it is actually mouth breathing that is causing the sensation of dry mouth. Data does not show a correlation between biochemical dehydration and the sensation of thirst or between actual hydration status and the perception of thirst in dying patients given intravenous hydration.[14-16] The sensation of a dry mouth can be easily and effectively relieved through ice chips, sips of favorite beverages, and meticulous mouth care.[11] Even if patients or families are able to accept that hunger and thirst can be effectively relieved and that ANH may be more physically burdensome, they may believe that the intervention prolongs survival. There is little evidence to support this contention and some to challenge it.[17,18]

These objective observations may not satisfy the emotional or moral concerns of practitioners or providers that they feel they are allowing a fellow human being to die of starvation and thirst. Subjective testimony may in this juncture be more persuasive. McCann, in a frequently quoted study, measured symptoms of hunger, thirst, and dry mouth, and their palliation through comfort care in terminally ill, competent patients in a hospice unit over a year until their death. A total of 63% of patients experienced no hunger, and another 34% were hungry only initially. A similar number (62%) of patients felt no thirst or only at the beginning of their illness. Any painful symptoms were easily satisfied with small amounts of favorite foods or fluids, and dry mouth was effectively alleviated with ice chips and good mouth care.[13]

Practice Scenario 39-1

Question: Is it ethically justifiable to forgo ANH in a terminally ill cancer patient? (Note: the term forgo refers to both withdrawing and withholding of treatment.)

Scenario: A nurse is caring for a decisionally capable patient with terminal esophageal cancer who is no longer able to swallow. The oncologist discussed the possibility of a percutaneous endoscopic gastrostomy (PEG) tube with the patient who made an informed refusal of ANH. The nurse tells the physician that ethically he must provide ANH despite the patient's wishes in order to prevent the patient from painfully dying of hunger and thirst rather than cancer. Is the nurse ethically justified in her concern? Can the nurse overrule the wishes of a patient with decision-making capacity? The physician consults the nutrition support professional on the ethics committee for advice.

Intervention: The nutrition support professional meets with the nurse and physician and provides an evidence-based answer that it is clinically appropriate and ethically justifiable to forgo ANH at the request of a terminal patient who has intact decisional capacity. She also reassures the nurse that with appropriate hospice care, the patient need not suffer.

Answer: The patient is not dying from lack of nutrition and hydration but from the underlying disease process, in this case cancer. As elucidated in the didactic section, with high-quality palliative care, patients do not suffer from hunger and thirst at the end of life due to metabolic alterations intrinsic to their dying process.[19]

Artificial Nutrition and Hydration in Advanced Dementia

The most critical aspect of advanced dementia that nutrition support professionals need to grasp—and that laypersons often find hard to understand and accept—is that advanced dementia is a terminal illness.[20] Patients with the most prevalent form of dementia, Alzheimer disease, have an average life expectancy of 5 to 7 years after diagnosis.[21] The second important aspect of the dementia diagnosis is that dysphagia, anorexia, apraxia with utensils, inability to self-feed, resistance to feeding by caregivers, and poor oral intake are all integral aspects of the natural course of the disorder.[22,23] These dysfunctions frequently result in malnutrition and substantial weight loss that are upsetting to family members and practitioners alike.

The need for, and efficacy of, PEG tubes in patients with advanced dementia is controversial. Nutrition support professionals[24] have a unique opportunity to dispel these misunderstandings, whether they are held by patients, families, or other health care professionals. Among the most controversial justifications for PEG tubes are that they prevent or reduce symptoms, improve functional and nutritional status, enhance comfort, or prolong survival.[25] As with the evidence for the use of ANH in terminal illness, the literature does not support, or even refutes, these contentions.

PEG tube use in advanced dementia does not reduce aspiration and prevent the pneumonia to which patients with dementia so often succumb; aspiration from oral and gastric secretions continues unabated.[26] Contrary to the logical assumption of many surrogate decision makers and even some health care professionals, feeding tubes do not extend survival. PEG tubes in advanced dementia, research shows, increases not only morbidity, but also mortality. PEG tube placement often requires concomitant use of physical or chemical restraints, exacerbating discomfort, increasing the risk of pressure sores, and further compromising patient comfort and human dignity.[26,27]

PEG tube placement does not extend and may actually shorten life. Not only are there no long-term proven benefits,[28] but short-term survival may be reduced after placement, especially when tubes are inserted in hospitalized patients who often have acute delirium superimposed upon chronic dementia.[27,29,30]

Just as with ANH in terminal illness, there are individual cases in which the use of PEG tubes in patients with advanced dementia may improve quality of life. Even the best research has limitations, and there are studies that suggest a more positive profile for feeding tubes in patients with dementia.[28,31]

Nutrition support professionals in command of this body of evidence can take several steps to discourage the placement of feeding tubes, especially in nursing home residents. For example, nutrition support professionals can recommend swallowing studies, and the results of these studies as well as of neuropsychiatric consultations can assist in formulating realistic goals for PEG placement.[31]

Even if not unequivocal, there is strong evidence that PEG tubes cause more harm than good in patients with end-stage dementia, so why are they often placed? Brody and colleagues underscore that there are family, physician, and administrative factors that serve as a force contravening the empirical data for ANH in both terminal illness and advanced dementia.[6] Surveys suggest that the physicians who ultimately order feeding tubes believe they reduce morbidity and mortality.[24,32] Nutrition support professionals can potentially and constructively educate clinicians regarding the data on the effect of feeding tubes on short- and long-term survival. As practitioners, nutrition support professionals can be aware and attuned to the complex and conflicting emotions of denial, guilt, fear, and responsibility that accompany ANH decisions.

Nutrition support professionals can facilitate policymaking and become involved in institutional ethics committees and specialty organizations that work to counter the financial and regulatory incentives for placing PEG tubes. Physicians are reimbursed for the actual procedures of inserting the tubes, but not for the hours of counseling and education often required to persuade families against feeding tubes as the preferred option. Physicians may also fear lawsuits if they do not accede to the demands of distraught or angry family members.

Yet perhaps the greatest obstacle to reducing the use of feeding tubes in patients with end-stage disease is the current regulation that both incentivizes and penalizes nursing homes if they feed patients via tube rather than by hand. Especially when done by family members or friends, hand-feeding has the added advantages of providing human touch, nurturing, and social stimulation.[25]

The Vegetative State

These disorders, as defined and classified by the Multi-Society Task Force in the Persistent Vegetative State in 1994, have been graphically depicted by Fine.[33,34] Regardless of the etiology—trauma, metabolic, degenerative, etc.—the spectrum of consciousness and awareness conditions range from normal to brain death.

The vegetative state has been described as a state of "eyes open unconsciousness" in contrast to "eyes closed unconsciousness" or coma. Patients remaining in a vegetative state for more than a month are considered to be in a PVS. Patients in a PVS, who continue to exhibit the same conditions of unconsciousness and unawareness beyond three months, if not caused by trauma, or one year if a result of trauma, are deemed to be in a permanent vegetative state.[33,34] These concepts are shown in Figure 39-1.The significant ethical point of these temporal distinctions is that the diagnosis does not always predict the outcome, which must be based on other clinical factors, especially etiology, that influence decision making.[35]

The potential for regaining some or all consciousness and awareness is present in the early stages of the vegetative state or coma, providing a precautionary note for the premature forgoing of ANH in these patients based solely on their neurologic status. The importance of accurate diagnosis and reassessment of the patient's neurologic status throughout this period of potential recovery cannot be overemphasized. Despite appearances to the contrary, patients in a PVS do not demonstrate emotive, purposeful, or reproducible responses to painful stimuli rendering them, at least clinically, incapable of experiencing suffering with regards to pain, thirst, or hunger.[36]

The question of whether patients in a PVS suffer is a common concern of surrogates and health care professionals dealing with the troubling trichotomy. Further evidence of the

FIGURE 39-1 Levels of Consciousness After Brain Injury

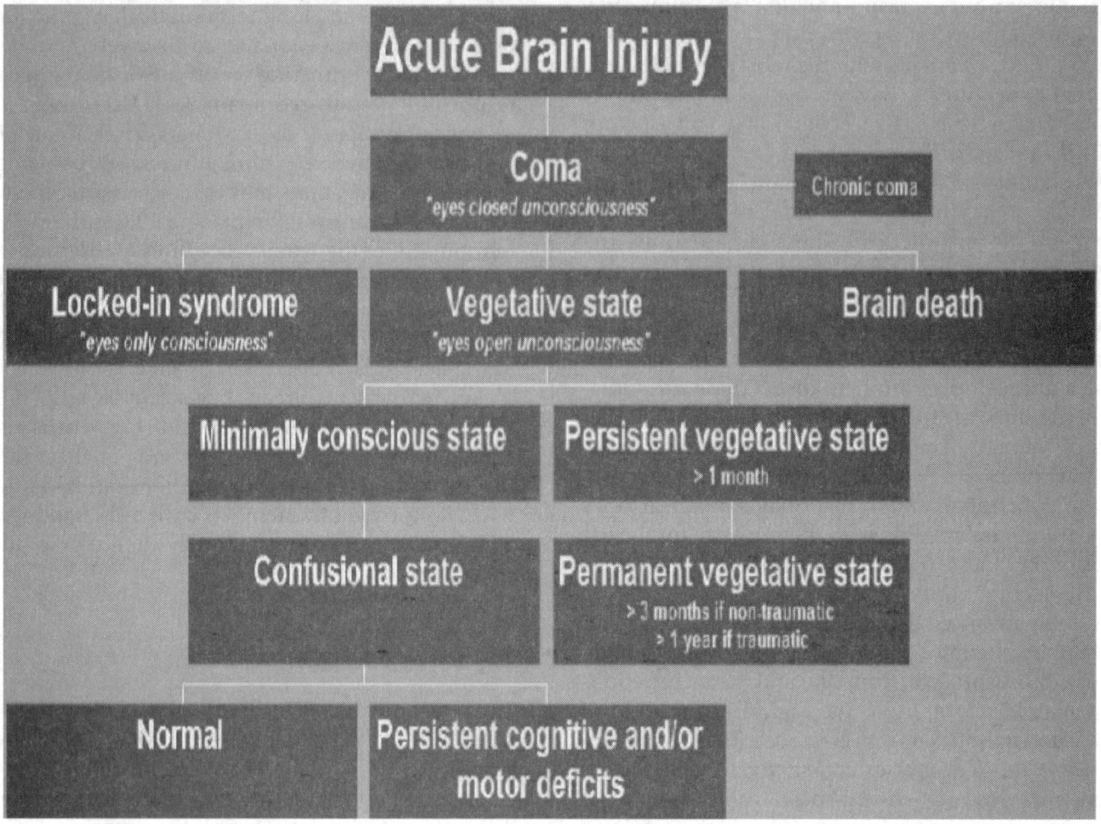

absence of suffering in patients in a PVS has been provided through sophisticated functional neuroimaging techniques such as position emission tomography scans[37] and functional magnetic resonance imaging, demonstrating which sections of the brain are functioning.[38] These techniques have established the disconnect between the thalamic and cortical areas necessary to experience pain in patients in a PVS compared to conscious patients. Neuroimaging has also demonstrated a return to normal functional imagery when the clinical picture demonstrates return of consciousness.[39]

In a functional magnetic resonance imaging of 54 patients initially classified as in a PVS, Monti and colleagues demonstrated brain activation reflecting some awareness and cognition in one, and only imaging activation in another.[40] The clinical significance of such neuroimaging findings has been questioned by Billings and colleagues and Ropper.[41,42] The study stressed the importance of accurate evaluation, classification, and reassessment of these patients because three of them or approximately 6% were found to be in a minimally conscious state rather than in a PVS.

When discussing the provision of ANH to patients in a PVS with surrogates, the health care team is often starved for credible, evidence-based medical information. The salient conclusions with respective references are summarized in Table 39-1.

Table 39-1 Persistent Vegetative State and Artifical Nutrition and Hydration

1. "Consciousness appears to be a pre-requisite to suffering."
2. "Solid neuroscience supports the clinical observation that comatose, brain dead, and vegetative patients do not suffer. Such patients experienc neither burdens nor benefits of any therapy."
3. "The experience of 'starvation' requires consciousness."
4. Artificial nutrition and hydration alone, though someitmes supportive, does not cure or reverse any terminal, irreversible diesease, injury, degenerative disease of the brain (Alzheimer, amyotrophic lateral sclerosis, multiple sclerosis, Parkinson, stroke, or organ failure).
5. Fasting can provide anesthesia secondary to the associated ketosis as well as increased endorphins.

Developed from Drane JF. Stopping nutrition and hydration technologies: a conflict between traditional Catholic ethics and church authority. *Christ Bioeth.* 2006;12(1):11–28; Hallenbeck J. *Fast Facts and Concepts #11 Tube Feed or Not Tube Feed?* 2nd ed. End-of-Life Physician Education Resource Center; August 2005.

One of the most difficult decisions facing health care professionals and surrogates of patients in a PVS is that of whether to place or remove a PEG tube. It is important to provide information of long-term outcomes and expectations as previously discussed, presented to the PVS surrogate decision maker. Alternatively, decisions to forgo PEG tubes in the early phase of the vegetative state, when persistent may not be permanent or may not be the correct diagnosis, may be premature and should trigger a consideration for a time-limited trial with frank discussions with the surrogate decision maker, other family, and significant others communicating specific goals and expectations.

The "Should" of Bioethics

Ethics refers to the "rules and standards governing the conduct of a person or members of a profession."[43] Bioethics is a broader and newer term that emerged in the 1960s in response to the rapid development of medical technology, the rise of the human rights movements, and the disclosure of abuses in scientific research.[44] Theoretical, clinical, regulatory, or policy and cultural ethics are four domains of bioethics,[45] each of which is relevant to the ethical issues examined in this chapter. Clinical ethics is the most important for nutrition support professionals and is the type of everyday ethics that engages practitioners in the care of patients.

Ethical Theory

Ethical theory is a general philosophical source of many ethical standards and is also the guide for how these standards are applied through ethical reasoning in specific situations such as the provision of ANH in patients in a PVS. Ethical theories are schools of thinking that form one of the bases of our moral decisions. A working familiarity with these schools can provide methods of analysis within which nutrition support professionals can contribute to the identification and resolution of ethical dilemmas.[46] Four of the most common ethical theories used in contemporary bioethics are principlism, deontology, utilitarianism, and virtue ethics. Each school is explicated through application to the sample care of Mr. L and discussed subsequently.

Mr. L is a 64-year-old who sustained a traumatic brain injury in a motorcycle accident in which he was not wearing a helmet. He has been in a vegetative state for a week, and the neurologists estimate the prognosis for meaningful recovery to be poor. His wife and young adult children believe he is a fighter and will improve. The intensive care physician consults the nutrition support professional regarding the clinical and ethical indications for placement of a feeding tube.

Beauchamp and Childress have developed principlism into one of the most widely employed modes of ethical analysis in contemporary bioethics.[47] This theory bases ethical decisions on general rules and principles that express broad moral considerations applied to particular situations. Dilemmas are resolved through the weighing, balancing, and specification of the basic principles of autonomy, beneficence, nonmaleficence, and justice. Definitions of these and other core ethics principles with applications to nutrition support are found in Table 39-2.

Deontology, or the ethics of duty, assumes the existence of absolute duties or judgments that are nearly unconditional in their application to particular circumstances. The philosopher Immanuel Kant is one of the most significant figures in deontological ethics.[48] For a decision to be ethical under the rubric of deontology, it must be universal, as expressed in Kant's famous categorical imperative as a philosophical formulation of the golden rule. The rightness or wrongness of decisions

Table 39-2 The Application of Core Ethical Principles to Nutrition Support Therapy

Principle	Definition	Application to ANH
Autonomy	The individual's right to self-determination as expressed in health care decision making. It is the predominant value in American bioethics and law.	A patient with intact decisional capacity may refuse ANH even if medically recommended.
Beneficence	The fundamental obligation of a health care professional to seek the good of the patient above all other priorities.	A nutrition support professional may recommend temporary placement of a (PEG) tube for patients undergoing chemotherapy and radiation for gastric cancer.
Nonmaleficence	"To do no harm" (primum non nocere), the prime directive of medicine to prevent, minimize, and relieve needless suffering and pain.	A nutrition support professional may recommend against using ANH in a patient with a PEG if it decreases quality of life and decreases outcomes.
Justice	Fairness requires specialized nutrition support professionals to equitably treat similar patients similarly and considers only clinical relevancy.	Lack of access to appropriate hospice and palliative care my lead to overuse of ANH in disadvantaged cohorts.

ANH, artificial nutrition and hydration; PEG, percutaneous endoscopic gastrostomy.
Developed from Brody H, Hermer LD, Scott LD, et al. Artificial nutrition and hydration: the evolution of ethics, evidence, and policy. *J Gen Intern Med.* 2011;26(9):1053–1058; Laureys S. Functional neuroimaging in the vegetative state. *NeuroRehabilitation.* 2004;19(4):335–341; Callahan D. Bioethics. In: Post SG, ed. *Encyclopedia of Bioethics.* Vol 1. 3rd ed. New York, NY: Thompson-Gale; 2004:278–286; Ferrie S. A quick guide to ethical theory in healthcare: solving ethical dilemmas in nutrition support situations. *Nutr Clin Pract.* 2006;21(2):113–117.

from the deontological perspective depends on the intentions of the agent, not on the consequences of the act. Deontological reasoning is the basis of the sanctity of life claims that ANH must be provided to all human beings, even those like Mr. L in a potential PVS.

Utilitarianism is an ethical theory that begins from the opposite premise: it is the consequences, not the intentions, of decisions that determine their ethical valence. This is an ethical theory most often associated with the English philosopher John Stuart Mill that is frequently used in health care economics, resource allocation, and policy.[49] Actions and obligations that maximize the good or benefit for the largest number of people are the most ethical. A policy that restricts feeding tubes for patents like Mr. L in a PVS because the patients have a low likelihood of recovering according to evidence-based criteria is an example of utilitarian thinking.

Virtue ethics is the moral theory that finds the locus of right and wrong in the character of the individual. Deriving from Aristotle,[50] virtue ethics is among the oldest theory of professional ethics and one many practitioners find the most natural. A clinician whose conduct displays habits of compassion, honesty, integrity, fidelity, and courage will develop a virtuous character from which will spring good clinical decisions. Such a decision about Mr. L might be to provide a time-limited trial of ANH as an expression of the fiduciary commitment to the patient and his family.

Key Ethico-Legal Concepts

The ethics of priniciplism, deontology, utilitarianism, and virtue provide the structure for decision making, but the process of these decisions is operationalized in clinical practice and law through a series of interrelated key ethico-legal concepts, as explicated in this section and summarized in Table 39-3.

Informed Consent

The legal and ethical doctrine of informed consent expresses the high valence of autonomy and respect for persons in Western bioethics. Informed consent is not the mere signing of a form but the outcome of a shared decision-making process between patient and/or surrogate and the health care professionals caring for the patient. Authentic informed consent consists of three main components. (1) The patient or surrogate is provided adequate information regarding the proposed treatment or procedure in understandable language. This includes, at a minimum, the diagnosis for which the treatment is clinically indicated, and the prognosis with and without the proposed intervention, the risks and benefits of the procedures, alternatives to the proposed intervention, including no treatment. (2) The patient or surrogate has intact decision-making capacity. (3) The patient possesses voluntarism, which is the ability to make a choice free of excessive internal or external coercion.[51]

Table 39-3 Key Ethico-Legal Concepts

Informed consent and refusal
Decisional capacity
Surrogates
Standards of surrogate decision making
Withholding and withdrawing
Futility/quality of life

Decisional Capacity

Advance directives are pivotal in the legal and ethical arena related to ANH and exemplify the intersection of law and bioethics on medical decision making. Discussion of the purpose of advance directives must be prefaced with a brief explanation of the terms decisional capacity and competence. Only a court can determine competence, but such determinations are often materially based on health care providers' judgments regarding the ability of the individual to comprehend and communicate health information, reason regarding aspects of treatment, appreciate the consequences of medical decisions for their lives and values, and freely choose a course of action.[51] Decision-making capacity is task-specific and not global in nature: a person may be able to make medical decisions but not manage his finances, or the reverse. Decision-making capacity can fluctuate particularly when the impairment is secondary to physical or mental illness. A patient may thus be more or less capable of making specific decisions at different times and under varying conditions.[52]

Surrogate Decision Making

Only a quarter of Americans are estimated to have completed an advance directive.[53] In response to what many experts consider a failure of advance directives to protect patient autonomy, all 50 states have legislation granting an order of priority in making decisions for patients who lack both capacity and an advance directive. Because of the differences in these laws, it is crucial for nutrition support professionals to be familiar with the content of the statutes in their own jurisdiction and to have access to expert legal advice. Generally, the hierarchy or priority for surrogacy is the following: spouse, adult children, siblings, other relatives, and in some states, friends. Divorce or legal separation may void the first order rank of the spouse as surrogate. Significant others including same-sex partners who are in long-standing relationships are considered the legal surrogate in some states, but not in others. Disputes among putative surrogates, especially in the absence of formal directives, are common and troubling and should be referred to the ethics committee or ethics consultant, hospital risk management, hospital attorney, or professional mediators to try and obtain consensus.[54]

Standards of Surrogate Decision Making

The surrogate is obligated to render decisions that are in accordance with legal criteria. When a patient's values and wishes are known, decisions are to be made in accordance with the standard called substituted judgment.[55] When the patient's wishes are not ascertainable, then the surrogate should make decisions in accordance with a best interest standard. The 1985 Conroy case[56]

Table 39-4 Standards of Surrogate Decision Making

Type of Test	Type of Evidence
• Subjective test • Most trustworthy	Clear and unequivocal evidence of the patient's wishes as expressed in an advance directive or oral instructions to a health care professional, family, or friend
Limited objective test	• Based on patient's best interests; trustworthy testimony that a patient would have refused treatment • Informal or casual expression or preferences in reaction to news reports or the condition of other persons
Pure objective test	When there is no trustworthy evidence of patient's wishes

presented guidelines for the exercise of substituted judgment for incompetent patients according to three levels of credibility. From most to least credible, these tests are summarized in Table 39-4.

Withholding versus Withdrawing Treatment

One of the major ethical decision points encountered in nutrition support practice is the decision to withhold or withdraw—the term forgoing refers to both actions—ANH. There is no ethical, legal, or moral distinction between withholding and withdrawing any treatment, including ANH. However, decisions to actively withdraw ANH are more psychologically charged for practitioners, patients, and families than decisions to passively withhold intervention. The potential benefits of a limited trial of ANH should not be eschewed in an effort to avoid the difficult emotional interactions of withdrawing nutrition support should those benefits not be realized.[8] A decisionally capable patient or his or her authorized surrogate may refuse any form of medical care including lifesaving treatments even if that inevitable result of that refusal is death.

Futility/Quality of Life

Health care professionals often invoke "futility" as the rationale for forgoing treatment or medical therapies. Levinsky described futility as "conferring technological immortality on dehumanized bodies."[57] In the U.S. Supreme Court deliberations regarding Nancy Cruzan, Associate Justice William Brenan opined, "medical technology has created a twilight zone of suspended animation where death commences while life, in some form, continues."[58] The Danaides pouring water from leaky vessels to leaky cisterns, the Greek mythological figures from which the word "futility" is derived, provide an imagery often seen in our critical care units when overutilization of precious resources are consumed like a sponge or sieve to no avail.[8]

While these scenarios are daily occurrences in our health care facilities, the recognition of the patients' severity of illness is shared by all; the same is not true for the acceptance that the medical interventions being rendered are "futile." The definitions of futility are value based, thus rendering them subject to varied interpretation leading to an inability to reach consensus about goals of care. There are a few clinical settings in which there is unanimity that any treatment is futile (eg, cardiopulmonary resuscitation on a decapitated individual). Religious beliefs, skepticism of a physician's ability to make a prognosis, and surrogates' need for a more experiential understanding of the patient's prognosis have been identified as grounds for objections to the medical futility rationale.[59] Two state court cases pertaining to the issue of whether doctors must continue to provide medical interventions that they consider medically unwarranted led to a controversy regarding the actual diagnosis and prognosis.[60,61]

The Education for Physicians in End of Life Care program[62] recommends substituting the term "low yield" rather than "futile" for interventions that are of questionable value and at the same time emphasizing the benefits/burdens/risk analysis in reaching decisions. The Education for Physicians in End of Life Care program prefers the designation of "medically inappropriate" treatment/intervention to facilitate better appreciation by surrogates of the severity of illness and prognosis, thus promoting open communications and understanding with less emotional upheaval in setting the stage for a time-limited trial of a potentially beneficial intervention.[62,63] Notwithstanding the previous discussion, if consensus is not reached regarding an intervention such as removal of a PEG tube, it is best to subscribe to the philosophy of "when in doubt, don't take it out" while continued dialogue including crucial conversations are held with all stakeholders. Such a discussion should include the option to transfer the patient's care to another practitioner willing and able to place or maintain the PEG tube.

Empirical Ethics Research

Empirical research suggests that shared decision making regarding ANH, especially PEG tubes, may not meet the ethical and legal criteria discussed previously. A retrospective study of 154 hospital patients receiving PEGs for serious illness found that only 1 patient had a documented discussion of risks and benefits of tube placement, and 12 of 33 patients providing signed consent had questionable or unclear decisional capacity.[64] A study of 1446 physicians and nurses found that 70% of attending physicians believed that even when all other forms of life support were forgone, nutrition and hydration should always be maintained.[65] Callahan analyzed the decisional process in 100 patients who received PEG tubes and physicians caring for these patients. Patients or surrogates reported discussing placement with multiple providers, being given incomplete information, and physicians, patients, and families experienced considerable distress around the ANH decision. Many involved in the process experienced it as one of "nondecision" because alternatives were not presented, and discussion seemed to focus on short-term acuity rather than long-term functional outcomes. Physicians perceived pressures both from families and other providers to place PEG tubes.[66] Recent research also shows that nurses, as the most direct deliverers of care for patients with dementia, experience considerable moral distress related to ANH.[67]

The tendency of health care professionals to favor the use of ANH and to view it as beneficial is in stark contrast to the opinions and choices of properly informed patients. Forty-nine decisionally capable nursing home residents were presented with a hypothetical scenario in which brain injury had damaged their ability to take oral nutrition. Thirty-three percent initially chose ANH, but after being educated that restraints might be necessary to keep the feeding tube in place, their preferences changed. Factors associated with desiring a feeding tube were the belief that nursing home staff would respect the choice, never having completed an advance directive or discussing health care preferences with family or providers, and being African American.[68] Hoeffler's review of numerous public opinion polls and scholarly studies, many done in the 1990s, found that the majority of Americans do not want a feeding tube at the end of life.[69]

General Ethical Analysis of Artificial Nutrition and Hydration

Beneficence and nonmaleficence—These principles support the goal of maximum benefit with minimum harm or burden. There are times when ANH can meet these goals and other times when this may not be the case. As the nutrition support professional is fully aware, inherent in this treatment are complications related to the tube or line placement, equipment, formula, and maintenance. In addition, ANH may not achieve the intended benefits of comfort or prolonged survival. Based on the ethical principles of beneficence and nonmaleficence, it is ethically appropriate to withhold or withdraw ANH when the benefits outweigh the burdens, provided there is appropriate consent from a patient with decisional capacity.

Justice (distributive justice)—Medical ethics has traditionally been focused on treatment decisions and advocacy for the individual patient. The rising cost of health care, the advent of managed care systems, a growing number of uninsured, and most important, a renewed emphasis on public health and the good of the community, have underscored issues of social and distributive justice. For nutrition support professionals, this means an obligation to responsibly and wisely utilize scarce resources, which may include considerations of cost. However, most ethicists would caution providers in employing bedside rationing when deciding on the appropriateness of ANH. Treatment decisions should be based on the clinical standard of care, evidence-based medicine, patient and family preferences, and institutional policy. It behooves nutrition support professionals to work through their professional organizations to influence the public and social debate on controversial questions involving ANH in a direction that balances the needs of individual patients with the duty to equitably use health care resources.

Cultural Values and Religious Beliefs

Food, even as a formula delivered through tubes, remains a source of life, a symbol of caring, and a social bond endowed with a spiritual and ritual significance no other medical treatment possesses.[70] Failure to appreciate the way in which the cultural values and religious beliefs of patients, families, and even other health care professionals impact health care decisions can trigger or amplify ethical conflicts. One of the most salient differences is that Asian, Native American, and Hispanic cultures often do not invest individual autonomy with the primacy it holds in Western bioethics. Instead, the family or community may be the accepted locus of decision making.[71–73] Practice Scenario 39-2 is an example of how decision making may be different in another culture.

Nutrition support professionals and other clinicians cannot realistically become experts in the diverse cultures and religions of our increasingly ethnically and spiritually diverse society. Therefore, practitioners should inquire to what degree any particular patient's wishes adhere to religious or cultural views. The most well-developed and debated positions on ANH belong to Judaism and Catholicism and will be examined in some detail.

Practice Scenario 39-2

Question: Is it ethical to allow a family to make decisions for a competent patient regarding ANH?

Scenario: An 83-year-old Asian woman has persistent dysphagia as the sequela of a stroke. She is unable to take in adequate oral nutrition but is otherwise recovering fairly well. The attending physician asks the patient whether she would be interested in ANH. The woman defers the decision to her eldest son, although the neurologist had documented that she is decisionally capable. The physician is uncomfortable allowing the woman's son to make the decision as he feels she has autonomy and can provide informed consent or refusal.

Intervention: The ethics consultation service is called. The ethics consultant speaks privately with the patient and finds no undue coercion is being exercised by the family and that the patient is voluntarily following her own cultural traditions that should be respected.[70]

Answer: The consultant understood the bioethics concept of familial autonomy that is normative in many cultures. Family autonomy locates the locus of medical decision making not in the individual but in the family or community. In this case, lack of knowledge and respect for non-Western cultural values led to an ethical conflict.

Judaism

Jewish bioethics derives from the Jewish Law, *Halacha*, developed from the Torah (Hebrew Bible) and Rabbinic commentary on the Torah contained in the Talmud. The infinite value and dignity of human life is the paramount consideration because life belongs to, and is a gift of, God. There are three main divisions of modern Judaism: the Orthodox, Conservative, and Reformed. Each branch follows Jewish law but differs in how strictly the law is observed especially when applied to contemporary dilemmas, with the Orthodox being the strictest and the Reformed the most flexible in their interpretations.

Hastening death is not permitted; for this reason, the active withdrawal of interventions may be seen as more morally problematic than passive withholding.[74] Jewish law does recognize a category of the actively dying "Goses," where death is imminent and irreversible. The period of Goses is often 3 days in duration, and a practitioner cannot act preemptively in anticipation of death. The Law of Goses does not require the continuation of life-sustaining interventions, particularly when they are especially burdensome to the patient. Dorff cites the decisive factors in making such a decision as the risk/benefit ratio and the patient's best interest and desires.[75] Gillick believes that even more traditional forms of Judaism may permit the withholding of ANH from patients with advanced dementia through an extension of the Goses category, thus permitting the forgoing of treatments that are only causing suffering but cannot bring about recovery.[27] Reformed Judaism would allow more room for individual autonomy and advance directives in making health care decisions.

The tension between dictates of religious law regarding the sanctity of life and secular medicine's respect for autonomy is evident in a recent law passed in Israel, the Israeli Dying Patient Act.[76] The act contains a legal requirement that family and physicians of a terminally ill patient try to persuade a competent patient to accept food and water including ANH in accordance with the duty of Jews to preserve life whenever possible. A competent patient can refuse these requests. The duty to protect life, however, outweighs the self-determination of an incompetent patient, and ANH must be provided even if this is against the previously expressed wishes of the patient.[77]

Catholicism

In 2004, Pope John Paul II issued a Papal allocution, "Life Sustaining Treatments and the Vegetative State."[78] The Pope describes the moral status of ANH in the following key passage:

> I should like particularly to underline how the administration of water and food, even when provided by artificial means, always represents a *natural means* of preserving life, not a medical act. Its use furthermore, should be considered, in principle ordinary and proportionate, and as such morally obligatory, insofar as and until it is seen to have attained its proper finality, which in the present case consists in providing nourishment to the patient and alleviation of his suffering.[78]

The Pope argues that the withdrawal of ANH in a patient with brain injury, even in a PVS, is the direct cause of death through starvation, not the underlying disease process, and as such is tantamount to euthanasia by omission.[78] It is important to recognize that the allocution discusses the role of ANH in a PVS and not advanced dementia or terminal illness, although the National Catholic Bioethics Center recently extended the argument that ANH is obligatory to patients with dementia.[79] The Pope himself did not accept life-sustaining treatments when he was dying. PVS is the subject because John Paul contends that the diagnosis, and hence, the prognosis, of the disorder are not nearly so certain or irreversible as the medical community claims.

The allocution caused such consternation among American Catholics that in 2005 the U.S. Conference of Catholic Bishops (USCCB) sought clarification of the meaning of the allocution from the Vatican. The USCCB posed two questions to the Church's teaching authority, and the current Pope Benedict XVI approved the responses issued in 2007. The responses reaffirmed that patients in a vegetative state are human beings who require basic care, and this includes nutrition and hydration even if provided through artificial means. The USCCB then extensively revised Directive 58 on Ethical and Religious Directives for Catholic Health Care Services in accordance with papal teaching.[80]

The Pope's original statement, the response to the USCCB, and the revised directive all turn upon a classic distinction in moral philosophy between ordinary and proportionate care that was morally obligatory, and extraordinary and disproportionate care that was morally permissible to refuse. Basic care such as keeping a patient clean, warm, and fed is considered "ordinary care."[80] Some Catholic ethicists would disagree with the USCCB on two key points with relevance for nutrition support. The first is that the papal teaching is not congruent with centuries of prior teaching that would view ANH as a medical treatment that could in some circumstances be considered an extraordinary treatment in terms of the burden of human suffering it imposes on patients and families.[81] Second, even within the hierarchy's own classification of ANH as ordinary care, there remains some room for interpretation. The allocution states ANH is morally obligatory "in principle," which some Catholic ethicists point out is a general statement that still leaves discretion to not use ANH in specific cases of PVS. Directive 58 also indicates that ANH would "become morally optional" when it cannot reasonably be expected to prolong life, is excessively burdensome to the patient, or causes significant physical discomfort."[82]

The significance of the USCCB action is to incorporate, or clarify, teaching regarding ANH that a person's life must never be considered worthless simply because the person is unconscious, or more specifically, in a PVS. Treatment decisions should be made based on the burdens and benefits of the treatment, not on the perceived burdens of the PVS itself. For example, repeated infection or treatment that causes significant physical discomfort, such as fluid overload from medically administered nutrition and hydration, might in Catholic moral theology be considered excessively burdensome. The directive obliges Catholic practitioners and administrators of Catholic institutions to offer ANH to patients and families, but it does not require either clinicians or health care facilities to overrule the wishes of patients as expressed through an advance directive or authorized surrogate decision maker. Informed consent still constitutes the foundation of respect for a person's dignity. However, clergy, patients, families, and health care institutions may hold varying interpretations of the directive that could lead to ethical conflicts warranting ethics consultation. Family members are thus encouraged to discuss their wishes for all forms of end-of-life treatment with their health care providers, family, and if appropriate, clergy, and to complete an advance directive that clearly states their preferences about medical treatment including ANH.[83] Practice Scenario 39-3 illustrates the dilemma when an advance directive is not available and there is religious conflict.

Table 39-5 summarizes the positions on ANH of other major world religions.

Practice Scenario 39-3

Question: Is it morally obligatory for Catholic parents to continue ANH in their daughter who is in a PVS from a diving accident?

Scenario: The treatment team at an academic medical center strongly recommends that the parents of a 25-year-old woman who has been in a PVS for 9 months discontinue ANH. The woman is breathing on her own but has shown no signs of neurological recovery. The team feels continued provision of nutrition and hydration is causing undue suffering with no prospect of benefit and calls for an ethics consultation. Being so young, the patient had not completed an advance directive, and the parents had never had a specific conversation with their daughter about end of life. Her parents did feel that their daughter's general values regarding being active and vital meant she would not likely wish to be kept alive when she could no longer meaningfully participate in life.

Intervention: The ethics consultation service meets with the parents, their parish priest, a hospital chaplain, and the health care team to discuss the situation. They discuss the daughter's values about an active life and the important role her religious beliefs had played in other major decisions she made. The family, with the support of their priest, refuses to withdraw ANH, stating it is against Catholic teaching. The ethics consultants arrange for transfer of the patient to a Catholic long-term care facility.

Answer: The Pope and USCCB, as explained previously, argue that food and water, even artificially provided, are a form of medical treatment that all human beings deserve. Administering nutrition and hydration to a patient in a PVS is morally obligatory, and failing to do so is a form of euthanasia.[82]

Conscience Clauses

The Catholic controversy reminds us that health care professionals and even institutions have their own religious and ethical beliefs and values that influence their decision making regarding ANH. These values should never be imposed on patients or families, as this violates the fundamental principle of respect for persons. Yet, there may be times in which a nutrition support professional or other practitioner feels in conscience they cannot participate in the care of a patient due to moral or religious objections. Historically, the federal government, some state statutes, and many health care organizations have granted contained conscience clause provisions that enable clinicians to be excused from a case as long as an equally qualified practitioner or facility is willing to assume the care of the patient. Until such time as an orderly transfer is completed, the clinician continues to be responsible for the care of the patient. The Bush administration expanded conscience clause protections to an extent many in medicine thought inappropriate. In 2011, President Obama reversed this trend, rescinding the majority of the Bush legislation, although extant federal laws remain in effect.[84]

Table 39-5 Position of World Religions on Artificial Nutrition and Hydration

World Religion	Position on ANH
Buddhism	• Preservation of life at all costs is not obligatory. • ANH is not mandatory to keep patients alive.
Greek Orthodox	• Prolongation of life is supreme goal. • ANH cannot be forgone even if there is no hope of recovery.
Islam	• Sanctity of life is the primary value. • Food and water are ordinary care. • ANH is obligatory if it can extend life.
Protestantism	• Life-sustaining therapies can be withheld/withdrawn if no hope of recovery.

ANH, artificial nutrition and hydration.
Developed from Brett AS, Rosenberg JC. The adequacy of informed consent for placement of gastrostomy tubes. *Arch Intern Med.* 2001;161(5):745–748; Bulow HH, Sprung CL, Reinhart K, et al. The world's major religions' points of view on end-of-life decisions in the intensive care unit. *Intensive Care Med.* 2008;34(3):423–430; Dorff EN. Applying traditional Jewish law to PVS. *NeuroRehabilitation.* 2004;19(4):277–283.

The "Must" of the Law

The duty of a health care professional to provide the most appropriate care with the most appropriate available technology is governed by the legal system—the must, or third component of "the troubling trichotomy." The U.S. legal system has its foundation in the federal and state constitutions, statutes, regulations, court decisions, and attorney general opinions.[84,85]

As depicted in Figure 39-2, the two major components of the law are criminal and civil. Civil law applies to the majority of cases involving health care professionals. Contract and tort (harm) are the two major components of civil law. While contract law may be occasionally implicated in cases of alleged abandonment, tort law dominates the legal concerns for the health care professional. Tort law includes intentional

FIGURE 39-2 The "Must": The U.S. Legal System

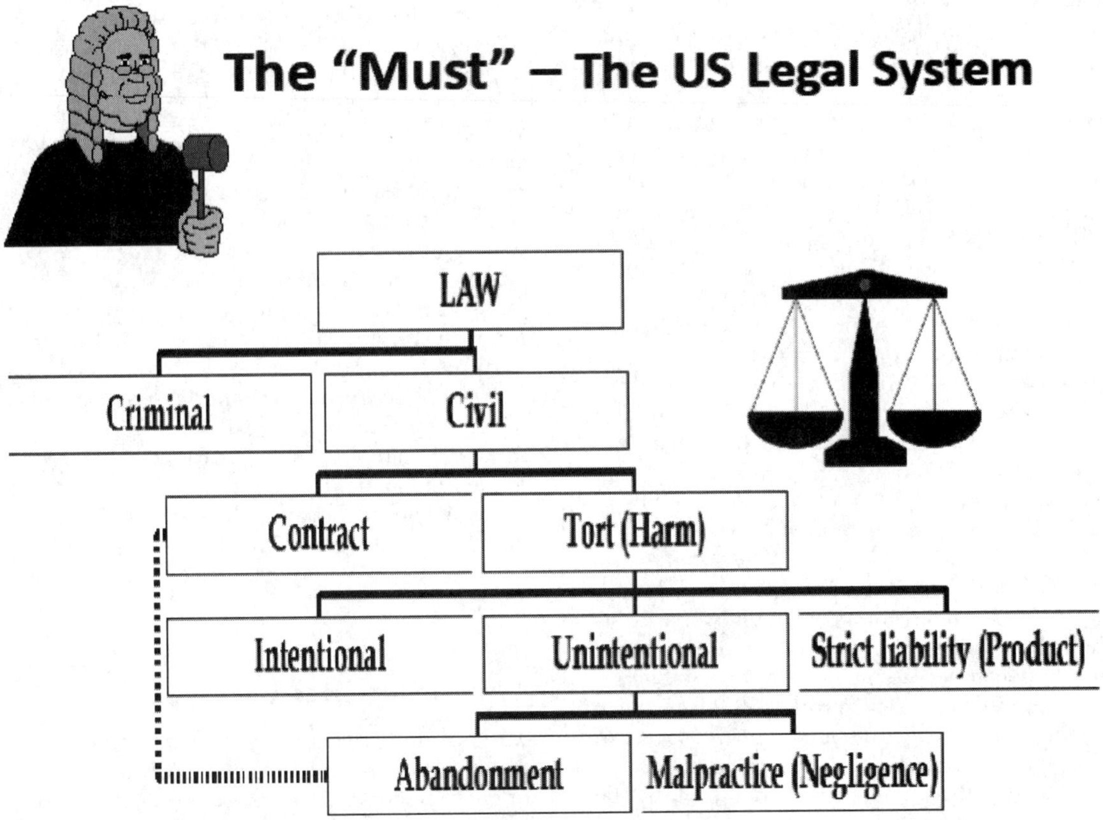

Reprinted from Barrocas A, Yarbrough G, Becnel PA, Nelson JE. Ethical and legal issues in nutrition support of the geriatric patient: the can, should and must of nutrition support. *Nutr Clin Pract.* 2003;18:37–47.

and unintentional harm as well as strict liability often associated with product liability and not involving health care professionals.

Intentional tort includes allegations of assault (attempt or threat to touch another without justification), battery (actual act of touching another), and invasion of privacy, defamation, misinterpretation, fraud, and false imprisonment. Violation of privacy rights and potential for alleged defamation may occur secondary to inattention to person, place, and type of communications. Assault and battery charges against health care professionals can be precipitated by the absence of appropriate informed consent when either or one of the following does not occur:

1. Consent is not for specific procedure (eg, PEG tube).
2. Patient was not provided with the information to give consent (eg, bleeding, peritonitis, and long-range outcomes regarding morbidity and mortality with PEG tube insertion).
3. Consent was not obtained for the individual(s) performing the procedure (eg, partner of gastroenterologists who obtained consent the previous day).
4. Consent was obtained from a patient with decisional incapacity (eg, a demented patient or a patient with recent intramuscular and intravenous narcotic).

Abandonment, an unintentional tort, refers to "the unilateral severance of the professional relationship without reasonable notice under the circumstances when continued attention is required." Refusal to treat, insufficient or delayed treatment, withdrawal without adequate notice, and premature discharge are potential triggers for allegations of abandonment.

The other unintentional tort that health care professionals are confronted with is malpractice (negligence). Palmisano proposed the ABCD rule as a quick reference to what constitutes a credible malpractice claim[86]: the health care practitioner has to *a*ccept the patient, establishing a legal relationship between the two; and conduct below the reasonable standard of care, indicating a *b*reach of duty that leads to a *c*ause which results in a specific alleged *d*amage. Appropriate communications and documentation provide useful prophylaxis charges of abandonment and/or malpractice (negligence).

Precedent Cases: Cruzan, Quinlan, and Schiavo

ANH has been the focus of a litany of legal decisions over the past three to four decades. The seminal case of Karen Ann Quinlan in 1976[87] set the stage for a cascade of additional cases, legal decisions, and statutes. Ms. Quinlan was in a PVS as a result of anoxic encephalopathy, rendering her ventilator dependent. Her parents, attempting to honor her previously expressed wishes, requested removal of the ventilator. The physicians caring for her were reluctant to comply, fearing criminal repercussions. The New Jersey Supreme Court ruled that the ventilator, a life-sustaining measure, could be removed if a prognosis existed of "no reasonable possibility of a patient returning to a cognitive, sapient state" and a hospital ethics committee could confirm such a conclusion. Additionally, the court provided for criminal and civil legal protection for all involved parties in the decision-making process. Interestingly, the patient lived without ventilator support for many years on enteral (tube) feedings that were never challenged by the health care team or family. The Quinlan case served as a stimulus for the establishment of hospital ethics committees and enactment of states' "living will" legislation.

In 1983, Nancy Cruzan was involved in an automobile accident resulting in anoxic brain injury.[58] Unable to swallow because of the brain damage, she would have died without ANH, but with a feeding tube placement could conceivably survive for years. After several years, and a confirmed diagnosis of a PVS, her parents requested permission from the courts to remove their daughter's feeding tube. The Missouri Supreme Court determined that the tube could only lawfully be removed if there was "clear and convincing evidence" that such removal was in accordance with Ms. Cruzan's wishes. Ms. Cruzan had not left an advance directive, and without this documentation, the court did not feel the family's views of their daughter's preferences to not receive ANH met the relatively stringent evidential standard they had set. The court required such evidence to override the state's compelling interest in preserving the life of a patient who lacked decisional capacity to make her own choices.[88]

The Cruzan family appealed the decision to the Supreme Court. While upholding the right of states to set their own evidential standards for withdrawal of feeding tubes, they established several salient ethical precedents related to ANH. Within a year of the Supreme Court decision, new testimony from friends of Ms. Cruzan was presented, which another court ruled met the Missouri criteria for clear and convincing evidence. The feeding tube was legally removed in 1990, with Ms. Cruzan dying peacefully shortly after.[88] Three outcomes of the Cruzan U.S. Supreme Court Decision are summarized as follows:

1. Affirmation of the authority of individual states to establish higher standards of evidence
2. Established ANH as life-sustaining no different than ventilators and hemodialysis
3. Stimulated increase in the use of health care proxies or Durable Power of Attorney for Health Care decisions and the enactment of the Patient Self-Determination Act of 1990 mandating advance directives[89]

In 1990, Terri Schiavo suffered a cardiac arrest; she was given cardiopulmonary resuscitation (CPR) but had already sustained severe brain damage. The hospital inserted a PEG tube in the 26-year-old woman, who was subsequently diagnosed as in a PVS, and her husband Michael was appointed guardian. In 1998, Michael filed a petition to have the feeding tube removed on the grounds that Terri would not wish to be maintained in a PVS. Her parents argued the opposite position, resulting in a contentious debate that spanned two removals and reinsertions of the feeding tube, four rejected appeals to the Supreme Court, and the unprecedented intervention of the Florida legislature, the governor, Congress, and the president. Finally in March of 2005, the federal district court refused to order reinsertion of the PEG for a third time, and Terri Schiavo died on the 31st of that month.[89]

The political reaction to the Schiavo experience eventuated in the refinement of living will legislation with regards to ANH in several states. In many instances, the forgoing of ANH is prohibited in a patient without decisional capacity unless clearly expressed in an advance directive. This trend goes against decades of legal and ethical opinion regarding the authority of a surrogate even without advance directives to make decisions about ANH.[90]

Advance Directives

Advance directives are documents that allow individuals to document their treatment preferences and identify a surrogate or proxy decision maker to act in the patient's stead when they lose the ability to do so. Usually the attending physician, or in some states two physicians, make the determination of incapacity. An advance directive is effectuated only if and when the patient loses the capacity to make his or her own decisions.[91] There are three main types of advance directives, and these are summarized in Table 39-6. In all states, court-appointed guardians for persons adjudicated as incompetent can make health care decisions for their wards. Increasingly, states and institutions are combining the types of directives onto one comprehensive form.

Data from a prospectively collected survey of 3302 Medicare beneficiaries who died between 1998 and 2007 found that advance directives specifying limitations of end-of-life care were associated with significantly lower levels of Medicare spending.[92] Additionally, the individuals in regions with higher levels of end-of-life care spending exhibited a lower likelihood of inhospital death and higher use of hospice. Advance directives may be especially important for ensuring medical treatment that is consistent with patients' preferences for those individuals who prefer less aggressive treatment at the end of life, but live in areas with a heathcare system that is characterized by high intensity of treatment.

Practice Scenario 39-4 shows the benefit of an advance directive when an individual does not want aggressive medical intervention at the end of life yet lives in a community where high intensity of treatment is the norm.

Table 39-6 Types of Advance Directives

Directive	Purpose
Living wills	Provide written instructions by a capable person regarding their end-of-life wishes in the event capacity is lost.
Durable powers of attorney for health care or medical powers of attorney or health care proxy	Designates a person who makes treatment decisions on behalf of the person once capacity is lost.
Surrogate decision maker	A person appointed in law or by policy to act as a surrogate in the absence of an advance directive.

Unfortunately in the United States, end-of-life care often does not reflect patients' values and preferences.[93] Yet, recent observational and interventional studies in selected patients suggest that advance directives substantially improve the patient-centered aspect of end-of-life care.[94,95] Surrogate decision makers may be reluctant to not provide aggressive medical therapies for patients and might experience substantial distress unless they are acting in accordance with an advance directive or an understanding of the patient's values. Perhaps the goal of advance care planning should not only be documenting the individual's treatment preferences for specific medical scenarios, but on preparing surrogates for in-the-moment decision making. The focus of such planning should include giving family members and physicians the tools they need to make appropriate treatment decisions for patients who lack decision-making capacity.[93]

Practice Scenario 39-4

Question: What is the benefit of an advance directive in a hospital in a region of high intensity health care use?

Scenario: An 88-year-old female with chest pains was admitted to a hospital in a region of the country identified with high intensity of health care use based on Medicare spending. She had completed an advance directive that identified her younger daughter as the decision maker and included specific information about not wanting any surgery, artificial nutrition, mechanical ventilation, or CPR. Although the younger daughter lived out of state, she spoke over the phone nearly every day with her mother, and they had discussed various scenarios about end-of-life issues.

The older daughter lived near her mother and dialed 911 when she came to visit her at home the day of the hospitalization and saw she was in distress. During the first evening of the hospitalization, a rapid response team was called to assess the patient due to decreased responsiveness. After the team leader's consultation with the physician, the patient was transferred to the intensive care unit (ICU). The patient was started on bilevel positive airway pressure, based on arterial blood gases, which exhibited respiratory acidosis with hypercapnia. The older daughter indicated she wanted her mother to be placed on a ventilator if her respiratory status continued to deteriorate despite use of bilevel positive airway pressure (which was very uncomfortable according to her mother) and she wanted her mother to receive nutrition through a feeding tube.

The younger daughter flew in the next day bringing with her a copy of her mother's advance directive. The patient also had given a copy of the advance directive that had been completed several years earlier to her primary care physician.

Intervention: The palliative care team was consulted to assist with helping the older daughter deal with issues related to accepting her mother's wishes for her end-of-life care. The patient was transferred out of the ICU to a comfort care room in the hospital with both of her daughters sitting by her bedside.

Answer: The focus is on providing patient-centered care based on the patient's wishes for quality of life goals. In this scenario, the advance directive with specific wishes and a decision maker that understood the patient's wishes were able to achieve patient-centered care during the end of life, despite potential areas of conflict: (1) family disagreement on mother's health care and (2) community with high intensity of health care use and patient desire to limit end-of-life therapies.

Resolving Ethical Conflicts Around Artificial Nutrition and Hydration: Crucial Conversations

If the health care team and patient and/or surrogate and family cannot reach consensus regarding any aspect of ANH, there are a number of resources available, and "if in doubt give a shout" is a wise approach. Several methodologies and templates[90] for analyzing and resolving ethical dilemmas such as Jonsen's famous four-box method or Barrocas's 12 C's[8] are accessible to clinicians and presented in Table 39-7. Practice Scenario 39-5 presents the role of the health care team in a crucial conversation using the 12 C's model.

Practice Scenario 39-5

Question: Is there a fair and systematic process for a health care team to approach the resolution of conflicts between the forces of the trichotomy?

Scenario: The adult children of a patient with advanced dementia and a recent stroke insists that their father receive a feeding tube despite the opinion of several neurologists that the patient will never recover any meaningful function. The health care team feels this is a low-yield/medically inappropriate procedure but is unable to persuade the children, who threaten legal action if the tube is not inserted. The patient had not executed an advance directive, but several of the grandchildren told the ethics consultant that, "Grandma had several times asked them to make sure that 'when my time comes, don't let my children keep me alive. Let me go to God.'"

Intervention: A transdisciplinary ethics committee meets with the family and health care team and uses the model of consensus-building found in Table 39-7.

Answer: Research[81] regarding end-of-life decision making has demonstrated the critical role of transdisciplinary teams in facilitating crucial conversations at the end of life.[90] Empathic and structured approaches to crucial conversations regarding the provision of life-sustaining treatments including ANH are among the most effective and satisfactory means of resolving ethical conflicts involving the use of life-sustaining treatments including ANH in life-limiting illnesses.[96]

Role of Nutrition Support Professionals in Ethical Decision Making for Artificial Nutrition and Hydration

Nutrition support professionals represent the bridge between a therapy that gives that sense of normalcy for patients, nourishment, and the technology-driven health care system. It is a slippery slope for many patients who start on a path without a known destination as to their future quality of life. This journey, including ANH, may result in patients, families, and significant others accepting therapies, such as mechanical ventilation, CPR, and other advanced procedures, that may not be in congruency with the patient's wishes if the patient had been informed of the benefit or excessive burden of the therapies.

Nutrition support professionals need to be a part of the multi-/inter-/transdisciplinary effort including physicians,

Table 39-7 Crucial Conversations and the 12 C's

Twelve C's	Application to Scenario
Common sense	What is important and the key to success is neither the advance directive nor the advance care plan, but rather the critical/crucial conversation(s) that precedes and continues after executing both of them.
Common decency	The voice of all stakeholders should be heard and respected.
Competence	Sound ethical decisions are founded upon solid science. Nutrition support professionals should bring to such conversations a command of the evidence base for ANH in particular conditions.
Commitment	Perhaps the most crucial counsel to all those struggling with ANH decisions is to continue the conversation so that the surrogate, family, and all practitioners involved in the case can keep the focus where it belongs on the values, interests, and welfare of the patient.
Communications	These often-difficult conversations/communications must be inclusive of all stakeholders, be patient-centered, provide evidence-based facts, arrange for adequate time for questions, and in language understood by all.
Consultation	Nutrition support professionals, chaplains, and other specialists relevant to a specific case can provide invaluable assistance as can the involvement of an ethics consultation service.
Collaboration	The concept of transdisciplinarity, while not often associated with nutrition support teams, is pivotal in the crucial conversations regarding ANH in the specific disease and states and entities discussed in this chapter. Thus, in addition to the adage that "There is no I in team," each member of the team needs to also realize that "There is no success without 'U.'"
Consent/consensus	To be successful, these conversations must incorporate the patient's, family's, and physician's medical goals of care, but also consider the cultural values and religious beliefs of family, patient, and professionals.
Concern	It is the conversation that is important as a sign and expression of mutual concern.
Care goals	These conversations, to be successful, must incorporate not just the medical goals of patient, family, and team, but also consider the cultural values and religious beliefs of family, patient, and professionals.
Compassion	Compassion for the suffering of the patient or even perception of suffering on the part of family must be the motivating force and remain at the center of these conversations.
Comfort	Comfort that can "always be provided" when cure is impossible and treatment is temporary and partial should be the unifying thread running through the discussion.

ANH, artifcial nutrition and hydration.

nurses, dietitians, social workers, palliative care team members, bioethics professionals, chaplains, and other health care professionals that focus on health literacy (the capacity to obtain, process, and understand basic health information and services needed to make appropriate health decisions). This involves incorporating cultural and religious diversity tailored information for patients, families, and significant others that promote understanding of aggressive life-sustaining treatments, including ANH. There are resources and initiatives in making decisions about advance care planning that are helpful to both the professional and the public including (1) National Healthcare Decision Day (www.nationalhealthcaredecisionsday.org); (2) Physician Orders for Life-Sustaining Treatment, which is available in many U.S. states and also known in some states as Medical Orders for Life-Sustaining Treatment (www.ohsu.edu/polst/); and (3) Speak Up campaign to support advance care planning in Canada (www.advancecareplanning.ca). These resources provide excellent tools that inform health care providers, patients, and their families/significant others that we all have responsibilities in this communication process.

The first step for health care providers is to become informed, then distribute this information, be a patient advocate, enhance their health literacy through patient education and teach-back method (asking that patients recall and restate what they have been told), and provide patient-centered care. Written documentation of advance directives should be encouraged throughout health care facilities designating a decision maker for the potential of the patient not always able to speak for him- or herself and specific directives as to what should be done in terms of advanced medical care, including ANH, mechanical ventilation, and CPR. Full disclosure of options for the patient, including benefits and excessive burdens of the therapies, should be the goal in this highly technologically capable health care environment. The first question for a nutrition support professional to address when providing patient care is not, "How well can we provide ANH?" Instead the following should be asked: "Should we provide ANH based on the informed patient or designated decision maker wishes for quality of life goals?"

Translating Ethical Decision Making for Artificial Nutrition and Hydration into Clinical Practice

Although numerous articles, book chapters, recommendations, and guidelines have been published on ethical decision making for ANH, it is the application that continues to remain inadequate, especially in the ICU. Reasons for the translation gap and actual application involve lack of communication by the patients, families, and health care clinicians. In some cultures, this is a taboo topic; families are unable to broach the subject with the family member and then the illness severity and therapies escalate. The patient at that point may be unable to speak and express his or her wishes for medical interventions. Unfortunately, if this subject is not dealt with before the individual reaches the hospital, it becomes the responsibility of the health care providers to advocate for patient-centered decision making in this ever-increasing technology-driven health care environment.

At Providence Saint Joseph Medical Center, an acute care facility, in Burbank, California, a survey was done in the two ICUs (total 38 beds). The results showed that only 12% of 323 patients had an advance directive (durable power of attorney for health care and/or physician orders for life-sustaining treatment) on the medical chart. Preferably, a patient would have both of these documents or a combined document in their medical record, designating a surrogate decision maker and use or forgoing of life-sustaining treatments. Of those ICU patients, 80 were 80 years of age or older; yet only 27% had an advance directive on their medical chart. Additional data were collected on family care conferences, palliative care involvement, bioethics consults, and patients' religious, cultural, and ethnic background. This survey created an awareness in the medical center that change was needed to improve patient-centered decision making for artificial nutrition and other life-sustaining treatments, where appropriate. The survey results were presented at the hospital's continuing medical education program. This process could serve as a tool for other facilities to identify the need to increase documentation of advanced care planning and provide an opportunity to develop a hospital policy and procedure for ethical decision making for artificial nutrition (Figure 39-3).

Development and implementation of this sample policy and procedure at other hospitals would require modifications indicative of the patient population, cultural diversity, and religious affiliation, where applicable. The published recommendations and guidelines from national organizations should be included as a foundation. Implementation of the policy and procedure would require education of all individuals involved in the process from admitting to the patients and their families.

Summary

In 2010, Geppert and Barrocas participated in the work of the American Society for Parenteral and Enteral Nutrition (A.S.P.E.N.) Ethics Position Paper Task Force. The A.S.P.E.N. ethics position paper[97] and the ethics toolkit supporting and expanding the paper are available online at www.nutritioncare.org/ethics. Together the paper, prior position statements and guidelines,[98-100] and the accompanying toolkit provide nutrition support professionals with what renowned clinical ethicist and palliative physician Robert Fine in another context describes as "navigation buoys on a stormy sea" of critical communications "uncertainty."[36]

This chapter not only provides a thorough review of the status of ethics and law, but should be used as an opportunity with readily accessible tools to move forward in a positive direction, with nutrition support professionals in this important effort of patient health literacy education and action on behalf of the people we serve.

FIGURE 39-3 Sample Hospital Policy and Procedure for Ethical Decision Making for Artificial Nutrition

Policy

The multi-/inter-/transdisciplinary health care team provides ethically and medically appropriate artificial nutrition, including to withhold or withdraw of artificial nutrition, based on published evidence-based guidelines and recommendations of recognized authorities. The focus of this policy is to translate these guidelines and recommendations into patient-centered clinical practice by providing compassionate service and honoring the dignity of every person.

Important Considerations

1. A.S.P.E.N. ethics position paper
   a. To the extent possible, decisions regarding artificial nutrition and hydration (ANH) should be based on evidenced-based medicine (EBM), best practices, and clinical experience and judgment in discussion with the patient, family, or significant others.
   b. From a scientific, ethical, and legal perspective, there should be no differentiation between withholding and withdrawing of ANH, thus this paper employs the term "forgoing" for both, recognizing that withdrawing is more emotionally laden than withholding, especially within specific cultures.
   c. Decisions regarding forgoing ANH should incorporate a benefit-risk-burden analysis based on EBM and best practices in discussion with the patient, family, or significant others.
   d. Limited time trails are an acceptable alternative when the benefits of ANH are questionable and the trial nature of ANH is communicated and consented to by the patients and family prior to its initiation.
   e. Scientific evidence on the physiology of patients with brain death, in a coma, or in a persistent vegetative state (PVS) indicates these patients do not experience thirst or hunger, and therefore are not likely to suffer.
   f. ANH may not provide benefit and may have associated risks in patients with severe dementia or in a PVS.
   g. Artificial hydration of terminally ill patients can lead to discomfort due to fluid overload, pulmonary and generalized edema, shortness of breath, etc., and may be discontinued on clinical and ethical grounds provided such discontinuation is not in conflict with existing laws, institutional policies, and consent/consensus of decision makers.
   h. Forgoing ANH in infants and children at the end of life may be ethically acceptable when competent parents and the medical team concur that the intervention no longer confers a benefit to the child or creates a burden that cannot be justified.
   i. The religious, cultural, and ethnic background of patients and families need to be respected to the extent it is consistent with other ethical principles and duties.
   j. Consent, respect, and preservation of dignity should be paramount during ethical and legal deliberations regarding ANH.
   k. Many states in the United States require "clear and convincing evidence" to forgo ANH in decisionally incapacitated patients without documented ANH preference.
   l. Patients with decision-making capacity and authority should be the appropriate moral agents to make choices regarding ANH based on evidence-based information qualified practitioners present to them.
   m. For patients lacking decision-making capacity, the health care professional has an ethical legal obligation to reference an advance directive or discussion with the authorized surrogate decision maker, whether appointed through mechanisms of a durable power of attorney for health care directive, court, or statutory processes.
   n. Surrogate decision makers (including but not limited to family members and/or significant others) should be given the same considerations as individual patients with decision-making capacity.
   o. Health care professionals should not be ethically obligated to offer ANH if in their clinical judgment there is not adequate evidence for the therapy, or the burden or risk of the intervention far outweighs its benefit.
   p. The establishment of interdisciplinary teams and conference with the patient and family is highly encouraged. Interdisciplinary ethics committees or panels should be consulted when the involved parties cannot resolve the ethical dilemma.
   q. Care should continue until the conflict regarding ANH is resolved. If unable to resolve conflicts, even with the ethics consultation, orderly transfer of care assuring continuity of care is recommended to an equally willing practitioner and or institution. At no time should patients or families feel abandoned.

2. American Medical Association (AMA) policy on provision of life-sustaining medical treatment
   a. Patients have a right to participate in decisions about their medical care. This fundamental principle of medical ethics holds true for all types of medical treatments.
   b. Patients can refuse treatments even when such refusal is likely to result in death.
   c. Life-sustaining treatments should provide medical benefits and should respect a patient's preferences, as communicated by the patient or a legally recognized surrogate.
   d. Treatments such as mechanical ventilation and ANH should be provided only with appropriate authorization from a patient, a surrogate, or a court.
   e. Once initiated, life-sustaining treatments may be ethically withdrawn upon request of the patient, or surrogate or court acting on the patient's behalf.

(continued)

FIGURE 39-3 Sample Hospital Policy and Procedure for Ethical Decision Making for Artificial Nutrition ***(continued)***

3. Position of the American Dietetic Association: ethical and legal issues in nutrition, hydration, and feeding
   a. Position statement: It is the position of the American Dietetic Association that individuals have the right to request or refuse nutrition and hydration as medical treatment. Registered dietitians should work collaboratively to make recommendations on providing, withdrawing, or withholding nutrition in individual cases and serve as active members of institutional ethics committees.
   b. Summary guidelines for feeding
      (1) Nutritional concept of "when in doubt, feed" is applicable to most patients.
      (2) Feeding should start immediately upon being medically stable and continue until the treatment is futile.
      (3) During feeding, it is essential to try to provide adequate nutrients and fluid to maintain or achieve a reasonable weight, maintain muscle mass, and achieve hydration.
      (4) Feeding can be discontinued if it is authorized by the patient or authorized surrogate, if the feeding is clinically contraindicated, or after the patient is diagnosed as permanently unconscious and the team has evidence of the patient's wish to stop nutrition and hydration.
      (5) In cases where the evidence in the case strongly suggest that feeding or hydration does not provide benefit, it is the responsibility of the team to explain this to the patient or authorized surrogate, but is it the patient or authorized surrogate that decides.
4. American Academy of Pediatrics 2009 clinical report
   a. Offered general principles designed to help practitioners decide when it is ethically permissible to forgo medically provided fluids and nutrients for infants, children, and adolescents.
   b. The American Academy of Pediatrics (AAP) report addressed the Child Abuse Prevention and Treatment Act as it applies in the case of infants only. AAP takes the position that although the language of Child Abuse Prevention and Treatment Act and the regulations "seem to advocate for the provision of appropriate fluids and nutrition in most cases," forgoing ANH is ethically acceptable with competent parents when the intervention no longer confers a benefit to the child or creates a burden that cannot be justified.
   c. In an earlier report from 1994, the AAP Committee on Bioethics provided a framework for documentation of medical futility, discussions with parents of treatment options, corroborating statements from other physicians, and the process of bioethics committee review to help protect the infant but also to provide the most humane treatment.
   d. Open communication with parents and realistic prognostic outlooks for their infant from the beginning is crucial to help avoid conflicts in providing or withdrawing care.
5. Consideration of ethical and legal aspects of delivering ANH first requires choosing therapy that is medically appropriate.
6. Clinicians are not obligated to provide futile treatments (ie, treatments for which evidence show no benefit from any perspective).
7. Code of medical ethics supports that clinicians are not obligated to provide disproportionate or futile treatment.
8. There is no ethical or legal difference between withholding or withdrawing life-sustaining treatments; therefore, treatment should not be withheld because of concern these therapies cannot be later withdrawn.
9. Crucial ethical responsibility is to ensure that the patient, not the family or institution, makes the decision about medical treatments, including artificial nutrition.
10. Psychologically competent patients who forcibly remove enteral or parenteral feeding tubes should be allowed to refuse this therapy.
11. Clinicians must be certain that patients who refuse or request the withdrawal of life-sustaining treatments, such as ANH, have adequate decision-making capacity and are informed of the consequences of their request.
12. Clinicians should discuss end-of-life values, goals, and preferences regarding life-sustaining treatments, including ANH, with patients when they possess decision-making capacity. Limited time trials of a therapy for a designated period of days (approximately 1 week or at the discretion of the physician in conjunction with the health care team and patient/family/surrogate decision maker to be reevaluated at the end of that period), with continued or cessation of use of the therapy based on the patient's defined response, either beneficial or negative response could be considered.
13. Patients and caregivers need to know the risk of the intervention as well as the evidence regarding use in selected populations. For example, patients with dementia who require gastrostomy tubes due to anorexia have a high 30-day and 1-year mortality.
14. Growing support in clinical literature for the position that neither nutrition nor hydration in terminal patients increases comfort or quality of life. Withholding nutrition has been studied closely and the majority of reports indicate that physiological adaptation allows patients not to suffer from the absence of food.

(continued)

FIGURE 39-3 Sample Hospital Policy and Procedure for Ethical Decision Making for Artificial Nutrition *(continued)*

15. The use of ANH may be incongruent with the patient's wishes to avoid prolongation of suffering. Withholding or withdrawing ANH often involves different considerations than other life-sustaining therapies in part due to emotional, religious, and symbolic meanings.
16. Withdrawal of ANH is ethically, morally, and legally appropriate when burden to the patient outweighs the benefit.
17. Age, religion, spirituality, cultural background, ethnicity, and socioeconomic aspects of the patient and his or her family should be considered in ethical decision making for artificial nutrition.

Procedure

1. The health care team determines patient's wishes as expressed directly and/or designated surrogate health care decision maker when the patient is not able to express desires for health care. These instructions are to be used for the provisions of ethically appropriate artificial nutrition.
2. Written documentation (advance directive) in the patient's medical record is encouraged throughout the health care system to help in the decision process with artificial nutrition, starting with admitting. Within the first 24 hours clarification of surrogate decision maker (nursing and social worker), determine if advance directive exists, copy should be placed in chart and reviewed by provider.
3. Clinical judgment based on a collaborative effort by the health care team including the patient and family, in conjunction with published guidelines, shall be used in the process to withhold or withdraw artificial nutrition, including dietitian involvement.
4. Family care conference is recommended for patients in the intensive care unit for 5 to 7 days to address plan of care, quality of life goals, and to determine decision maker if advance directive not on chart to provide direction for treatment from patient or an appropriate surrogate decision maker (ie, completing physician orders for life-sustaining treatment or durable power of attorney for health care for appropriate patients and placed in patient's chart). Written documentation of family care conference discussion and decisions should be included in the medical record.
5. Palliative care team consult is recommended early in the process to assist with clarification of goals of care for the patient and assist with family, including artificial nutrition. Palliative care team member should be present at family care conferences. Patients in the intensive care unit for 3 or more days should be screened for support care needs by palliative care team members.
6. Bioethics committee consult is recommended when there is a conflict in the process to withhold or withdraw of artificial nutrition.

References

1. AMA Policy on Provision of Life-Sustaining Medical Treatment. www.ama-assn.org/ama/...life.../ama-policy-provision-life-sustaining-medical.shtml. Accessed January 2011.
2. American Society for Parenteral and Enteral Nutrition Board of Directors and Task Force. Standards for specialized nutrition support: adult hospitalized patients. *Nutr Clin Prac.* 2002;17:384–391.
3. American Society for Parenteral and Enteral Nutrition Board of Directors and Task Force. Standards for specialized nutrition support: hospitalized pediatric patients. *Nutr Clin Prac.* 2005;20:103–116.
4. Barrocas A, Geppert C, Durfee SM, et al., and A.S.P.E.N. Board of Directors. A.S.P.E.N. Ethics Position Paper. *Nutr Clin Pract.* 2010;35:1–8.
5. Barrocas A, Bivona BB, Schwartz DB. Medical legal and ethical aspects of nutritional support. In: Buchman A, ed. *Nutrition in Gastrointestinal Disease. Thorofare,* NJ: Slack, Inc.; 2006:559–581.
6. U.S. Conference of Catholic Bishops. *Ethical and Religious Directives Issued by the United States Conference of Catholic Bishops.* 5th ed.: U.S. Conference of Catholic Bishops; 2009.
7. Geppert CMA, Andrews MR, Druyan ME. Ethical issues in artificial nutrition and hydration: a review. *J Parenter Enteral Nutr.* 2010;34:79–88.
8. McMahon MM, Hurley DL, Kamath PS, et al. Medical and ethical aspects of long-term enteral tube feeding. *Mayo Clin Proc.* 2005;80:1461–1476.
9. Mueller PS, Hook CC, Fleming KC. Ethical issues in geriatrics: a guide for clinicians. *Mayo Clin Proc.* 2004;79:554–562.
10. O'Sullivan Maillet J. Position of the American Dietetic Association: Ethical and legal issues in nutrition, hydration, and feeding. *J Am Diet Assoc.* 2008;108:873–882.
11. Preedy VR, ed. *Diet and Nutrition in Palliative Care.* Boca Raton, FL: CRC Press; 2011.
12. Schwartz DB. Ethical/legal issues. In: Matarese LE, Mullin G, eds. *Gastrointestinal Nutrition.* Chicago, IL: American Dietetic Association; 2012 (in press).

Approval

Committee/Approval Date

Used with permission from Denise Schwartz.

References

1. Sampson EL, Candy B, Jones L. Enteral tube feeding for older people with advanced dementia. *Cochrane Database Syst Rev.* 2009;(2): CD007209.
2. Drane JF. Stopping nutrition and hydration technologies: a conflict between traditional Catholic ethics and church authority. *Christ Bioeth.* 2006;12(1):11–28.
3. Andrews M, Bell ER, Smith SA, et al. Dehydration in terminally ill patients. Is it appropriate palliative care? *Postgrad Med.* 1993; 93(1):201–203,206–208.
4. Barrocas A. Nutrition support and the troubling trichotomy: a call to action. *Nutr Clin Pract.* 2006;21(2):109–112.
5. Hallenbeck J. *Fast Facts and Concepts #11 Tube Feed or Not Tube Feed?* 2nd ed. End-of-Life Physician Education Resource Center; August 2005.
6. Brody H, Hermer LD, Scott LD, et al. Artificial nutrition and hydration: the evolution of ethics, evidence, and policy. *J Gen Intern Med.* 2011;26(9):1053–1058.
7. Monturo C. The artificial nutrition debate: still an issue... after all these years. *Nutr Clin Pract.* 2009;24(2):206–213.
8. Barrocas A, Yarbrough G, Becnel PA 3rd, et al. Ethical and legal issues in nutrition support of the geriatric patient: the can, should, and must of nutrition support. *Nutr Clin Pract.* 2003;18(1):37–47.
9. Andrews MR, Levine AM. Dehydration in the terminal patient: perception of hospice nurses. *Am J Hosp Care.* 1989;6(1):31–34.
10. Zerwekh JV. The dehydration question. *Nursing.* 1983;13(1):47–51.
11. Zerwekh JV. Do dying patients really need i.v. fluids? *Am J Nurs.* 1997;97(3):26–30,quiz 31.
12. Printz LA. Is withholding hydration a valid comfort measure in the terminally ill? *Geriatrics.* 1988;43(11):84–88.
13. McCann RM, Hall WJ, Groth-Juncker A. Comfort care for terminally ill patients. The appropriate use of nutrition and hydration. *JAMA.* 1994;272(16):1263–1266.
14. Musgrave CF, Bartal N, Opstad J. The sensation of thirst in dying patients receiving i.v. hydration. *J Palliat Care.* 1995;11(4):17–21.
15. Ellershaw JE, Sutcliffe JM, Saunders CM. Dehydration and the dying patient. *J Pain Symptom Manage.* 1995;10(3):192–197.
16. Burge FI. Dehydration symptoms of palliative care cancer patients. *J Pain Symptom Manage.* 1993;8(7):454–464.
17. Burge FI. Dehydration and provision of fluids in palliative care. What is the evidence? *Can Fam Physician.* 1996;42:2383–2388.
18. Lang F, Quill T. Making decisions with families at the end of life. *Am Fam Physician.* 2004;70(4):719–723.
19. Ganzini L. Artificial nutrition and hydration at the end of life: ethics and evidence. *Palliat Support Care.* 2006;4(2):135–143.
20. Curtis JR, Levine S, Rocker G, et al, eds. *The Hospice and Palliative Medicine Approach to Selected Chronic Illnesses: Dementia, COPD, and CHF.* 3rd ed. Glenview, IL: American Academy of Hospice and Palliative Medicine; 2008. Storey CP, Levine S, Shega J, W., eds. Hospice and Palliative Care Training for Physicians: A Self-Study Program; No. 9.
21. Wolfson C, Wolfson DB, Asgharian M, et al. A reevaluation of the duration of survival after the onset of dementia. *N Engl J Med.* 2001;344(15):1111–1116.
22. Chernoff R. Tube feeding patients with dementia. *Nutr Clin Pract.* 2006;21(2):142–146.
23. Finucane TE, Christmas C, Travis K. Tube feeding in patients with advanced dementia: a review of the evidence. *JAMA.* 1999; 282(14):1365–1370.
24. Shega JW, Hougham GW, Stocking CB, et al. Barriers to limiting the practice of feeding tube placement in advanced dementia. *J Palliat Med.* Dec 2003;6(6):885–893.
25. Li I. Feeding tubes in patients with severe dementia. *Am Fam Physician.* 2002;65(8):1605–1610,1615.
26. Cervo FA, Bryan L, Farber S. To PEG or not to PEG: a review of evidence for placing feeding tubes in advanced dementia and the decision-making process. *Geriatrics.* 2006;61(6):30–35.
27. Gillick MR. Rethinking the role of tube feeding in patients with advanced dementia. *N Engl J Med.* 2000;342(3):206–210.
28. Kaw M, Sekas G. Long-term follow-up of consequences of percutaneous endoscopic gastrostomy (PEG) tubes in nursing home patients. *Dig Dis Sci.* 1994;39(4):738–743.
29. Meier DE, Ahronheim JC, Morris J, et al. High short-term mortality in hospitalized patients with advanced dementia: lack of benefit of tube feeding. *Arch Intern Med.* 2001;161(4):594–599.
30. Murphy LM, Lipman TO. Percutaneous endoscopic gastrostomy does not prolong survival in patients with dementia. *Arch Intern Med.* 2003;163(11):1351–1353.
31. Peck A, Cohen CE, Mulvihill MN. Long-term enteral feeding of aged demented nursing home patients. *J Am Geriatr Soc.* 1990; 38(11):1195–1198.
32. Vitale CA, Hiner T, Ury WA, et al. Tube feeding in advanced dementia: an exploratory survey of physician knowledge. *Care Manag J.* 2006;7(2):79–85.
33. Medical aspects of the persistent vegetative state (1). The Multi-Society Task Force on PVS. *N Engl J Med.* 1994;330(21):1499–1508.
34. Medical aspects of the persistent vegetative state (2). The Multi-Society Task Force on PVS. *N Engl J Med.* 1994;330(22):1572–1579.
35. Celesia GG. Persistent vegetative state: clinical and ethical issues. *Theoretical Medicine.* 1997;18(3):221–236.
36. Fine RL. Ethical issues in artificial nutrition and hydration. *Nutr Clin Pract.* 2006;21(2):118–125.
37. Laureys S, Faymonville ME, Peigneux P, et al. Cortical processing of noxious somatosensory stimuli in the persistent vegetative state. *Neuroimage.* 2002;17(2):732–741.
38. Antognini JF, Buonocore MH, Disbrow EA, et al. Isoflurane anesthesia blunts cerebral responses to noxious and innocuous stimuli: a fMRI study. *Life Sci.* 1997;61(24):349–354.
39. Laureys S. Functional neuroimaging in the vegetative state. *NeuroRehabilitation.* 2004;19(4):335–341.
40. Monti MM, Vanhaudenhuyse A, Coleman MR, et al. Willful modulation of brain activity in disorders of consciousness. *N Engl J Med.* 2010;362(7):579–589.
41. Ropper AH. Cogito ergo sum by MRI. *N Engl J Med.* 2010;362 (7):648–649.
42. Billings JA, Churchill LR, Payne R. Severe brain injury and the subjective life. *Hastings Cent Rep.* 2010;40(3):17–21.
43. *The American Heritage Dictionary of the English Language.* 4th ed. Boston, MA: Houghton Mifflin; 2006.
44. Rothman DJ. *Strangers at the Bedside.* New York, NY: Basic Books; 1991.
45. Callahan D. Bioethics. In: Post SG, ed. *Encyclopedia of Bioethics.* Vol 1. 3rd ed. New York, NY: Thompson-Gale; 2004:278–286.
46. Ferrie S. A quick guide to ethical theory in healthcare: solving ethical dilemmas in nutrition support situations. *Nutr Clin Pract.* 2006;21(2):113–117.
47. Beauchamp TL, Childress JF. *Principles of Biomedical Ethics.* 6th ed. New York, NY: Oxford University Press; 2009.
48. Kant I. In: Friedrich CJ, ed. *The Philosophy of Kant: Immanuel Kant's Moral and Political Writings.* New York, NY: Modern Library; 1949.
49. Burtt EA, ed. *The English Philosophers From Bacon to Mill.* New York, NY: Random House Modern Library; 1939.
50. Aristotle. *The Ethics of Aristotle: The Nicomachean Ethics.* Thomson JAK, trans. New York, NY: Penguin Books; 1976:244.
51. Appelbaum PS. Clinical practice. Assessment of patients' competence to consent to treatment. *N Engl J Med.* 2007;357(18): 1834–1840.

52. Ganzini L, Volicer L, Nelson WA, et al. Ten myths about decision-making capacity. *J Am Med Dir Assoc.* 2004;5(4):263–267.
53. Kemp KR, Emmons E, Hayes J. Advance directives and do-not-resuscitate orders on general medical wards versus the intensive care unit. *Mil Med.* 2004;169(6):433–436.
54. DuVal G, Sartorius L, Clarridge B, et al. What triggers requests for ethics consultations? *J Med Ethics.* 2001;27(Suppl 1):i24–29.
55. Sulmasy DP, Snyder L. Substituted interests and best judgments: an integrated model of surrogate decision making. *JAMA.* 2010;304(17):1946–1947.
56. *In re Conroy,* 486 A. 2d 1209(1985).
57. Levinsky NG. The doctor's master. *N Engl J Med.* 1984;311(24):1573–1575.
58. *Cruzan v. Director Missouri Department of Health,* 497 261(1990).
59. Schneiderman LJ, Jecker NS, Jonsen AR. Medical futility: its meaning and ethical implications. *Ann Intern Med.* 1990;112(12):949–954.
60. *Hawkins v. Dekalb Medical Center* (Georgia Court of Appeals 2011).
61. *Betancourt v. Trinitas Regional Hospital* (Superior Court of New Jersey 2009).
62. Emanuel L, von Gutnen C, Ferris FD, eds., *The Education for Physicians on End-of-Life Curriculum.* No. Module 9. Princeton, NJ: Robert Wood Johnson Foundation; 1999.
63. Fine RL, Mayo TW. Resolution of futility by due process: early experience with the Texas Advance Directives Act. *Ann Intern Med.* 2003;138(9):743–746.
64. Brett AS, Rosenberg JC. The adequacy of informed consent for placement of gastrostomy tubes. *Arch Intern Med.* 2001;161(5):745–748.
65. Solomon MZ, O'Donnell L, Jennings B, et al. Decisions near the end of life: professional views on life-sustaining treatments. *Am J Public Health.* 1993;83(1):14–23.
66. Callahan CM, Haag KM, Buchanan NN, et al. Decision-making for percutaneous endoscopic gastrostomy among older adults in a community setting. *J Am Geriatr Soc.* 1999;47(9):1105–1109.
67. Bryon E, Dierckx DECB, Gastmans C. "Because we see them naked"—nurses' experiences in caring for hospitalized patients with dementia: considering artificial nutrition or hydration (ANH). *Bioethics.* Epub Feb 14 2011.
68. O'Brien LA, Siegert EA, Grisso JA, et al. Tube feeding preferences among nursing home residents. *J Gen Intern Med.* 1997;12(6):364–371.
69. Hoefler JM. Making decisions about tube feeding for severely demented patients at the end of life: clinical, legal, and ethical considerations. *Death Stud.* 2000;24(3):233–254.
70. Caspar R. Food and water: symbol and reality. *Health Prog.* 1988;69(4):54–58.
71. Bedolla M. Patient Self-Determination Act: a Hispanic perspective. *Camb Q Healthc Ethics.* 1994;3(3):413–417.
72. Fetters MD. The family in medical decision making: Japanese perspectives. *J Clin Ethics.* 1998;9(2):132–146.
73. Carrese JA, Rhodes LA. Western bioethics on the Navajo reservation. Benefit or harm? *JAMA.* 1995;274(10):826–829.
74. Bulow HH, Sprung CL, Reinhart K, et al. The world's major religions' points of view on end-of-life decisions in the intensive care unit. *Intensive Care Med.* 2008;34(3):423–430.
75. Dorff EN. Applying traditional Jewish law to PVS. *NeuroRehabilitation.* 2004;19(4):277–283.
76. Steinberg A, Sprung CL. The dying patient act, 2005: Israeli innovative legislation. *Isr Med Assoc J.* 2007;9(7):550–552.
77. Ravitsky V. A Jewish perspective on the refusal of life-sustaining therapies: culture as shaping bioethical discourse. *Am J Bioeth.* 2009;9(4):60–62.
78. Pope John Paul II. Life-sustaining treatments and the vegetaive state: scientific advances and ethical dilemmas. *Address to the Participants in the International Congress on Life-Sustaining Treatments and the Vegetative State: Scientific Advances and Ethical Dilemmas.* 2004.
79. Howland J. A defense of assisted nutrition and hydration in patients with dementia. *National Catholic Bioethics Quarterly.* 2009;9:697–710.
80. Congregation for the Doctrine of the Faith. *Responses to Certain Questions of the United States Conference of Catholic Bishops Concerning Artificial Nutrition and Hydration.* 2007. www.vatican.va/roman_curia/congregations/cfaith/documents/rc_con_cfaith_doc_20070801_risposte-usa_en.html. Accessed May 29, 2011.
81. Shannon TA. Nutrition and hydration: an analysis of the recent papal statement in the light of the Roman Catholic bioethical tradition. *Christ Bioeth.* 2006;12(1):29–41.
82. Sulmasy DP. Are feeding tubes morally obligatory. *St. Anthony Messenger.* 2006;113:28–32.
83. Alliance of Catholic Health Care. *Ethical and Religious Directive 58: How Does it Affect Patients in a Catholic Acute Care Hospital.* www.thealliance.net/. Accessed November 19, 2011.
84. Henry TA. Obama voids Bush conscience rule in favor of decades-old protections. *American Medical News.* March 7, 2011.
85. Barrocas A, Bivona B, Schwartz DB. Medical, ethical, legal aspects. In: Buchman AL, ed. *Clinical Nutrition in Gastrointestinal Disease.* Thorofare, NJ: Slack; 2006.
86. Barrocas A, Farquharson J, Fernandez M. Legal considerations in nutritional support. *Nutr Support Serv.* 1986;6:13–15.
87. *In re Quinlan,* 355 A.2d 647(70 N.J. 10 1976).
88. Pence GE. *Classic Cases in Medical Ethics.* 5th ed. Boston, MA: McGraw-Hill; 2008.
89. Omnibus Reconciliation Act of 1990. Vol 101-508: Pub. L; 1990.
90. Jonsen AR, Seigler M, Winslade WJ. *Clinical Ethics: A Practical Approach to Ethical Decisions in Clinical Medicine.* 7th ed. New York, NY: McGraw-Hill, Inc.; 2010.
91. Tulsky JA. Beyond advance directives: importance of communication skills at the end of life. *JAMA.* 2005;294(3):359–365.
92. Nicholas LH, Langa KM, Iwashyna TJ, et al. Regional variation in the association between advance directives and end-of-life Medicare expenditures. *JAMA.* 2011;306(13);1447–1453.
93. White DB, Arnold RM. The evolution of advance directives. *JAMA.* 2011;306(13);1485–1486.
94. Silveira MJ, Kim SY, Langa KM. Advance directives and outcomes of surrogate decision making before death. *N Engl J Med.* 2010;362(13);1211–1218.
95. Detering KM, Hancock AD, Reade MC, et al. The impact of advance care planning on end of life care in elderly patients: randomised controlled trial. *BMJ.* 2010;340:c1345.
96. Back AL, Arnold RM. Dealing with conflict in caring for the seriously ill: "it was just out of the question." *JAMA.* 2005;293(11):1374–1381.
97. Barrocas A, Geppert C, Durfee SM, et al. A.S.P.E.N. ethics position paper. *Nutr Clin Pract.* 2010;25(6):672–679.
98. Bacon D, Williams MA, Gordon J. Position statement on laws and regulations concerning life-sustaining treatment, including artificial nutrition and hydration, for patients lacking decision-making capacity. *Neurology.* 2007;68(14):1097–1100.
99. American Academy of Hospice and Palliative Medicine. *Statement on the Use of Nutrition and Hydration.* Glenview, IL: American Academy of Hospice and Palliative Medicine; 2005.
100. Maillet JO, Potter RL, Heller L. Position of the American Dietetic Association: ethical and legal issues in nutrition, hydration, and feeding. *J Am Diet Assoc.* 2002;102(5):716–726.

40 Quality Improvement

Naomi E. Cahill, RD, MSc

CONTENTS

Background . . . 678
What Is Quality Improvement? . . . 679
The Current State of Quality in American Health Care . . . 679
Measuring Quality . . . 681
Quality Indicators . . . 682
Data Collection . . . 682
Data Analysis . . . 683
Measuring Quality of Nutrition Care . . . 683
Quality Improvement Strategies in Nutrition Support . . . 684
Clinical Practice Guidelines . . . 684
Care Pathways . . . 684
Bundles . . . 685
Health Information Technology . . . 685
Quality Improvement Methodologies . . . 686
Plan-Do-Study-Act Cycle . . . 686
Step 1: Setting Aims . . . 686
Step 2: Establishing Measures . . . 686
Step 3: Selecting Change . . . 686
Step 4: Implementing and Testing Changes . . . 687
Step 5: Implementing Changes . . . 687
Step 6: Spreading Changes . . . 687
Six Sigma . . . 688
Lean Methodology . . . 688
Step 1: Identify Value . . . 688
Step 2: Identify and Visualize the Value Stream . . . 688
Step 3: Create Flow . . . 688
Step 4: Establish Pull . . . 688
Step 5: Seek Perfection . . . 689
The Focus-Analyze-Develop-Execute-Evaluate Model . . . 689
Step 1: Focus . . . 689
Step 2: Analyze . . . 689
Step 3: Develop . . . 689
Step 4: Execute and Evaluate . . . 690
Quality Assurance Versus Quality Improvement . . . 690
Clinical Research Versus Quality Improvement . . . 690
Knowledge Translation Versus Quality Improvement . . . 690
Summary . . . 690
Acknowledgments . . . 691
References . . . 691

Objectives

1. Identify why quality of care is a high priority when providing nutrition therapy in today's health care system.
2. Explain the differences between structure, process, and outcome indicators.
3. Describe methods for measuring nutrition performance and assessing the quality of nutrition care.
4. Apply quality improvement models to analyze and improve a nutrition care process within the clinical setting.

Test Your Knowledge Questions

1. What U.S. non-profit organization led by Don Berwick was established to promote change in the health care system?
   A. The Joint Commission on Accreditation of Health care Organizations (JCAHO)
   B. The Institute of Healthcare Improvement (IHI)
   C. The Leapfrog Group
   D. The Institute of Medicine (IOM)
2. What government legislation mandated the creation of a national quality strategy?
   A. The Affordable Care Act of 2010
   B. The Food and Drug Act of 1906
   C. The Patient Safety and Quality Improvement Act of 2005
   D. The Social Security Act Amendment of 1966
3. Which of the following would be a valid quality indicator for assessing the effectiveness of the provision of nutrition support?
   A. The prevalence of malnutrition in the study population
   B. The total number of patients who receive enteral nutrition and/or parenteral nutrition
   C. The mortality rate in the population
   D. The proportion of patients assessed as requiring nutrition support who receive >80% of prescribed calories
4. Which of the following is the best example of a quality improvement project?
   A. Randomized controlled trial evaluating the effect of a new postpyloric feeding tube
   B. A patient survey to assess satisfaction with the hospital meal service
   C. A reduction in the inappropriate ordering of parenteral nutrition following an educational intervention targeted at residents and fellows
   D. A prospective study to assess the incidence of aspiration pneumonia in enterally fed patients

Test Your Knowledge Answers

1. The correct answer is **B.** The IHI was founded by Dr. Don Berwick in 1991. This non-profit organization campaigns for health care changes in the United States and worldwide, sponsoring collaborative initiatives such as the 100,000 Lives Campaign. JCAHO provides voluntary accreditation of hospitals based on defined minimum quality standards, and uses information on sentinel events to establish and update National Patient Safety Goals for accredited health care organizations on a yearly basis. The Leapfrog Group is a private association that uses its collective purchasing power to promote health care quality. The IOM is a non-profit independent scientific advisor, the goal of which is to improve the nation's health.
2. The correct answer is **A.** In 2010, the Obama administration introduced the Affordable Care Act, legislation that focused on improving the quality of health care in the United States. This act mandated the creation of national aims and priorities to inform quality improvement (QI) efforts. The Food and Drug Act of 1906 was primarily concerned with the accurate labeling of drugs and led to the creation of the U.S. Food and Drug Administration. The Patient Safety and Quality Improvement Act established a confidential, voluntary reporting system in which physicians and other health care providers could submit information on medical errors. The Social Security Act Amendment mandated that health care organizations must meet the JCAHO standards to participate in Medicaid and Medicare programs.
3. The correct answer is **D.** A valid quality indicator should be a direct measure of the outcome of interest or the process that is associated with the outcome. Although the overall goal of nutrition support may differ for each patient (eg, correct malnutrition, weight gain, wound healing), a quality indicator that reflects if all patients received the therapy they were intended to receive might be the proportion of prescribed calories received. The prevalence of malnutrition provides information on the magnitude of the problem in the hospital but does not provide any information about the effectiveness of the nutrition support. It is difficult to attribute a change in the mortality rate in the population to the effectiveness of nutrition support due to other variables that may also affect mortality such as severity of illness, age, other interventions, etc. Finally, the total number of patients who receive nutrition support provides information on the use of the therapy, but without a denominator (ie, total number of patients requiring nutrition support), any inferences regarding its effectiveness cannot be made.
4. The correct answer is **C.** A quality improvement project involves identifying the problem and setting goals (ie, inappropriate ordering of parenteral nutrition), finding a solution to the problem (ie, increase the knowledge of residents), and implementing and evaluating the change (ie, educational intervention). Randomized controlled trials where individual patients are randomized to receive a novel therapy or a control therapy is clinical research and not quality improvement. A patient survey to assess patient satisfaction or a prospective study to evaluate the incidence of aspiration pneumonia might be completed as part of a QI project either to identify if a problem exists or to evaluate the effectiveness of an intervention, but the survey or prospective study alone is not considered a quality improvement project.

Background

Over the past 2 decades, there have been significant advances in understanding the role of nutrition in the treatment of patients,[1,2] with the emergence of evidence demonstrating that nutrition therapy is associated with significant reductions in length of stay, infectious complications, and mortality,[1–3] and the subsequent development of Clinical Practice

Guidelines (CPGs),[4–8] providing recommendations for practice. Consequently, the role of nutrition in patient care has transitioned from supporting patients while they recover from their underlying illness to modulating their disease response and improving their chances of survival. However, despite these advances in our knowledge, the provision of nutrition therapy to our patients is not synonymous with best practices as defined by guideline recommendations.[9] Observational studies in hospitalized patients demonstrate that the quality of nutrition care received varies considerably by geographic region, the type of institution (ie, teaching versus nonteaching), and patient case mix.[10–13] Consequently, there is a need to reduce this variation in nutrition practice to achieve the highest quality of care possible.

This observation of significant and persistent gaps between evidence-based and actual practice is not isolated to the provision of nutrition therapy but permeates the health care system. It is estimated that 35% to 55% of patients are not receiving care according to scientific evidence, and 20% to 25% of care provided is not needed or could cause harm.[14,15] The recognition of this problem, together with a heightened focus on evidence informed practice, has stimulated interest in the science and practice of quality improvement (QI). Improving the quality of care requires an understanding of the reasons for the current gaps in care and an appreciation of the complex environment in which clinical decisions are made. Ironically, the evidentiary basis for QI pales in comparison to the foundation of knowledge arising from clinical research. Comparatively few resources are channeled into optimizing the implementation of research evidence compared to the investment in developing new drugs and technologies. For example, the Agency for Healthcare Research and Quality (AHRQ), responsible for QI research in the United States, attracts only 1% of the resources allocated to the National Institutes for Health (NIH), the primary federal agency for supporting medical research. Furthermore, the AHRQ budget is equal to the amount that the pharmaceutical industry spends on developing just a single medication.[16] Nonetheless, attempts to close the quality gap are warranted and are being actively pursued.

What Is Quality Improvement?

As health care providers working in today's complex health care system, it is imperative that one understands the fundamental basics of QI and the importance of engaging in quality initiatives. With employers, insurance companies, and consumers all demanding higher quality and efficient services, in the future, QI will undoubtedly affect the daily practice of health care providers in unprecedented ways, regardless of clinical specialty or professional role.

The conceptual underpinnings of QI are not dissimilar to a clinical assessment routinely undertaken in our hospitals, with which clinicians are extremely familiar. A patient presents with a set of symptoms, a series of tests are completed where the results are compared to normal or healthy ranges, abnormalities are identified, and a treatment plan to correct the abnormality is developed and implemented. A QI process parallels these steps but instead of a physiological system, the context is the health care system and the focus is on the improvement of this system and not on the performance of individuals. A practice or process is evaluated, problems are identified (ie, overuse, underuse, or misuse of services), and a corrective strategy is developed and implemented, and the process is monitored or re-evaluated. Much like the vital signs of our patients, quality is a tangible thing that can be measured and changed.

The Institute of Medicine (IOM) defines quality as "the degree to which health services for individuals and populations increase the likelihood of desired health outcomes and [the degree to which they] are consistent with current professional knowledge".[17] Quality was first studied as an industrial process and this knowledge was then applied to the health care system. The history of quality in health care in the United States is outlined in Table 40-1.

The Current State of Quality in American Health Care

The U.S. health system is the most expensive in the world, but comparative analyses consistently show that the United States underperforms relative to other countries on any one of the many measures of quality. A recent report from the Commonwealth Foundation observed that "compared with five other nations—Australia, Canada, Germany, New Zealand, the United Kingdom—the U.S. health care system ranks last or next-to-last on five dimensions of a high performance health system: quality, access, efficiency, equity, and healthy lives."[18] This report also included results of an international survey of primary care physicians that showed that the United States is lagging in the adoption of information technology and national policies that promote QI.[18] These findings clearly indicate that change is needed.

Consequently, health care reform was a key issue addressed by both major political parties during the presidential election in 2008. Health care reform was enacted in 2010 in the form of the Patient Protection and Affordable Care Act (PPACA) and the Health Care and Education Reconciliation Act of 2010, which subsequently amended the PPACA.[19,20] The law includes numerous health-related provisions intended to increase access to high quality, affordable health care for all Americans, which are to be implemented over a 4-year period beginning in 2010. To this end, the Affordable Care Act called for the creation of national aims and priorities to guide local, state, and national efforts to improve the quality of health care in the United States. On March 21, 2011, a year after the act was passed, the U.S. Department of Health and Human Services released the National Strategy for Quality Improvement in Health Care (National Quality Strategy).[21]

The intention of the National Quality Strategy is to promote quality health care that is focused on the needs of patients, families, and communities. At the same time, the strategy is designed to move the system to work better for physicians and other health care providers by reducing their administrative burdens and helping them collaborate to improve care. The strategy presents three aims for the health care system:

1. Better Care: Improve the overall quality by making health care more patient-centered, reliable, accessible, and safe.
2. Healthy People and Communities: Improve the health of the U.S. population by supporting proven interventions to address behavioral, social, and environmental determinants of health in addition to delivering higher quality care.

TABLE 40-1 History of the Quality Improvement Movement in the United States

Year	Event
1906	President Theodore Roosevelt signed the **Food and Drug Act**, also known as the Wiley Act, which was enacted in response to national concern about the quality of foods and drugs that Americans consumed.
1910	**Dr. Ernest Codman**, a physician at Massachusetts General Hospital, proposed the "end result system," a system for hospitals to track the effectiveness of patient care and improve practice.
1918	Dr. Codman inspired the American College of Surgeons (ACS) to establish **minimum quality standards for hospitals**. When on-site inspections of hospitals began, only 89 (13%) of the 692 hospitals with at least 100 beds surveyed passed the minimum quality standards.
1924	**Walter A. Shewhart**, a statistician for Bell Laboratories and often considered the father of modern quality control, invented the **control chart,** a statistical tool allowing managers to focus on process redesign. A control chart is a run chart that uses success as the numerator and total opportunities as the denominator to evaluate performance over time. An average line together with upper and lower control limit lines are used to chart movement of data away from the average. The process is assumed to be in control if the data points plot within the two control limits.[54]
1945	Beginning in the mid 1940s, **Joseph Juran** and **Edwards Deming** were prominent figures in pioneering QI as a formal approach to the management of quality within industry. With their work largely ignored in America, following World War II, they were invited to Japan where they helped to restructure Japanese production methods.
1952	The ACS formed a coalition with other medical and hospital organizations and formed the **Joint Commission on the Accreditation of Hospitals (JCAH),** a not-for-profit organization providing voluntary accreditation of hospitals based on defined minimum quality standards. (In 1987, the name changed to Joint Commission on Accreditation of Healthcare Organizations [JCAHO].)
1966	With the initiation of the Medicaid and the Medicare programs, the federal government's interest in health care quality grew, and Congress passed the **Social Security Act Amendments**, which mandated that health care organizations must meet the JCAH standards to participate in the Medicaid and Medicare programs.
1966	**Avedis Donabedian**, MD, published *Evaluating the Quality of Medical Care*, a significant article proposing the "structure, process, and outcome" construct for evaluating the quality of health care.[24] (Refer to the Measuring Quality section.)
1970	The National Academies of Science established the **Institute of Medicine (IOM)**, a non-profit independent scientific advisor to improve the nation's health.
1979	The **Accreditation Association for Ambulatory Healthcare** was formed to assist ambulatory health care organizations improve the quality of care provided to patients.
1979	The **National Committee for Quality Assurance (NCQA)** was established.
1989	Congress formed the **Agency for Health Care Policy and Research**, a health service agency in the Department of Health and Human Services supporting QI research. (This agency later became the Agency for Healthcare Research and Quality [AHRQ].)
1990	The NCQA was given a mandate to offer **accreditation programs** for managed care organizations and assumed responsibility for the Health Plan Employer Data and Information Set.
1991	The **Institute of Healthcare Improvement** was founded by Dr. Don Berwick. This non-profit organization campaigns for health care changes in the United States and worldwide.
1996	The **National Patient Safety Foundation** was established to provide a voice for the patient as a consumer of health care.
1996	The IOM launched its comprehensive **Quality Initiative**, which focused on assessing and improving the nation's quality of care.
1996	JCAHO established the **Sentinel Event Policy** to mandate that an organization must report any significant unexplained/unanticipated patient outcome (eg, death or serious physical or psychological injury).
1998	The **Leapfrog Group** was founded by a group of employers dedicated to improving the quality of health care for their employees.
1999	The IOM published ***To Err is Human: Building a Safer Health System***. This report highlighted widespread and serious care problems and brought public attention to the issue, thus prompting a number of regulatory and legislative initiatives aimed at documenting errors and seeking solutions.
1999	The AHRQ and the **National Quality Forum** (a non-profit organization including a wide variety of health care stakeholders including providers, payers, and consumers) joined to form a public–private partnership to promote a national health care quality agenda.
2001	The IOM published ***Crossing the Quality Chasm: A New Health System for the 21 Century***. This publication again highlighted current problems in the health care system and called for major reform. It proposed six overarching aims of quality care, namely: 1. Safety: Avoid injuries to patients from care that is intended to help them. 2. Effectiveness: Provide evidence-based care, and avoid both overuse and underuse of services.

(continued)

TABLE 40-1 History of the Quality Improvement Movement in the United States *(continued)*

Year	Event
	3. Patient centeredness: Provide respectful, responsive, and individualized care. 4. Timeliness: Reduce waiting time and harmful delays in care. 5. Efficiency: Minimize wasteful use of resources (eg, equipment, supplies, personnel). 6. Equity: All individuals should receive the same care regardless of personal characteristics, gender, ethnicity, geographic location, and socioeconomic status.
2001	JCAHO mandated the establishment of **specific standards for patient safety**.
2001	The AHRQ and NQF published ***Making Healthcare Safer: A Critical Analysis of Patient Safety Practices***. This report reviewed 79 practices and rated them as to the likelihood of impact, thus identifying practices that should be used (when appropriate) to reduce the risk of harm to patients. Preventing malnutrition and preventing central line infections were 2 of the 30 recommended safe practices.
2002	JCAHO announced significant changes to the accreditation process through the **Shared Visions-New Pathways** initiative, which was designed to progressively sharpen the focus of the accreditation process on operational systems critical to patient care safety and quality.
2003	JCAHO announced the first set of National Patient Safety Goals for improving the safety of patient care in health care organizations. The listed goals included: • Improve the accuracy of patient identification. • Improve the effectiveness of communication among caregivers. • Improve the safety of using high-alert medications. • Eliminate wrong-site, wrong-patient, and wrong-procedure surgery. • Improve the safety of using infusion pumps. • Improve the effectiveness of clinical alarm systems.
2005	President George W. Bush signed the Patient Safety and Quality Improvement Act into law establishing a confidential, voluntary reporting system in which physicians and other health care providers could submit information on errors to patient safety organizations without fear of lawsuits or punishments.
2005	The Centers for Medicare and Medicaid Services published the Quality Improvement Roadmap, a structured Quality Improvement Organization (QIO) Program consisting of a national network of 53 QIOs. QIOs work with consumers and physicians, hospitals, and other caregivers to refine care delivery systems to make sure patients (particularly those from underserved populations) get the right care at the right time.
2010	The Obama administration introduced the **Affordable Care Act**, legislation that focused on improving the quality of health care in the United States. This act mandated the creation of national aims and priorities to inform QI efforts.

QI, quality improvement.

3. Affordable Care: Reduce the cost of quality health care for individuals, families, employers, and the government.

To help achieve these aims, the strategy also establishes six priorities to help focus efforts by public and private partners. These priorities include:

1. Making care safer by reducing harm caused in the delivery of care.
2. Ensuring that individuals and families are engaged as partners in their care.
3. Promoting effective communication and coordination of care.
4. Promoting the most effective prevention and treatment practices for the leading causes of mortality, starting with cardiovascular disease.
5. Working with communities to promote the wide use of best practices to enable healthy living.
6. Making quality care more affordable for individuals, families, employers, and governments by developing and spreading new health care delivery models.

The strategy was developed both through evidence-based results of the latest research and consultation with a wide range of stakeholders across the health care system, including federal and state agencies, local communities, provider organizations, clinicians, patients, businesses, employers, and payers. The National Quality Strategy will be updated continually as the Affordable Care Act is implemented. The AHRQ is tasked with supporting and coordinating the implementation, planning, and further development, and for updating the strategy.

The National Quality Strategy is just one piece of a broader effort by the Obama administration to improve the quality of health care. Other initiatives include the recently formed Innovation Center at the Center for Medicine and Medicaid Services,[22] which intends to evaluate models of safer care delivery and promote implementation of best practices in patient safety; and the Partnership for Patients,[23] a new public–private partnership that brings together leaders of major hospitals, employers, physicians, nurses, and patient advocates along with state and federal governments in a shared effort to make hospital care safer, more reliable, and less costly.

Measuring Quality

Performance measurement is integral to QI. More than 30 years ago, Avedis Donabedian[24] proposed a framework for evaluating health care quality based on three components of the system, namely, structure, process, and outcome. He defined structure as the environment in which health care is provided (ie, physical equipment and facilities), process as the method by which health care is provided, and outcome as the consequence of the health care provided (ie, health status). He recognized that all three components are linked, with structure influencing the process, and both structure and process influencing the outcome, and thus all three components should be measured to evaluate the quality of care. Figure 40-1 provides examples of structure, process, and outcome measures in nutrition therapy.

Quality Indicators

One of the biggest challenges of measuring quality is identifying objective and quantifiable measures that accurately reflect the quality of care provided. Validity, reliability, sensitivity, clinical relevance, and the ease with which data can be obtained are some of the key attributes required for quality or performance indicators.[25] Indicators related to structure are often easy to define and measure, whereas process and outcome are more dynamic concepts, and therefore, related indicators are more difficult to quantify.[26] Outcomes are often believed to be the most valid indicator of quality, especially because clinicians are motivated to achieve the best outcome for patients, such as preventing complications and reducing the length of stay. However, the requirement for long-term patient follow-up to measure outcomes may preclude the collection of this data, and outcomes are not only determined by the care provided but also by genetic, environmental, and behavioral factors. For example, mortality is an important outcome measure, but it is difficult to determine a causal link between the medical intervention and mortality, especially if the cause of death is not determined. One of the significant limitations of comparing mortality rates is that some institutions or specific providers, such as in large teaching hospitals, may treat patients with a higher severity of illness and therefore may have higher mortality rates. Consequently, various methods are used to adjust for case severity, comorbidities, and other patient/hospital characteristics in an attempt to reduce the influence of these factors and enable comparison between groups and across time points.[27] However, although risk adjustment is recommended, there may always be residual differences or unmeasured factors that cannot be accounted for in an analysis.[28] Due to these difficulties in defining, measuring, and analyzing process and outcome indicators, proxy measures are often relied upon to evaluate quality.[26] A proxy indicator is a process measure that is used when it is not practical to evaluate the outcome of interest or when the process being evaluated cannot be measured directly. Proxy measures should be selected based on evidence from other research studies demonstrating that changes in the proxy measure are associated with changes in the outcome or process of interest.

Regardless of which type of quality indicator is selected, to evaluate the quality of a specific aspect of care, indicators must be compared to an established criterion and the degree of deviation from this criterion assessed. The degree of deviation from a criterion that represents the threshold between an acceptable and a nonacceptable quality may be determined by established standards (eg, clinical practice guidelines, clinical literature) but in the event that standards are lacking, the threshold may be defined by current norms (ie, usual or average performance).

Data Collection

After deciding what to measure as an indicator of quality, the next step is to acquire the necessary information on the indicator. This process involves defining how the data will be acquired (ie, study design or existing data source), on whom (ie, study population), from where (ie, location), and when (ie, time frame). Data collection may be retrospective, concurrent, or prospective depending on the moment in time the data were derived. The studies may be observational in nature and should purely record what is happening or has happened in the past; examples are cross-sectional, cohort, and case-control studies. Alternatively, QI studies may be experimental in nature, whereby an intervention is evaluated and the change or effect on the outcome of interest is described. Experimental designs include pretest-posttest, time series, and the randomized controlled trial. Observational studies may be further classified as descriptive or analytic. In the former, the clinical indicators are measured and described, whereas the latter goes one step further and incorporates an analysis comparing indicators between specific subgroups of clinical patients or units, or evaluates associations between factors and quality indicators.

It is often not feasible to collect data on the whole population of interest; therefore, sampling is used to select

FIGURE 40-1 Quality Indicators. Examples of Structure, Process, and Outcomes Measures Related to Nutrition Support

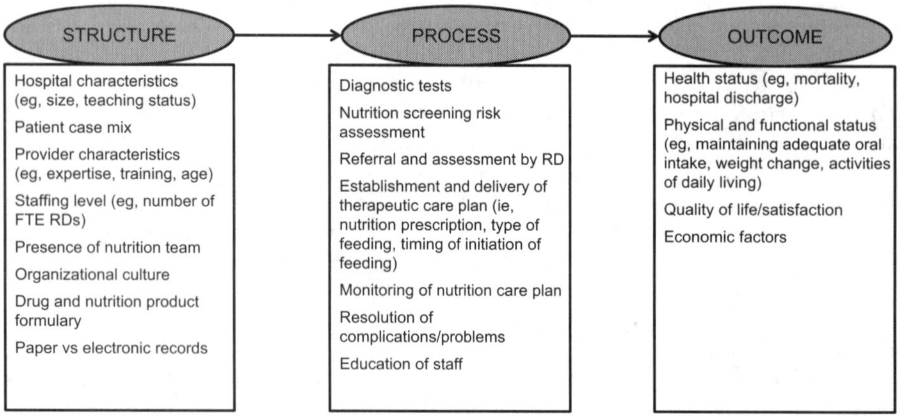

FTE, full-time equivalent; RD, registered dietitian.

individuals to be included in the study. If statistical rules are applied to select a random sample, the observations made on this smaller sample should be representative of the population. However, when conducting QI projects obtaining a sampling frame of the population of interest may be problematic and, in such cases, a convenience sample may be used. Although more readily obtained, a convenience sample may not be representative of the whole group and this should be kept in mind when interpreting the results of QI studies.

Data sources for QI studies may include data collected routinely as part of clinical care, such as electronic health records, or may require the collection of additional data. The methods for collecting data, including a clear description of each variable required, how often each should be collected, and how or where to record the abstracted data should be clearly outlined in a study manual or protocol.

Data Analysis

Data collected on quality indicators must be analyzed and interpreted with validity. Data can be presented in various ways including tabulation of counts, visual representations (eg, bar charts, histograms, pie charts, control charts), descriptive statistics (eg, means, medians, percentiles, proportions), or statistical tests (eg, chi-square, t-test, analysis of variance, regression analysis).

Comparing quality indicators with established criteria or standards highlight if the quality of care is acceptable or not. If problems are identified, appropriate improvement strategies must be sought and implemented. This process of selecting change strategies may involve "brainstorming" with a wide range of stakeholders to identify feasible solutions to the problem, or alternatively can involve using various QI models and/or theoretical frameworks to inform which interventions may be most successful.[29]

Measuring Quality of Nutrition Care

In our hospitals, artificial nutrition is often provided to seriously ill patients who are unable to achieve adequate nutrition intake orally. They often have an underlying disease process and/or clinical complications that further compromise their nutritional status, resulting in a lack of improvement in nutritional or clinical outcomes following the provision of enteral nutrition (EN) or parenteral nutrition (PN). In such cases, it is not always appropriate to measure outcomes as an indicator of quality. Process measures are, therefore, more commonly used to assess the effectiveness of nutrition support.[30] Table 40-2 provides examples of goals of nutrition care, outcome or process indicators of these goals, and standards or criteria by which the indicators might be compared. Practice Scenario 40-1 provides an example of measuring the quality of nutrition care.

TABLE 40-2 Measuring the Quality of Nutrition Care: Examples of Goals, Outcome and Process Indicators, and Comparison Criteria

Goal	Quality Indicator	Comparison Criteria
Identify patients who require nutrition support	Proportion of admitted patients screened for nutrition risk	90%
	Proportion of screened patients identified as high risk on screening subsequently assessed by RD/nutrition team for nutrition support	90%
Initiate nutrition therapy in a timely manner	In patients assessed to require nutrition support, the mean time from admission to the initiation of nutrition support	96 hours
	In patients assessed to require nutrition support, the proportion in which EN/PN/oral is initiated within 2 hours of ordering nutrition support	90%
Deliver nutrition therapy by the most appropriate route	Of the total number of patients that receive PN, the proportion who receive appropriately indicated PN	90%
	Of the total number of patients at high risk of malnutrition, the proportion excluding patients who received appropriately indicated PN or oral supplements	90%
Ensure patients are prescribed and receive an appropriate quantity of calories and protein	Proportion of patients receiving nutrition support that receive >80% of prescribed calories and protein	75%
Prevent further deterioration of nutrition status	Proportion of patients receiving nutrition support who maintain or gain body weight	75%
	Proportion of patients receiving nutrition support with positive nitrogen balance	75%
Minimize the risks and prevent complications associated with nutrition support	Proportion of patients with hyperglycemia in patients on PN	10%
	Proportion of patients with high gastric residuals prescribed motility agents	90%
	Proportion of patients receiving EN diagnosed with aspiration pneumonia	10%
	Incidence of catheter-related infections in patients receiving PN	5 per 1000 catheter days

RD, registered dietitian; EN, enteral nutrition; PN, parenteral nutrition.

Practice Scenario 40-1

Question: How do you assess the appropriate use of PN in your hospital?

Scenario: The manager of the pharmacy reports that spending on parenteral solutions has increased by over 30% during the previous quarter and questions the Nutrition Support Team about the reasons for this increase. He asks them to reduce the future use of parenteral solutions in order to remain within budget.

Intervention: Conduct a clinical audit of PN use in the hospital.

Answer: The charts of all patients who received PN over the previous 3 months were reviewed and information was abstracted on the reasons PN was initiated. The results of this data collection were then compared with evidence-based standards. Of the 32 patients who received PN, 29 (90%) had a contraindication to receiving EN and therefore PN was provided appropriately. For the remaining 3 patients, the team identified reasons why the standards may not have been met. In 2 of the cases, the patients were severely malnourished and were receiving care in the ICU while awaiting upper gastrointestinal (GI) surgery. In the final case, PN was initiated by the surgical team over the weekend but transitioned to EN following an assessment by the Nutrition Support Team on Monday. Following the clinical audit, the results were reported to the manager of the pharmacy; after further discussions, it was decided that no action was required at this time to reduce the use of PN. The Nutrition Support Team planned to repeat the audit annually.

Rationale: The use of parenteral solutions may have high cost implications for the pharmacy's budget, but implementing changes to reduce the use of PN may not be appropriate if patients require nutrition via this route to meet and maintain their nutritional needs. Consequently, the first step is to evaluate whether the current use is appropriate by comparing practices with evidence-based standards (ie, conduct a clinical audit). The American Society for Parenteral and Enteral Nutrition (A.S.P.E.N.) Standards for Nutrition Support in Adult Hospitalized Patients states that "the route selected to provide nutrition support therapy shall be appropriate to the patient's medical condition and that PN should only be provided if there is a contraindication to EN" (ie, intestinal, obstruction, ileus, peritonitis, bowel ischemia, intractable vomiting and diarrhea), or if the provision of EN is inadequate due to intolerance. The A.S.P.E.N. Guidelines for the Provision and Assessment of Nutrition Support Therapy in the Adult Critically Ill Patient recommends that if a patient is expected to undergo major upper GI surgery and EN is not feasible, PN should be provided preoperatively if the patient is malnourished. Therefore, in this scenario, data was collected, compared with these standards, and compliance was found to be high. No action was taken to change current practice, but a plan to monitor the use of PN was developed.

Quality Improvement Strategies in Nutrition Support

Clinical Practice Guidelines

Clinical practice guidelines (CPGs) are "systematically developed statements to assist practitioner and patients [in making] decisions about appropriate health care for specific clinical circumstances."[31] They are tools that operationalize the implementation of evidence-based care and improve the quality of care received by patients by reducing variations in practice and improving effectiveness and efficiency. Guidelines are typically internationally or nationally developed broad statements of best practice. Guideline recommendations are a function of the underlying evidence coupled with a valuation of other aspects pertinent to the topic of the recommendation such as safety, cost, feasibility, and patient preferences. The development of CPGs have increased dramatically in recent years with professional and government bodies producing guidelines on a diverse range of clinical topics including the publication of CPGs for nutrition support.[4–8] These guidelines may be targeted to specific health care provider groups (eg, physicians, nurses, physiotherapists, dietitians) working within specific settings (eg, hospitals, primary care practices, specialist units). To ensure guideline recommendations remain pertinent to current clinical practice, there must be a process for appraising and incorporating new evidence and revising these documents. The heightened emphasis on guidelines has led to the establishment of specific programs for developing, collating, and critically appraising CPGs, such as the National Guideline Clearing House in the United States.

As is common with changes in health care, the growth in CPGs as a QI tool has not escaped controversy. Critics of guidelines condemn them as cookbook medicine,[32,33] whereas advocates argue that they facilitate the integration of individual expertise with the best available clinical evidence.[34] Despite this controversy, there is evidence that CPGs improve the quality of care provided.[35]

Care Pathways

Care pathways are sometimes referred to as clinical pathways, critical pathways, integrated care pathways, multidisciplinary pathways of care, collaborative care plans, and care maps. Despite the lack of one accepted definition, care pathways are one of the main tools applied to manage the quality of care through the standardization of care processes across different disciplines and settings.[36]

Care pathways were first introduced in the United States in the early 1990s and have been increasingly used over the past 2 decades. Essentially, care pathways assist the health care team in the day-to-day delivery of care. Care pathways are structured, locally agreed, multidisciplinary plans of care that are based on guidelines or evidence where available. They provide detailed guidance for each stage in the management of a specific patient group with a predictable clinical course and include details on the expected progress and outcomes.

They are most commonly formatted as a flow chart, highlighting decisions to be made and the care to be provided for a given condition in a stepwise sequence. Hill[37] described the four main components of care pathways as (1) a timeline, (2) the categories of care or activities and associated interventions, (3) long-term and intermediate outcome criteria, and (4) the variance record (to permit deviations to be evaluated).

Evidence suggests that care pathways reduce the cost of care and the length of stay in hospitals, as well as increase patient satisfaction and education.[38] (Refer to Practice Scenario 40-2 for an example of a QI initiative involving the implementation of a care pathway.)

Practice Scenario 40-2

Question: How do you ensure that all patients are screened for nutritional risk on admission to the hospital?

Scenario: To comply with the Joint Commissions standards for nutrition care,[62] in 1986, the nutrition services department of a 350-bed, nonteaching hospital developed a policy document stating that nutritional risk screening should be conducted on all hospital patients, and patients at high risk should be referred to the dietitian. To support the policy, a care pathway coupled with a paper-based nutritional screening tool was developed. However, since its implementation, use of these tools have not been monitored and, anecdotally, it has been observed that nutrition screening is not routinely completed on admission to the hospital.

Intervention: The FADE model is adopted to update the care pathway and the nutritional screening tool and to implement it at the bedside.

Answer: FOCUS – A literature review is conducted so that the team clearly understands the evidence for nutrition screening and can update the tools accordingly.

ANALYZE – A chart review is conducted on a convenience sample of all inpatients on the medical floor to audit the conduct of nutrition screening. As suspected, nutrition screening was not completed on any of the 45 patients whose charts were reviewed. A project steering group is established to identify the root causes of the problem and potential solutions. It is identified that very few paper-based forms have been used after the introduction of an electronic health record in 2010; therefore, the care pathway and tool were no longer easily accessible to nursing staff and weren't part of the routine admission assessment.

DEVELOP – An action plan is developed to integrate the care pathway and tool into the electronic patient admission assessment form and to educate nurses on them. The steering group identifies resources required, develops actions, and sets timelines.

EXECUTE and EVALUATE – The developed plan is first implemented on the medical floor on which the baseline audit was conducted. After a 3-month implementation and education phase, the chart review is repeated. Adherence to the care pathway and completion of the nutrition screening tool is now 85%. The electronic tools are consequently implemented hospital-wide. A monitoring component is incorporated into the electronic system to produce a monthly report of the proportion of admitted patients who are screened. The steering group plans to review the evidence for nutrition screening and the content of the current tools annually. They also plan an annual hospital-wide nutrition day to maintain awareness of the importance of nutrition and screening.

Rationale: A previous QI initiative to implement nutritional screening at hospital admission did not incorporate a strategy for continuous monitoring and evaluation. Consequently, over the years, the care pathway and screening tool became outdated and compliance waned. Using the four steps of the FADE model, the project steering group was able to successfully increase compliance with nutritional screening on admission. The group could have adopted any of the QI methodologies or used a combination of the different models to achieve the same goal.

Bundles

Bundles are a QI strategy introduced by the Institute for Healthcare Improvement (IHI) to describe a collection of processes needed to effectively care for patients undergoing particular treatments with a specific set of risks.[39–41] A bundle is typically a small set of evidence-based practices (usually three to five) that, when implemented together, will achieve significantly better outcomes than when implemented individually. Examples of bundles related to nutrition support include the IHI ventilator bundle (ie, elevation of the head of the bed; daily "sedation vacations"; an assessment of readiness to extubate, peptic ulcer disease prophylaxis, deep venous thrombosis prophylaxis; and daily oral care with chlorhexidine) used in intensive care units (ICUs) for the prevention of ventilator-associated pneumonia[42] and the IHI central line bundle (ie, hand hygiene, maximal barrier precautions upon insertion, chlorhexidine skin antisepsis, optimal catheter site selection, daily review of the line) for the prevention of catheter-related bloodstream infections.[43]

Health Information Technology

In recent years, health care researchers and policymakers have proposed that health information technology is a key factor in reforming the health care system. Health information technology is the application of computer-related technologies in health care. Examples of such technologies include patient electronic medical records, decision support systems, and computerized physician order entry. A systematic review of such technologies on the quality, efficiency, and costs of medical care concluded that they improve quality by increasing adherence to guidelines, enhancing disease surveillance, and decreasing medication errors.[44] However, much of this evidence comes from four benchmark research institutions and relates to preventative care; therefore, the generalizability of these findings remains unclear. Regardless, in theory, the benefits of health information technology over traditional paper-based information management are clear.

Adherence to guidelines is enhanced by embedding decision support functions in electronic health records or provider order entry systems. These functions are usually in the form of computerized reminders or algorithms. A reminder is when the system is programmed to detect and alert the provider about a clinical event that might need corrective action (eg, triggering a reminder to order insulin when untreated hyperglycemia is detected in patients on PN). Algorithms are similar to care pathways that illustrate the decision-making process in a stepwise fashion and that incorporate management strategies to consider. (Refer to Practice Scenario 40-3 for an example of how a paper-based care pathway can be embedded into the electronic health record to improve nutrition screening.)

Chapter 41 provides more detailed explanations of evidence-based resources that can be integrated into practice to improve quality.

Practice Scenario 40-3

Question: How do you improve the timeliness of EN initiation in your ICU?

Scenario: A clinical audit of nutrition practice in the medical ICU reveals that the mean time to initiation of EN in mechanically ventilated patients is 54 hours, and enteral feeding is started early (within 24 to 48 hours) in only 45% of patients. These observations in 30 patients reveal a gap between what the A.S.P.E.N. guidelines recommend and what is actually happening in practice.

Intervention: The PDSA cycle is adopted to help achieve the desired goal of improving the timeliness of EN initiation.

Answer: PLAN – The dietitian organizes a meeting with the ICU team to identify the reasons that EN is not initiated early, and to brainstorm potential solutions to the problem. Discussions reveal that nutrition is usually not addressed on rounds until day 3 of ICU admission. The team discusses several suggestions for improving the timeliness of EN:

- Add EN initiation order to the electronic ICU admission order set
- Add nutrition category to the bedside daily rounding checklist
- Dietitian to attend rounds
- Educate staff on the importance of nutrition during critical illness

It is agreed that a nutrition category will be added to the rounding checklist and the dietitian will attend rounds when available.

DO – The nutrition category is added to the checklist, circulated to the ICU team for comments, and the revised checklist is disseminated at the bedside.

STUDY – After 2 months the dietitian reviews the checklists and determines that the nutrition category is complete in less than 60% of patients, and that due to her work schedule, she is only able to attend rounds on Tuesday and Thursdays.

ACT – The team decides to proceed with the current changes and, in addition, to work toward adding EN initiation to the ICU admission order set. They support this change with staff education.

A second PDSA cycle is initiated to implement and evaluate this change. A subsequent clinical audit reveals that the mean time to the initiation of EN has been reduced to 49 hours and 60% of patients are now receiving EN within 24 to 48 hours.

Rationale: A problem with the quality of nutrition practice in the ICU had been highlighted. Any of the QI methodologies could have been adopted to propose, implement, and evaluate a solution to the problem. One of the most widely adopted methodologies is the PDSA cycle. In this process, the quality issues to be addressed are identified and analyzed to form a plan of action. In the second phase, proposed solutions are created, and implemented on a trial basis under limited circumstances. The next phase consists of an evaluation of the trial to see if the proposed standards and processes result in improvements in the process. If they do not, new solutions will be developed, and the testing process will begin again until the desired goal is achieved.

Quality Improvement Methodologies

Several QI methodologies have been developed to improve the quality and safety of health care. The most commonly used are the plan-do-study-act (PDSA) cycle, Six Sigma, Lean, and focus-analyze-develop-execute-evaluate (FADE) models. There are several similarities between the different strategies, with each involving an analysis, an implementation, and an evaluation. The choice of the QI methodology depends on the nature of the QI project and no one method is best for each situation. Principles from several of these methodologies may be employed in a single QI project.

Plan-Do-Study-Act Cycle

The PDSA cycle is a rapid cycle improvement strategy, and is one of the most commonly used approaches to improve health care quality. This method involves proposing a solution to a problem that is then tested on a small scale using the PDSA cycle. The results are then used to decide whether to implement, modify, or abandon the proposed solution. If the tested solution does not achieve desired results, another change is selected, implemented, and evaluated. If the results are achieved, the solution is implemented on a larger scale and monitored over time for continuous improvement.[45] (Figure 40-2 and refer to Practice Scenario 40-3 for applied examples of using the PDSA cycle to improve the timeliness of EN.)

Step 1: Setting Aims

By asking "What are we trying to accomplish?" the aim or goal of the improvement activity is established. The aim should be time-specific, measurable, and should clearly define the specific population of patients that will be affected. For example, if the focus of the activity is to improve the timeliness of nutrition support, the aim might be to reduce the time from the order of nutrition support to its initiation to 2 hours. Aims that are clearly defined and relentlessly pursued increase the chance of success in QI initiatives.[46]

Step 2: Establishing Measures

By asking "How will we know that a change is an improvement?" measures are selected to evaluate if a change leads to a quantitative improvement. (Refer to section on quality indicators.)

Step 3: Selecting Change

By asking "What changes can we make that will result in improvement?" a plan for change is developed. Although all

FIGURE 40-2 The Plan-Do-Study-Act Cycle (PDSA) for Change

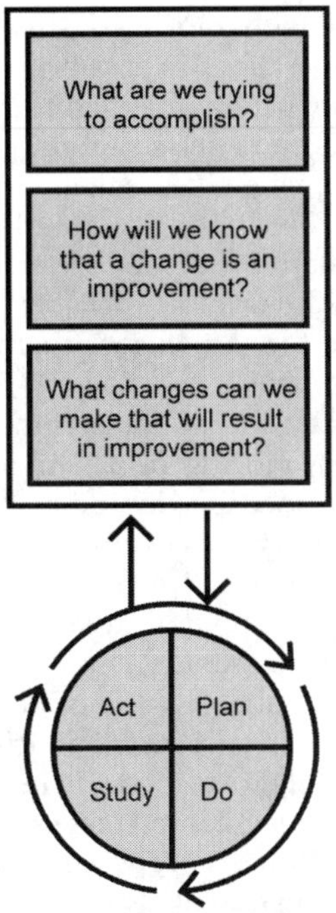

Reproduced with permission from Langley GJ, Moen RM, Nolan KM, Nolan TW, Norman CL, Provost LP. *The Improvement Guide: A Practical Approach to Enhancing Organizational Performance*. 2nd ed. San Francisco, CA: Jossey-Bass; 2009.

improvements require making changes, not all changes result in improvement.[47] Therefore, teams must identify the changes that are most likely to result in the desired improvement within their local setting. This involves having an understanding of barriers to changing practices and selecting strategies that will overcome these barriers.

Step 4: Implementing and Testing Changes

Any change or solution must be tested in the real work setting to see whether it yields an improvement. No matter how effective a change is in one setting, it must be adapted to the local environment. Testing helps determine how much improvement can be expected from a change and helps to assess the cost and other effects of the proposed change. The PDSA cycle systematically tests changes for QI.

Plan: In the planning phase, the team plans the change and lists the objective of the proposed change. They make predictions about the results of the proposed change. Focus groups, brainstorming, fishbone diagrams, Pareto charts, and affinity diagrams are some quality tools that may be helpful during the planning stage.[48]

A critical part of the planning phase is deciding what and how data will need to be collected. The data management process must be manageable for busy clinicians, so data collection should be simple and use available data if possible. If new data need to be gathered, small samples should be used. Teams who build data collection, analysis, and display into the daily patterns and rhythms of work and whose job descriptions and performance reviews include data management have more success with data management.[49]

Do: In this action phase, teams try out the test on a small scale on a trial basis. During this phase, teams collect data and also document problems and unexpected observations. Testing the solution on a small scale helps to decide whether the proposed change will work on a bigger scale and allows the team to evaluate the cost and impact of the change on the process and other parts of the system. Trying out solutions on a small scale also helps gain buy-in from stakeholders and minimize resistance upon implementation. Check sheets, parking lots, and run charts are useful quality tools during the "Do" phase.[45,48]

Study: In this evaluation phase, the team analyzes the data and interprets the results to determine if the proposed solution addressed the quality issue. By examining the accumulated data, teams can identify current performance, patterns, or trends. They can then compare current findings with the previous status, intervention, or reference standards and draw conclusions. It is important to determine how the results of the test did or did not agree with the predictions made at the beginning of the cycle.[45] Because the purpose of the data is to stimulate constructive change, the data analysis must be simple enough for everyone in the care process to understand.

Act: In the last phase, the team takes action to ensure that improvement will have the maximum effect over time. The team may refine the change based on what was learned from the test. If the test is not as successful as anticipated, they may revise the theory tested and prepare a new plan for the next test, and so the cycle is repeated. If the test was successful, the team determines how the process will be implemented on a broader scale. Quality tools that may be used in this phase are brainstorming, affinity diagrams, and interrelationship digraphs.[48] Even if the test was successful, new aims and goals may have been highlighted during the cycle and the process begins again at Step 1 with these new aims (Figure 40-3).

Step 5: Implementing Changes

This step involves implementing the change on a broader scale—for example, from one ward to the entire hospital. Implementing the change on a permanent basis involves another cycle to build the change into the organization's infrastructure of policies, documentation, training, and so forth.

Step 6: Spreading Changes

This final step involves expanding the change to a different area either within or outside the organization. Spreading also refers to building on previous PDCA cycles, with each new cycle beginning with a new and slightly more complex project. The process is referred to as moving up the "ramp of improvement" as new knowledge is gained and new improvements are implemented over time with each completed cycle (Figure 40-3).[50,51]

FIGURE 40-3 The Ramp of Improvement. Spreading Change by Repeating the Plan-Do-Study-Act Cycle (PDSA) Cycle

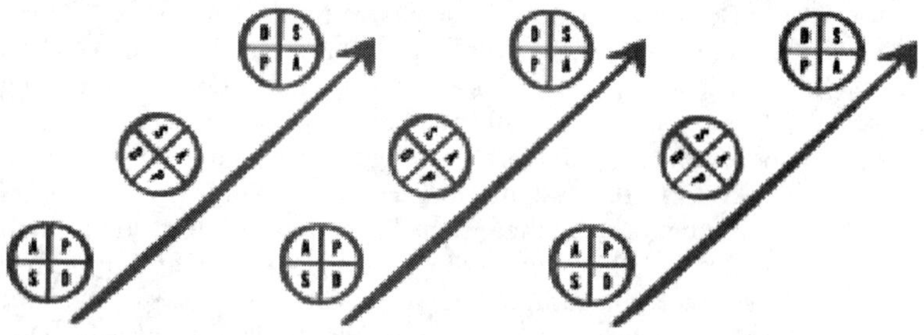

Reproduced with permission from Langley GJ, Moen RM, Nolan KM, Nolan TW, Norman CL, Provost LP. *The Improvement Guide: A Practical Approach to Enhancing Organizational Performance.* 2nd ed. San Francisco, CA: Jossey-Bass; 2009.

Six Sigma

Six Sigma is another model for QI. Six Sigma uses a structured approach and sophisticated statistical techniques to strive for near perfection. Adapted from techniques used by Motorola, Six Sigma is a disciplined, data-driven methodology for eliminating defects in any process.[52] The term comes from the use in statistics of the Greek letter sigma to denote a standard deviation from the mean. Six sigma is equivalent to 3.4 defects or errors per million.[53]

The goal of Six Sigma is not to eliminate all failures of quality but to reduce them to the extent that it is no longer cost-effective to pursue any further reduction.[54] This is accomplished through the use of the DMAIC model[55]:

- D: Define the goals to be reached.
- M: Measure the current performance levels to establish a baseline for comparison.
- A: Analyze the current performance regarding what factors are present that effect quality.
- I: Improve these factors through the implementation of appropriate performance improvement strategies.
- C: Control mechanisms are implemented to prevent errors before they occur.

Six Sigma has been criticized as unrealistic in the health care setting because in many of the services and procedures performed, errors in performance do not follow standard deviation curves. Also, the statistical techniques have not been validated outside of the manufacturing industry. In spite of these limitations, use of the Six Sigma model is expanding in the health care industry.[54]

Lean Methodology

Lean is another QI approach that overlaps with Six Sigma but focuses on the identified needs of the customer and aims to improve processes and to eliminate inefficiency.[55] The methodology was first developed by Toyota in the early 1950s and has been adopted by many other industries, including health care.

Lean thinking focuses on what the customer values; so in health care, any activity that does not contribute to improving patient outcomes, quality of life, or satisfaction with care is classified as waste. Seven different types of waste have been identified[56]:

1. Overproduction or underproduction (eg, requesting tests and referrals to outpatient clinics just in case the patient needs them)
2. Wasted inventory (eg, ordering excess tube feed from pharmacy or food service because the supply at the ward level is unreliable)
3. Waiting (eg, patients waiting to be seen at clinic appointments)
4. Transportation (ie, transporting patients unnecessarily [eg, moving the patient off the ward/unit for tests or to see the physiotherapist])
5. Defects (ie, mistakes along the process)
6. Staff movement (ie, poor work area ergonomics [eg, no computer at the bedside to check biochemistry results])
7. Unnecessary processing (eg, using complex equipment to undertake simple tasks, outdated policies and procedures)

Identifying wasteful processes can help staff understand the root cause of a problem and implement strategies to eliminate waste. Womack and Jones[57] proposed a five-step process for guiding the implementation of Lean techniques.

Step 1: Identify Value

The first step is to understand what the patient values. The opposite of this is waste. This simple analysis should include patients so that their perspectives can be understood and everyone can evaluate if waste exists in an organization.

Step 2: Identify and Visualize the Value Stream

One of the commonly used tools in Lean methodology is called value stream mapping. The technique helps to visualize all the steps in the patient's pathway from when he or she enters to when the patient leaves the system. This mapping informs decisions about how best to improve the process.

Step 3: Create Flow

Achieving continuous flow is central to Lean thinking. This is where the patient moves from one step along the pathway to the next without delay. It is the most efficient way to manage any process because it reduces waste to a minimum. In this third step, any obstacles that prevent continuous flow are identified and solutions to overcome them are proposed.

Step 4: Establish Pull

Pull is delivering care in line with demand, where the next part of the process pulls patients from the previous one (ie, discharge pulls patients from wards, wards pull patients from surgery and the emergency room).

Step 5: Seek Perfection

Continue the first four steps until a state of perfection is reached in which perfect value is created with no waste.

The Focus-Analyze-Develop-Execute-Evaluate Model

Another common model for QI is the FADE model.[58] The four steps in this model cover a broad area and are easy to apply. (Figure 40-4 and refer to Practice Scenario 40-2 for an applied example of using FADE to improve nutrition screening.)

Step 1: Focus

The first step involves defining and verifying the process to be targeted for improvement. Establishing a defined focus requires having a clear understanding of what should be happening and how the process might be improved.

Step 2: Analyze

This step involves collecting and analyzing data in order to establish baseline performance, to identify the root causes of the problem for which a solution is being sought, and to assist in identifying possible solutions.

Step 3: Develop

Based on the data generated in step 2, action plans for improvement are developed. These plans outline what needs to occur for the required changes to take effect, and encompass implementation, communication, and the measuring and monitoring of progress.

FIGURE 40-4 The Focus, Analyze, Develop, Execute, Evaluate (FADE) Model

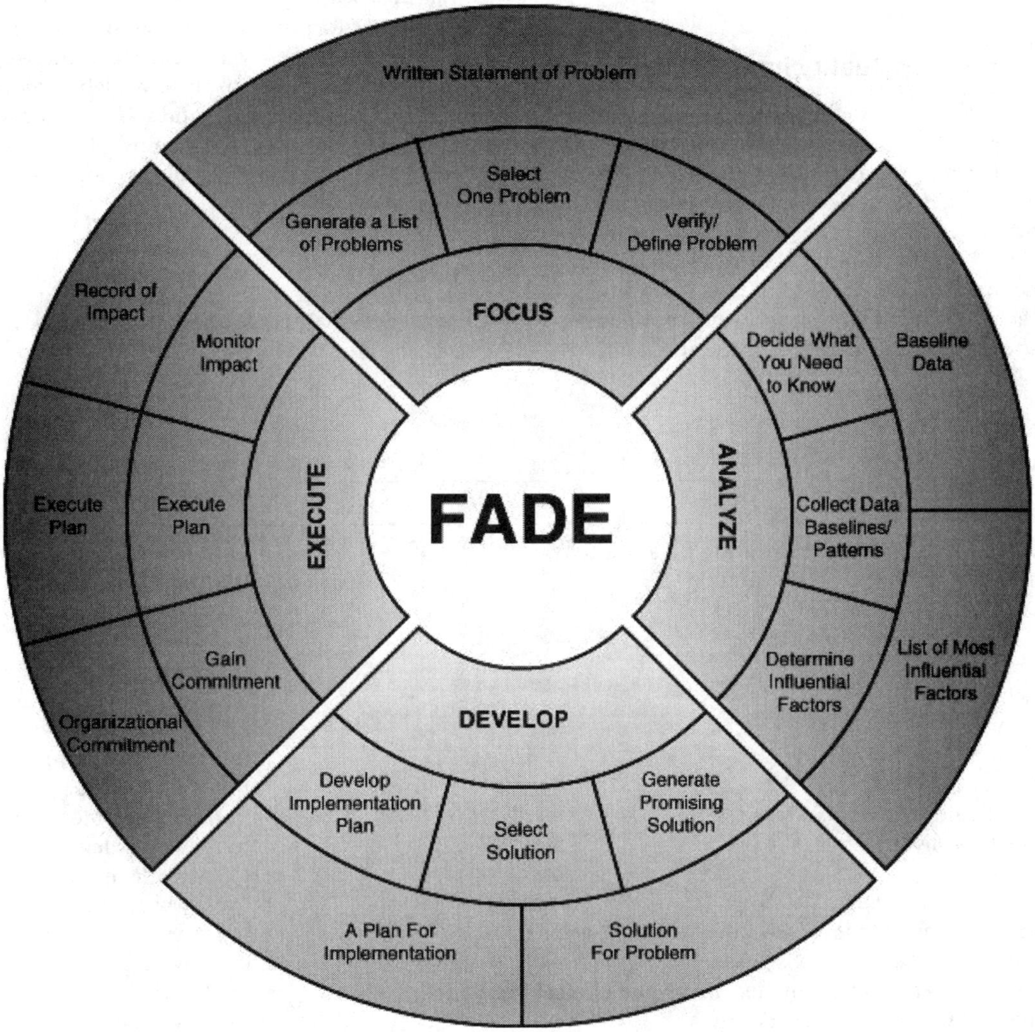

Reproduced with permission from The FADE Model in Your Quality Action Teams. ODI. Billerica, MA.

Step 4: Execute and Evaluate

Finally, the action plans are implemented. This may first be as a pilot, so the action plans can be tested and further changes made if necessary. The implementation of the plans is then evaluated, and ongoing measuring and monitoring systems are installed to ensure success.

Quality Assurance Versus Quality Improvement

Quality assurance (QA) is a planned program used to ensure that all products and services conform to established requirements. QA methods were first used extensively in World War II to address the need for tremendous volumes of high quality, lower cost materials and focused on inspecting products at the end of the process. Actual processes and/or outcomes are compared to predefined criteria or preselected requirements, and corrective action is taken if performance falls below these acceptable standards. QI, on the other hand, focuses on designing and redesigning systems to meet the needs of patients. Philosophically, QA is based on human effort being the source of performance problems, whereas QI focuses on systems being the source of the problem.

Clinical Research Versus Quality Improvement

Confusion often exists about whether a project is categorized as QI or clinical research.[59] QI projects aim to integrate new knowledge into practice, whereas the purpose of clinical research is to discover new knowledge. QI projects target the local setting, whereas research aims to generate results that are generalizable across settings. In improvement projects, teams generally conduct many small, short-term tests that build on each other and accelerate the rate of improvement. Improvement teams gather only enough data to learn and complete another cycle before moving on to the next test. Clinical research, on the other hand, focuses on one large "blind" test where as much data as possible are collected and as many biases as possible are controlled.[47] (Refer to Chapter 41 for more detail regarding research design.)

However, there are circumstances in which QI projects may be considered research, namely if (1) the tested intervention is novel and involves a deviation from established practices, (2) randomization or blinding of individual patients is conducted, (3) patients or staff are exposed to additional risks beyond standard practice, (4) collected data are being transferred to an external organization, and (5) the results of the project will be published.

Knowledge Translation Versus Quality Improvement

Knowledge translation (KT) is defined as "a dynamic and iterative process that includes the synthesis, dissemination, exchange and sound application of knowledge to improve health, provide more effective health services and products and strengthen the health care system".[60] Therefore, KT has many similarities with QI, in that they both aim to improve care. However, KT focuses on ensuring that current practice is synonymous with the best available evidence. Although QI projects also aim to use the best available evidence, the overall goal of a QI project is wider and seeks to address problems that are perceived to affect the quality of care, including safety, effectiveness, patient centeredness, timeliness, efficiency, and equity.[61]

Summary

Closing the quality gap in nutrition support practice is the responsibility of every nutrition care practitioner. The

Additional Information: Useful Links

Organization	URL
Joint Commission on Accreditation of Healthcare Organizations	http://www.jointcommission.org/
The Health Resources and Services Administration	http://www.hrsa.gov/index.html
The Centers for Medicare and Medicaid Services	http://www.cms.gov/
National Committee for Quality Assurance	http://www.ncqa.org/
Agency for Healthcare Research and Quality	http://www.ahrq.gov/
Institute of Medicine	http://www.iom.edu/About-IOM.aspx
National Quality Forum	http://www.qualityforum.org/Home.aspx
Institute for Healthcare Improvement	http://www.ihi.org/ihi
Leapfrog Group	http://www.leapfroggroup.org/
U.S. Department of Health and Human Services	http://www.healthcare.gov/index.html
National Guideline Clearinghouse	http://www.guideline.gov/
Lean Enterprise Institute	http://www.lean.org/
Organizational Dynamics Institute	http://www.orgdynamics.com/
National Health Service, Institute for Innovation and Improvement	http://www.institute.nhs.uk/
AGREE collaboration	http://www.agreecollaboration.org/
National Health Service National Institute for Health and Clinical Excellence	http://www.nice.org.uk/
Scottish Intercollegiate Guidelines Network	http://www.sign.ac.uk/

measurement and improvement of quality are achievable goals. Success is dependent on adopting QI methodologies to identify the root cause of the problem and to develop solutions that are specific to the local context and designed to address local barriers to change.

Acknowledgments

Quality improvement material from the previous *Core Curriculum* was contributed by Janet Skates, MS, RD and Lillian Harvey-Banchik, MD, FACS, CNSP.

References

1. Heyland DK. Nutritional support in the critically ill patient: a critical review of the evidence. *Crit Care Clin.* 1998;14(3):423–440.
2. Heyland DK, Heyland J, Dhaliwal R, Madden S, Cook D. Randomized trials in critical care nutrition: look how far we've come! (and where do we go from here?). *JPEN J Parenter Enteral Nutr.* 2010;34(6):697–706.
3. Alberda C, Gramlich L, Jones N, et al. The relationship between nutritional intake and clinical outcomes in critically ill patients: results of an international multicenter observational study. *Intensive Care Med.* 2009;35(10):1728–1737.
4. Heyland DK, Dhaliwal R, Drover JW, et al. Canadian clinical practice guidelines for nutrition support in mechanically ventilated, critically ill adult patients. *JPEN J Parenter Enteral Nutr.* 2003; 27(5):355–373.
5. American Society for Parenteral and Enteral Nutrition (A.S.P.E.N.) Board of Directors. Clinical guidelines for the use of parenteral and enteral nutrition in adult and pediatric patients, 2009. *JPEN J Parenter Enteral Nutr.* 2009 May 1;33(3):255–259.
6. Lochs H, Valentini L, Schütz T, et al. ESPEN Guidelines on Adult Enteral Nutrition. *Br J Nutr* 2007; 98: 253–259.
7. American Dietetic Association. ADA Evidence Based Nutrition Practice Guidelines 2006. http://www.adaevidencelibrary.com/category.cfm?cat=0&cid=14. Accessed 15 June 2011.
8. Doig GS, Simpson F. *Evidence-Based Guidelines for Nutritional Support of the Critically Ill: Results of A Bi-National Guideline Development Conference.* Sydney, Australia: EvidenceBased.net; 2005.
9. Cahill NE, Dhaliwal R, Day AG, Jiang X, Heyland DK. Nutrition therapy in the critical care setting: what is "best achievable" practice? An international multicenter observational study. *Crit Care Med.* 2010;38(2):395–401.
10. Rice TW, Swope T, Bozeman S, Wheeler AP. Variation in enteral nutrition delivery in mechanically ventilated patients. *Nutrition.* 2005;21(7–8):786–792.
11. Heyland DK, Schtoter-Noppe D, Drover JW. Nutrition support in the critical care setting: Current practice in Canadian ICUs - Opportunities for improvement. *JPEN J Parenter Enteral Nutr.* 2003;27:74–83.
12. De Jonghe B, Appere-De-Vechi C, Fournier M. A prospective survey of nutritional support practices in intensive care unit patients: what is prescribed? What is delivered? *Crit Care Med.* 2001;29:8–12.
13. O'Meara D, Mireles-Cabodevila E, Frame F, et al. Evaluation of delivery of enteral nutrition in critically ill patients receiving mechanical ventilation. *Am J Crit Care.* 2008 January 1;17(1):53–61.
14. Schuster M, McGlynn E, Brook R. How good is the quality of healthcare in the United States? *Millbank Q.* 2003;76:517–563.
15. McGlynn EA, Asch SM, Adams J. The quality of healthcare delivered to adults in the United States. *N Engl J Med.* 2003;483: 2635–2645.
16. Woolf SH, Johnson RE. The break-even point: when medical advances are less important than improving the fidelity with which they are delivered. *Ann Fam Med.* 2005;3(6):545–552.
17. Kohn LT, Corrigan JM, Donaldson MS. Committee on quality of healthcare in America, Institute of Medicine. *To Err is Human—Building a Safer Health System.* Washington, DC: National Academy Press; 2000.
18. Davis K, Schoen C, Schoenbaum SC, et al. *Mirror, Mirror on the Wall: An International Update on the Comparative Performance of American Health Care.* New York: The Commonwealth Fund; May 2007.
19. *Compilation of the Patient Protection and Affordable Care Act,* 111th Cong, 2nd Sess (2010) (http://docs.house.gov/energycommerce/ppacacon.pdf. Accessed June 15, 2010).
20. US Department of Health and Human Services. *Understanding the Affordable Care Act.* http://www.healthcare.gov/law/introduc-tion/index.html. Accessed June 15, 2011.
21. U.S. Department of Health and Human Services. *Report to Congress: National Strategy for Quality Improvement in Health Care.* http://www.healthcare.gov/center/reports/nationalquality strategy032011.pdf. Published March 2011. Accessed June 15, 2011.
22. U.S. Department of Health and Human Services. Center for Medicare & Medicaid Innovation Web site. http://innovations.cms.gov/. Accessed June 15, 2011.
23. U.S. Department of Health and Human Services. Partnerships for Patients: A Common Commitment Web site. http://www.health-care.gov/center/programs/partnership/about/index.html Accessed June 15, 2011.
24. Donabedian A. Explorations in quality assessment and monitoring. *The Definition of Quality and Approaches to its Assessment,* Vol I. Ann Arbor, MI: Health Administration Press; 1980.
25. Mainz J. Developing clinical indicators. *Int J Qual Health Care.* 2003;15(Suppl. 1):i5–i11.
26. Mainz J. Defining and classifying clinical indicators for quality improvement. *Int J Qual Health Care.* 2003;15(6):523–530.
27. Iezzoni LI. The risks of risk adjustment. *J Am Med Assoc.* 1997;278: 1600–1607.
28. Thomas WJ, Hofer TP. Accuracy of risk-adjusted mortality rate as a measure of hospital quality of care. *Med Care.* 1999;37(1): 83–92.
29. McLaughlin CP, Kaluzny AD. *Continuous Quality Improvement in Health Care: Theory, Implementation, and Applications.* 2nd ed. Sudbury, MA: Jones & Bartlett; 2004.
30. Schneider PJ. Nutrition support teams: an evidence-based practice. *Nutr Clin Pract.* 2006;21:62–67.
31. Field MJ, Lohr KN, eds. *Clinical Practice Guidelines: Directions for a New Program.* Washington, DC: National Academy Press; 1990.
32. Mead P. Clinical guidelines: promoting clinical effectiveness of a professional minefield? *J Adv Nurs.* 2000;31:110–116.
33. Haycock A, Bagust A, Walley T. Clinical guidelines: the hidden cost. *BMJ.* 1999;318:391–393.
34. Sackett DL, Rosenburg WMC, Gray JAM, Haynes RB, Richardson WS. Evidence based medicine: what it is and what it isn't. *BMJ.* 1996;312:71–72.
35. Woolf SH, Grol R, Hutchinson A, Eccles M, Grimshaw J. Potential benefits, limitations, and harms of clinical guidelines. *BMJ.* 1999;318:527–530.
36. Vanhaecht K, Panella P, van Zelm R, Sermeus W. An overview on the history and concept of care pathways as complex interventions. *Intl J Care Pathw.* 2010;14(3):117–123.
37. Hill M. The development of care management systems to achieve clinical integration. *Adv Pract Nurs Q.* 1998;4(1):33–39.
38. Renholm M, Leino-Kilpi H, Suominen T. Critical pathways. A systematic review. *J Nurs Adm.* 2002 Apr;32(4)196–202.

39. Joint Commission on Perspectives on Patient Safety. Raising the bar with bundles: treating patients with an all-or-nothing standard. *Joint Commission Perspect Patient Safety.* 2006 Apr; 6(4):5–6.
40. Fulbrook P, Mooney S. Care bundles in critical care: a practical approach to evidence-based practice. *Intensive Crit Care Nurs.* 2003;8:249–255.
41. Resar R, Pronovost P, Haraden C, et al. Using a bundle approach to improve ventilator care processes and reduce ventilator-associated pneumonia. *Jt Comm J Qual Patient Saf.* 2005;31(5): 243–248.
42. Institute for Healthcare Improvement. *Implement the IHI ventilator bundle.* http://www.ihi.org/IHI/Topics/CriticalCare/IntensiveCare/Changes/ImplementtheVentilatorBundle.htm. Accessed June 15, 2010.
43. Institute for Healthcare Improvement. *Implement the central line bundle.* http://www.ihi.org/IHI/Topics/CriticalCare/IntensiveCare/Changes/ImplementtheCentralLineBundle.htm. Accessed June 15, 2010.
44. Chaudry B, Wang J, Wu S, et al. Systematic review: impact of health information technology on quality, efficiency, and costs of medical care. *Ann Intern Med.* 2010;144(10):742–752.
45. Langley GJ, Nolan KM, Nolan TW, et al. *The Improvement Guide: A Practical Approach to Enhancing Organizational Performance.* San Francisco, CA: Jossey-Bass; 1996.
46. Leape L, Kabcenell AI, Gandhi TK, et al. Reducing adverse drug events: lessons from a breakthrough collaborative. *Jt Comm J Qual Improv.* 2000;26:321–331.
47. Berwick DM. Harvesting knowledge from improvement. *JAMA.* 1996;275:877–878.
48. Mears P. *Quality Improvement Techniques and Tools.* New York, NY: McGraw-Hill; 1995.
49. Nelson EC, Splaine ME, Batalden PB, Plume SK. Building measurement and data collection into medical practice. *Ann Intern Med.*1998;128(6):460–466.
50. Massoud MR, Nielsen GA, Nolan K, et al. *A Framework for Spread: From Local Improvements to System-Wide Change.* IHI Innovation Series white paper. Cambridge, MA: Institute for Healthcare Improvement; 2006.
51. Nolan K, Schall MW, Erb F, Nolan T. Using a framework for spread: the case of patient access in the Veterans Health Administration. *Jt Comm J Qual Patient Saf.* 2005;31(6):339–347.
52. Chassin MR. Is healthcare ready for Six Sigma quality? *Millbank Q.* 1998; 76(4):565–591.
53. Varkey P, Reller MK, Resar RK. Basics of quality improvement in healthcare. *Mayo Clin Proc.* 2007;82(6):735–739.
54. Vonderheide-Liem DN, Pate B. *Applying Quality Methodologies to Improve Healthcare: Six Sigma, Lean Thinking, Balanced Scorecard, and More.* Marblehead, MA: HCPro, Inc.; 2004.
55. Barry R, Murcko AC, Brubaker CE. *The Six Sigma Book for Healthcare: Improving Outcomes by Reducing Errors.* Chicago, IL: Health Administration Press; 2003.
56. Endsley S, Magill MK, Godfrey MM. Creating a lean practice. *Fam Pract Manag.* 2006;13(4):34–38.
57. Womack J, Jones D. *Lean Thinking.* New York: Simon and Schuster; 1996.
58. Organizational Dynamics Institute Web site. http://orgdynamics.com/tqci.html. Published 2006. Accessed June 15, 2011.
59. Lynn J. When does quality improvement count as research? Human subject protection and theories of knowledge. *Qual Safe Health Care.* 2004;13:67–70.
60. Canadian Institutes of Health Research. About Knowledge Translation. http://www.cihr-irsc.gc.ca/e/29418.html. Published May 8, 2009. Accessed June 15, 2011.
61. Corrigan JF, Donaldson MS, Cohn L, et al., Committee on Quality of Health Care in America. *Crossing the Quality Chasm: A New Health System for the 21st Century.* Washington, DC: National Academy Press; 2001.
62. Joint Commission on Accreditation of Healthcare Organizations. *Comprehensive Accreditation Manual for Hospitals.* Chicago, IL: Joint Commission on Accreditation of Healthcare Organizations; 2007.

41 Application of Research, Derivation of Guidelines, and Evidence-Based Practice

Kelly A. Tappenden, PhD, RD

CONTENTS

Background 694
The Purpose of Evidence-Based Practice 694
How Should Evidence-Based Practice Be Used? 695
How and Where Can Evidence-Based Research Be Found? 696
Clinical Guidelines 696
Challenges of Evidence-Based Practice 697
What Can Be Done to Improve Evidence-Based Practice? 697
References 698

Objectives

1. Describe the essential need for evidence-based practice in the routine care provided by health care professionals.
2. Identify sources of evidence-based research and select those relevant for use in evidence-based practice with specific patients.
3. Distinguish low- and high-quality evidence and how each is used in developing clinical guidelines.
4. Outline the attributes of trustworthy clinical guidelines.

Test Your Knowledge Questions

1. Which of the following are incorporated into evidence-based practice?
   A. Evidence-based research
   B. Clinical expertise
   C. Patient values
   D. All of the above
2. What is the most significant challenge evidence-based practice faces?
   A. Patient concerns are not incorporated.
   B. The best quality evidence is not always obtained.
   C. Time constraints do not allow clinicians to effectively search for evidence.
   D. Randomized, placebo-controlled trials (RCTs) cannot be related to clinical practice.
3. Which of the following evidence is deemed the highest quality?
   A. Case-controlled retrospective review
   B. Randomized, double-blind, placebo-controlled trial
   C. Professional opinion of well-regarded primary physician
   D. Well-documented case series

Test Your Knowledge Answers

1. The correct answer is **D**. Evidence-based practice improves clinical decision making by combining clinical judgment and experience, best available scientific evidence, and patient preferences to improve medical decision making.[1] Interestingly, the definition of evidence-based practice may reflect the manner in which professionals use the process. Some individuals believe clinical expertise should take a higher priority than both evidence and patient values when making a clinical decision.[2] In that case, a definition of clinical expertise must be formulated, which undoubtedly would include both research evidence and patient concerns. Therefore, evidence-based practice relies on the essential integration of these three factors into practice in order to maximize the efficiency of patient care.[3]
2. The correct answer is **C**. Both A and B are actually strengths of evidence-based practice. As the process unfolds, only high quality evidence can be used and patient concerns are an essential aspect of evidence-based practice.[4] Randomized controlled trials (RCTs) are the gold standard of evidence-based research. The results of RCTs are often directly applicable to patients unless methodological flaws, investigator bias, or conflicting evidence are present within the trials.[5] Clearly, time constraints present the most significant challenge; some clinicians believe evidence-based practice is time consuming or they have not invested the time to learn the necessary skills to effectively incorporate evidence-based practice into their daily routine.[6] However, this is a limitation in achieving the best outcomes for their patient(s).
3. The correct answer is **B**. The best form of evidence is a prospective randomized, double-blind, placebo-controlled trial. Considering the enormous amount of research evidence available, electronic sources may be considered the "current best" because of search options, high speed, and accessibility.[7] Looking in a textbook or a journal for the answer to a detailed question could require multiple volumes of research as well as hours, if not days, of reading, and this information may not even represent the most updated research available. Typing keywords into a search engine, on the other hand, can retrieve thousands of abstracted articles, and publish dates and contact information. Ultimately, using well-developed, trustworthy clinical guidelines provides a peer-reviewed strategy for determining evidence-based best practices.

Background

Although clinical trials have been conducted for decades, interest in evidence-based practice (EBP) has grown exponentially since its formal introduction in 1992,[8] and the definition continues to evolve. EBP (also called evidence-based medicine) requires integration of the best research evidence with clinical expertise, and the patient's unique values and circumstances.[7] However, more specific descriptions of EBP not only stress the importance of examining evidence from clinical research trials, but at the same time, discouraging methods that rely on intuition, unsystematic clinical experience, and pathophysiologic rationale as sufficient grounds for clinical decision making.[9] Clearly, one definition cannot perfectly elucidate the critical meaning of EBP to all members of the health care team, including clinicians, patients, researchers, policy makers, and payers. However, as Figure 41-1 demonstrates, this process provides each stakeholder with a method for incorporating valid scientific evidence, clinical expertise, and patients' values.[10]

FIGURE 41-1 Components of Evidence-Based Practice (EBP).[10]

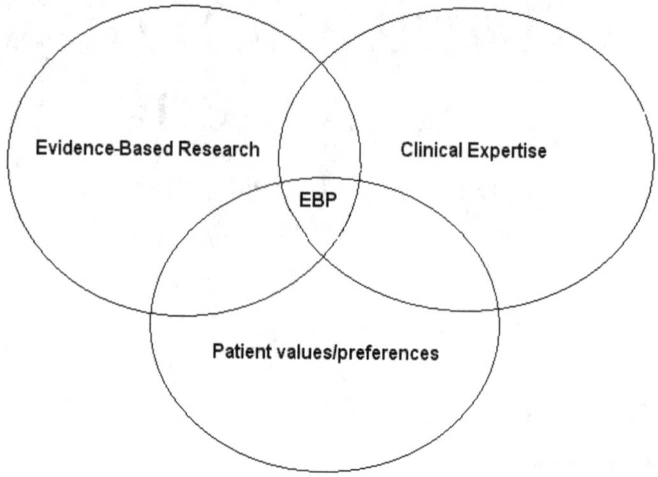

The Purpose of Evidence-Based Practice

EBP aims to improve patient outcomes by providing clinicians with the highest grade evidence available, which facilitates informed decisions regarding the distribution of limited resources and the application of clinical practice techniques.[9] The consistent flow of new research into the clinical setting allows for the application of new therapies to patients and reduces the reliance on long-standing, but sometimes suboptimal, treatment methods. Therefore, EBP helps clinicians maximize their *effectiveness* (adequacy to accomplish a purpose) and *efficiency* (production of the desired effect with minimal waste of time, effort, or skill) both clinically and economically. The advantages garnered by the use of EBP have increased the demand for high quality research, online databases, and Internet search engines that provide access to quality evidence libraries for the convenient incorporation of EBP into clinicians' daily routines.

EBP has influenced the science and practice of clinical nutrition. Various evidence-based clinical practice guidelines for the provision of nutrition support have been developed and can be found published in the *Journal of Parenteral and Enteral Nutrition*. A recent report evaluating the impact of routine administration of these evidence-based clinical guidelines indicates that intensive care units that adhered more consistently to the Canadian Clinical Practice Guidelines were more likely to feed patients successfully with enteral nutrition (EN).[3] The prevalence of EBP in specialized nutrition support is not well studied. However, among pediatric dietitians working in Australian teaching hospitals, survey results indicate that although the majority of dietitians strongly believe in the philosophy of EBP, almost three-quarters of them failed to integrate the principles into their practice.[6] Within the field of clinical nutrition, leadership is needed to enhance the teaching and implementation of EBP.

How Should Evidence-Based Practice Be Conducted?

To properly implement EBP, Straus and colleagues[7] developed a system of steps that serve as a basis for the following process (Table 41-1).

Step 1: ***Ask.*** To find relevant clinical research, the desired answers must be defined by concise, searchable questions. These questions fall into one of two categories that address either background or foreground information. Background questions involve general knowledge; for example, the history of the patient, disease, and available treatments. The questions can be answered by studying the patient history or by consulting a review paper or textbook that addresses the patient's medical condition. Foreground questions demand more specific knowledge and require the formulation of a question with four parts: the patient, intervention, comparison, and outcomes. Given the vast body of scientific literature that exists, it is essential for this knowledge to be distilled down to the smallest number of studies that hold relevance to the care of the individual patients. As such, a critical feature of the literature review involves formulating relevant, focused questions that identify key factors that impact clinical outcomes, as well as any potential interactions between factors that might exist.[11]

Step 2: ***Find quality evidence.*** Armed with the right questions, clinicians should stratify the evidence within the scientific literature based on the quality of study design within each report. The highest quality of evidence must be used (Table 41-2). Evidence obtained from properly randomized, controlled trials (RCTs) minimizes bias and is least likely to be misleading, thus it is considered the gold standard for EBP.[9] Evidence obtained from well-designed controlled trials without randomization is the next grade of evidence. Data obtained from well-designed cohort or case-control analytic studies, preferably from more than one center or research group, fall farther down the hierarchy. The lowest quality of evidence, among primary reports of new data, is that from multiple time series or uncontrolled experiments. Finally, reports that synthesize or reflect on the collection of other primary reports (ie, meta-analysis, cost-benefit analyses, review articles, consensus statements) or expert opinion should be viewed as a separate class of evidence with the least substantiation for application in EBP.

Step 3: ***Assess.*** Equally important as finding good evidence-based research is assessing the validity and quality of the information.[12] The validity can be assessed by examining the existence of fundamental criteria within the study design such as an independent blind comparison, a relevant and appropriate patient population, a reference standard, and repetition (by independent groups) of the study. The sensitivity and specificity of the intervention should be considered wherein *sensitivity* refers to the proportion of the patients with the disease who show a positive result and *specificity* is the proportion of patients without the disease who have a negative result.

Step 4: ***Integrate.*** Central to EBP is the integration of clinical expertise, patient values, and the best research evidence into the decision-making process. At this point, the clinician must decide if the evidence is applicable to the patient. Clearly, the evidence being contemplated must be relevant to your clinical scenario—one must ensure that the inclusion and exclusion criteria of the evidence apply to the clinical care of the specific patient in question.

Step 5: ***Evaluate.*** Keeping in mind the intentions of EBP—to allow clinicians to find answers to questions that are not readily available and to keep up to date with scientific advances in clinical care[13]—it is essential to continually review one's own implementation of EBP. Essential elements of this review involve a self-assessment of both the process and the outcomes of EBP. To evaluate the *effectiveness* of an intervention, clinicians should keep summaries available to determine if outcomes are improving with a change in practice. Whereas an evaluation of *efficiency* of the EBP process should include an assessment of the clinician's skill in asking critical questions; finding valid and important evidence; and integrating their expertise with research and patient preference.

TABLE 41-1 Evidence-Based Practice Steps

Step 1	**Ask** clinical questions that will be answered with evidence-based research.
Step 2	**Find** the best evidence-based research relating to the specific concern.
Step 3	**Assess** the research for validity, impact, and applicability.
Step 4	**Integrate** the research with clinical expertise and patient circumstances.
Step 5	**Evaluate** both the effectiveness and efficiency of the steps.

TABLE 41-2 Grading the Quality of Evidence[a]

Levels of Evidence	Type of Evidence
I	Large randomized trials with clear-cut results; low risk of false-positive and/or false-negative error
II	Small randomized trials with uncertain results; moderate risk of false-positive and/or false-negative error
III	Nonrandomized cohort with contemporaneous controls
IV	Nonrandomized cohort with historical controls
V	Case series, uncontrolled studies, and expert opinion

[a]Table 2. Grading System. Used with permission from Dellinger RP, Carlet JM, Masur H. Introduction. *Crit Care Med.* 2004;32(suppl 11):S446.

To enhance their implementation of the EBP process, clinicians may benefit from reviewing the information found at the Centre for Evidence Based Medicine based at the University of Oxford (http://www.cebm.net/). This Web-based resource aims to promote evidence-based health care by offering overviews on study design, statistics, and asking focused clinical questions. A particularly useful resource is entitled "EBM Tools," which includes educational resources and step-by-step processes for:

- Asking focused clinical questions
- Finding the evidence
- Critical appraisal
- Making a decision
- Evaluating performance
- Designing research

TABLE 41-3 Grading of Guidelines[a]

Grade	Criteria
A	Supported by at least 2 Level I[b] investigations
B	Supported by one Level I[b] investigation
C	Supported by at least one Level II[b] investigation
D	Supported by one Level III[b] investigation
E	Supported by Level IV[b] or V[b] evidence

[a]Table 2. Grading System. Used with permission from Dellinger RP, Carlet JM, Masur H. Introduction. *Crit Care Med.* 2004;32(suppl 11):S446.
[b]Level of evidence as outlined in Table 41-2.

How and Where Can Evidence-Based Research Be Found?

When searching for evidence to apply in the clinical setting, quality, accessibility, and clinical relevance are essential factors. The current gold standard of evidence, as previously discussed, is the RCT. The key question centers on where can this evidence be easily and quickly located in order to effectively apply it in a clinical setting? To bridge the gap between research and practice, evidence must be readily available for use in practice. Keeping up with the literature is time consuming. Estimates suggest that to keep up to date with the current research, clinicians must read approximately 200 articles per month from 10 specialized journals.[14] After evidence is found, clinicians must then take time to determine if it is applicable to individual patients, an essential step that is often overlooked.

In the most ideal situation, relevant evidence will be attached to patient records or available before the patient visit. This would enable clinicians to quickly obtain the best evidence, assess it, and decide whether or not to use it in a case-by-case process. The only foreseeable option for this process would entail electronic patient records and compatible electronic databases that could sort and assess evidence in relation to patient relevance.[7] An electronic system, as described previously, is not yet available; however, many alternative strategies for searching for evidence exist, such as is available at *pubmed.gov*.

Clinical Guidelines

The movement toward evidence-based practice has resulted in the proliferation of clinical guidelines (CGs) such that there were 2700 clinical practice guidelines in the Agency for Healthcare Research and Quality's National Guideline Clearinghouse in spring 2011. Worldwide, the Guidelines International Network's Database contained more than 7000 CG documents at that time. As such, users were faced with the decision regarding which CG to trust and implement within their own practice.

The Institute of Medicine (IOM) released a consensus report titled, "Clinical Practice Guidelines We Can Trust" in the spring of 2011.[15] The committee contends that the *development process* is a serious weakness of most guidelines in clinical use. Further, to be trustworthy, the authors contend that CG development should:

- Be based on a systematic review of the literature
- Be developed by a group of multidisciplinary experts, including representatives of key affected groups
- Consider patient subgroups and preferences, as appropriate
- Use an explicit and transparent process aimed to minimize distortions, biases, and conflicts of interest
- Discuss alternative care options and health options, including ratings for both the quality of evidence (Table 41-2) and the strength of recommendations (Table 41-3)
- Be reconsidered and revised as warranted by new evidence

The A.S.P.E.N. CG and Standard initiative are strongly aligned with these criteria. Rather than publishing a single, all-encompassing compendium of guideline recommendations, A.S.P.E.N. now publishes CGs focused on specific nutrition support practices in age and diagnostic groups. Further, the American Society for Parenteral and Enteral Nutrition (A.S.P.E.N.) has adopted the recommendations of a working group for the Grading of Recommendations, Assessment, Development, and Evaluations (GRADE),[16] with modifications needed for nutrition support research while continuing A.S.P.E.N.'s multidisciplinary working team approach. The inclusion of patient-level opinions regarding some key guideline questions should be considered for future CGs.

Based on the IOM report criteria, the CG process should include ratings for both the quality of evidence (Table 41-2) and the strength of each recommendation (Table 41-3). A rigorous review and approval process safeguards the quality of the process. Poor quality evidence can result in recommendations that are not in the patients' best interests; therefore, users know the strength of a recommendation before implementing it. Although many systems exist for grading evidence and recommendations, a particularly strong system has been developed by the GRADE working group.[16] This system is an excellent resource for those seeking to use EBP, as it is freely available for use at http://www.gradeworkinggroup.org/ and includes tutorials and software resources that directly interact with the Cochrane Collaboration (http://www.cochrane.org/). The Cochrane Collaboration is an international network whose vision is to provide the best evidence for health care.

Challenges of Evidence-Based Practice

Although the benefits of EBP are well established, potential downfalls do exist. The limitations of EBP fall into two general categories: quality and restrictions. Quality of EBP relates to both evidence and patient care. The ever-expanding bank of evidence requires an ongoing critical analysis of the quality of the obtained evidence. Key examples of questionable evidence include outdated or unrevised evidence, irreproducible protocols, missing references, incomplete trials, and unsupported claims.[7] Furthermore, not every subspecialty has sufficient high-quality evidence available to support a thorough search.

Patient care quality concerns also arise when contemplating EBP. Critics of the process argue that EBP is a step further away from patient-centered practice.[17] Although an imbalance between evidence, expertise, and patient concerns could potentially have a negative impact on patient care, clinicians must strive to integrate each of these essential components equally when implementing EBP. EBP begins with a patient-centered question and ends with a decision about whether or not the available evidence applies in the specific clinical circumstances surrounding the patient. These steps help to ensure that EBP does not lose sight of the patient.

Other clinicians find that EBP restricts both clinical freedom and time.[18] Clinical freedom, doing all that is medically necessary without interference, can be restricted by EBP. As evidence suggests changes in practice, some techniques and treatments must be abandoned. Clinicians and patients may not be able to freely choose which procedure to follow, but rather, evidence will drive the decisions. Some believe that as clinicians face large amounts of research without sufficient time to review all of it, they will be forced to selectively choose evidence that agrees with their beliefs. Clearly, this is not the goal of EBP, but is indeed a reality of the process that must be guarded against.

To be widely adopted, implementation of nutrition guidelines should be done with a strategy recognizing the institutional culture and the characteristics of the patient, provider, and guideline. To this end, investigations are necessary to enhance our understanding regarding how institutional culture influences guideline implementation, and which organizational change strategies might be most effective in optimizing nutrition therapy.[19]

What Can Be Done to Improve Evidence-Based Practice?

To maximize the efficiency of EBP, more directly relevant sources are needed. The quality of the evidence needs to be filtered, and the specificity of clinical topics needs to increase. The sources also need to be readily available to clinicians. Computers, books, journals, and online sources must be located where they will be used in the clinical setting. Further, restrictions of sources, such as the costs of subscription, need to be lifted to make evidence available to the public and professionals. Although EBP has been a topic of increasing discussions for nearly 20 years, advancements occur every year and diligent leadership is needed among researchers and clinicians for both the teaching and the practice of EBP.

Practice Scenarios 41-1 and 41-2 present clinical questions and scenarios whereby the EBP application of nutrition support practice interventions are the basis for clinical nutrition interventions.

Practice Scenario 41-1

Question: In adult patients following a massive small bowel resection, what are the goals of nutrition therapy?

Scenario: A 29-year-old female with a history of irritable bowel syndrome followed by a diagnosis of Crohn's disease (see Chapter 26) 3 years ago has been prescribed regimens of azulfidine, corticosteroids, antibiotics, and most recently, azathioprine. She presented with complaints of nausea and vomiting, fever, constipation, and abdominal pain. At that time, she admitted that she did not always follow her prescribed regimen and feels it is only necessary when she experiences discomfort. Her height is 152 cm. The patient reports an unwanted weight loss of 18 pounds from a weight of 115 pounds 8 months ago. A physical examination revealed abdominal tenderness in the upper left quadrant and audible bowel sounds. A computed tomography (CT) scan and an esophagogastroduodenoscopy revealed a small bowel obstruction and exacerbation of Crohn's disease. She underwent an enterectomy of 200 cm of distal jejunum and ileum with the preservation of her ileocecal valve and the entire colon. A jejunostomy tube was placed. Following surgery, parenteral nutrition was initiated, and the nutrition support team was consulted.

Intervention: A review of the literature needs to be conducted to identify the available evidence-based guidelines relevant to the question posed in this scenario.

Answer: Although the beginning steps of the research process should be broad and should survey many available sources, the ultimate goal should be to obtain the best possible evidence that is relevant to this patient. The advanced search options within online database resources include many categories including publication type, focus area, language, gender, age groups, grade of evidence, and animal study type. In order to most efficiently carry out the proposed search, the results should be limited using these filtering options. For example, at the time of publication, using the search terms "nutrition" and "short bowel syndrome" in pubmed.gov yielded 479 reports. Clearly, this is too many reviews and many of them do not apply to the specific patients, are original research reports of limited scope, or are opinion pieces that have not used defined methodology for assessing the quality of the evidence. However, refining the search to use more specific search terms, such as "tube feeding," "short-bowel syndrome," and "evidence-based guidelines" reduces the articles cited to just 4, from which the ESPEN Guidelines on Enteral Nutrition: Gastroenterology[20] are easily found. Within this document, evidence-based guidelines outlining the goals of nutrition therapy and relevant best practices are easily found.

Rationale: After reviewing the most appropriate evidence-based guidelines for optimizing nutrition support in adult patients with a massive small bowel resection, efforts can now be focused on developing a care plan and consulting the colleagues necessary to educate and support the patient as she transitions onto her new therapeutic diet.

Practice Scenario 41-2

Question: In adult patients with acute pancreatitis secondary to alcohol intake, what form of nutrition support will optimize the clinical outcome?

Scenario: A 32-year-old African American male is diagnosed with acute pancreatitis. He has a family history of pancreatitis, and both his father and grandfather suffer from chronic abdominal pain and recurrent bouts of pancreatitis. He is currently not on medications and has no allergies to medications. The patient complains of epigastric pain, nausea, vomiting, diarrhea, anorexia, and unintentional weight loss of 20 pounds from 1 year ago. A physical examination reveals a temperature of 100.6°F, a height measured at 6 feet and 1 inch, a current weight of 150 pounds, and abdominal tenderness. Following a biochemical assessment, he is diagnosed with acute pancreatitis secondary to alcohol intake.

Intervention: Discussions with several colleagues reveal various opinions on the appropriate approach ranging from no nutrition support, the initiation of nasojejunal feedings, to parenteral nutrition. However, clinicians committed to evidence-based practice will review the evidence to answer the question posed, rather than survey their colleagues. As clinicians become proficient with evidence-based practice, navigating online databases and identifying relevant specialty journals becomes easier. Using focused search terms, as outlined in the example previously, and reviewing the current available evidence by experts within this field, the clinician determines that trustworthy practice guidelines for acute pancreatitis are in the Guidelines for the Provision and Assessment of Nutrition Support Therapy in the Adult Critically Ill Patient.[21] Therefore, following admission, the team initiates early enteral nutrition with continuous infusion (Grade: C) of a partially hydrolyzed low triglyceride elemental formula (Grade: E) via a nasojejunal (Grade: C) feeding tube, armed with the assurance that an excellent clinical choice has been made based on the best available evidence.

Answer: Using focused search terms and reviewing the current available evidence by experts within this field, the clinician determines that trustworthy practice guidelines for acute pancreatitis are in the Guidelines for the Provision and Assessment of Nutrition Support Therapy in the Adult Critically Ill Patient.[21] Therefore, following admission, the team initiates early enteral nutrition with continuous infusion (Grade: C) of a partially hydrolyzed low triglyceride elemental formula (Grade: E) via a nasojejunal (Grade: C) feeding tube, armed with the assurance that an excellent clinical choice has been made based on the best available evidence.

Rationale: Review of current guidelines clearly indicates the appropriate course of action and allows the clinician to proceed with confidence that the proposed care plan is consistent with the best available evidence.

References

1. Rizzo JD. Evidence-based medicine: Can it be applied to stimulation of erythropoiesis for patients with malignancy? *Best Pract Res Clin Haematol.* 2005;18:439–448.
2. Haynes RB, Devereaux PJ, Guyatt GH. Clinical expertise in the era of evidence-based medicine and patient choice. *Vox Sang.* 2002; 83(Suppl 1):383–386.
3. Heyland DK, Dhaliwal R, Day A, et al. Validation of the Canadian clinical practice guidelines for nutrition support in mechanically ventilated, critically ill adult patients: Results of a prospective observational study. *Crit Care Med.* 2004;32: 2260–2206.
4. Sackett DL, Rosenberg WM, Gray JA. Evidence based medicine: What it is and what it isn't. *BMJ.* 1996;312:71–72.
5. Feagan BG, Sachar D. What do I do in my practice that isn't evidence based? *Inflamm Bowel Dis.* 2002;8:422–425.
6. Thomas DE, Kukuruzovic R, Martino B, et al. Knowledge and use of evidence-based nutrition: A survey of paediatric dietitians. *J Hum Nutr Diet.* 2003;16:315–322.
7. Straus S, Richardson WS, Glasziou P, Haynes RB. *Evidence-Based Medicine: How to Practice and Teach EBM.* 3rd ed. London, England: Elsevier Churchill Livingstone; 2005.
8. Evidence-Based Medicine Working Group. Evidence-based medicine. A new approach to teaching the practice of medicine. *JAMA.* 1992;268:2420–2425.
9. Jennings BM, Loan LA. Misconceptions among nurses about evidence-based practice. *J Nurs Scholarsh.* 2001;33:121–127.
10. Haynes RB. What kind of evidence is it that evidence-based medicine advocates want health care providers and consumers to pay attention to? *BMC Health Serv Res.* 2002;2:3.
11. Scientific Affairs and Research. *American Dietetic Association Evidence Analysis Manual, Edition IV.* Chicago, IL: American Dietetic Association; 2003.
12. Concato J, Shah N, Horwitz RI. Randomized, controlled trials, observational studies, and the hierarchy of research designs. *N Engl J Med.* 2000;342:1887–1892.
13. Zakowski L, Seibert C, VanEyck S. Evidence-based medicine: Answering questions of diagnosis. *Clin Med Res.* 2004;2:63–69.
14. Straus SE, Sackett DL. Bringing evidence to the clinic. *Arch Dermatol.* 1998;134:1519–1520.
15. Institute of Medicine. *Clinical Practice Guidelines We Can Trust.* Washington, D.C.: National Academies Press; 2011.
16. Guyatt GH, Oxman AD, Vist G, et al. GRADE: an emerging consensus on rating quality of evidence and strength of recommendations. *BMJ.* 2008;336:924–926.
17. Nolan MR. Reconciling tensions between research, evidence-based practice and user participation: time for nursing to take the lead. *Int J Nurs Stud.* 2005;42:503–505.
18. Wormald R, Oldfield K. Evidence based medicine, the Cochrane Collaboration, and the CONSORT statement. *Br J Ophthalmol.* 1998;82:597–598.
19. Dodek P, Cahol NE, Heyland DK. The relationship between organizational culture and implementation of clinical practice guidelines: a narrative review. *JPEN J Parenter Enteral Nutr.* 2010;34(6): 669–674.
20. Van Gossum A, Cabre E, Hébuterne X, et al. ESPEN Guidelines on Parenteral Nutrition: gastroenterology. *Clin Nutr.* 2009;28: 415–427.
21. McClave SA, Martindale, RG, Vanek VW, et al. Guidelines for the provision and assessment of nutrition support therapy in the adult critically ill patient. *J Parenter Enteral Nutr.* 2009;33: 277–316.

Index

Page numbers followed by *f* or *t* indicate figures or tables, respectively.

A
AAD. *See* antibiotic-associated diarrhea
abdominal distention, 220
absorption, 17. *See also* digestion
  apparent, 305
  carbohydrate, 17, 39–40, 40*f*
  electrolyte, 18
  lipid, 17–18
  mechanisms, 17
  medium-chain triglyceride, 18
  mineral, 18
  protein, 17, 87–88, 87*f*
  short-chain fatty acid (SCFA), 18
  vitamin, 18
  water, 18
access devices. *See* enteral access devices; parenteral access devices
ACDs. *See* automated compounding devices
acid–base balance, 114–115, 115*t*, 503
acid–base disorders
  analysis, 115
  characteristics, 117*t*
  compensation, 117*t*
  high anion-gap acidosis, 117
  metabolic acidosis, 116, 116*t*
  metabolic alkalosis, 116*t*, 118
  normal anion-gap acidosis, 117
  respiratory acidosis, 115, 116*t*
  respiratory alkalosis, 116, 116*t*
  saline-responsive metabolic alkalosis, 118
  saline-unresponsive metabolic alkalosis, 118
acid-base monitoring, pregnancy, 340
acidosis
  high anion-gap, 117
  hyperchloremic, 117
  metabolic, 116, 116*t*
  normal anion-gap, 117
  respiratory, 115, 116*t*
acute hypocalcemia, treatment, 111*t*
acute kidney injury (AKI), 493–494, 493*t*
acute lung injury (ALI), 414
acute pancreatitis. *See* pancreatitis, acute
acute pulmonary failure, 414
acute respiratory distress syndrome (ARDS), 196–197, 197*t*, 414, 417*f*
acute wound healing, 350–351, 350*f*, 351*f*
acutely ill patients, energy expenditure, 30
adjunctive therapies, critical injury, 404–405
admixtures
  preparation, quality control, 255
  total nutrient, intravenous fat emulsion and, 256–258
  total nutrient *vs.* dextrose-amino acids, 252–253, 253*t*
adolescent females, energy requirements
  lactation, 341*t*
  pregnancy, 334*t*
adult females, energy requirements
  lactation, 341*t*
  pregnancy, 334*t*
advance directives, 668–669, 669*t*
advanced dementia, 623, 627, 659
adverse event reporting, 321–322
advertising, 320–321
aerobic exercise, HIV-associated lipodystrophy syndrome and, 555
afferent limb syndrome, 430
AKI. *See* acute kidney injury
alcohol content, common libations, 482*t*
alcoholic hepatitis, 457–458
alcoholic liver disease (ALD), 457
ALI. *See* acute lung injury
alkaline reflux gastritis, 430
alkalosis
  metabolic, 116*t*, 118
  respiratory, 116, 116*t*
  saline-responsive metabolic, 118
  saline-unresponsive metabolic, 118
aloe vera, 322
alternative nutrients, liver disease, 465–467
aluminum contamination control, 259–262
aluminum toxicity, 294
amino acids, 84–85, 86*t*
  absorption, 89*f*
  branched-chain, liver disease and, 467
  conditionally essential, 95
  functions, 86*t*
  parenteral nutrition (PN) and, 247*t*, 250
  structures, 85*f*
  supplements, wound healing, 356
  wound healing, 356
anabolic steroids, 570
anabolic–androgenic steroids, 548–550
anemia, 430
ANH. *See* artificial nutrition/hydration
anorexia nervosa, 159
anthropometrics
  critical injury, 396–397
  liver disease, 462
  nutrition assessment, 162
antibiotic-associated diarrhea (AAD), 57
antidumping diet, 429*t*
antimicrobial technology, catheters, 275–276
antioxidants
  critical injury, 404–405
  liver disease and, 465–466
  sepsis and, 387
antiretroviral medications, 540–541, 541*t*
apparent absorption, 305
appetite changes, cancer, 566
appetite stimulants, cancer therapy, 570–571
ARDS. *See* acute respiratory distress syndrome
arginine
  critical injury, 404
  in sepsis, 386–387
  in wound healing, 353–356
arteriovenous amino acid differences across organs, 91

artificial nutrition/hydration (ANH)
advanced dementia, 659
analysis, 664
palliative care, 658
practice scenario, 658
precedent cases, 668
vegetative state, 659–661, 660*f*, 660*t*
ascites, 159–160, 632–633
ascorbic acid, 131
aspiration
enteral nutrition (EN), 179, 224–226
ventilator-associated pneumonia (VAP), 420–422, 421*f*, 422*t*
atrophy, mucosal, 18–19
automated compounding devices (ACDs), 254–255
azotemia, 287

B
bacterial overgrowth, small bowel (SBBO), 436–437, 437*t*
bag characteristics, drug-nutrient interactions, 305
bariatric enteral formulations, 200–201
bariatric surgery, 610–611
indications, contraindications, 610*f*
nutritional assessment, 611–612, 612*t*
supplementation, 612*t*
basal metabolic rate (BMR), 23–24
basal-bolus insulin therapy, 589*t*, 591–592, 591*f*
behavioral treatment, obesity, 609
betaine, 466
bezoars, 434
bile secretion, 14–15
biochemical measures, critical injury, 397
bioethics, 661
biosynthesis, eicosanoid, 73–74
biotin, 136
blood circulation, splanchnic, 15–16
blood gas values, normal, 114–115, 115*t*
bloodstream infections, parenteral access devices, 276–279
BMR. *See* basal metabolic rate
body composition assessment tools, 162, 163–164*t*
body fluids. *See* fluid(s)
body weight, nutrition assessment, 162
bolus feeding, 176
bone disease, metabolic, 292–293, 431
bone loss-associated diseases, 293*t*
bowel rest, 18–19
β-oxidation, fatty acid, 68
brain, central nervous system role, protein breakdown, 93
branched-chain amino acids, 467
bundles. *See* care bundles
burn patient, *practice scenario*, 397–399
burns, 406

C
calcium
hypercalcemia, 112
hypocalcemia, 111–112, 111*t*
intravenous, shortage, *practice scenario*, 249
metabolic bone disease and, 293
phosphate and, 258–259, 258*t*
in renal failure (RF), 503
supplements, 112*t*
calorie malnutrition, chronic pancreatitis and, 482–483
calories
impaired intake with cancer, 566–567
requirements
Crohn's disease, 440
diabetes mellitus, 593
estimates, accuracy factors, 25*t*
pregnancy, 333–334
cancer
malnutrition with
etiology, 565
impaired caloric intake, 566–567
malabsorption, 567
maldigestion, 567
metabolic alterations, 565–566
prevalence, 564–565
significance, 565
nutritional therapies
colon, rectal cancer, 574–575
enteral, 568–569
esophageal cancer, 112–114, 573
graft-*vs.*-host disease (GVHD), 576
gynecologic cancer, 575
head, neck cancer, 572–573
hematopoietic stem cell transplantation, 575–576
during palliative care, 576–577
pancreatic cancer, 574
parenteral nutrition (PN), 240
practice scenarios, 112–114, 573, 576
stomach cancer, 573–574
total parenteral, 569
tumor growth effect, 572
taste changes with, 566
trends, impact, 564
cancer pharmacotherapy, 569
appetite stimulants
corticosteroids, 570–571
cytokine inhibitors, 571–572
symptom relief drugs, 572
hormones, 569–570
cannabinoids, 571
carbamazepine, 309
carbohydrate metabolism
with cancer, 565
gluconeogenesis, 42–43
gluconeogenic pathway, 44*f*
glucose transporters, 40–41
glycogenesis, glycogenolysis and, 43–45
glycolysis, 41
glycolytic pathway, 42*f*
precursor formation, other metabolites, 45
pyruvate–lactate pathway, 41–42
sepsis, 379–380
tricarboxylic acid cycle, 41
carbohydrate(s), 37
absorption, 17, 39–40, 40*f*
background, 37
classification, 37–39
critical injury requirements, 400–401
digestion, 16, 39–40, 39*f*
enteral formulations, 186
exercise requirements, 49
gestational diabetes mellitus and, *practice scenario*, 47
healthy adult requirements, 48–49
illness, injury requirements, 49
parenteral nutrition (PN) risk factor, 290
plasma glucose homeostasis, 45–48, 45*f*, 46*f*
pregnancy requirements, 334–335
sepsis, requirements, 385
cardiovascular disease, 555–557
care bundles, 278, 685
care pathways, 684–685
carnitine
parenteral nutrition (PN) formulations, 252
parenteral nutrition (PN) risk factor, 291
renal replacement therapy (RRT), 505
cART. *See* combination antiretroviral therapy
catheter-related bloodstream infection (CRBSI), 266
catheter-related bloodstream infection (CRBSI), *practice scenario*, 278–279
catheters
antimicrobial technology, 275–276
care, postinsertion, 213
central venous, 271*f*, 272*f*, 274*t*, 275
hub care, 274
infections, 277*t*
insertion, 272–273
insertion site maintenance, 273–274
materials, 275–276
occluded central, *practice scenario*, 280
patency, 274–275, 280
percutaneous nontunneled, 268, 270*f*
stabilization, 275
technology, 275–276
vascular access, 269*t*
Catholic values, beliefs, 665–666

celiac disease (CD), 437–438
associated disorders, 438*t*
clinical features, 438*t*
dermatitis herpetiformis, 438
diagnosis, 438
nutrition implications, 438
nutritional management, 439–440
patient management, 439*t*
refractory, 439
resources, 440*t*
similar symptom conditions, 439*t*
small bowel biopsy, 438–439
central parenteral nutrition (CPN), 236
central venous access, 268, 273*f*
central venous catheters, 271*f*, 272*f*, 274*t*, 275
central *vs.* peripheral access, 268
chemical buffers, acid-base balance, 114–115
cholestasis, 291–292
cholestatic liver disease, 460
choline, 136–137, 291
chromium, 145–146
chronic critical illness, 415
chronic disease–associated malnutrition syndrome, 159–160
chronic kidney disease (CKD), 494–495, 495*t*
chronic liver disease
energy expenditure, 461
malnutrition and, 460–461
metabolism, 461–462
practice scenario, 463–464
chronic pancreatitis. *See* pancreatitis, chronic
chronic pulmonary failure, 414–415
chronic wound healing, 351–352, 351*f*
chyle, 631, 632*t*, 633–634
chylothorax, 632
background, 631
etiology, 632, 633*t*
lymphatic system, 631–632
nutrition management, 634–635
chylous ascites, 632–633
background, 631
etiology, 633, 633*t*
lymphatic system, 631–632
nutrition management, 634–635
practice scenario, 635–636
chylous effusions, 635
cirrhosis, 456. *See also* liver disease
malnutrition causes in, 460*t*
nutritional therapy, 464*t*
practice scenario, 159–160
vitamin, mineral deficiencies complicating, 467
CKD. *See* chronic kidney disease
clinical monitoring, home nutrition support, 649
clinical practice guidelines (CPGs), quality improvement (QI), 684
clinical research *vs.* quality improvement (QI), 690
clinician's role
dietary supplements, 324–325
home nutrition support, 651–652
micronutrient management, 147–148
clogging prevention, catheter, 213
cobalamin, 134–135
colitis, ulcerative, 441
colon, disorders. *See* small bowel, colon diseases/disorders
colon, rectal cancer, 574–575
colorectal motility, 10
combination antiretroviral therapy (cART), 537
compensated liver disease, 462–463
compensation, acid–base disorders, 117*t*
complementary nutrients, liver disease, 465–467
complex trauma patient, 397–399
compounded sterile parenteral nutrient preparations, 253–254, 254*t*
compounding devices, 254–255
compounding limitations, *practice scenario*, 257–258
computed tomography grading system, 474*t*
computed tomography severity index, 475*t*
conditionally essential amino acids, 95
conscience clauses, 666
constipation, 13
enteral nutrition (EN) and, 224
pregnant trauma patient, *practice scenario*, 343
contamination
aluminum, 259–262
enteral nutrition (EN), 180–181, 222–223
continuous infusion, 175
copper, 142–143, 294
corticosteroids, 570–571
CPGs. *See* clinical practice guidelines
CPN. *See* central parenteral nutrition
Cr. *See* chromium
CRBSI. *See* catheter-related bloodstream infections
critically ill patient
adjunctive therapies, 403–405
background, 393
burns, 406
carbohydrate requirements, 400–401
chronic, 415
complex burn, *practice scenario*, 397–399
energy expenditure, 29–30
energy requirements, 396*f*, 398–399*t*, 399–400
enteral nutrition (EN), *practice scenario*, 178
fat requirements, 401
feeding access, 403
fluid, electrolyte requirements, 401–402, 401*t*
formula selection/immunonutrition, 405–406
malnutrition, 395–396
mineral requirements, 402
nutrition assessment
biochemical measures, 397
practice scenario, 405
screening, anthropometrics and, 396–397
nutrition requirements, 399
nutrition support route, 402–403
obese
impact, 613
intensive care unit mortality, 612–613
nutrition delivery impact, 614–615
nutritional assessment, 613–614
parenteral nutrition (PN), 240
perioperative nutrition provision, 406
probiotics, 57–58
protein requirements, 94–95, 396*f*, 400
protein requirements, *practice scenario*, 90–91
selenium, 144–145
selenium, practice scenario, 144–145
severity, 394
trace element requirements, 402
transitioning to oral, 403
traumatic brain injury (TBI), *practice scenario*, 368–369
vitamin requirements, 402
Crohn's disease, 440–442
Cruzan case, artificial nutrition/hydration (ANH), 668
Cu. *See* copper
cultural values, 664
cyclic feeding, 175
cyclic infusion, hepatobiliary complications, 292
cyproheptadine, 571
cytokine inhibitors, 571–572

D

dating guidelines, compounded sterile parenteral nutrient preparations, 254*t*
decisional capacity, 662
decompensated liver disease, 464
dehydration, enteral nutrition (EN) and, 229–230
delayed gastric emptying. *See* gastroparesis (GP)

delivery environment, drug-nutrient interactions, 306–307
delivery methods, enteral nutrition (EN), 175–176
delivery site factors, drug-nutrient interactions, 305–306
dementia, 623, 627, 659
depression with cancer, 566–567
dermatitis herpetiformis, 438
dextrose-amino acids *vs.* total nutrient admixtures, 252–253, 253*t*
diabetes insipidus, causes, 106*t*
diabetes mellitus, 47, 581–582
  classification, 582–583
  diagnosis, 582, 582*t*
  enteral nutrition (EN), 594–595, 595*t*
    continuous feeding, 596
    delivery, 595–596
    formulations, 189–190, 191*t*
    insulin therapy during, 596–597
    intermittent feeding, 596–597
    nutrition, 594–595, 595*t*
    practice scenarios, 190–192, 597
  gestational, 47, 583, 584*t*
  hospitalized patients, medications, 587–588
    intravenous insulin therapy, 588–590, 590*t*, 591*f*
    subcutaneous insulin injections, 589*t*, 590–592
  hyperglycemia and, complications, 585
    glycemia measurement, 585
    glycemic control, 585–586, 587*t*
    hospitalized patient outcomes, 586
    hospitalized patient targets, 586–587, 587*t*
  hypoglycemia, 587
  nutrition assessment, 592–593
    calorie requirements, 593
    electrolytes, 593
    gastroparesis, 594
    oral diet, 593–594
    protein requirements, 593
  parenteral nutrition (PN), 598–599, 600*t*
  pathophysiology, 582
    prediabetic conditions, 583–584
    stress-induced hyperglycemia, 584–585
  treatment during transitions, 599–600
  type 1, 582–583
  type 2, 190–192, 195*t*, 583
diarrhea, 11–12
  antibiotic-associated (AAD), 57
  enteral nutrition (EN) and, 219*f*, 221–222, 224*t*
  enterally tube-fed patient, *practice scenario*, 57
  postvagatomy, 430
  severe, *practice scenario*, 12
dietary data, nutrition assessment, 162–165, 165*t*
dietary fatty acids in oils, 71*t*
dietary reference intakes, trace elements, 138*t*
dietary reference intakes, vitamin, 124*t*
Dietary Supplement Health and Education Act of 1994 (DSHEA), 314
dietary supplements/supplementation, 314
  adverse event reporting, 321–322
  advertising, promotion, 320–322
  bariatric surgery, 612*t*
  burns, 402*t*
  calcium, 112*t*
  clinician's role, 324–325
  Crohn's disease and, *practice scenario*, 322
  current use, 314
  definitions, 314–318
  efficacy, 322
  for enterocutaneous (EC) fistulas, 449
  Federal Trade Commission (FTC) and, 320
  gastric bypass surgery and, *practice scenario*, 325
  health claims, 320
  heart failure and, *practice scenario*, 325
  herbal, 317*t*
  high blood pressure and, *practice scenario*, 321
  labeling requirements, 319–320
  nutrient content claims, 320
  nutrient supplement ingredients, 316*t*
  nutritional support statements, 320
  popular ingredients, 318*t*
  product quality, 321
  regulation, 319
  resources, 315*t*
  risk *vs.* benefit, 323*t*
  safety, 322–324
  selenium, *practice scenario*, 144–145
  structure/function claims, 320
  trace elements, parenteral, 147*t*
  U.S. Food and Drug Administration authority, 319
  weight loss, *practice scenario*, 321
  wound healing, 356
dieting, obesity and, 608–609
digestion. *See also* absorption
  bowel rest, 18–19
  carbohydrate(s), 16, 39–40, 39*f*
  fat, 16–17
  low flow states, 18–19
  mucosal atrophy, 18–19
  nucleic acids, 17
  protein, 16, 87–88, 87*f*
  starvation, 18–19
  thermogenic effect, 24
direct calorimetry, 24–25
discharge planning, 642–646
disease-associated malnutrition, 161
disease-related factors, drug-nutrient interactions, 308
disease-specific parenteral nutrition (PN) formulations, 249–252
dosage forms, drug-nutrient interactions, 303–304
dosing, enteral nutrition (EN), 173
doubly labeled water, 27
drug-induced diarrhea, enteral nutrition (EN), 221–222, 221*t*, 222*t*
drug-induced hyperkalemia, 109*t*
drug-induced hypokalemia, 107*t*
drug-nutrient interactions
  administration-related factors, 305–307
  background, 299–300
  delayed gastric emptying, 306*t*
  disease-related factors, 308
  drug-related factors, 307–308
  formula-related factors, 308
  macronutrients, 308
  micronutrients, 308
  pharmaceutical, 303–305
  pharmaceutical, *practice scenario*, 304
  pharmacokinetic, 305
  physical, 300
    enteral nutrition (EN), 301–302
    occlusion prevention, *practice scenario*, 303
    parenteral nutrition (PN), 301
    preventing, mitigating, 302–303
    vascular access device (VAD) occlusion, *practice scenario*, 301
  specific drugs, 309
    carbamazepine, 309
    fluoroquinolones, 309–310
    phenytoin, 309
    warfarin, 310
    warfarin, *practice scenario*, 310–311
  types, 300, 300*t*
drugs, symptom relief, cancer therapy, 571–572
DSHEA. *See* Dietary Supplement Health and Education Act of 1994
dumping syndrome (DS), 13, 429
dysphagia diet, 366*t*

E

EBP. *See* evidence-based practice
EC fistulas. *See* enterocutaneous (EC) fistulas
eicosanoid biosynthesis, 73–74
1800 Rule, 592
elderly. *See* older adults

electrolyte disorders
hypercalcemia, 112
hyperkalemia, 107–108
hypermagnesemia, 110–111
hypernatremia, 104, 106*f*
hyperphosphatemia, 114
hypocalcemia, 111–112
hypokalemia, 106–107, 107*t*, 108*t*
hypomagnesemia, 109–110
hyponatremia, 102–104, 105*f*
hypophosphatemia, 112–113
management, 102, 103*f*
electrolyte salts, 248*t*
electrolytes, 99
absorption, 18
background, 99
daily requirements, 248*t*
diabetes mellitus, 593
enteral formulations, 188
enterocutaneous (EC) fistulas, 449
esophageal cancer patient, *practice scenario*, 112–114
fluids and, disorders, 101–102
gastrointestinal (GI) secretions, 102*t*
imbalances, enteral nutrition (EN) and, 228–229
intravenous, shortage, 250*t*
parenteral nutrition (PN) complications and, 287
parenteral nutrition (PN) formulations, 248
requirements, critical injury, 401–402, 401*t*
requirements, renal failure (RF), 502
wasting syndrome/disease and, 550–551
emulsions, lipid, fat composition, 67*t*
EN. *See* enteral nutrition (EN)
energy
background, 23
intake, parenteral nutrition (PN) risk factor, 290
wasting syndrome/disease and, 550–551
energy expenditure
assessing metabolic response, 30–31
avoiding underfeeding, overfeeding, 31–32
basal metabolic rate (BMR), 23–24
with cancer, 565
chronic liver disease, 461
components, 23
digestion thermogenic effect, 24
illness, 24
measurement, 24, 27
direct calorimetry, 24–25
doubly labeled water, 27
indirect calorimetry, 25–27, 25*t*
reverse Fick equation, 27
obesity, 614
physical activity, 24
predictive equations
acutely ill patients, 31
critically ill patients, 29–31
healthy individuals, 27–29, 28*f*
sepsis, 381
energy metabolism, 23
energy requirements
critical injury, 396*f*, 398–399*t*, 399–400
lactation, 341*t*
organ transplantation, 529–530
pregnancy, 334*t*
renal failure (RF), 499–501, 501*f*
sepsis, 385
wound healing, 353
energy substrates, parenteral nutrition (PN), 247
enteral access, critical injury, 403
enteral access devices, 173–174, 174*f*, 207
complications, 214–215
enterostomy, 211
enterostomy tubes, 214–215, 214*t*
gastrojejunal tubes, 212, 215
gastrostomy, 211–212, 211*f*
head, neck cancer, *practice scenario*, 208
jejunal tubes, 215
jejunostomy, 212
nasal tubes, 209–211, 214
postinsertion catheter care, 212–213
selection, 207–208
skin-level, 212
tube selection
nasal, 209–211
physical characteristics, 208, 208*t*
types, 208–209, 209*f*, 209*t*
enteral delivery, metabolism and, lipids, 66–67
enteral formulas/formulations, 186
acute respiratory distress syndrome, 196–197, 197*t*
bariatric, 200–201
carbohydrate, 186
chronic pancreatitis, 485*t*
classification, terms, definitions, 186*t*
critical injury, 406
developing formulary, 202
diabetes/glucose intolerance, 189–190, 191*t*
diarrhea and, *practice scenario*, 221
electrolytes, 188
evaluation considerations, 189*t*
fat, 187–188
fat composition, 70*t*
fiber, 187
fluid restriction, 199*t*
food allergies, intolerances, 189
gastrointestinal disorders/ malabsorption, 192, 193–194*t*, 436
hepatic failure, 192
high protein, 201*t*
immune modulating, 192–196
macronutrient sources, 187*t*
modular products, 201–202
obese patients, 202*t*
open *vs.* closed systems, 202
oral products, 189
osmolality, 188–189
protein, 188
pulmonary failure, 196–197, 197*t*
renal failure, 198, 198*t*
safety, 203, 203*t*
type 2 diabetes, *practice scenario*, 190–192, 195*t*
vitamins, minerals, 188
wasting conditions, 199–200
water content, 188
wound healing, 200, 200*t*
enteral nutrition (EN), 171
acute pancreatitis, 476*t*, 478–479, 478*t*
alcoholic hepatitis and, *practice scenario*, 457–458
aspiration, 179
background, 171
benefits, 171–173
cancer, 568–569
contraindications, 173, 173*t*
critical illness, *practice scenario*, 178
Crohn's disease and, 441
delivery methods, 175–176
diabetes mellitus, 594–597
dosing, 173
drug-nutrient interactions, 301–302
feeding tube placement, 176–177
fluid-restricted regimen, 179*f*
formulations, 176
gastrointestinal issues, 178–179
gastroparesis (GP), 435, 436*t*
home nutrition support, 641*t*, 650*t*
indications, 171–173
intravenous *vs.* tube feeding, *practice scenario*, 181
medication administration, 177
meeting nutritional goals, 177–178
metabolic monitoring, 179–180
obese patient, 614–615
order sets, protocols, 174–175
outcomes, 181–182
patient selection, 171, 172*t*
prebiotic therapy and, 59
pregnancy, 336–337
prescription calculation, 175*f*
pulmonary failure and, 419–420, 419*t*, 420*t*

aspiration, ventilator-associated pneumonia (VAP) and, 420, 421*f*, 422*t*
ventilator-associated pneumonia (VAP), *practice scenario*, 422
renal failure (RF), 505
safety, 180–181
safety, *practice scenario*, 181
sepsis, *practice scenario*, 382
short bowel syndrome (SBS) and, 447, 517
timing, 173
vitamins, mineral adequacy, 147
ω-3 fatty acid effects, 74–75
wasting syndrome/disease and, 551
enteral nutrition (EN), complications, 220
abdominal distention, 220
aspiration, 224–226
background, 219
constipation, 224
contamination, 222–223
dehydration, 229–230
diarrhea, 57, 219*f*, 221–222, 224*t*
diarrhea, *practice scenario*, 57
fluid requirements, 230–231
gastrointestinal diseases, 223–224
intestinal ischemia, 223
intestinal tract bacterial overgrowth, 222
intolerance, *practice scenario*, 226
maldigestion/malabsorption, 220–221
metabolic alterations, 226–227, 227–228*t*
electrolyte imbalances, 228–229
hyperglycemia, 229
nausea, 220
prevention, home nutrition support, 650–651
vomiting, 220
enteral nutrition (EN) formulas/formulations
pregnancy, 336–337
enterocutaneous (EC) fistulas
associated conditions, 448*t*
closure, 449*t*
complications, 448*t*
diagnosis, 448
etiology, 447–448
nutrient issues, 449
nutrition intervention, 448
enterostomy tubes, 211
complications, 214–215, 214*t*
sizes, 209*t*
environmental factors, obesity, 606
esophageal cancer, 573
esophageal cancer, *practice scenario*, 112–114
essential fatty acids
deficiency, parenteral nutrition (PN) and, 286
deficiency prevention, *practice scenario*, 73
lipids and, recommendations
healthy population, 68–69, 69*f*
propofol use, *practice scenario*, 71–72
specialized nutrition support (SNS) patients, 69–73, 70*t*
ethical conflicts, 669–670, 670*t*
ethical decision making
clinical practice translation, 671
hospital policy, procedure, 672–674*f*
support professionals' role, 670–671
ethical theory, 661–662, 661*t*
ethics, cultural values, religious beliefs and, 664
Catholicism, 665–666
conscience clauses, 666
Judaism, 664
practice scenarios, 664–665, 666
world religions, positions, 666*t*
ethics, law and
advance directives, 668–669, 669*t*
artificial nutrition, hydration (ANH), 658–659
background, 657
bioethics, 661–662
concepts, 662, 662*t*
decisional capacity, 662
futility/quality of life, 663
informed consent, 662
surrogate decision making, 662–665, 663*t*
withholding *vs.* withdrawing treatment, 663
empirical research, 663–664
nutrition support technology and, 657–661
practice scenario, 669
precedent cases, 668
United States law, 666–668, 667*f*
evidence-based practice (EBP)
background, 694
challenges, 697
clinical guidelines, 696, 696*t*
components, 694*f*
evidence quality grading, 695*t*
implementation, 695–696, 695*t*
improvement, 697–698
practice scenarios, 697–698
purpose, 694–695
evidence-based research, 696
exercise
aerobic, HIV-associated lipodystrophy syndrome and, 555
aerobic, progressive resistance and, wasting syndrome/disease, 550
carbohydrate requirements, 49

F

F. *See* fluoride
FADE. *See* focus-analyze-develop-execute-evaluate model
family history, wasting syndrome/disease and, 547
fasting adaptation, protein and, 93
fasting state glucose metabolism, 46*f*
fasting state glucose regulation, 45–46
fat(s). *See also* lipids
composition, enteral formulas, 70*t*
composition, lipid emulsions, 67*t*
digestion, 16–17
enteral formulations, 187–188
maldigestion, 429
maldigestion, gastric resections and, 429
pregnancy and, 335
requirements, critical injury, 401
fat-soluble vitamins, 123–131, 504
fatty acids
β-oxidation, 68
requirements, wound healing, 356
short-chain, 76
short-chain (SCFA), absorption, 18
ω-3, 73–75
ω-6, 73–74
ω-9, 76
fatty liver disease, nonalcoholic, 458
Fe. *See* iron
fed state glucose metabolism, 45*f*
fed state glucose regulation, 45–46
Federal Trade Commission (FTC), dietary supplements and, 320
feeding access, critical injury, 403
feeding formula. *See* enteral formulas/formulations
feeding, hypocaloric, clinical indications, 31*t*
feeding tube placement, 176–177
ferritin, 433
fetal growth, 333
fiber
clinical nutrition role, 48
Crohn's disease and, 440
enteral formulations, 187
fibrates, 556
Fick equation, reverse, 27
1500 Rule, 592
filter, parenteral nutrition (PN) formulations, 259
fish oil, 442
fistulas. *See* enterocutaneous (EC) fistulas

fluid(s), 99
background, 99
balance, 100–101
compartments, 99–100, 100*f*
critical injury, requirements, 401–402
electrolytes and, disorders, 101–102
enteral nutrition (EN) requirements, 230–231
heart failure patient, *practice scenario*, 101
intravenous, short bowel syndrome (SBS) and, 447
older adults, requirements, *practice scenario*, 624–625
organ transplantation, requirements, 530
parenteral nutrition (PN) complications and, 287
recommendations, short bowel syndrome (SBS), 516*t*
renal failure (RF), requirements, 502
restriction, enteral nutrition (EN), 179*f*, 199*t*
restriction, parenteral nutrition (PN) formulation, 261*f*
short bowel syndrome (SBS), *practice scenario*, 516–517
volume, electrolyte content, gastrointestinal secretion, 102*t*
fluoride, 146
fluoroquinolones, 309–310
focus-analyze-develop-execute-evaluate (FADE) model, 689–690, 689*f*
folacin. *See* folic acid
folate deficiency, 430–431
folic acid, 135–136
food allergies, intolerances, 189
food aversions with cancer, 566
food intake influence, gut hormones, 6*t*
formula. *See* enteral formulas/formulations; parenteral formulas/formulations
formula selection/immunonutrition, critical injury, 405–406
formula-related factors, drug-nutrient interactions, 308
formulary, enteral, developing, 202
frailty, older adults, 622
Frazier Free Water Protocol guidelines, 625
FTC. *See* Federal Trade Commission
futility *vs.* quality of life, 663

G
GALT. *See* gut-associated lymphoid tissue
gastrectomy. *See* gastric resections
gastric bypass surgery, dietary supplements and, *practice scenario*, 325
gastric emptying, 434
gastric emptying, delayed. *See* gastroparesis (GP)
gastric feeding access, critical injury, 403
gastric motility, 9
gastric resections
afferent limb syndrome, 430
alkaline reflux gastritis, 430
antidumping diet, 429*t*
dumping syndrome, 429
fat maldigestion, 429
gastric stasis, 429–430
lactose intolerance, 430
metabolic bone disease, 431
nutrient deficiencies, 430–431
nutrition management following, 432*t*
nutritional assessment, 429
partial (PG), 428
postgastrectomy syndrome, 429
postvagatomy diarrhea, 430
Roux-en-Y total, 429
treatment after, 430
vagotomy, 428–429
gastric secretions, 14
gastric stasis, 429–430
gastritis, alkaline reflux, 430
gastrointestinal (GI) blood circulation, 15–16
gastrointestinal (GI) disease/disorders. *See also* stomach disorders
background, 428
bacterial overgrowth, 436–437, 437*t*
bezoars, 434
celiac disease (CD), 437–440
Crohn's disease, 440–441
enteral nutrition (EN) for, 178–179, 192, 193–194*t*, 223–224
enterocutaneous (EC) fistulas, 447–449
factors affecting oral intake, 434
ferritin and, 433
inflammatory bowel disease, 440–442
intestinal urinary diversions, 449
laboratory data, 433–434
parenteral nutrition (PN) for, 238
protein-losing enteropathy (PLE), 442–443, 443*t*
short bowel syndrome (SBS), 443–447, 444*t*
gastrointestinal (GI) function, parenteral nutrition (PN) and, 238
gastrointestinal (GI) motility, 7
colorectal, 10
constipation, 13
diarrhea, 11–12
dumping syndrome (DS), 13
gastric, 9
gastroparesis, 12–13
ileus, 10–11
practice scenario, 11
pseudo-obstruction, 11
small bowel obstruction, 10–11
small intestine, 10
types, 7–8
gastrointestinal (GI) secretions, 13–15, 102*t*
gastrointestinal (GI) tract
background, 4
disturbances with cancer, 567
fluid volume secreted, electrolyte content, 102*t*
immunity and, 19
role, protein breakdown, 92
gastrojejunal tubes, 212, 215
gastrojejunostomy feeding ports, 210*f*
gastroparesis (GP), 10, 12–13, 306*t*, 432
associated conditions, 433*t*
associated factors, 306*t*
clinical symptoms, 433*t*
diabetes mellitus and, 594
feeding tube occlusion prevention, 303
nutritional assessment, 432–433
nutritional management, 434–436
practice scenarios, 10, 303
small bowel bacterial overgrowth (SBBO) and, 434
gastrostomy tubes, 209*f*, 210*f*, 211–212
genetics, obesity and, 605–606
gestation, multiple, 332–333, 333*t*
gestational diabetes mellitus, 583, 584*t*
carbohydrates and, *practice scenario*, 47
pregnancy and, practice scenario, 47
GI. *See* gastrointestinal tract
gluconeogenesis, 42–43
gluconeogenic pathway, 44*f*
glucose
alterations, organ transplantation, 528–529
intolerance, enteral formulations, 189–190, 191*t*
metabolism, fasting state, 46*f*
metabolism, fed state, 45*f*
regulation, fasting, fed states, 45–46
transporters, 40–41
glucose tolerance diagnosis, 582*t*. *See also* diabetes mellitus
glutamine
critical injury, 404
parenteral nutrition (PN), 251, 251*t*
sepsis, 386–387
glutathione prodrugs, 465–466
glycemia measurement, 585
glycemic control, 585–586, 587*t*
glycemic index, 49*t*
glycogenesis, glycogenolysis and, 43–45
glycolysis, 41
glycolytic pathway, 42*f*
glycoproteins, cancer and, 566

graft-*vs.*-host disease (GVHD), cancer and, 576
gravity drip feeding, enteral nutrition (EN), 176
growth, energy expenditure and, 24
growth hormone releasing factor analog, HIV virus, 556–557
gut. *See also* gastrointestinal tract
  microbiota, 52–53 (*See also* prebiotics; probiotics; synbiotics)
  microbiota, obesity and, 59–60
gut hormone action, 5*f*
gut hormones, peptides and, 6*t*
gut-associated lymphoid tissue (GALT), 19
GVHD. *See* graft-*vs.*-host disease
gynecologic cancer, 575

H

Harris-Benedict predictive equations, 28, 28*f*
head cancer, 572–573
head, neck cancer, enteral feeding, *practice scenario*, 208
health claims, dietary supplements, 320
health information technology, quality improvement (QI), 685–686
healthy individuals
  carbohydrate requirements, 48–49
  energy expenditure predictive equations, 27–29
  essential fatty acid recommendations, 68–69, 69*f*
heart failure, dietary supplements and, 325
heart failure, *practice scenarios*, 101, 325
height, nutrition assessment and, 162
hematopoietic stem cell transplantation, 575–576
hemochromatosis, hereditary, 459
hemodialysis, *practice scenario*, 506
hemoglobin A1C, 433
hepatic failure, 192
hepatitis. *See also* liver disease
  alcoholic, *practice scenario*, 457–458
  viral, 459
hepatobiliary complications, parenteral nutrition (PN), 289
  disorder types, 289
  managing, 291–292, 291*t*
  prevalence, 289–290
herbal supplements, 317*t*. *See also* dietary supplements//supplementation
hereditary hemochromatosis, 459
high anion-gap acidosis, 117
high blood pressure, weight loss supplements and, *practice scenario*, 321
high output ileostomy, *practice scenario*, 117
high-protein enteral formulations, 201*t*
high-protein hypocaloric feeding, 614
HIV infection
  background, 537–538
    antiretroviral medications, 540–541, 541*t*
    clinical manifestation, 540
    diagnosis, 539, 539*t*
    immunopathogenesis, 539–540
    nutritional metabolism in cART era, 542
    pandemic epidemiology, 538–539
    replication cycle, 542*f*
    statistics, 538*t*
    transmission, 539, 539*t*
  cardiovascular disease and
    background, 555
    clinical evaluation, 556
    etiology, 555–556
    fibrates and, 556
    growth hormone releasing factor analog, 556–557
    HMG CoA reductase inhibitors, 556
    Mediterranean diet and, 556
    omega-3 fatty acids, 556
  wasting syndrome/disease and
    anabolic–androgenic steroids, 548–550
    case definition, 543
    clinical management, 547–548
    compared to uncomplicated starvation, 543
    diagnosis, 543
    electrolytes and, 550–551
    encounter, assessment, 546, 546*f*, 547*t*
    energy and, 550–551
    enteral nutrition (EN) and, 551
    epidemiology, 542–543
    etiology, pathogenesis, 543–545
    history, 542
    management, 547–548, 548*t*
    medication, 547, 549*t*
    omega-3 fatty acid enrichment, 551
    orexigenic agents, 548
    osteopenia, osteoporosis and, 552–553
    parenteral nutrition (PN), 551–552
    physical examination, 546–547
    practice scenario, 545, 550
    progressive resistance, aerobic exercise, 550
    protein and, 550–551
    recombinant human growth hormone (rhGH) and, 550
    sarcopenia, 552, 552*t*
    social, family history, 547
    thalidomide, 550
    tube feeding, 551
    vitamin D and, 551
HIV-associated lipodystrophy syndrome, 553
  epidemiology, 553
  etiology, 553–554
  evaluation, diagnosis, 554–555
  liposuction, 555
  management, 555
  metformin, 555
  other lipodystrophies, 553
  pathogenesis, 553–554
  resistance, aerobic exercise, 555
  soft tissue fillers, 555
  thiazolidinediones, 555
HMG CoA reductase inhibitors, 556
home nutrition support, 640
  advantages, benefits, 640
  care improvement, 652–653
  care plan, 646–647
  clinical monitoring, 649–651, 651*t*
  clinical monitoring, *practice scenario*, 650
  clinician role, 651–652
  complications prevention, 651
  discharge planning, 642
    hospital personnel role, 642*t*
    needs assessment, 645
    practice scenarios, 643, 645
    provider services selection, 646
    reimbursement eligibility, 642–643
    safety evaluation, 643–645
  enteral (EN), 641*t*, 650*t*
  medical necessity documentation, 643, 643*t*, 644*t*
  outcomes tracking, 652–653
  parenteral (PN), 240, 241*t*, 641*t*
  patient education, 647–648
    learning assessment, 648
    materials, 648, 648*t*
    teaching, evaluation strategies, 648–649, 649*t*
  patient selection, indications, 640–642
  patient support, 653, 653*t*
  provider services selection, 646
  quality of life, 652–653
  total parenteral (PN), cancer, 569
homeostasis, plasma glucose, hormonal regulation, 46
hormones
  cancer therapy, 569–570
  gut, action, 5*f*
  gut, peptides, food intake influence, 6*t*
  regulation, plasma glucose homeostasis, 46
hospital personnel role, home nutrition support, 642*t*

hospital policy, procedure, ethical decision making, 672–674*f*
hospital-acquired dehydration, 229
hospitalized patients, diabetes mellitus
  intravenous insulin therapy, 588–590, 590*t*, 591*f*
  medications, 587–588
  subcutaneous insulin injections, 589*t*, 590–592
host immunity, sepsis, 387–388
hub care, catheters, 274
human immunodeficiency virus infection. *See* HIV infection
hydration
  enterocutaneous (EC) fistulas, 449
  requirements, wound healing, 356
  short bowel syndrome (SBS), 446*t*
hydrazine sulfate, 571
hydrogen ion concentration regulation, 114
hypercalcemia, 112
hyperchloremic acidosis, 117
hyperemesis gravidarum, 341–342, 342*f*
hyperemesis gravidarum, *practice scenario*, 337
hyperglycemia
  diabetes mellitus and, 585
    control, 585–586, 587*t*
    hospitalized patient targets, 586–587, 587*t*
    measurement, 585
    outcomes, hospitalized patient, 586
  enteral nutrition (EN) and, 229
  parenteral nutrition (PN) and, 285–286
  during stress, inflammation, 395*f*
  stress-induced, 47–48, 584–585
hyperkalemia, 107–108
hypermagnesemia, 110–111
hypernatremia, 104, 106*f*
hyperphosphatemia, 114
hypertonic feeding solutions, diarrhea and, 222
hypertriglyceridemia, 286–287, 482
hypocalcemia, 111–112, 111*t*
hypocaloric feeding, 31*t*, 614
hypoglycemia, 286, 587
hypokalemia, 106–107, 107*t*, 108*t*
hypomagnesemia, 109–110, 446*t*
hyponatremia, 102–104, 105*f*
hypophosphatemia, 112–113

I

I. *See* iodine
IDPN. *See* intradialytic parenteral nutrition
ileostomy, *practice scenario*, 117
ileus, 10–11
illness, carbohydrate requirements, 49
illness, critical. *See* critically ill patient
illness, energy expenditure and, 24
immune modulating formulations (IMF), 192–196
immunity, gastrointestinal tract (GI) and, 19
immunity of host, sepsis, 387–388
immunonutrition
  critical injury, 405–406
  neurologic impairment, 371*t*
  pulmonary failure, 422
immunopathogenesis, HIV Infection, 539–540
immunosuppression, organ transplantation, 524, 525*t*
impaction, pregnant trauma patient, *practice scenario*, 343
implanted catheters, 269–270
indirect calorimetry, 25, 25*t*
  accuracy improvement, 26*t*
  clinical indications, 25
  conducting frequency, 27
  factors decreasing accuracy, 26*t*
  pulmonary failure, 417–418
  technical aspects, 25
infections, bloodstream, 276–279
inflammatory bowel disease, 440–442
informed consent, 662
infusion delivery, parenteral access devices, 281
infusion routes, parenteral nutrition (PN), 236
injury
  carbohydrate requirements, 49
  malnutrition and, 161
  spinal cord (SCI), *practice scenario*, 369
injury, critical. *See* critically ill patient
injury, neurologic. *See* neurologic impairment
insertion, catheters, 272–274
insulin therapy during enteral feeding, 596–597
insulin therapy during parenteral feeding, 598–599
intensive care unit mortality, obesity effect, 612–613
interferon gamma, 566
interleukin 1, 566
interleukin 6, 566
intermittent feeding, 175–176
intestinal adaptation, 513
intestinal ischemia, 223
intestinal rehabilitation, short bowel syndrome (SBS), 518
intestinal tract bacterial overgrowth, 222
intestinal transplant, *practice scenario*, 527
intestinal urinary diversions, 449
intestine, small, gastrointestinal motility, 10
intradialytic parenteral nutrition (IDPN), 508
intravenous alimentation. *See* parenteral nutrition (PN)
intravenous fat emulsion (IVFE)
  liver disease and, data, 77
  parenteral delivery, metabolism, 67–68
  parenteral nutrition (PN) risk factor, 290
  shortage, 249*t*
  total nutrient admixture stability, 256–258
intravenous feeding. *See* parenteral nutrition (PN)
intravenous fluids, short bowel syndrome (SBS), 447
intravenous lipid emulsions, 480
iodine, 145
Ireton-Jones predictive equations, 29–30
iron, 137–141
iron deficiency, 141, 431
IVFE. *See* intravenous fat emulsion

J

jejunal tubes, 215
jejunostomy tubes, 212
Judaism, values, beliefs, 664

K

kidney disease, chronic (CKD), 494–495, 495*t*
kidney failure. *See* renal failure (RF)
kidney injury, acute (AKI), 493–494
kidneys. *See also* renal entries
  acid-base balance role, 114–115
  acid-base physiology, 115
  protein breakdown role, 92–93
knowledge translation (KT) *vs.* quality improvement (QI), 690
KT. *See* knowledge translation

L

labeling requirements, dietary supplements, 319–320
laboratory data, studies, nutrition assessment, 162, 163–164*t*
laboratory measurements, liver disease, 462
laboratory values, pregnancy, 339*t*
lactation, 341, 341*t*
lactose, Crohn's disease and, 440
lactose intolerance, 222, 430
large bowel secretions, 15
law. *See also* ethics, law and
  United States, 666–668, 667*f*
Lean methodology, 688–689
lipid emulsions, fat composition, 67*t*
lipid metabolism with cancer, 565–566

lipid-free parenteral nutrition (PN) regimen, *practice scenario,* 73
lipids, 64. *See also* fat(s)
- absorption, 17–18
- alterations, organ transplantation, 529
- background, 64
- biochemistry, 65–66
- eicosanoid biosynthesis, 73–74
- enteral delivery, 66–67
- essential fatty acids and, recommendations, 68–69, 69*f*
- essential fatty acids and, specialized nutrition support (SNS), 69–73, 70*t*
- fatty acid β-oxidation, 68
  - intravenous fat emulsions (IVFEs), associated liver disease (PNALD) and, 77
  - intravenous fat emulsions (IVFEs), metabolism, 67–68
  - medium-chain triglycerides, 76–77
- metabolism, 66–67, 380
- nomenclature, 65–66
- sepsis and, 380, 385–386
  - short-chain fatty acids, 76
- structure, 64–65
  - structured, 77
    - ω-3 fatty acids, 73–75
    - ω-6 fatty acids, 73–74
    - ω-9 fatty acids, 76

lipodystrophy syndrome, 553–555
liposuction, 555
liver disease
- alcoholic (ALD), 457
- alcoholic hepatitis, *practice scenario,* 457–458
- background, 455–456
- causes, 456*t*
- cholestatic, 460
- chronic
  - energy expenditure, 461
  - malnutrition, 460–461
  - metabolism, 461–462
  - *practice scenario,* 463–464
- complications, 467–468
- decompensated, 461
- hereditary hemochromatosis, 459
- malnutrition and, 456–457
- nonalcoholic fatty, 458
- nonalcoholic steatohepatitis, 458
- nutrient provision
  - compensated liver disease, 462–463
  - complementary, alternative, 465–467
  - decompensated liver disease, 464
  - malnourishment, *practice scenario,* 464–465
  - micronutrients, 465–467
- nutritional aspects, 456–457
- nutritional assessment, 462, 462*t*, 463*t*
- parenteral nutrition-associated (PNALD), intravenous fat emulsions (IVFEs) and, 77
- pathogenesis, 456–457
- viral hepatitis, 459
- Wilson disease, 459–460

liver failure, 192
liver, protein breakdown role, 92
low-flow states, 18–19, 394–395
lungs
- acid–base balance role, 114–115
- acid–base physiology, 115
- acute injury (ALI)/respiratory distress syndrome (ARDS), 414, 417*f*

lymphatic system, 631–632, 632*f*
lymphoid tissue, gut-associated (GALT), 19

M

macronutrients
- drug-nutrient interactions, 308
- pregnancy, 333–335
- pulmonary failure, 419
- sources, enteral formulations, 187*t*

magnesium
- deficiency, metabolic bone disease and, 294
- fluid, electrolyte balance and, 109
- hypermagnesemia, 110–111
- hypomagnesemia, 109–110, 110*t*
- oral replacement products, 110*t*

malabsorption
- with cancer, 567
- enteral formulations, 192, 193–194*t*
- enteral nutrition (EN), 220–221

maldigestion
- with cancer, 567
- enteral nutrition (EN), 220–221
- fat, 429

malnourishment, liver disease, *practice scenario,* 464–465
malnutrition
- with cancer, 564–567
- chronic liver disease, 460–461
- chronic pancreatitis and, 482–483
- pretransplant, *practice scenario,* 526–527
- short bowel syndrome (SBS) and, *practice scenario,* 518
- stress response, 395–396

malnutrition syndromes, 156–157, 157–159*t*
- acute disease- or injury-associated, 161
- chronic disease–associated, 159–160
- starvation–associated, 159

manganese, 143–144
maternal weight gain, pregnancy, 333, 333*t*
mechanical ventilation hierarchy, 416*t*
medical necessity documentation, home nutrition support, 643, 643*t*, 644*t*
medication(s)
- additives, parenteral nutrition (PN), 256*t*, 259
- administration, enteral nutrition (EN), 177
- consideration, pulmonary failure, 417
- delaying gastric emptying, 434*t*
- diarrhea-associated, 221–222, 221*t*, 222*t*
- history, nutrition assessment, 161
- neurologic impairment, 370*t*
- short bowel syndrome (SBS), 518
- wasting syndrome/disease, 547, 549*t*

Mediterranean diet, 556
- medium-chain triglycerides, 18, 76–77

metabolic acidosis, 116, 116*t*
metabolic alkalosis, 116*t*, 118
metabolic alterations
- with cancer, 565–566
- enteral nutrition (EN) and, 226–227, 227–228*t*
  - electrolyte imbalances, 228–229
  - hyperglycemia, 229

metabolic bone disease, 292–293, 431
metabolic rate, 23–24
metabolic response, assessing, 30–31
metabolic syndrome diagnosis, 584*t*
metabolism
- aberrations, organ transplantation, 528
- abnormalities, acute kidney injury (AKI), 494
- abnormalities, chronic kidney disease (CKD), 495
- apparent absorption and, 305
- chronic liver disease, 461–462
- complications, renal failure (RF), 494*t*
- intravenous fat emulsions (IVFEs), 67–68
- lipids and, 66–67
- monitoring, enteral nutrition (EN), 179–180
- neurologic impairment, 364–365, 365*t*
- nutritional, combination antiretroviral therapy (cART) era, 542
- pharmacokinetic interactions, 305
- presystemic, drug-nutrient interactions, 308
- sepsis and, 379–380

metabolism, carbohydrates and
- gluconeogenesis, 42–43
- glucose transporters, 40–41
- glycogenesis, glycogenolysis and, 43–45
- glycolysis, 41
- precursor formation, other metabolites, 45

pyruvate–lactate pathway, 41–42
tricarboxylic acid cycle, 41, 43*f*
metabolites, 45
metformin, 555
microbial etiology, pathogenesis, parenteral access devices, 276–278
micronutrients
drug-nutrient interactions, 308
liver disease, 465–467
management, 147–148
organ transplantation, 530, 531*t*
pregnancy, 335–336
pulmonary failure and, 419
wound healing and, 352*t*, 356–357
Mifflin-St. Jeor predictive equations, 28*f*, 29
minerals. *See also* trace elements; ultratrace elements
absorption, 18
deficiency, cirrhosis, 467
deficiency, Crohn's disease, 441–442
enteral formulations, 147, 188
intravenous, shortage, 250*t*
requirements
critical injury, 402, 404–405
pregnancy, 336*t*
renal failure (RF), 502
wound healing, 356–357
supplementation, burns, 402*t*
supplementation, enterocutaneous (EC) fistulas, 449
mirtazapine, cancer therapy, 571
misconnections, enteral nutrition (EN), 181
mixed acid–base disorders, 115
Mn. *See* manganese
Mo. *See* molybdenum
modified amino acid, 247*t*, 250
modular products, enteral formulations, 201–202
molybdenum, 146
monitoring, pregnancy
acid-base, 340
laboratory values, 339*t*
serum analysis, 338–340
transitional feeds, 340
urinalysis, 340
monosaccharide chemical structures, 38*f*
motility
colorectal, 10
gastric, 9
gastrointestinal, 7
abnormalities, 10–13
types, 7–8
small intestine, 10
mucosal atrophy, 18–19
multiple gestation, 332–333, 333*t*
multivitamin products, 147*t*
multivitamins
muscle, skeletal, protein breakdown and, 92

N
nasal tubes, 209–211, 209*t*, 214
nasogastric *vs.* nasojejunal support, 479
nausea, 220, 434
neck cancer, 572–573
neck cancer, enteral feeding device, *practice scenario*, 208
nephron, 493*f*
neuroendocrine pathophysiology, 606–607
neuroendocrine response to stress, 394, 395*f*
neurologic impairment
background, 364
complications, monitoring, 370–371
dysphagia diet, 366*t*
immunonutrients, 371*t*
medication, 370*t*
metabolism, 364–365, 365*t*
nutrition assessment, 366–368
nutrition support
advances, 371–372
complications affecting, 365–366
route, 369–370
nutritional consequences, 365*t*
spinal cord injury (SCI), *practice scenario*, 369
traumatic brain injury (TBI), *practice scenario*, 368–369
neuropeptides, 566
niacin, 133
nitrogen balance, protein and, 90
nitrogen-energy relationships, protein and, 94
nonalcoholic fatty liver disease, 458
nonoliguric acute kidney injury (AKI), *practice scenario*, 506–507
nonsterile powdered amino acids, *practice scenario*, 254
nonthrombotic catheter occlusion, 280
nontunneled catheters, percutaneous, 268, 270*f*
normal anion-gap acidosis, 117
nucleic acids, digestion, 17
nutrient content claims, dietary supplements, 320
nutrient deficiencies, gastric resections, 430–431
nutrient intake, appetite and, 4–7
nutrient supplements, 316*t*. *See also* dietary supplements/supplementation
nutrition assessment/screening, 156, 161
anthropometrics and, 162, 396–397
bariatric surgery, 611–612, 612*t*
body composition assessment tools, 162, 163–164*t*
concepts, 156
critical injury, 396–397
critically ill obese patient, 613–614
Crohn's disease, 440
dietary data, 162–165, 165*t*
functional outcomes, 165
gastroparesis (GP), 432–433
laboratory, other studies, 162, 163–164*t*
liver disease, 462, 462*t*, 463*t*
medical, surgical data, 161
medication history, 161
neurologic impairment, 366–368
older adults, 623
physical examination, 161–162
pulmonary failure, 419*t*
renal failure (RF), 498*t*
short bowel syndrome (SBS), 513–514
stomach disorders, 429
tools, 165–167, 166*t*
weight history, 161
wound healing, 353
nutrition consult form, 239*f*
nutrition deficiency. *See also* individual nutrients
bariatric surgery, 612
gastric resections, 430–431
nutrition intervention
Crohn's disease, 440
enterocutaneous (EC) fistulas, 448
older adults, 625, 626*f*
nutrition management algorithm, acute pancreatitis, 477*f*
nutrition support statements, dietary supplements, 320

O
ω-3 fatty acids, 73–74
clinical effects, enteral nutrition (EN), 74–75
clinical effects, parenteral nutrition (PN), 75
ω-6 fatty acids, 73–74
ω-9 fatty acids, 76
obesity, 604
ambulatory patient, 607
behavioral treatment, 609
dieting, 608–609
evaluation, 607–608
pharmacological treatment, 610
physical activity, 609
weight loss methods, 608
bariatric surgery, 610–611
indications, contraindications, 610*f*
nutrition assessment, 611–612, 612*t*
supplementation, 612*t*
classification, 605*f*
comorbidities, 607

critically ill patient
impact, 613
intensive care unit mortality, 612–613
nutrition delivery impact, 614–615
nutritional assessment, 613–614
practice scenario, 613
enteral formulations, 202*t*
environmental factors, 606
epidemiology, 604–605
genetics, 605–606
gut microbiota and, 59–60
neuroendocrine pathophysiology, 606–607
pulmonary failure and, 419
occlusion, catheter, 279–280, 279*t*
occlusion prevention, *practice scenario*, 303
oils, dietary fatty acids in, 71*t*
olanzapine, cancer therapy, 571
older adults
advanced dementia, 623
advanced dementia, *practice scenario*, 627
background, 621–622
fluid needs, *practice scenario*, 624–625
frailty, 622
Frazier Free Water Protocol guidelines, 625
functional assessment, 623*t*
malnutrition, 621*t*
nutrient requirements, 624, 624*t*
nutrition interventions, 625, 626*f*
nutrition screening, assessment, 623
nutrition support, 625–627
obese, *practice scenario*, 160–161
sarcopenia, 622
omega-3 fat emulsions, 251–252
omega-3 fatty acid metabolism, 423*f*
omega-3 fatty acids
cardiovascular disease and, 556
critical injury, 404
pulmonary failure, 422–424, 423*f*
wasting syndrome/disease and, 551
omega-6 fat emulsions/structured lipids, 251, 252*t*
omega-6 fatty acid metabolism, 423*f*
omega-9 fat emulsions, 251–252
open *vs*. closed systems, 202
oral diet. *See* oral nutrition
oral fluids, short bowel syndrome (SBS), 515–517, 515*t*
oral intake, gastrointestinal disease, 434
oral intake resumption, acute pancreatitis, 480
oral magnesium replacement products, 110*t*
oral nutrition
cancer, 567–568
chronic pancreatitis, 483–484
diabetes mellitus, 593–594
gastroparesis (GP), 434–435, 435*t*
hepatobiliary complications, 292
products, enteral formulations, 189
renal failure (RF), 505
short bowel syndrome (SBS), 446–447, 514–515
transitioning to, critical injury, 403
oral phosphate replacement products, 113*t*
oral potassium replacement products, 108*t*
order sets, 174–175
orexigenic agents, 548
organ transplantation
complications, 530–531
contraindications, 524
hepatobiliary complications, 292
immunosuppression, 524, 525*t*
indications, 524
metabolic aberrations, 528–529
nutrient requirements, 529–530, 531*t*
nutrition monitoring, 533, 533*t*
nutrition status determination, 529, 529*t*
nutrition support route selection, 530, 533*t*
phases, 526
acute posttransplant, 527–528
chronic posttransplant, 528
intestinal, *practice scenario*, 527
malnutrition pretransplant, *practice scenario*, 526–527
posttransplant complications, *practice scenario*, 530–531
posttransplant nutrition, *practice scenario*, 528
pretransplant, 526–527
prevalence, 524
osmolality, 188–189
osteopenia, 552–553
osteoporosis, 295*t*, 552–553
overfeeding
avoiding, 31–32
consequences, 31*t*
pulmonary failure assessment, 418

P

palliative care, 576–577, 658
pancreatic cancer, 574
pancreatic enzyme replacement, 485*t*, 486*t*
pancreatic insufficiency, 484–486
pancreatic rest, 476
pancreatic secretions, 15
pancreaticoduodenectomy, 431–432
pancreatitis
background, 473
nutritional status deterioration, 475*t*
pancreatitis, acute, 474, 698
computed tomography grading system, 474*t*
computed tomography severity index, 475*t*
differentiating severe, mild, moderate, 474*t*
etiology, 474–475
incidence, 474
nutritional implications, 475–476
nutritional management algorithm, 477*f*
nutritional support
enteral, 476*t*, 478–479, 478*t*
oral intake resumption, 480
parenteral, 479–480
practice scenario, 480
pathophysiology, 474
pancreatitis, chronic, 480–481
clinical presentation, 482
epidemiology, 481
etiology, 481, 481*t*
malnutrition, 482–483, 482*t*
pathophysiology, 482
treatment, 483
enteral formulas, 485*t*
nutrition support, 484
oral diet, 483–484
practice scenario, 484
pantothenic acid, 136
parenteral access devices, 266
catheters
antimicrobial technology, 275–276
central venous, 271*f*, 272*f*, 274*t*, 275
hub care, 274
implanted, 269–270
infections, 277*t*
insertion, 272–273
insertion site maintenance, 273–274
materials, 275–276
patency, 274–275, 280
percutaneous nontunneled, 268, 270*f*
stabilization, 275
technology, 275–276
vascular access, 269*t*
central venous access, 268, 273*f*
central *vs*. peripheral access, 268
complications, 276
bloodstream infections, 276–279
care bundles, 278
catheter-related bloodstream infection (CRBSI), *practice scenario*, 278–279
microbial etiology, pathogenesis, 276–278, 277*f*
occlusion, 279–280, 279*t*
occlusion, *practice scenario*, 280
infusion delivery, 281

patient assessment, 270–271
risk reduction, 278
selection, 270
parenteral fluids, short bowel syndrome (SBS), 517
parenteral nutrition (PN)
acute pancreatitis, 479–480
advancing, *practice scenario*, 242–243
approaches, 237
background, 235–236
central (CPN), 236
Crohn's disease and, 441
delivery, intravenous fat emulsions (IVFEs), 67–68
diabetes mellitus, 598–599, 600*t*
discontinuing, *practice scenario*, 243
drug-nutrient interactions, 301
gastroparesis (GP), 436
glutamine, selenium and, *practice scenario*, 144–145
indications, 237*t*
cancer, 240
clinical conditions, 240*f*
clinical status, 238
intradialytic (IDPN), 508
lipid-free regimen, *practice scenario*, 73
monitoring, 242*t*
multivitamin products, 147*t*
peripheral (PPN), 236, 236*t*
pregnancy, 337–338
product shortages, 248–249, 249*t*, 250*t*
renal failure (RF), 506–507
sepsis, *practice scenario*, 382–383
short bowel syndrome (SBS), 447, 517–518, 518*t*, 519*t*
system, 241
trace elements, 147, 147*t*
vitamins, 146–147
wasting syndrome/disease and, 551–552
parenteral nutrition (PN) complications
azotemia, 287
background, 285
essential fatty acid deficiency, 286
hepatobiliary, 289
managing, 291–292, 291*t*
prevalence, 289–290
types, 289
hyperglycemia, 285–286
hypertriglyceridemia, 286–287
hypoglycemia, 286
metabolic bone disease, 292–293
aluminum toxicity and, 294
associated diseases, conditions, 293*t*
calcium role, 293
copper deficiency and, 294
magnesium deficiency and, 294
management, 294–295, 295*t*
prevalence, 293
prevention, 294–295, 295*t*
vitamin D role, 293–294
micronutrient-related, 287–288
preventing, *practice scenario*, 287
refeeding syndrome, 288–289
refeeding syndrome, *practice scenario*, 289
risk factors, 290–291
sepsis, 384
parenteral nutrition (PN) formulas/formulations
components, 246–247, 248*t*
disease-specific/specific nutrients
carnitine, 252
glutamine, 251, 251*t*
lipid emulsions comparison, 252*t*
modified amino acid, 247*t*, 249–250
omega-3, omega-9 fat emulsions, 251–252
omega-6 fat emulsions/structured lipids, 251
electrolyte salts, 248*t*
electrolytes, 248, 248*t*
energy substrates, 247
premixed, 255–256
preparation
admixtures, 252–253, 253*t*, 255
automated compounding devices (ACDs), 254–255
compounded sterile, 253–254, 254*t*
nonsterile powdered amino acids, *practice scenario*, 254
premixed formulations, 255–256
protein, 247
stability/compatibility, 256
aluminum contamination control, 259–262
calcium, phosphate, 258–259, 258*t*
calculation, 260*f*, 262
calculation, fluid-restricted, 261*f*
compounding limitations, *practice scenario*, 257–258
filter use, 259
intravenous fat emulsion, total nutrient admixture, 256–258
medication additives, 256*t*, 259
trace elements, 248
vitamins, 248, 248*t*
parenteral nutrition-associated liver disease (PNALD), 77
partial gastrectomy (PG), 428
patency, catheter, 274–275, 280
pathophysiology, sepsis, 379
patient assessment, parenteral access devices, 270–271
patient education, home nutrition support, 647–648
patient selection, enteral nutrition (EN), 171, 172*t*
patient selection, indications, home nutrition support, 640–642
patient support, home nutrition support, 653, 653*t*
PDSA. *See* plan-do-study-act cycle
PEG. *See* percutaneous endoscopic gastrostomy
Penn State predictive equations, 30
peptides, 86, 89*f*
percutaneous endoscopic gastrojejunostomy feeding ports, 209, 210*f*
percutaneous endoscopic gastrostomy (PEG) tubes, 210–211, 210*f*
percutaneous nontunneled catheters, 268, 270*f*
perioperative malnutrition, parenteral nutrition (PN) and, 238–240
perioperative nutrition, critical injury, 406
peripheral parenteral nutrition (PPN), 236
peripheral venous access, 267–268
pernicious anemia, gastric resection, 430
persistent vegetative state, 659–661, 660*f*, 660*t*
PG. *See* partial gastrectomy
pharmacokinetic drug-nutrient interactions, 305
pharmacological treatment, hepatobiliary complications, 292
pharmacological treatment, obesity, 610
phenytoin, 309
phosphate, calcium and, stability/compatibility, parenteral nutrition (PN), 258–259, 258*t*
phosphate replacement products, oral 113*t*
phosphorus
fluid, electrolyte balance and, 112
hyperphosphatemia, 114
hypophosphatemia, 112–113
requirements, renal failure (RF), 502–503
physical activity, energy expenditure and, 24
physical activity, obesity and, 609
physical examination, nutrition assessment, 161–162
physiological changes, short bowel syndrome (SBS), 443–444
physiological principles, 266–267
plan-do-study-act (PDSA) cycle, 686–687, 687*f*, 688*f*
plasma glucose homeostasis, 45
diabetes mellitus, 47
glucose metabolism, fasting state, 46*f*
glucose metabolism, fed state, 45*f*
glucose regulation, 45–46

hormonal regulation, 46
stress hyperglycemia, 47–48
PLE. *See* protein-losing enteropathy
PN. *See* parenteral nutrition (PN)
PNALD. *See* parenteral nutrition-associated liver disease
pneumonia, ventilator-associated (VAP), *practice scenario,* 422
portal hypertension, *practice scenario,* 159–160
postgastrectomy syndrome, 429
postinsertion catheter care, 212–213
postvagatomy diarrhea, 430
potassium, fluid, electrolyte balance and, 104
hyperkalemia, 107–108, 109*t*
hypokalemia, 106–107, 107*t*, 108*t*
oral replacement products, 108*t*
PPN. *See* peripheral parenteral nutrition
prebiotics, 54–56
candidates for use, 56
characteristics, 55*t*
contraindications, 56
critical injury, 405
provision, clinical evidence, 58
safety, 56
therapy, enteral nutrition (EN) and, 59
type, timing, dosing, 56
precedent cases, artificial nutrition/hydration (ANH), 668
precursor formation, metabolites, 45
prediabetic conditions, 583–584
predictive equations
energy expenditure, 29
acutely ill patients, 30
critically ill patients, 29–30
healthy individuals, 27
Harris-Benedict, 28, 28f
Mifflin-St. Jeor, 28f, 29
new equations, 29
validity testing, 27–28
pulmonary failure, 417–418
pregnancy
background, 332
constipation, trauma patient, *practice scenario,* 343
diabetes and, 344
eating disorders and, 343–344
energy requirements, 334*t*
enteral nutrition (EN) and, 336
access, 337
complications, 337
contraindications, 336
formula composition, 336–337
hyperemesis gravidarum, *practice scenario,* 337
indications, 336
fetal growth, 333
gestational diabetes and, *practice scenario,* 47
hyperemesis gravidarum, 341–342, 342*f*
impaction, trauma patient, *practice scenario,* 343
macronutrients, 333
calories, 333–334
carbohydrate, 334–335
fat, 335
protein, 335
maternal weight gain, 333, 333*t*
micronutrients, 335–336, 335*t*, 336*t*
monitoring
acid-base, 340
laboratory values, 339*t*
serum analysis, 338–340
transitional feeds, 340
urinalysis, 340
multiple gestation, 332–333, 333*t*
parenteral nutrition (PN) and, 337–338
trauma and, 342–343
premixed parenteral nutrition (PN) formulations, 255–256
prescription calculation, enteral nutrition (EN), 175*f*
pressure ulcers, healing, 351–352, 354–355*t*
pressure ulcers, *practice scenario,* 358–359
presystemic metabolism, drug-nutrient interactions, 308
probiotics, 53. *See also* gut microbia
action mechanisms, 53–54, 54*t*
candidates for use, 56
commercially available, 55*t*
contraindications, 56
criteria, 53*t*
critical injury, 405
dosing, 56
provision, clinical evidence, 56–57
antibiotic-associated diarrhea (AAD), 57
critical illness, 57–58
safety, 56
sources, 54
timing, 56
type, 56
progestagens, 570–571
progressive resistance, wasting syndrome/disease and, 550
proinflammatory cytokines, 566
prolonged mechanical ventilation (PMV), 414–415
propofol, 71–72
protein, 84
absorption, 17, 87–88, 87*f*
alterations, organ transplantation, 529
amino acids, 84–85, 85*f*, 86*t*, 89*f*
conditionally essential amino acids, 95
content in food, 94
critical illness requirements, 94–95
critical injury requirements, 90–91, 400
Crohn's disease requirements, 440
diabetes mellitus requirements, 593
digestion, 16, 87–88, 87*f*, 88*t*
enteral formulations, 188
fasting, starvation adaptation, 93
functions, 86, 86*t*
liver role, protein breakdown, 92
malnutrition, chronic pancreatitis and, 482–483
metabolism, sepsis, 380
metabolism, with cancer, 565
obesity requirements, 614
optimizing nitrogen-energy relationships, 94
organ transplantation requirements, 530
parenteral nutrition (PN) formulations, 247
parenteral nutrition (PN) risk factor, 290
peptides, 86
pregnancy and, 335
quality, 93–94
renal failure (RF) requirements, 501–502
sepsis requirements, 386
signaling, 87
structure, 86–87
synthesis, 89–90
transport, 87
turnover measurement, breakdown, 90, 90*t*
arteriovenous amino acid differences across organs, 91
brain, central nervous system role, 93
gastrointestinal tract role, 92
kidney role, 92–93
liver role, 92
nitrogen balance, 90
skeletal muscle role, 92
tracer methodology, 91
wasting syndrome/disease and, 550–551
wound healing requirements, 353
protein-losing enteropathy (PLE), 442–443, 443*t*
proteolysis-inducing factor, 566
protocols, enteral nutrition (EN), 174–175
pseudo-obstruction, gastrointestinal (GI) tract, 11

pulmonary failure, 413
  acute, 414
  acute lung injury (ALI)/respiratory distress syndrome (ARDS), 414, 417*f*
  chronic, 414–415
  enteral formulations, 196–197, 197*t*
  enteral nutrition (EN), 419–420, 419*t*
    aspiration, ventilator-associated pneumonia (VAP) and, 420–422, 421*f*, 422*t*
    ventilator-associated pneumonia (VAP), *practice scenario*, 422
  immunonutrition, 422
  medication consideration, 417
  nutrition assessment, 419*t*
    history, physical exam, 417
    indirect calorimetry, 417–418
    obesity, 419
    overfeeding, 418
    predictive equations, 417–418
    underfeeding, 418
  nutrition considerations, 415–417
  nutrition support, 419
  omega-3 fatty acids, 422–424, 423*f*
  parenteral nutrition (PN), 420*t*, 422
  prolonged mechanical ventilation (PMV), 414–415
  sources, 416*t*
  terminology, 415*t*
  types, 414–417
pulmonary function, 413–414, 414*f*, 416*t*
pyridoxine, 133–134
pyruvate–lactate pathway, 41–42

Q
QI. *See* quality improvement
quality
  control, admixtures, 255
  current state in healthcare, 679–681
  measuring, 681–682
    data analysis, 683
    data collection, 682–683
    indicators, 682, 682*f*
    nutrition care, 683–684, 683*t*
    practice scenario, 684
quality improvement (QI), 679
  background, 678–679
  clinical research *vs.*, 690
  history, 680–681*t*
  knowledge translation (KT) *vs.*, 690
  methodologies, 686
    focus-analyze-develop-execute-evaluate (FADE) model, 689–690, 689*f*
    Lean, 688–689
    plan-do-study-act cycle (PDSA), 686–687, 687*f*, 688*f*
    Six Sigma, 688
  quality assurance *vs.*, 690
  strategies
    bundles, 685
    care pathways, 684–685
    clinical practice guidelines (CPGs), 684
    health information technology, 685–686
    practice scenarios, 685–686
quality of life, home nutrition support, 652
quality of life *vs.* futility, 663
Quinlan case, artificial nutrition/hydration (ANH), 668

R
recombinant human growth hormone (rhGH), 550
rectal cancer, 574–575
refeeding syndrome, 288–289
refractory celiac disease, 439
regimen factors, drug-nutrient interactions, 307
regulation, dietary supplements, 319
rehospitalization prevention, home nutrition support, 647
reimbursement eligibility, home nutrition support, 642–643
religious beliefs, 664
renal disease. *See also* acute kidney injury (AKI); chronic kidney disease (CKD)
  background, 492
  nutrition assessment, 497–499, 498*t*
renal failure (RF)
  enteral formulations, 198*t*
  metabolic complications, 494*t*
  nutrition assessment, monitoring, 498*t*
  nutrition requirements, 499, 500*t*
    acid–base balance, 503
    calcium, 503
    electrolytes, 502
    energy, 499–501, 501*f*
    fluid, 502
    minerals, 502
    phosphorus, 502–503
    protein, 501–502
    sodium, 502
    trace elements, 503
    vitamins, 503–504
  nutrition therapy
    enteral, 505
    hemodialysis, *practice scenario*, 506
    intradialytic parenteral (IDPN), 508
    nonoliguric acute kidney injury (AKI), *practice scenario*, 506–507
    oral diets, 505
    parenteral, 506–507
renal function, normal, 492–493, 493*f*
renal replacement therapy (RRT), 495
  continuous (CRRT), 496–497
  hemodialysis, 496
  methods, 495*t*
  peritoneal dialysis (PD), 496
  trace elements, 504–505
reobstruction after surgery, *practice scenario*, 11
reperfusion injury/low-flow states, 394–395
replication cycle, HIV Infection, 542*f*
resistance, progressive, wasting syndrome/disease and, 550
respiratory acidosis, 115, 116*t*
respiratory alkalosis, 116, 116*t*
respiratory distress syndrome, 414
respiratory quotient interpretation, 26–27, 27*t*
resting metabolic rate (RMR), 23–26
reverse Fick equation, 27
RF. *See* renal failure
rhGH. *See* recombinant human growth hormone
riboflavin, 132–133
risk classification, compounded sterile parenteral nutrient preparations, 254*t*
risk reduction, parenteral access devices, 278
RMR. *See* resting metabolic rate
Roux-en-Y total, 429
RRT. *See* renal replacement therapy

S
s-adenosylmethionine (SAM)/betaine, 466
safety
  dietary supplements, 322–324
  enteral formulations, 203, 203*t*
  enteral nutrition (EN), 180–181
  enteral nutrition (EN), *practice scenario*, 181
  evaluation, home nutrition support, 643–645
  prebiotics, 56
  probiotics, 56
saline-responsive metabolic alkalosis, 118
saline-unresponsive metabolic alkalosis, 118
sarcopenia, 552, 622
SBBO. *See* small bowel bacterial overgrowth
SBS. *See* short bowel syndrome
Schiavo case, artificial nutrition/hydration (ANH), 668
SCI. *See* spinal cord injury
Se. *See* selenium
secretions
  bile, 14–15
  gastric, 14

pancreatic, 15
small, large bowel, 15
secretory diarrhea, enteral nutrition (EN) and, 224*t*
selenium, 144–145
seniors. *See* older adults
sepsis
antioxidant requirements, 387
arginine requirements, 386–387
background, 378
carbohydrate requirements, 385
definitions, 378–379
energy expenditure, 381
energy requirements, 385
enteral feeding complications, 384
glutamine requirements, 386–387
host immunity, 387–388
lipid requirements, 385–386
metabolic responses during, 379–380
nutrition support
assessment, 380–381
practice scenarios, 382–383
route, 381–382
timing, 383–384
parenteral feeding complications, 384
pathophysiology, 379
protein requirements, 386
serological testing, celiac disease, 438
serum analysis, pregnancy, 338–340
serum glucose, 433
short bowel syndrome (SBS), 443–444
anatomic, physiologic considerations, 512–513
assessment/monitoring, 445–446
background, 512
complications, 520–521, 520*t*
Crohn's disease and, *practice scenario*, 441
diet, 447*t*, 515*t*
etiology, 444*t*
hydration, 446*t*
hypomagnesemia treatment, 446*t*
intestinal adaptation, 513
nutrition, other interventions, 446–447, 514
enteral (EN), 517
fluid recommendations, 516*t*
fluids, *practice scenario*, 516–517
intestinal rehabilitation, 518
malnutrition, *practice scenario*, 518
medications, 518–519
oral diet, 514–515
oral fluids, 515–517, 515*t*
parenteral fluids, 517
parenteral (PN), 517–518, 518*t*, 519*t*
surgery, 519–520
trophic factors, 519
nutritional assessment, 513–514
outcomes, 521
physiological changes, 444–445
short-chain fatty acids (SCFAs), 18, 76
signaling, protein, 87
silymarin, 466–467
SIRS. *See* systemic inflammatory response syndrome
Six Sigma model, 688
skeletal muscle, protein breakdown and, 92
skin folds, nutrition assessment, 162
skin, postinsertion catheter care, 212–213
skin, wound healing and, 349–350
skin-level enteral access devices, 212
sliding-scale insulin therapy, 590
small bowel
biopsy, celiac disease (CD), 438–439
feeding access, critical injury, 403
obstruction, 10–11
resection, 697
secretions, 15
small bowel bacterial overgrowth (SBBO), 436–437, 437*t*
small bowel, colon diseases/disorders
celiac disease (CD), 437–440
Crohn's disease, 440–441
enterocutaneous (EC) fistulas, 447–449
inflammatory bowel disease, 440–442
intestinal urinary diversions, 449
protein-losing enteropathy (PLE), 442–443, 443*t*
short bowel syndrome (SBS), 443–447
ulcerative colitis, 442
small intestine motility, 10
SNS. *See* specialized nutrition support
social history, wasting syndrome/disease, 547
sodium
fluid, electrolyte balance and, 102
hypernatremia, 104, 106*f*
hyponatremia, 102–104, 105*f*
requirements, renal failure (RF), 502
soft tissue fillers, HIV-associated lipodystrophy syndrome, 555
sorbitol, diarrhea and, 221, 221*t*
specialized nutrition support (SNS), essential fatty acids, lipids and, 69–73, 70*t*
specialized nutrition support (SNS), propofol use, *practice scenario*, 71–72
spinal cord injury (SCI), *practice scenario*, 369
splanchnic blood circulation, 15–16
stabilization, catheters, 275
starch chemical structures, 38*f*
starvation, 18–19
adaptation, protein and, 93
uncomplicated, wasting syndrome/disease comparison, 543
starvation-associated malnutrition, 159
statins, 556
steatohepatitis, nonalcoholic. *See* nonalcoholic fatty liver disease
stomach anatomy, 9*f*
stomach cancer, 573–574
stomach disorders. *See also* gastric entries
gastric resections, 428–431
gastroparesis (GP), 432–433
pancreaticoduodenectomy, 431–432
stress
hyperglycemia, 47–48, 584–585
malnutrition and, 395–396
neuroendocrine response, 394, 395*f*
reperfusion injury/low-flow states, 394–395
systemic inflammation, 394, 395*f*
structured lipids, 77
subjective global assessment, liver disease, 463*t*
supplements/supplementation. *See* dietary supplements/supplementation
support professionals' role, ethical decision making, 670–671
surgery
bariatric, 610–612, 610*f*, 612*t*
data, nutrition assessment, 161
gastric bypass, dietary supplements and, *practice scenario*, 325
reobstruction after, *practice scenario*, 11
short bowel syndrome (SBS), 519–520
surgical wound, micronutrients and, 359
surrogate decision making, 662–665, 663*t*
Swinamer predictive equations, 30
symptom relief drugs, cancer therapy, 572
synbiotics, 56, 405
systemic inflammatory response syndrome (SIRS), 394, 395*f*, 476

T

tachycardia, weight loss supplements and, *practice scenario*, 321
taste changes with cancer, 566
TBI. *See* traumatic brain injury
teaching strategies, home nutrition support, 649–651
TG. *See* total gastrectomy
thalidomide, 550
therapeutic index, 308
thiamin, 131–132
thiazolidinediones, 555
thoracic duct, 632*f*
thrombotic catheter occlusion, 279–280
tolerable upper intake level (UL), 128*t*

total gastrectomy (TG), 428
total nutrient admixtures, 252–253, 253*t*
total parenteral nutrition (PN), 569
toxicity, micronutrients, pregnancy, 336
trace elements, 137
  background, 122–123
  chromium, 145–146
  copper, 142–143
  critical injury and, 404–405
  dietary reference intakes, 138*t*
  fluoride, 146
  iodine, 145
  iron, 137–141
  iron deficiency, *practice scenario*, 141
  manganese, 143–144
  molybdenum, 146
  parenteral nutrition (PN) and
    complications, 288
    formulations, 248
    product shortage, *practice scenario*, 250*t*
    supplementation recommendations, 147, 147*t*
  requirements, critical injury, 402
  requirements, renal failure (RF), 503
  selenium, 144
  selenium, *practice scenario*, 144–145
  status, 139–140*t*
  tolerable upper intake level (UL), 128*t*
  zinc, 141–142
trace minerals. *See* trace elements
tracer methodology, protein turnover, 91
transitional feeding, 176, 340
transplantation. *See* organ transplantation
transport, protein, 87
trauma. *See also* critically ill patient; stress
  practice scenario, 30–31
  pregnancy, *practice scenario*, 343
  sepsis, *practice scenario*, 382
trauma, complex, *practice scenario*, 405
traumatic brain injury (TBI), *practice scenario*, 368–369. *See also* neurologic impairment
tricarboxylic acid cycle, 41, 43*f*
triglycerides, medium-chain, 18, 76–77
trophic factors, short bowel syndrome (SBS), 519
tube exchange, removal, 213
tube feeding. *See* enteral nutrition (EN)
tubing, drug-nutrient interactions and, 305
tumor growth, 572
tumor necrosis factor alpha, 566
tunneled catheters, 268–269
turnover measurement, breakdown, protein, 90–92, 90*t*
12 C's, ethical conflicts, 670*t*
type 1 diabetes mellitus, 582–583
type 2 diabetes mellitus, 190–192, 195*t*, 583

U
UL. *See* upper intake level
ulcerative colitis, 442
ulcers
  diabetic, 352
  pressure, 351–352, 354–355*t*
  pressure, *practice scenario*, 358–359
  venous, 352
ultratrace elements, 122–123, 146
uncomplicated starvation, 543
underfeeding
  avoiding, 31–32
  consequences, 31*t*
  pulmonary failure nutrition assessment, 418
United States law, 666–668, 667*f*
upper intake level (UL), 129*t*
urinalysis, pregnancy, 340

V
vagotomy, 428–429
validity testing predictive equations, 29
vascular access, catheters, 269*t*
vascular access device (VAD) occlusion, *practice scenario*, 301
vascular anatomy, 267, 267*f*
vegetative state, 659–661, 660*f*, 660*t*
venous ulcers, 352
ventilator modes, 413–414, 416*t*
ventilator-associated pneumonia (VAP), *practice scenario*, 422
viral hepatitis, 459
vitamin A, 123–125, 356
vitamin B_1. *See* thiamin
vitamin B_2. *See* riboflavin
vitamin B_{12}, 434
vitamin C, 131, 356
vitamin D, 125–128
  gastrointestinal disease and, 434
  metabolic bone disease and, 293–294
  optimal requirement, *practice scenario*, 129
  wasting syndrome/disease and, 551
vitamin E, 129–130, 356, 465
vitamin K, 130–131
vitamins
  absorption, 18
  burns and, 402*t*
  critical injury and, 402
  deficiencies
    cirrhosis, 467
    Crohn's disease and, 441–442
  dietary reference intakes, select sources, 124*t*
  enteral formulations, 147, 188
  enterocutaneous (EC) fistulas and, 449
  fat-soluble, 123–131, 504
  parenteral nutrition (PN) and, 146–147
    complications, 288
    formulations, 248, 248*t*
    products, 147*t*
  pregnancy and, 335*t*
  renal failure (RF) and, 503
  status, 126–127*t*
  tolerable upper intake level (UL), 128*t*, 129*t*
  water-soluble, 131–137, 503
vomiting, 220, 434

W
warfarin, 310–311
wasting conditions, enteral formulations and, 199–200
wasting syndrome/disease
  anabolic-androgenic steroids, 548–550
  case definition, 543
  clinical management, 547–548
  diagnosis, 543
  electrolytes and, 550–551
  encounter, assessment, 546, 546*f*, 547*t*
  energy and, 550–551
  enteral feeding, 551
  enteral nutrition (EN) and, 551
  epidemiology, 542–543
  etiology, pathogenesis, 543–545
  history, 542
  management, 547–548, 548*t*
  medication, 547, 549*t*
  omega-3 fatty acid enrichment, 551
  orexigenic agents, 548
  osteopenia, osteoporosis and, 552–553
  parenteral nutrition (PN), 551–552
  parenteral nutrition (PN), *practice scenario*, 545–546
  physical examination, 546–547
  practice scenario, 545, 550
  progressive resistance, aerobic exercise, 550
  protein and, 550–551
  recombinant human growth hormone (rhGH) and, 550
  sarcopenia, 552, 552*t*
  social, family history, 547
  thalidomide, 550
  uncomplicated starvation comparison, 543
  vitamin D and, 551
water absorption, 18
water content, enteral formulations, 188

water-soluble vitamins, 131–137, 503
weight loss
  methods, obesity, 608
  practice scenario, 321
  pregnancy, gestational diabetes and, *practice scenario*, 47
  supplements, *practice scenario*, 321
weight, nutrition assessment, 161, 162
Whipple procedure, 431–432
Wilson disease, 459–460
withholding *vs.* withdrawing treatment, 663
world religions, artificial nutrition and hydration (ANH) and, 666*t*
wound healing, 349
  acute, phases, 350–351, 350*f*, 351*f*
  acute surgical wound, *practice scenario*, 359
  chronic wounds, 351–352, 351*f*
  delayed, etiology, 352–353
  diabetic ulcers, 352
  enteral formulations, 200, 200*t*
  hydration, 356
  micronutrients, role, 352*t*, 356–357
  monitoring, outcomes, 358, 358*f*
  nutrition requirements, 353, 356–357
  nutrition screening, assessment, 353
  nutrition support, 357–358
  pressure ulcers, 351–352, 354–355*t*
  pressure ulcers, *practice scenario*, 358–359
  skin as organ, 349–350
  venous ulcers, 352

Z
zinc, 141–142, 356, 466